W0081046

MBBS
DE-CODE

Semi-solved Series

Second Professional Examination

Second Edition

(2019–2007)

INCLUDES Recent Papers of 2019-2018 & Previous Years' Papers of Guru Gobind Singh Indraprastha University as Model Papers (see pg. no. RP-1 to RP-68)

Contributors

Swati Mehra

Mansi Midha

Swati Mishra

Mrinalini Bakshi

Edited by
Sudhir Kumar Singh

Reviewed by
J Magendran

Praveen Kumar Gupta

Vandana Puri

Ranjan Kumar Patel

Malathi Murugesan

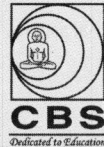

CBS
Dedicated to Education

CBS Publishers & Distributors Pvt Ltd

• New Delhi • Bengaluru • Chennai • Kochi • Kolkata • Mumbai
• Hyderabad • Nagpur • Patna • Pune • Vijayawada

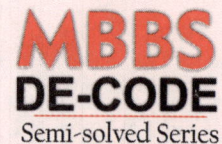

MBBS
DE-CODE
Semi-solved Series

ISBN: 978-81-945234-2-0

Copyright © Publishers

Second Edition: 2020

All rights reserved. No part of this book may be reproduced or transmitted in any form or by any means, electronic or mechanical, including photocopying, recording, or any information storage and retrieval system without permission, in writing, from the publishers.

Published by **Satish Kumar Jain** and produced by **Varun Jain** for

CBS Publishers & Distributors Pvt Ltd

4819/XI Prahlad Street, 24 Ansari Road, Daryaganj, New Delhi 110 002, India.
Ph: +91-11-23289259, 23266861, 23266867   Website: www.cbspd.com
Fax: 011-23243014
e-mail: delhi@cbspd.com; cbspubs@airtelmail.in.

Corporate Office: 204 FIE, Industrial Area, Patparganj, Delhi 110 092
Ph: +91-11-4934 4934   Fax: 4934 4935
e-mail: feedback@cbspd.com; bhupesharora@cbspd.com

Branches

- **Bengaluru:** Seema House 2975, 17th Cross, K.R. Road, Banasankari 2nd Stage, Bengaluru 560 070, Karnataka
  Ph: +91-80-26771678/79   Fax: +91-80-26771680   e-mail: bangalore@cbspd.com

- **Chennai:** 7, Subbaraya Street, Shenoy Nagar, Chennai 600 030, Tamil Nadu
  Ph: +91-44-26680620, 26681266   Fax: +91-44-42032115   e-mail: chennai@cbspd.com

- **Kochi:** 68/1534, 35, 36-Power House Road, Opp. KSEB, Cochin-682018, Kochi, Kerala
  Ph: +91-484-4059061-65   Fax: +91-484-4059065   e-mail: kochi@cbspd.com

- **Kolkata:** 6/B, Ground Floor, Rameswar Shaw Road, Kolkata-700 014, West Bengal
  Ph: +91-33-22891126, 22891127, 22891128   e-mail: kolkata@cbspd.com

- **Mumbai:** 83-C, Dr E Moses Road, Worli, Mumbai-400018, Maharashtra
  Ph: +91-22-24902340/41   Fax: +91-22-24902342   e-mail: mumbai@cbspd.com

Representatives

- **Hyderabad**   +91-9885175004
- **Pune**   +91-9623451994
- **Patna**   +91-9334159340
- **Vijayawada**   +91-9000660880

Printed at: Rashtriya Printers, 27/487, Zulfe Bengal Industrial Area, Dilshad Garden, Delhi-110 095

Reviewers' List

We appreciate and thanks all the reviewers for providing their valuable inputs and suggestions, and devoting their precious time in reviewing the text. It is our proud privilege to include the name of the students in the reviewers' list of the book.

NAMES OF STUDENTS	CURRENT PROFESSIONAL YEAR
MAULANA AZAD MEDICAL COLLEGE, NEW DELHI	
Aadhyayan	
Anika Saini	
Ankit Jindal	2nd Year
Ankur	3rd Year
Asif	
Khushagra Jain	2nd Year
Mohd. Hasim	
Ojasvini	2nd Year
Prattyusha	
Priyanka	
LADY HARDINGE MEDICAL COLLEGE, NEW DELHI	
Arju	2nd Year
Lalita	2nd Year
Lori Thakur	
Manvi	2nd Year
Sakshi Rao	
Sanidhya	
Shreyasi Raje	
Shubhi	
VARDHMAN MAHAVIR MEDICAL COLLEGE, NEW DELHI	
Ayan Agarwal	2nd Year
Jitender Singh	3rd Year
Manav Yadav	3rd Year
UNIVERSITY COLLEGE OF MEDICAL SCIENCES, NEW DELHI	
Ishita Singh	2nd Year
Lalit Yadav	2nd Year
Sahil	3rd Year
Sudhanshu Sharma	2nd Year
DR BABA SAHEB AMBEDKAR MEDICAL COLLEGE AND HOSPITAL, NEW DELHI	
Amrish Kumar	Final Year
Shristi Choudhary	Final Year
NORTH DMC MEDICAL COLLEGE & HINDU RAO HOSPITAL, NEW DELHI	
Abhishek goel	2nd Year
Ankush	Final Year
Lakshay	2nd Year
ALL INDIA INSTITUTE OF MEDICAL SCIENCES, NEW DELHI	
Alen Joe Joseph	

We have tried our level best to include all the names of the reviewers in the list, but if inadvertently any name(s) is left to mention in the list we apologize for the same.

Request to Readers

Dear Readers,

'No work is complete without the support of our readers'.

The book *MBBS De-Code Semi-Solved Series*, 2nd edition, is published on the demand of our readers. We really appreciate their support by sharing question papers and updates related to the exams.

This is our privilege to thank all those students who have made this endeavor successful. We hope, this book will help you to develop the approach and skills of answer writing.

In the pursuit of providing the forthcoming titles of semi-solved series for the undergraduates, we request our readers to share the recent questions of upcoming exams or any previous exam papers which are not covered in this edition at **feedback@cbspd.com** or WhatsApp the questions on + 91-9555590180.

Your contribution will be highly appreciated and acknowledged in the upcoming title(s) of this series. Any students who share the latest question paper or the additional papers at the earliest with us will get the complimentary copy of MBBS DE-CODE Semi-solved Series IIIrd Prof/Final Prof book along with our other CBS books (optional).

Publishers

From the Publisher's Desk

Dear Readers,

It is our pleasure to publish the second edition of this highly-acclaimed book. We are extremely grateful to our readers and extend heartily thanks for accepting and appreciating the 1st edition of *MBBS DE-CODE Semi-solved Series.*

In this 2nd edition, we have focused on four subjects—Pathology, Pharmacology, Microbiology and Forensic Medicine & Toxicology of IInd Prof. Questions of last 12 years (2019–2007) of Delhi University have been presented, subject-wise. In writing the answers, special care has been taken to make them appropriate, authentic and up to the mark. Each answer is referenced from the standard textbooks of its relevant subjects.

The standardized answers presented in the book have been strategized after various brainstorming sessions. The answers given here have been checked and cross-checked several times by the subject experts, and finally reviewed and edited for enhancing the quality of content and authentication of the answers. All the suggestions provided by the reviewers have been critically evaluated and properly incorporated in the answers to make them as standard model answers. We believe that by going through the questions and answers, the students can develop good command over writing well-framed answers.

Apart from the solved questions of the last 12 years, the special feature of this book is "Extra Edge Section" in fully colored format, and with valuable additions like, "Model Papers" and Clinical Pattern Multiple Choice Questions. Extra Edge includes—Subject-wise important Spotters, Tables and MCQs from the exam point of view. This section is the compilation of content from CBS Exam Books of the relevant subject. Tables included in the book carry important information related to the subject, which will help you revise the important facts before the examination. For better recall and visualization, the colored spotters play an important role in this book. Important MCQs from the related subjects are given for the purpose of revision and quick recall of the facts before examination. Another important feature is the inclusion of subject-wise Clinical Multiple Choice Questions, in order to increase the understanding of clinical cases and their application. It also includes previous IInd year MBBS papers of Guru Gobind Singh Indraprastha University as model papers to make the students aware of new questions and topics asked in the university examination.

Hope this book would prove quite handy and very useful in developing your skills and will enhance your style of answer writing!

I am grateful to **Mr Satish Kumar Jain** (*Chairman*) and **Mr Varun Jain** (*Managing Director*), M/s CBS Publishers and Distributors Pvt Ltd for believing in us and providing us a platform for the project.

The job of developing this title was tedious and the people involved in it need special appreciation. I would like to extend my special thanks to all the contributors—**Dr Swati Mehra, Dr Mansi Midha, Dr Mrinalini Bakshi** and **Dr Swati Mishra** who played a vital role for developing this title throughout. Their inputs were valuable and much appreciated. They have given the realistic meaning to the line that *Team Work makes Dreams Work*. I also appreciate the efforts taken by **Ms Nitasha Arora** (Production Head & Content Strategist) for managing the task and accomplishing it on time.

My special thanks to **Dr Sudhir Kumar Singh**, who take out the time from his busy academic schedule in editing this book.

My special thanks to **Dr J Magendran** for providing valuable inputs in Forensic Medicine & Toxicology.

My heartfelt thanks to **Dr Praveen Kumar Gupta, Dr Vandana Puri, Dr Ranjan Kumar Patel, Dr Malathi Murugesan and Dr Sudhir Kumar Singh** for providing content support in drafting the Extra Edge section and Clinical Pattern Multiple Choice Questions.

I would also like to thank Dr Anju Dhir (Project Manager & Senior Scientific Coordinator), Shivendu Bhushan Pandey (Senior Editor), Mr Ashutosh Pathak (Senior Proof Reader) and all the production team members Mr Bunty Kashyap, Mr Phool Kumar, Mr Chaman Lal, Mr Prakash Gaur, Mr Chander Mani, Ms Tahira Parveen, Ms Babita Verma, Ms Manorama Gupta, Mr Raju Sharma, Mr Manoj Chaudhary, Mr Vikram Chaudhary, Mr Manoj Malakar, Mr Arun Kumar and Mr Rahul Negi for devoting laborious hours in designing and typesetting of the book.

Last but not the least, my special thanks to Ms Shagufta Khan (Sr Marketing Manager, PGMEE & Nursing) and entire sales team for their efforts in collecting the previous year question papers of Delhi University from the students.

I would like to end my thoughts with one very old saying *"If you like this book tell others and if you don't like this book tell me."* You can contact me at below given email id/mobile number.

All the best!

Bhupesh Arora
Vice President – Publishing & Marketing
(PGMEE Division)
Email: bhupesharora@cbspd.com
Mobile: (+91) 9555590180

Contents

PHARMACOLOGY

MICROBIOLOGY

FORENSIC MEDICINE & TOXICOLOGY

EXTRA EDGE

Pathology

Pharmacology

Microbiology

Forensic Medicine & Toxicology

Subject-wise cum Topic-wise Content List

Although this book is based on year-wise pattern, for a quick glance over important topics,
this list has been prepared alphabetically under each subject, respectively

PATHOLOGY

PHARMACOLOGY

MICROBIOLOGY

FORENSIC MEDICINE & TOXICOLOGY

Clinical Pattern
Multiple Choice Questions

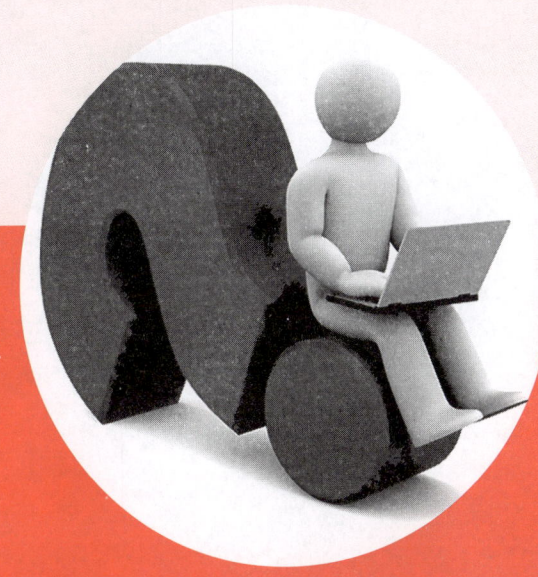

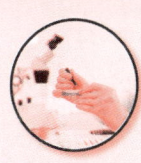 Pathology

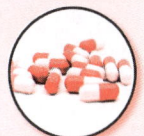 Pharmacology

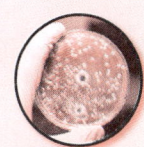 Microbiology

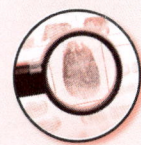 Forensic Medicine & Toxicology

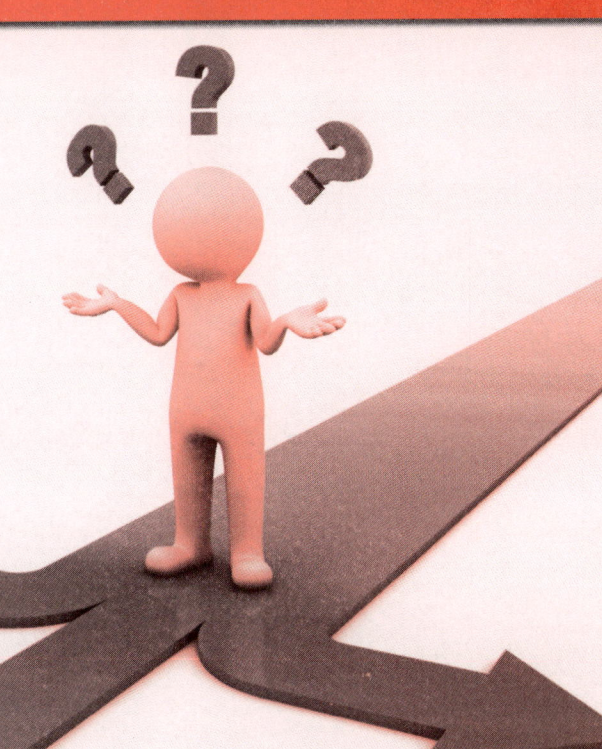

Pathology

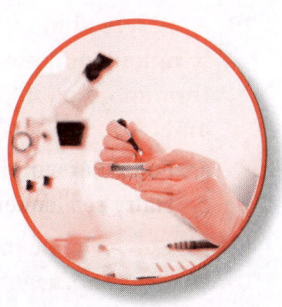

1. A 45-year-old female patient presented with vaginal discharge. Her pap smear revealed HSV infection. What inclusions do you suspect in this case:
   a. Cowdry A bodies
   b. koilocytosis
   c. Guarnieri bodies
   d. Warthin-Finkeldey giant cells
   e. Ground-Glass Change
   f. Atypical lymphocytes

2. A patient presents with biventricular failure and narrow pulse pressure. His CXR was suggestive of Dilated cardiomyopathy. Which of the following statements tell correctly about etiology:
   1. Idiopathic (most common)
   2. Genetic (most common)
   3. Postpartum state can be a causative
   4. Alcohol can cause direct toxicity to cause DCM
   5. Most common cause of sudden death in young athletes
   a. Option 1, 3, 4 are true
   b. Option 2 and 5 are true
   c. Option 5 is true, all others are false
   d. All options are false

3. A 1-year-old boy presented with hepatosplenomegaly and delayed milestones. The liver biopsy and bone marrow biopsy revealed presence of histiocytes with PAS-positive Diastase resistant material in the cytoplasm. Electron microscopic examination of these histiocytes is most likely to reveal the presence of:
   a. Birbeck granules in the cytoplasm
   b. Myelin figures in the cytoplasm
   c. Parallel rays of tubular structures in lysosomes
   d. Electron dense deposit in the mitochondria

4. A 50-year old post menopausal woman comes with complaints of bleeding per vaginum. Which one of the following investigations is NOT required:
   a. Endometrial biopsy
   b. Diagnostic laparoscopy
   c. Hysteroscopy
   d. Pap smear

5. In a 40-year-old woman, pap smear shows atypical glandular cells, The next step of management should be:
   a. Repeat pap smear after three months
   b. Colposcopic directed cervical biopsy
   c. Colposcopy: cervical biopsy, endocervical curettage and endometrial biopsy
   d. Hysteroscopy and directed endometrial biopsy

6. A patient develops skin necrosis 3 days after being started on warfarin for deep vein thrombosis. What is the most likely cause?
   1. Antiphospholipid antibody syndrome
   2. Protein C deficiency
   3. Disseminated intravascular coagulation
   4. Thrombotic thrombocytopenic ....
   a. Only 1   b. Only 3
   c. 1 and 3   d. 1, 2, 3

7. Children with germ line retinoblastoma are more likely to develop other primary malignancies in their later lifetime course. Which of the following can occur in such patients?
   a. Osteosarcoma of lower limbs and soft tissue sarcoma
   b. Thyroid carcinoma
   c. Seminoma
   d. Squamous cell carcinoma

8. A person is having painless lymphadenopathy. On biopsy, binucleated owl shaped nuclei with clear vacuolated area is seen. On IHC CD 15 and CD 30 were positive. What is the most probable diagnosis?
   a. Nodular sclerosis
   b. Large granular lymphocytic lymphoma
   c. Lymphocyte depletion type
   d. Lymphocyte predominant HD

9. A 10-year-old boy with mass in the abdomen. On imaging the para-aortic LN is enlarged. On biopsy starry sky appearance is seen. What is the underlying abnormality?
   a. p53 gene mutation   b. RB gene mutation
   c. Translocation involving BCR-ABL genes
   d. Translocation involving MYC gene

10. A 60-year-old male presents with generalized lymphadenopathy and hepatosplenomegaly. Immunophenotype: CD5 and CD19 are positive and CD10 negative. Diagnosis:
   a. Follicular lymphoma b. Burkitt lymphoma
   c. Hairy cell leukemia d. CLL

11. An elderly male presents with anemia and fatigue. O/E splenomegaly-2 cm palpable below costal margin. Hemogram showed Pancytopenia. Which is the most common etiology?
   a. Hairy cell leukemia b. CML
   c. Thalassemia d. Follicular lymphoma

12. A 55-year-old gentleman presented with history of right upper quadrant discomfort, jaundice, pruritis, fever, fatigue and weight loss. His serum bilirubin and alkaline phosphatase levels are raised and he also gives history of treatment for inflammatory bowel disease. He is most likely to be suffering from:
   a. Benign bile duct stricture with cholangitis
   b. Biliary worms
   c. Bile duct malignancy
   d. Primary sclerosing cholangitis

13. A 2-year-old child presents with scattered lytic lesions in the skull. Biopsy revealed Langerhans giant cells. The most commonly associated marker with this condition will be:
   a. CD la b. CD57
   c. CD3 d. CD68

14. True about BCR-ABL 'traits' are all except?
   a. P190 has an indolent course
   b. P190 is a bad prognostic factor
   c. P230 is positive in chronic neutrophilc leukemia
   d. P230 has an indolent course

15. 45/m presented with leuko-erythroblastic blood picture with dacrocytes. What is bone marrow finding?
   a. Fatty degeneration with erythroid cell hyperplasia with megakaryocytes
   b. Abundant fat cells
   c. Focal cellular marrow with hypocellular areas and atypical megakaryocytes
   d. Hypercellular marrow with prominent blasts

16. A 25-year-old female came to OPD 1 year after postpartum. She was treated for iron deficiency anemia while pregnancy. Now she is pale and her Hb was 5% and reticulocyte count was 9%. Her corrected retic count is?
   a. 6 b. 4.5
   c. 3 d. 1

17. A 25-year-old patient presents with the history of dyspnea on exertion for 3 weeks. Investigations revealed Hb–7g/dl, reticulocyte count 18% and positive coomb's test. Diagnosis:
   a. Autoimmune hemolytic anemia
   b. Paroxysmal nocturnal hemoglobimuria
   c. Sickle cell anemia
   d. Hereditary spherocytosis

18. A 17/F underwent FNAC for a lump in the breast which was non-tender, firm and mobile. Which of the following features would suggest finding of a benign breast disease?
   a. Dyscohesive ductal epithelial cells without cellular fragments
   b. Tightly arranged ductal epithelial cells with bare nuclei
   c. Stromal predominance with spindle cells
   d. Polymorphism with single or arranged ductal epithelial cells

19. A 25-year-old male presented with swelling in the wrist joint. Histopathological examination showed spindle cells and Verocay bodies. What is the most likely diagnosis?
   a. Neurofibroma
   b. Schwannoma
   c. Lipoma
   d. Squamous cell carcinoma

20. 70 M presented to AIIMS OPD with fatigue. Fasting sugar was 110 mg%, PP was 180 mg%, Hba1c was 6.1%. What is your diagnosis?
   a. Prediabetes
   b. Stress induced
   c. Normal
   d. Diabetes

21. 2-year-old child presents with short stature and café-au-lait spots. Bone marrow aspiration yields a little material and mostly containing fat. What is your diagnosis:
   a. Fanconi anemia
   b. Dyskeratosis congenita
   c. Tuberous sclerosis
   d. Osteogenesis imperfect

22. A female presents with history of progressive breathlessness. Histology shows heterogenous patchy fibrosis with several fibroblastic foci. The most likely diagnosis is:
   a. Cryptogenic organizing pneumonia
   b. Non specific interstitial pneumonia
   c. Usual interstitial pneumonia
   d. Desquamative interstitial pneumonia

23. A trauma patient presents at emergency department. There is no time for cross matching. FFP of which blood group can be transfused safely?

a. O RH D positive
b. O RH D negative
c. AB RH D positive
d. AB RH D negative

24. 25-year-old female presented with swelling in front of neck. TSH levels were elevated. Biopsy showed lymphocytic infiltration and Hurthle cells. Which of the following is the possible diagnosis?

a. Graves' disease
b. Hashimoto's thyroiditis
c. Medullary carcinoma thyroid
d. Papillary carcinoma thyroid

25. 11. A 8-year-old child presented with history of recurrent infections. The child had rashes. Investigations revealed low platelets. What could be the probable cause?

a. Job syndrome
b. Wiskott-Aldrich syndrome
c. Henoch-Schonlein purpura
d. Hyper IgM syndrome

26. A 23-year-old lady presented with diarrhoea, vomiting and poor appetite. Biopsy showed crypt hyperplasia, villous atrophy and CD8+ cells in the lamina propria. What could be the diagnosis?

a. Whipple's disease
b. Chronic pancreatitis
c. Environmental enteropathy
d. Celiac disease

27. A 25-year-old female presented with swelling around the knee joint. Biopsy showed giant cells interspersed with mononuclear cells. What is your diagnosis?

a. Rheumatoid arthritis b. Osteosarcoma
c. Aneurysmal bone cyst d. Giant cell tumor

28. A 30-year-old female presented with 4 cm mass in the right breast. Biopsy showed densely packed cells with bland nuclei and mucin infiltrating the stroma. What is your diagnosis?

a. Invasive papillary carcinoma
b. Medullary carcinoma
c. Apocrine carcinoma
d. Colloid carcinoma

29. Patient came with swelling in midline of neck measuring 2 cm in size. Histopathological examination showed Orphan Annie eye nuclei. What is the most likely diagnosis?

a. Medullary carcinoma
b. Papillary carcinoma thyroid
c. Toxic nodular goitre
d. Follicular thyroid carcinoma

30. A 55-year-old male presents with severe chest pain radiating to the left arm. ECG shows ST segment elevation in the V4, V5 and V6 leads. CK-MB and troponin levels are found to be increased. The most likely cause for the increase in enzyme in serum is:

a. Clumping of nuclear chromatin
b. Lysosomal Autophagy
c. Mitochondrial swelling
d. Cell membrane defects

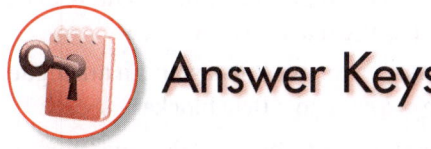 Answer Keys

1. a	2. a	3. c	4. b	5. c	6. b	7. a	8. a	9. d	10. d
11. a	12. d	13. a	14. a	15. c	16. c	17. a	18. b	19. b	20. a
21. a	22. c	23. d	24. b	25. b	26. d	27. d	28. d	29. b	30. d

Pharmacology

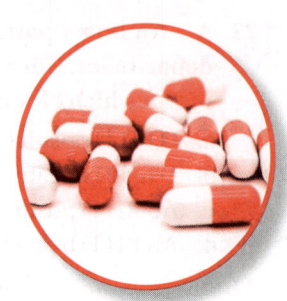

1. **A patient came to casualty with acute attack of asthma after starting treatment of glaucoma. The causative drug is:**
   - a. Timolol
   - b. Betaxolol
   - c. Clonidine
   - d. Acetazolamide

2. **A treatment naive 13-year-old patient of rheumatoid arthritis with deformity given in picture. How will you start treatment?**
   - a. 3 months of NSAID
   - b. Single TNF alpha inhibitors
   - c. Start methotrexate and short course of steroids
   - d. Start Leflunomide

3. **A patient of rheumatoid arthritis is not responding to NSAIDs and methotrexate for 6 months. What will you do next?**
   - a. Start single DMARD
   - b. Increase dose of methotrexate
   - c. Replace leflunomide with methotrexate
   - d. Add sulfasalazine and hydroxychloroquine

4. **You have to give 180 mg of ceftriaxone to a patient in 2 mL syringe which has 10 divisions per mL. Concentration of this drug in vial is 500mg/5ml. How many divisions should be filled in 2 mL syringe to give 180 mg?**
   - a. 18
   - b. 1.8
   - c. 2
   - d. 20

5. **A patient comes 6 hours after consuming morphine and presents with pin point pupils and respiratory depression. T ½ of morphine is 3 hours and Volume of distribution (Vd) is 200 L. Plasma concentration is 0.5 microgram/ml. Calculate the initial morphine dose consumed.**
   - a. 100 mg
   - b. 400 mg
   - c. 10 mg
   - d. 50 mg

6. **A patient was administered 200 mg of a drug. 75 mg of the drug is eliminated in 90 minutes. If the drug follows first order kinetics how much drug will remain after 6 hours?**
   - a. 6.25 mg
   - b. 12.5 mg
   - c. 25 mg
   - d. 50 mg

7. **An 80 kg man is in shock. Vasopressor has to be started at 10 microg/kg/min. One vial has 200 mg in 5 mL and 2 vials were diluted to 250 mL. If 16 drops = 1ml, calculate drops per min required.**
   - a. 4
   - b. 8
   - c. 16
   - d. 24

8. **A person has given 0.175 g oral digoxin with bioavailability 70%. The amount of drug reaching in systemic circulation is:**
   - a. 0.175
   - b. 0.175×0.7
   - c. 0.175/7
   - d. 0.175 + 0.7
   - e. 0.175 + 1/0.7

9. **An anticancer drug is given by continuous intravenous infusion. If the plasma concentration at steady state is 10 mg/mL and clearance is 20 mL/hour, what would be the infusion rate if half-life is 2 minutes?**
   - a. 200 mg/hour
   - b. 400 mg/hour
   - c. 800 mg/hour
   - d. 1600 mg/hour
   - e. 3200 mg/hour

10. **A Male with insulin dependent diabetes having macular edema develops glaucoma. Which drug should be used as the least resort to treat?**
    - a. Alpha agonist
    - b. Prostaglandin analogue
    - c. Pilocarpine
    - d. Beta blocker

11. **A child presented with history of ingestion of some unknown plant and developed mydriasis, tachycardia, dry mouth, warm skin and delirium. Which of the following group of drugs is likely to be responsible for the symptoms of this child?**
    - a. Anticholinergic
    - b. Sympathomimetic
    - c. Opioid
    - d. Benzodiazepine

12. **A 28-year-old woman has been treated with several autonomic drugs for about a month. Which of the following signs would distinguish between an overdose of muscarinic blocker and a ganglionic blocker?**
    - a. Blurred vision
    - b. Dry mouth and constipation
    - c. Mydriasis
    - d. Postural hypotension

13. A new drug effect was compared as compared to placebo in phase I trial in healthy volunteers. The effect of the new drug is predominantly on which receptors

    Placebo New   BP 120/80 100/50
    HR 70/mm 110/mm
    a. α_1 and α_2 b. $\beta1$ and $\beta2$
    c. α_1, α_2 and β_1 d. α_2 and β_2

14. Primary action of nitrates in a patient of angina is:
    a. Coronary vasodilation
    b. Decreases preload
    c. Decreases afterload
    d. Decreases heart rate

15. A man presents with chest pain. ECG shows ST segment depression in leads V1-V4. Which of the following should not be given?
    a. Beta blocker   b. Thrombolytic
    c. Morphine   d. Aspirin

16. A patient was started on fluphenazine. After few weeks of treatment, he started developing tremors, rigidity, bradykinesia and excessive salivation. First line of management for this patient is
    a. Trihexyphenidyl   b. Pramipexole
    c. Amantadine   d. Selegiline

17. A patient of CAD with history of MI 2 months back, diabetes mellitus with LDL 126, HDL 32 and triglycerides 236. What should be given:
    a. Atorvastatin 80 mg
    b. Rosuvastatin 10 mg
    c. Fenofibrate
    d. Fenofibrate and rosuvastatin

18. A female developed a feeling of an insect crawling on her legs at night which was relieved by shaking her legs. Which of the following is the drug of choice for her condition?
    a. Pramipexole   b. Gabapentin
    c. Vit B12   d. Iron tablets

19. A 34-year-old male presents to the outpatient department with a complaint of pain in the right sided jaw pain. Each episode of pain is lasting for around 30 seconds. The present complaint was present for the past one month but the increased in the number of episodes per day brought her to the clinic. Those episodes are increasing especially when she walks out in the cold. The mechanism of action of drug of choice in this patient is?
    a. Prevention of Na^+ influx
    b. Increase the time of Cl^- channel opening
    c. Increase the frequency of Cl^- channel opening
    d. Decrease in the Ca_{+2} influx

20. A 59-year-old female patient taking medications for hypertension and congestive cardiac failure. She suddenly develops skin rashes along with swelling of tongue, lips as well as eyes, causing her breathing difficulty. Which one of the following medications is the reason for the untoward effects?
    a. Propranolol   b. Hydrochlorthiazide
    c. Captopril   d. Clonidine

21. A 16-year-old girl was on antiepileptic for treatment of seizure episodes while asleep. She had no seizure for 6 months and NCCT and EEG was normal. What is further management?
    a. Stop treatment
    b. Continue for 2 years
    c. Lifelong treatment
    d. Stop treatment and follow up with 6 monthly EEG

22. A female with history of previous pregnancy associated with neural tube defect. What should be the prophylactic dose of folic acid given in microgram?
    a. 4   b. 40
    c. 400   d. 4,000

23. A patient presented with right lower quadrant pain. He was already treated for right renal stone disease. Which of the following opioid is partial agonist at mu and full agonist at kappa?
    a. Pentazocin
    b. Buprenorphine
    c. Tramadol
    d. Fentanyl

24. A patient an antipsychotic drugs develops temperature of 104°C, BP about 150/100 and abnormal behavior. What is the likely diagnosis?
    a. Aggravation of psychosis
    b. Dystonia
    c. Neuroleptic malignant syndrome
    d. Akathisia

25. A 15-year-old boy needs to go for a long distance in bus. Which of the following drugs would be useful for him?
    a. Desloratiadine   b. Cetirizine
    c. Diphenhydramine   d. Promethazine

26. A bed ridden female patient with catheter related UTI by beta lactamase producing klebsiella pneumoniae. Which of the following drug will you choose?
    a. Ampicillin
    b. Beta lactams and beta lactamase inhibitors
    c. 2nd generation cephalosporins
    d. 3rd generation cephalosporins

PHARMACOLOGY

27. A patient is on indinavir, zidovudine, lamivudine and ketoconazole. He developed breast hypertrophy, nephrolithiasis, hyperlipidemia and central obesity; identify the drug causing these side effects amongst all:

   a. Lamivudine
   b. Indinavir
   c. Ketoconazole
   d. Zidovudine

28. A patient, diagnosed with rheumatoid arthritis, was on medications. After 2 years, developed blurring of vision and was found to have corneal opacity. Which of the following drug most likely causes that?

   a. Sulfasalazine   b. Chloroquine
   c. Methotrexate   d. Leflunomide

29. A patient on lithium therapy developed hypertension. After being started on thiazides for hypertension, he suffered from coarse tremors and other symptoms suggestive of lithium toxicity. Explain the likely mechanism of this interaction.

   a. Thiazide inhibits metabolism of lithium
   b. Thiazides increases tubular reabsorption of lithium
   c. Thiazides acts as add on drug for lithium
   d. Thiazides and lithium both cause tremors

30. In an orthopedic surgery, a patient was given acetyl choline receptor competitive blocker drug. Which of the following could be used as recovery against this blockade?

   a. Neostigmine   b. Physostigmine
   c. Pyridostigmine   d. Succinylcholine

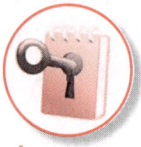 ## Answer Keys

1. a	2. c	3. d	4. a	5. b	6. d	7. b	8. b	9. a	10. b
11. a	12. d	13. b	14. b	15. b	16. a	17. a	18. a	19. a	20. c
21. c	22. d	23. a	24. c	25. d	26. b	27. b	28. b	29. b	30. a

Microbiology

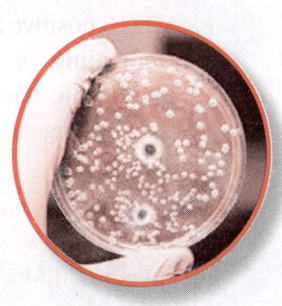

1. A 5-year-old child presented to the OPD with complaints of rectal prolapse. On examination stunting and growth retardation was documented; What is the parasitological cause for this clinical feature?
   a. Trichuris trichiura
   b. Trichinella spiralis
   c. Giardia Lamblia
   d. Enterobius vermicularis

2. A 35-year-old man presented with dry cough and rusty coloured sputum. He has history of eating in Chinese restaurant very often with consumption of crabs often; What is the probable causative agent in this condition?
   a. Diphyllobothrium latum
   b. Pneumocystis jirovecii
   c. Paragonimus westermani
   d. Strongyloides stercoralis

3. A child is suffering from recurrent chronic infections with encapsulated bacteria; Which subclass of IgG does the child has deficiency?
   a. IgG1
   b. IgG2
   c. IgG3
   d. IgG4

4. An AIDS patient presented to OPD with dyspnoea and respiratory illness; Which of the following is suitable to diagnose the opportunistic infection commonly seen in AIDS patient?
   a. Sputum microscopy
   b. Broncho alveolar lavage
   c. Chest X-ray
   d. CT scan

5. 12-year-old presents with vomiting within 3 hours of consumption of food at a party. What is the likely organism responsible for the symptoms:
   a. Staphylococcus aureus
   b. Salmonella
   c. Clostridium botulinum
   d. Clostridium perfringens

6. A farmer presents to the emergency department with painful inguinal lymphadenopathy and history of fever and flu like symptoms. Clinical examination reveals an ulcer in the leg. Which of the following strains should be used to detect suspected bipolar stained organisms:
   a. Albert's stain   b. Wayson's stain
   c. Ziehl Neelson stain d. Mc Fayden's stain

7. A patient has prosthetic valve replacement and he develops endocarditis 8 months later. Organism responsible is:
   a. *Staph aureus*   b. *Strep viridans*
   c. *Staph epidermidis* d. HACEK

8. An HIV positive patient with CD4 count 300/cu.mm presents with mucosal lesion in the mouth. On microscopy budding yeast cells and pseudohyphae are seen. What is the likely diagnosis?
   a. Candidiasis   b. Oral hairy leukoplakia
   c. Lichen planus   d. Diphtheria

9. A child presents with sepsis. Bacteria isolated showed beta hemolysis on blood agar, resistance to bacitracin, and a positive CAMP test. The most probable organism causing infection is:
   a. *Streptococcus pyogenes*
   b. *Streptococcus agalactiae*
   c. Enterococcus
   d. Streptococcus pneumonia

10. In a school, child had abscess on lower leg. Swab taken revealed Gram-positive β-hemolytic streptococci, and these were bacitracin sensitive. School physician observed that similar organism was isolated from throats of many other children. Which of the following is true statement with regards to this patient:
    a. Difference in surface protein can differentiate the pathogenic bacteria from the pharyngeal culture bacteria
    b. Component C carbohydrate can differentiate the pathogenic bacteria from the throat culture bacteria

c. MEG 3 positive are throat culture streptococci

d. Depending on the M protein the cutaneous pathogenic bacteria can be differentiated from the pharyngeal culture bacteria

11. A child presents with infective skin lesion of the leg. Culture was done which showed Gram-positive cocci in chains which were hemolytic colonies. The test to confirm the organism is:

a. Bile solubility   b. Optochin sensitivity

c. Bacitracin sensitivity d. Catalase positive

12. A boy with skin ulcer on leg, culture reveals beta hemolysis. Culture from school children with sore throat some days back also revealed beta hemolysis. What is the similarity between both:

a. Mec A gene is related to it

b. M protein is same

c. Carbohydrate antigen is same

d. Strains causing both are same

13. A 11-year-old child presented with sore throat since 3 days, which medium is used to culture the throat swab:

a. Blood agar   b. LJ medium

c. Stewart medium   d. Chocolate agar

14. A beta hemolytic bacteria is resistant to vancomycin. It shows growth in 6.5% NaCl, is non bile sensitive. It is likely to be:

a. *Streptococcus agalactiae*

b. *Streptococcus pneumoniae*

c. *Enterococcus*

d. *Streptococcus bovis*

15. A patient presents with signs of pneumonia. The bacterium obtained from sputum was a Gram-positive cocci which showed alpha hemolysis on sheep agar. Which of the following test will help to confirm the diagnosis?

a. Bile solubility   b. Coagulase test

c. Bacitracin test   d. cAMP test

16. A person presents with pneumonia. His sputum was sent for culture. The bacterium obtained was Gram-positive cocci in chains and alpha-hemolytic colonies on sheep agar. Which of the following will help in confirming the diagnosis:

a. Novobiocin   b. Optochin

c. Bacitracin   d. Oxacillin

17. A chronic alcoholic is presenting with clinical features of meningitis. Most likely organism which will grow on CSF culture:

a. *Streptococcus pneumoniae*

b. *N. meningitidis*

c. *Listeria monocytogenes*

d. *E. coli*

18. A young lady complains of sore throat for 3 days along with fever and headache. On examination, she was severely dehydrated, her BP was found to be 90/50 mm Hg and on the distal aspect of the cuff, small red spots were noted. What could be the most probable etiological agent responsible for causing these symptoms:

a. Brucella abortus

b. Brucella suis

c. *Neisseria meningitidis*

d. *Staphylococcus aureus*

19. An intern while doing phlebotomy spilled blood in the floor accidentally. What is the next ideal step in the disinfection of blood?

a. Pour 1% hypochlorite solution

b. Cover with a cloth/material

c. Mop the floor

d. Call infectious control unit

20. Patient presenting with abdominal pain, diarrhea is taking clindamycin for 5 days. Treated with metronidazole, the symptoms subsided. What is the causative agent:

a. *Clostridium difficile*

b. *Clostridium perfringens*

c. *Clostridium welchii*

d. *Clostridium marneffi*

21. A 52-year-old man has undergone lung transplantation. Two months after transplantation, he developed pulmonary symptoms and diagnosed as having bilateral diffuse interstitial pulmonary pneumonitis and bron-chiolitis. Which of the following etiological agent is responsible in this condition?

a. Cytomegalovirus   b. Herpes simplex virus

c. Epstein Barr virus   d. Varicella zoster virus

e. Rhino virus

22. A 70-year-old lady refused to take influenza vaccine and developed influenza. She died due to pneumonia 1 week after contracting influenza. Which is the most common cause of acute post influenza pneumonia:

a. Cytomegalovirus

b. Legionella

c. Staphylococcus aureus

d. Measles

23. A 35-years-old female with h/o fever for five days, headache, back ache with rash in the back and fore arm presents with decreased platelet count; Which test is helpful at this stage for diagnosis?

a. NS1 antigen detection

b. IgM ELISA

c. IgG ELISA   d. PCR

24. A patient presents with headache, high fever and meningismus. Within 3 days he become unconscious. Most probable causative agent:
    a. Naegleria fowleri
    b. Acanthamoeba castellani
    c. Entamoeba histolytica
    d. Trypanosoma cruzi

25. A patient presenting from West Bengal with fever, lymphadenopathy. Serological test showed rk39 positive. What is the treatment of choice?
    a. Sodium stibogluconate
    b. Artemesinin
    c. Chloroquine
    d. Dapsone

26. A 48-year-old immunocompromised patient attended the emergency block with complaints of abdominal pain, vomiting and dyspnea. On examination and baseline investigation, he was diagnosed as gastro-intestinal perforation with paralytic ileus. The most common cause of this disseminated infection in immunocompromised patient is due to the following. Identify it:
    a. Rhabditiform larvae of S. stercoralis
    b. Filariform larvae of S. stercoralis
    c. Adult female worm of S. stercoralis
    d. Adult male worm of S. stercoralis
    e. Egg of S. stercoralis

27. A patient coming from Himachal Pradesh, presents with multiple skin lesions. Microscopy reveals cigar shaped yeast cells and asteroid bodies. Microscopy of culture shows flower like pattern. Identify the agent:
    a. Candida sp.
    b. Sporothrix schenckii
    c. Epidermophyton floccosum
    d. Rhizopus

28. A 5-year-old child presented with fever, rashes all over her body, head ache and altered sensorium. Which is the best method for diagnosis of this encephalitis?
    a. PCR
    b. Viral culture
    c. ELISA
    d. Tzanck smear

29. A 19-year-old female college student has fever, sore throat and lymphadenopathy accompanied by lymphocytosis with atypical cells and an increase in sheep cell agglutinins. Diagnosis is most likely?
    a. Infectious hepatitis
    b. Infectious mononucleosis
    c. Chicken pox
    d. Herpes simplex infection

30. A 48-year-old woman develops fever and focal neurological signs. MRI shows a left temporal lobe lesion. Most appropriate test that can be used to confirm the diagnosis of HSV encephalitis is:
    a. Brain biopsy
    b. Tzanck smear
    c. PCR assay for viral DNA in CSF
    d. Serum IgM antibody detection

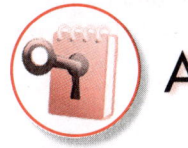 Answer Keys

1. a	2. c	3. b	4. b	5. a	6. b	7. c	8. a	9. b	10. d
11. c	12. c	13. a	14. c	15. a	16. b	17. a	18. c	19. b	20. a
21. a	22. c	23. a	24. a	25. a	26. a	27. b	28. a	29. b	30. c

Forensic Medicine & Toxicology

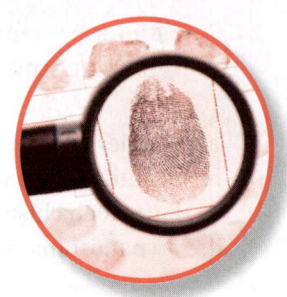

1. **A circular bullet wound, erythema seen around the margin, blackening & tattooing present. What is the range?**
   a. Close shot entry wound
   b. Close shot exit wound
   c. Distant shot entry wound
   d. Distant shot exit wound

2. **A person in alleged to have been dead and body is not found. Proof is produced that the same person has not been heard of for seven years by his friend and relative, death is presumed under:**
   a. S. 107 IEA
   b. S. 108 IEA
   c. S. 105 IEA
   d. S. 106 IEA

3. **A rugby player hit his head on the post whilst involved in a tackle. He was unconscious for 5 min but regained full consciousness and sat on the sideline until the end of the game. He was then noted to be drowsy and over the past 30 min became confused and no longer obeyed commands. Most likely diagnosis is:**
   a. Extradural hematoma
   b. Subdural hematoma
   c. Subarachnoid hematoma
   d. Cerebral edema

4. **A farmer ingested unknown poisonous seeds and had pain and vomiting. Soon he developed paralysis of lower limb which ascends till it affected the respiratory muscles and he died within two days. The poisoning is due to:**
   a. Dhatura
   b. Strychnos nux vomica
   c. Conium maculatum
   d. Opium

5. **As per Mental health care act, an individual with a known psychotic disorder on treatment and is not a minor, can choose to decide the caretaker and the course of treatment. This is called as:**
   a. Advance directive
   b. Treatment directive
   c. Mental will
   d. Future directive

6. **An adult came to casualty with complaints of rapid heart rate. On examination everything else was normal except for episodic tachycardia and occasional extra systole and ambylopia. Which of the following is the cause of it?**
   a. Nicotine
   b. Cannabis
   c. Atropine
   d. Cocaine

7. **Heera lals's 10-year-old child presented in casualty with snake bite since six hours. On examination no systemic signs are found and lab investigations are normal except localized leg swelling <5 cm. Next step in management.**
   a. Incision and suction of local swelling
   b. IV anti-snake serum
   c. S/c anti snake serum at local swelling
   d. Observe the patient for progression of symptoms wait for antivenom therapy

8. **Man hit by car is thrown up and hits road divider and falls on the ground, sustains head injury then run over by another car. Cause of head injury:**
   a. Primary impact injury
   b. Secondary impact injury
   c. Primary injury
   d. Secondary injury

9. **Patient's relative gives a history of tattoo, however it was not found during autopsy. What should be dissected to find it:**
   a. Lymph node
   b. Skin
   c. Spleen
   d. Kidney

10. **A 16-year-old girl come to a doctor with fractured forearm. She told she tripped and fell but cigarette burns were observed on her forearm. What will be your next step?**
    a. To infrom higher authorities
    b. To do a complete physical examination
    c. To tell or discuss with colleagues that she is a case of abuse
    d. To call local social worker for help

11. **A small girl with neuropsychiatry symptoms has a habit of licking paint in walls. Symptoms due to inhibition of:**
    a. ALA dehydratase
    b. ALA synthase
    c. Heme oxygenase
    d. CPG oxidase

12. **An 18 year-old girl was brought to OPD, labia major separated, labia minora flabby, fourchette tear present and vaginal is roomy but Hymen is intact. What could be possible?**
    a. True virgin
    b. False virgin
    c. Premenstrual stage
    d. Molestation

13. **An infant is brought to casualty with reports of violent shaking by parents. Most characteristic injury is:**
    a. Long bone fracture
    b. Ruptured spleen
    c. Subdural haematoma
    d. Skull bone fracture

14. **In the skeletal remains in a building suspected to be of a male, the length of humerus is 24.5 cm. The stature of the person will be:**
    a. 130.095 cm
    b. 93.59 cm
    c. 143.00 cm
    d. 110.00 cm

15. **A person falsely perceives that his close friend has been replaced by an exact double. This phenomenon is referred to as:**
    a. Cotard syndrome
    b. Fregoli syndrome
    c. Capgras syndrome
    d. Delusional perception

16. **A 14-year-old raped girl coming with 22 weeks pregnancy. What should not be done in this case?**
    a. Male doctor can examine in the presence of female attendant
    b. No need for vaginal swab
    c. No need to confirm pregnancy
    d. Termination of pregnancy can be done with her consent by a gynecologist

17. **23 years female was cheated in name of marriage & a man was in contact with her belongs to:**
    a. Sec. 492 IPC
    b. Sec. 493 IPC
    c. Sec. 494 IPC
    d. Sec. 495 IPC

18. **A person 'X' hits another person 'Y' with a wooden stick on provocation. This leads to formation of a bruise 3 cm x 3 cm on the forearm. No other injuries are noted. Which of the following is true, regarding his punishment:**
    a. Imprisonment for one year and/or fine of ₹ 1,000
    b. Imprisonment for two year and/or fine of ₹ 5,000
    c. Imprisonment for one month and/or fine of ₹ 500
    d. Rigorous imprisonment for six months

19. **Two farmers were brought dead, autopsy done revealed viscera that had the smell of bitten almonds. The most likely poisoning is due to:**
    a. Organophosphorus
    b. Morphine
    c. Atropine
    d. Hydrocyanic acid

20. **A person a brought by police from the railway platform. He is talking irrelevent and having dry mouth with hot skin, dilated pupils, staggering gait and slurred speech. The possible diagnosis is:**
    a. Alcohol intoxication
    b. Carbamate poisoning
    c. Organophosphorus poisoning
    d. Datura poisoning

21. **A dead body is found to have marks like branching of a tree in front of the chest. The most likely cause of death is:**
    a. Firearm
    b. Lightening injury
    c. Injuries due to bomb blast
    d. Road traffic accident

22. **A lady died due to natural death within seven year after her marriage. The inquest in this case will be done by:**
    a. Forensic expert
    b. Deputy superintendent of police
    c. Sub-divisional magistrate
    d. Coroner

23. **A middle aged man presents with paresthesia of hand & feet. Examination reveals presence of 'mees' lines in the nails and rain drop pigmentation in hands. The most likely causative toxin is:**
    a. Lead
    b. Arsenic
    c. Thallium
    d. Mercury

24. **A-25-year old person sustained injury in right eye. He developed right corneal opacity following injury. Left eye was already having poor vision. Corneoplasty of right eye was done and vision was restored. Medicolegally such injury is labeled as:**
    a. Grievous
    b. Simple
    c. Serious
    d. Dangerous

25. **A boy has 20 permanent and 8 temporary teeth. His age is more likely to be:**
    a. 8 years
    b. 9 years
    c. 11 years
    d. 10 years

 Answer Keys

1. a	**2.** b	**3.** a	**4.** c	**5.** a	**6.** a	**7.** d	**8.** d	**9.** a	**10.** b
11. a	**12.** b	**13.** c	**14.** a	**15.** c	**16.** d	**17.** b	**18.** c	**19.** d	**20.** d
21. b	**22.** c	**23.** b	**24.** a	**25.** c					

Model Papers

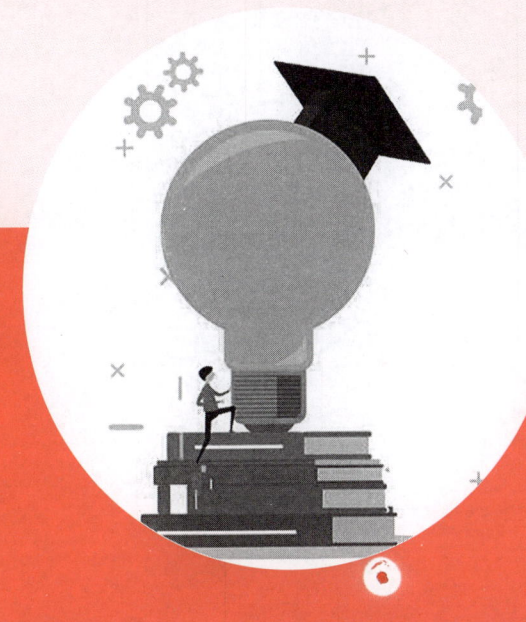

Guru Gobind Singh Indraprastha University

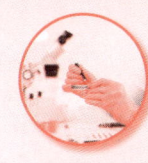 Pathology

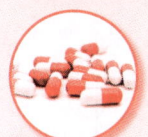 Pharmacology

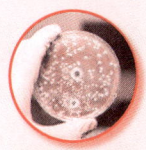 Microbiology

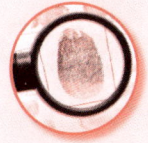 Forensic Medicine & Toxicology

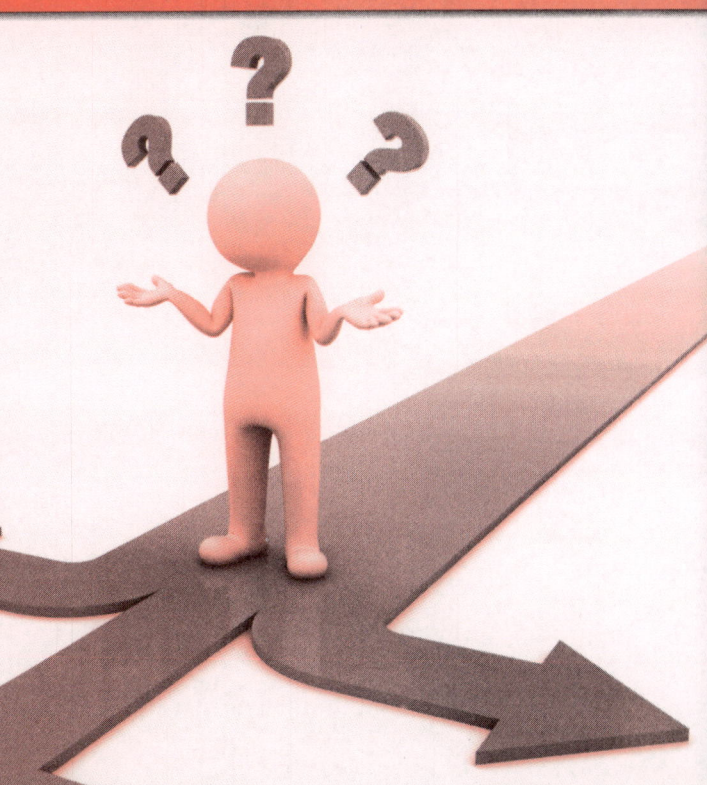

Model Paper: Pathology-I
Second Prof [MBBS] 2018

Time: 3 Hours   **M.M.: 40**

Instructions

Note: Attempt all questions from section-I and section-II directed. Draw neat and labeled diagrams wherever necessary

---

PART-I

1. **Enumerate chemical carcinogens. Describe steps involved in chemical carcinogenesis. Differentiate between initiator and promoter carcinogens** [6]

ANSWER

For answer refer 2017 paper-I, Q. 2(c), Pg. 6

2. **Differentiate between:** [8]
   a. Antemortem and postmortem thrombus
   b. Healing by primary and secondary intention
   c. Benign and malignant tumors

ANSWER

For answer refer 2015 paper-I, Q. 1(b), Pg. 51
   d. Caseous and coagulative necrosis

3. **Write short note on:** [6]
   a. Role of HPV in neoplasia

ANSWER

For answer refer 2018 paper-I, Q. 2(a), Pg. RP-97
   b. Mechanism of graft rejection

ANSWER

For answer refer 2015 paper-I, Q. 2(a), Pg. 51
   c. Abnormalities in immune function in AIDS

ANSWER

For answer refer 2017 paper-I, Q. 2(b), Pg. 5

4. **Discuss the etiopathogenesis and laboratory diagnosis of sickle cell anaemia** [6]

ANSWER

For answer refer 2013 paper-I, Q. 5(b), Pg. 89

5. **Give the peripheral smear and bone marrow findings in:** [8]
   a. Megaloblastic anemia

ANSWER

For answer refer 2018 paper-I, Q. 3(a), Pg. RP-99

    b.   Thalassemia major

ANSWER

For answer refer 2013 paper-I, Q. 3(a), Pg. 86

    c.   Acute myeloid leukemia

    d.   Chronic lymphoblastic leukemia

6. Differentiate between: [6]

    a.   Extravascular and intravascular hemolysis

ANSWER

For answer refer 2014 paper-I, Q. 1(d), Pg. 70

    b.   Acute and chronic immune thrombocytopenic purpura

    c.   Chronic myeloid leukemia and leukemoid reaction

ANSWER

For answer refer 2017 paper-I, Q. 1(c), Pg. 4

Model Paper: Pathology-II
Second Prof [MBBS] 2018

Time: 3 Hours   **M.M.: 40**

Instructions

Note: Attempt all questions from section-I and section-II directed. Draw neat and labeled diagrams wherever necessary

PART-I

1. Classify cirrhosis. Write briefly on the morphology and complications of micronodular cirrhosis.   [6]

2. Write briefly on: [10]

    a.   Giant cell tumor of bone

ANSWER

For answer refer 2018 paper-II, Q. 5(a), Pg. RP-112

    b.   Intraductal carcinoma breast

    c.   Papillary carcinoma thyroid

ANSWER

For answer refer 2018 paper-II, Q. 2(a), Pg. RP-108

    d.   Barrett's oesophagus

ANSWER

For answer refer 2012 paper-II, Q. 5(c), Pg. 112

    e.   Pleomorphic adenoma

ANSWER

For answer refer 2019 paper-II, Q. 4(a), Pg. RP-89

 f. Rapidly progressive glomerulonephritis

ANSWER

For answer refer 2015 paper-II, Q. 3(a), Pg. 62
 g. Asbestosis lung

ANSWER

For answer refer 2017 paper-II Q. 6(c), Pg. 25

PART-II

3. Give the etiology, laboratory lindings and morphological changes in myocardial infarction [6]

ANSWER

For answer refer 2008 paper-II, Q. 6(a), Pg. 168, and 2014 paper-II, Q.4(b), Pg. 80

4. Differentiate between: [18]

 a. Hodgkin's lymphoma and non-Hodgkin's lymphoma

 b. Tubercular and pyogenic meningitis

 c. Crohn's and ulcerative colitis

ANSWER

For answer refer 2018 paper-II, Q. 1(a), Pg. RP-107

 d. Nephrotic and Nephritic syndrome

ANSWER

For answer refer 2013 paper-II, Q. 1(c), Pg. 94

 e. Adult and Infantile polycystic disease of kidney

 f. Type I and Type II endometrial carcinoma

 g. Hemolytic and Obstructive Jaundice.

ANSWER

For answer refer 2014 paper-II, Q. 1(d), Pg. 77

Model Paper: Pathology-I

Second Prof [MBBS] 2017

Time: 3 Hours   **M.M.: 40**

Instructions

Note: Attempt all questions from section-I and section-II directed. Draw neat and labeled diagrams wherever necessary

PART-I

1. Explain vascular and cellular events in acute inflammation. Give the sequelae of acute inflammation.   [6]

ANSWER

For answer refer 2015 paper-I, Q. 4(a), Pg. 55

2. Differentiate between: [8]
   a. Hyperemia and congestion
   b. Necrosis and apoptosis

ANSWER

For answer refer 2013 paper-I, Q. 1(b), Pg. 85

   c. Metastatic and dystrophic calcification

ANSWER

For answer refer 2014 paper-I, Q. 1(a), Pg. 70

   d. Metaplasia and dysplasia.

ANSWER

For answer refer 2011 paper-I, Q. 1(b), Pg. 116

3. Write short notes on: [6]

   a. Pathogenesis of septic shock

ANSWER

For answer refer 2016 paper-I, Q. 3 (a), Pg. 29 and 2015 paper-I, Q. 4 (b), Pg. 56

   b. Type IV hypersensitivity reaction
   c. Tumor markers.

ANSWER

For answer refer 2017 paper-I, Q. 5(c), Pg. 10

PART-II

4. Give the morphological classification on anemia. Write pathogenesis and laboratory investigations in Iron Deficiency anemia.   [10]

ANSWER

For answer refer 2012 paper-I, Q. 4(a), Pg. 104

5. **Differentiate between:** [6]

    a.   Extravascular and Intravascular hemolysis

ANSWER

For answer refer 2014 paper-I, Q. 1(d), Pg. 70

    b.   Lymphoblast and myeloblast

ANSWER

For answer refer 2013 paper-I, Q. 1(a), Pg. 85

    c.   Chronic myeloid leukemia and leukemoid reaction

ANSWER

For answer refer 2017 paper-I, Q. 1(c), Pg. 4

    d.   Acute and chronic immune thrombocytopenic purpura.

6. **Write briefly on:** [6]

    a.   Rh incompatibility

    b.   Peripheral smear findings in hemolytic anaemia

    c.   Bence Jones proteins.

Model Paper: Pathology-II
Second Prof [MBBS] 2017

Time: 3 Hours   **M.M.: 40**

Instructions

Note: Attempt all questions from section-I and section-II directed. Draw neat and labeled diagrams wherever necessary

PART-I

1. **Classify gastric tumors. Discuss the etiopathogenesis and morphology of gastric carcinoma.** [6]

2. **Differentiate between:** [6]

    a.   Primary and secondary biliary cirrhosis

    b.   Hodgkins and non Hodgkins lymphoma

    c.   Ulcerative colitis and Crohn's disease.

ANSWER

For answer refer 2018 paper-II, Q. 1(a), Pg. RP-107

3. **Write briefly on:** [8]

    a.   Prognostic factors in carcinoma breast

ANSWER

For answer refer 2008 paper-II, Q. 2(a), Pg. 130

    b.   Alcoholic liver disease

ANSWER

For answer refer 2011 paper-II, Q. 4(b), Pg. 126

c. Giant cell tumor of bone

ANSWER

For answer refer 2018 paper-II, Q. 5(a), Pg. 128

d. Seminoma testis.

PART-II

4. Classify glomerulonephritis. Give the pathogenesis and morphological features of rapidly progressive glomerulonephritis. [6]

ANSWER

For answer refer 2015 paper-II, Q. 3(a), Pg. 62 and refer 2010 paper-II, Q. 3(b), Pg. 141

5. Write briefly on: [14]
   a. Hashimoto's thyroditis
   b. Malignant small round cell tumor of childhood
   c. Emphysema lung

ANSWER

For answer refer 2010 paper-II, Q. 2(c), Pg. 139

d. Laboratory diagnosis of myocardial infarction

ANSWER

For answer refer 2008 paper-II, Q.6(a), Pg. 168, and 2014 paper-II, Q.4(b), Pg. 80

e. Pyogenic meningitis

ANSWER

For answer refer 2011 paper-I, Q. 5(a), Pg. 118

f. Primary tuberculosis of lung

ANSWER

For answer refer 2016 paper-I, Q. 5(d), Pg. 34

g. Rheumatic nodule.

Model Paper: Pathology-I

Second Prof [MBBS] 2016

Time: 3 Hours   **M.M.: 40**

Instructions

Note: Attempt all questions from section-I and section-II directed. Draw neat and labeled diagrams wherever necessary

---

PART-I

1. **Briefly comment on:**   [10]
    a. Thrombogenesis
    b. Ghon complex

ANSWER

For answer refer 2016 paper-I, Q. 5(d), Pg. 34
    c. Necrosis
    d. Type I hypersensitivity

ANSWER

For answer refer 2012 paper-I, Q. 5(b), Pg. 106
    e. Amniotic fluid embolism.

2. **Define inflammation. Describe the role of chemical mediators of inflammation.**   [10]

ANSWER

For answer refer 2019 paper-I, Q. 2(a), Pg. RP-75

PART-II

3. **Differentiate between:**   [10]
    a. Exudate and transudate

ANSWER

For answer refer 2017 paper-I, Q. 1(b), Pg. 4
    b. CML and leukemoid reaction

ANSWER

For answer refer 2017 paper-I, Q. 1(c), Pg. 4
    c. Hypertrophy and hyperplasia
    d. Hyperemia and congestion
    e. Dystrophic and metastatic calcification.

ANSWER

For answer refer 2014 paper-I Q. 1(a), Pg. 70

4. Classify anaemia and discuss in detail the etiology and diagnosis of iron deficiency anaemia. **[10]**

ANSWER

For answer refer 2012 paper-I, Q. 4(a), Pg. 104

Model Paper: Pathology-II
Second Prof [MBBS] 2016

Time: 3 Hours   M.M.: 40

Instructions

Note: Attempt all questions from section-I and section-II directed. Draw neat and labeled diagrams wherever necessary

---

PART-I

1. Write short note on: **[8]**

   a. Type I and Type II diabetes mellitus

ANSWER

For answer refer 2018 paper-II, Q. 1(b), Pg. 123
   b. Squamous cell carcinoma of cervix

ANSWER

For answer refer 2017 paper-II, Q. 4(a), Pg. 20 and refer 2013 paper-II, Q. 6(b), Pg. 100
   c. Seminoma

ANSWER

For answer refer 2013 paper-II, Q. 5(d), Pg. ??
   d. Chronic osteomyelitis.

2. Describe pathogenesis, morphology and clinical features of adenocarcinoma colon.   **[8]**

PART-II

3. Write briefly on: **[8]**

   a. Renal cell carcinoma

ANSWER

For answer refer 2009 paper-II, Q. 6(b), Pg. 158
   b. Diabetic nephropathy

ANSWER

For answer refer 2016 paper-II, Q. 6(c), Pg. 48
   c. Emphysema

ANSWER

For answer refer 2010 paper-II, Q. 2(c), Pg. 139

    d.   Osteogenic sarcoma.

ANSWER

For answer refer 2017 paper-II Q. 3(a), Pg. 19

4. Describe the etiology, pathogenesis and complications of pneumonia.

    Or

    Define cirrhosis of liver and write its pathogenesis, clinical features and complications.   [8]

5. Differentiate between: [8]

    a.   True and false aneurysm

    b.   Nephritic & nephrotic syndrome

ANSWER

For answer refer 2013 paper-II, Q. 1(c), Pg. 94

    c.   Rheumatic & infective endocarditis vegetations

ANSWER

For answer refer 2017 paper-II, Q. 1(b), Pg. 15

    d.   Viral & pyogenic meningitis

Model Paper: Pathology-I
Second Prof [MBBS] 2015

Time: 3 Hours   **M.M.: 40**

Instructions

Note: Attempt all questions from section-I and section-II directed. Draw neat and labeled diagrams wherever necessary

PART-I

1. **Define carcinogenesis. Write briefly on steps in chemical carcinogenesis.**   [8]

ANSWER

For answer refer 2017 paper-I, Q. 2(c), Pg. 6

2. **Differentiate between:**   [8]

    a.   Carcinoma and sarcoma

    b.   Transudate and exudate

ANSWER

For answer refer 2017 paper-I, Q. 1(b), Pg. 4

    c.   Dystrophic and metastatic calcification

ANSWER

For answer refer 2014 paper-I Q. 1(a), Pg. 70

    d.   B and T lymphocytes.

3. Write briefly on: [8]

a. Stains for amyloid

ANSWER

For answer refer 2010 paper-I, Q. 2(a), Pg. 131

b. Tumour metastasis

c. Renal edema

ANSWER

For answer refer 2010 paper-I, Q. 3(a), Pg. 132

d. Fine needle aspiration cytology.

4. Write short notes on: [8]

a. Laboratory investigation of megaloblastic anaemia

ANSWER

For answer refer 2018 paper-I, Q. 3(a), Pg. 115

b. Type III hypersensitivity

ANSWER

For answer refer 2013 paper-I Q. 2(b), Pg. 86

c. Hyerplasia

d. Factor VIII deficiency.

5. Enumerate the causes of microcytic hypochromic anaemia. Write briefly on etiology and laboratory diagnosis of iron deficiency anaemia. [8]

ANSWER

For answer refer 2013 paper-I, Q. 3(a), Pg. 86 and refer 2012 paper-I, Q. 4(a), Pg. 104

Model Paper: Pathology-I
Second Prof [MBBS] 2014

Time: 3 Hours   **M.M.: 40**

Instructions

Note: Attempt all questions from section-I and section-II directed. Draw neat and labeled diagrams wherever necessary

---

PART-I

1. **Write differences between:**   **[10]**

    a. Necrosis and apoptosis

    ANSWER

    For answer refer 2016 paper-I, Q. 1(b), Pg. 27

    b. Reversible and irreversible cell injury

    ANSWER

    For answer refer 2012 paper-I, Q. 1(b), Pg. 102

    c. Infarction and gangrene

    d. Congestion and hyperemia

    e. T and B cells.

2. **Describe cell derived mediators of acute inflammation.**   **[5]**

3. **Describe the genesis and complications of peptic ulcer.**   **[5]**

PART-II

4. **Write briefly on the following:**   **[10]**

    a. Laboratory diagnosis of Cancer

    b. Pathogenesis of Septic Shock.

    ANSWER

    For answer refer 2016 paper-I Q. 3(a), Pg. 29 and 2015 paper-I Q. 4(b), Pg. 56

5. **Write briefly on the following:**   **[10]**

    a. Rh incompatibility

    b. Caseous necrosis

    ANSWER

    For answer refer 2016 paper-I, Q. 3(b), Pg. 30

    c. Hemophilia

    ANSWER

    For answer refer 2018 paper-I, Q. 5(b), Pg. RP-102

    d. Atrophy

    e. PBF and Bone marrow findings in megaloblastic anaemia.

Model Paper: Pathology-I

Second Prof [MBBS] 2013

Time: 3 Hours **M.M.: 40**

Instructions

Note: Attempt all questions from section-I and section-II directed. Draw neat and labeled diagrams wherever necessary

---

PART-I

1. Write briefly on: [8]
   a. Basal cell carcinoma (Rodent Ulcer)
   b. Teratoma

ANSWER

For answer refer 2016 paper-II Q. 6(a), Pg. 47

   c. Premalignant oral lesion
   d. Osteogenic sarcoma.

ANSWER

For answer refer 2017 paper-II Q. 3(a), Pg. 19

2. Describe the etiopathogenesis and morphology of rheumatic carditis. [8]

PART-II

3. Write briefly on: [8]
   a. Tophi
   b. Bronchiectasis

ANSWER

For answer refer 2018 paper-II, Q.2(c), Pg. RP-109

   c. Diabetic foot.

4. What is the glomerulonephritis? Describe the etiopathogenesis, types and its features. [8]

Or

ANSWER

For answer refer 2010 paper-II, Q. 3(b), Pg. 141

   What is atherosclerosis? Describe the etiopathogenesis and its complication. [8]

ANSWER

For answer refer 2007 paper-II, Q. 4(b), Pg. 178

5. Differentiate between: **[8]**

   a.   Lobar and lobular pneumonia

ANSWER

For answer refer 2014 paper-II, Q. 1(c), Pg. 77

   b.   Exudative and proliferative retinopathy
   c.   Extravascular and intravascular haemolytic anaemia
   d.   Physiological and pathological proteinuria.

Model Paper: Pathology-I
Second Prof [MBBS] 2012

Time: 3 Hours   **M.M.: 40**

Instructions

Note: Attempt all questions from section-I and section-II directed. Draw neat and labeled diagrams wherever necessary

PART-I

1. Write briefly on: [10]
   a. Chemical mediators of Inflammation
   b. Stem cells
   c. Growth Factors
   d. Mutation
   e. Complications of Blood Transfusion.

2. Classify Hypersensitivity Reactions and give example. Describe the pathogenetic mechanisms in detail and clinicopathological manifestations of each type. [10]

ANSWER

For answer refer 2013 paper-I, Q. 2(b) Pg. 86 and 2012 paper-I, Q. 5(b), Pg. 106

PART-II

3. Differentiate between: [10]
   a. Necrosis and Apoptosis

ANSWER

For answer refer 2016 paper-I, Q. 1(b), Pg. 27
   b. Dystrophic and metastatic calcification

ANSWER

For answer refer 2014 paper-I, Q. 1(a), Pg. 70
   c. Oncogenes and anti oncogenes
   d. Hyperemia and congestion
   e. Myeloid and Lymphoid leukemoid reaction.

ANSWER

For answer refer 2017 paper-I, Q. 1(c), Pg. 4

4. Write the etiologic classification of megaloblastic anaemia. Describe the clinical features, pathogenesis and laboratory diagnosis. [10]

Model Paper: Pathology-I

Second Prof [MBBS] 2011

Time: 3 Hours   **M.M.: 40**

Instructions

Note: Attempt all questions from section-I and section-II directed. Draw neat and labeled diagrams wherever necessary

---

PART-I

1. Define Embolism. Enumerate its types. Discuss the pathogenesis and fate of pulmonary thromboembolism.   **[8]**

2. Write short notes on: **[6]**

    a. Metaplasia

ANSWER

For answer refer 2011 paper-I, Q. 1(b), Pg. 116

    b. Sequelae of acute inflammation

    c. Coomb's test.

ANSWER

For answer refer 2016 paper-I, Q. 5(a), Pg. 32

3. Differentiate between: **[6]**

    a. Lymphoblast and Myeloblast

    b. Necrosis and Apoptosis

ANSWER

For answer refer 2016 paper-I, Q. 1(b), Pg. 27

    c. Metastatic and dystrophic calcification.

ANSWER

For answer refer 2014 paper-I, Q. 1(a), Pg. 70

PART-II

4. Enumerate the causes of macrocytic anemia. Give the peripheral blood picture and bone marrow findings in a case of megaloblastic anemia.   **[6]**

5. Write short notes on the following: **[8]**

    a. Staining properties of amyloid

    b. Dysplasia

ANSWER

For answer refer 2011 paper-I, Q. 1(b), Pg. 116

c. Erythroblastosis fetalis

ANSWER

For answer refer 2016 paper-I, Q. 6(c), Pg. 13

    d.   Primary complex.

ANSWER

For answer refer 2016 paper-I, Q. 5(d), Pg. 34

6. **Differentiate between:**   [6]

    a.   ABO and Rh blood group

    b.   Marasmus and Kwashiorkar

ANSWER

For answer refer 2016 paper-I, Q. 1(c), Pg. 27

    c.   Innate and adaptive immunity.

Model Paper: Pathology-II
Second Prof [MBBS] 2011

Time: 3 Hours   **M.M.: 40**

Instructions

Note: Attempt all questions from section-I and section-II directed. Draw neat and labeled diagrams wherever necessary

PART-I

1. **Describe in brief:**   [8]

    a.   Giant cell tumour of bone

ANSWER

For answer refer 2018 paper-II, Q. 5(a) Pg. RP-112

    b.   Classification on ovarian tumours

    c.   Barrett's esophagus

ANSWER

For answer refer 2012 paper-II, Q. 5(c), Pg. 112

    d.   Gilbert syndrome.

2. **Describe gross and microscopic changes as they evolve during 1st week after myocardial infarction and its complications.**   [8]

ANSWER

For answer refer 2008 paper-II, Q. 6(a), Pg. 168 and 2014 paper-II, Q. 4(b), Pg. 80

3. **Write short notes on:** [8]
   a. Crescentic Glomerulonephritis

ANSWER

For answer refer 2017 paper-II, Q. 6(a), Pg. 23
   b. Hashimoto's Thyroiditis
   c. Pathogenesis of type II diabetes Mellitus
   d. Polyarteritis Nodosa.

ANSWER

For answer refer 2017 paper-II, Q. 6(b), Pg. 24

4. **Describe aetiopathogenesis of colorectal carcinoma and its gross and microscopic patterns.** [8]

Or

ANSWER

For answer refer 2011 paper-II, Q. 3(a), Pg. 123

   Describe predisposing factors, pathogenesis and morphology of bronchogenic carcinoma.

ANSWER

For answer refer 2008 paper-II, Q. 5(a), Pg. 167

5. **Differentiate between:** [8]
   a. Chronic bronchitis vs bronchial asthma
   b. Laboratory diagnosis of acute and chronic pancreatitis
   c. CSF findings of aseptic and tubercular meningitis

ANSWER

For answer refer 2011 paper-II, Q. 1(b), Pg. 123
   d. Nephritic and nephrotic syndrome.

ANSWER

For answer refer 2013 paper-II, Q. 1(c), Pg. 94

Model Paper: Pathology-I

Second Prof [MBBS] 2010

Time: 3 Hours   **M.M.: 40**

Instructions

Note: Attempt all questions from section-I and section-II directed. Draw neat and labeled diagrams wherever necessary

---

PART-I

1. **Differentiate between:**   [10]

   a. Benign and malignant tumors

   ANSWER

   For answer refer 2015 paper-I, Q. 1(b), Pg. 51

   b. IDA and beta thalassemia trait

   c. Necrosis and apoptosis

   ANSWER

   For answer refer 2016 paper-I, Q. 1(b), Pg. 27

   d. Marasmus and Kwashiorkor

   ANSWER

   For answer refer 2016 paper-I, Q. 1(c), Pg. 27

   e. Acute and Chronic ITP.

2. **Comment briefly on:**   [10]

   a. Fatty change liver

   ANSWER

   For answer refer 2012 paper-I, Q. 2(c), Pg. 102

   b. Pathogenesis of renal edema

   ANSWER

   For answer refer 2010 paper-I, Q. 3(a), Pg. 132

   c. G6PD deficiency

   ANSWER

   For answer refer 2013 paper-I, Q. 2(a), Pg. 85

   d. Factors predisposing to thrombosis

   e. Type I hypersensitivity reaction.

   ANSWER

   For answer refer 2012 paper-I, Q. 5(b), Pg. 106

3. Differentiate between: [10]

   a. Bleeding due to platelet defect and coagulation factor deficiency

ANSWER

For answer refer 2016 paper-I, Q. 1(d), Pg. 27

   b. Rickets and osteomalacia

   c. Lymphoblast and myeloblast

ANSWER

For answer refer 2013 paper-I, Q. 1(a), Pg. 85

   d. Hyperplasia and neoplasia

   e. Chronic myeloid leukemia and leukemoid reaction.

ANSWER

For answer refer 2017 paper-I, Q. 1(c), Pg. 4

4. Comment on: [10]

   a. Cellular events is acute inflammation

ANSWER

For answer refer 2019 paper-I, Q. 2(a), Pg. RP-75

   b. Paraneoplastic syndrome

ANSWER

For answer refer 2013 paper-I, Q. 5(a), Pg. 88

   c. Down's syndrome

ANSWER

For answer refer 2012 paper-I, Q. 5(a), Pg. 105

   d. Oncogenic viruses

ANSWER

For answer refer 2014 paper-I, Q. 4(a), Pg. 72

   e. Hemolytic transfusion reaction.

Model Paper: Pharmacology-I

Second Prof [MBBS] 2018

Time: 3 Hours   **M.M.: 40**

Instructions

Note: Attempt all questions from section-I and section-II directed. Draw neat and labeled diagrams wherever necessary

PART-I

1. a. Enumerate the drugs used in congestive heart failure. Describe the mechanism of action of Digitalis using diagram and write uses and adverse effects of Digitalis.   [5]

ANSWER

For answer refer 2014 paper-I, Q. 3(b), Pg. 233, and 2013 paper-I, Q. 3(a) Pg. 244

   b. Enumerate the drugs used in glaucoma using diagram showing sites of action of ocular hypotensive drugs. Write the advantages of topical beta blockers over miotics.   [5]

2. Describe the mechanisms of action, therapeutic use and important adverse effects of the following: [10]

   a. Nitrodilators
   b. Centrally acting muscle relaxants
   c. Furosemide

ANSWER

For answer refer 2015 paper-I, Q. 5(b), Pg. 219

   d. Niacin
   e. Proton pump inhibitors.

ANSWER

For answer refer 2008 paper-II, Q. 4(b), Pg. 319-320

PART-II

3. Write the rationale for: [10]

   a. Use of zinc in diarrhea
   b. Modification of doses of certain drugs in elderly patients
   c. Loading dose to start treatment with some drugs in elderly patients
   d. Using metoclopramide in gastroparesis
   e. Erythropoietin in renal failure.

4. Describe in brief: [10]

   a. Plateau principle
   b. Prokinetic drugs
   c. Non cardiac uses of beta blockers
   d. Thrombolytic drugs
   e. Compare and contrast competitive and non-competitive antagonism.

Model Paper: Pharmacology-II

Second Prof [MBBS] 2018

Time: 3 Hours   M.M.: 40

Instructions

Note: Attempt all questions from section-I and section-II directed. Draw neat and labeled diagrams wherever necessary

---

PART-I

1. a. Write classification of anti-tubercular drugs. Discuss the drugs for the treatment of multidrug resistant tuberculosis (MDR) according to new RNTCP guidelines. [5]

ANSWER

For answer refer 2007 paper-II, Q. 4(b), Pg. 332

   b. Enumerate anti-epileptic drugs. Write mechanism of action using diagram, therapeutic uses and important adverse effects of phenytoin. [5]

ANSWER

For answer refer 2017 paper-I, Q. 5(a), Pg. 191

2. Describe the mechanisms of action, therapeutic use and adverse effects of the following: [10]

   a. Status asthamaticus

ANSWER

For answer refer 2015 paper-I, Q. 4(b), Pg. 219

   b. Migraine
   c. Thyrotoxicosis
   d. Depression
   e. Post exposure prophylaxis of HIV.

PART-II

3. Write the rationale for the use of: [10]

   a. Thiopentone sodium for induction of general anesthesia

ANSWER

For answer refer 2018 paper-I, Q. 3(c), Pg. RP-138

   b. Propylthiouracil in hyperthyroidism

ANSWER

For answer refer 2019 paper-II, Q. 3(a), Pg. RP-130

   c. Bisphosphonates in osteoporosis

ANSWER

For answer refer 2007 paper-II, Q. 5(a), Pg. 332

    d.   Low dose aspirin in post MI patients

ANSWER

For answer refer 2019 paper-I, Q. 1(a), Pg. RP-120

    e.   Albendazole in neurocysticercosis.

ANSWER

For answer refer 2010 paper-II, Q. 3(b), Pg. 294

4. **Write short notes on the following:**   **[10]**

    a.   DPP-IV inhibitors

    b.   Retinoids

    c.   Allopurinol

ANSWER

For answer refer 2013 paper-II, Q. 3(d), Pg. 253

    d.   Cyclosporine

ANSWER

For answer refer 2016 paper-II, Q. 3(c), Pg. 211

    e.   COMT-inhibitors.

Model Paper: Pharmacology-I

Second Prof [MBBS] 2017

Time: 3 Hours   **M.M.: 40**

Instructions

Note: Attempt all questions from section-I and section-II directed. Draw neat and labeled diagrams wherever necessary

---

PART-I

1. **Explain why:**   [10]

    a. Loading dose is given with some drugs

    b. Tamsulosin is preferred over prazosin for the treatment of benign prostate hypertrophy

ANSWER

For answer refer 2014 paper-I, Q. 3(a), Pg. 232

    c. Felypressin, instead of adrenaline can be added to local anesthetics

    d. Hydrochlorthiazide in low dose is usually prescribed as antihypertensive

    e. Purgatives should not be used concomitantly with activated charcoal in poisoning.

2. **Describe the mechanism of action, therapeutic uses and important adverse effects of the following:**   [10]

    a. Atorvastatin

ANSWER

For answer refer 2009 paper-I, Q. 6(a), Pg. 302-303

    b. Enoxaparin

    c. Ranolazine

    d. Clonidine.

PART-II

---

3. **Write the rationale for the use of:**   [10]

    a. Folinic acid in methotrexate toxicity

    b. Beta blocker in myocardial infarction

ANSWER

For answer refer 2014 paper-I, Q. 3(b), Pg. 233

    c. Oximes in organophosphate poisoning

ANSWER

For answer refer 2010 paper-I, Q. 3(d), Pg. 287

    d. Zinc in diarrhea

    e. Potassium sparing diuretics in congestive heart failure.

4. Describe in brief: [10]
   a. Fixed dose combinations

ANSWER

For answer refer 2011 paper-I, Q. 6(c), Pg. 277
   b. Ionotropic receptors
   c. Levobupivacaine
   d. Iron chelating agents
   e. Bioequivalence and therapeutic equivalence.

ANSWER

For answer Bioequivalence refer 2019 paper-I, Q. 6(b), Pg. RP-125

Model Paper: Pharmacology-II
Second Prof [MBBS] 2017

Time: 3 Hours   M.M.: 40

Instructions

Note: Attempt all questions from section-I and section-II directed. Draw neat and labeled diagrams wherever necessary

PART-I

1. **Explain why:** [10]
   a. Morphine is contraindicated in head injury

ANSWER

For answer refer 2012 paper-I, Q. 2, Pg. 258
   b. Potassium iodide/Lugol's iodine is used prior to thyroid surgery
   c. Anastrazole is indicated in Breast cancer
   d. Thalidomide is used in the management of lepra reactions

ANSWER

For answer refer 2007 paper-II, Q. 1(c), Pg. 329
   e. Fluoroquinolones should be avoided in extremes of age.

2. **Describe in brief the pharmacological management of:** [10]
   a. Post exposure prophylaxis of HIV
   b. Multi drug resistant tuberculosis

ANSWER

For answer refer 2007 paper-II, Q. 4(b), Pg. 332
   c. Osteoporosis

ANSWER

For answer refer 2018 paper-II, Q. 4(b), Pg. RP-127

    d.   Insomnia

ANSWER

For answer refer 2012 paper-I Q. 4(b), Pg. 260

    e.   Acute gout.

PART-II

3. **Write the rationale for the use of:**   **[10]**

    a.   Cyclosporine in organ transplantation

ANSWER

For answer refer 2016 paper-II, Q. 3(c), Pg. 211

    b.   Neomycin in hepatic coma

    c.   Ciclesonide in bronchial asthma

    d.   Anticholinergics in drug induced parkinsonism

    e.   Hormone replacement therapy (HRT) in women.

4. **Discuss the mechanism of action, therapeutic uses and adverse effects of:**   **[10]**

    a.   Metronidazole

    b.   Olanzapine

ANSWER

For answer refer 2017 paper-I, Q. 5(b), Pg. 191

    c.   Pentazocine

    d.   Retinoids.

Model Paper: Pharmacology-II

Second Prof [MBBS] 2016

Time: 3 Hours   **M.M.: 40**

Instructions

Note: Attempt all questions from section-I and section-II directed. Draw neat and labeled diagrams wherever necessary

PART-I

1. **Explain why:**   **[10]**

    a.   Therapeutic drug monitoring is needed for patients on theophylline therapy

    b.   Clomiphene is used for the treatment of infertility

ANSWER

For answer refer 2016 paper-I, Q. 4(b), Pg. 205

    c.   Alendronate is used for the treatment of osteoporosis

ANSWER

For answer refer 2016 paper-II, Q. 4(b), Pg. 212

d. Alcohol is used as an antiseptic
   e. Atypical antipsychotics are preferred over classical antipsychotics.

2. **Discuss the pharmacological management of:** [10]
   a. Vancomycin resistant staphylococcal aureus infection
   b. Thyroid storm

ANSWER

For answer refer 2014 paper-II, Q. 4(a), Pg. 239
   c. Scabies
   d. Type II diabetes mellitus

ANSWER

For answer refer 2017 paper-II, Q. 2, Pg. 196
   e. Acute attack of Bronchial asthma.

PART-II

3. **Comment on following:** [10]
   a. Rizatriptan in treatment of migraine
   b. Raltegravir in HIV infection
   c. Infliximab as an immunomodulator
   d. Hormone replacement therapy
   e. Methotrexate in cancer chemotherapy.

ANSWER

For answer refer 2017 paper-II, Q. 5(a), Pg. 199

4. **Discuss mechanism of action, therapeutic uses and adverse effects of:** [10]
   a. Ceftriaxone
   b. Phenytoin

ANSWER

For answer refer 2017 paper-I, Q. 5(a), Pg. 191
   c. Metronidazole
   d. Alprazolam
   e. Lignocaine.

ANSWER

For answer refer 2015 paper-I, Q. 5(a), Pg. 219

Model Paper: Pharmacology-I

Second Prof [MBBS] 2015

Time: 3 Hours   M.M.: 40

Instructions

Note: Attempt all questions from section-I and section-II directed. Draw neat and labeled diagrams wherever necessary

---

PART-I

1. **Explain why:**   [10]
   a. Close monitoring is required in patients in whom quinidine and digoxin are co-administered
   b. Therapeutic drug monitoring is not required for all the drugs
   c. Multiple doses of activated charcoal can speed elimination of absorbed drugs
   d. Glucagon is useful in management of beta-adrenergic blocker toxicity
   e. ACE inhibitors are contraindicated in patients with bilateral renal artery stenosis.

2. **Describe the mechanisms of action, therapeutic use and adverse effects of the following:**   [10]
   a. Dobutamine
   b. Spironolactone

ANSWER

For answer refer 2014 paper-I, Q. 5(a), Pg. 234
   c. Nicotinic acid
   d. Clopidogrel
   e. Aprepitant.

PART-II

3. **Describe in brief:**   [10]
   a. Drugs offering mortality benefits in heart failure
   b. Importance of pharmacogenetics to variability in drug response
   c. Drug treatment of open angle glaucoma

ANSWER

For answer refer 2015 paper-I, Q. 3(c), Pg. 218
   d. Uroselective alpha adrenergic blockers
   e. Compare and contrast competitive and non-competitive neuromuscular blockers.

4. **Write short notes on:**   [10]
   a. Ligand and voltage gated ion channels
   b. Parenteral iron therapy
   c. Third generation beta blockers
   d. Low molecular weight heparins

ANSWER

For answer refer 2017 paper-II, Q. 1(d), Pg. 195
   e. Hit and run drugs.

Model Paper: Pharmacology-I

Second Prof [MBBS] 2014

Time: 3 Hours   **M.M.: 40**

Instructions

Note: Attempt all questions from section-I and section-II directed. Draw neat and labeled diagrams wherever necessary

---

PART-I

1. **Explain the following:**   [10]
   a. Co-administration of aspirin with ibuprofen results in failure of antiplatelet effects of aspirin
   b. Phenobarbitone is used for treatment of kernicterus in failure of levodopa therapy in patients of parkinsonism
   c. While physotigmine is effective in atropine poisoning neostigmine is not
   d. Morphine is effective in acute LVF.

2. **Discuss the drug treatment of:**   [10]
   a. Hypertensive emergency

ANSWER

For answer refer 2009 paper-I, Q. 4(a), Pg. 301
   b. Peptic ulcer disease.

ANSWER

For answer refer 2019 paper-II, Q. 4(b), Pg. RP-131

PART-II

3. **Write the pharmacological basis of therapeutic use of:**   [10]
   a. Thiopentone sodium for induction of general anacsthesia

ANSWER

For answer refer 2018 paper-I, Q. 3(c), Pg. RP-138
   b. GTN in angina pectoris

ANSWER

For answer refer 2017 paper-I, Q. 2, Pg. 187
   c. Propranolol in anxiety
   d. Captopril in CHF.

4. **Write in brief on the following:**   [10]
   a. Plasma half life and its clinical significance

ANSWER

For answer refer 2019 paper-I, Q. 6(a), Pg. RP-125

b. Oral anti coagulants

c. Statins

ANSWER

For answer refer 2007 paper-I, Q. 5(b), Pg. 326

d. Loop diuretics.

ANSWER

For answer refer 2007 paper-I, Q. 1(a), Pg. 323

Model Paper: Pharmacology-II

Second Prof [MBBS] 2014

Time: 3 Hours   M.M.: 40

Instructions

Note: Attempt all questions from section-I and section-II directed. Draw neat and labeled diagrams wherever necessary

PART-I

1. **Explain the following:**   [10]

   a. Cotrimoxazole contains sulphamethoxazole and Trimethoprim in ration of 5:1

   b. Finasteride is effective in Benign hypertrophy of prostate

ANSWER

For answer refer 2007 paper-II, Q. 3(d), Pg. 331

   c. Levodopa along with carbidopa is used in parkinsonism

ANSWER

For answer refer 2008 paper-I, Q. 3(c), Pg. 311

   d. Cilastatin is used in combination with imipenem

ANSWER

For answer refer 2008 paper-II, Q. 5(b), Pg. 320

   e. Corticosteroids are useful in Bronchial asthma.

2. **Discuss the drug treatment of:**   [10]

   a. Chloroquine resistant malaria

ANSWER

For answer refer 2008 paper-II, Q. 6(b), Pg. 321

   b. Migraine.

ANSWER

For answer refer 2013 paper-II, Q. 3(c), Pg. 252-253

3. **Write the pharmacological basis of therapeutic use of:** [10]

   a. Diazepam in status epilepticus

ANSWER

For answer refer 2010 paper-I, Q. 2, Pg. 286

   b. Rosiglitazone in Diabetes mellitus
   c. Montelukast in bronchial asthma.

ANSWER

For answer refer 2017 paper-I, Q. 3(d), Pg. 189

4. **Write in brief on the following:** [10]

   a. Tocolytics
   b. Propylthiouracil
   c. Fluconazole
   d. Mini pill.

Model Paper: Pharmacology-I

Second Prof [MBBS] 2013

Time: 3 Hours   M.M.: 40

Instructions

Note: Attempt all questions from section-I and section-II directed. Draw neat and labeled diagrams wherever necessary

PART-I

1. **Explain why:** [10]

   a. "Drug holidays" are useful during long-term treatment of angina pectoris with nitrates
   b. Pentazocine is not used in patients of acute MI
   c. Folic acid should not be given alone in undiagnosed megaloblastic anaemia
   d. β-agonists increase the peak force of contraction of myocardium but also increase its rate of relaxation
   e. Digoxin in therapeutic dose causes bradycardia but in toxic dose produces ventricular tachyarrhythmia.

2. **Describe the mechanism of action, therapeutic use and dose limiting adverse effect of the following:** [10]

   a. Clopidogrel
   b. Atorvastatin

ANSWER

For answer refer 2009 paper-I, Q. 6(a), Pg. 302-303

   c. Dopamine
   d. Febuxostat
   e. Prochlorperazine.

3. **Describe in brief:** [10]

    a.   Competitive antagonism and its therapeutic application

    b.   Role of beta blockers in long term management of CHF

ANSWER

For answer refer 2014 paper-I, Q. 3(b), Pg. 233

    c.   Advantages of low molecular weight heparins over conventional heparin

    d.   Therapeutic uses of prostaglandin analogues

    e.   Anorectic agents.

4. **Write short notes on:** [10]

    a.   Pharmacovigilance

ANSWER

For answer refer 2013 paper-I, Q. 6(a), Pg. 248

    b.   Enzyme linked receptors

    c.   Essential drugs

ANSWER

For answer refer 2012 paper-I, Q. 6(b), Pg. 261

    d.   Drug treatment of Glaucoma

ANSWER

For answer refer 2013 paper-I, Q. 4(a), Pg. 246

    e.   High ceiling diuretics.

ANSWER

For answer refer Furosemide 2015 paper-I, Q. 5(b), Pg. 219

Model Paper: Pharmacology-I

Second Prof [MBBS] 2012

Time: 3 Hours   **M.M.: 40**

Instructions

Note: Attempt all questions from section-I and section-II directed. Draw neat and labeled diagrams wherever necessary

---

PART-I

1. **Explain why:**   [10]

   a. Low dose aspirin is used in management of myocardial infarction

   ANSWER

   For answer refer 2019 paper-I, Q. 1(a), Pg. RP-120

   b. Beta blockade should not be attempted prior to alpha blockade in patients of pheochromocytoma

   c. Physostigmine and not neostigmine is used in the treatment of atropine poisoning

   d. Furosemide is used in the treatment of acute pulmonary edema

   ANSWER

   For answer refer 2019 paper-I, Q. 1(d), Pg. RP-120

   e. Propranolol is contraindicated in patients with peripheral arterial disease.

2. **Discuss the pharmacological management of the following:**   [10]

   a. Acute congestive glaucoma

   b. Peptic ulcer

   ANSWER

   For answer refer 2015 paper-II, Q. 4(b), Pg. 227

   c. Congestive cardiac failure

   ANSWER

   For answer refer 2011 paper-I, Q. 4(a), Pg. 274

   d. Organophosphate poisoning.

   ANSWER

   For answer refer 2010 paper-I, Q. 3(d), Pg. 287

PART-II

3. **Write briefly on the following:**   [10]

   a. Pharmacovigilance

   ANSWER

   For answer refer 2013 paper-I, Q. 6(a), Pg. 248

b. Bisphosphonates

ANSWER

For answer refer 2007 paper-II, Q. 5(a), Pg. 332

c. Hepatic enzyme inducers

d. Half life

ANSWER

For answer refer 2015 paper-I, Q. 6(c), Pg. 220

e. Atracurium.

4. **Describe in brief, the mechanism of action, indications and adverse effects of the following:** [10]

a. Propranolol

b. Atropine

c. Digoxin

d. Low molecular weight heparins.

Model Paper: Pharmacology-II
Second Prof [MBBS] 2012

Time: 3 Hours   M.M.: 40

Instructions

Note: Attempt all questions from section-I and section-II directed. Draw neat and labeled diagrams wherever necessary

---

PART-I

1. **Explain why:** [10]

a. Glucocorticoids are not effective alone in acute anaphylactic reaction

b. Phenytoin is contraindicated in pregnancy

c. Therapeutic effect of anti-depressants is delayed for few weeks after starting the drug therapy

d. Benzodiazepines are not suitable for long term treatment of epilepsy

e. Clomiphene is preferred over tamoxifen for treatment of infertility.

ANSWER

For answer refer 2010 paper-II, Q. 6(a), Pg. 296-297

2. **Discuss briefly the drug treatment of following:** [10]

a. Diabetic ketoacidosis

ANSWER

For answer refer 2012 paper-II, Q. 4(a), Pg. 267

b. Bipolar disorder

ANSWER

For answer refer 2010 paper-I, Q. 4(b), Pg. 288

c. MRSA infection

d. Kala-azar.

3. Describe the rationale for the use of: [10]

   a. Halotha halothane and nitrous oxide co-administration for general anesthesia

   b. Aspirin for cardio protective role

   c. Gentamicin as single bolus dose instead of divided doses

   d. Methotrexate in rheumatoid arthritis

   e. Dexamethasone as diagnostic agent

4. Discuss briefly on: [10]

   a. 3rd generation cephalosporins

ANSWER

For answer refer 2019 paper-II, Q. 6(c), Pg. RP-133

   b. Cyclosporine

   c. Drug treatment of migraine

ANSWER

For answer refer 2013 paper-II, Q. 3(c), Pg. 252-253

   d. MDR tuberculosis.

Model Paper: Pharmacology-I
Second Prof [MBBS] 2011

Time: 3 Hours   **M.M.: 40**

Instructions

Note: Attempt all questions from section-I and section-II directed. Draw neat and labeled diagrams wherever necessary

PART-I

1. Explain why: [10]

   a. Spironolactone is used in the treatment of congestive heart failure

ANSWER

For answer refer 2017 paper-I, Q. 3(a), Pg. 188

   b. Alterplase is used in the treatment of myocardial infarction

ANSWER

For answer refer 2011 paper-II, Q. 5(a), Pg. 282

   c. Tamsulosin is used in the treatment of benign hypertrophy of prostate

ANSWER

For answer refer 2014 paper-I, Q. 3(a), Pg. 232

   d. Physostigmine and not neostigmine, is used in the treatment of atropine poisoning

e. Furosamide is used in the treatment of acute pulmonary oedema.

ANSWER

For answer refer 2019 paper-I, Q. 1(d), Pg. RP-120

2. **Discuss the drug treatment along with the pharmacological bans of drugs used in:** [10]

    a. Acute congestive glaucoma

    b. Vomiting.

PART-II

3. **Discuss the rationale for the use of:** [10]

    a. Epoetin in anaemia of chronic renal failure

    b. Calcium disodium edetate in lead poisoning

    c. Atenolol in hypertension

    d. Omeprazole in peptic ulcer.

ANSWER

For answer refer 2010 paper-II, Q. 2, Pg. 293

4. **Write short notes on:** [10]

    a. Bioavailability and bioequivalence

ANSWER

For answer refer 2017 paper-I, Q. 6(a) Pg. 191-192 and 2019 paper-I, Q. 6(b) Pg. RP-125

    b. Drug antagonism

    c. Lignocaine

ANSWER

For answer refer 2015 paper-I, Q. 5(a), Pg. 219

    d. Milrinone.

Model Paper: Pharmacology-I
Second Prof [MBBS] 2010

Time: 3 Hours   M.M.: 40

Instructions

Note: Attempt all questions from section-I and section-II directed. Draw neat and labeled diagrams wherever necessary

---

PART-I

1. **Explain why?**   [10]
   a. Sublingual glyceral trinitrate is used in the treatment of acute attack of angina
   b. Neostigmine is administered to reverse the action of non-depolarizing neuromuscular –blocking drugs at the end of an operation
   c. Oxytocin is preferred over ergometrine to augment labour
   d. Disulfiram is used as a pharmacologic adjunct in the treatment of alcoholism

ANSWER

For answer refer 2017 paper-I, Q. 4(b), Pg. 190

   e. Use of multivitamin preparations for the treatment of vitamin B_{12} deficiency can be dangerous.

2. **Discuss the drug treatment along with pharmacological basis of drugs used is:**   [10]
   a. Open angle glaucoma

ANSWER

For answer refer 2013 paper-I, Q. 4(a), Pg. 246

   b. Dyslipidaemia.

ANSWER

For answer refer 2007 paper-I, Q. 5(b), Pg. 326

PART-II

3. **Discuss the rationale for the use of:**   [10]
   a. β blockers in myocardial infarction
   b. Amiloride with hydrochlorothiazide
   c. Low molecular weight heparins in deep vein thrombosis
   d. Antibiotics in peptic ulcer disease
   e. ACE inhibitors in congestive heart failure.

ANSWER

For answer refer 2007 paper-I, Q. 5(a), Pg. 326

4. **Write short notes on:**   [10]
   a. Latrogenic disease
   b. First pass metabolism

c. Spinal anaesthesia
d. Therapeutic index

ANSWER

For answer refer 2016 paper-I, Q. 6(b), Pg. 206

e. Genetic polymorphism in drug metabolism.

Model Paper: Pharmacology-II
Second Prof [MBBS] 2010

Time: 3 Hours   M.M.: 40

Instructions

Note: Attempt all questions from section-I and section-II directed. Draw neat and labeled diagrams wherever necessary

---

PART-I

1. **Explain why:**   [10]
   a. Drug combination therapy is used in treatment of tuberculosis
   b. Sodium valproate is used in treatment of epilepsy
   c. Lesna is usually coadministered with cyclophosphamide
   d. Inhaled corticosteroids are preferred is long term prophylaxis of bronchial asthma
   e. Folinic acid is given with high dose methotrexate therapy.

2. **Discuss the therapeutic status of:**   [10]
   a. Aromatase inhibitors in breast cancer
   b. Benzodiazepines in epilepsy
   c. Clozapine in psychosis
   d. Sodium cromoglycate in bronchial asthma

ANSWER

For answer refer 2008 paper-I, Q. 5(a), Pg. 312

   e. Albandazole in neurocysticercosis.

PART-II

3. **Give the rationale for the use of:**   [10]
   a. Raloxifene in osteoporosis

ANSWER

For answer refer 2016 paper-II, Q. 4(b), Pg. 212

   b. Benzodiazepines in epilepsy
   c. Clozapine in psychosis
   d. Sodium chromoglycate in bronchial asthma

ANSWER

For answer refer 2008 paper-I, Q. 5(a), Pg. 312

e. Albandazole in neurocysticercosis.

4. Discuss the drug treatment of: [10]

a. Diabetic ketoacidosis

ANSWER

For answer refer 2012 paper-II, Q. 4(a), Pg. 267

b. Leprosy

ANSWER

For answer refer 2016 paper-II, Q. 4(a), Pg. 211

c. Status epilepticus

ANSWER

For answer refer 2008 paper-I, Q. 1(a), Pg. 309

d. Typhoid fever

ANSWER

For answer refer 2015 paper-II, Q. 4(a), Pg. 227

e. Hyperprolactinemia.

Model Paper: Microbiology-I

Second Prof [MBBS] 2019

Time: 3 Hours   M.M.: 40

Instructions

Note: Attempt all questions from section-I and section-II directed. Draw neat and labeled diagrams wherever necessary

PART-I

1. What is complement? Explain classical complement pathway. List complement deficiency diseases.   [10]

ANSWER

For answer of Classical Complement Pathway refer 2016 paper-I, Q. 2(a), Pg. 355

2. Write in brief about   [10]

   a. Draw a labelled diagram of the structure of flagella in a gram negative bacteria
   b. Laboratory diagnosis of whooping cough
   c. Methicillin resistant staphylococcus aureus (MRSA)

ANSWER

For answer refer 2013 paper-I, Q. 6, Pg. 391

   d. Plasma sterilization
   e. Enrichment media.

PART-II

3. A 3 year old boy presented to the Emergency Department with the complaint of fever and difficulty in breathing. On examination a pseudomembrane was observed in his throat. Give your diagnosis and name the causative agent. Elaborate the laboratory diagnosis for the case.   [10]

4. Write short notes on: [10]

   a. Leptospirosis

ANSWER

For answer refer 2008 paper-I, Q. 4(a), Pg. 440

   b. HACEK group of bacteria
   c. Laboratory diagnosis of cholera.

ANSWER

For answer refer 2016 paper-I, Q. 4(a), Pg. 357

Model Paper: Microbiology-I
Second Prof [MBBS] 2018

Time: 3 Hours   M.M.: 40

Instructions

Note: Attempt all questions from section-I and section-II directed. Draw neat and labeled diagrams wherever necessary

---

PART-I

1. **Enumerate antigen-antibody reactions. Describe agglutination reaction with appropriate examples.**   [10]

ANSWER

For Agglutination Reaction refer 2018 paper-I, Q. 2(a), Pg. RP-171

2. **Write briefly about the following:**   [10]
   a. Monoclonal antibody

ANSWER

For answer refer 2017 paper-I, Q. 2(a), Pg. 389

   b. Type-III hypersensitivity

ANSWER

For answer refer 2011 paper-I, Q. 2(b), Pg. 412

   c. IgM

ANSWER

For answer refer 2019 paper-I, Q. 2(a), Pg. RP-153

   d. Bacterial capsule

ANSWER

For answer refer 2018 paper-I, Q. 2(b), Pg. RP-172

   e. Differences between active and passive immunity.

PART-II

3. **Classify anaerobic bacteria. Write about the methods of anaerobiosis.**   [10]

ANSWER

For answer Methods of Anaerobiosis refer 2013 paper-I, Q. 1, Pg. 389

4. **Write short notes on:**   [10]
   a. VDRL test   b. Atypical Mycobacteria
   c. TRIC agent

ANSWER

For answer refer 2007 paper-I, Q. 4(a), Pg. 449

   d. Group B streptococcus   e. DPT vaccine.

Model Paper: Microbiology-II

Second Prof [MBBS] November 2018

Time: 3 Hours   **M.M.: 40**

Instructions

Note: Attempt all questions from section-I and section-II directed. Draw neat and labeled diagrams wherever necessary

---

PART-I

1. Describe for life cycle, pathogenesis and methods of laboratory diagnosis of plasmodium parasite infection in Homo sapiens.   [10]

ANSWER

For answer refer Life Cycle refer 2013 paper-II, Q. 1, Pg. 393

2. Write in brief about: [10]
   i.   NIH swab
   ii. Laboratory diagnosis of hydatid cyst disease

ANSWER

For answer refer 2017 paper-II, Q. 2(b), Pg. 346 and 2007 paper-II, Q. 2(b), Pg. 453

   iii. Laboratory diagnosis of toxoplasmosis

ANSWER

For answer refer 2017 paper-II, Q. 2(a), Pg. 346

   iv. Acanthamoeba

ANSWER

For answer refer 2016 paper-II, Q. 1, Pg. 362

   v.   PKDL (Post kala-azar dermal leishmaniasis).

PART-II

3. Describe laboratory diagnosis of a case of influenza virus infection. Write in brief about antigenic shift and drift in influenza. Add a note on prevention of influenza including vaccines.   [10]

4. Write short notes on: [10]
   i.   Histoplasmosis
   ii. Treatment and method of disposal of biomedical waste

ANSWER

For answer refer 2018 paper-I, Q. 5, Pg. RP-175

   iii. Germ tube test
   iv. NACO strategies for HIV testing.

ANSWER

For answer refer 2013 paper-II, Q. 6, Pg. 397

Model Paper: Microbiology-I
Second Prof [MBBS] 2017

Time: 3 Hours   **M.M.: 40**

Instructions

Note: Attempt all questions from section-I and section-II directed. Draw neat and labeled diagrams wherever necessary

---

PART-I

1. a. i. **Write down differences between exotoxin and endotoxin**   **[6]**

ANSWER

For answer refer 2016 paper-I, Q. 2(b), Pg. 356

    ii. **Anaerobic culture methods.**

ANSWER

For answer refer 2013 paper-I, Q. 1, Pg. 389

   b. **Short notes on:**   **[4]**

    i. Bacterial capsule

ANSWER

For answer refer 2018 paper-I, Q. 2(b), Pg. RP-172

    ii. Gaseous disinfectants.

2. a. **Write the differences between T-Lymphocyte and B-Lymphocyte.**   **[2]**

   b. **Write briefly:**   **[8]**

    i. Principle of immunofluorescent test

ANSWER

For answer refer 2008 paper-I, Q. 2(b), Pg. 439

    ii. Adjuvant

ANSWER

For answer refer 2007 paper-I, Q. 2(b), Pg. 448

    iii. Type II hypersensitivity

    iv. IgM.

ANSWER

For answer refer 2019 paper-I, Q. 2(a), Pg. RP-153

3. **Classify streptococci. Enumerate the toxins and enzymes produced by streptococcus pyogenes. Discuss the laboratory diagnosis of non-suppurative complications of streptococcus pyogenes infection.** [10]

ANSWER

For answer Toxins and Enzymes Produced by Streptococcus Pyogenes refer 2015 paper-I, Q. 4(b), Pg. 370

4. **Write short notes on:** [10]

   a. Chlamydia trachomatis

ANSWER

For answer refer 2014 paper-I, Q. 4(a), Pg. 382

   b. Enterotoxins of Escherichia coli

   c. Leptospirosis.

ANSWER

For answer refer 2008 paper-I, Q. 4(a), Pg. 440

Model Paper: Microbiology-II

Second Prof [MBBS] 2017

Time: 3 Hours   **M.M.: 40**

Instructions

Note: Attempt all questions from section-I and section-II directed. Draw neat and labeled diagrams wherever necessary

PART-I

1. Describe the life cycle, pathogenesis and laboratory diagnosis of Echinococcosis.   [10]

2. Write short notes on the following: [10]
   a. Laboratory diagnosis of tapeworm infection
   b. Post kala azar dermal leishmaniasis
   c. Laboratory diagnosis of intestinal amoebiasis
   d. Larva migrans

ANSWER

For answer refer 2019 paper-II, Q. 2(b), Pg. RP-165 and 2008 paper-II, 2(b) Pg. 444
   e. Viviparous nematode.

PART-II

3. Describe the pathogenesis, laboratory diagnosis and prevention of Hepatitis B virus infection.   [10]

ANSWER

For Prophylaxis refer 2017 paper-II, Q. 4(b), Pg. 349

4. Write in brief about: [10]
   a. Dengue virus
   b. Aspergillosis

ANSWER

For answer refer 2016 paper-II, Q. 4(b), Pg. 364
   c. Dermatophytes.

ANSWER

For answer refer 2015 paper-II, Q. 3 Pg. 375 and 2010 paper-II, Q. 3, Pg. 428

Time: 3 Hours   **M.M.: 40**

Instructions

Note: Attempt all questions from section-I and section-II directed. Draw neat and labeled diagrams wherever necessary

PART-I

1. a. Draw a labeled diagram of bacterial cell wall. Describe the difference between cell wall of gram positive and gram negative bacteria.   [6]

   b. Write briefly about the following: [4]

      i. Pili

      ii. Hot air oven.

ANSWER

For answer refer 2019 paper-I, Q. 1, Pg. RP-152

2. Write briefly about the following: [10]

   a. Alternate complement pathway

   b. Type III hypersensitivity reaction

ANSWER

For answer refer 2011 paper-I, Q. 2(b), Pg. 412

   c. Structure and function of IgA

   d. Transformation

ANSWER

For answer refer 2012 paper-I, Q. 1, Pg. 400

   e. Multiplex PCR.

PART-II

3. Define PUO and enumerate the causes of PUO. Describe the laboratory diagnosis of Enteric fever.   [10]

ANSWER

For answer refer 2016 paper-I, Q. 5 Pg. 358 and 2017 paper-I, Q. 3, Pg. 340

4. Write briefly about: [10]

   a. Non-tuberculous mycobacteria (NTMs)

   b. Difference between diphtheria and diphtheroids

   c. Methods of anaerobiosis.

ANSWER

For answer refer 2013 paper-I, Q. 1, Pg. 389

Model Paper: Microbiology-II
Second Prof [MBBS] 2016

Time: 3 Hours

M.M.: 40

Instructions

Note: Attempt all questions from section-I and section-II directed. Draw neat and labeled diagrams wherever necessary

---

PART-I

1. Enumerate vector borne parasitic diseases. Describe life cycle, pathogenesis and laboratory diagnosis of plasmodium falciparum. **[10]**

ANSWER

For answer refer 2013 paper-II, Q. 1, Pg. 394

2. Write briefly about the following: **[10]**

   a. Cysticercus cellulosae

ANSWER

For answer refer 2013 paper-II, Q. 2(a), Pg. 394

   b. Visceral larva migrans

ANSWER

For answer refer 2019 paper-II, Q. 2(b), Pg. RP-165

   c. Microfilaria

ANSWER

For answer refer 2017 paper-II, Q. 1, Pg. 345

   d. Life cycle of hookworm

ANSWER

For answer refer 2013 paper-II, Q. 2(b), Pg. 393

   e. Difference between amoebic and bacillary dysentery.

PART-II

3. Name the arboviruses common in India. Describe pathogenesis, complications and laboratory diagnosis of dengue fever. **[10]**

ANSWER

For answer refer 2014 paper-II, Q. 6, Pg. 387

4. Write briefly about the following: **[10]**

   a. Dermatophytes

ANSWER

For answer refer 2015 paper-II, Q. 3 Pg. 375 and 2010 paper-II, Q. 3, Pg. 428

   b. Mycetoma

   c. Mycotoxicosis.

Model Paper: Microbiology-II

Second Prof [MBBS] 2015

Time: 3 Hours   **M.M.: 40**

Instructions

Note: Attempt all questions from section-I and section-II directed. Draw neat and labeled diagrams wherever necessary

PART-I

1. Name the parasite/s causing filariasis in India. Describe the life cycle of the parasite & write about the laboratory diagnosis of Filariasis. [10]

ANSWER

For answer refer 2017 paper-II, Q. 1, Pg. 345

2. Write short notes on: [10]

    a. Toxoplasmosis

ANSWER

For answer refer 2017 paper-II, Q. 2(a), Pg. 346

    b. Casoni test

ANSWER

For answer refer 2007 paper-II, Q. 2(b), Pg. 453

    c. Cryptosporidium parvum

ANSWER

For answer refer 2009 paper-II, Q. 2(b), Pg. 435

    d. Trichomonas vaginalis

    e. Difference between bacillary and amoebic dysentery.

PART-II

3. Classify viruses and give three (3) examples in each group. Write briefly about the various methods for laboratory diagnosis of viral infection [10]

ANSWER

For answer refer 2016 paper-II, Q. 6, Pg. 365

4. Write short notes on: [10]

    a. Dengue haemorrhagic fever   b. Mycetoma

    c. Dimorphic fungus

ANSWER

For answer refer 2014 paper-II, Q. 3, Pg. 385

    d. Mycotic keratitis   e. Chikungunya.

Model Paper: Microbiology-I

Second Prof [MBBS] 2014

Time: 3 Hours   **M.M.: 40**

Instructions

Note: Attempt all questions from section-I and section-II directed. Draw neat and labeled diagrams wherever necessary

---

PART-I

1. a. **Describe the mechanism of transduction.**   [5]

ANSWER

For answer refer 2012 paper-I, Q. 1, Pg. 400

   b. **Write briefly on the following:**   [5]

   i.   Sterilization by filtration
   ii. Bacterial capsule.

ANSWER

For answer refer 2018 paper-I, Q. 2(b), Pg. RP-172

2. **Write short notes on the following:**   [10]

   a. Louis Pasteur
   b. Autoclave .

ANSWER

For answer refer 2010 paper-I, Q. 1, Pg. 421

   c. Dark ground microscopy
   d. Difference between active and passive immunity
   e. Structure of IgG.

PART-II

---

3. **Classify spirochetes causing disease in man. Write briefly the laboratory diagnosis of primary syphilis.**   [5]

ANSWER

For Laboratory Diagnosis of Primary Syphilis refer 2019 paper-I, Q. 3, Pg. RP-155

4. **Briefly outline the diagnosis of pulmonary tuberculosis.**   [5]

ANSWER

For answer refer 2007 paper-I, Q. 3, Pg. 448

5. **Write short notes on the following:**   [10]

   a. Camp test
   b. DPT vaccine
   c. Difference between streptococcus pneumonia and streptococcus viridans.

Model Paper: Microbiology-II

Second Prof [MBBS] 2014

Time: 3 Hours   M.M.: 40

Instructions

Note: Attempt all questions from section-I and section-II directed. Draw neat and labeled diagrams wherever necessary

---

PART-I

1. a. A patient, resident of Bihar suffering from fever, developed hepatosplenomegaly. He was admitted to a hospital with a provisional diagnosis of Kala azar. Differentiate the two morphological forms of its causative agent with diagram. Briefly describe the laboratory diagnosis of Kala azar under the following headings: (a) Specimen, (b) Direct examination (c) Rapid diagnostic tests. [10]

OR

Enumerate malarial parasites pathogenic to man. Describe with the help of a diagram the life cycle of the malarial parasite. Describe the laboratory diagnosis of malaria.

ANSWER

For answer refer 2013 paper-II, Q. 1, Pg. 393 and 2010 paper-II, Q. 1, Pg. 425

2. Write short notes on the following: [10]

   a. Casoni test

ANSWER

For answer refer 2007 paper-II, Q. 2(b), Pg. 453

   b. Cutaneous larva migrans

ANSWER

For answer refer 2008 paper-II, Q. 2(b), Pg. 444

   c. Diagnosis of Filariasis
   d. Cryptosporidium.

ANSWER

For answer refer 2009 paper-II, Q. 2(b), Pg. 435

PART-II

3. A 30 year old man develops fever, chills, headache, and backache. Five days later he develops petechial hemorrhage and a sudden drop in the platelet count to 30,000/mm^3. Name the causative agent and briefly describe the pathogenesis. Identify the specific tests for its laboratory diagnosis. [10]

4. Write in brief about the following: [10]

   a. Enumerate opportunistic infections in patient with HIV

ANSWER

For answer refer 2008 paper-II, Q. 3, Pg. 444

b.   Cryptococcosis
c.   Classification of superficial mycoses with examples
d.   Polio vaccine.

ANSWER

For answer refer 2011 paper-II, Q. 6, Pg. 419

Model Paper: Microbiology-I

Second Prof [MBBS] 2013

Time: 3 Hours   **M.M.: 40**

Instructions

Note: Attempt all questions from section-I and section-II directed. Draw neat and labeled diagrams wherever necessary

---

PART-I

1. a. **Draw a labeled diagram of bacterial cell. Describe the bacterial growth curve.**   [6]

   b. **Write briefly about the following:**   [4]
      i. Plasmid
      ii. Autoclave.

ANSWER

For answer refer 2010 paper-I, Q. 1, Pg. 421

2. **Write briefly about the following:**   [10]
   a. Properties of complement
   b. Delayed hypersensitivity
   c. Structure and function of IgG
   d. Transduction

ANSWER

For answer refer 2012 paper-I, Q. 1, Pg. 400

   e. Principle of Polymerase chain reaction.

ANSWER

For answer refer 2007 paper-I, Q. 6, Pg. 450

PART-II

3. **Name the causative agents of Enteric fever. Describe the laboratory diagnosis of enteric fever.**   [10]

ANSWER

For answer refer 2017 paper-I, Q. 3, Pg. 340

4. **Write the differences between the following:**   [10]
   a. Classical and El tor biotypes of Vibrio cholerae
   b. Streptococcus pneumonia and Streptococcus viridans
   c. Mycobacterium tuberculosis and mycobacterium bovis.

Model Paper: Microbiology-II
Second Prof [MBBS] 2013

Time: 3 Hours   **M.M.: 40**

Instructions

Note: Attempt all questions from section-I and section-II directed. Draw neat and labeled diagrams wherever necessary

PART-I

1. Describe the life cycle, pathogenesis and laboratory diagnosis of filariasis.   **[10]**

2. Write short notes on the following: **[10]**
   a. Toxoplasmosis

ANSWER

- -

For answer refer 2017 paper-II, Q. 2(a), Pg. 346
   b. Isospora belli
   c. Laboratory diagnosis of Malaria

ANSWER

- -

For answer refer 2015 paper-II, Q. 2(a), Pg. 374
   d. Laboratory diagnosis of extraintestinal amoebiasis
   e. Casoni Test.

ANSWER

- -

For answer refer 2007 paper-II, Q. 2(b), Pg. 453

PART-II

3. Describe the pathogenesis, laboratory diagnosis and prevention of poliomyelitis.   **[10]**

4. Write short notes on the following: **[10]**
   a. Cryptococcosis
   b. Non-albicans candida
   c. Rota virus.

ANSWER

- -

For answer refer 2014 paper-II, Q. 5, Pg. 386

Model Paper: Microbiology-II
Second Prof [MBBS] 2012

Time: 3 Hours   M.M.: 40

Instructions

Note: Attempt all questions from section-I and section-II directed. Draw neat and labeled diagrams wherever necessary

PART-I

1. Enumerate the cestodes causing diseases in humans. Write briefly on hydatid cyst and laboratory diagnosis of hydatid disease in man.   [10]

ANSWER

For answer refer 2017 paper-II, Q. 2(b), Pg. 346

2. Write briefly on: [10]
   a. Serological diagnosis of visceral leishmaniasis

ANSWER

For answer refer 2011 paper-II, Q. 1, Pg. 416

   b. Laboratory diagnosis of toxoplasmosis

ANSWER

For answer refer 2017 paper-II, Q. 2(a), Pg. 346

   c. Primary amoebic meningoencephalitis
   d. Life cycle of Ancylostoma duodenale

ANSWER

For answer refer 2013 paper-II, Q. 2(b), Pg. 396

   e. Cysticercus cellulosae.

PART-II

3. Enumerate arboviruses prevalent in India. Describe the pathogenicity and laboratory diagnosis of dengue virus.   [10]

ANSWER

For answer refer 2014 paper-II, Q. 6, Pg. 387

4. Write short notes on the following: [10]
   a. Rhinosporidiosis

ANSWER

For answer refer 2011 paper-II, Q. 4(a), Pg. 418

b.   Histoplasmosis

ANSWER

For answer refer 2010 paper-II, Q. 4(a), Pg. 428

c.   Cryptococcosis

d.   Classification of fungi

e.   Kuru.

Model Paper: Microbiology-II
Second Prof [MBBS] 2011

Time: 3 Hours   M.M.: 40

Instructions

Note: Attempt all questions from section-I and section-II directed. Draw neat and labeled diagrams wherever necessary

---

PART-I

1. a.   **Describe the life cycle and laboratory diagnosis of Leishmania donovani. Draw labeled diagram.**   [6]

ANSWER

For answer refer 2016 paper-II, Q. 2(a), Pg. 362 and 2011 paper-II, Q. 1, Pg. 416

   b.   **Enumerate free living amoebae. Describe their morphology with suitable labeled diagrams. List the diseases caused by them.**   [4]

ANSWER

For answer refer 2016 paper-II, Q. 1, Pg. 362

2.   **Write in brief about:**   [10]

a.   Cryptosporidium parvum- morphology, disease and lab. Diagnosis

ANSWER

For answer refer 2009 paper-II, Q. 2(b), Pg. 435

b.   Laboratory diagnosis of toxoplasmosis

ANSWER

For answer refer 2017 paper-II, Q. 2(a), Pg. 346

c.   Differentiate between plasmodium vivax and plasmodium falciparum

ANSWER

For answer refer 2008 paper-II, Q. 2(a), Pg. 443

d.   Life cycle of Taenia saginata with labeled diagrams

e.   Lab diagnosis of extra-intestinal amoebiasis.

3. Draw labeled diagram of HIV. Describe its modes of transmission and pathogenicity. How do you diagnose AIDS patient? What type of opportunistic infections are seen in AIDS patients? [10]

ANSWER

For answer refer 2017 paper-II, Q. 5, Pg. 349 and 2008 paper-II, Q. 3, Pg. 444

4. Write short notes on the following: [10]

   a. Aspergillosis

ANSWER

For answer refer 2016 paper-II, Q. 4(b), Pg. 364

   b. Rhinosporidiosis

ANSWER

For answer refer 2011 paper-II, Q. 4(a), Pg. 418

   c. Mycetoma foot
   d. Candida albicans

ANSWER

For answer refer 2016 paper-II, Q. 3 Pg. 363 and 2013 paper-II, Q. 3, Pg. 396

   e. Histoplasmosis.

ANSWER

For answer refer 2010 paper-II, Q. 4(a), Pg. 428

Model Paper: Microbiology-II

Second Prof [MBBS] 2010

Time: 3 Hours   M.M.: 40

Instructions

Note: Attempt all questions from section-I and section-II directed. Draw neat and labeled diagrams wherever necessary

PART-I

1. a. Enumerate the human infections caused by protozoa. Describe in brief the life cycle of Plasmodium. Add a note on laboratory diagnosis of malaria. [6]

ANSWER

For answer Life Cycle of Plasmodium refer 2013 paper-II, Q. 1 Pg. 393 and Laboratory Diagnosis of Malaria 2015 paper-II, Q. 2(a) Pg. 374

   b. Briefly write about the different techniques used for examination of a stool specimen for ova and cysts giving advantages and disadvantages of each method. [4]

2. Write in brief about: [10]
   a. Hydatid disease

ANSWER

For answer refer 2017 paper-II, Q. 2(b), Pg. 346
   b. Laboratory diagnosis of kala-azar

ANSWER

For answer refer 2016 paper-II, Q. 2(b), Pg. 362
   c. Cutaneous larva migrans

ANSWER

For answer refer 2008 paper-II, Q. 2(b), Pg. 444
   d. Cryptosporidiosis
   e. Amoebic dysentery.

PART-II

3. Enumerate the arthropod borne virus infections. Describe the complications and laboratory diagnosis of dengue fever. [8]

ANSWER

For answer refer 2014 paper-II, Q. 6, Pg. 387

4. Write in brief about: [12]
   a. Cryptococcosis
   b. Mycetoma
   c. Opportunistic fungal infections

ANSWER

For answer refer 2019 paper-II, Q. 3, Pg. RP-165
   d. Staining methods for fungi

ANSWER

For answer refer 2008 paper-II, Q. 4(b), Pg. 445
   e. Postexposure prophylaxis in rabies

ANSWER

For answer refer 2017 paper-II, Q. 6, Pg. 351
   f. Enumerate the viruses causing respiratory tract infections. Write in brief about lab diagnosis of influenza.

Model Paper: Microbiology-II

Second Prof [MBBS] 2008

Time: 3 Hours   M.M.: 40

Instructions

Note: Attempt all questions from section-I and section-II directed. Draw neat and labeled diagrams wherever necessary

---

PART-I

1. a. Describe, in brief, life cycle and laboratory diagnosis of plasmodium parasite infection with suitable labeled diagrams.   [6]

ANSWER

For answer refer 2013 paper-II, Q. 1, Pg. 393 and 2015 paper-II, Q. 2(a), Pg. 374

   b. Define definitive host and intermediate host with suitable examples. Mention their importance in study of parasitic diseases.   [4]

2. Write briefly on: [10]

   a. Hydatid cyst disease and steps of its laboratory diagnosis

ANSWER

For answer refer 2017 paper-II, Q. 2(b), Pg. 346

   b. Larva migrans-Types and its clinical effects

ANSWER

For answer refer 2008 paper-II, Q. 2(a), Pg. 444

   c. Giardiasis and its detection in laboratory
   d. Methods used for detection of Microfilariae from blood
   e. Ova and cysts commonly seen in routine stool examination.

PART-II

3. List Hepatitis viruses. Mention important routes of transmission of hepatitis B virus infection. Briefly, outline the steps of laboratory diagnosis of hepatitis B virus infection.   [10]

ANSWER

For answer refer 2018 paper-II, Q. 3, Pg. RP-182

4. Write in brief about: [10]

   a. Culture media employed, in routine, for primary isolation of fungi from clinical specimens
   b. Dimorphic fungi of medical importance

ANSWER

For answer refer 2011 paper-II, Q. 3, Pg. 417

   c. Mycotoxicosis and its prevention
   d. Yeast like fungal infections commonly seen in hospital settings
   e. 'In use' vaccine for pulse polio immunization program.

Model Paper: Forensic Medicine & Toxicology

Second Prof [MBBS] 2017

Time: 3 Hours   **M.M.: 40**

Instructions

Note: Attempt all questions from section-I and section-II directed. Draw neat and labeled diagrams wherever necessary

---

PART-I

1. **What are the findings, interpretations and medicolegal importance when it is stated that:**   **[10]**

   a.   A child is battered

   ANSWER

   For answer refer 2017 paper, Q. 1(c), Pg. 461

   b.   There is a case of partial hanging
   c.   Opisthotonus posture is seen
   d.   A bruise is 5 days old
   e.   A person is in lucid interval state

   ANSWER

   For answer refer 2012 paper, Q. 1(d), Pg. 501

2. **Write short notes on:**   **[10]**

   a.   Examination of a witness in the court of law

   ANSWER

   For answer refer 2016 paper, Q. 6(a), Pg. 475

   b.   Privileged communication

   ANSWER

   For answer refer 2015 paper, Q. 2(b), Pg. 480

   c.   Plumbism
   d.   Saponification
   e.   Diatoms test

   ANSWER

   For answer refer 2007 paper, Q. 1(d), Pg. 534

3. **Differentiate between:**   **[10]**

   a.   Arsenic poisoning and cholera

   ANSWER

   For answer refer 2013 paper, Q. 4(b), Pg. 495

   b.   Male and female pelvis

   ANSWER

   For answer refer 2017 paper, Q. 4(a), Pg. 463

c. True and false virgin

d. Poisonous and nonpoisonous snakes

ANSWER

For answer refer 2012 paper, Q. 4(b), Pg. 502

e. Antemortem and postmortem injury

ANSWER

For answer refer 2016 paper, Q. 4(c), Pg. 474

4. **Classify injuries. Describe in detail the injuries caused to a pedestrian in a road traffic accident. Discuss the Patho-physiology and MLI of whiplash injury.** [10]

ANSWER

For answer refer 2014 paper, Q. 5, Pg. 488

Model Paper: Forensic Medicine & Toxicology

Second Prof [MBBS] 2016

Time: 3 Hours

M.M.: 40

Instructions

Note: Attempt all questions from section-I and section-II directed. Draw neat and labeled diagrams wherever necessary

PART-I

1. **What are the findings and medicolegal importance when it is stated that:** [10]

   a. Skull is showing ring fracture

ANSWER

For answer refer 2007 paper, Q. 1(a), Pg. 533

   b. Hesitation cuts are present in a person

ANSWER

For answer refer 2012 paper, Q. 1(c), Pg. 500

   c. Fetus is dead born

ANSWER

For answer refer 2010 paper, Q. 1(c), Pg. 512

   d. Person is having hatters' shake

   e. Girl is 18 years of age.

ANSWER

For answer refer 2017 paper, Q. 1(a), Pg. 500

2. **Write short notes on:** [10]
   a. Grievous hurt
   b. Joule burn

ANSWER

For answer refer 2012 paper, Q. 6(c), Pg. 505
   c. Delusion

ANSWER

For answer refer 2008 paper, Q. 6(b), Pg. 531
   d. Treatment of a snake bite
   e. Entry wound of point blank range rifle bore firearm.

ANSWER

For answer refer 2017 paper, Q. 5, Pg. 464

PART-II

3. **Differentiate between:** [10]
   a. Male and female sacrum
   b. Rigor mortis and cadaveric spasm
   c. Seeds of Dhatura and capsicum

ANSWER

For answer refer 2007 paper, Q. 4(a), Pg. 534
   d. Ligature mark of hanging and strangulation

ANSWER

For answer refer 2008 paper, Q. 4(c), Pg. 530
   e. True and false virgin.

4. **Define and classify medical negligence. Describe in details the various medicolegal issues involved in case of such negligence.** [10]

Model Paper: Forensic Medicine & Toxicology

Second Prof [MBBS] 2015

Time: 3 Hours   **M.M.: 40**

Instructions

Note: Attempt all questions from section-I and section-II directed. Draw neat and labeled diagrams wherever necessary

---

PART-I

1. **What are the findings and medico-legal importance when it is stated that:**   **[10]**

    a. Child is a case of battered baby syndrome

    ANSWER

    For answer refer 2017 paper, Q. 1(c), Pg. 461

    b. Age of the boy is 21 years

    ANSWER

    For answer refer 2014 paper, Q. 1(a), Pg. 485

    c. Death is due to traumatic asphyxia

    ANSWER

    For answer refer 2010 paper, Q. 1(c), Pg. 512

    d. The person is suffering from delirium tremens

    ANSWER

    For answer refer 2017 paper, Q. 6(a), Pg. 465

    e. The women is a false virgin.

    ANSWER

    For answer refer 2014 paper, Q. 1(d), Pg. 486

2. **Write short notes on:**   **[10]**

    a. Res lpsa loquitur
    b. Section 320 IPC
    c. Treatment of acute cyanide poisoning
    d. Lab diagnosis of chronic lead poisoning
    e. Dactylography.

    ANSWER

    For answer refer 2012 paper, Q. 6(b), Pg. 504

PART-II

3. **Differentiate between:**   **[10]**

    a. Poisonous and non poisonous snakes

For answer refer 2012 paper, Q. 4(b), Pg. 502

b.   Hanging and ligature strangulation

ANSWER

For answer refer 2008 paper, Q. 4(c), Pg. 530

c.   Tetanus and strychnine poisoning

ANSWER

For answer refer 2015 paper, Q. 4(b), Pg. 482

d.   True and feigned insanity

ANSWER

For answer refer 2018 paper, Q. 4(b), Pg. RP-203

e.   Male and female skull.

ANSWER

For answer refer 2015 paper, Q. 4(c), Pg. 482

4.   **Define rape. How will you proceed to examine a girl victim of rape? What samples you will preserve? Discuss their medicolegal importance.**   **[10]**

ANSWER

For answer refer 2013 paper, Q. 6(b), Pg. 497

Model Paper: Forensic Medicine & Toxicology

Second Prof [MBBS] 2014

Time: 3 Hours   **M.M.: 40**

Instructions

Note: Attempt all questions from section-I and section-II directed. Draw neat and labeled diagrams wherever necessary

---

PART-I

1. **Write down findings and medicolegal importance in the following:**   [10]
   a. Death is due to drowning
   b. Sixteen weeks pregnancy
   c. Brain stem death

   ANSWER

   For answer refer 2017 paper, Q. 2(a), Pg. 461

   d. Death due to starvation
   e. Joule burn.

   ANSWER

   For answer refer 2012 paper, Q. 6(c), Pg. 505

2. **Write short notes on the following:**   [10]
   a. Hanging

   ANSWER

   For answer refer 2018 paper, Q. 6(b), Pg. RP-206

   b. Plumbism   c. I.P.C. 320
   d. Anaphylactic shock   e. Food poisoning

PART-II

---

3. **Write down signs, symptoms, and management and post mortem findings in a case of acute arsenic poisoning.**
                                                                                                       [10]

4. **Differentiate between the following:**   [10]
   a. Rigor Mortis and cadaveric spasm
   b. Strangulation and smothering
   c. Cobra and vipers snake bite

   ANSWER

   For answer refer 2010 paper, Q. 4(a), Pg. 516

   d. Common and expert witness
   e. True and False bruise.

   ANSWER

   For answer refer 2015 paper, Q. 4(a), Pg. 482

Model Paper: Forensic Medicine & Toxicology

Second Prof [MBBS] 2013

Time: 3 Hours   **M.M.: 40**

Instructions

Note: Attempt all questions from section-I and section-II directed. Draw neat and labeled diagrams wherever necessary

PART-I

1. **What are the findings and medicolegal importance when it is state that:**   **[10]**
   a. The patient is brain dead
   b. Washer woman's sign in a dead body
   c. Presence of spalding sign

ANSWER

For answer refer 2010 paper, Q. 1(c), Pg. 512
   d. Adipocere formation in a dead body
   e. Person has feigned insanity.

2. **Write short notes on:**   **[10]**
   a. Privileged communication

ANSWER

For answer refer 2015 paper, Q. 2(b), Pg. 480
   b. Management of organophosphorous poisoning

ANSWER

For answer refer 2019 paper, Q. 3, Pg. RP-194
   c. Superimposition
   d. Diatoms

ANSWER

For answer refer 2007 paper, Q. 1(d), Pg. 534
   e. Methods of criminal abortion.

ANSWER

For answer refer 2019 paper, Q. 5, Pg. RP-196

PART-II

3. **Differentiate between:**   **[10]**
   a. Male and female skull

ANSWER

For answer refer 2015 paper, Q. 4(c), Pg. 482

    b.   Dry and wet burns

    c.   Poisonous and Non Poisonous snakes

ANSWER

For answer refer 2012 paper, Q. 4(b), Pg. 502

    d.   Coup and contrecoup injuries

    e.   Human and animal hair.

ANSWER

For answer refer 2010 paper, Q. 4(b), Pg. 510

4.   **Define Rape. Describe the findings that are seen on medical examination in case of rape of a 16 year old girl. Enumerate biological evidences of medico legal importance that can be preserved and recent amendments**   **[10]**

ANSWER

For answer refer 2007 paper, Q. 5, Pg. 535

Model Paper: Forensic Medicine & Toxicology
Second Prof [MBBS] 2008

Time: 3 Hours   M.M.: 40

Instructions

Note: Attempt all questions from section-I and section-II directed. Draw neat and labeled diagrams wherever necessary

PART-I

1.   **What are the findings and medicolegal importance when it is stated that:**   **[10]**

    a.   The girls is 18 years of age

ANSWER

For answer refer 2017 paper, Q. 1(a), Pg. 500

    b.   The women is a false virgin

ANSWER

For answer refer 2014 paper, Q. 1(d), Pg. 486

    c.   Hesitation cuts are present over the neck

ANSWER

For answer refer 2012 paper, Q. 1(c), Pg. 500

    d.   The dead body is showing marbling

    e.   The person is in lucid interval.

ANSWER

For answer refer 2012 paper, Q. 1(d), Pg. 501

2. **Write short notes on:**   **[10]**
   a. Grievous hurt
   b. Delirium tremens

ANSWER

For answer refer 2017 paper, Q. 6(a), Pg. 465

   c. Dying declaration

ANSWER

For answer refer 2016 paper, Q. 2(c), Pg. 470

   d. Management of barbiturate poisoning
   e. Functions of medical council of India

ANSWER

For answer refer 2010 paper, Q. 5, Pg. 516

PART-B

3. **Differentiate between:**   **[10]**
   a. Male and female pelvis

ANSWER

For answer refer 2017 paper, Q. 4(a), Pg. 463

   b. Strychnine poisoning and tetanus

ANSWER

For answer refer 2015 paper, Q. 4(b), Pg. 482

   c. Postmortem staining and contusion
   d. Antemortem and postmortem burns

ANSWER

For answer refer 2016 paper, Q. 4(c), Pg. 474

   e. Police and magistrate's inquest.

4. **Classify violent asphyxia deaths. Discuss the postmortem findings in a case of drowning. Which are the findings suggestive of ante mortem drowning?**
                                                                          [10]

Recent Papers
2019-2018

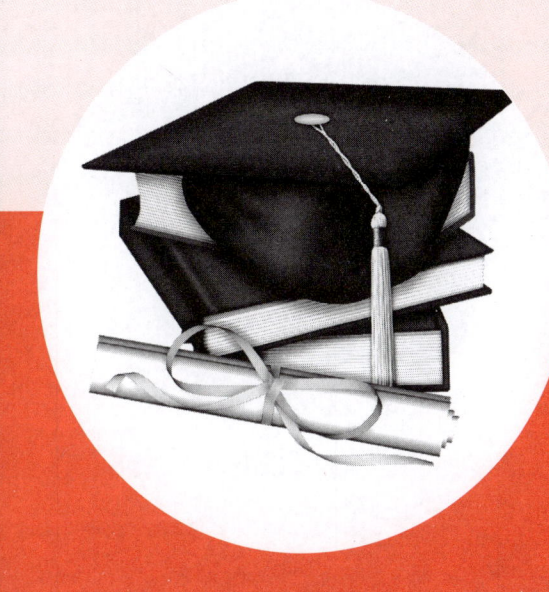

Delhi University

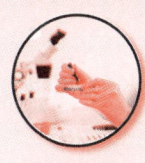 Pathology

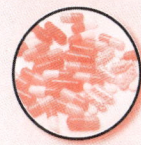 Pharmacology

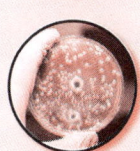 Microbiology

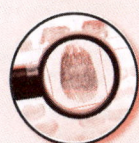 Forensic Medicine & Toxicology

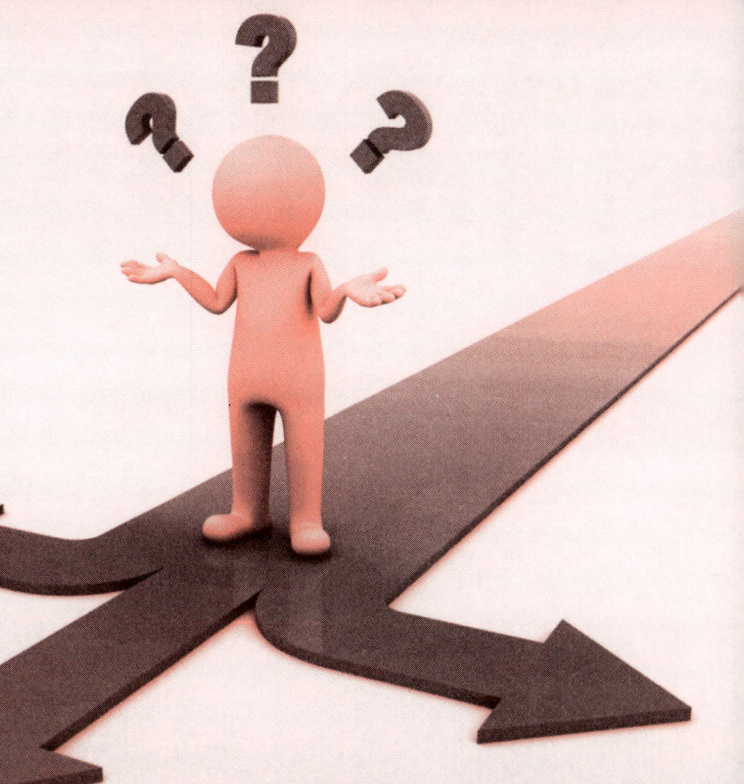

Recent Papers
2019-2018

Pathology

Pharmacology

Microbiology

Forensic Medicine &
Toxicology

Pathology

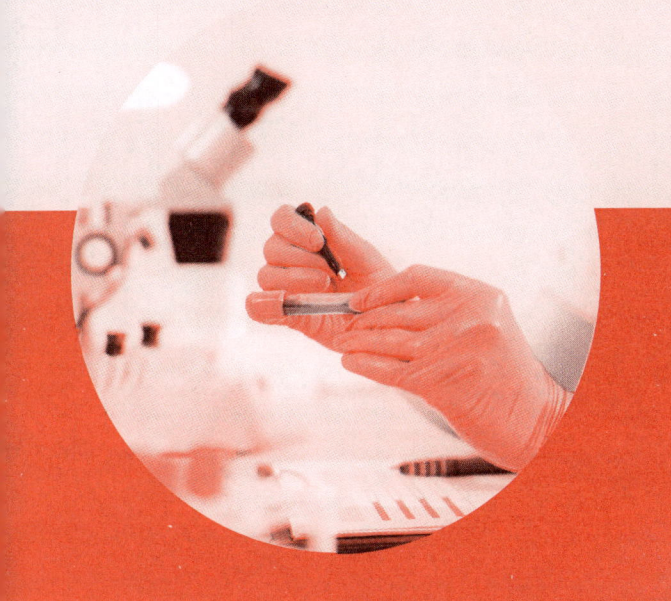

References Taken From:

○ *Textbook of Pathology, Harsh Mohan, 8th edition*
○ *Robbins & Cotran Pathologic Basis of Disease-South Asia edition*

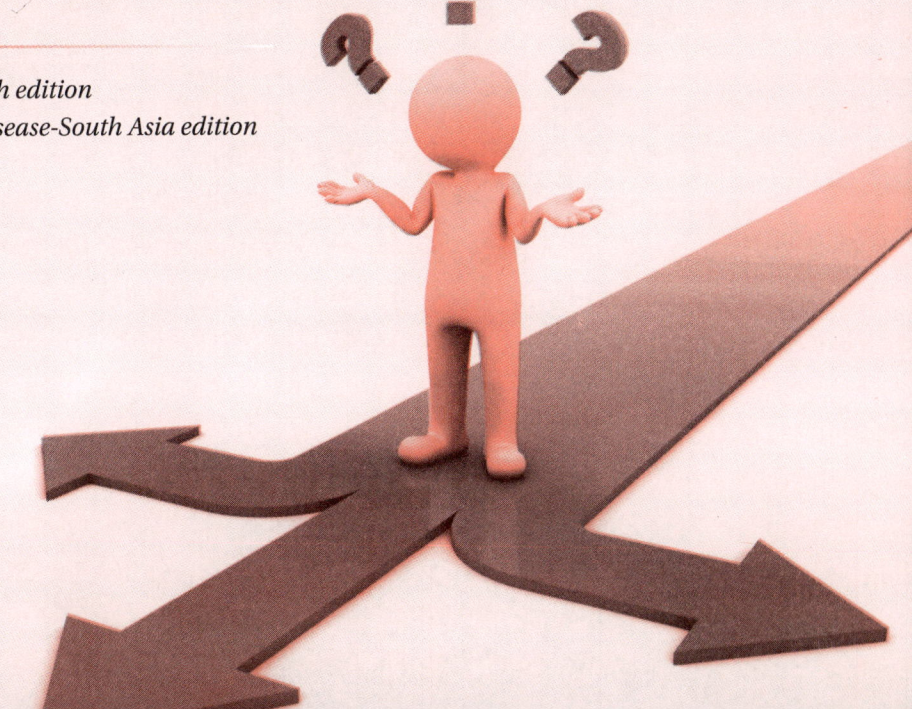

Name of the Paper	:	**Pathology Paper-I**
Name of the Course	:	**MBBS-2019**
Semester	:	**Annual**

Time: 3 Hours   **M.M.: 40**

INSTRUCTIONS

1. Write your Roll No. on the top immediately on receipt of this question paper
2. All questions are to be attempted
3. Answers to Parts I, II and III should be written in separate answer sheets provided
4. Attempt parts of a question in sequence

PART-I

1. **Differentiate between:**   [8]

   a. Reversible and irreversible cell injury
   b. Type III and type IV hypersensitivity
   c. Metaplasia and dysplasia
   d. Normoblast and megaloblast.

2. **Write briefly on:**   [6]

   a. Mediators of acute inflammation
   b. Fate of thrombus
   c. Antiglobulin test.

PART-II

3. **Write briefly on:**   [6]

   a. Niemann-Pick disease
   b. Von Willebrand disease.

4. **Write briefly on:**   [6]

   a. Laboratory diagnosis of acute lymphoblastic leukemia
   b. Tumor markers.

PART-III

5. **Write short note on:**   [8]

   a. Protein energy malnutrition
   b. Acute graft rejection
   c. Classification of Hodgkin's lymphoma
   d. Acute radiation injury.

6. **Write short notes on:**   [6]

   a. Classification of thalassemia syndromes
   b. Lepromatous leprosy
   c. Pathogenesis of renal oedema.

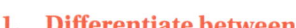

1. **Differentiate between:**

a. **Reversible and irreversible cell injury**

(Ref: Textbook of Pathology, Harsh Mohan, 8th ed. pg. 43)

ANSWER

Irreversible and Reversible Cell Injury

Irreversible cell injury	Reversible cell injury
Structural and functional changes induced by an injurious stimulus which cannot be reversed even after removal of stimulus	Structural and functional changes induced by an injurious stimulus can be reversed back to normal on removal of the stimulus
Bleb formation and defect in cell membrane is absent	Bleb formation and defect in cell membrane is present
Swelling and lysis is present in endoplasmic reticulum	Swelling is present in endoplasmic reticulum
Ribosomes are dispersed and destroyed	Ribosomes are dispersed
Rupture of lysosomes and autolysis of cell	Autophagy of organelles by lysosomes, no rupture
Nucleus shows pyknosis, karyolysis and karyorrhexis	Nucleus shows clumping of nuclear chromatin
Swelling of mitochondria with presence of large densities	Swelling of mitochondria with presence of small densities
Fate of cell is permanent change that is Cell death	Fate of cell is that it changes to normal if the stimuli is removed
Dystrophic Calcification is present	Calcification is absent

b. **Type III and Type IV hypersensitivity**

(Ref: Textbook of Pathology, Harsh Mohan, 8th ed. pg. 140)

ANSWER

Type III and Type IV Hypersensitivity

Characteristic	Type III Hypersensitivity	Type IV Hypersensitivity
Results from	Deposition of antigen-antibody complexes on tissues	T-cell mediated slow and prolonged response
Reaction type	Serum sickness and Arthus reaction	Delayed type hypersensitivity
Etiology	Due to persistence of low-grade infection, environmental antigens, autoimmune process	Microbial antigens, self-antigens
Mediated by	IgG, IgM antibodies	T-cell mediated
Pathogenesis	Circulating immune complex-mediated cell injury; local immune complex injury (Arthus reaction)	Classic DTH mediated by CD T cells; Direct CD8+ T cell mediated lysis
Examples	SLE; Immune complex glomerulonephritis; Rheumatoid arthritis; Arthus reaction; serum sickness; reactive arthritis; PAN; Farmer's lung; drug-induced vasculitis; reactive arthritis	Contact dermatitis; organ transplant reaction; rheumatoid arthritis; multiple sclerosis; reaction against mycobacterial antigen (tuberculin reaction), inflammatory bowel disease; reaction against virus infected cells

PATHOLOGY

c. Metaplasia and dysplasia

(Ref: Textbook of Pathology, Harsh Mohan, 8th ed. pg. 39)

ANSWER

Metaplasia and Dysplasia

Metaplasia	Dysplasia
Change of one type of epithelial or mesenchymal cell to another type of adult epithelial or mesenchymal cell usually in response to inciting stimulus	Disordered cellular development, may be accompanied with hyperplasia or metaplasia, usually in response to inciting stimulus
Types of metaplasia are Squamous (bronchus, uterine cervix etc.), Columnar (Barrett's esophagus, gastric ulcer etc.), Osseous (myositis ossificans, arteriosclerosis etc.)	Types of dysplasia - Epithelial (uterine cervix, bronchus, oral cavity etc.)
Cellular development is mature – from specialized to less specialized and resistant cells	Disordered cellular development – increased layers, loss of polarity, pleomorphism, nuclear hyperchromasia, mitoses
Reprogramming of precursor stem cells triggered by exogenous stimuli to another pathway	Abnormal cell growth by mutations in genes as in neoplasia
Reversible on withdrawal of stimulus, persistence of stimuli may cause progression to dysplasia	Mild and moderate grades on removal of inciting stimulus, severe grade and persistence of stimuli may cause progression to carcinoma in situ and invasive cancer

d. Normoblast and megaloblast

ANSWER

Normoblast and Megaloblast

Normoblast	Megaloblast
Size is normal (78-100 fl)	Size larger than normal (>100 fl)
Seen in normal red cells	Formed in vitamin B12 and folic acid deficiency
Nucleus is small with clumped chromatin. Nucleoli is absent	Nucleus is three-fourth of the cell volume with "opened" chromatin. Nucleoli present (2-3 in number)
Cytoplasm is less basophilic	Cytoplasm is deeply basophilic

2. Write briefly on:

a. Mediators of acute inflammation

(Ref: Textbook of Pathology, Harsh Mohan, 8th ed. pg. 70, Robbins, 1st SA ed. pg. 70)

ANSWER

Introduction

○ Acute inflammation is mediated by large endogenous chemical substance which are increasing in number

Properties of Chemical Mediators of Inflammation

○ Released either from cells or from plasma proteins
  - Mediators released from cells – derived either from cell granules storage or synthesised in the cells
  - Mediators released from plasma proteins – synthesised in the liver and require activation after releasing from liver
○ Released in response to a stimulus which can be-
  - Injurious agent
  - Dead or damaged tissue
  - One mediator stimulating other – called as secondary mediators
○ Action on different targets
  - Similar action on different targets or different action on different target cells
○ Range of actions–
  - Increased vascular permeability
  - Vasodilatation
  - Chemotaxis
  - Pain
  - Tissue damage
○ Lifespan is short after releasing
  - Various mechanisms removing the mediators immediately after releasing are
    ◆ Enzymatic inactivation
    ◆ Antioxidants
    ◆ Regulatory proteins
    ◆ Decaying

Chemical mediators of inflammation are:

○ Cell derived mediators – sources are – mast cells, basophils, platelets, inflammatory cells
  - Vasoactive amines
    ◆ Histamine
    ◆ 5-Hydroxytryptamine
    ◆ Neuropeptides
  - Arachidonic acid metabolites or Eicosanoids
    ◆ Via Cyclo-oxygenase pathway
      □ Prostaglandins
      □ Thromboxane A2

PATHOLOGY

- Prostacyclin
- Resolvins
- Via Lipo-oxygenase pathway
  - 5-HETE
  - Leukotrienes
  - Lipoxins
- Lysosomal components
  - From PMNs
  - Macrophages
- Platelet activating factor
- Cytokines
  - IL-1
  - IL-6
  - IL-8
  - IL-12
  - IIL-17
  - TNF-alpha
  - TNF-beta
  - IFN-gamma
  - Chemokines
- Free radicals
  - Oxygen metabolites
  - Nitric oxide
- Plasma protein derived mediators or plasma proteases – products of:
  - The Kinin system
  - The Clotting system
  - The Fibrinolytic system
  - The Complement system

b. Fate of thrombus

(Ref: Textbook of Pathology, Harsh Mohan, 8th ed. pg. 183, Robbins, 1st SA ed. pg. 101)

Answer

Fate of Thrombus

The fate of thrombus is:

Resolution

- Lysis and removal of thrombus by the fibrinolytic activity
- Effective in recently formed thrombus
- Older thrombus resistant to lysis due to extensive fibrin polymerization

Organization and Recanalization

- If thrombus is not removed, ingrowth of endothelial cells, smooth muscle cells, fibroblasts and formation of fibrin rich thrombus organization.

- New vascular channels may be formed re-establishing the blood flow

Propagation

- Obstruction of vessel due to accumulation of blood constituents resulting in large size of thrombus

Thromboembolism

- Thrombi may get dislodged and produce ill-effects at the site of thrombi

c. Antiglobulin Test

(Ref: Textbook of Pathology, Harsh Mohan, 8th ed. pg. 324)

Answer

Antiglobulin Test

Introduction

- Also known as Coomb's Test
- Discovered by Coomb's et al.

Principle

- During centifugation, Red cells sensitized with IgG or complement don't directly agglutinate
- An additional antibody is required that reacts with Fc portion of the IgG antibody, or with the C3b or C3d component of complement for agglutination.
- A "bridge" is formed between the antibodies or complement coating the red cells resulting in agglutination.

Methods: 2 types:

- **Direct Coomb's test:**
  - Detection of incomplete antibodies coated on the surface of red cells (in vivo), like as in hemolytic disease of newborn
  - Indications:
    - Autoimmune hemolytic anemia
    - Hemolytic disease of newborn
    - Transfusion reactions
- **Indirect Coomb's test:**
  - Detection of incomplete antibodies in vitro (person's sera)
  - Indications:
    - In case of Rh positive child of a Rh negative mother and mother wants second conception
    - In cross matching of blood for detection of incomplete antibodies in donar's serum

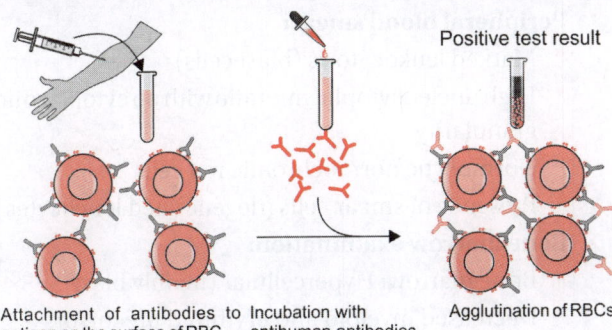

Fig. Direct Coomb's test

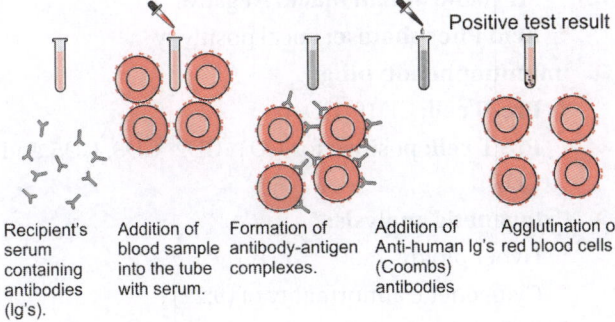

Fig. Indirect Coomb's test

PART-II

3.   Write briefly on:

a.   Niemann-Pick Disease

(Ref: Textbook of Pathology, Harsh Mohan, 8th ed. pg. 294)

ANSWER

Niemann-Pick Disease

Introduction

○ Autosomal recessive disorder that exhibits accumulation of cholesterol and sphingomyelin

○ As a result of defect in acid sphingomyelinase

○ Usually, liver, spleen, bone marrow, lungs and brain is involved

Types: two types

○ **Type A: Classic infantile form**
   ■ Common
   ■ Commonly seen in infancy (within first few months of life)
   ■ Clinical features:
      ♦ Lymphadenopathy
      ♦ Hepatosplenomegaly
      ♦ CNS deterioration

♦ Cherry-red spot in the eye (amaurosis)
♦ Poor muscle tone
♦ Feeding problems

○ **Type B: Visceral juvenile form**
   ■ Appear in late childhood or adolescence
   ■ Impaired lung function
   ■ Mental retardation
   ■ Peripheral nerve problems
   ■ Delayed growth and short stature
   ■ High blood lipids

○ **Type C:** Subacute or juvenile form
   ■ Abnormal posture of limbs, head, trunk, face
   ■ Seizures
   ■ Jaundice
   ■ Speech irregularity
   ■ Dementia
   ■ Sleep disorders, bipolar disorder, etc.
   ■ Sudden loss of muscle tone, etc.

Diagnosis

○ **Type A and B:**
   ■ Measurement of ASM in white blood cell
   ■ DNA test (to determine the type)

○ **Type C:**
   ■ DNA test
   ■ Biopsy of skin

○ **Other test:**
   ■ Bone marrow examination
   ■ Liver biopsy, etc.

b.   Von Willebrand disease

(Ref: Textbook of Pathology, Harsh Mohan, 8th ed. pg. 352)

ANSWER

Von Willebrand Disease

Introduction

○ Most common hereditary coagulation disorder

○ Occurs due to qualitative or quantitative defect in von Willebrand's factor (vWF) in ratio of 1:1000 in either sex

○ Also known as "angiohemophilia", "pseudohemophilia"

Synthesis of Von Willebrand Factor (vWF)

○ Endothelial cells

○ Platelets

○ Megakaryocytes

Function of Von Willebrand Factor (vWF)

○ Adhesion of platelet to subendothelial collagen

Clinical Features

○ Mucosal and cutaneous bleeding, GIT bleeding, etc.

○ Hemarthroses, intramuscular hematoma

Types: 3 types

1. **Type I:**
   ▪ Most common
   ▪ Mild to moderate deficiency of vWF (approx. 50%)

2. **Type II:**
   ▪ Less common
   ▪ Functional/qualitative defect in vWF

3. **Type III:**
   ▪ Most severe form
   ▪ Inherited as Autosomal recessive trait

Laboratory Diagnosis

○ Normal platelet count

○ Prolonged BT

○ Platelet aggregation with ristocetin is defective

○ Decreased factor VIII activity

○ Decreased plasma vWF concentration

○ Serum electrophoresis: vWF multimers reduced in type 1 and 3

Treatment

○ Desmopressin- sudden rise in vWF and factor VIII

○ FFP (Fresh frozen plasma)

---

4. **Write briefly on:**

   a. **Laboratory diagnosis of acute lymphoblastic leukemia**

   (Ref: Textbook of Pathology, Harsh Mohan, 8th ed. pg. 392)

ANSWER

Laboratory Diagnosis of Acute Lymphoblastic Leukemia

Introduction

○ Malignancy of immature B (pre-B) or T(pre-T) cells

○ Most common cancer of children (under 4 years of age)

Laboratory Diagnosis

○ **Complete blood count:**
   ▪ Decreased hemoglobin
   ▪ Hematocrit: Decreased
   ▪ Platelet count: Reduced
   ▪ RBC count: Decreased
   ▪ TLC: Markedly increased

○ **Peripheral blood smear:**
   ▪ Marked leukocytosis (blast cells)
   ▪ High nucleocytoplasmic ratio with no cytoplasmic granularity
   ▪ Normocytic normochromic red cells
   ▪ Presence of smear cells (degenerated leucocytes)

○ **Bone marrow examination:**
   ▪ Bone marrow: Hypercellular (mainly blast)
   ▪ Decreased myeloid and erythroid precursors
   ▪ Dyserythropoiesis

○ **Cytochemistry:**
   ▪ **PAS:** Positive
   ▪ **MPO and Sudan black:** Negative
   ▪ **Acid Phosphatase:** Focal positivity

○ **Immunophenotyping:**
   ▪ **Pre-B cell:** CD19, CD10
   ▪ **Pre T cell:** positive for CD1, CD2, CD3, CD5 and CD7

○ **Cytogenetic analysis:**
   ▪ Hyper ploidy
   ▪ Cytogenetic abnormality of (9;22)
   ▪ Philadelphia positive

○ **Serum markers:**
   ▪ **LDH:** Increased
   ▪ **Uric acid:** Increased
   ▪ **Phosphate:** Increased
   ▪ **Calcium:** Decreased

○ **Radiology:**
   ▪ Leukemic lines in long bones

   b. **Tumor markers**

   (Ref: Textbook of Pathology, Harsh Mohan, 8th ed pg. 245)

ANSWER

Tumor Markers

Introduction

○ Biological substances present in or synthesized by tumor itself or produced by host in response to a tumor

○ Usually proteins

○ Found in blood, urine or body tissues

Ideal Properties

○ Should be highly sensitive and specific

○ Should have high positive and negative predictive value

○ It should be able to differentiate between neoplastic and non-neoplastic disease

○ Should predict early recurrence and

○ Should have prognostic value

○ Clinically sensitive i.e., detectable at early stage of tumor
○ It should be easily assayable

Clinically Useful Tumor Markers

Alpha-fetoprotein (AFP)	Hepatoma, non-seminomatous testicular germ cell tumors, Yolk sac (endodermal sinus) tumor
Beta human chorionic gonadotropin (hCG)	Hydatidiform moles, Trophoblastic tumors, choriocarcinoma, Dysgerminoma
Calcitonin	Medullary carcinoma of the thyroid (alone and in MEN2A, MEN2B).
Carcinoembryonic antigen (CEA)	• **Major associations:** Colorectal and pancreatic cancers. • **Minor associations:** Gastric, breast, and medullary thyroid carcinomas.
CA-125	Malignant ovarian epithelial tumors
CA19-9	Malignant pancreatic adenocarcinoma
Placental Alkaline Phosphatase (ALP)	Seminoma, Metastases to bone or liver, Paget disease of bone
Prostate specific antigen (PSA)	Prostate cancer
Chromogranin	Neuroendocrine tumors
CA 15–3/CA 27–29	Breast cancer

PART-III

5. Write short notes on:

a.   Protein energy malnutrition

(Ref: Textbook of Pathology, Harsh Mohan, 8th ed. pg. 276, Robbins, 1st SA ed. pg. 324)

ANSWER

Protein Energy Malnutrition

Introduction

○ Insufficient consumption of protein and energy due to primary dietary deficiency or conditioned deficiency causing loss of body mass and adipose tissue, leading to protein energy malnutrition

Clinical Syndromes

○ **Kwashiorkar**
   ▪ Deficiency of protein with sufficient calorie intake
   ▪ Also known as protein malnutrition, protein-calorie malnutrition or malignant malnutrition
   ▪ Clinical Features
      ◆ Age: Children between 6 months and 3 years of age

◆ Retardation of growth
◆ Early signs include, fatigue, irritability and lethargy
◆ Skeletal muscles are spared
◆ Loss of muscle mass
◆ Visceral protein compartment markedly reduced, thus sometimes life threatening
◆ Hair changes: Thin, dry, brittle, easily pluckable and sparse hair. "Flag sign" (alternate band of light and dark hair) evident.
◆ Skin changes: "Flaky paint" dermatosis
◆ Edema: Pitting edema (due to low albumin level)
◆ Poor appetite: Apathy, listlessness
◆ Large protuberant belly (pot belly)
◆ Hepatomegaly with fatty changes
◆ Thymic and lymphoid atrophy: Marked
◆ Severe infections with delayed recovery (reduced secretory IgA)
◆ Psychomotor changes

▪ **Complications**
   ◆ Anemia (low red blood cell count)
   ◆ Frequent infections
   ◆ Physical disability
   ◆ Poor wound healing
   ◆ Shock
   ◆ Skin pigmentation changes
   ◆ Fatty liver

▪ **Treatment**
   ◆ Gradual increase in dietary protein
   ◆ Gradual increases in dietary calories from carbohydrates, sugars and fats
   ◆ Intravenous fluids to correct fluid and electrolyte imbalances
   ◆ Vitamin and mineral supplements to treat deficiencies
   ◆ Antibiotics to treat infections

○ **Marasmus**
   ▪ Starvation in infants with overall lack of calories
   ▪ **Clinical features**
      ◆ Occurs in infants under 1 year of age
      ◆ Growth failure
      ◆ Wasting of all tissues including muscle and adipose tissue
      ◆ Oedema is absent
      ◆ No hepatic enlargement is seen
      ◆ Serum proteins are low
      ◆ Anaemia
      ◆ Monkey like face
      ◆ Protuberant abdomen
      ◆ Thin limbs
   ▪ **Morphology**
      ◆ No fatty liver

◆ Atrophy of different tissues and organs including subcutaneous fat

b. Acute graft rejection

(Ref: Textbook of Pathology, Harsh Mohan, 8th ed. pg. 130)

ANSWER

Acute Graft Rejection

Introduction

○ It occurs more frequently from cellular rejection but may also occur by antibody-mediated rejection reaction too in non-sensitised individual

○ It generally becomes apparent within a few days to a few months of transplantation

Morphology

Microscopic appearance:

Characteristics of the 2 forms are as follows:

1. Acute cellular rejection
   ■ Characterized by extensive infiltration in the interstitium of the transplant by lymphocytes (mainly T cells), a few plasma cells, monocytes and a few polymorphs
   ■ Damage to the blood vessels is evident and foci of necrosis in the transplanted tissue are seen
2. Acute humoral rejection
   ■ Presented owing to poor response to immunosuppressive therapy
   ■ Marked by acute rejection vasculitis and foci of necrosis in small vessels
   ■ Mononuclear cell infiltrate is less visible as compared to acute cellular rejection and consists majorly of B lymphocytes

c. Classification of Hodgkin's Lymphoma

(Ref: Textbook of Pathology, Harsh Mohan, 8th ed. pg. 400)

ANSWER

Classification of Hodgkin's Lymphoma

○ Classic Hodgkin's disease
   ■ Nodular sclerosis – 70%
      ◆ RS cells – abundant, lacunar type, CD15+, CD30+
      ◆ Morphology – lymphoid nodules, collagen bands
      ◆ Prognosis – very good
   ■ Mixed cellularity – 22%
      ◆ RS cells – plentiful, classic type, CD15+, CD30+
      ◆ Morphology – mixed infiltrate
      ◆ Prognosis – good

   ■ Lymphocyte predominance – 5%
      ◆ RS cells – scarce, classic and polypoid type, CD15-, CD30-, CD20+
      ◆ Morphology – proliferating lymphocytes, few histiocytes
      ◆ Prognosis – excellent
   ■ Lymphocyte depletion type (Diffuse fibrotic and reticular variants) – 1%
      ◆ RS cells – abundant, pleomorphic type, CD15+, CD30+
      ◆ Morphology – few lymphocytes, atypical histiocytes, fibrosis
      ◆ Prognosis – poor
○ Nodular lymphocyte predominant Hodgkin's disease
   ■ Occurs in 2% cases
   ■ RS cells – scarce number, CD45+, CD15-, CD30-, EMA+
   ■ Morphology – proliferation of small lymphocytes, nodular growth pattern
   ■ Prognosis – chronic relapsing, may transform into large B cell NHL

d. Acute radiation injury

(Ref: Harsh Mohan, 8/e, P. 45)

ANSWER

Acute Radiation Injury

Introduction

○ Also known as "acute radiation syndrome"
○ DNA damage by ionizing radiation
○ Usually reversible (acute injuries)

Sign and Symptoms

○ Depend on the degree or dose of radiation exposure
○ Onset of symptoms depends on the dose of radiation

Phases

○ Prodromal or initial
○ Latent phase
○ Manifest illness
○ Recovery

Manifestations

○ Hematopoietic syndrome
○ Gastrointestinal syndrome
○ Neurovascular syndrome

Hematopoietic Syndrome

○ Nausea, vomiting, hemorrhage, weakness, neutropenic fever, sepsis etc.

Gastrointestinal Syndrome

○ Loss of absorptive capacity

○ Severe nausea, vomiting, fever, diarrhea, weakness

○ Bloody diarrhea, anemia, cardiovascular collapse, shock, etc.

Neurovascular Syndrome

○ Hypotension

○ Loss of balance

○ Confusion

○ Respiratory distress

○ Gross CNS sign, etc.

Low doses: Onset within 1–6 hours, medium doses: onset within minutes, high doses: immediate onset of symptoms

Small doses: Nausea, vomiting, anorexia, diarrhea, fever, abdominal pain, low blood counts and bleeding.

Large dose: Headache, neurological symptoms, seizures, ataxia, severe fever and death.

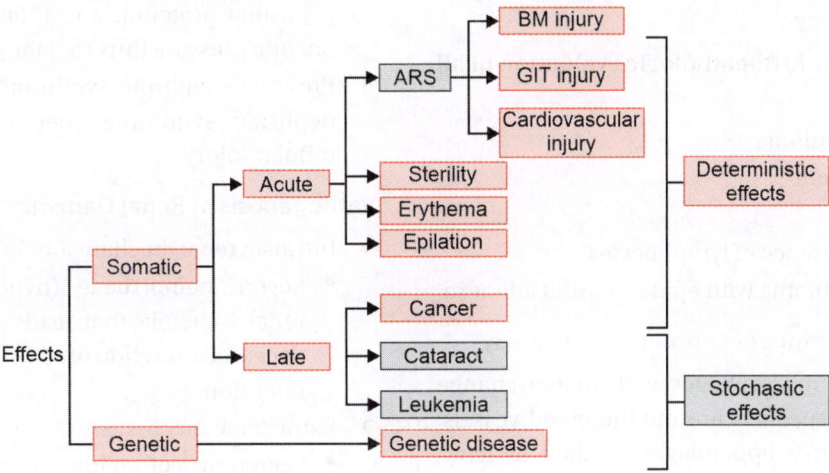

Fig. Human health effects of radiation exposure

Diagnosis

○ History of radiation exposure

○ Clinical symptoms.

○ Blood test—to assess white blood cell count, especially if present with nausea and vomiting.

Treatment

○ Blood transfusions—increase white blood cell count

○ Antibiotics—to control infection

○ Stem cell transplants

---

6. Write short notes on:

a. Classification of Thalassemia Syndromes

(Ref: Textbook of Pathology, Harsh Mohan, 8th ed. pg. 336)

ANSWER

Classification of Thalassemia Syndromes

Classification of Thalassemias

○ Alpha-thalassemias

   ▪ Hydrops fetalis

      ♦ HB – 3-10 g/dL

      ♦ HB-electrophoresis – Hb Bart's (g4) (100%)

      ♦ Genotype – Deletion of four alpha-genes

      ♦ Clinical syndrome–fatal in utero or in early infancy

   ▪ Hb-H disease

      ♦ HB - 2-12 g/dL

      ♦ Hb-electrophoresis – HbF (10%), HbH (2-4%)

      ♦ Genotype – Deletion of three alpha-genes

      ♦ Clinical syndrome – Hemolytic anemia

   ▪ Alpha-thalassemia trait

      ♦ HB – 10-14 g/dL

      ♦ HB-electrophoresis – almost normal

      ♦ Genotype – Deletion of 2 alpha genes

      ♦ Clinical syndrome – Microcytic hypochromic blood picture but no anemia

○ Beta – thalassemias

   ▪ Beta- thalassemia major

      ♦ HB - <5 g/dL

      ♦ HB-electrophoresis – HbA (0-50%), HbF (50-98%)

      ♦ Genotype – Beta(thal)/Beta(thal)

      ♦ Clinical syndrome – Severe congenital hemolytic anemia, requires blood transfusion

   ▪ Beta-thalassemia intermedia

      ♦ HB – 5-10 g/dL

      ♦ HB-electrophoresis – variable

      ♦ Genotype – multiple mechanisms

      ♦ Clinical syndrome – severe anemia, but regular blood transfusions not required

○ Beta-thalassemia minor
  ▪ HB - 10-12 g/dL
  ▪ HB-electrophoresis – HbA2 (4-9%), HbF (1-5%)
  ▪ Genotype – Beta(A)/Beta(thal)
  ▪ Clinical syndrome – Generally asymptomatic

b. Lepromatous Leprosy

(Ref: Textbook of Pathology, Harsh Mohan, 8th ed. pg. 103)

ANSWER

Lepromatous Leprosy

General features for histopathologic evaluation of all types of leprosy:

○ Cell type of granuloma
○ Nerve involvement
○ Bacterial load
○ Presence and absence of lymphocytes
○ Relation of granuloma with epidermis and adenexa

Microscopic Appearance of Lepromatous Leprosy

○ Proliferation of macrophages with foamy change in the dermis, especially around the blood vessels, nerves and dermal appendages – called as lepra cells or Virchow cells
○ Lepra cells are profoundly laden with acid-fast bacilli revealed with AFB staining
○ AFB appear as compact globular masses or organised in parallel fashion like Cigarettes in pack
○ Dermal infiltrate of lepra cells does not invade basal layer of epidermis separating it by a clear zone

○ Overlying epidermis is thin, flat and may even ulcerate

c. Pathogenesis of renal oedema

(Ref: Textbook of Pathology, Harsh Mohan, 8th ed. pg. 165, Robbins, 1st SA ed. p. 98)

ANSWER

Renal Oedema

○ Renal oedema is characterized by heavy and persistent proteinuria resulting in reduced plasma oncotic pressure thus causing generalized oedema
○ Present in nephrotic syndrome (nephrotic oedema), nephritic syndrome (nephritic oedema), acute tubular injury

Pathogenesis of Renal Oedema

○ Intrinsic renal mechanism:
  ▪ Severe hemorrhage (hypovolemia) results in renal ischemia that leads to reduced GFR and deceased excretion of sodium resulting in sodium retention
○ Extra-renal mechanism:
  ▪ Secretion of aldosterone by the renin-angiotensin– aldosterone system
  ▪ Increased tubular reabsorption of sodium and decreased excretion
○ ADH mechanism:
  ▪ Anti-diuretic hormone (ADH) influences the retention of sodium and water
  ▪ Increased sodium concentration in the plasma stimulates ADH release

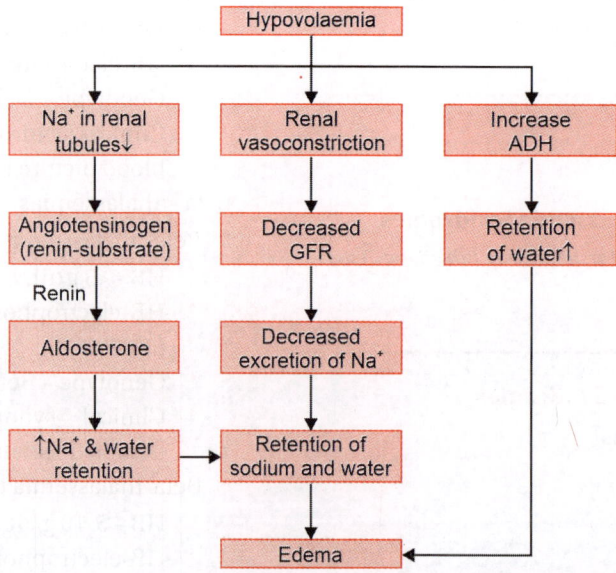

Name of the Paper	:	**Pathology Paper-II**
Name of the Course	:	**MBBS-2019**
Semester	:	**Annual**

Time: 3 Hours   **M.M.: 40**

INSTRUCTIONS

1. Write your Roll No. on the top immediately on receipt of this question paper
2. All questions are to be attempted
3. Answers to Parts I, II and III should be written in separate answer sheets provided
4. Attempt parts of a question in sequence

PART-I

1. **Differentiate between:**   **[8]**
   a. Ulcerative colitis and Crohn's disease
   b. Bronchiectasis and emphysema
   c. Nephrotic and nephritic syndrome
   d. Benign and malignant peptic ulcer.

2. **Write briefly on:**   **[6]**
   a. Infective endocarditis
   b. Ewing's sarcoma
   c. Medullary carcinoma thyroid.

PART-II

3. **Write briefly on:**   **[6]**
   a. Benign prostatic hyperplasia
   b. Etiopathogenesis of cirrhosis.

4. **Write briefly on:**   **[6]**
   a. Pleomorphic adenoma of parotid gland
   b. Etiopathogenesis of carcinoma breast.

PART-III

5. **Write short note on:**   **[8]**
   a. Krukenberg tumor
   b. Pneumoconiosis
   c. Renal cell carcinoma
   d. Rheumatoid arthritis.

6. **Write short notes on:**   **[6]**
   a. Pathogenesis of uterine cervical carcinoma
   b. Tubercular meningitis
   c. Retinoblastoma.

PART-I

1. **Differentiate between:**

   a. **Ulcerative colitis and Crohn's disease**

   (Ref: Textbook of Pathology, Harsh Mohan, 8th ed. pg. 590; Robbins, 1st SA ed. pg. 624)

ANSWER

Ulcerative Colitis and Crohn's Disease

Characteristic	Crohn's disease	Ulcerative colitis
• Site of origin	• Distal ileum, proximal colon	• Rectum
• Thickness of pathology	• Transmural	• Mucosa and submucosa only
• Progression	• Irregular (skip lesions)	• Proximal, continuous from rectum; no skipped areas
• Location	• From mouth to anus	• Involves colon and rectum; rarely extends to ileum
• Change in bowel habits	• Obstruction, abdominal pain	• Bloody diarrhoea
• Classic lesions	• Fistulas or abscesses, cobblestoning, string sign on barium radiographs	• Pseudopolyps, leadpipe colon on barium radiographs, toxic • Megacolon
• Colon cancer risk	• Slightly increased	• Markedly increased
• Surgery cures bowel disease?	• No (can worsen it)	• Yes (Proctocolectomy with ileoanal anastomosis)

   b. **Bronchiectasis and emphysema**

   (Ref: Textbook of Pathology, Harsh Mohan, 8th ed. pg. 501; Robbins, 1st SA ed. pg. 499)

ANSWER

Bronchiectasis and Emphysema

Characteristic	Bronchiectasis	Emphysema
Location	Bronchus	Acinus
Age of the patient at diagnosis	Adults	Adults
Cause	Infection or obstruction	Tobacco Smoking or air pollution
Pathogenesis	Damaged airways	Deficiency of alpha-1 antitrypsin
Gross appearance	Dilated bronchi and bronchioles	Distended air sacs
Histologic feature	Inflamed bronchi	Broken alveolar septa
Clinical feature	Copious foul-smelling expectoration, fever, cough	Exertional dyspnea

c. **Nephrotic and nephritic syndrome**

(Ref: Textbook of Pathology Harsh Mohan, 8th ed. pg. 690)

ANSWER

Nephritic and Nephrotic Syndrome

Nephrotic syndrome	Nephritic syndrome
Presents mild edema	Presents generalised peripheral edema
Marked proteinuria present	Mild proteinuria
Hyperlipidemia present	Hyperlipidemia absent
Hematuria/RBC cast not evident or mild in certain cases	Hematuria/RBC cast is evident
Oliguria and uremia absent	Presence of oliguria and uremia

d. **Benign and malignant peptic ulcer**

(Ref: Textbook of Pathology Harsh Mohan, 8th ed. pg. 584)

ANSWER

Benign and Malignant Peptic Ulcer

Characteristic	Benign	Malignant
Occurs in	Mostly in males at younger age	Commonly in males at older age
Duration of ailment	Weeks to years	Weeks to months
Located at	Usually lesser curvature of pylorus and antrum	Usually greater curvature of pylorus and antrum
Gross appearance	Small, regular in shape with radiating mucosal folds, hemorrhagic ulcer bed	Large, irregular shaped with interrupted mucosal folds, necrotic ulcer bed
Barium studies	Punched out ulcer	Irregular filling defect
Acidity	Generally, normal to low	May be normal to even achlorhydria
Therapy	Responds well to medical therapy	Does not respond to medical therapy usually

2. **Write briefly on:**

a. **Infective endocarditis**

(Ref: Textbook of Pathology Harsh Mohan, 8th ed. pg. 467)

ANSWER

Infective Endocarditis

Introduction

○ Different types of microorganisms cause serious infection of the valvular and mural endocardium with characteristic feature as typical infected and friable vegetations

○ Based on the severity of infection, can be classified into

- Acute bacterial endocarditis (ABE)—caused by highly virulent bacteria, fulminant and destructive acute infection in previously normal heart, runs a rapidly fatal course in a period of 2-6 weeks

- Subacute bacterial endocarditis (SABE)—caused by less virulent bacteria in a previously affected heart, has a gradual course of period of 6 weeks to few months or years

Incidence

○ Occurs at any age but more common in 50 years and above

○ Males are more commonly affected

Etiology

○ Infective agents—90% are due to streptococci and staphylococci

○ **Predisposing factors**

- Bacteraemia, septicaemia and pyaemia— periodontal infections, genitourinary infections, infections of biliary tract or GIT, surgery of bowel, skin infections, URTI, cardiac catheterisation

- Underlying heart disease—previously affected heart valves, chronic rheumatic valvular disease, congenital heart diseases, subaortic stenosis,

PATHOLOGY

bicuspid aortic valve, coarctation of aorta, syphilitic aortic valve disease, floppy mitral valve
- Impaired host defense—lymphomas, leukaemias, cytotoxic therapy in cancers and transplants

Vegetations of Infective Endocarditis

- Aortic and mitral valve get affected
- Vegetations present on valve cusps (on one side)
- Usually large, irregular, friable vegetations
- Microscopically, composed of platelets and fibrin
- Deeper parts show bacterial colonies along with granulation tissue present at the base
- Underlying endocardium present abscesses in ABE and inflammatory granulation in SABE

Complications

- **Cardiac complications**
  - Valvular stenosis/insufficiency
  - Myocardial abscesses
  - Perforation, rupture or aneurysm of valvular leaflets
  - Valvular ring abscesses
  - Suppurative pericarditis
  - Cardiac failure
- **Extracardiac complications**
  - Being characteristically friable, vegetations have tendency to get dislodged owing to rapid blood stream and result in embolism and leads to complications such as
    - Emboli arises from left side of heart and enter the systemic circulation affecting organs such as kidneys, spleen and brain thereby resulting in abscesses, infarcts and mycotic aneurysms
    - Emboli which originates from right side of heart enters the pulmonary circulation thereby giving rise to pulmonary abscesses
    - Due to emboli or toxic injury to capillaries, skin and conjunctiva may present with petechiae
    - Osler's nodes are seen on finger tips of hands and feet in SABE whereas Janeway's lesions are found on pulp of fingers in ABE
    - Focal necrotising glomerulonephritis is present frequently in SABE
    - Death may occur due to cardiac failure, embolism to vital organs, persistent infection, rupture of mycotic aneurysm of cerebral arteries or renal failure

b. Ewing sarcoma

(Ref: Textbook of Pathology, Harsh Mohan, 8th ed. pg. 891, Robbins, 1st SA ed. pg. 812)

ANSWER

Ewing's Sarcoma

Introduction

- Highly malignant small round cell tumor affecting patients of 5–20 years of age with preference for females
- Three types of Ewing's sarcoma are:
  1. Classic (skeletal) Ewing's sarcoma
  2. Soft tissue Ewing's sarcoma
  3. Primitive neuroectodermal tumor (PNET)
- All three types are linked together by common neuroectodermal origin and by a common cytogenetic translocation abnormality t(11; 22) (q24; 12)
- Skeletal Ewing's sarcoma begins in medullary canal of diaphysis or metaphysis

Clinical Features

- Pain
- Tenderness
- Swelling of affected part
- Fever
- Leucocytosis
- Raised ESR

Diagnosis

- Radiographic examination shows predominantly osteolytic lesion with patchy subperiosteal reactive bone formation producing typical onion-skin appearance

Morphology

- **Gross appearance:**
  - Located in medullary cavity and affected diaphysis or metaphysis expands commonly extending to adjacent soft tissues
  - Appearance of tumor tissue is grey-white, soft and friable
- **Microscopic appearance:**
  - Small round cell tumors involving other tumors such as PNET, neuroblastoma, embryonal rhabdomyosarcoma, lymphoma-leukemias and metastatic small cell carcinoma
    - Pattern—fibrous septa divides the tumor into irregular lobules of closely packed tumor cells which are characteristically organised around capillaries forming pseudorosettes
    - Tumor cells—small, uniform tumor cells similar to lymphocytes and have indefinite cytoplasmic outlines, scanty cytoplasm

- and round nuclei having salt and pepper chromatin and recurrent mitoses
  - Also known as round cell tumor or small blue cell tumor
  - Cytoplasm contains glycogen which stains with periodic acid-Schiff (PAS) reaction
  - Frequently expressed cell surface marker by tumor cells of ES/PNET group is CD99 which is a product of MIC-2 gene located on X and Y chromosome

c. **Medullary carcinoma thyroid**

(Ref: Textbook of Pathology Harsh Mohan, 8th ed. pg. 855)

ANSWER

Medullary Carcinoma Thyroid

Introduction

- Less common type originated from parafollicular or C-cells present in the thyroid
- Comprises of 5% of thyroid carcinomas
- Equally present in males and females

Pathogenesis

- **Familial occurrence**
  - Mostly occurs sporadically with 10% having a genetic background with point mutation in RET – protooncogene located on chromosome 10q
  - Familial type is associated with pheochromo-cytoma and parathyroid adenoma (multiple endocrine neoplasia, neoplasia, MEN II A) or with pheochromocytoma and multiple mucosal neuromas (MEN II B)
  - Sporadic cases are seen in the middle and old age (5th -6th decades) and are usually unilateral whereas the familial cases are seen in younger age (2nd – 3rd decades)
  - Generally bilateral and multicentric
- **Secretion of calcitonin and other peptides**
  - Tumor cells of medullary carcinoma secrete calcitonin, the hypocalcemic hormone like normal cells
  - Tumor may also elaborate prostaglandins, histaminase, somatostatin, vasoactive intestinal peptide (VIP) and ACTH
  - Such hormone elaborations are responsible for a number of clinical syndromes such as carcinoid syndrome, Cushing's syndrome and diarrhea
- **Amyloid stroma**
  - Majority of medullary carcinomas have amyloid deposits in the stroma which stains positively with usual amyloid stains such as Congo red

- Amyloid deposits are believed to represent stored calcitonin derived from neoplastic C-cells in the form of prohormone
- Most cases of medullary carcinoma present as solitary thyroid nodule but sometimes an enlarged cervical lymph node may be first manifestation

Morphology

Gross Appearance

- Tumor may either be exhibited as unilateral solitary nodule (sporadic form) or have bilateral and multicentric involvement (familial form)
- Sporadic neoplasms eventually spread to the contralateral lobe
- Cut surface of tumor in both forms shows well defined tumor areas which are firm to hard grey-white to yellow brown with areas of hemorrhages and necrosis

Microscopic Appearance

- **Tumor cells**
  - Neuroendocrine tumors (e.g. carcinoid, islet cell tumor, paraganglioma etc. medullary carcinoma of thyroid too has a well-defined organoid pattern, forming nests of tumor cells separated by fibrovascular septa
  - Sometimes tumor cells may be arranged in sheets, ribbons pseudopapillae or small follicles
  - Tumor cells are uniform and have structural and functional characteristics of C cells
  - Some times neoplastic cells are spindle shaped
- **Amyloid stroma**
  - Separated by amyloid stroma originated from altered calcitonin which can be demonstrated by immunostain for calcitonin
  - The staining properties of amyloid are similar to that seen in systemic amyloidosis any may have areas of irregular calcification but without regular laminations seen in psammoma bodies
- **C-cell hyperplasia**
  - Familial cases usually have C-cell hyperplasia as a precursor lesion but not in sporadic cases

PART-II

3. **Write briefly on:**

a. **Benign prostatic hyperplasia**

(Ref: Textbook of Pathology Harsh Mohan, 8th ed. pg. 698)

ANSWER

Benign Prostatic Hyperplasia

Introduction

○ BPH is a part of natural aging process

○ Characterized by hyperplasia of epithelial and stromal cells of prostate

Pathogenesis

○ Increased epithelial cells and stromal component in the periurethral area

○ Responsible hormone: Dihydrotestosterone (DHT)

○ Production of growth factors due to action of DHT

○ Growth factors induces proliferation of fibroblast and epithelial cells as well as decreased loss of epithelial cells

○ Thus, epithelial and stromal cells increased resulting in enlarged prostate

Clinical Features

○ Usually seen in older people (over 50 years of age)

○ **Due to urethra compression:**
  ▪ Nocturia
  ▪ Painful micturition
  ▪ Increased frequency
  ▪ Dribbling or leaking after urination
  ▪ Decrease in urine stream

○ **Due to urine retention in the bladder:**
  ▪ Infection
  ▪ Hypertrophy
  ▪ Cystitis, etc.

Morphology

Gross Appearance

○ **Early nodules:** Usually composed of stromal cells but later epithelial cells predominate

○ No true capsule but plane of cleavage present

○ **In glandular proliferation:** consistency is soft and milky white prostatic fluid oozes out

Microscopic Features

○ Composed of fibromuscular nodule to fibroepithelial nodules with dominant glandular tissue

○ Glandular tissue composed of inner layer of columnar cells and outer layer of cuboidal or flattened epithelial cells

○ Stromal component exhibits muscular and fibrous proliferation

Diagnosis

○ Assessment of symptoms

○ Digital rectal examination

○ Ultrasonography-PV determination

○ Urodynamic analysis

○ Prostate specific antigen (PSA) measurement: prognostic marker for BPH

b. Etiopathogenesis of cirrhosis

(Ref: Textbook of Pathology Harsh Mohan, 8th ed. pg. 645)

ANSWER

Cirrhosis of Liver

Introduction

○ Irreversible end stage of several diffuse diseases causing hepatocellular injury

○ **Typical features are:**
  ▪ Involves entire liver
  ▪ Normal lobular architecture of hepatic parenchyma is disorganized
  ▪ Formation of nodules separated from one another by irregular bands of fibrosis
  ▪ Occurs after hepatocellular necrosis of erratic aetiology and has alternate areas of necrosis and regenerative nodules

Pathogenesis

○ Undergoes a combination of few processes – hepatocellular necrosis, healing by fibrosis, formation of regenerative nodules and changes in vascular pattern of hepatic parenchyma

Classification of Cirrhosis

○ **Morphologic**
  ▪ Micronodular—nodules less than 3 mm
  ▪ Macronodular—nodules more than 3 mm
  ▪ Mixed

○ **Etiologic**
  ▪ Alcoholic cirrhosis – most frequent (60–70%)
  ▪ Post necrotic cirrhosis – 10%
  ▪ Biliary cirrhosis – 5–10%
  ▪ Pigment cirrhosis in haemochromatosis – 5%
  ▪ Cirrhosis in Wilson's disease
  ▪ Cirrhosis in alpha-1-antitrypsin deficiency
  ▪ Cardiac cirrhosis
  ▪ Indian childhood cirrhosis
  ▪ Cirrhosis in autoimmune hepatitis
  ▪ Cirrhosis in non-alcoholic steatohepatitis
  ▪ Miscellaneous forms – metabolic, infectious, GI, infiltrative diseases
  ▪ Cryptogenic cirrhosis

4. Write briefly on:

a. Pleomorphic adenoma of parotid gland

(Ref: Textbook of Pathology Harsh Mohan, 8th ed. pg. 560)

ANSWER

Pleomorphic Adenoma of Parotid Gland

Introduction

○ Also known as mixed salivary tumor

○ Most frequent tumor in parotid gland, seen mostly in women of 30-50 years of age

○ Painless, slow growing, solitary, smooth surfaced or nodular tumor located below and in front of ear

○ Presents both epithelial and mesenchymal differentiation hence known as mixed salivary tumor

Morphology

○ **Gross appearance:**
  ▪ Circumscribed, pseudoencapsulated, round, or multilobulated firm tumor of 2–5 cm in diameter with soft and mucoid consistency
  ▪ Cut surface exhibits grey white or bluish, variegated, semitranslucent, solid or cystic spaces

○ **Microscopic appearance:**
  ▪ Epithelial element forms patterns such as ducts, acini, tubules, sheets and strands of ductal or myoepithelial origin
  ▪ Stromal elements present as loose connective tissue and as myxoid, mucoid and chondroid matrix simulating cartilage

Prognosis

○ Recurrent, sometimes after several years

○ Factors responsible for recurrence
  ▪ Incomplete surgical removal owing to proximity of facial nerve
  ▪ Multiple tumor foci
  ▪ Implantation in the surgical field
  ▪ Pseudoencapsulation

b. Etiopathogenesis of carcinoma breast
(Ref: Textbook of Pathology, Harsh Mohan, 8th ed. pg. 804, Robbins, 1st SA ed. pg. 739)

ANSWER

Introduction

○ CA breast is the most common cancer among the cancers occuring in female.

○ Ca breast is common among the perimenopausal women and uncommon below the age group of 25 years.

○ The development of triple assessment technique has led to increased frequency of detection of Ca breast.

Risk Factors

Geographical factor	It is common among women of developed countries
Race factors	Breast cancer occurs at earliest age in African Americans and Hispanics
Family history	Increased risk for women with first degree relatives diagnosed to have ca breast
Menstrual history	Early menarche and late menopause are the risk factor for development of Ca breast
Obstetric factor	Nulliparity and late first childbirth also predispose to Ca breast
Fibrocystic disease	Presence of atypical epithelial hyperplasia has increased risk of developing breast cancer
Other factors	Increased intake of animal fats and high calorie diet Cigarette smoking Alcohol consumption Breast augmentation surgery High breast density Radiation exposure

Etiopathogenesis

Hormonal factors	• Ca breast is a hormone dependent disease. • Increased duration and high activity of the estrogen hormone predisposes to Ca breast like
	▪ Women with early menarche ▪ Women late menopause ▪ Nulliparous women ▪ Women late child birth ▪ Hormone secreting ovarian tumor ▪ Hormone replacement therapy ▪ Hormonal contraceptive pills. ▪ This proves the role of hormone in development of Ca breast. • Breast feeding and lactation provides protection against the breast cancer
Genetic factors	• BRCA 1 gene located in chromosome 17 is a DNA repair gene. • Any mutation in BRCA1 gene mutation predisposes to ca breast. • BRCA 2 gene located in chromosome 14 is also a DNA repair gene, its mutation cause increased incidence of breast cancer and prostate cancer. • P53 gene located in chromosome 17 is a tumor suppressor gene. Mutation of this gene predisposes to many tumor including breast. • Li-fraumeni syndrome, is characterized by P53 gene mutation results in development of several cancers. • CHEK2 gene mutation also predisposes to ca breast. • Ataxia tlengiectasia gene and PTEN gene mutation also predisposes to breast cancer.

Molecular Mechanism

○ Development of carcinoma of breast is a complex mechanism affecting various cellular pathways involved in cell growth and proliferations like MAPK, RB/E2F, P13K/AKTmTOR AND TP53 pathways.

○ The molecular mechanism is regulated by changes in various oncogenes like HER 2, c-MYC and RAS, ER gene and other tumor suppressor genes like P53, PTEN and BRCA 1 & BRCA 2.

Prognostic and Predictive Factors

○ **Potentially precancerous lesions**

▪ Atypical ductal hyperplasia—linked with 4–5 times increased risk than woman of same age; frequent in 45–55 years of age

▪ Clinging carcinoma—associated lesion in the duct but differs from carcinoma in situ and has lower risk of progression

♦ Fibroadenoma—long term risk factor (after over 20 years) for invasive breast cancer with 2 times increased risk

○ **Breast carcinoma in situ**

▪ Ductal carcinoma in situ (comedo and non-comedo types) is diagnosed depending on 3 histologic features

♦ Nuclear grade
♦ Nuclear morphology
♦ Necrosis

▪ Breast conservative therapy – more common and requires three factors to be considered
  1. Margins
  2. Extent of disease
  3. Biological markers

▪ Biological markers such as p53 and BCL-2 have low positivity in high grade in situ carcinoma and have chances of recurrence

○ **Invasive breast cancer:** Prognostic and predictive factors are studied by univariate analysis and multivariate analysis

Factor	Favourable prognosis	Poor prognosis
• Routine Histopathology Criteria		
▪ Tumor size (two dimensions)	<1 cm size tumor; 10 years survival 90% in node negative	Size >1 cm
▪ Histologic type	Medullary ca., tubular c., mucinous (colloid) ca.; lobular ca. of low grade	Inflammatory ca
▪ Histologic (Nottingham)grading (Score range of 3–9) based on degree of tubule formation 1–3 score, regularity of nuclei-1–3 score, and mitoses-1–3 score	Low grade (grade I) tumor = score 3–5, moderate grade (grade II) tumor = score 6–7	High grade (grade III) tumor = score 8–9
• Axillary nodal status	Node negative: recurrence after 10 years 10–30%;	Node positive: recurrence after 10 years 70%; number of nodes: more than 4; sentinel node positive
• Hormone receptor status		
▪ Oestrogen-progesterone receptors (ER-PR)HER-2/neu (C-erb B-2)	ER-PR positive cases respond better to adjuvant therapy Underexpression	ER-PR negative cases respond poorly to adjuvant therapy Overexpression (predictive of response to herceptin)
• Lymphatic and/or vascular invasion (both extratumoral)	Number of nodes: less than 4; sentinel node negative Negative for both: good	Positive for one or both: poor
▪ Others:		
♦ Skin involvement	Absence good	Presence poor
♦ Tumor circumscription	Good	Poor
♦ Inflammatory reaction	May have some role	Controversial
♦ Intraductal component	Presence good	Absence poor
♦ Stromal elastosis	Absence good	Presence poor
• Biological indicators		
▪ DNA ploidy analysis (aneuploidy, diploidy)	Not related	Not related
▪ Oncogene disregulation		
♦ BRCA1, BRCA2	BRCA negative	BRCA positive
♦ p53	P53 positive respond better to chemotherapy and radiotherapy	P53 negative respond poorly to chemotherapy and radiotherapy BCL2 negative poor
♦ BCL2	BCL2 positive good	Presence poor prognosis
♦ Cathepsin D	Absence good prognosis	
▪ Mitotic index (by Ki67, MIB-1)	Low mitotic count	High mitotic count
▪ Angiogenesis (VEGF, CD31, CD34, microvessel density counts)	Angiogenic activity low	High angiogenic activity

PART-III

5. Write short notes on:

a. Krukenberg tumor

(Ref: Textbook of Pathology, Harsh Mohan, 8th ed. pg. 786, Robbins, 1st SA ed. pg. 729)

ANSWER

Krukenberg tumor

Introduction

- It is a bilateral metastatic ovarian malignancy
- **Common primary sites for metastasis:**
  - Gastrointestinal tract (gastric carcinoma)
  - Other sites- breast, colon, appendix, etc.
- Metastasis-by trans coelomic spread

Clinical Features

- Common in 30–40 years of age
- Clinically, silent
- Abdominal pain or pelvic pain
- Ascites
- Bloating
- Vaginal bleeding or change in menstrual habits

Morphology

Gross Appearance

- Multinodular mass in both ovaries that are round to kidney shaped, firm, grey-white to yellow in color with areas of necrosis and hemorrhage
- Cut surface exhibits grey-white to yellow, firm fleshy tumor having areas of necrosis and hemorrhage

Microscopic Findings

- Presence of signet ring cells filled with mucin and proliferation of ovarian stromal cells

Diagnosis

- Laparotomy
- CT scan
- Ovarian biopsy

b. Pneumoconiosis

(Ref: Textbook of Pathology, Harsh Mohan, 8th ed. pg. 510, Robbins, 1st SA ed. pg. 508)

ANSWER

Pneumoconiosis

Introduction

- Occupational Lung diseases caused due to inhalation of dust (usually at work)

- Depending upon the nature of inhaled dust particle, type of lung disease occurs
- Factors determining the extent of damage caused sue to inhaled dust
  - Size and shape of particles
  - Their solubility and physicochemical composition
  - Amount of dust retained in lungs
  - Additional effect of other irritants such as tobacco smoke
  - Host factors such as efficiency of clearance mechanism and immune status of the host
- Tissue response to inhaled dust may be one of the following three types:
  1. Fibrous nodules—coal workers' pneumoconiosis and silicosis
  2. Interstitial fibrosis—asbestosis
  3. Hypersensitivity reaction—berylliosis

Classification

- **Inorganic (Mineral) dusts**
  - Coal dust
    - Simple coal-workers' pneumoconiosis
    - Progressive massive fibrosis
    - Caplan's syndrome
  - Silica
    - Silicosis
    - Caplan's syndrome
  - Asbestos
    - Asbestosis
    - Pleural diseases
    - Tumors
  - Beryllium
    - Acute berylliosis
    - Chronic berylliosis
  - Iron oxide
    - Pulmonary siderosis
- **Organic (biologic) dusts**
  - Mouldy hay
    - Farmer's lungs
  - Bagasse
    - Bagassosis
  - Cotton, flax, hemp dust
    - Byssinosis
  - Bird droppings
    - Bird breeders' (bird fancier's) lung
  - Mushroom compost dust
    - Mushroom-workers' lung
  - Mouldy barley, malt dust
    - Malt-workers' lung
  - Mouldy maple bark
    - Maple-bark disease
  - Silage fermentation
    - Silo-fillers' disease

PATHOLOGY

Silicosis

- Type of pneumoconiosis caused by prolonged inhalation of silica (silicon dioxide)
- Occurs in persons engaged in occupations which has exposure to siliceous rocks or sand and products manufactured from them such as:
  - Miners (granite, sandstone, slate, coal, gold, tin and copper)
  - Quarry workers
  - Tunnellers
  - Sandblasters
  - Grinders
  - Ceramic workers
  - Foundry workers
  - Manufacture of abrasives containing silica

Clinical Picture

- Dyspnoea
- Obstructive or restrictive pattern of disease may develop
- **Complications such as**
  - Pulmonary tuberculosis
  - Rheumatoid arthritis
  - Cor pulmonale

Morphologic Features

- **Gross appearance:**
  - Chronic silicotic lung is embossed with well circumscribed, hard, fibrotic nodules – 1 to 5 mm in diameter which are dispersed throughout the lung parenchyma but more commonly located in upper regions of the lungs
  - Gross thickness and adherence of pleura to the chest wall
  - Ischemic necrosis and cavitation of lesions which may get complicated by tuberculosis and rheumatoid pneumoconiosis
- **Microscopic examination:**
  - Silicotic nodules in the region of respiratory bronchioles, adjacent alveoli, pulmonary arteries, in the pleura and the regional lymph nodes
  - They comprise of central hyalinized material with scanty cellularity and some amount of dust
  - Hyalinized center is encircled by concentric laminations of collagen which in turn is enclosed by more cellular connective tissue, dust filled macrophages and a few lymphocytes and plasma cells
  - Collagenous nodules present with cleft like spaces between the lamellae of collagen which on examination polariscopically may exhibit numerous birefringent particles of silica
  - Coalescence of adjacent nodules is seen in severe and progressive form of disease
  - Emphysema or hyperinflation of intervening lung parenchyma

Coal workers' Pneumoconiosis

- Most frequent type of pneumoconiosis and caused by inhalation of coal dust particles generally in coal miners engaged in handling soft bituminous coal for many years, around 20–30 years

Predisposing Factors

- Old age of miners
- Severity of coal dust burden engulfed by macrophages
- Prolonged duration of exposure to coal dust
- Concomitant tuberculosis
- Additional role of silica dust

Morphology

Gross Appearance

- Coal macules—small, black focal lesions of size less than 5 mm in diameter evenly distributed throughout the lung especially in the upper lobes, palpable macules are called nodules Dilated air spaces with little destruction of alveolar walls
- Black pigmentation on the pleural surface and regional lymph nodes

Microscopic Appearance

- Coal macules comprises of aggregates of dust laden macrophages present in alveoli and bronchiolar and alveolar walls
- Increase in the network of reticulin and collagen in coal macules
- Distention of respiratory bronchioles and alveoli without any noticeable destruction of alveolar walls

Clinical Picture

- Chronic cough with black expectoration
- Radiological findings—nodularity in the lungs

c. **Renal cell carcinoma**

(Ref: Textbook of Pathology, Harsh Mohan, 8th ed. pg. 724; Robbins, 1st SA ed. pg. 578)

ANSWER

Renal Cell Carcinoma

Introduction

- Adenocarcinoma originating from tubular epithelium comprising 70–80% of all RCCs
- Affects usually males in the age of 50–70 years
- Associated genes are VHL, MET

- Has tendency to invade renal vein
- Prognosis is poor
- Paraneoplastic syndrome is very frequent

Microscopic Appearance of Renal Cell Carcinoma

- **Clear cell type (70%)**
  - Most frequent pattern
  - Clear cytoplasm owing to removal of glycogen and lipid from cytoplasm during processing of tissues
  - Various patterns of tumor cells—solid, trabecular, tubular, separated by delicate vasculature
  - Well differentiated tumors
- **Papillary cell type (15%)**
  - Organisation of tumor cells in papillary pattern over fibrovascular stalks
  - Cuboidal cells with round small nuclei
  - Psammoma bodies may appear
- **Granular cell type (8%)**
  - Tumor cells possess acidophilic cytoplasm in abundance
  - More marked nuclear pleomorphism, hyperchromatism and cellular atypia
- **Chromophobe type (5%)**
  - Exhibits admixture of pale clear cells with perinuclear halo and acidophilic granular cells
  - Cytoplasm contains many vesicles
- **Sarcomatoid type (1.5%)**
  - Most anaplastic and poorly differentiated type
  - Characterised by whorls of atypical spindle tumor cells
- **Collecting duct type (0.5%)**
  - Rare form which occurs in medulla
  - Consists of a single layer of cuboidal tumor cells organised in tubular and papillary pattern

d. Rheumatoid arthritis

(Ref: Textbook of Pathology, Harsh Mohan, 8th ed. pg. 895, Robbins, 1st SA ed. pg. 818)

Answer

Rheumatoid Arthritis

Introduction

- Abnormal fibrovascular tissue or granular tissue layer seen in cornea, rheumatoid arthritis, prosthetic heart valve
- In Rheumatoid arthritis, cytokines are released due to activation of macrophages resulting in damage to joint tissues and vascularisation of cartilage known as Pannus formation

- Characteristic finding of rheumatoid arthritis is diffuse proliferative synovitis with pannus formation

Morphologic changes seen in rheumatoid arthritis due to pannus formation are:

- Involvement of small joints of hands, feet, elbows, wrists, knees, ankles
- **Microscopic changes are**
  - Pannus formation
  - Numerous folds of large villi of synovium
  - Thickening of synovial membrane owing to oedema, congestion and multi-layered synoviocytes
  - Synovial membrane is filled with inflammatory infiltrate—lymphocytes, plasma cells, macrophages
  - Fibrinoid necrosis and fibrin deposition
  - Destruction of underlying cartilage and subchondral bone due to progressive pannus formation
  - Demineralisation and cystic resorption of underlying bone
  - Opposing joint surfaces may be united due to fibrous adhesions and bony ankylosis
  - Tendons may get weak and ruptured due to persistent inflammation

---

6. **Write short notes on:**

   a. **Pathogenesis of uterine cervical carcinoma**

   (Ref: Textbook of Pathology Harsh Mohan, 8th ed. pg. 762)

Answer

Pathogenesis of Uterine Cervical Carcinoma

Etiopathogenesis in Uterine Cervical Carcinoma

- **Epidemiology—depending on epidemiology, risk factors identified are**
  - Women with early age of sexual activity
  - Women with multiple sex partners
  - Women having persistent HPV infection with high risk type oncogenic virus
  - Potential role of high-risk male sex partner such as promiscuous male with multiple sex partners, males with history of penile condyloma or males who had previous spouse with cervical cancer
  - **Other epidemiologic studies**
    - Lower socioeconomic status
    - Multiparous women
    - Cigarette smoking
    - Oral contraceptive use
    - HIV infection and immunosuppression

PATHOLOGY

○ **Virologic studies—human papilloma virus infection**
  ▪ High risk type HPV—most common types are types 16 and 18 in 70% cases and less common types are 31, 33, 52 and 58 in 70-100% cases
  ▪ Low risk type HPV—HPV types 6 and 11 seen in condylomas
  ▪ Mixed high and low risk types seen in dysplasias

○ **Molecular studies**
  ▪ According to immunohistochemical, cytogenetic and molecular studies, low risk HPV types do not integrate in host cell genome whereas high risk HPV types are integrated into nucleus of cervical epithelial cells

○ **Immunologic studies**
  ▪ Circulating tumor specific antigens and antibodies are found

○ **Ultrastructural studies**
  ▪ Increased mitochondria and free ribosomes with depletion of normally accumulated glycogen in surface cells

Morphologic Changes

○ **Gross appearance**
  ▪ Three types of patterns are fungating, ulcerating and infiltrating
  ▪ Arises from squamocolumnar junction
  ▪ Advanced stage is distinguished by extensive destruction and infiltration into adjacent structures including urinary bladder, rectum, vagina and regional lymph nodes
  ▪ Lungs, liver, bone marrow and kidneys exhibit distant metastases

○ **Microscopic appearance**
  ▪ **Epidermoid (squamous cell) carcinoma—70%**
    ♦ Most frequent is moderately-differentiate non-keratinising large cell type with better prognosis
    ♦ Well differentiated keratinising epidermoid carcinoma is next in frequency
    ♦ Less commonly seen is small cell undifferentiated carcinoma (neuroendocrine or oat cell carcinoma) with poor prognosis
  ▪ **Adenocarcinoma—20-25%**
    ♦ Well differentiated mucus secreting adenocarcinoma or clear cell type containing glycogen but no mucin
  ▪ **Others—5%**
    ♦ Variety of other patterns such as adenosquamous carcinoma, verrucous carcinoma and undifferentiated carcinoma

b. **Tubercular meningitis**

(Ref: Textbook of Pathology Harsh Mohan, 8th ed. pg. 922)

ANSWER

Tubercular Meningitis

Introduction

○ Inflammatory involvement of the meninges and may involve the dura (Pachymeningitis) or the leptomeninges (leptomeningitis)

○ Leptomeningitis is more frequent and occurs as a result of infection but less commonly chemical meningitis and carcinomatous meningitis may occur due to infiltration of subarachnoid space by cancer cells

Types of Meningitis

○ Acute pyogenic
○ Acute lymphocytic - viral, aseptic
○ Chronic—bacterial (tuberculous) and fungal (cryptococcal)

Tuberculous or Tubercular Meningitis

○ Occurs in children and adults
○ Route of spread—haematogenous from tuberculosis elsewhere in the body or may occur as manifestation of military tuberculosis. It may also occur directly from tuberculosis of a vertebral body

Morphology

Gross Appearance

○ Subarachnoid space consists of thick exudate especially abundant in the sulci and the base of the brain
○ Tubercles of 1-2 mm diameter may be visible particularly adjacent to the blood vessels

Microscopic Appearance

○ Exudate of acute and chronic inflammatory cells and granulomas with or without caseation necrosis and giant cells
○ Acid-fast bacilli may be revealed
○ Late cases present dense fibrous adhesions in the subarachnoid space and resultant hydrocephalus

Clinical Features

○ Headache
○ Malaise
○ Confusion
○ Vomiting

Diagnosis CSF findings are as follows

○ Naked eye appearance of a clear or slightly turbid CSF forming web on standing

- Increased CSF pressure (above 300 mm water)
- Mononuclear leukocytosis consisting majorly of lymphocytes and some macrophages (100–1000 cells/mL)
- Increased protein content
- Decreased glucose concentration
- Tubercle bacilli may be seen on microscopy of centrifuged deposits by ZN staining in tuberculous meningitis

c. Retinoblastoma

(Ref: Textbook of Pathology Harsh Mohan, 8th ed. pg. 537)

ANSWER

Retinoblastoma

Introduction

- Malignant eye tumor commonly present in childhood
- Origin: From retinal neurons
- May be sporadic (approximately 60%) or familial
- Familial- multifocal and transmission as autosomal dominant trait

Clinical Features

- Age: <15 years (Commonly present 2 years of age)
- Retina is commonly involved
- Poor vision
- Whitish hue to the pupil
- Pain in eye
- Strabismus

Morphological Features

Gross Appearance

- White nodular mass within the retina that is partly solid and partly necrotic and it may be exophytic or endophytic

Microscopic Features: Consists of:

- Undifferentiated retinal cells and differentiated tumor cells in rosettes form
- **Two types of rosettes:**
1. Flexner–Wintersteiner rosette composed of clusters of tumor cells arranged around a lumen with nuclei placed away from the lumen
2. Homer Wright rosette consist of tumor cells that are radially arranged around the central neurofibrillary structure

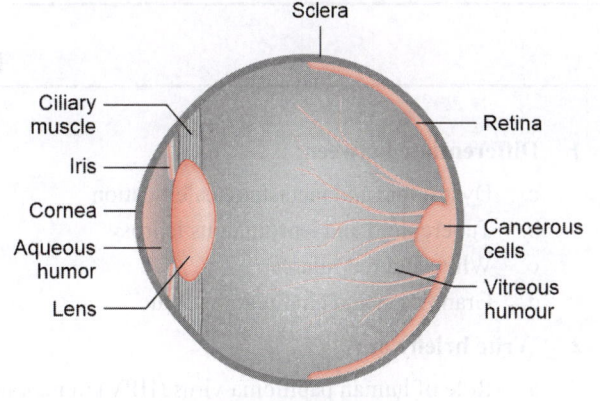

Fig. Retinoblastoma

Your Roll No. ....

Name of the Paper	:	**Pathology Paper-I**
Name of the Course	:	**MBBS-2018**
Semester	:	**Annual**

Time: 3 Hours   **M.M.: 40**

INSTRUCTIONS

1. Write your Roll No. on the top immediately on receipt of this question paper
2. All questions are to be attempted
3. Answers to Parts I, II and III should be written in separate answer sheets provided
4. Attempt parts of a question in sequence

PART-I

1. **Differentiate between:** [8]
   a. Dystrophic and metastatic calcification
   b. Tuberculoid and lepromatous leprosy
   c. White and red infarct
   d. Granuloma and Granulation tissue.

2. **Write briefly on:** [6]
   a. Role of human papilloma virus (HPV) in neoplasia
   b. Risk factors for arterial thrombosis
   c. Skeletal changes in rickets.

PART-II

3. **Write briefly on:** [6]
   a. Causes of macrocytic anemia and lab findings in vitamin B12 deficiency anemia
   b. Lab Diagnosis of chronic myeloid leukemia.

4. **Write briefly on** [6]
   a. Pathogenesis of septic shock
   b. Paraneoplastic syndrome.

PART-III

5. **Write short notes on:** [8]
   a. Blood components
   b. Down syndrome
   c. Clinical features and lab diagnosis of haemophilia
   d. Radiation carcinogenesis.

6. **Write short notes on:** [6]
   a. Type I hypersensitivity reaction
   b. Leukemoid reaction
   c. Mechanism of T cell depletion in HIV infection.

2018 PAPER-I

PART-I

1. Differentiate between:

a. Dystrophic and metastatic calcification

(Ref: Textbook of Pathology Harsh Mohan, 8th ed. pg. 990)

ANSWER

Dystrophic and Metastatic Calcification

Dystrophic calcification	Metastatic calcification
Deposition of calcium salts in dead and degenerated tissue	Deposition of calcium salts in living/normal tissue
Serum calcium level normal	Elevated serum calcium level
Can lead to organ dysfunction	No usual clinical dysfunction of the organs is evident
Generally, not reversible	Can be reversed (depends upon correction of disorder)
Due to infarcts, haematomas, necrosis, dead parasites, atheromas, certain tumours, cysts, etc.	Due to Hyperparathyroidism, multiple myeloma, vitamin D related disorders, Milk-alkali syndrome, vitamin A toxicity, etc.

b. Tuberculoid and lepromatous leprosy

(Ref: Textbook of Pathology Harsh Mohan, 8th ed. pg. 104)

ANSWER

Tuberculoid and Lepromatous Leprosy

Tuberculoid Leprosy	Lepromatous Leprosy
Asymmetrical, macular, erythematous, hypopigmented may be single or few skin lesions	Symmetrical, multiple, hypopigmented, maculopapular skin lesion
Lepromin test positive	Negative lepromin test
Immune response is good	Immunity is suppressed
Few lepra bacilli in granular or beaded form	Lepra cells present with numerous lepra bacilli exhibiting "globi" or "cigarettes-in-pack" appearance
Histopathologically, hard tubercle – similar to granulomas with no clear zone	Histopathologically, lepra cells or Virchow cells in the dermis and separated from epidermis by a clear zone

c. White and red infarct

(Ref: Textbook of Pathology Harsh Mohan, 8th ed. pg. 194)

ANSWER

White and Red Infarct

White infarct	Red infarct
Occurs due to arterial occlusion	Occurs due to pulmonary arterial obstruction or venous or arterial occlusion
Seen in compact organs	Seen in soft loose tissues
Occurs in organs with dual blood supply	Occurs in end arterial supply
Examples – Kidneys, heart, spleen	Examples – lungs, intestine

d. Granuloma and Granulation tissue

(Ref: Textbook of Pathology Harsh Mohan, 8th ed. pg. 91)

ANSWER

Granuloma and Granulation Tissue

Granuloma	Granulation tissue
Circumscribed, tiny lesion made up of collection of modified macrophages (epithelioid cell) and rimmed at the periphery by lymphoid cells	Characteristic of healing, there is acute inflammatory response to clear necrotic debris, followed by angiogenesis and fibrous tissue formation
Chronic inflammatory reactions like leprosy, tuberculosis, syphilis etc.	Typical physiological response after any injury
Causes damage to host	Not pathological
Proliferation is not significant	Significant proliferation
Microscopically, accumulation of epithelioid cells, giant cell, histiocytes, macrophages and lymphocytes	Microscopically, newly formed blood vessels embedded in loose, edematous matrix with neutrophils, monocytes and plasma cells
Not highly vascularised as no angiogenesis occurs	Highly vascularised owing to angiogenesis
Growth factors are cytokines such as IL-1, IL-2 and gamma-IFN	Growth factors are angiogenic and fibrogenic PDGF, FGF, TNF, VEGF

2. Write briefly on:

a. Role of human papilloma virus (HPV) in neoplasia

(Ref: Textbook of Pathology Harsh Mohan, 8th ed. pg. 233)

ANSWER

Role of Human Papilloma Virus (HPV) in Neoplasia

Introduction

○ First to be involved in etiology of any human tumor

○ Replicate in the layers of stratified squamous epithelium

○ Above 100 types have been recognised and individual types are related to different tumors

Types of HPV causing benign and malignant tumors are:

○ Low risk HPV – types 6 and 11 are associated with etiology of genital warts (condylomata accuminata)

○ Viral DNA of high risk HPV – types 16, 18, 31 33 and 45 is seen in 75-100% cases of invasive cervical cancer and its precursor lesions

○ High risk HPV – also associated with squamous cell carcinomas and dysplasias of other sites such as of anus, perianal region, vagina, vulva, penis and oral cavity

○ HPV types 5 and 8 are associated with infrequent autosomal recessive condition – epidermodysplasia verruciformis

○ Some types also cause multiple juvenile papillomas of the larynx

Mechanism

○ Due to the occurrence of infection with high risk HPV types, viral DNA is integrated into target epithelial cells

○ It leads to genomic instability of the host cell resulting in loss of E2 viral repressor and overexpression of viral oncoproteins E6 and E7

○ These oncoproteins from high risk HPV have high affinity for target host cells than these oncoproteins from low risk HPVs

○ Transforming effects of HPV are mainly owing to alterations in genes encoding for E6 and E7 oncoproteins as follows:

▪ Oncogenic effects of E6

♦ It degrades p53 thereby inhibiting its tumor suppressor effect

♦ Degradation of p53 causes blockage in apoptosis as p53 generally activates BAX (a proapoptotic gene)

♦ It stimulates expression of TERT catalytic sub-unit thereby contributing to immortalisation of the cell

▪ Oncogenic effects of E7

♦ It binds to RB protein and displaces its E2F transcription factor thereby removing brake in the cell cycle

♦ It inactivates CDK inhibitors p21 and p27 thereby promoting cell proliferation

○ Some cofactors play role in development of cervical cancer such as

▪ Cigarette smoking

▪ Immunosuppression

▪ Other coexisting infections

▪ Hormonal changes

▪ Dietary deficiency

b. Risk factors for arterial thrombosis

(Ref: Textbook of Pathology Harsh Mohan, 8th ed. pg. 183)

ANSWER

Risk Factors for Arterial Thrombosis

Modifiable risk factors	Non-modifiable risk factors	Other risk factors
• Dyslipidaemia	• Age – increasing age	• Infection (C. pneumoniae, Herpesvirus, CMV)
• Hypertension	• Sex – males are commonly affected	• Environmental influences
• Diabetes mellitus	• Family history	• Obesity
• Cigarette smoking	• Genetic factors	• Hormones – oestrogen deficiency, oral contraceptives
• Physical inactivity	• Stress	• Alcohol consumption
• Inflammation	• Racial factors – Whites are more commonly affected than Blacks	• Homocystinuria

c. Skeletal changes in rickets

(Ref: Textbook of Pathology Harsh Mohan, 8th ed. pg. 279)

ANSWER

Skeletal Changes in Rickets

Introduction

○ It is due to deficiency of vitamin D in children

○ Primary defects in rickets are

▪ Interference with mineralisation of bone

▪ Deranged endochondral and intramembranous bone growth

Skeletal changes seen are:

○ **Craniotabes**

▪ Earliest bony lesion resulting from small unossified areas in the membranous bones of skull, disappearing with 12 months of birth

▪ The skull appears square and box like

○ Harrison's sulcus – occurs due to indrawing of soft ribs on inspiration

○ Rachitic rosary – deformity of chest due to cartilaginous overgrowth at costochondral junction

○ Pigeon chest deformity – anterior protrusion of sternum owing to action of respiratory muscles

○ Bow legs – in ambulatory children caused by weak bones of lower legs

○ Knocked knees – due to enlarged ends of femur, tibia and fibula

○ Lower epiphyses of radius may be enlarged

○ Lumbar lordosis – due to involvement of spine and pelvis

PART-II

3. Write briefly on:

a. Causes of macrocytic anemia and lab findings in vitamin B12 deficiency anemia

(Ref: Textbook of Pathology, Harsh Mohan, 8th ed. pg. 317, Robbins, 1st SA ed. pg. 456)

ANSWER

Macrocytic Anemia

Introduction

○ Disorders due to impaired DNA synthesis caused by deficiency of vitamin B12 and/or folate characterised by distinctive abnormality in the haemopoietic precursors in the bone marrow where maturation of nucleus is delayed relative to that of cytoplasm

Causes and Classification

○ Vitamin B12 deficiency
  ▪ Inadequate dietary intake—strict vegetarians, breast fed infants
  ▪ Malabsorption
    ♦ Gastric causes—pernicious anaemia, gastrectomy, congenital lack of intrinsic factor
    ♦ Intestinal causes—tropical sprue, ileal resection, Crohn's disease, intestinal blind loop syndrome, fish tapeworm infestation

○ Folate deficiency
  ▪ Inadequate dietary intake—alcoholics, teenagers, infants, old age, poverty
  ▪ Malabsorption—tropical sprue, coeliac disease, partial gastrectomy, jejunal resection, Crohn's disease

▪ Excess demand
  ♦ Physiological—pregnancy, lactation, infancy
  ♦ Pathological—malignancy, increased haematopoiesis, chronic exfoliative skin disorders, tuberculosis, rheumatoid arthritis
▪ Excess urinary folate loss – in active liver disease, congestive heart failure

○ Other
  ▪ Impaired metabolism – inhibitors of dihydrofolate (DHF) reductase such as methotrexate and pyrimethamine, alcohol, congenital enzyme deficiencies

Unknown causes—in Di Guglielmo's syndrome, congenital dyserythropoietic anaemia, refractory megaloblastic anaemia

Laboratory Diagnosis

○ CBC
  ▪ RBC count – decreased
  ▪ Hb – low
  ▪ TLC – decreased
  ▪ Platelet – Normal/decreased
  ▪ MCV - >100 fl indicative of megaloblastic anaemia, if >110 fl is indicative of megaloblastic anaemia than any liver disease, aplastic anemia
  ▪ MCH – increased
  ▪ MCHC – normal/decreased
  ▪ Reticulocyte – decreased/normal
  ▪ Severe megaloblastic anaemia is associated with pancytopenia

○ Peripheral blood smear
  ▪ Macrocytosis – macrocytes are larger in diameter, thickness and volume, Hb content is increased and hence MCHC remains normal
  ▪ Anisopoikilocytosis - Moderate to marked
  ▪ Red cells – variable in size
  ▪ Tear drop cells
  ▪ Evidence of dyserythropoiesis like elongated cells with inclusion like Howell-Jolly bodies, basophilic stippling and Cabot's ring
  ▪ Rare large hypersegmented neutrophils

Bone Marrow Picture

○ Hypercellular predominance
○ M:E ratio = decreased upto 1:1 (normal 3:1)
○ Megaloblasts are abnormal, large, nucleated, having nuclear cytoplasmic maturation asynchrony, nuclear chromatin failing to mature due to impaired DNA synthesis, whereas cytoplasm gets hemoglobinized, nuclear chromatin more dispersed than expected
○ Degenerated erythroid precursor cells (ineffective erythropoiesis)
○ Abundant stainable iron found

PATHOLOGY

- Megakaryocytes—large, multilobulated nuclei
- Giant form of metamyelocytes and band cells may be present
- Increase in number and size of iron granules in erythroid precursor cells (Prussian blue staining)

b. Lab Diagnosis of chronic Myeloid leukemia

(Ref: Textbook of Pathology Harsh Mohan, 8th ed. pg. 371)

ANSWER

Lab Diagnosis of Chronic Myeloid Leukemia

Laboratory Findings

- Blood picture:
  - Normocytic normochromic anemia (moderate)
  - Marked leukocytosis (approx. 200, 000/µL or more)
  - Basophilia
  - Blast phase/blast crisis- ≥20%
- Bone marrow examination:
  - Hypercellular
  - Myeloid: Erythroid ratio increased (myeloid cells predominate)
  - Increased, small dysplastic form of megakaryocytes
  - Sea blue histiocytes/pseudo-Gaucher cells
  - Reduced erythropoietic cells
  - Blasts less than 5%
- Cytogenetics:
  - Philadelphia chromosome present

- Cytochemistry:
  - LAP/NAP score reduced (helps to differentiate it from myeloid leukemoid reaction, in which LAP is elevated)
- Other investigations:
  - Hyperuricaemia
  - Raised serum B12 and vitamin B12 binding capacity

4. Write briefly on:

a. Pathogenesis of septic shock

(Ref: Textbook of Pathology, Harsh Mohan, 8th ed. pg. 178, Robbins, 1st SA ed. pg. 115)

ANSWER

Pathogenesis of Shock

Pathogenesis

- Macrophage-monocyte activation: Results in liberation of free radicals and increased synthesis of nitric oxide resulting in vasodilatation and hypotension
- Activation of inflammatory cascade, like complement pathway, coagulation system, mast cells, kinin system
- Results in vasodilatation and increased vascular permeability thus causing hyperdynamic circulation and inflammatory edema
- Organ dysfunction as a result of hypotension and inadequate perfusion of cells and tissues

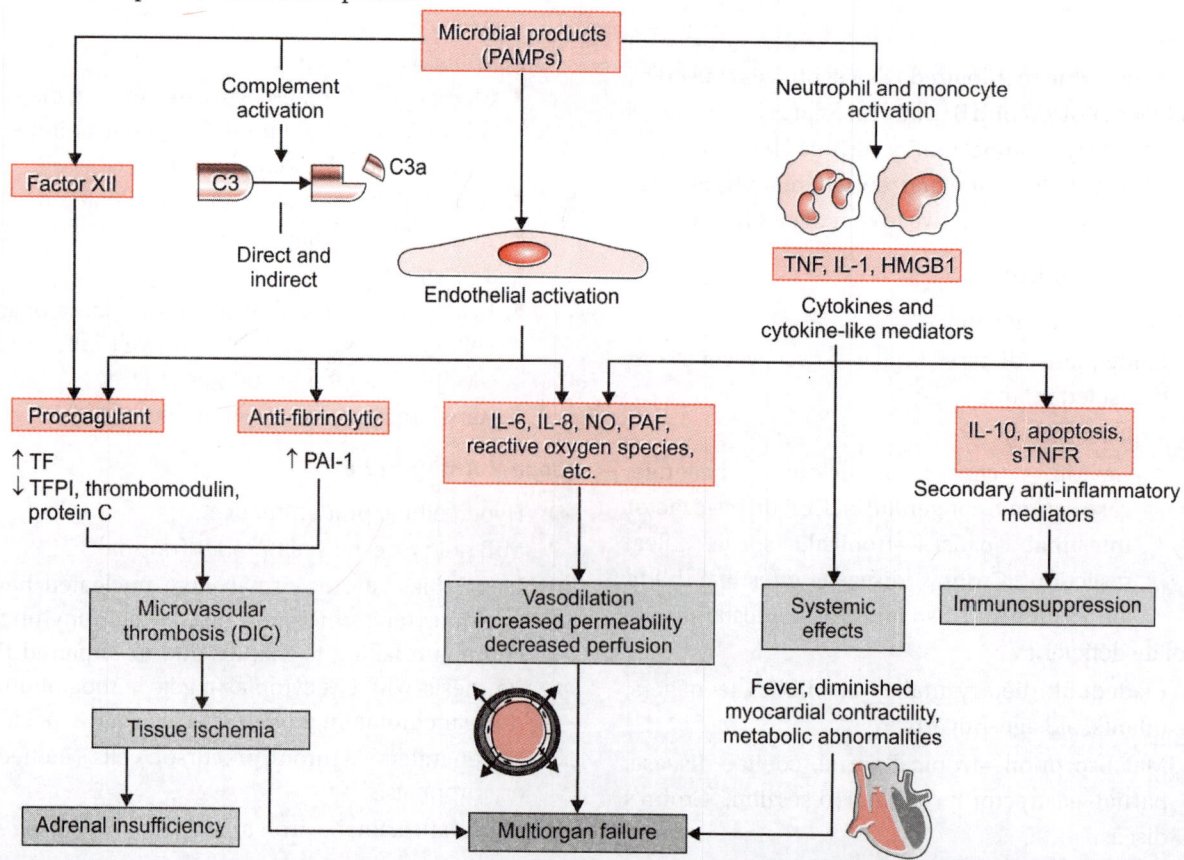

b. **Paraneoplastic syndromes**

(Ref: Textbook of Pathology Harsh Mohan, 8th ed. pg. 239)

ANSWER

Paraneoplastic Syndromes

Introduction

○ Group of disorders that develops in cancer bearing patients and that cannot be explained by direct or distant spread of tumor and nor by hormonal elaboration of the tumor (tissue of origin)

○ Triggered by an altered immune system response

○ Prevalent in middle-aged to older people

○ Commonly seen in lung, ovarian, lymphatic, or breast cancer.

Clinical Features

○ Difficulty in walking or swallowing

○ Decrease muscle tone and fine motor coordination

○ Memory loss, sleep disturbances, dementia and seizures

○ Loss of limb sensation and vertigo/dizziness.

○ Commonly seen in patients with undiagnosed cancer, patients with active cancer, or those in remission.

Syndromes included in the PNS are as follows:

Syndrome	Form of cancer	Mechanism
Endocrine syndrome		
• Hypercalcaemia	Sq.cell car. of lung, kidney,breast, Adult T cell leukemia-lymphoma	Paratharmone like protein, vitamin D
• Cushing's syndrome	Small cell ca of lung, pancreas	ACTH or ACTH like substance
• Carcinoid syndrome	Bronchial carcinoid tumor, ca pancreas, stomach	Serotonin, bradykinin
• Polycythaemia	Kidney, liver	Erythropoietin
Neuromuscular syndrome		
• Myasthenia gravis	Thymoma	Immunologic
Hematologic syndromes		
• Thrombophlebitis	Pancreas, lungs. GIT	Hypercoagulability
• DIC	Adenocarcinoma, AML	Chronic thrombotic phenomenon
• Anemia	Thymoma	
Gastrointestinal syndromes		
• Malabsorption	Small bowel lymphoma	Hypoalbuminaemia
Renal syndrome		
• Nephrotic syndrome	Advanced cancer	Renal vein thrombosis
Cutaneous syndromes		
• Acanthosis nigricans	Gastric ca	Immunologic
• Exfoliative dermatitis	Lymphoma	
Osseous, joint and soft tissue		
• Hypertrophic osteoarthropath, clubbing of fingers	Bronchogenic carcinoma	

PART-III

5 Write short notes on:

a. **Blood components**

(Ref: Textbook of Pathology Harsh Mohan, 8th ed. pg. 356)

ANSWER

Blood Components

Introduction

○ Blood received from donors in collected as whole blood in a suitable anticoagulant and divided into components in blood bank

▪ Packed RBCs

▪ Platelets

▪ Fresh frozen plasma

▪ Cryoprecipitates

○ Procedure involves initial centrifugation at low speed to separate whole blood into 2 parts—packed RBCs and platelet rich plasma

○ Subsequently, PRP is centrifuged at high speed to produce 2 parts—random donor platelets and FFP (Fresh frozen plasma)

○ Cryoprecipitates are obtained by thawing of FFP followed by centrifugation

○ Apheresis – technique of direct collection of large excess of platelets from a single donor

Clinical Applications of Blood Components

○ Packed RBCs

  ▪ To raise oxygen-carrying capacity of blood

  ▪ Used in normovolaemic patients of anemia without cardiac disease

  ▪ 1 unit of packed RBCs may raise haemoglobin by 1 g/dl

○ Platelets

  ▪ Platelet transfusion is done in patients of thrombocytopenia with haemorrhage

  ▪ Can be given to patient with platelet count below 10,000/micro l

  ▪ Each unit of platelets can raise platelet count by 5000-10000/micro l

○ Fresh frozen plasma

  ▪ Contains plasma proteins and coagulation factors that include albumin, protein C and S and antithrombin

  ▪ Given in patients of coagulation failure and TTP

  ▪ Each unit of FFP raises coagulation factors by about 2%

○ Cryoprecipitate

  ▪ Source of insoluble plasma proteins, fibrinogen, factor VIII and vWF

  ▪ Indications – patients requiring fibrinogen, factor VIII and vWF

  ▪ Each unit produces around 80IU of factor VIII

b. Down syndrome

(Ref: Harsh Mohan, 8/e, P. 289)

ANSWER

Down Syndrome

Introduction

○ Also known as Trisomy 21

○ Most common chromosomal abnormality

○ Caused by maternal nondisjunction

Epidemiology

○ Influenced with maternal age (increases with increasing maternal age)

Clinical Features

○ Mental Retardation

○ Short stature

○ Brachycephaly

○ Protruding tongue

○ Depressed nasal bridge, hypotonia

○ Open, wide fontanelle, flat occiput

○ Brush field spots in iris

○ Congenital heart defects

○ Single palmar crease- simian crease

○ Clinodactyly – 5th figure

○ Sandle gap between 1st and 2nd toes

○ Increased incidence of leukemia, Alzheimer's disease

○ Intestinal stenosis, anal atresia

Diagnosis

○ Antenatal screening:

  ▪ Nuchal thickness, dual marker (non-invasive) during first trimester

○ Triple test, quadruple test (non-invasive) during second trimester

○ Invasive:

○ Chorionic villus sampling for karyotype in first trimester (9-11 weeks)

○ Amniocentesis in 2nd trimester (14-16 weeks)

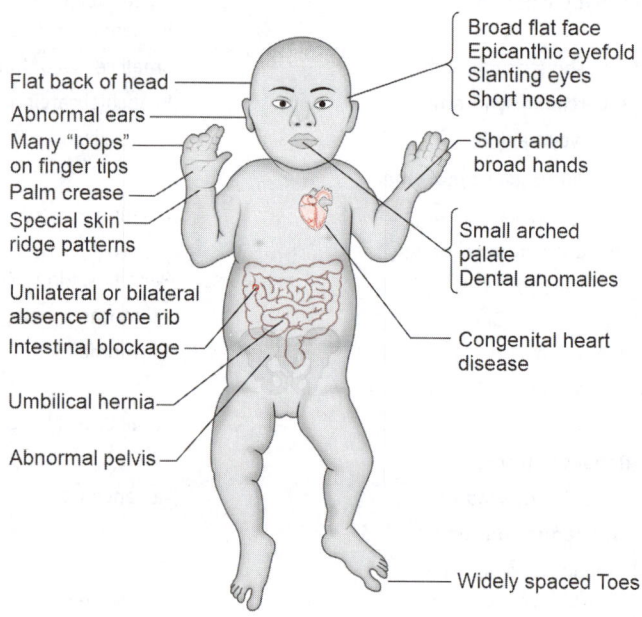

Fig. Down syndrome

c. Clinical features and lab diagnosis of haemophilia

(Ref: Textbook of Pathology Harsh Mohan, 8th ed. pg. 351, Robbins, 1st SA ed. P. 492)

ANSWER

Haemophilia

Introduction

○ A disorder of coagulation factor

○ Common heredity coagulation disorders are – hemophilia A, hemophilia B and von Willebrand's factor

○ Haemophilia A is also known as Classic Haemophilia and Haemophilia B is known as Christmas disease

Haemophilia A

Pathogenesis

- Deficiency of factor VIII (anti-hemophilic factor) because of mutation in F8 gene
- Due to quantitative reduction of factor VIII (90%) cases and qualitative dysfunction of factor VIII (10%) cases
- Sex (X) recessive trait

Epidemiology

- Most of the clinical manifestation in males, females are carrier

Clinical Features

- Massive bleeding after trauma or injury (bleeding continues for hours to days)
- Painful, recurrent hemarthroses, hematomas commonly occur as a result of spontaneous hemorrhage

Laboratory Findings

- Whole blood coagulation time: Prolonged Prothrombin time: Normal
- APTT or PTTK: Prolonged
- Confirmatory test:
  - Factor VIII assay: Reduced plasma level or reduced function
  - Cytogenetics: Mutations in X chromosome, like deletion, splicing defect, inversion, etc.

Treatment

- Symptomatic cases:
  - Factor VIII replacement therapy

Haemophilia B

- Due to deficiency of factor IX (Christmas factor or plasma thromboplastin component)
- Less common than hemophilia A

Treatment

- Fresh frozen plasma infusion or plasma enriched with factor IX infusion (mainly in symptomatic cases)

     d. Radiation Carcinogenesis

(Ref: Harsh Mohan, 8/e, P. 230)

ANSWER

Radiation Carcinogenesis
Introduction

- UV light and ionising radiation are 2 major forms of radiation carcinogens which can cause cancer in experimental animals and are involved in producing some forms of human cancers

- Appearance of mutations followed by long period of latency after initial exposure (usually 10-12 years later) is the property common between both types of radiation carcinogens
- Radiation carcinogens may enhance the effect of another carcinogen (co-carcinogens)
- Radiation agents also have sequential stages of initiation, promotion and progression in their evolution, just like chemical carcinogens

UV Light

Introduction

- Main source of UV radiation is sunlight, others being UV lamps and welder's arcs
- It penetrates the skin for a few millimetres only so that its effect is limited to epidermis
- Efficiency of UV light ass carcinogen depends on the extent of light absorbing protective melanin pigmentation of the skin
- In humans, excessive exposure to UV rays can cause various forms of skin cancers—squamous cell carcinoma, basal cell carcinoma and malignant melanoma

Mechanism

- Most important effect of UV radiation on cells is induction of mutation
- Other effects are inhibition of cell division, inactivation of enzymes and sometimes causing cell death
- Most important biochemical effect of UV radiation is formation of pyrimidine dimers in DNA
- UV induced damage in normal individuals is repaired whereas such damages remain unrepaired in predisposed persons who are excessively exposed to sunlight

Examples

- Xeroderma pigmentosum is predisposed to skin cancers at young age (below 20 years of age)
- Ataxia telangiectasia is predisposed to leukemia
- Bloom's syndrome is predisposed to all types of cancers
- Fanconi's anemia with increased risk to develop cancer

Ionising Radiation

Introduction

- All kinds of ionising radiation such as X-rays, alpha, beta and gamma rays, radioactive isotopes, protons and neutrons can cause cancer in humans and animals
- Most commonly radiation induced cancers are all types of leukemias

- Other forms are thyroid cancer, skin, breast, ovarian, uterine, lung, myeloma and salivary gland cancers
- Risk is increased by higher dose and with high LET such as in neutrons and alpha rays than with low LET as in X-rays and gamma rays

Mechanism

- May directly alter the cellular DNA
- May dislodge ions from water and other molecules of the cell and cause the formation of reactive oxygen species which may damage the DNA
- Damage to the DNA causes mutagenesis and is the most important action of ionising radiation
- It may result in chromosomal breakage, point mutation or translocation
- Effect depends on number of factors such as type of radiation, dose, dose-rate, frequency and various host factors such as age, immune competence, individual susceptibility, hormonal influences and type of cells irradiated

Examples

- Higher incidence of radiation dermatitis and other malignant tumors of skin was observed in X-ray workers and radiotherapists who did not take any safety measures
- High incidence of osteosarcoma was seen in young American watch working girls engaged in painting the dials with luminous radium who unknowingly ingested radium while using lips to point their brushes
- High incidence is seen in miners in radioactive elements

---

6. Write short notes on:

a. Type I Hypersensitivity reaction

(Ref: Textbook of Pathology Harsh Mohan, 8th ed. pg. 139, Robbins, 1st SA ed. P. 132)

ANSWER

Type I Hypersensitivity Reaction
Introduction

- State of immediately developing or anaphylactic type of immune response to an antigen to which the individual is previously sensitised (anaphylaxis is the opposite of prophylaxis)
- Reaction appears within 15-30 minutes of exposure to antigen
- Also known as Anaphylactic or Atopic reaction

Etiology

- Genetic basis
- Environmental pollutants
- Concomitant factors
- IgE antibodies mediated hypersensitivity reaction

Pathogenesis

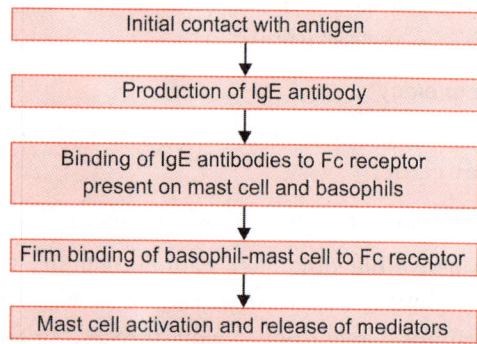

Mediators

- Primary Mediators:
  - Histamine
  - Adenosine
  - Eosinophil chemotactic factor
  - Proteases, etc.
- Secondary Mediators:
  - Leukotrienes B4, C4
  - Cytokines
  - Prostaglandin

Examples

- Bronchial asthma
- Hay fever
- Food allergy
- Systemic anaphylaxis- administration of drugs, antisera, etc.

b. Leukemoid reaction

(Ref: Textbook of Pathology Harsh Mohan, 8th ed. pg. 367)

ANSWER

Leukemoid Reaction
Definition

- Reactive excessive leucocytosis in the peripheral blood which appears same as that of leukaemia in a person who is not suffering from leukaemia
- The usual clinical features of leukaemia like haemorrhages, splenomegaly and lymphadenopathy are not present and characteristics of underlying disease resulting in leukaemoid reaction are apparent.

Types of Leukemoid Reaction

- Myeloid Leukaemoid reaction
  - In most of the reactions, granulocyte series are included and may be associated with various diseases such as
    - Infections—meningitis, sepsis, endocarditis, diphtheria, plague, staphylococcal pneumonia etc.
    - Intoxication—severe burns, eclampsia, mercury poisoning etc.
    - Malignant diseases—multiple myeloma, bone metastasis, Hodgkin's disease
    - Severe haemorrhages and severe haemolysis
  - Laboratory findings
    - Leucocytosis—moderate, not more than 100,000 (mu)l
    - Immature cells—mild to moderate, consisting of metamyelocytes, myelocytes (5-15%), blasts less than 5%
    - Toxic granulation and Dohle bodies are seen in cytoplasm of neutrophils in infective cases
    - Neutrophil (or leucocyte) alkaline phosphatase score (NAP or LAP score) – in cytoplasm of mature neutrophils in leukaemoid reaction is markedly high and is beneficial for distinguishing it from chronic myeloid leukaemia in suspicious cases
    - Cytogenic studies is valuable in cases which detect negative Philadelpphia chromosome i.e. t (9; 22) or BCR-ABL fusion gene in myeloid leukaemoid reaction but positive in cases of CML
    - Additional characteristics are – anemia, platelet count (normal to high), myeloid hyperplasia of bone marrow and absent infiltration of immature cells in organs and tissues
- Lymphoid Leukaemoid reaction
  - Found in certain conditions such as
    - Infections – cytomegalovirus infection, pertussis, infectious mononucleosis, chickenpox, tuberculosis, measles
    - Malignant diseases—may infrequently produce lymphoid reaction
  - Laboratory findings
    - Leucocytosis not more than 100,000 (mu)l
    - Differential white cell count majorly detects mature lymphocytes

c. **Mechanism of T cell depletion in HIV infection**

(Ref: Textbook of Pathology Harsh Mohan, 8th ed. pg. 135)

ANSWER

Mechanism of T cell Depletion in HIV Infection

Introduction

- HIV viremia and CD4+ T cells depletion in the host are correlated i.e higher the number of copies of HIV, more profound is the destruction of CD4+ T cells

Mechanism of CD4+ T Cell Depletion

- Usually, it is owing to direct virus-induced cytolysis of host CD4+ T cells
- Loss of integrity pf plasma membrane of the host cell during viral budding of viral particles may result in death of host CD4+ T cells
- HIV infected CD4+ T cells may fuse to form syncytial giant cells which have abundant expression of gp 120 and gp 41 molecules and bind more and more uninfected CD4+ T cells. Syncytia are intended to die of apoptosis
- Activation of inflammasome pathway (by release of proinflammatory cytokine may result in CD4+ T cells by pyroptosis
- Continuing destruction of architecture of lymphoid tissue ultimately causes burnt out lymphoid organs and depleted lymphoid population in these organs
- Other indirect mechanisms of CD4+ T cells depletion are aberrant intracellular signalling, T cell activation-induced cell death and autoimmune destruction of T cells

Name of the Paper   : Pathology Paper-II

Name of the Course   : MBBS-2018

Semester   : Annual

Time: 3 Hours   **M.M.: 40**

INSTRUCTIONS

1. Write your Roll No. on the top immediately on receipt of this question paper
2. All questions are to be attempted
3. Answers to Parts I, II and III should be written in separate answer sheets provided
4. Attempt parts of a question in sequence

PART-I

1. **Differentiate between:**   [8]
    a. Crohn's disease and ulcerative colitis
    b. Type I and Type II diabetes mellitus
    c. Poststreptococcal glomerulonephritis and membranous nephropathy
    d. Complete and partial hydatidiform mole.

2. **Write briefly on:**   [6]
    a. Papillary carcinoma thyroid
    b. Benign prostatic hyperplasia
    c. Etiopathogenesis and morphology of bronchiectasis.

PART-II

3. **Write briefly on:**   [6]
    a. Classification and etiopathogenesis of bronchogenic carcinoma
    b. Laboratory diagnosis of acute myocardial infarction.

4. **Write briefly on:**   [6]
    a. Causes of nephrotic syndrome and laboratory diagnosis of minimal change disease
    b. Sequence of serologic changes of hepatitis B infection.

PART-III

5. **Write short notes on:**   [8]
    a. Giant cell tumor bone
    b. Meningioma
    c. Etiopathogenesis of acute osteomyelitis
    d. Prognostic factors in breast carcinoma.

6. **Write short notes on:**   [6]
    a. Amoebic colitis
    b. Etiopathogenesis and complications of portal hypertension
    c. Burkitt's lymphoma.

PART-I

1. Differentiate between:

a. Crohn's disease and ulcerative colitis

(Ref: Textbook of Pathology Harsh Mohan, 8th ed. pg. 594)

ANSWER

Differences between Crohn's Disease and Ulcerative Colitis

Characteristic	Crohn's disease	Ulcerative colitis
• Site of origin	• Distal ileum, proximal colon	• Rectum
• Thickness of inflammation	• Transmural	• Mucosa and submucosa only
• Progression	• Irregular (skip lesions)	• Proximal, continuous from rectum; no • Skipped areas
• Location	• From mouth to anus	• Involves colon and rectum; rarely extends to ileum
• Change in bowel habits	• Obstruction, abdominal pain	• Bloody diarrhoea
• Classic lesions	• Fistulas or abscesses, cobblestone appearance, string sign on barium • Radiographs	• Pseudopolyps, lead pipe colon on barium radiographs, toxic megacolon
• Colon cancer risk	• Slightly increased	• Markedly increased
• Effect of Surgery on bowel disease	• Can worsen it	• Effective (Proctocolectomy with ileoanal anastomosis)

b. Type I and Type II Diabetes Mellitus

(Ref: Textbook of Pathology Harsh Mohan, 8th ed. pg. 864)

ANSWER

Type I and Type II Diabetes Mellitus

Characteristic	Type DM	Type II DM
Type of onset	Sudden and severe	Gradual and insidious
Age at onset	Early (under 35 years)	Late (above 40 years)
Frequency	10-20%	80-90%
Weight	Normal	Obese/non-obese
HLA	Associated with HLA DR3, HLA DR4, HLA DQ	No HLA linkage has been found
Genetic locus	Not known	Chromosome 6
Family history	<20%	Around 60%
Occurrence of Diabetes in identical twins	50% concordance	80% concordance
Pathogenesis	Autoimmune destruction of beta cells	Insulin resistance, impaired insulin secretion
Islet cell antibodies	Present	Absent
Blood insulin level	Reduced insulin	Normal to increased insulin
Islet cell changes	Insulitis, beta cell depletion	No insulitis, later fibrosis of islets
Amyloidosis	Uncommon	Common in chronic cases
Clinical management	Insulin and diet	Diet, exercise, oral drugs and insulin
Complications	Ketoacidosis	Hyperosmolar coma

PATHOLOGY

c. **Poststreptococcal glomerulonephritis and membranous nephropathy**

(Ref: Textbook of Pathology Harsh Mohan, 8th ed. pg. 693)

ANSWER

Poststreptococcal Glomerulonephritis and Membranous Nephropathy

Characteristic	Poststreptococcal glomerulonephritis	Membranous nephropathy
Etiology	Group A beta hemolytic streptococci	Idiopathic, infection (such as malaria, syphilis, hepatitis), drugs (such as gold, penicillamine, NSAIDs), autoimmune (such as SLE), neoplasms (such as lung and colon), metabolic disorders (such as Diabetes Mellitus)
Pathogenesis	Ab-mediated against circulating or planted Ag like endostreptosin, proteinase	Ag-Ab-mediated, in situ immune complex formation
Light Microscopy	Diffused hypercellular glomeruli owing to proliferation of endothelial and mesangial cells, and in-filtration of neutrophils and monocytes	Diffused thickening of Glomerular Basement Membrane, scarcity of neutrophils and macrophages in glomeruli
Electron microscopy	Subepithelial humps are seen	Subepithelial deposits, irregular silver stained spikes are observed
IFM	Granular deposits of IgM, IgG and C3 in Glomerular Basement Membrane and mesangium	Granular deposits of IgG and C3
Clinical	Nephritic syndrome	Nephrotic syndrome, selective proteinuria

d. **Complete and partial hydatidiform mole**

(Ref: Textbook of Pathology Harsh Mohan, 8th ed. pg. 788, Robbins, 1st SA ed. pg. 733)

Characteristic	Partial	Complete
Ploidy	Triploid	Diploid
No. of chromosomes	69, XXX; 69, XXY	46, XX or rarely 46, XY
hCG levels	Low	High
Chorionic villi	Some are hydropic	All are hydropic
Trophoblast proliferation	Focal	Marked
Fetal tissue	Present	Absent
Invasive mole	2%	10%
Choriocarcinoma	Rare	2%
Components	2 sperm + 1 egg	Most commonly enucleated egg + single sperm egg + single sperm (subsequently duplicates paternal DNA)

2. **Write briefly on:**

a. **Papillary carcinoma thyroid**

(Ref: Textbook of Pathology Harsh Mohan, 8th ed. pg. 850)

ANSWER

Morphologic Features of Papillary Carcinoma–Thyroid

Introduction

- Most frequent type of thyroid carcinoma (75-85%)
- Affects people of all ages including children and young adults with predilection for advancing age
- More common in females (female/male ratio is 3:1)
- Characteristically slow growing tumour presenting as asymptomatic solitary nodule
- Prognosis is good
- 10-year survival rate is 80-95%

Morphology

- Gross appearance:
  - Ranging from small, multifocal nodules to 10 cm in diameter
  - Poorly delineated
  - Cut surface exhibits grey-white, hard and scar like tumour

- Tumour may transform into a cyst into which numerous papillae project
- ○ Microscopic appearance:
  - Papillary pattern
    - ◆ Composed of fibrovascular stalk and covered by single layer of tumour cells
    - ◆ Papillae are accompanied with follicles
  - Tumour cells
    - ◆ Ground glass or optically clear appearance due to dispersed nuclear chromatin
    - ◆ Clear, oxyphilic cytoplasm
    - ◆ Apart from covering the papillae, tumour cells may form follicles and solid sheets
  - Invasion
    - ◆ Invasion of capsule and intrathyroid lymphatics by tumour cells is seen but not of blood vessels
  - Psammoma bodies
    - ◆ Half of papillary carcinomas exhibit typical small, concentric, calcified spherules in the stroma

b.   Benign prostatic hyperplasia

(Ref: Textbook of Pathology Harsh Mohan, 8th ed. pg. 698)

ANSWER

Benign Prostatic Hyperplasia

For answer, refer 2019 paper-II Q. 3(a), Pg. RP-87, RP-88

c.   Etiopathogenesis and morphology of bronchiectasis

(Ref: Textbook of Pathology Harsh Mohan, 8th ed. pg. 507)

ANSWER

Bronchiectasis

Introduction

- ○ Bronchiectasis is the chronic necrotizing infection of the bronchi and bronchioles that results in abnormal permanent dilatation of the airways

Etiopathogenesis

- ○ Endobronchial obstruction due to foreign body, neoplastic growth or enlargement of lymph nodes resulting in resorption of air distal to the obstruction with atelectasis and retention of secretions
- ○ Infection
  - Secondary to local obstruction and weakened systemic defense mechanism encouraging bacterial growth
  - Primary – emerging in suppurative necrotising pneumonia

Predisposing Factors

- ○ Hereditary and congenital factors
  - Congenital bronchiectasis due to developmental defect of bronchial system
  - Cystic fibrosis—generalised defect of exocrine gland leading to obstruction, infection and bronchiectasis
  - Hereditary immune deficiency diseases are usually linked with high incidence
  - Immotile cilia syndrome characterised by ultrastructural changes in microtubules causing immotility of cilia of the respiratory tract epithelium, sperms and other cells
  - Atopic bronchial asthma—patients with history of allergic diseases
- ○ Obstruction
  - Post obstructive bronchiectasis is localised and confined to one part of bronchial system
  - Causes include—foreign bodies, endobronchial tumours, compression by enlarged hilar lymph nodes and post inflammatory scarring
- ○ Secondary complication
  - Necrotising pneumonia such as in staphylococcal suppurative pneumonia and tuberculosis

Morphology

- ○ Gross changes:
  - Diffuse or segmental involvement of lungs
  - Bilateral involvement of lower lobes especially vertical air passages of left lower lobe
  - Fibrotic and thickened pleura with adhesions to chest wall
  - Dilated airways are classified as:
    - ◆ Cylindrical – tube like bronchial dilatation
    - ◆ Fusiform – spindle shaped
    - ◆ Saccular – rounded sac like
    - ◆ Varicose – irregular enlargements
  - Cut surface shows honey comb appearance
  - Extensive dilation of bronchi, with mucus filled lamina
- ○ Microscopic appearance:
  - Normal, ulcerated or presenting squamous metaplastic epithelium
  - Infiltration of bronchial walls by chronic inflammatory cells and destruction of normal muscle and elastic tissue with replacement by fibrosis
  - Intervening lung parenchyma appears fibrotic whereas surrounding lung tissue presents interstitial pneumonia
  - Pleura is adherent and presents bands of tissue between the bronchus and pleura

Complications

- Recurrent infection, breathing difficulty and increased sputum production:
  - Because lungs are not able to mobilize the secretions
- Pulmonary hypertension:
  - Constriction of the pulmonary arteries as a result of decreased oxygen supply results in raised pressure in the arteries
- Cor pulmonale:
  - Thickening of right ventricle
- Haemoptysis
- Heart failure and respiratory failure:
  - Cause of death in patients with bronchiectasis
- Fibrosis of the bronchial and bronchiolar wall
  - Amyloidosis
  - Lung abscess
  - Peribronchiolar fibrosis
  - Metastatic brain abscess
  - Empyema of thorax

PART-II

3. Write briefly on:

a. Classification and etiopathogenesis of bronchogenic carcinoma

(Ref: Textbook of Pathology Harsh Mohan, 7th ed. pg. 520)

ANSWER

Bronchogenic Carcinoma

Introduction

- Commonly known as "lung cancer"
- Characterized by carcinoma of the respiratory epithelium lining bronchi, bronchioles and alveoli
- Most common primary malignant tumour

Classification of Bronchogenic Carcinoma

- Squamous cell carcinoma
- Small cell carcinoma
  - Pure
  - Combined
- Adenocarcinoma
  - Acinar predominant
  - Papillary predominant
  - Lepidic predominant
  - Solid predominant with mucin formation
  - Micropapillary predominant
- Large cell carcinoma
- Adenosquamous carcinoma

Etiology

- Smoking (tobacco smoking) – most common
- Pollution
- Radiation exposure
- Dietary factors, like- vitamin A deficiency
- Occupational, example- workers exposed to asbestos, arsenic, nickel, beryllium, etc.

Clinical Features

- Common in middle age with peak incidence between 55–65 years of age
- Local symptoms: Cough, chest pain, dyspnoea, haemoptysis
- Fever
- Pleural effusion
- Weight loss
- Painful bony lesion, paralysis of recurrent nerve, superior vena caval syndrome (as a result of metastasis)
- Paraneoplastic syndromes, like-polymyositis, peripheral neuropathy, calcitonin producing hypocalcaemia, etc.

Morphology

Two main types:

1. **Hilar type:** Involves main bronchus or its branches in the hilar part, chiefly right side
2. **Peripheral type:** Single or multiple nodular tumour present in the lung periphery exhibiting pneumonia like consolidation of a large part of the lung

Microscopic Findings

Five main histologic subtypes:

- Squamous cell carcinoma:
  - Most common type, frequently seen in males
  - Microscopically, exhibits keratinization or intercellular bridges
- Adenocarcinoma:
  - Common in females
  - Categorized into preinvasive, minimally invasive and invasive adenocarcinoma
- Small cell carcinoma:

Two subtypes:

- Pure small cell carcinoma: Consists of small, round, oat-like cells arranged in the form of cords, ribbons forming pseudo rosettes
- Combined small cell carcinoma: Consist of a definite component of small cell carcinoma along with component of non-small lung carcinoma
- Large cell carcinoma: Undifferentiated carcinomas and composed of tumour cells with large nuclei, abundant cytoplasm, prominent nucleoli and well-defined borders
- Adenosquamous carcinoma: Exhibit keratinization and glandular differentiation

Diagnosis

○ Sputum examination (cytological)
○ Radiological examination of the chest
○ Bronchioalveolar lavage and bronchial washing

b. Laboratory diagnosis of acute myocardial infarction

(Ref: Textbook of Pathology Harsh Mohan, 8th ed. pg. 451, Robbins, 1st SA ed. pg. 409)

ANSWER

Acute Myocardial Infarction

Introduction

○ Life threatening condition resulting from coronary artery disease
○ Establishment of collateral circulation through anastomotic channels over a period of time may prevent myocardial damage
○ Incidence: Causes 10-25% of all deaths in developed countries
○ Age: Occurs at all ages, incidence being higher in old age especially with risk factors such as hypertension, diabetes mellitus, smoking, dyslipidemia
○ Sex: Males are more prone than females

Laboratory Diagnosis

○ Electrocardiogram changes–ST segment elevation, T wave inversion, appearance of wide deep Q waves
○ Laboratory Findings: Serum cardiac markers
  ▪ Creatinine phosphokinase (CK) and CK-MB–3 types are CK-MM (from skeletal muscle), CK-BB (from brain and lungs), CK-MB (from cardiac muscles and extracardiac tissue)
    ♦ Increased CK-MB is indicative of myocardial damage
    ♦ Ratio of CK-MB2: CK-MB1 above 4:1 is highly suggestive of acute MI after 4-6 hours of onset
    ♦ After 48 hours, it disappears from blood
  ▪ Lactate dehydrogenase (LDH)–2 isoforms–LDH 1 and LDH 2
    ♦ Ratio of LDH 1: LDH 2 more than 1 is suggestive of MI
    ♦ LDH levels rise after 24 hours, reach to peak in 3-6 days, returns to normal in around 14 days
  ▪ Cardiac-specific troponins (cTn)–2 types are cardiac troponin T (cTnT), cardiac troponin I (cTnI)
    ♦ cTnT and cTnI levels increase after myocardial injury
    ♦ cTnT remains elevated for 7-10 days and cTnI for 10-14 days
  ▪ Myoglobin–first cardiac marker to increase after MI, gets excreted rapidly in urine
○ Returns to normal after 24 hours of MI

4. Write briefly:

a. Causes of nephrotic syndrome and laboratory diagnosis of minimal change disease

(Ref: Textbook of Pathology Harsh Mohan, 8th ed. pg. 690, 696, Robbins, 1st SA ed. pg. 550)

ANSWER

Nephrotic Syndrome

Introduction

○ Constellation of features in different diseases with different pathogenesis
○ Characteristic features are:
  ▪ Heavy proteinuria
  ▪ Hypoalbuminaemia
  ▪ Oedema
  ▪ Hyperlipidaemia

Causes

○ Primary glomerulonephritis
  ▪ Minimal change disease – most frequent in children
  ▪ Membranous GN – most frequent in adults
  ▪ Membranoproliferative GN
  ▪ Focal segmental glomerulosclerosis
  ▪ Focal and diffuse proliferative GN
  ▪ IgA nephropathy
○ Systemic diseases
  ▪ Diabetes mellitus
  ▪ Amyloidosis
  ▪ SLE
○ Systemic infections
  ▪ Viral infections – HCV, HBV, HIV
  ▪ Bacterial infections – bacterial endocarditis, syphilis, leprosy
  ▪ Protozoa and parasites – P. falciparum malaria, filariasis
○ Hypersensitivity reactions
  ▪ Drugs – heavy metal compounds such as gold and mercury, other drugs such as penicillamine, trimethadione and tolbutamide, heroin addiction
  ▪ Bee stings, snake bite, poison ivy
○ Malignancy
  ▪ Carcinomas
  ▪ Myeloma
  ▪ Hodgkin's disease

○ Pregnancy
  ▪ Toxaemia of pregnancy
○ Circulatory disturbances
  ▪ Renal vein thrombosis
  ▪ Constrictive pericarditis
○ Hereditary diseases
  ▪ Alport's disease
  ▪ Fabry's disease
  ▪ Nail-patella syndrome

Laboratory Diagnosis of Minimal Change Disease

Lab findings are:

○ Proteinuria - >3 g daily and sometimes 15-20 g /day
○ Hypoalbuminemia – usually <2 g/dL
○ Hyperlipidemia
○ Microcytic hematuria – common in adults, 20-25% in children
○ Hypertension – 40-50% have at the time of diagnosis
○ Creatinine – increased level – typically 30-40% >baseline

  b. **Sequence of Serologic changes of Hepatitis B infection**

  (Ref: Textbook of Pathology Harsh Mohan, 8th ed. pg. 636)

ANSWER

Sequence of Serologic Changes of Hepatitis B Infection

○ HBsAg
  ▪ Appears early in blood after 6 weeks of infection
  ▪ Presence is suggestive of active HBV infection
  ▪ Disappears in 3-6 months
  ▪ If persists for more than 6 months – carrier state
○ Anti-HBs
  ▪ Appears late after 3 months of infection
  ▪ Response may be both IgM and IgG type
○ HBeAg
  ▪ Derived from core protein
  ▪ Present momentarily (3-6 weeks) during an attack
  ▪ If persists for more than 10 weeks suggests development of chronic liver disease and carrier state
○ Anti-HBe
  ▪ Appears after HBeAg disappears
  ▪ For resolution of infection during acute stage, seroconversion from HBeAg to anti-HBe is a prognostic sign
○ HBcAg
  ▪ Derived from core protein cannot be distinguished in blood

  ▪ Can be verified in nuclei of hepatocytes in carrier state and in chronic hepatitis patients
○ Anti-HBc
  ▪ Can be seen in serum of acute hepatitis B patients during pre- jaundice stage
  ▪ Initially, it is IgM class antibody persisting for 4-6 months and later followed by IgG anti-HBc
○ HBV-DNA
  ▪ Detection of HBV-DNA by molecular hybridisation using Southern blot technique is most sensitive index

---

PART-III

5. **Write short notes on:**

  a. **Giant cell tumour of bone**

  (Ref: Textbook of Pathology Harsh Mohan, 8th ed. pg. 839)

ANSWER

Giant Cell Tumour of Bone

Introduction

○ Also known as osteoclastoma
○ Benign locally aggressive tumour
○ Origin: Fusion of stromal mononuclear cells
○ Molecular genetics: Expression of RANK (factor responsible for osteoclastic proliferation) in stromal cells. RANK/RANKL signaling pathway may be responsible for formation of giant osteoclastic cells

Clinical Features

○ Common between 20 and 40 yrs. of age and no sex predilection
○ Common sites: lower end of femur and upper end of tibia, lower end of radius and upper end of fibula
○ Pain usually on movement
○ Pathologic fracture and swelling
○ Arthritic symptoms (joints are involved)

Morphology

Gross Appearance

○ Well-circumscribed, dark-tan and covered by a thin shell of subperiosteal bone

Microscopic Findings

○ Composed of osteoclast–like tumour giant cells scattered throughout the stroma
○ Stroma composed of sparse collagen fibres, spindle-shaped, plump, uniform mononuclear cells with areas of haemorrhage, macrophages and rich vascularity

Radiographic Findings

- Appears as lobulated, large, osteolytic lesion usually solitary with "soap bubble" appearance

Prognosis

- Recurrent and aggressive tumour
- Mostly shows recurrence after curettage (40-60%)
- Metastases to lungs is rare (approximately 4%)

b. Meningioma

(Ref: Harsh Mohan,8/e, P. 938, Robbins, 1st SA ed. pg. 885)

ANSWER

Meningioma

Introduction

- Slow growing benign tumor of adults
- Origin from the meningothelial cell of the arachnoid
- Molecular genetics: loss of chromosome 22q (NF2 gene)
- Positive for epithelial membrane antigens

Clinical Features

- Common in females as compared to males (3:2)
- Common sites involved are lateral cerebral convexities, midline along the falx cerebri, olfactory groove
- Less common sites are foramen magnum, cerebellopontine angle, cerebral ventricles and spinal cord
- Usually solitary
- May be present in patients with neurofibromatosis 2

Morphology

- Gross appearance
  - Present as masses in the well-defined dural base resulting in compression of underlying brain
  - Bosselated polypoid appearance
  - Hyperostosis of overlying bone
  - Cut surface is fibrous and firm with foci of calcification
- Microscopic findings: Five types—
  1. Fibrous (fibroblastic) meningioma:
     - Parallel or interlacing bundles of tumor cells
     - Psammoma bodies and whorled pattern are less common
  2. Transitional (mixed) meningioma:
     - Combination of syncytial and fibroblastic features with whorled appearance of tumor cells present around capillary sized blood vessel present in the centre

- Psammoma bodies may be present at some places in whorls
  3. Meningotheliomatous (syncytial) meningioma:
     - Resemblance to normal arachnoid cap cells
     - Solid masses of polygonal tumor cells with poorly defined cell membranes (called as syncytial appearance)
     - Granular cytoplasm with round to oval, central nuclei
  4. Angioblastic meningioma:
     - Consist of two patterns
       - Hemangioblastic pattern
       - Hemangiopericytic pattern
     - High recurrence rate
  5. Anaplastic (malignant) meningioma:
     - Exhibits extraneural metastases, usually to lungs

Diagnosis

- Neurological, vision, and hearing tests
- Stereotactic neurosurgery/biopsy
- Imaging tests: Includes MRI, CT scan, cerebral angiogram

Factors Determining the Prognosis

- Histology of tumor:
  - Type of tumor, its grade and molecular features helps in determining treatment outcome
- Patient's age:
  - Younger the adult better is the prognosis
- Extent of residual tumor:
  - Removal of all the tumor- better prognosis
- Location of tumor:
  - Tumor can be formed in any part of CNS
  - Difficult removal if location is not easily accessible
- Functional neurologic status:
  - Neurologic status is assessed using Karnofsky Performance scale, a higher score-better prognosis
- Metastatic spread:
  - Rare spread to other parts of the body

c. Etiopathogenesis of acute Osteomyelitis

(Ref: Harsh Mohan, 8/e, P. 873)

ANSWER

Etiopathogenesis of Acute Osteomyelitis

Etiology

- It is caused by Staphylococcus aureus (80-90%), E. coli, Pseudomonas, Klebsiella

Pathogenesis

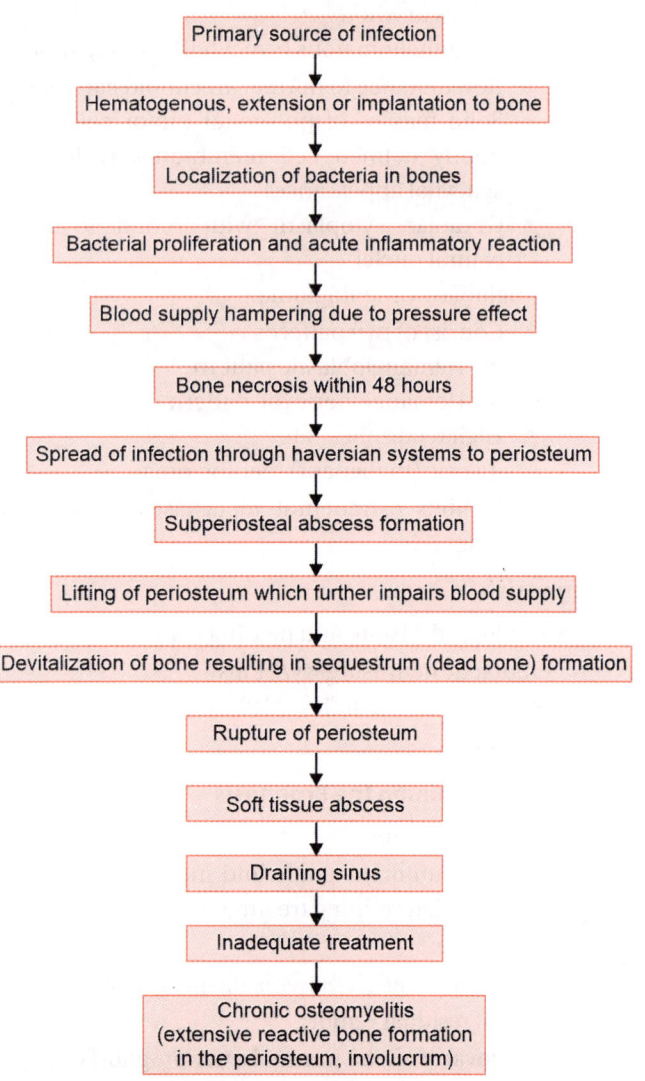

ANSWER

Prognostic Factors in Breast Carcinoma

- ○ Potentially precancerous lesions
  - Atypical ductal hyperplasia – linked with 4-5 times increased risk than woman of same age; frequent in 45-55 years of age
  - Clinging carcinoma – associated lesion in the duct but differs from carcinoma in situ and has lower risk of progression
  - Fibroadenoma – long term risk factor (after over 20 years) for invasive breast cancer with 2 times increased risk
- ○ Breast carcinoma in situ
  - Ductal carcinoma in situ (comedo and non comedo types) is diagnosed depending on 3 histologic features
    - ◆ Nuclear grade
    - ◆ Nuclear morphology
    - ◆ Necrosis
  - Breast conservative therapy – more common and requires three factors to be considered
    1. Margins
    2. Extent of disease
    3. Biological markers
  - Biological markers such as p53 and BCL-2 have low positivity in high grade in situ carcinoma and have chances of recurrence
- ○ Invasive breast cancer – Prognostic and predictive factors are studied by univariate analysis and multivariate analysis

d.   Prognostic factors in breast carcinoma

(Ref: Textbook of Pathology Harsh Mohan, 8th ed. pg. 799)

Factor	Favourable prognosis	Poor prognosis
• Routine Histopathology Criteria		
▪ Tumour size (two dimensions)	<1 cm size tumour; 10 years survival 90% in node negative	Size >1 cm
▪ Histologic type	Medullary ca., tubular c., mucinous (colloid) ca.; lobular ca. of low grade	Inflammatory ca
▪ Histologic (Nottingham)grading (Score range of 3–9) based on degree of tubule formation 1–3 score, regularity of nuclei-1–3 score, and mitoses-1–3 score	Low grade (grade I) tumour = score 3–5, moderate grade (grade II) tumour = score 6–7	High grade (grade III) tumour = score 8–9
• Axillary nodal status	Node negative: recurrence after 10 years 10–30%;	Node positive: recurrence after 10 years 70%; number of nodes: more than 4; sentinel node positive
• Hormone receptor status		
▪ Oestrogen-progesterone receptors (ER-PR)HER-2/neu (C-erb B-2)	ER-PR positive cases respond better to adjuvant therapy Underexpression	ER-PR negative cases respond poorly to adjuvant therapy Overexpression (predictive of response to herceptin)

Factor	Favourable prognosis	Poor prognosis
• Lymphatic and/or vascular invasion (both extratumoural)	Number of nodes: less than 4; sentinel node negative Negative for both: good	Positive for one or both: poor
■ Others:		
◆ Skin involvement ◆ Tumour circumscription ◆ Inflammatory reaction ◆ Intraductal component ◆ Stromal elastosis	Absence good Good May have some role Presence good Absence good	Presence poor Poor Controversial Absence poor Presence poor
• Biological indicators		
■ DNA ploidy analysis (aneuploidy, diploidy)	Not related	Not related
■ Oncogene disregulation		
◆ BRCA1, BRCA2 ◆ p53 ◆ BCL2 ◆ Cathepsin D	BRCA negative P53 positive respond better to chemotherapy and radiotherapy BCL2 positive good Absence good prognosis	BRCA positive P53 negative respond poorly to chemotherapy and radiotherapy BCL2 negative poor Presence poor prognosis
■ Mitotic index (by Ki67, MIB-1)	Low mitotic count	High mitotic count
■ Angiogenesis (VEGF, CD31, CD34, microvessel density counts)	Angiogenic activity low	High angiogenic activity

6. Write short notes:

a. Amoebic colitis

(Ref: Textbook of Pathology Harsh Mohan, 8th ed. pg. 641)

ANSWER

Amoebic Colitis

Introduction

○ Also known as amebiasis

Causative Organism

○ Entamoeba histolytica

Clinical Features

○ Present at any age, common in children
○ Causative organism: entamoeba histolytica
○ Spread through fecal-oral route
○ Generalized involvement of large intestine or localized to cecum, ascending colon, sigmoid, rectum and appendix
○ Abdominal pain
○ Diarrhea (may be bloody)
○ Fever, vomiting, weakness, unintentional weight loss
○ Ulcers:
  ■ Discrete and flask-shaped ulcers with broad base and narrow neck along with normal mucosa
  ■ Size is pinhead to >2.5 cm in diameter
  ■ Ulcer extends deep or may be superficial
  ■ No evidence of pseudopolyps

Morphology

○ Gross appearance: Lesion exhibits elevated mucosal surface advanced lesion exhibits flask-shaped ulcer with broad-base
○ Microscopic findings: Lesion consist of chronic inflammatory cell infiltrate composed of lymphocytes, plasma cells, macrophages, etc. trophozoites of Entamoeba present and usually present in the margins of the lesion

Differential Diagnosis

○ Giardiasis—no bloody stool
○ Ulcerative colitis—no abdominal pain
○ Crohn's disease—barium enema studies help to rule out both ulcerative colitis and amebiasis
○ Shigellosis—presence of high number of fecal leukocytes in the stool

Complications

○ Perforation
○ Hemorrhage
○ Amoebic abscess or hepatitis
○ Amoeboma formation

Diagnostic Tests

○ **Stool test:** Presence of ameboid protozoan in the patient's stool

PATHOLOGY

○ ELISA antigen tests

○ **Complete blood count:** Determination of the patient if become anemic due to bloody diarrhea

○ **Metabolic profile:** To assess electrolyte status of the patient

○ **Colonoscopy:** In case if stool test is negative for E. histolytica

○ **Tissue samples:** Shows trophozoites and flask shaped ulcer (characteristic finding)

b. Etiopathogenesis and complications of portal hypertension

(Ref: Textbook of Pathology Harsh Mohan, 8th ed. pg. 656)

ANSWER

Etiopathogenesis and Complications of Portal Hypertension

Introduction

○ Increased pressure to the portal system occurring after obstruction to the portal blood anywhere along its course

○ Portal veins have no valves and therefore obstruction anywhere in the portal system increases pressure in all veins proximal to the obstruction

○ Normal portal venous pressure is quite low – 10-15 mm saline

○ It occurs when the portal pressure is above 30 mm saline

○ Measurement of intrasplenic pressure imitates pressure in the splenic vein, percutaneous transhepatic pressure provides measure of pressure in the main portal vein, wedged hepatic venous pressure represents sinusoidal pressure

Etiology of Portal Hypertension

○ Intrahepatic
  ▪ Cirrhosis
  ▪ Metastatic tumors
  ▪ Budd-Chiari syndrome
  ▪ Hepatic veno-occlusive disease
  ▪ Diffuse granulomatous disease
  ▪ Extensive fatty change

○ Posthepatic
  ▪ Congestive heart failure
  ▪ Constrictive pericarditis
  ▪ Hepatic veno-occlusive disease
  ▪ Budd-Chiari syndrome

○ Prehepatic
  ▪ Portal vein thrombosis
  ▪ Neoplastic obstruction of portal vein
  ▪ Myelofibrosis
  ▪ Congenital absence of portal vein

Complications

○ Ascites

c. Burkitt's Lymphoma

(Ref: Textbook of Pathology Harsh Mohan, 8th ed. pg. 396)

ANSWER

Burkitt's Lymphoma

Introduction

○ Infrequent tumor found in adults but 30% of them comprises of childhood NHLs

○ It corresponds to L3 ALL of FAB grouping

○ It is a high grade, rapidly progressive human tumor

Subgroups of Burkitt's Lymphoma

○ African endemic
  ▪ At first described in African children, chiefly appearing as jaw tumor extending to extranodal sites such as bone marrow and meninges

○ Sporadic
  ▪ Tumor cells are similar to those of Burkitt's lymphoma but are more pleomorphic and may sometimes be multinucleated
  ▪ It has a propensity to infiltrate the CNS and is more aggressive than true Burkitt's lymphoma

○ Immunodeficiency associated Burkitt's lymphoma
  ▪ It includes cases associated with HIV infection

Morphology

○ Histologically, all 3 types of Burkitt's lymphoma are similar

○ Tumor cells are intermediate in size, non-cleaved and homogenous in size and shape

○ Nuclei are round to oval and contain 2-3 nucleoli

○ Cytoplasm – basophilic, contains lipid vacuolation

○ Mitotic rate of tumor cells is very high so high cell death occurs

○ Numerous macrophages are present in the background of the tumor containing phagocytosed tumor debris giving it a starry sky appearance

○ It is recognised as classical appearance of monomorphic medium sized cells having round nuclei, frequent mitoses, multiple nucleoli and basophilic cytoplasm with vacuoles

○ Immunophenotypically, tumor cells are positive for CD 19 and CD 10 and surface immunoglobulin IgM

○ Typical cytogenic abnormalities in the tumor cells are t(8;14) and t(8;22) involving MYC gene on chromosome 8, with overexpression of MYC protein having transforming activity

Pharmacology

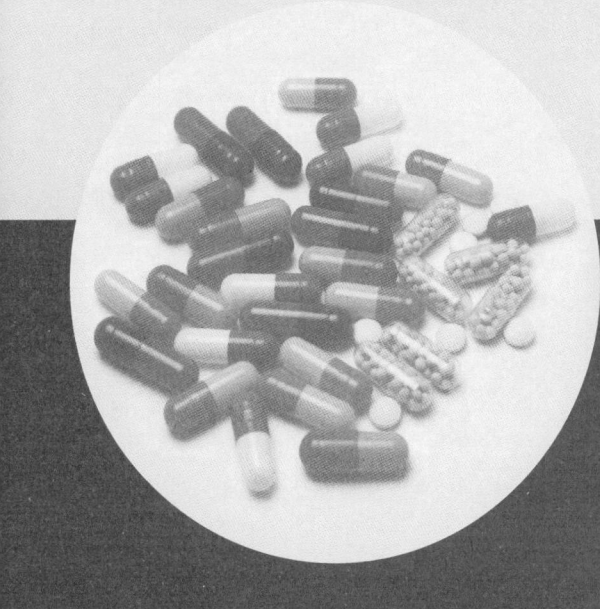

References Taken From:

O *Essentials of Medical Pharmacology, KD Tripathi, 7th and 8th edition*

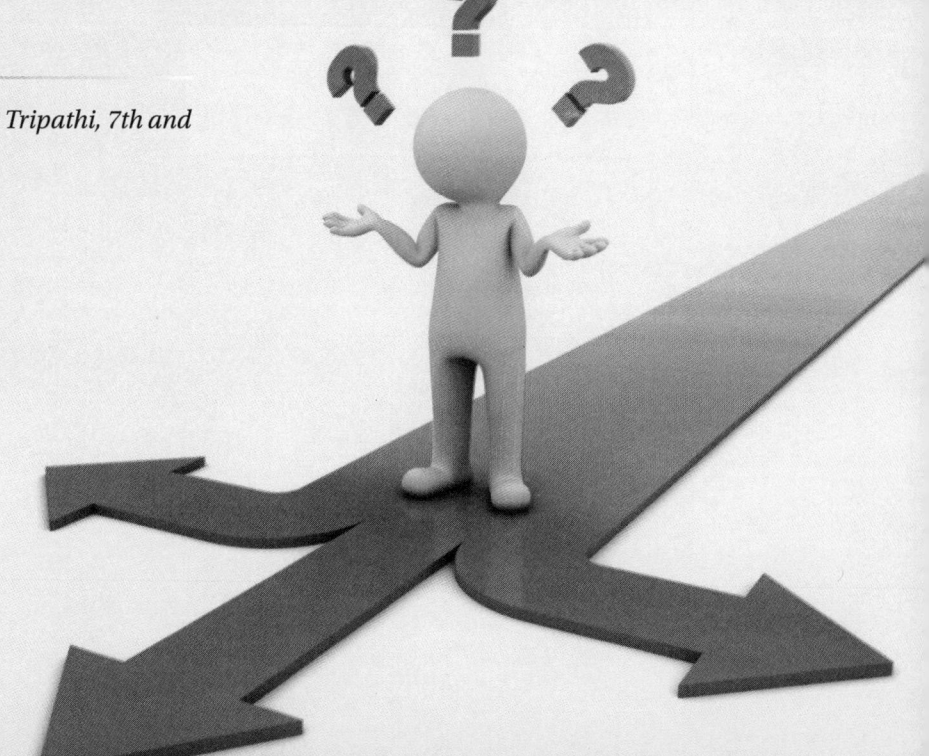

Your Roll No. ....

Name of the Paper	:	**Pharmacology Paper-I**
Name of the Course	:	**MBBS-2019**
Semester	:	**Annual**

Time: 3 Hours   M.M.: 40

INSTRUCTIONS

1. Write your Roll No. on the top immediately on receipt of this question paper
2. All questions are to be attempted
3. Answers to Parts I, II and III should be written in separate answer sheets provided
4. Attempt parts of a question in sequence

PART-I

1. **Explain Why?**   [8]
   a. Low dose aspirin is given for postmyocardial infarction prophylaxis
   b. Entacapone is prescribed as adjuvant to levodopa-carbidopa for the treatment of advanced parkinsonism
   c. Abrupt withdrawal of beta blockers may precipitate acute attack of angina
   d. Furosemide is given in pulmonary oedema.

2. **Classify and enumerate antianginal drugs. Discuss the mechanism of action, uses and adverse effects of nitrates.**
                                                                                                       [6]

PART-II

3. **Discuss the therapeutic status of:**   [8]
   a. Acetazolamide in angle closure glaucoma
   b. Tricyclic antidepressants in depression
   c. Carbamazepine in epilepsy
   d. Ezetimibe in hyperlipidemia.

4. **Discuss the drug treatment of:**   [6]
   a. Anaphylactic shock
   b. Methyl alcohol poisoning.

PART-III

5. **Discuss the therapeutic uses and adverse effects of:**   [6]
   a. Amiodarone
   b. Anticholinesterase inhibitors.

6. **Write short notes on:**   [6]
   a. Plasma half life
   b. Bioequivalence
   c. Drug synergism.

PART-I

1. Explain Why?

a. Low dose aspirin is given for postmyocardial infarction prophylaxis

ANSWER

Aspirin

- Cardioprotective effects are mediated through irreversible inhibition of platelet cyclooxygenase (COX) 1 and subsequent blockade of the production of thromboxane A2 (TXA2), reducing thrombus formation
- Prolongation of bleeding time is induced to last for 5–7 days

Low Doses of Aspirin is Used as an Antiplatelet Agent

- Effects of aspirin at any given time are influenced by the aspirin doses as well as plasma exposure and rate of platelet renewal in body
- Doses as low as 40 mg/day affects platelet aggregation
- In the clinical settings, aspirin is used at doses from 75 to 1500 mg/day. Daily doses at or below 162 mg are usually referred as "low-dose" aspirin
- Maximal inhibition of platelet function occurs at 75–150 mg aspirin given per day
- Also at low doses, there is possibility of selective suppression of TXA2 formation, whereas higher doses (>900 mg/day) may cut both TXA2 and prostacyclin (PGI2) production.

b. Entacapone is prescribed as adjuvant to levodopa-carbidopa for the treatment of advanced parkinsonism

ANSWER

- Entacapone is a COMT inhibitor
- Catechol-O-methyl transferase (COMT) enzyme breaks down levodopa
- COMT inhibitors do not help to manage the symptoms of Parkinson's on their own
- They have to be used with levodopa as an adjuvant to help prevent its breakdown by COMT enzyme
- Other example include tolcapone, etc.

c. Abrupt withdrawal of beta blockers may precipitate acute attack of angina.

(Ref: Essentials of Medical Pharmacology, KD Tripathi, 8th ed. pg. 597-598)

ANSWER

Beta Blockers

- Beta blockers lowers myocardial oxygen demand by reducing heart rate and blood pressure and reducing myocardial contractility
- Beta blockers exert their therapeutic effects in angina pectoris due to inhibition of beta1 receptor mediated stimulation of heart rate and myocardial contractility, which results in an enhanced oxygen supply-demand balance in the myocardium

Rationale Not to Suddenly Stop use of Beta Blockers in a Patient of Angina Pectoris

- On abrupt discontinuation, there is a possibility of rebound effect and also a risk of precipitating arrhythmias, worsening angina, or even causing myocardial infarction
- Patients with ischemic heart disease may have exacerbation of angina or acute ischemic events
- Known as beta blocker withdrawal syndrome.

d. Furosemide is given in pulmonary oedema

ANSWER

Rationale to Prefer Furosemide in Treatment of Pulmonary Edema

- Furosemide is a loop diuretic; are indicated for patients with fluid overload
- Furosemide acts by reducing preload and hence provide relief in edema
- Should be withheld or judiciously employed in patients presenting with intravascular volume depletion
- **Mechanism of action:** It inhibits NaCl reabsorption in the thick ascending limb of the loop of Henle; and since a significant proportion of filtered NaCl is absorbed by the thick ascending limb of loop of Henle, thus diuretics acting at this location are highly efficacious
- No significant downstream compensatory reabsorption mechanisms seen; loop diuretics like furosemide are highly effective and are called high ceiling diuretics.

2. **Classify and enumerate antianginal drugs. Discuss the mechanism of action, uses and adverse effects of nitrates.**

ANSWER

Classification of Antianginal Drugs

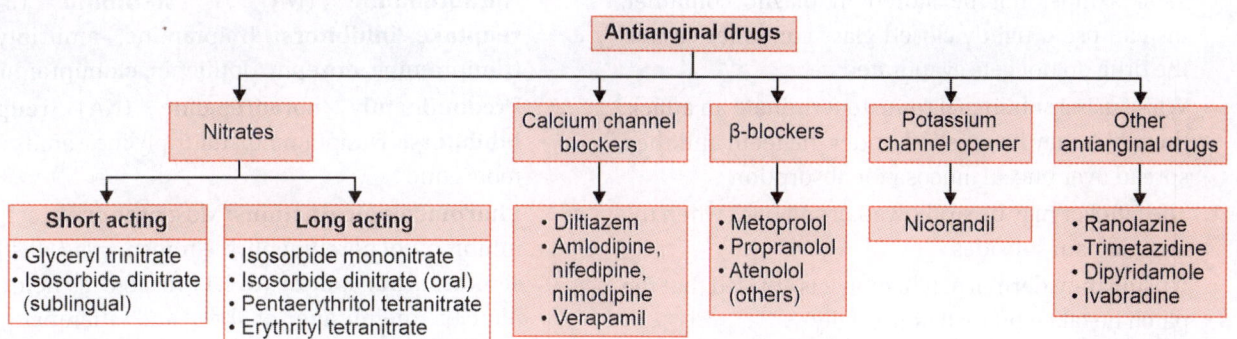

Clinical Classification

○ **Those that are used to abort or terminate attack:** GTN, Isosorbide dinitrate (sublingually).

○ **Those that are used for chronic prophylaxis:** Rest of the drugs.

Nitroglycerine

○ **Mechanism of action:** The mechanism of action revolves around major action being direct nonspecific smooth muscle relaxation

Rapid denitration of organic nitrates enzymatically in the smooth muscle cell

↓

Release of the reactive free radical *nitric oxide (NO)*

↓

Activation of cytosolic guanylyl cyclase and leads to increased cGMP

↓ cGMP dependent protein kinase

Dephosphorylation of myosin light chain kinase

↓

Decreased availability of phosphorylated (active) MLCK which interferes with activation of myosin

↓

Failure of myosin to interact with actin to cause contraction, thus relaxation occurs

↓

Relaxation effect is also enhanced by elevated intracellular cGMP leading to decline in calcium ions entry

↓

Nitrates causes generation of NO that activates cGMP production in platelets as well

↓

Beneficial in unstable angina.

Therapeutic Uses

Nitroglycerine (NTG)

○ Nitroglycerine undergoes significant first pass metabolism by nitrate reductase and hence is not effective by oral route.

○ Sublingual Nitroglycerine is the drug of choice for treatment of an acute attack of stable and Prinzmetal (variant) angina, for which a buccal spray can also be used. To prevent an acute attack in case of expected stress, sublingual NTG should be taken five minutes before.

○ Sublingual Nitroglycerine is also drug of choice for treatment of pain associated with MI.

○ Buccal and transdermal route can be used for prophylaxis. Transdermal NTG is preferred for prophylaxis of nocturnal angina.

○ Intravenous nitroglycerine is used for treatment of pulmonary edema associated with acute CHF and for hypertensive emergency.

Isosorbide Dinitrate (IDN)

○ IDN also undergoes first pass metabolism but lesser than NTG. IDN is metabolized by denitration into IMN (Isosorbide mononitrate), the active form.

○ It is administered by sublingual route for an acute attack and by oral route for long term prophylaxis of angina.

○ By oral route it is also used along with hydrazine for treatment of chronic CHF.

Adverse Effects

○ Fullness in head and throbbing headache

○ Continued use results in tolerance

○ Lying down causes flushing, weakness, sweating; also causes palpitation, dizziness and fainting

PHARMACOLOGY

○ **Methemoglobinemia:** Significant in severe anemia, this can further decrease O_2 carrying capacity of blood

○ Rarely, rashes, though relatively more common with pentaerythritol tetranitrate.

Precaution and Clinical Considerations

○ Tablets must not be stored in plastic container, instead use a tightly closed glass container so that the drug do not gets evaporated

○ While using sublingual route to terminate an attack, the tablet may be crushed under the teeth and then spread over buccal mucosa for absorption

○ The leftover may be swallowed or spit back when the anginal pain subsides

○ If using transdermal patch, then it is advised that the patch be taken off for 8 hours daily

○ If using a transmucosal dosage form, then to be stuck to the gums under the upper lip.

PART-II

3. Discuss the therapeutic status of:

a. Acetazolamide in angle closure glaucoma

(Ref: KD Tripathi, Essentials of Medical Pharmacology, 7th ed, pg. 586-87, 8th ed, pg. 634, 637)

ANSWER

○ Acetazolamide is a Carbonic anhydrase inhibitors

○ A sulfonamide derivative that acts as a weak or adjunct diuretic

○ Dose of 0.25 g 6–12 hourly taken orally

○ **Use:** Supplement ocular hypotensive drugs for angle closure, before and after ocular surgery/laser therapy.

○ **Mechanism of action**

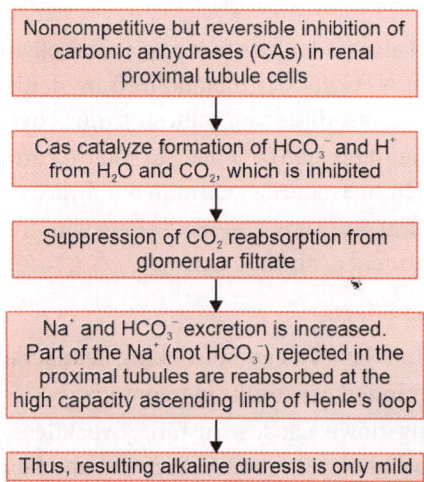

Noncompetitive but reversible inhibition of carbonic anhydrases (CAs) in renal proximal tubule cells

↓

Cas catalyze formation of HCO_3^- and H^+ from H_2O and CO_2, which is inhibited

↓

Suppression of CO_2 reabsorption from glomerular filtrate

↓

Na^+ and HCO_3^- excretion is increased. Part of the Na^+ (not HCO_3^-) rejected in the proximal tubules are reabsorbed at the high capacity ascending limb of Henle's loop

↓

Thus, resulting alkaline diuresis is only mild

b. Tricyclic antidepressants in depression

(Ref: KD Tripathi, 8th ed. pg. 454-59)

ANSWER

Tricyclic Antidepressants

○ **Noradrenaline (NA) + serotonin (5-HT) reuptake inhibitors:** Imipramine, amitriptyline, trimipramine, doxepin, dothiepin, clomipramine

○ **Predominantly noradrenaline (NA) reuptake inhibitors:** Desipramine, nortriptyline, amoxapine, reboxetine

○ **Pharmacological actions:** Most prominent action is inhibition of norepinephrine transporter (NET) and serotonin transporter (SERT) located at neuronal/platelet membrane at low and therapeutically attained concentrations

  ▪ Inhibition of monoamine reuptake and interaction with a variety of receptors *viz.* muscarinic, α adrenergic, histamine H1, 5-HT1, 5-HT2 and occasionally dopamine D2

  ▪ **CNS:** Different effects in normal individuals and in the depressed ones

    ♦ Induction of a peculiar clumsy feeling, tiredness, light-headedness, sleepiness, difficulty in concentrating and thinking, unsteady gait in *normal individuals*; no mood elevation or euphoria

    ♦ Little acute effects except sedation *in depressed patients*

    ♦ TCAs are not euphorients; act only antidepressants

    ♦ It has been proposed that TCAs indirectly facilitate dopaminergic transmission in forebrain. This may add to the mood elevating action

    ♦ Inhibition of NA and 5-HT uptake is associated with antidepressant action

    ♦ None of the TCAs, except amoxapine, block DA receptors or possess antipsychotic activity.

c. Carbamazepine in epilepsy

(Ref: KD Tripathi, 8th ed. pg. 415-16)

ANSWER

Carbamazepine

○ This drug is chemically related to imipramine

○ **Mechanism of action:** Modification of maximal electroshock seizures along with raising threshold to PTZ and electroshock convulsions

  ▪ Similar to phenytoin, action on Na^+ channels (prolongation of inactivated state)

  ▪ A lithium-like therapeutic effect in mania and bipolar mood disorder

  ▪ Also exhibits antidiuretic action

○ **Therapeutic uses**: Most effective drug for complex partial seizures (CPS)

- Most common drug for generalized tonic-clonic seizures (GTCS) and simple partial seizures (SPS)
- Drug of choice in *trigeminal and related neuralgias.* Carbamazepine do not act as an analgesic, but has a specific action. Around 60% patients respond well
- **Note:** Not useful in diabetic, traumatic and other forms of neuropathic pain
- As an alternative to lithium to treat *Manic depressive illness and acute mania.*

○ **Adverse effects:**

- Dose-related neurotoxicity—vertigo, sedation, dizziness, diplopia and ataxia. Vomiting, diarrhoea, worsening of seizures seen with higher doses
- Acute intoxication results in coma, convulsions and cardiovascular collapse
- Hypersensitivity reactions that include rashes, photosensitivity, hepatitis, lupus like syndrome, rarely agranulocytosis and aplastic anaemia
- In elderly people, water retention and hyponatremia
- Increased incidence of minor fetal malformations.

d. Ezetimibe in hyperlipidemia

ANSWER:

○ **Ezetimibe** acts by selective inhibition of intestinal cholesterol absorption, leading to the reduced delivery of cholesterol to the liver, a decline in hepatic cholesterol content, and an up-regulation of hepatic LDL receptors.

○ It is used alone or with other medication to treat hyperlipidemia

○ Lowers bad (LDL) cholesterol levels by approximately 20%

○ Very useful as add on therapy when statin therapy is not sufficient or in patients intolerant to statins.

○ **Mechanism of action of lipid-lowering drugs:**

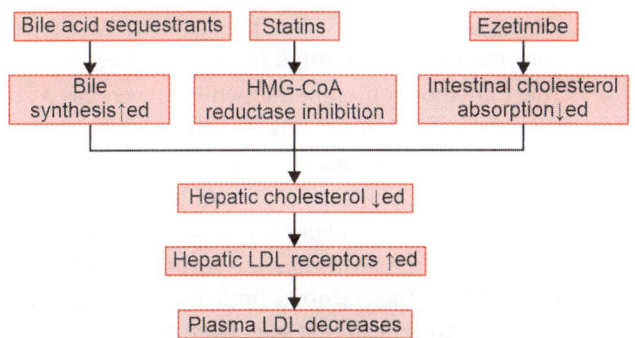

Abbreviation: HMG-CoA, 3-hydroxy-3-methylglutaryl coenzyme A; LDL, low density lipoprotein

4. Discuss the drug treatment of:

a. Anaphylactic shock

ANSWER

○ **Anaphylactic shock:** Severe allergic reaction

○ **Treatment and drugs used:** Removal of the cause, if possible

- Intramuscular (IM) injection of epinephrine, followed by additional epinephrine by IM or intravenous (IV) routes
- Placement in the supine position with the legs elevated, unless there is prominent upper airway swelling prompting the patient to remain upright (and often leaning forward)
- Place pregnant patients on their left side
- Supplemental oxygen
- Volume resuscitation with intravenous fluids.

b. Methyl alcohol poisoning

(Ref: KD Tripathi, 8th ed. pg. 422-423)

ANSWER

Methyl Alcohol Poisoning

Uncommon and massively lethal intoxication; presenting with headache, epigastric pain, vomiting, tachypnea, bradycardia, acidosis, retinal damage, and disorientation, etc.

Drug Treatment

○ Patient to be kept in a quiet, dark room to provide protection from light to the eyes

○ Within 2 hours of methanol ingestion, gastric lavage with sodium bicarbonate; maintenance of BP and ventilation by supportive measures

○ Acidosis to be countered by intravenous sodium bicarbonate infusion. Large amounts may be needed. Serves as a significant measure as combats retinal damage and other symptoms

○ If alkali therapy results in hypokalemia, potassium chloride infusion is required

○ Ethanol (10% in water) administered through a nasogastric tube. Loading dose 0.7 mL/kg, followed by 0.15 mL/kg/h

○ **How ethanol works?**

- Preferential metabolism of ethanol over methanol by the enzyme alcohol dehydrogenase.
- **Continuation of treatment for long**

○ Hemodialysis can clear off methanol and recovery is hastened

○ *Fomepizole* (4-methylpyrazole); drug of choice

- Specifically inhibits alcohol dehydrogenase

PHARMACOLOGY

- Loading dose of intravenous 15 mg/kg, followed by 10 mg/kg every 12 hours till methanol levels in serum fall below 20 mg/dL
- Not available commercially in India
- **Folate therapy:** Injection calcium leucovorin in a dose of 50 mg given 6 hourly is an adjuvant approach; enhances oxidation of blood formate.

Methanol Poisoning

- Uncommon form of poisoning, however, a massively lethal intoxication.
- Methanol is a multipurpose fuel. It has increasing use in an energy-driven society, thus high index of suspicion and immediate laboratory confirmation is required to manage the symptoms.
- Methanol poisoning manifests as:
  - Headache
  - Epigastric pain
  - Vomiting
  - Uneasiness
  - Tachypnea
  - Dyspnea
  - **Bradycardia:** Hypotension also occurs in most cases.
  - **Disorientation:** Delirium and seizures may occur. The patient may also suddenly pass into coma.
  - **Acidosis:** There is production of formic acid. This is very significant.
  - **Retinal damage:** This results as a specific toxicity of formic acid.
  - Blurring of vision and congestion of optic disc, and finally followed by blindness before demise.
  - Death due to respiratory failure.

Rationale for Ethanol to be used in Methanol Poisoning

- Preferential metabolism of ethanol over methanol by the enzyme alcohol dehydrogenase.
- This enzyme gets saturated by concentration 100 mg/dl of ethanol in blood. This slows down methanol metabolism and the rate of generation of formaldehyde and formic acid (conversion of methanol to these compounds is responsible for toxic manifestations) is reduced.

Dose

- Ethanol (10% in water) administered through a nasogastric tube.
- Loading dose 0.7 mL/kg, followed by 0.15 mL/kg/h.
- **Note**: The enzyme saturating concentration of ethanol yields to intoxication and thus can lead to hypoglycemia.

PART-III

5. Discuss the therapeutic uses and adverse effects of:

a. Amiodarone

(Ref: KD Tripathi, 8th ed. pg. 573)

ANSWER

Amiodarone in Arrhythmias

- Efficacious in a wide range of ventricular and supraventricular arrhythmias that includes paroxysmal supraventricular tachycardia (PSVT), nodal and ventricular tachycardia, atrial fibrillation, etc.
- Most significant indications include resistant VT and recurrent VF
- Intravenous injection can rapidly terminate ventricular (VT and VF) and supraventricular arrhythmias
- Also employed to maintain sinus rhythm in AF after failure of other drugs
- Also suited for chronic prophylactic therapy since it has long duration of action
- In addition, long term use reduces sudden cardiac death
- Organ toxicity (pulmonary alveolitis and fibrosis, goiter, photosensitization, etc.) is caused; but its high and broad spectrum efficacy and relatively low proarrhythmic potential makes it among drugs most commonly employed in arrhythmias.

b. Anticholinesterases or AChE inhibitors

ANSWER

- AChE inhibitors or anti-cholinesterases inhibit the cholinesterase enzyme from breaking down ACh, and thus increasing both the level and duration of the neurotransmitter action
- Basis the mode of action, they can be classified into two groups:
  - Irreversible and
  - Reversible.
- Reversible inhibitors can be again of two types- competitive or noncompetitive.
- These are mostly therapeutic, while irreversible AChE activity modulators are linked with toxic effects.
- Some examples include:
  - *Donepezil:* A selective, reversible AChE inhibitor which binds to the peripheral anionic site
  - *Rivastigmine:* A strong, slow-reversible carbamate inhibitor. This inhibits both BuChE and AChE, unlike donepezil that selectively inhibits AChE.
  - Diisopropyl fluorophosphates: A parasympatho-mimetic drug, irreversible anti-cholinesterase,

and has been used locally as a miotic agent in treating glaucoma.

6. Write short notes on:

a. Plasma half-life

(Ref: KD Tripathi, 8th ed. pg. 39-40)

ANSWER

○ Defined as the time duration in which the plasma concentration of any drug falls by 50% of the initial value.
○ **Therapeutic applications:** on dosing schedules
  ▪ Drugs having very short half-life given by constant intravenous infusion, e.g., dopamine
  ▪ Drugs having short half-life (30 minutes–2 hours) given at 6–8 hourly interval, e.g., cephalexin
  ▪ Drugs having medium half-life given at 12-hour interval
  ▪ Drugs having longer half-life, loading dose is followed by a maintenance dose, e.g., digoxin
○ Dose adjustments and change in intervals needed in renal/liver diseases
  ▪ Due to alteration in half-life

b. Bioequivalence

ANSWER

Bioequivalence

○ Two drugs are considered bioequivalent if they are pharmaceutically equivalent, and if they have similar bioavailability, so that the efficacy and safety are principally the same
○ If two medicines are bioequivalent there is no clinically significant difference in their bioavailability
○ Bioequivalence is measured based on the relative bioavailability of the innovator medicine versus the generic medicine
○ Determined by relating the ratio of the pharmacokinetic variables for innovator drug versus the generic medicine, wherein equality comes to be 1
  Note: Drugs that are not listed as bioequivalent should not be substituted for each other.

c. Drug synergism

ANSWER

○ **Synergism:** Pharmacologic action of one drug is expedited or increased by the other drug, this type of positive interaction is called synergism, and the drugs are said to be synergistic. It is possible that either drug when given alone is inactive, but it may still enhance the action of other drug when taken together.

It can be further classified as:

○ **Additive:** The two drugs act in the same direction and just simply adds up to the effect. The components in an additive combination exhibit their side effects separately and do not add up. This makes this pair better tolerated than higher dose. Examples include Analgesic action of aspirin and paracetamol
  ▪ General anaesthetic activity of nitrous oxide and halothane
  ▪ Antidiabetic action of metformin and glibenclamide
○ **Supraadditive:** The effect of the drug combination is higher than the individual components used in isolation. It is different from additive interactions in a way that it is always certain that one drug is inactive when given alone, but always enhances the effect of other drug. Examples include Acetylcholine + physostigmine
  ▪ Levodopa + carbidopa
  ▪ Sulfamethoxazole + trimethoprim.

Your Roll No. ....

Name of the Paper : **Pharmacology Paper-II**

Name of the Course : **MBBS-2019**

Semester : **Annual**

Time: 3 Hours   M.M.: 40

INSTRUCTIONS

1. Write your Roll No. on the top immediately on receipt of this question paper
2. All questions are to be attempted
3. Answers to Parts I, II and III should be written in separate answer sheets provided
4. Attempt parts of a question in sequence

PART-I

1. **Explain Why?** [8]
   a. Ergometrine is preferred over oxytocin for postpartum haemorrhage
   b. Liposomal amphotericin B is preferred over conventional amphotericin B in the treatment of fungal infection
   c. Folinic acid is used for toxicity of methotrexate
   d. Alendronate is used in treatment of osteoporosis.

2. **Classify and enumerate the drugs for diabetes mellitus. Discuss the mechanism of action, uses and adverse effects of Metformin.** [6]

PART-II

3. **Discuss the therapeutic status of:** [8]
   a. Valacyclovir in herpes simplex infection
   b. Propylthiouracil in hyperthyroidism
   c. Corticosteroids in tuberculosis
   d. Artesunate in malaria.

4. **Discuss the drug treatment of:** [6]
   a. Multibacillary leprosy
   b. Peptic ulcer with H. pylori infection.

PART-III

5. **Discuss the therapeutic uses and adverse effects of:** [6]
   a. Warfarin
   b. Ketoconazole.

6. **Write short notes on:** [6]
   a. Fibrinolytic agents
   b. Vitamin C
   c. Third generation cephalosporins.

PART-I

1. Explain Why?

a. Ergometrine is preferred over oxytocin for postpartum haemorrhage

ANSWER

Ergotamine

Belongs to a group of drugs ergot alkaloids

Mechanism of Action

○ Works by partial agonist and antagonist action at α adrenergic and all subtypes of 5-HT$_1$ and 5-HT$_2$ receptors

Ergotamine in Postpartum Hemorrhage (PPH)

○ Uterotonics are used to prevent PPH during the third stage of labor

○ Oxytocin is recommended, but in settings if it is not available, ergotamine can be used

○ This drug produces continued and sustained vasoconstriction and contraction of visceral smooth muscle

○ It has specific action on uterus; contractions are tetanic and do not resemble normal physiological contractions, unlike oxytocin

○ It has moderate onset and long duration of action
  ▪ Since the spasms are very powerful, therefore should not be used before delivery; should be used only to control late uterine bleeding.

b. Liposomal amphotericin B is preferred over conventional amphotericin B in the treatment of fungal infection

ANSWER

○ Liposomal amphotericin B is preferred over conventional amphotericin B due to its greatly improved tolerability profile compared with conventional amphotericin B.

○ Usage of conventional amphotericin B is limited by substantial toxicity (either infusion-related or linked with renal failure).

○ Liposomal amphotericin B is less nephrotoxic and maintains a broad antifungal spectrum.

○ Liposomal amphotericin B is associated with fewer infusion-related and kidney-related reactions.

c. Folinic acid is used for toxicity of methotrexate

ANSWER

○ **Folinic acid**: A reduced folic acid

○ Generic name: Leucovorin

○ Used in combination with other chemotherapy drugs to either improve effectiveness, or serve as a "chemoprotectant"

○ It is used for toxicity of methotrexate (Mtx) as Mtx blocks some of the effects of folic acid; this drug-induced folate deficiency may result in mouth sores, nausea or abdominal pain, liver problems, or problems with producing blood cells. These side effects can interfere with continuation of the therapy

○ Folinic acid decreases the toxic effects of methotrexate and pyrimethamine

○ **Note:** Contact with physician is a must if shortness of breath, wheezing, difficulty breathing, closing up of the throat, swelling of facial features, hives are experienced.

d. Alendronate is used in treatment of osteoporosis.

ANSWER

○ Alendronate is a potent 2nd generation amino-bisphosphonates, effective orally

○ Mainly used for prevention and treatment of osteoporosis both in males and females and also for Paget's disease

○ These are the most effective antiresorptive drugs

○ **Mechanism of action in Osteoporosis**

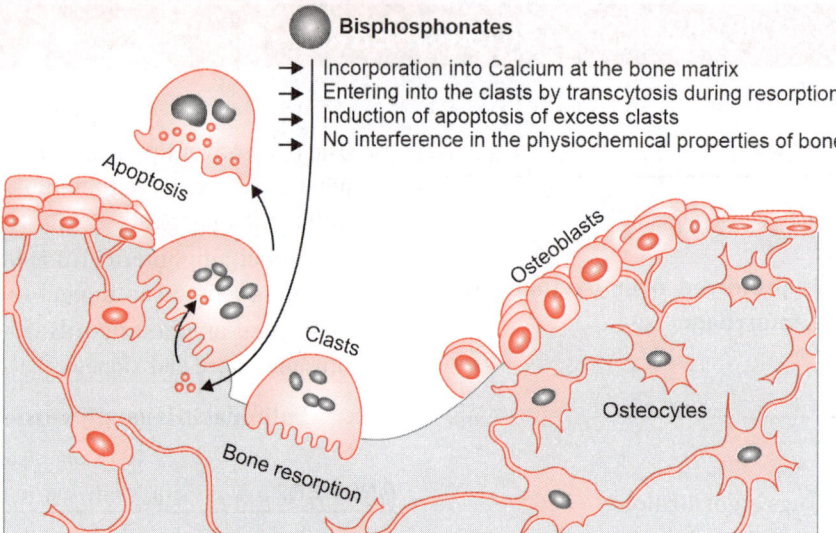

○ **Note: Patients need to be adequately instructed before starting therapy since**

- Patient should be instructed to take the dose on empty stomach in the morning with a full glass of water
- Instruction should also be given to not lie down or take food for at least 30 minutes after the dose
- These are important to prevent drug coming in contact with esophageal mucosa which can cause esophagitis
- Also, calcium, iron, antacids, tea, coffee, even mineral water, fruit juice, interferes with absorption of alendronate

○ **Note:** NSAIDs cause accentuation of gastric irritation caused by alendronate.

2. **Classify and enumerate the drugs for Diabetes Mellitus. Discuss the mechanism of action, uses and adverse effects of Metformin.**

ANSWER

Oral Hypoglycemic Drugs (OHAs)

Drugs employed to lower blood glucose levels in blood when diet and exercise are not sufficient to maintain the recommended levels.

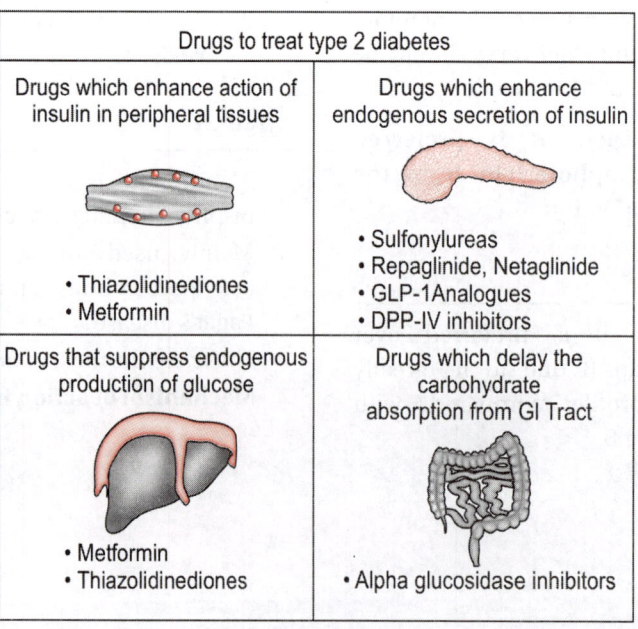

Abbreviation: GLP-1, glucagon-like peptide-1; DPP-4, dipeptidyl-peptidase-4; GI, gastrointestinal

Pharmacology of Major OHAs

OHA class	Pharmacological effects	Mechanism of action	Adverse effects
Sulfonylureas	• These drugs cause blood glucose lowering in normal subjects and in type 2 DM, but not in type 1 DM	• They exert their hypoglycemic effects by stimulating insulin secretion from the pancreatic β-cell • There is closure of ATP-sensitive K-channels in the β-cell plasma membrane • Thus initiate a chain of events resulting into insulin release	• Hypoglycemia • Nausea • Vomiting • Flatulence • Diarrhea or constipation • Mild headache and paresthesias • Hypersensitivity symptoms like rashes, purpura, transient leukopenia
Meglitinide analogues	• These are indicated only in those type 2 DM patients who suffer marked postprandial hyperglycemia, or supplementing metformin/ long-acting insulin • These drugs are administered before each major meal to control postprandial glucose excursion	• Binding to sulfonylurea receptor leads to closure of ATP dependent K^+ channels • Depolarization occurs → insulin release	• Mild headache • Dyspepsia • Arthralgia • Weight gain
GLP-1 receptor agonists	• GLP-1 based therapy is the most effective measure for preserving β cell function in type 2 diabetics	• Induces insulin release from pancreatic β cell • Inhibits release of glucagon • Suppresses appetite by activating specific GLP-1 receptors expressed on β and α cells, central and peripheral neurons, gastrointestinal mucosa, etc.	• Nausea and diarrhea infrequently • Weight loss • Hypoglycemia is rare with monotherapy, but can occur when combined with sulfonylureas/ metformin.
DPP-4 inhibitors	• Mostly employed as adjuvant drugs in type 2 DM not well-controlled by metformin/insulin/ sulfonylureas/ pioglitazone	• Competitive and selective DPP-4 inhibitor • Boosts postprandial insulin release • Decreases glucagon secretion and lowers meal-time as well as fasting blood glucose in type 2 DM	• Nausea • Loose stools • Headache • Rashes • Allergic reactions and edema • Nasopharyngitis and cough
Biguanides	• Metformin is the first choice drug for all type 2 diabetics • Not effective in pancreatectomized animals and in type 1 DM	• Suppresses gluconeogenesis in liver and • Glucose output • Enhances insulin-mediated glucose uptake in peripheral tissues • Glycogen storage in skeletal muscle • Decreased lipogenesis in adipose tissue and enhanced fatty acid oxidation	• Frequent, but generally not serious • Abdominal pain • Anorexia • Bloating • Nausea • Metallic taste • Mild diarrhea and tiredness • Hypoglycemia in overdose. • Vit B12 deficiency • Lactic acidosis (not as pronounced as with phenformin which was banned in 2003)
Alpha-glucosidase inhibitors	• They may be used as an adjuvant to diet (with or without metformin/SU) in obese diabetics • Doses are taken at the start of each major meal.	• Reversibly inhibit α-glucosidases, which is the final enzyme for the digestion of carbohydrates in small intestine • It slows down and decreases digestion and absorption of polysaccharides • Postmeal glycemia declines without significant rise in insulin levels	• Flatulence • Abdominal discomfort • Loose stool
Thiazolidinedi-ones	• They are indicated in type 2 diabetics, but not in type 1 diabetics • Primarily used as supplement to SUs/ metformin and in insulin resistance cases	• Act as selective agonists for the nuclear peroxisome proliferator-activated receptor γ which is expressed mostly in fat cells, but also in muscle and some other cells • Augments transcription of several insulin responsive genes • Entry of glucose into muscle and fat is improved. • Suppression of hepatic gluconeogenesis	• Greater fluid retention • Weight gain • Precipitation of CHF if using glitazones with insulin • Pioglitazone should not be used during pregnancy

PHARMACOLOGY

Therapeutic Uses of Metformin

○ **Type 2 diabetes:** Employed in first choice treatment of type 2 diabetes cases

○ **Complications of type 2 diabetes:** Useful in preventing complications related to cardiovascular, ophthalmic, and renal complications in patients that are long-term cases of type 2 diabetes

○ **PCOS:** Also employed in treatment of polycystic ovarian syndrome

○ **Anti-cancer drug:** Metformin has demonstrated ability to slow tumor cells growth in vitro. This effect is also observed when metformin is used in combination with other anticancer treatments in breast cancer cells.

Contraindications of Metformin

○ If serum concentration of creatinine higher than 150 micromols/L (cutoff point for renal failure)

○ Periods when suspecting tissue hypoxia (MI, sepsis cases)

○ Use of intravenous contrast dye medium (3 days after iodine has been given)

○ Cases of alcohol abuse sufficient to cause acute hepatic toxicity

○ History of lactic acidosis.

PART-II

3. **Discuss the therapeutic status of:**

   a. **Valacyclovir in herpes simplex infection**

        (Ref: KD Tripathi, 8th ed. pg.800)

ANSWER

○ **Valacyclovir:** An ester prodrug of acyclovir

○ It exhibits an improved oral bioavailability (55–70%) due to active transport by peptide transporters in the intestine

○ Higher plasma levels of acyclovir are obtained and clinical efficacy is improved in herpes zoster since it is completely converted to acyclovir in the first passage by esterases while passing through intestine and liver

○ ***Dose:***

   ▪ For genital herpes simplex: 1st episode 0.5–1.0 g BD × 10 days; recurrent episode 0.5 g BD × 3 days; suppressive treatment 0.5 g OD × 6–12 months.

   ▪ For orolabial herpes 2 g BD × 1 day; in immunocompromised patient 1 g BD × 5 days.

   ▪ For herpes zoster 1 g TDS × 7 days.

b. **Propylthiouracil in hyperthyroidism**

ANSWER

○ **Propylthiouracil:** Propylthiouracil is an antithyroid drug

○ **Mechanism of action:**

   ▪ Bind to the thyroid peroxidase and oxidation of iodide/iodotyrosyl residues is prevented

   ▪ Inhibiting tyrosine residues iodination in thyroglobulin

   ▪ Inhibition of iodotyrosine residues coupling to form T3 and T4.

   ▪ Peripheral conversion of T4 to T3 is inhibited by D1 type of 5'DI, but not by D2 type.

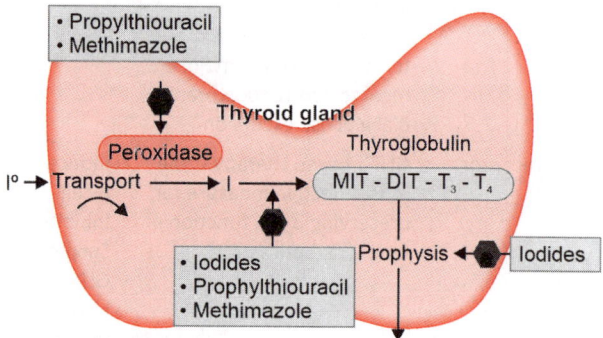

○ **Clinical uses:**

   ▪ Therapy of Graves' disease and toxic nodular goitre

   ▪ Treating thyroid storm. Dose: Oral 200–300 mg 6 hourly. Synthesis of hormone and peripheral conversion of T4 to T3 both are reduced

   ▪ Dose: Oral 200–300 mg 6 hourly

   ▪ Synthesis of hormone and peripheral conversion of T4 to T3 both are reduced

> **Thyroid Storm**
> Referred as thyrotoxic crisis; emergency condition arising due to decompensated hyperthyroidism

c. **Corticosteroids in tuberculosis**

ANSWER

○ Corticosteroids are frequently used as an adjunctive therapy for treating various forms of tuberculosis and for preventing complications, like constrictive pericarditis, intestinal strictures, hydrocephalus, focal neurological deficits, and pleural adhesions.

○ The risk of pleural thickening in patients with tubercular pleural effusion is significantly decreased by corticosteroids use.

○ Many studies have stated that using adjunctive corticosteroids may decrease mortality from all forms of tuberculosis by 17%, irrespective of the organ group was affected.

Note: Reactivation of tuberculosis is a risk among patients taking inhaled corticosteroids as it decreases local immunity of the lung.

d. Artesunate in malaria

ANSWER

Artesunate

An artemisinin derivative; water soluble while

Mechanism of Action

○ It possess potent schizonticidal action

○ Lethal damage to malarial gametes at early stage; but not mature ones

○ Release of highly reactive free radical species, which binds to membrane proteins, leading to lipid peroxidation, damage to endoplasmic reticulum, and eventually parasite lysis

Artesunate in Malaria

○ Reduction but no complete interruption in disease transmission

○ No cross resistance with any other antimalarial class

○ Short-acting or drug

○ Can be administered orally, or as an intramuscular as well as intravenous injection.

4. **Describe the drug treatment of:**

   a. Multibacillary leprosy

   (Ref: KD Tripathi, Essentials of Medical Pharmacology, 7th ed, pg. 783, 8th ed, pg. 835-36)

ANSWER

○ **Leprosy has been categorized by WHO into:**
  - *Paucibacillary leprosy (PBL):* Patient has few bacilli and is non-infectious
  - *Multibacillary leprosy (MBL):* Patient has large bacillary load and is infectious

○ **Multidrug therapy (MDT) of Multibacillary leprosy**

Rifampin	600 mg once a month supervised
Dapsone	100 mg daily self administered
Clofazimine	300 mg once a month supervised and 50 mg daily self administered

○ Duration 12 months

○ Doses need to be reduced suitably for children.

   b. Peptic ulcer with H. pylori infection

ANSWER

Peptic Ulcer with *H. pylori*

○ Gets attached to the surface epithelium

○ Maintains a neutral microenvironment around bacteria so as to protect against highly acidic gastric secretions

○ Around 90% cases of gastric and duodenal ulcers demonstrated positive test for *H. pylori*

Drug Treatment

○ *H. pylori* eradication therapy should be employed in all cases tested positive

○ H2 blockers and proton pump inhibitors (PPIs) form mainstay of treatment

○ Antibiotic therapy is mandatory, though no single antibiotic can be preferred as the organism develops resistance very rapidly

○ Antimicrobials used: Amoxicillin, Clarithromycin, tetracycline, and metronidazole/tinidazole

○ Combination regimens should include bismuth to be employed in case of double resistance to metronidazole and clarithromycin

○ H2 blockers/PPIs enhance efficacy antimicrobials active against *H. pylori* infections due to acid suppression

○ 1-week regimen may be sufficient; in some cases, high eradication rates with 2-week regimen

○ **Approved regimen:**
  - Lansoprazole 30 mg + Amoxicillin 1000 mg + clarithromycin 500 mg, BD for 2 weeks
  - Omeprazole 40 mg OD + Metronidazole 400 mg TDS + Amoxicillin 500 mg TDS
  - For ulcers (>10 mm in diameter) or presence of bleeding/perforation: Continue till complete healing
  - In case of eradication failure: Quadruple therapy with CBS 120 mg QID + tetracycline 500 mg QID + metronidazole 400 mg TDS + omeprazole 20 mg BD.

PART-III

5. **Discuss the therapeutic uses and adverse effects of:**

   a. Warfarin

ANSWER

○ Warfarin is an oral anticoagulants acting only *in vivo,* not *in vitro*

PHARMACOLOGY

○ **Mechanism of action:**

Act as competitive antagonists of vitamin K

↓

Interfere with the synthesis of vitamin K dependent clotting factors in liver

○ Heparin and warfarin are started together in acute thromboembolic states

○ Heparin is administered parenterally and used for *swift and short-lived action*

○ Warfarin is administered orally and suited for *maintenance therapy*

○ The objective of using these two anticoagulants is to impart immediate and fast action as well as prevent further thrombus extension and embolic complications by decreasing the rate of fibrin formation

○ However started together, heparin is withdrawn after 4–7 days when warfarin has taken effect.

○ **Adverse effects:**
   ▪ Bleeding
   ▪ Alopecia
   ▪ Diarrhea
   ▪ Dermatitis

> **Did you know?**
> *Warfarin* was initially used as rat poison while it is now a commonly employed oral anticoagulant.

b. Ketoconazole

(Ref: KD Tripathi, Essentials of Medical Pharmacology, 7th ed, pg. 792, 8th ed, pg. 844)

ANSWER

Ketoconazole

○ Belongs to a class of antifungals called imidazoles

○ Broad-spectrum antifungal drug

○ **Mechanism of action:** Works by slowing the growth of fungi, which cause infections

Clinical Profile

○ Used to treat dermatophytosis and deep mycosis; ineffective in fungal meningitis

○ Useful in seborrhea of scalp and dandruff

○ Used in recurrent cases of monilial vaginitis or those who have not responded to topical agents

○ **Note:** Contraindicated in pregnant and lactating women

○ Should not be used to treat fungal meningitis or fungal nail infections

○ **Also used in Cushing syndrome:** High doses are employed in Cushing's syndrome to reduce synthesis of corticosteroid

○ Effect is reported to be mediated by inhibiting adrenal 11 beta-hydroxylase and 17, 20-lyase

○ Prevents the expected upsurge in ACTH secretion in patients with Cushing's disease

○ In effect for long term control of hypercortisolism of either pituitary or adrenal origin

Side Effect Profile

Common side effects include following:

○ Headache

○ Diarrhea

○ Constipation

○ Stomach pain

○ Numbness, burning, or tingling of the hands or feet

○ Muscle pain

○ Hair loss

○ Heartburn

○ Dry mouth

○ Difficulty to fall asleep or stay asleep

○ Nervousness

○ Flushing

○ Chills

○ Sensitivity to light

○ Nosebleeds

○ Decline in sexual ability

○ **Note:** Decrease in the number of sperms produced, in particular if taken at high doses

Uncommon side effects include:

○ Rash and itching

○ Hives

○ Swelling of eyes, face, lips, tongue, hands, feet, ankles, or lower legs

○ Hoarseness

○ Tiredness or weakness.

6. Write short notes on:

a. Fibrinolytic agents

ANSWER

Fibrinolytic Agents

○ Drugs employed to lyse thrombi/clot to recanalize occluded blood vessels (mainly coronary artery)

○ Therapeutic effect rather than prophylactic

○ Activates the natural fibrinolytic system

○ Important ones include streptokinase, alteplase (rt-PA), urokinase, etc.

- **Uses:**
  - **For MI:** An accelerated regimen of alteplase
    - Alternative first line approach to emergency percutaneous coronary intervention (PCI) with stent placement
    - Achievement of recanalization of thrombosed coronary artery
  - **For pulmonary embolism:** Dose of 100 mg IV infused over 2 hours
  - **For ischaemic stroke:** Dose of 0.9 mg/kg by IV infusion over 60 minutes
  - **Deep vein thrombosis:** Leads to decrease in pain and swelling
    - Chief use is preservation of venous valves and may be a reduced risk of pulmonary embolism
- All cases with STEMI are indicated for reperfusion therapy
- No consistent clinical value in non-STEMI cases
- Careful patient identification is important.

  b. Vitamin C

ANSWER

Vitamin C

- Vitamin C (also known as Ascorbic acid) is a water soluble vitamin. Increasing proportions are excreted in urine with higher intakes.
- Citrus fruits (lemons, oranges) and black currants are the richest sources; others are tomato, potato, green chillies, and other vegetables
- **Note:** Human milk is richer source of vitamin C than cow's milk.
- Body is not able to store more than 2.5 g.
- **Major uses:**
  - Prevention of ascorbic acid deficiency
  - Treatment of scurvy: 0.5–1.5 g/day.
  - Postoperatively (500 mg daily) to guard against suboptimal healing

- Accelerate healing of bedsores and chronic leg ulcers
- Anaemia: Enhances iron absorption and is frequently combined with ferrous salts
- Acidification of urine (1 g TDS–QID) in urinary tract infections.

  c. Third generation cephalosporins

ANSWER

- **Third Generation Cephalosporins**
  - Enhanced and highly augmented activity against gram-negative Enterobacteriaceae
  - Some few members cause inhibition of *Pseudomonas* as well
  - Less active on gram-positive cocci and anaerobes
- **Cefotaxime:** Prototype of this group
  - Exhibits potent action on both aerobic gram-negative and some gram-positive bacteria
  - Inactive on anaerobes (particularly *Bact. fragilis*), *Staph. aureus* and *Ps. Aeruginosa*
  - Valuable in meningitis caused by gram-negative bacilli, life-threatening resistant/hospital acquired infections
  - Beneficial in septicemias and infections in immunocompromised patients
  - Potent alternative for typhoid fever, utilized for single dose therapy in PPNG urethritis
- **Ceftriaxone:** Distinctive feature its longer duration of action
  - Highly effective extensively in serious infections including bacterial meningitis (particularly **in children**), **multiresistant typhoid fever,** complicated urinary tract infections
  - In addition, inhibition of *B. fragilis* also.
- **Cefixime:** Is the oral drug of choice for thyroid and is preferred in ambulatory medicine.

Name of the Paper	:	**Pharmacology Paper-I**
Name of the Course	:	**MBBS-2018**
Semester	:	**Annual**

Time: 3 Hours   **M.M.: 40**

INSTRUCTIONS

1. Write your Roll No. on the top immediately on receipt of this question paper
2. All questions are to be attempted
3. Answers to Parts I, II and III should be written in separate answer sheets provided
4. Attempt parts of a question in sequence

PART-I

1. **Explain Why?**   [8]
   a. Furosemide is used for the treatment of acute left ventricular failure
   b. Atracurium is preferred skeletal muscle relaxant in patients with compromised hepatorenal function
   c. Tadalafil is used in the treatment of erectile dysfunction
   d. Atypical antipsychotics are preferred over typical antipsychotic drugs for the treatment of schizophrenia.

2. **Enumerate drugs used for the treatment of hypertension. Discuss the mechanism of action, therapeutic uses and adverse effects of telmisartan.**   [6]

PART-II

3. **Discuss the therapeutic status of:**   [8]
   a. Inhaled salbutamol in the treatment of bronchial asthma
   b. Zolpidem in the treatment of insomnia
   c. Thiopentone for the induction of anesthesia
   d. Paracetamol for the management of osteoarthritis.

4. **Discuss the drug treatment of:**   [6]
   a. Chronic simple glaucoma
   b. Nicotine addiction.

PART-III

5. **Discuss the therapeutic uses and adverse effects of:**   [6]
   a. Amitryptline
   b. Sodium valproate.

6. **Write short notes on:**   [6]
   a. Zero order kinetics
   b. Inverse agonist
   c. Drug tolerance.

PART-I

1. Explain Why?

a. Furosemide is used for the treatment of acute left ventricular failure

ANSWER

○ Furosemide is a loop diuretic
○ **Rationale to use in acute left ventricular failure:**
  ▪ It can effectively **treat** the sodium and water retention
  ▪ When given intravenously, **furosemide** provides rapid symptomatic relief. This effect precedes the increase in urinary sodium and water output by up to half a hour.
  ▪ **Mechanism of action:** It inhibits NaCl reabsorption in the thick ascending limb of the loop of Henle; and since a significant proportion of filtered NaCl is absorbed by the thick ascending limb of loop of Henle, thus diuretics acting at this location are highly efficacious.

b. Atracurium is preferred skeletal muscle relaxant in patients with compromised hepatorenal function

ANSWER

Atracurium

○ A bisquaternary competitive blocker that is four times less effective than pancuronium
○ Reversal is mostly not needed
○ **Preferred skeletal muscle relaxant in patients with altered hepatic and renal function:**
  ▪ The unique feature of atracurium is that it undergoes spontaneous degradation via a process known as Hofmann elimination as well as ester hydrolysis
  ▪ As a result, its duration of action is not altered by either renal or hepatic insufficiency
  ▪ Thus, it is the preferred muscle relaxant for liver/ kidney disease patients as well as for neonates and the elderly
  ▪ Because of these properties, it rapidly gained favor for providing neuromuscular blockade in intensive care unit patients
  ▪ For this purpose, it is most commonly used by continuous infusion.

c. Tadalafil is used in the treatment of Erectile dysfunction

(Ref: KD Tripathi, Essentials of Medical Pharmacology, 8th ed, pg. 327-29)

ANSWER

○ **Rationale to use tadalafil in the treatment of Erectile dysfunction:**
  ▪ Tadalafil is a selective Phosphodiesterase-5 (PDE-5) inhibitors, that forms first-line therapy for ED
  ▪ Selectively inhibits PDE-5 and enhances nitric oxide (NO) action in corpus cavernosum
  ▪ Thus erection of penis during sexual activity is improved, however, no such effect occur in the sexual arousal is absent.

d. Atypical antipsychotics are preferred over typical antipsychotic drugs for the treatment of schizophrenia

ANSWER

○ **Atypical antipsychotics:** Clozapine, risperidone, olanzapine, quetipine, aripiprazole, ziprasidone, amisulpiride, quetiapine, zotepine
○ **Preferred in the treatment of schizophrenia over typical antipsychotics:**
  ▪ Serves broad spectrum efficacy in schizophrenia; both positive and negative symptoms appear to be benefited
  ▪ At least as effective as conventional agents, with most producing fewer extrapyramidal symptoms
○ Adjunctive treatment of depression
○ Can also be employed to treat acute mania and anxiety
○ Relief in post-traumatic stress disorder and behavioural disturbances associated with dementia

2. Enumerate drugs used for the treatment of Hypertension. Discuss the mechanism of action, therapeutic uses and adverse effects of telmisartan.

ANSWER

Hypertension

○ According to WHO and JNC 7, hypertension (HTN) is described as systolic pressure above 140 mmHg and diastolic 90 mmHg

- According to JNC 8, 150/90 mm Hg is normal pressure for the age above 60
- The higher the pressure is directly related to greater risk of cardiovascular disease
- The first antihypertensive treatment was evidenced using Primaquine (antimalarial)
- Goal of treatment is to prevent the complications of hypertension heart attack
    - Stroke
    - Heart failure
    - Chronic kidney disease.

Antihypertensive Drugs

- Drugs used to lower BP in hypertension

Classification

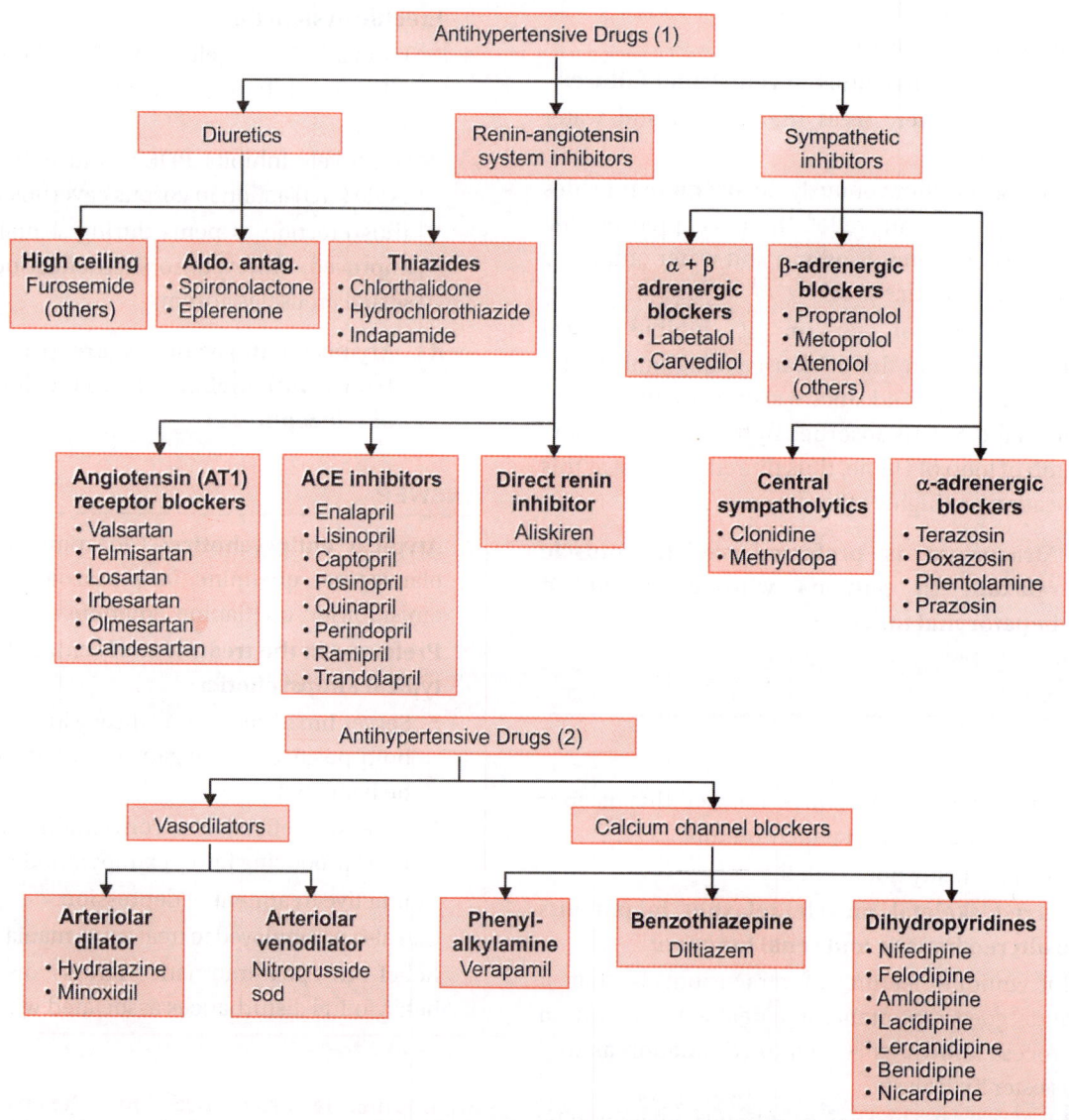

Telmisartan

- Belongs to angiotensin receptor blockers (ARBs)

Mechanism of action:

- Reduce the action of the hormone, angiotensin II

- Work by blocking receptors that the hormone acts on, specifically AT1 receptors
- Blocking the action of angiotensin II helps to lower blood pressure and prevent damage to the heart and kidneys

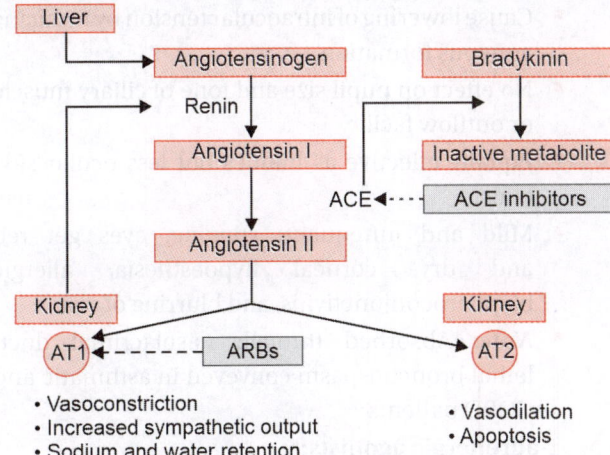

ACE, angiotensin converting enzyme
ARBs, sngiotensin receptor blockers
AT1, angiotensin 1; AT2, angiotensin 2

Therapeutic Indications

○ Treatment of essential hypertension in adults and in children and adolescents 6–18 years of age

○ Treatment of renal disease in patients with hypertension and type 2 diabetes mellitus with proteinuria ≥0.5 g/day as part of an antihypertensive treatment.

○ Reduced risk of stroke in hypertensive patients with left ventricular hypertrophy documented by ECG.

Adverse Effects

○ Symptomatic hypotension: especially after the first dose: Risk is higher in patients who are volume and/or sodium depleted by vigorous diuretic therapy, dietary salt restriction, diarrhoea or vomiting.

○ Back pain

○ Diarrhea

○ Nasal congestion

○ Sinus pain.

PART-II

3. **Discuss the therapeutic status of:**

    a. **Inhaled salbutamol in the treatment of bronchial asthma**

    (Ref: KD Tripathi, Essentials of Medical Pharmacology, 8th ed, pg. 252)

ANSWER

Salbutamol

Prototype drug of the group short-acting beta-2 receptor agonist

○ Salbutamol in bronchial asthma:

- Predominantly selective for beta-2 adrenergic receptors, and poorly selective for beta-1 receptors

- *Mechanism of action:* Stimulation of beta 2 receptors stimulates formation of cAMP, thus relaxation of smooth muscles of airways, from trachea to the terminal bronchi

- Administered preferably by inhalation through a pressurized metered dose inhaler, nebulizers, and dry powder inhalers; as this is not only effective but also reduces systemic toxicity

- Bronchodilation starts within 1–5 minutes after inhalation

- It is used in terminating mild, moderate and severe acute asthmatic attacks

- Used in exercise induced asthma

- Also employed in mild intermittent asthma as needed basis

- Side effects include palpitations, restlessness, nervousness, throat irritation, at times angioedema, etc.

- **Note:** While prescribing an inhaler, the patient must be taught synchronization of actuation of inhaler with inspiration or breathing to maximize drug delivery to lungs.

b. **Zolpidem in the treatment of Insomnia**

(Ref: KD Tripathi, Essentials of Medical Pharmacology, 8th ed, pg. 433-34)

ANSWER

Zolpidem

A selective BZD receptor agonist, but structurally non-BZD

○ **Zolpidem in insomnia**:

- Marked hypnotic effect

- Shortens sleep latency, duration of sleep is prolonged in insomniacs

- Indicated for short-term (1–2 weeks) use in sleep onset insomnia, also includes intermittent awakenings

- Morning sedation or extension of reaction time can ensue if taken late at night

- Few side effects reported; respiration not depressed even by large doses

- One of the most commonly recommended hypnotics currently

Benefits

- Relative lack of effect on stages of sleep

- Residual daytime sedation is nominal

- When discontinued, no or very less rebound insomnia seen
- Doses to be reduced to half in elderly and patients of liver disease.

c. Thiopentone for the induction of anesthesia

(Ref: KD Tripathi, Essentials of Medical Pharmacology, 8th ed, pg. 373-384)

ANSWER

○ Thiopentone is fast-acting anaesthetic that are usually used for induction

○ Thiopentone is a poor analgesic and painful procedures if performed under its influence without an opioid or N_2O, can cause the patient to struggle, shout and show reflex changes in BP and respiration

○ Respiratory depression with large doses can be severe

○ Cardiovascular collapse may also happen if hypovolemia, shock or sepsis are present.

d. Paracetamol for the management of Osteoarthritis

ANSWER

○ Paracetamol is extensively recommended for analgesia at an early stage of osteoarthritis

○ The use has derived its root from the analgesic and antipyretic actions

○ Offers symptomatic relief in osteoarthritis

○ May be used on 'as and when required' (SOS) basis

○ Generally considered to be safer than other commonly used analgesics such as NSAIDs or opiates.

4. Discuss the drug treatment of:

a. Chronic simple glaucoma

ANSWER

Open Angle Glaucoma

○ A degenerative disease which affects patency of the trabecular meshwork and gradually lost past middle age

○ Progressive increase in intraocular tension

Drug Treatment

○ **β-adrenergic blockers:**
  - First line drugs till recently, replaced by PG F2α analogs

- Cause lowering of intraocular tension by reducing aqueous formation
- No effect on pupil size and tone of ciliary muscle or outflow facility
- Equally effective as miotics but less ocular side effects
- Mild and infrequent; stinging, eyes get red and dry, corneal hypoesthesia, allergic blepharoconjunctivitis, and blurring of vision
- *Note:* Absorbed through nasolacrimal duct; lethal bronchospasm conveyed in asthmatic and COPD patients

○ α-**adrenergic agonists:**
  - Dipivefrine, Apraclonidine, Brimonidine, etc., used
  - Dipivefrine, though better tolerated than adrenaline, leads to marked ocular burning and other side effects
  - **Use of apraclonidine:** Short-term control of intraocular tension spikes after laser
  - **Use of brimonidine:** Both short-term and long-term use in glaucoma; commonly used as add on therapy only

○ **Prostaglandin analogs:**
  - Increases uveoscleral outflow by increasing permeability of tissues in ciliary muscle or by acting on episcleral vessels
  - Current treatment approach starts with these drugs
  - **Latanoprost:** Effect well-sustained over long-term
    - **Use:** Reduces intraocular tension in normal pressure glaucoma also
    - Due to better effectiveness and absence of systemic complications, forms the first choice drugs for open angle glaucoma cases despite side certain effects

○ **Carbonic anhydrase inhibitors**
  - **Acetazolamide:** Dose of 0.25 g 6–12 hourly oral
    - **Use:** Supplement ocular hypotensive drugs for angle closure, before and after ocular surgery/laser therapy
    - Dorzolamide is also used

○ **Miotics**
  - Now added only as the last option; due to several adverse effects.

b. Nicotine addiction

ANSWER

○ **Nicotine addiction:** A pattern of uncontrollable drug use characterized by irresistible involvement with the use of a drug.

○ FDA has approved bupropion and varenicline for treating nicotine addiction

○ Studies have indicated that smokers who receive a combination of behavioral treatment and cessation medications have higher quit rates than the people who receive minimal or no intervention.

○ Bupropion can help around 1 in 5 smokers to stop smoking

○ Bupropion use is generally associated with mainly insomnia and a dry mouth, that are closely linked to the nicotine withdrawal syndrome.

PART-III

5. Discuss the therapeutic uses and adverse effects

 a. Amitryptline

ANSWER

○ **Amitriptyline:** A tricyclic antidepressant (TCA); the plasma half-life of amitriptyline, range between 16–24 hours

○ **Therapeutic uses:**

- **Major depression:** To relieve symptoms of depression and restore normal social behaviour.

- **Obsessive-compulsive and phobic states:** Help reduce compulsive eating in *bulimia*, and help patients with *body dysmorphic disorder, compulsive buying* and *kleptomania,* though these habits may not completely die.

- **Neuropathic pain:** Affords considerable relief in diabetic and some other types of chronic pain.

- **Post-herpetic neuralgia:** Reduces intensity of post-herpetic neuralgia in around half of the patients.

- **Migraine:** Some prophylactic value, particularly in patients with mixed headaches.

Adverse Effects

○ **Anticholinergic:** Dry mouth, bad taste, constipation, urinary retention (particularly in males with enlarged prostate), blurred vision, palpitation.

○ Sedation, mental confusion and weakness

○ Increased appetite

○ Weight gain

○ Abrupt '*switch over*' to a dysphoric agitated state or to mania.

 b. Sodium valproate

(Ref: KD Tripathi, Essentials of Medical Pharmacology, 8th ed, pg. 417-418)

ANSWER

○ **Sodium valproate:** It is a broad spectrum anticonvulsant drug.

○ **Mechanism of action:**

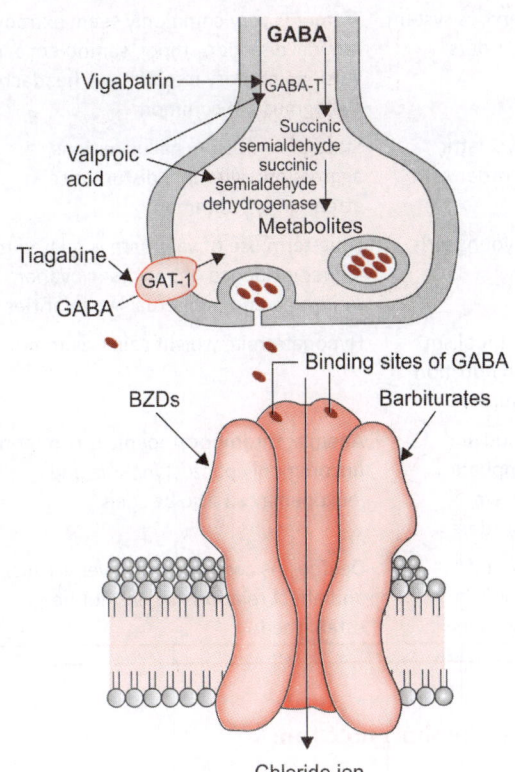

Chloride ion
BZDs, benzodiazepines

○ **Therapeutic uses:**

- Sodium valproate is the drug of choice for absence seizures

- Acts as adjuvant drug for generalized tonic-clonic seizures (GTCS), simple partial seizures (SPS), and complex partial seizures (CPS)

- Often incomplete control, but still drug of choice in myoclonic and atonic seizures

- Mania and bipolar illness: as alternative therapy to lithium

- Also been employed in panic attacks

- Some prophylactic efficacy in migraine has also been noted.

Adverse Effects

Hepatobiliary disorders	Severe liver damage, can occur, including hepatic failure sometimes resulting in death, has been reported. Increased liver enzymes are commonly noticed, particularly early in treatment, and may be temporary
	A rare but serious adverse effect is fulminant hepatitis; this occurs only in children (in particular below 3 years of age)
During pregnancy	If this is taken by pregnant women, it can cause spina bifida and other neural tube defects in the fetus

Gastrointestinal disorders	Nausea is very commonly seen; vomiting, gingival hyperplasia, stomatitis, gastralgia, diarrhea are commonly seen; these issues can generally be overcome by taking sodium valproate with or after food
Nervous system disorders	Tremor is very commonly seen; extrapyramidal disorder, stupor, somnolence, convulsion, memory impairment, headache, nystagmus are common
Psychiatric disorder	State of confusion, hallucinations, aggression, agitation, disturbance in attention are common
In young girls	Long-term use of valproate is related to higher incidence of polycystic ovarian syndrome and menstrual irregularities
Metabolism and nutrition disorders	Hyponatremia, weight gain is common
Blood and lymphatic system disorders	Anemia, thrombocytopenia is common; uncommonly pantoctyopenia and leukopenia can also be seen
Ear and labyrinth disorders	Deafness is common; however, a cause and effect relationship has not been established.

6. Write short notes on:

a. Zero order kinetics

ANSWER

- **Zero order kinetics:** An elimination kinetics that refers to a constant amount of drug is eliminated/ per unit time
- This refers to a state at which an enzyme reaction rate is independent of the concentration of the substrate/drug administered
- Examples inlcude ethanol, phenytoin, salicylates, cisplatin, fluoxetine, omeprazol
- A graphic presentation is given in the figure:

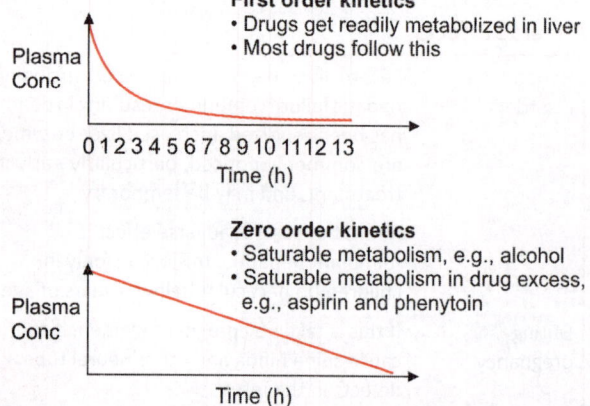

c. Inverse agonist

(Ref: KD Tripathi, Essentials of Medical Pharmacology,8th ed, pg .49)

ANSWER

- **Inverse agonist:** An inverse agonist is an agent that stimulates a receptor to generate a pharmacological effect in the opposite direction to that of the agonist
- Exhibits affinity, however, intrinsic activity presents a minus sign (IA between 0 and –1)
- Examples include chlorpheniramine (on H1 histamine receptor)
- Simple example for easy understanding, if agonism of the receptor led to sedation, an inverse agonist might cause wakefulness.

d. Drug tolerance

ANSWER

- **Drug tolerance:** It is defined as a phenomenon when it takes a higher dose of the drug to achieve the same level of response that is achieved initially
- This occurs when a person no longer responds to the drug in the same way that he/she initially responded
- Example, In case of morphine, tolerance develops rapidly to the analgesic effects
- **Also know**
  - Tolerance development does not refer to addiction, although many drugs that produce tolerance also have addictive potential.
- **Mechanism of tolerance development:** A change in either the density or affinity of its receptor: One potential mechanism for tolerance to opioids is receptor desensitization. This is caused by a decrease in functional opioid receptors after chronic opioid administration.
- Drugs that need occupancy of a smaller number of receptors for producing a therapeutic effect (example, fentanyl) less likely produce tolerance than the drugs that are less potent (example, codeine, butorphanol, meperidine).
- Drug tolerance can develop acutely (within hours) or chronically (over days, weeks, months)
- Irrespective of the cause, drug tolerance presents a significant problem in the pain treatment
- May result in discontinuation of therapy and implementation of an alternative analgesic therapy
- **Two types of tolerance:**
  1. **General/Nonspecific:** All the effects of a particular drug are diminished to a same extent
  2. **Specific:** Tolerance develops specific to one or some effects of a particular drug. This develops independent of other tolerance mechanisms.

PHARMACOLOGY

Name of the Paper : **Pharmacology Paper-II**

Name of the Course : **MBBS-2018**

Semester : **Annual**

Time: 3 Hours   M.M.: 40

INSTRUCTIONS

1. Write your Roll No. on the top immediately on receipt of this question paper
2. All questions are to be attempted
3. Answers to Parts I, II and III should be written in separate answer sheets provided
4. Attempt parts of a question in sequence

PART-I

1. **Explain Why?**   [8]
   a. Artemisinin derivatives are administered in combination for treatment of malaria
   b. Oxytocin is used for induction of labour
   c. Alteplase is used in management of acute myocardial infarction
   d. Imipenem is combined with cilastatin for treatment of infections.

2. **Enumerate corticosteroids. Discuss the mechanism of action, therapeutic uses and adverse effects of Prednisolone.**   [6]

PART-II

3. **Discuss the therapeutic status of:**   [8]
   a. Acyclovir in the treatment of herpes virus infection
   b. Pantoprazole in the treatment of acid peptic disorders
   c. Ofloxacin in the treatment of enteric fever
   d. H_2 blockers in peptic ulcer.

4. **Discuss the drug treatment of:**   [6]
   a. Anaerobic infection
   b. Osteoporosis.

PART-III

5. **Discuss the therapeutic uses and adverse effects of:**   [6]
   a. Heparin
   b. Metforrnin.

6. **Write short notes on:**   [6]
   a. Combination therapy of tuberculosis
   b. Anti-snake venom
   c. Immunomodulators.

PART-I

1. **Explain Why?**

   a. **Artemisinin derivatives are administered in combination for treatment of Malaria**

ANSWER

Artemisinin in Malaria

- Active against *P. falciparum* resistant to all other antimalarial agents; also includes sensitive strains and other malarial species
- **Mechanism of action:** In the erythrocytic schizogony cycle, acting on ring forms to early schizonts; exerts schizonticidal action
- These drugs are also fatal to early stage malarial gametes but not mature ones; decreasing the population of gametes
- Thus, disease transmission reduced but not totally interrupted
- Primary liver forms or vivax hypnozoites are not killed
- Their short acting action mandates monotherapy to be extended even after parasites disappear to prevent recrudescence
- Can be totally prevented by combining 3 day artemisinin with a long-acting antimalarial drug
- Examples include artesunate and artemether, etc.

   b. **Oxytocin is used for induction of labor**

(Ref: KD Tripathi, Essentials of Medical Pharmacology, 8th ed, pg. 283, 308-17)

ANSWER

Rationale to use Oxytocin in Induction of Labor

- Actions resemble normal physiological contractions
- Control in intensity of action is better afforded by oxytocin (as compared to ergometrine) due to its short half-life and slow intravenous infusion
- Foetal oxygenation has not to be suffered
- Provides consistent augmentation of uterine contractions.

   c. **Alteplase is used in management of acute Myocardial infarction**

ANSWER

Alteplase in Myocardial Infarction

- Used to lyse thrombi/clot to recanalize blocked blood vessels (mainly coronary artery), thus significantly employed in subjects with myocardial infarction
- It work by activating the natural fibrinolytic system
- Therapeutic action profile than prophylactic
- Produced from human tissue culture by using recombinant DNA technology, it shows moderate specificity to fibrin-bound plasminogen, thus lowering circulating fibrinogen only by around 50%
- An accelerated regimen is used in cases of myocardial infarction; 15 mg bolus intravenous injection followed by 50 mg over 30 minutes, then 35 mg administered over the next 1 hour
- Heparin coadministration is often required
- Can also be used for ischemic stroke and pulmonary embolism.

   d. **Imipenem is combined with cilastatin for treatment of infections**

(Ref: KD Tripathi, 8th ed. pg. 782)

ANSWER

Imipenem

- A thienamycin derivative
- An extremely potent and broad-spectrum β-lactam antibiotic
- Inhibition of some MRSA, not reliable for treatment of such infections

Rationale to Use with Cilastatin

- Imipenem undergoes rapid hydrolysis by the enzyme dehydropeptidase I, which is located on the brush border of renal tubular cells
- Cilastatin (a reversible inhibitor of dehydropeptidase I)
- Thus, it protects imipenem from hydrolysis
- Combination of imipenem-cilastatin 0.5 g intravenously every 6 hours is effective in a wide range of severe hospital-acquired respiratory, abdominal, urinary, pelvic, and skin and soft tissue infections
- Patients in neutropenia, cancer and AIDS included
- Though may induce diarrhea, vomiting, rashes on skin, etc., as side effects.

2. Enumerate Corticosteroids. Discuss the mechanism of action, therapeutic uses and adverse effects of Prednisolone.

(Ref: KD Tripathi, 7th ed. pg. 288, 8th ed. pg. 306)

ANSWER

Classification of Corticosteroids

- **Functional classification:**
  - **Glucocorticoids:** Regulate carbohydrates, lipids, and proteins metabolism, e.g., hydrocortisone
  - **Mineralocorticoids:** Control electrolytes and water balance, e.g., aldosterone
- **Based on duration of action:**
  - **Short-acting:** Hydrocortisone, cortisone, fludrocortisone
  - **Intermediate-acting:** Methyl-prednisolone, prednisolone, triamcinolone
  - **Long-acting:** Betamethasone, dexamethasone.

Pharmacological Actions of Glucocorticoids

- **Carbohydrate and protein metabolism:**
  - Promoting gluconeogenesis and glycogen deposition (in liver)
  - Inhibition of peripheral glucose utilization by tissues
  - Increased release of glucose from liver
  - Breakdown of proteins and mobilization of amino acids, thus can cause muscle wasting, etc.
- **Fat metabolism:**
  - Promote lipolysis due to glucagon, growth hormone, adrenaline, and thyroxine
  - Redistribution of fat in body: fats lost by extremities gets deposited over face, neck and shoulder
  - Characteristic feature producing "moon face", "buffalo hump", and "fish mouth"
- **Calcium metabolism:**
  - Inhibition of intestinal absorption
  - Enhancement of renal excretion of calcium
- **Water excretion:**
  - Enhancement of secretory activity of renal tubules
- **Cardiovascular system:**
  - Maintain tone of arterioles and contractility of myocardium
  - Restriction of capillary permeability, etc.
- **Skeletal muscles:**
  - Excessive action of mineralocorticoid leads to hypokalemia, and eventually weakness
  - Excessive action of glucocorticoid cause wasting of muscles and myopathy, leading to weakness

- **Central nervous system:**
  - Mild euphoria when administered with pharmacological doses
  - Level of sensory perception and neurons excitability maintained
- **Stomach:**
  - Increase in secretion of gastric acid and pepsin
- **Lymphoid tissue and blood cells:**
  - Increase in the number of RBCs, neutrophils, and platelets
  - Lymphocytes, eosinophils and basophils are decreased
- **Inflammatory responses:**
  - Suppression of inflammation
  - **All stages of inflammation:** Raised capillary permeability, exudation, etc. all are tempered
- **Immunological and allergic responses:** Allergies and hypersensitivity reactions are subdued

Indications (Corticoste)

- **C:** Collagen disorders
- **O:** Osteoarthritis
- **R:** Rheumatoid arthritis
- **T:** Thyroid storm
- **I:** Intestinal disease (Ulcerative colitis, Crohn's disease)
- **C:** Cerebral edema
- **O:** Organ transplantation
- **S:** Skin disorders and allergic reactions
- **T:** Testing functioning of adrenal pituitary axis
- **E:** Eye diseases
- **R:** Rheumatic fever
- **O:** Other lung diseases, bronchial asthma
- **I:** Inflammatory and infective diseases; and immunosuppression
- **D:** Dermatitis (Atopic)
- **S:** Septic shock

Side Effects

- Central obesity, supraclavicular hump, characteristic rounded face and narrow mouth (Cushing's habitus)
- Purple striae on thighs and lower abdomen
- Skin becomes fragile
- Weakness in muscles
- Hyperglycemia
- **Hirsutism:** Unwanted growth of coarse hairs in women (male pattern)
- Wound healing is deferred
- Osteoporosis in vertebrae and other flat spongy bones
- Bleeding and perforation of peptic ulcers may occur
- Children may exhibit growth retardation when given for long periods
- Glaucoma may also develop, etc.

Therapeutic Uses

○ Used to treat certain types of allergies, inflammatory conditions, and autoimmune disorders

○ Some of conditions include rheumatoid arthritis, dermatitis, asthma, adrenocortical insufficiency, inflammation in the eyes, multiple sclerosis, etc.

○ It can be used as oral dose, intravenously, as skin preparations, and eye drops

○ Used for long-term treatment of asthma and to control severe exacerbations of asthmatic attack with inhaled steroids

Adverse Effects

• Blood and lymphatic system disorders	• Leukocytosis
• Immune system disorders	• Increased susceptibility and severity of infections with suppression of clinical symptoms and signs, opportunistic infections, recurrence of dormant tuberculosis
• Endocrine disorders	• Cushingoid facies, growth suppression in infancy, hirsutism, impaired carbohydrate tolerance with increased requirement for antidiabetic therapy, suppression of the hypothalamo-pituitary adrenal axis, and weight gain
• Metabolism and nutrition disorders	• Hypokalaemic alkalosis, potassium loss, sodium and water retention.
• Psychiatric disorders	• Marked euphoria leading to dependence; aggravation of epilepsy, behavioural disturbances, irritability, nervousness, anxiety, sleep disturbances, and cognitive dysfunction
• Nervous system disorders	• Intracranial pressure with papilloedema in children (pseudotumour cerebri) usually after treatment withdrawal
• Eye disorders	• Corneal or scleral thinning, scleral perforation, papilledema
• Cardiac disorders	• Risk of congestive heart failure in susceptible cases
• Vascular disorders	• Hypertension, thromboembolism
• Gastrointestinal disorders	• Abdominal distension, dyspepsia, nausea, increased appetite, oesophageal candidiasis, oesophageal ulceration, peptic ulceration with perforation and hemorrhage
• Skin and subcutaneous tissue disorders	• Acne, bruising, impaired healing, purple striae
• Musculoskeletal and connective tissue disorders	• Muscle weakness, wasting and loss of muscle mass.
• Renal and urinary disorders	• Nocturia, scleroderma renal crisis (frequency unknown).
• General disorders and administration site conditions	• Hypersensitivity including anaphylaxis, malaise.

PART-II

3. Discuss the therapeutic status of:

a. Acyclovir in the treatment of Herpes virus infection

ANSWER

Acyclovir

○ Acyclovir is effective only against herpes group of viruses

○ Varicella-zoster virus is responsible for causing herpes zoster

○ Symptomatic relief is provided and healing of lesions is also promoted by use of acyclovir

○ It cannot prevent postherpetic neuralgia, but its duration may be reduced

○ When compared to other herpes virus, for example, herpes simplex virus (HSV)-1, VZV is less susceptible to acyclovir

○ Thus, higher doses are required and should be used only in immunodeficient individuals or in severe cases.

Mechanism of Action

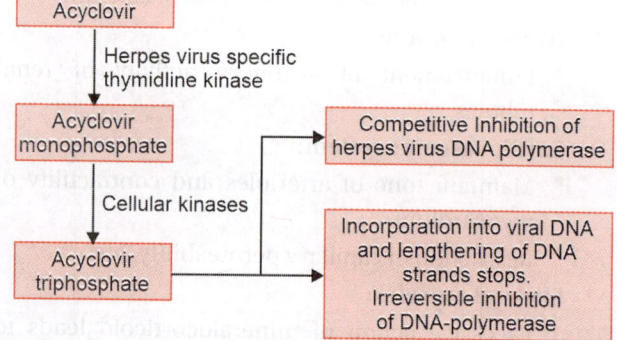

b. Pantoprazole in the treatment of acid peptic disorders

ANSWER

Mechanism of Action

Dose dependent suppression of gastric acid secretion; without anticholinergic or H_2 blocking action

↓

HCl secretion, both resting as well as that stimulated by food or any of the secretagogues, can be abolished without considerable effect on pepsin, intrinsic factor, and gastric motility

Indications in Acid Peptic Disorders

- Eradication of *H. pylori* (combined with antimicrobial drugs)
- Resistant severe peptic ulcer (4 to 8 weeks) and prevent bleeding from ulcers

Side Effect Profile: (Minimal)

- Nausea
- Loose stools
- Headache and pain abdomen
- Muscle and joint pain
- Rashes, leukopenia, and hepatic dysfunction infrequently
- Atrophic gastritis on prolonged treatment.

c. Ofloxacin in the treatment of Enteric fever

ANSWER

- An increase in use of fluoroquinolones such as ofloxacin and ciprofloxacin has been seen due to the high rates of multidrug-resistant (MDR) strains and the use of ampicillin, chloramphenicol and cotrimoxazole has decreased
- Ofloxacin has excellent plasma and intracellular penetrations with enhanced bactericidal action
- However, susceptibility of *Salmonella enterica* subsp. *enterica* serovar Typhi (*S.* Typhi) to fluoroquinolones has reduced and in fact is on the rise and of major concern in many developing nations.
- 3rd-generation cephalosporins, such as cefixime and ceftriaxone, or azithromycin are the alternative for treating *S.* Typhi infection with reduced susceptibility to ciprofloxacin.

d. H_2 blockers in peptic ulcer

ANSWER

- H_2 antihistamines act in peptic ulcer by reduction of Gastric Acid Secretion

- **Drugs include** Cimetidine, ranitidine, famotidine, Roxatidine
- **Mechanism of action:**
  - *H2 blockade:* The main action is blockade of histamine-H_2 receptors, and thus inhibit gastric secretion. Other effects include cardiac stimulation (prominent in isolated preparations and bronchial relaxation
  - Inhibition of gastric secretion: Suppressed all phases of secretion (basal, psychic, neurogenic, gastric) dose-dependently
  - Reduction in the volume, content of pepsin and intrinsic factor secretion, but the most prominent impact is on acid secretion
- **Notes:** H_2 blockers cause more reduction in acid secretion in evening since they cause more significant basal nocturnal acid secretion
- No effect on H_1 mediated responses highly selective.

4. Describe the drug treatment of:

a. Anaerobic infection

ANSWER

- Anaerobic bacteria forms the major flora in the normal human skin and mucous membranes
- These infections are generally polymicrobial, implying that anaerobic and aerobic organisms are mixed, thus potential therapy should cover both types of pathogens
- Most effectual antibiotics that act against anaerobic organisms include metronidazole, carbapenems (imipenem, meropenem and ertapenem), chloramphenicol, combinations of penicillin and beta-lactamase inhibitor (ampicillin or ticarcillin + clavulanate, and piperacillin + tazobactam), tigecycline and clindamycin
- Also include beta-lactam/beta-lactamase combinations (for example, amoxicillin/ clavulanate, piperacillin/tazobactam, ampicillin/ sulbactam)
- In required, ancillary susceptibility testing can be done for antibiotics cefoxitin, tigecycline, and moxifloxacin.

b. Osteoporosis

ANSWER

Osteoporosis

- A condition in which bones become fragile, accompanied by an increased susceptibility to fracture

Drug Treatment

- **Bisphosphonates:**
  - Most efficacious antiresorptive drug therapy
  - BPNs cause hastening of osteoclasts apoptosis
  - Osteoclasts differentiation is inhibited and interference with cytoskeleton
  - 2nd and 3rd generation BPNs (alendronate, risedronate) proven efficacious in osteoporosis in postmenopausal women
  - Also effective in osteoporosis cases due to age, idiopathic and steroid-induced in both genders
  - Bone mineral density is conserved and reduce the risk of vertebral and hip fractures significantly
- **Raloxifene:**
  - Leads to preventing bone loss in postmenopausal women
  - Forms second line therapy in postmenopausal women for preventing and treating osteoporosis
  - Can be alternatively used in vertebral fractures for secondary prevention and treatment
  - Not approved for primary prevention fractures due to osteoporotic bone loss
- **Calcium:**
  - Calcium and vitamin D_3 plays adjuvant role to drugs employed
  - Enhances benefits of raloxifene in prevention and treatment of osteoporosis
  - No reported effects in fracture prevention in healthy controls.

PART-III

5. Discuss the therapeutic status of:

a. Heparin

(Ref: KD Tripathi, Essentials of Medical Pharmacology, 8th ed, pg. 663-64)

ANSWER

- **Heparin:** A powerful and promptly acting anticoagulant to be administered by intravenous or deep subcutaneous routes
- Effective both in vivo and in vitro anticoagulation: Chief reason is that it inhibits reactions that lead to the blood clotting and formation of fibrin clots both in vivo and in vitro
- Indirect action by activation of plasma antithrombin III

↓

Binding of heparin-AT III complex to clotting factors of the intrinsic and common pathways

↓

Inhibition of factor Xa and thrombin (IIa) mediated conversion of fibrinogen to fibrin

- Not absorbed orally as it is a large and highly ionized molecule.
- **Note:** Heparin and Warfarin are started together in Acute Thromboembolic States
  - The objective of using these two anticoagulants is to impart immediate and fast action as well as prevent further thrombus extension and embolic complications by decreasing the rate of fibrin formation
  - However started together, heparin is withdrawn after 4–7 days when warfarin has taken effect.

b. Metformin

ANSWER

For answer, refer 2019 paper-II Q. 2 Pg. RP-130

6. Write short notes on:

a. Combination therapy of Tuberculosis

ANSWER

Rationale to Use Combination of Antitubercular Drugs in Tuberculosis

- **For preventing emergence of drug-resistant tuberculosis:**
  - One most important step to ensure complete and effective treatment of tuberculosis is to prevent further emergence of drug-resistant tuberculosis
  - Any inappropriate selection of antitubercular agent and monotherapy with any one drug has showed up risk of developing drug-resistant tuberculosis
  - Drug resistance have been predominantly occurring due to multiple disruptions of treatment
  - Also, if single dose preparations are given, patients are more likely to continue one drug and negligence towards others
  - Use of fixed dose combinations of antitubercular agents results in limiting the risks of drug-resistant cases
- Use of combinations also make prescription of drugs and management of drug supply simpler

○ **Overcoming limitations of treatment centers:**

  ▪ At times, drugs being out-of-stock in treatment facilities, may lead to continuation of some drugs, while new stocks of the others are awaited

  ▪ This epitomizes another possible source of monotherapy.

b. **Anti-snake venom**

(Ref: KD Tripathi 7th ed. pg. 927)

ANSWER

Antisnake Venom (ASV) Serum Polyvalent

○ Available as purified, enzyme refined and concentrated equine globulins in lyophilized vials with 10 ml ampule of distilled water.

○ *Dose:* 20 ml intravenously repeated at 1–6 hourly intervals till symptoms of envenomation disappear: upto 300 ml may be required in viper bites, while upto 900 ml have been used in cobra bites

○ Important to continue ASV treatment till evidence of envenomation persists.

○ After reconstitution, each ml neutralizes:

  ▪ 0.6 mg of standard Cobra venom.

  ▪ 0.6 mg of standard Russells viper venom.

  ▪ 0.45 mg of standard Saw scaled viper venom.

  ▪ 0.45 mg of standard Krait venom.

c. **Immunomodulators**

ANSWER

○ **Immunomodulators:** Medicines that are used to facilitate regulate or normalize the immune system.

○ Can be used as add-on therapy to treat asthma and hereditary angioedema.

○ **Example: Leflunomide is** an immunomodulatory, that inhibits proliferation of stimulated lymphocytes in patients with active RA.

○ **Types of immunomodulators:**

  ▪ **Immunostimulants:** That stimulates the immune system

  ▪ **Immunosuppressants:** That suppress the immune system

PHARMACOLOGY

Notes

Microbiology

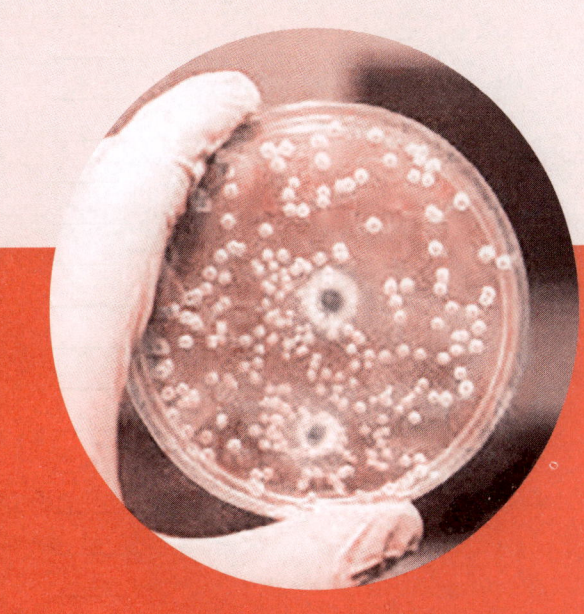

References Taken From:

- *Textbook of Microbiology, Ananthanarayan and Paniker's, 10th edition*
- *Medical Parasitology, DR Arora & Brij Bala Arora, 5th edition*

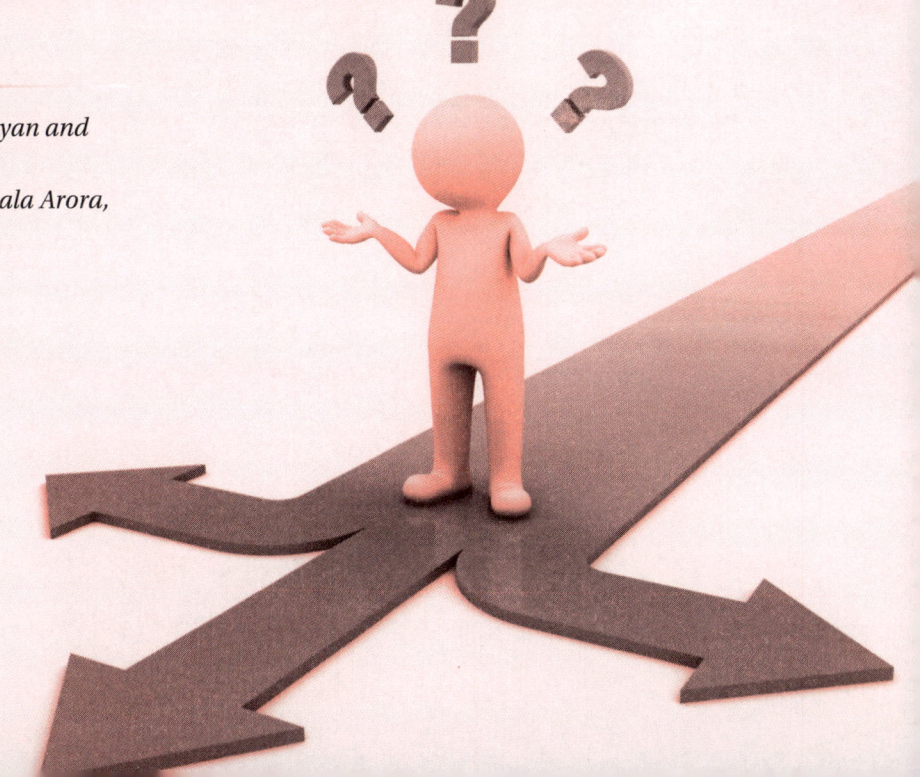

Your Roll No. ....

Name of the Paper	:	**Microbiology Paper-I**
Name of the Course	:	**MBBS-2019**
Semester	:	**Annual**

Time: 3 Hours   M.M.: 40

INSTRUCTIONS

1. Write your Roll No. on the top immediately on receipt of this question paper
2. All questions are to be attempted
3. Answers to Parts I, II and III should be written in separate answer sheets provided
4. Attempt parts of a question in sequence

PART-I

1. Define sterilization. Enumerate the methods of sterilization. Write briefly the principle of hot air oven.   [5]

2. Write short notes on: [10]
   a. IgM
   b. Transposons.

PART-II

3. Enumerate the bacteria causing sexually transmitted diseases. Describe the laboratory diagnosis of syphilis.   [5]

4. Write briefly on: [10]
   a. Scrub typhus
   b. Helicobacter pylori.

PART-III

5. Enumerate the bacterial diseases spread by water. Discuss the bacteriological examination of water.   [5]

6. Describe the laboratory diagnosis of fever of unknown origin (FUO).   [5]

PART-I

1. Define sterilization. Enumerate the methods of sterilization. Write briefly the principle of hot air oven.

(Ref: Ananthanarayan and Paniker's, Textbook of Microbiology 10th ed, pg. 28-30)

ANSWER

Sterilization

- ○ Sterilization is defined as a process that destroys or eliminates all forms of microbial life like bacteria, spores, fungi and viruses such as hepatitis virus and HIV.
- ○ Sterilization is done to preserve the substance for a long time without decay.
- ○ The efficacy of any sterilization process will depend on the nature of the product, the extent and type of any contamination, and the conditions under which the final product has been prepared.
- ○ Classical sterilization techniques using saturated steam under pressure whenever possible. Other sterilization methods include filtration, ionizing radiation (gamma and electron-beam radiation), and gas (ethylene oxide, formaldehyde).

Methods used for Sterilization

Method	Types	Use
Dry heat	Flaming	Inoculating loop/wire, tip of forceps, searing spatulas
	Hot-air oven	Glassware, all glass syringes, sharp instruments, liquid paraffin, dusting powder, fats and grease
Moist heat	**100°C:** • Boiling • Tyndallisation or intermittent sterilisation at 100°C intermittently for three consecutive days	Media containing sugars or gelatin Material used for domestic appliances, baby bottle, teats and caps
	Below 100°C: • Pasteurisation • Vaccine baths • Inspissation	Milk Lowenstein–Jensen medium, Loeffler's serum slope Vaccines and sera
	Steam at atmospheric pressure: • Steam sterilisers (Koch or Arnold steamer)	Culture media sensitive to higher temperature

	Steam under pressure:
	• Autoclave
	  ■ Gravity displacement type
	  ■ High vacuum type
		Instruments, laboratory ware, hospital linen, media and pharmaceutical products

Cold sterilization	**Radiation:**
	• **Ionising:**
	  ■ X-rays
	  ■ Gamma rays
	  ■ Cosmic rays
	• **Non-ionising:**
	  ■ Infrared
	  ■ Ultraviolet
		Swabs, plastics, syringes, catheters, oils, grease industrial use: animal feeds, fabric and metal foils
		Mass pre-packed: plastic syringes, catheters
		Laboratory cabinets, closed chambers

Filtration	Sintered glass filters Asbestos filters candle filters Membrane filters	Water purification and analysis, sterilization and sterility testing of liquids Solutions for parenteral use

Hot Air Oven

Introduction

- Hot air oven is the most widely used method of sterilization
- Uses dry heat for sterilization and it is achieved by conduction.

Principle

- Inside the chamber, the air flows in a forced circulation manner that allows appropriate heat distribution in the chamber.
- As the air becomes hot inside the chamber, it becomes lighter and moves in upward direction. As it reaches the top, the fan inside pushes it back to the bottom.
- This creates a circular motion inside the cabinet and a consistent flow of the air is maintained. Eventually, with this process, optimum temperature is reached.
- The heat is absorbed by the outside surface of the item, then passes towards the center of the item, layer by layer. The entire item will eventually reach the temperature required for sterilization to take place.
- The commonly used temperatures and time that hot air ovens need to sterilize materials is 180°C for 30 minutes, 170°C for 60 minutes, and 160°C for 120 minutes.

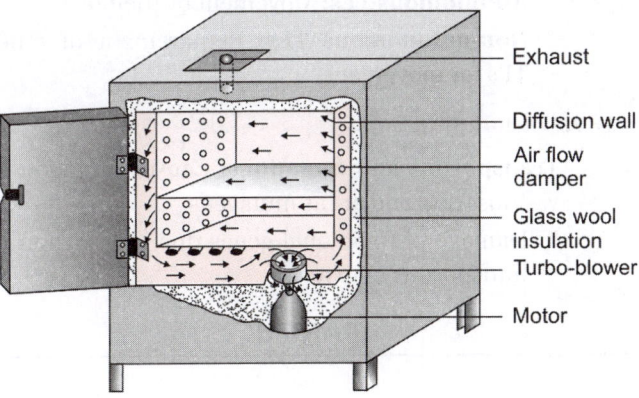

- Exhaust
- Diffusion wall
- Air flow damper
- Glass wool insulation
- Turbo-blower
- Motor

Fig. Hot air oven

Functions

- Mainly used for the sterilization of glass syringes, test tubes, pipettes, flasks, petri dishes, forceps, scissors, scalpels, sealed oils, jellies, powders (impervious to steam)
- Not used for materials destroyed by heat, like-fabrics.

2. **Write short notes on:**

   a. **IgM**

(Ref: Ananthanarayan and Paniker's, Textbook of Microbiology 10th ed, pg. 98)

ANSWER

Immunoglobulin

- Antibody or immunoglobulin is a substance produced in the body in response to an antigen and reacts with it specifically.

IgM

- IgM is the largest antibody and the first immunoglobulin that is produced on exposure.
- It is responsible for complement activation and forms ABO antibodies.
- The molecular wt. of IgM is 900,000–1,000,000 and hence, it is called a millionaire molecule.
- Serum IgM exists as a pentamer in mammals and comprises approximately 10% of normal human serum Ig content.
- It predominates in primary immune responses to most antigens and is the most efficient complement-fixing immunoglobulin.
- It also present as a component of secretory immunoglobulins at the mucosal surfaces and in breast milk.
- IgM is also expressed on the plasma membrane of B lymphocytes as a monomer. In this form, it is a B cell antigen receptor, with the H chains each containing an additional hydrophobic domain for anchoring in the membrane.
- Monomers of serum IgM are bound together by disulfide bonds and a joining (J) chain.

Role in Immune Response

- Immunoglobulin M is the third most common serum Ig and takes one of two forms:
  1. A pentamer where all heavy chains are identical and all light chains are identical
  2. A monomer (e.g., found on B lymphocytes as B cell receptors)
- The large pentameric structure allows for building of bridges between encountered epitopes on molecules that are too distant as to be connected by smaller IgG antibodies.

MICROBIOLOGY

○ It is responsible for agglutination and cytolytic reactions since in theory, its pentameric structure gives it 10 free antigen-binding sites as well as it possesses a high avidity

○ Due to conformational constraints among the 10 Fab portions, IgM only has a valence of 5. Additionally, IgM is not as versatile as IgG

○ However, it is of vital importance in complement activation and agglutination

○ IgM is predominantly found in the lymph fluid and blood and is a very effective neutralizing agent in the early stages of disease

○ Elevated levels can be a sign of recent infection or exposure to antigen.

Properties of IgM

Molecular weight	900,000
Heavy chain	M (65000)
Serum concentration (mg/mL)	1.2
Half-life (days)	5
Percent of total immunoglobulin 10%	10%
Placental transport	Absent
Glycosylation (by weight)	12%
Distribution	Mostly intravascular
Present in mother's milk	Absent
Function	Primary response

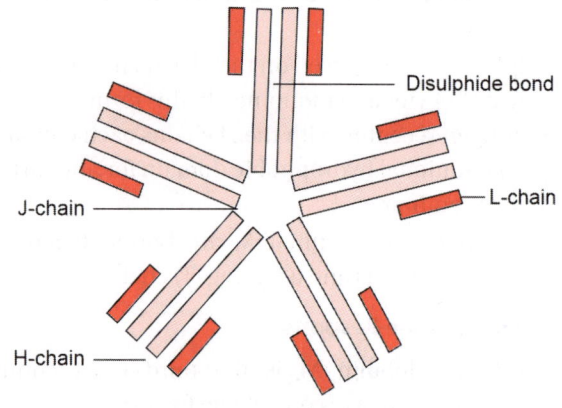

Fig. Structure of IgM

b. Transposons

(Ref: Ananthanarayan and Paniker's, Textbook of Microbiology 10th ed, pg. 63)

ANSWER

Introduction

○ Transposons are segments of DNA that can move around to different positions in the genome of a single cell.

○ First identified by geneticist Barbara McClintock

○ These mobile segments of DNA are sometimes called "jumping genes".

○ In the process, they may results in mutations and increase (or decrease) the amount of DNA in the genome of the cell, and if the cell is the precursor of a gamete, in the genomes of any descendants.

Types

There are two types:

1. **Class I transposons:**
   - Known as retrotransposons.
   - Movement by "copy and paste" mechanism in which copy is made up of RNA and in the presence of reverse transcriptase these RNA copies are transcribed back into DNA and are lodged into new locations in the genome.

2. **Class II transposons:**
   - Comprises of DNA that moves directly from place to place.
   - Movement by "copy and paste" mechanism insertion into new location in the presence of enzyme transposase-present within some of these transposons

Autonomous and Nonautonomous Transposons

○ Both class I and class II transposons can be - autonomous or non-autonomous.
   - **Autonomous TEs:** Movement by their own
   - **Non-autonomous TEs:** Requirement of other TEs for movement

Role of Jumping Gene

○ **Transposons and mutations:** Causes mutation in various ways and act as mutagens.
   - Damage of functional genes due to insertion of transposons in to it.

PART-II

3. **Enumerate the bacteria causing sexually transmitted diseases. Describe the laboratory diagnosis of syphilis.**

(Ref: Ananthanarayan and Paniker's, Textbook of Microbiology 10th ed, pg. 380)

ANSWER

Bacteria Causing Sexually Transmitted Diseases

○ Treponema pallidum (syphilis)
○ Neisseria gonorrhoeae (gonorrhea)
○ Chlamydia trachomatis (lymphogranuloma venereum)

- Gardnerella vaginalis (bacterial vaginosis)
- Haemophilus ducreyi (chancroid)
- Klebsiella granulomatis (granuloma inguinale)

Laboratory Diagnosis of Syphilis

- Serological testing is the mainstay in the laboratory diagnosis and follow-up of syphilis
- Definitive diagnosis is achieved by identifying spirochetes by microscopic dark field examination
- Direct fluorescent antibody tests of lesion exudate or tissue
- Most cases of syphilis are diagnosed serologically
- Presumptive diagnosis is possible using two types of serologic tests, i.e., non-treponemal tests and treponemal tests
- Neither type of test alone is sufficient for diagnosis
- **Serological tests fall into two categories:**
  1. Nontreponemal tests for screening
  2. Treponemal tests for confirmation.
  - **Nontreponemal tests:** They measure both immunoglobulin (IgG and IgM) antiphospholipid antibodies formed by the host in response to lipoidal material released by damaged host cells early in infection and lipid from the cell surfaces of the treponeme itself.
  - **Commonly used nontreponemal tests:**
    - **Rapid plasma reagin (RPR) test**:
      - Can be rapidly performed
      - Result is neatly evident and clear cut
      - Can be performed with plasma or unheated serum
      - Demerit: can not be used for CSF testing
    - **Venereal disease research laboratory (VDRL):**
      - It is a slide flocculation test
      - Rapid test
      - Inactivated serum drop is mixed with drop of VDRL antigen and rotation of slides for 4 minutes and in case of nonreactivity uniform distribution of fusiform crystals are seen and if reactive, medium to large antigen antibody complexes in the form of clumps are present
      - Present with quantitative result
      - Can test CSF but not plasma.
  - **Cardiolipin tests are nonspecific:** They may become false-positive in a variety of autoimmune diseases or in those involving substance tissue destruction or liver involvement, such as lupus erythematosus, viral hepatitis, infectious mononucleosis, and malaria.

- False-positive results can also occur occasionally in pregnancy and in patients with HIV infection.
- Non-treponemal tests are thus used as screening procedures for diagnosis and are confirmed by one of the treponemal tests.
- **Treponemal tests:** Treponemal tests are used as confirmatory tests to verify reactivity in non-treponemal tests.
- **Commonly used treponemal tests:**
  - **Fluorescent treponemal antibody absorption test (FTA-ABS) test:**
    - An indirect immunofluorescence test
    - Long shelf life of slides- can be stored in deep freeze for months
    - Used as a standard reference test
    - Not used in routine testing
  - **Treponema pallidum immobilisation:**
    - It was the most specific test used in the diagnosis
    - Not used commonly (rarely use) because of its complex nature
  - **Treponema pallidum hemagglutination assay (TPHA):**
    - TPHA is a good primary screening test for syphilis at all stages beyond the early primary stage.
    - TPHA test is a passive hemagglutination assay based on hemagglutination of erythrocytes sensitized with *T. pallidum* antigen by antibodies found in the patient's serum or plasma.
    - It is used for both qualitative and semi-quantative detection of anti-treponemal antibodies.
    - Simple and economical test
    - No requirement of special equipment.
- Diagnosis of primary syphilis can be made based on the presence of chancre and a proceeding history of sexual contact within the last 3 months
- During the period; dark field microscopy of PCR or DFA-TP can be used to confirm the diagnosis
- Humoral antibody response can be detected by treponemal or non treponema tests 1–4 weeks after the chancre has formed
- Sensitivites of various tests during this stage: VDRL/RPR–70–90%, TPPA–94%
- Most sensitive test in monitoring treatment is VDRL
- For mass screening VDRL is used
- For primary syphilis most sensitive test is western blot and enzyme immunoassay
- For latent syphilis all treponemal test are sensitive.

Table: Laboratory diagnosis of syphilis

Microscopy:
- Direct fluorescent antibody staining for T. pallidum (DFA-TP-Sensitivity is 100%)
- Silver impregnation method: (i) Levaditi stain (for tissue section), (ii) Fontana stain (smear)
- Dark ground microscopy:
  - Bacteria appear as slender, spirally coiled bacill, flexible and tapering ends
    Three types of motility seen- corkscrew motility, flexion extension type and rotational type

Culture:
- In artificial culture media, pathogenic treponemes cannot be grown
- Smith noguchi media is used for nonpathogenic treponemes (e.g Reiter treponemes)

Serology (antibody detection)

A. Nontreponemal or nonspecific tests or (standard tests for syphilis):

i.	Venereal disease research laboratory (VDRL) test	Complement fixation test (CFT)
ii.	Rapid plasma regain (RPR)	Slide flocculation
iii.	Wassermann test	Complement fixation test (CFT)
iv.	Kahn Test	Tube flocculation
v.	Unheated serum regain test (USR)	Slide flocculation
vi.	Toluidine red unheated serum test (TRUST)	Slide flocculation

B. Treponemal/Specific tests:

i.	FTA-ABS (Fluorescent treponemal antibody absorption test)
ii.	TPA (T. pallidum agglutination test)
iii.	TPIA (T. pallidum immune adherence test)
iv.	TPI (Treponema pallidum immobilization test)
v.	TPHA (T. pallidum hemagglutination test)
Vi.	TPPA (T. pallidum particle agglutination test)
Vii.	Enzyme immunoassay (EIA)
viii.	Western blot

C. Group specific: RP CFT (Reiter protein complement fixation test)

Polymerase chain reaction (PCR)

4. Write briefly on:

a. Scrub typhus
(Ref: Ananthanarayan and Paniker's, Textbook of Microbiology 10th ed, pg. 415)

ANSWER

Scrub Typhus
- Scrub typhus is an acute febrile illness caused by orientia tsutsugamushi, transmitted to humans by the bite of the larva of trombiculid mites.
- It causes a disseminated vasculitis and perivascular inflammatory lesions resulting in significant vascular leakage and end-organ injury.
- It affects people of all ages and even though scrub typhus in pregnancy is uncommon, it is associated with increased fetal loss, preterm delivery, and small for gestational age infants.
- After an incubation period of 6–21 days, onset is characterized by fever, headache, myalgia, cough, and gastrointestinal symptoms.
- A primary popular lesion which later crusts to form a flat black eschar, may be present. If untreated, serious complications may occur involving various organs.
- Laboratory studies usually reveal leukopenia, thrombocytopenia, deranged hepatic and renal function, proteinuria and reticulonodular infiltrate.
- Owing to the potential for severe complications, diagnosis, and decision to initiate treatment should be based on clinical suspicion and confirmed by serologic tests

Infections Caused by Rickettsiae and Close Relatives

Group disease	Bacterium	Arthropod vector	Reservoir host
Rocky mountain spotted fever	R. rickettsii	Ticks	Ticks, dogs, rodents
Epidemic typhus	R. prowazekii	Human louse	Humans
Endemic typhus	R. typhi	Fleas	Rodents

Contd...

Group disease	Bacterium	Arthropod vector	Reservoir host
Scrub typhus	*Orientia tsutsugamushi*	Mites	Rodents
Ehrlichiosis	*E. chaffeensis A. phagocytophilum*	Tick	Small mammals

b. Helicobacter pylori

(Ref: Ananthanarayan and Paniker's, Textbook of Microbiology, 10th ed, pg. 407)

ANSWER

Introduction

- Helicobacter pylori (H. pylori) is a Gram-negative, curved or spiral shaped bacteria
- It is the major cause of peptic ulcer disease and gastritis.

Epidemiology

Approximately two-thirds of the world's population is infected with H. pylori.

Pathogenesis

- Colonization of H. pylori in the stomach
- Certain strains bind to mucosal epithelium by expression of adherence associated lipoprotein
- Virulence genes: cagA, vacA genes causes induction of pathological changes, like formation of vacuoles in the cytoplasm
- Certain environmental factors like-smoking increases the risk of ulcers and cancer and high salt diet and preserved food also increases the chances of cancer risk
- Molecular factor: H. pylori LPS cross reacts with Lewis blood group antigen leading to chronic active gastritis

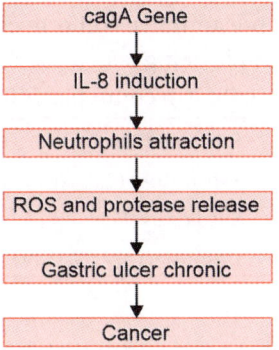

Clinical Manifestation

- Peptic ulcer disease: Gastric ulcers approx. 60% and duodenal ulcers approx. 80% are associated with H. pylori infection
- Chronic atrophic gastritis
- Acute gastritis: Most commonly antrum is involved, no involvement of cardiac end.
- Pernicious anemia initiation
- Pan gastritis, antral gastritis, autoimmune gastritis
- Adenocarcinoma of stomach

Diagnosis

- Various tests are available to diagnose H. pylori infection.
- These tests can be categorized into those that are based on direct assessment of gastric biopsies (endoscopic testing) and indirect tests (nonendoscopic testing) that detect an immunological response (i.e. antibodies against *H. pylori*) or metabolic products (i.e. urease activity) of *H. pylori*
- **Invasive test:**
  - **Urease test:** Urease indicator medium is used for treating biopsy and revels positive result
- **Microscopic examination using silver stain:** Revels spiral bacilli
- **Culture:** Enriched medium is used, growth at 37°C in microaerophilic conditions. Oxidase and catalase positive
- **Non-invasive test:**
  - **ELISA**
  - **Urease breath test:** Carbon labeled urea solution is used and can be detected in the breath. Reliable and sensitive method.
  - **Stool antigen (Coproantigen) assay**

Treatment

- Bismuth subsalicylate, tetracycline and metronidazole combination for 2 weeks
- Omeprazole and clarithromycin–alternative treatment.

PART-III

---

5. **Enumerate the bacterial diseases spread by water. Discuss the bacteriological examination of water.**

(Ref: Ananthanarayan and Paniker's, Textbook of Microbiology, 10th ed, pg. 630)

Answer

Bacterial Diseases Spread Through Water

Bacterial diseases (community acquired)
• Cholera
• Enteric fever
• Bacillary dysentery
• Leptospiremia, leptospiruria

Bacterial diseases (hospital acquired)
• Pneumonia
• Otitis and nasal septum cellulitis
• Bacteremia, folliculitis and skin infections
• Diarrhea

Bacteriological Examination of Water

○ Presumptive coliform count(Multiple tube method)
○ Eijkman test (Differential coliform count)
○ Plate count
○ Membrane filtration method
○ Clostridium perfringens detection
○ Fecal streptococci detection.

Multiple Tube Method (Presumptive Coliform Count)

Introduction

○ Multiple tube technique is used for presumptive coliform count
○ Method is used for bacteriological examination of water.

Principle

○ Test is presumptive because presence of other bacteria other than coliform bacteria may sometimes be responsible for the reaction so the presence of coliform bacteria need to be confirmed
○ Bile salt lactose peptone water (with an acidity indicator) is used and added with different quantity of water (0.1–50 mL) and incubated at required temperature
○ **Alternate medium:** MacConkey's broth
○ Formation of acid and gas provide indication of the presence of coliform bacteria.

Method

○ **Usually, following range of quantity is prepared:**
   ▪ Five 10 mL quantity each to 10 mL double strength medium
   ▪ One 50 mL of water added to 50 mL double strength medium
   ▪ Five 1 mL quantity each to 5 mL single strength medium
   ▪ Five 0.1 mL quantity each to 5 mL single strength.

○ Modified MacConkey's fluid medium is used
○ Range of quantity also depends on the intensity of contamination
○ In case of high level of contamination- small quantity is tested
○ Incubation of bottles at 37°C and examination after 18–24 hours
○ Record the reading of presumptive positive and re-incubation of negative bottles again for 24 hours.

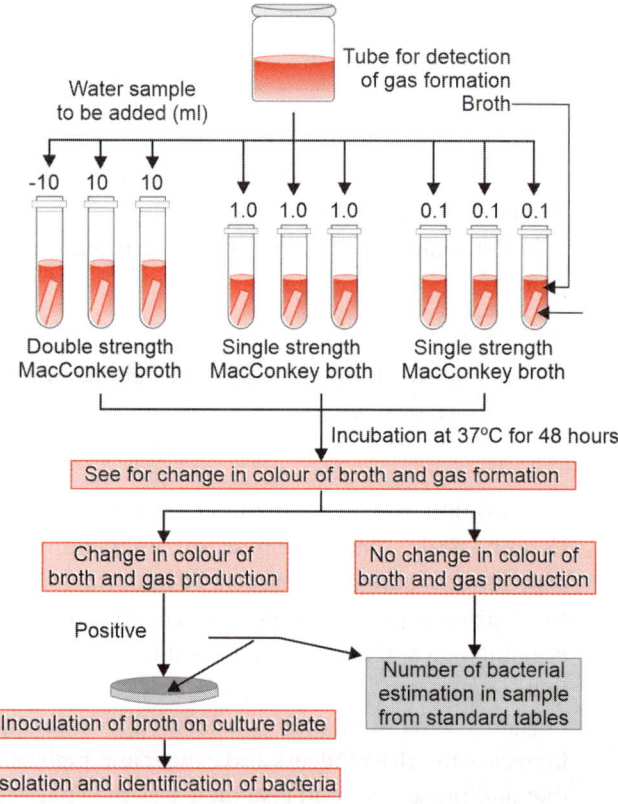

Fig. Method for bacteriological analysis of water

Interpretation

○ Probability table of McCrady is used for interpreting the probable number of coliforms count/100 mL. It is called as "presumptive coliform count" present in the water sample being tested.
○ Presumptive coliform count per 100 mL

0	Excellent (Class I)
1–3	Satisfactory (Class II)
4–10	Suspicious (Class III)
More than 10	Unsatisfactory (Class IV)

Eijkman Test

○ This test is done to confirm that the coliform bacilli detected in the presumptive test are E.coli

Detection of Fecal Streptococci

○ Detection of fecal streptococci (Enterococcus species) in water sample suggests recent fecal contamination of water but for short duration

Detection of Clostridium Perfringens

○ Presence of clostridium perfringens in water sample demonstrate fecal contamination that is not recent but present for a long duration.

6. Describe the laboratory diagnosis of fever of unknown origin (FUO).

(Ref: Ananthanarayan and Paniker's, Textbook of Microbiology, 10th ed. pg. 689-691)

ANSWER

Introduction

Temperature above 38°C for more than three weeks and without any diagnosis even after one week of investigations is known as pyrexia of unknown origin (PUO).

Various Causes of Pyrexia of Unknown Origin (PUO)

Infectious Causes

Bacterial	Fungal	Parasitic	Viral
• M. tuberculosis • Leptospira spp • Rickettsia spp • Brucella spp • Chlamydia psittaci • Salmonella spp • Atypical mycobacteria • Coxiella burnetii • Mycoplasma spp	• Candida albicans • Cryptococcus neoformans • Histoplasma capsulatum • Aspergillus spp • Coccidioides immitis	• Plasmodium spp • Leishmania spp • Trypanosoma spp • Toxoplasma gondii • Wuchereria bancrofti • Brugia malayi	• Cytomegalovirus • Epstein – Barr virus • Arboviruses • Enteroviruses • HIV

Noninfectious Causes

Connective tissue disorder	Neoplasms	Granulomatous diseases
• Systemic lupus erythematosus (SLE) • Polyarteritis nodosa	• Lymphoma • Leukemia • Myeloma • Gout • Porphyria • Renal cancer • Colon cancer • Liver cancer • Metabolic disorders	• Rheumatoid arthritis • Crohn's disease • Polymyositis • Sarcoidosis

Laboratory Diagnosis

To assess and confirm the cause of fever of unknown origin

○ **Complete blood count and erythrocyte sedimentation rate:**
  ▪ Marked increase in neutrophil count (neutrophilic leukocytosis) suggestive of pyogenic infection
  ▪ Raised ESR suggestive of tubercular infection

○ **Blood film examination:**
  ▪ Demonstration of microfilariae or trypanosome
  ▪ Gram stained film demonstrate gram negative bacilli-brucella species

  ▪ Ziehl-Neelsen stain for demonstration of mycobacterium species
  ▪ Giemsa stain for fungus demonstration

○ **Blood culture:** Performed for enteric Salmonella or for organisms responsible for infective endocarditis

○ **Urine culture:** Demonstration of pyogenic bacteria or tubercle bacilli

○ Bone marrow culture for fungus demonstration

○ **Serological test:**
  ▪ **ELISA:** To diagnose viral diseases—HIV, CMV or Epstein Barr virus
  ▪ **Complement fixation test (CFT):** For bacterial diseases like- tularaemia (Francisella tularensis), lymphogranuloma venereum (C. trachomatis serotypes L1-L3)
  ▪ Weil—Felix for rickettsia
  ▪ Widal test for typhoid
  ▪ ASO titre for rheumatic fever
  ▪ RA factor for rheumatoid arthritis
  ▪ Paul Bunnell test—infectious mononucleosis

○ **Skin test:**
  ▪ **Delayed hypersensitivity reaction:** For demonstration of tuberculosis (Mantoux skin test) or fungal infection like-histoplasmosis (histoplasmin skin test)

MICROBIOLOGY

- Anti nuclear antibody or anti-DNA antibody – suggesting SLE
- Thyroglobulin antibody- for subacute thyroiditis

○ **Biopsy:** For detection of leukemia, Hodgkin's disease-bone marrow biopsy is performed. Endoscopy for gastrointestinal structures, etc.

○ **Imaging studies:**

- X-ray chest for demonstration of pulmonary tuberculosis
- ECHO for demonstration of infective endocarditis or rheumatic fever
- Upper and lower gastrointestinal tract barium study
- CT and MRI
- Intravenous urogram, lung, bone scan—for detection of neoplastic processes or collagen vascular disease.

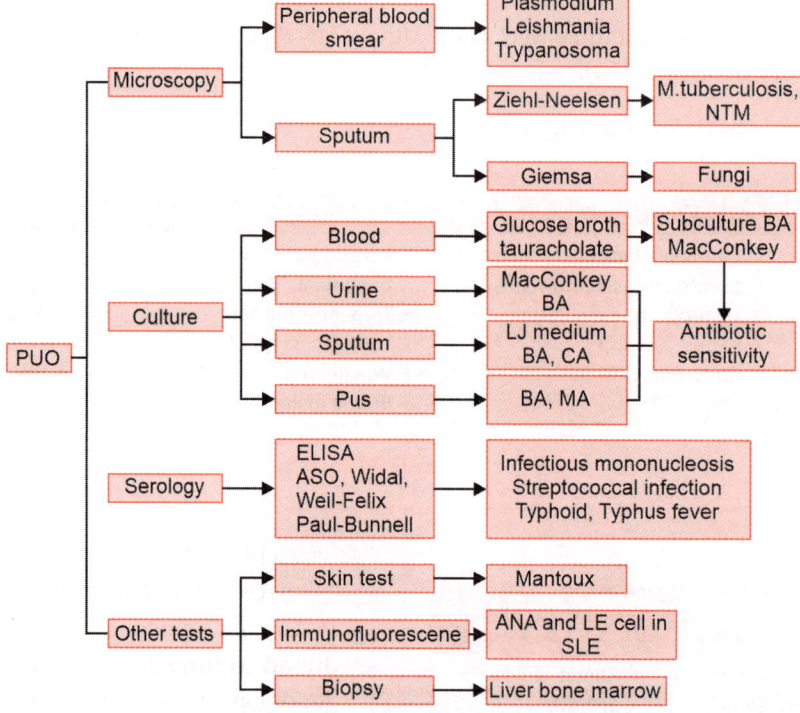

Fig. Diagnosis of pyrexia of unknown origin

Your Roll No. ....

Name of the Paper : **Microbiology Paper-II**

Name of the Course : **MBBS-2019**

Semester : **Annual**

Time: 3 Hours   M.M.: 40

INSTRUCTIONS

1. Write your Roll No. on the top immediately on receipt of this question paper
2. All questions are to be attempted
3. Answers to Parts I, II and III should be written in separate answer sheets provided
4. Attempt parts of a question in sequence

PART-I

1. **Name the species of filarial worms that infect humans. Describe briefly the life cycle and laboratory diagnosis of**
    W. bancrofti.   [5]

2. **Write short notes on:**   [10]
    a. Life cycle of T. solium
    b. Visceral larva migrans.

PART-II

3. **Enumerate the opportunistic fungal infections. Describe briefly the laboratory diagnosis of any one of them.** [5]

4. **Write briefly on:**   [10]
    a. Rabies vaccine
    b. Japanese encephalitis.

PART-III

5. **Describe briefly the laboratory diagnosis of amoebic liver abscess.**   [5]

6. **Write briefly on postexposure prophylaxis in HIV infection.**   [5]

PART-I

1. **Name the species of filarial worms that infect humans. Describe briefly the life cycle and laboratory diagnosis of *W. bancrofti*.**

(Ref: Arora Parasitology, 5th ed. pg. 199)

ANSWER

Species of Filarial Worms that Infect Humans

Parasite	Location in the body		Vector
	Adults	**Microfilaria**	
Subcutaneous Filariasis			
Loa loa	Subcutaneous connective tissue, subconjunctival tissue	Blood	*Chrysops*
Onchocerca volvulus	Subcutaneous connective tissue	Skin	*Simulium*
Mansonella streptocerca	Dermis	Skin	*Culicoides*
Lymphatic Filariasis			
Wuchereria bancrofti	Lymphatics	Blood	*Culex, Anopheles, Aedes*
Brugia malayi	Lymphatics	Blood	*Mansonia, Anopheles, Aedes*
Brugia timori	Lymphatics	Blood	*Anopheles*
Serous Cavity Filariasis			
Mansonella ozzardi	Body cavities	Blood	*Culicoides*
Mansonella perstans	Body cavities	Blood	*Culicoides*

Wuchereria Bancrofti

Wuchereria bancrofti, a tissue nematode is commonly associated with lymphatic filariasis

Life Cycle of Wuchereria Bancrofti

○ During a blood meal, an infected mosquito introduces third-stage filarial larvae onto the skin of the human host, where they penetrate into the bite wound.

○ They develop in adults that commonly reside in the lymphatics.

○ The female worms measure 80 to 100 mm in length and 0.24 to 0.30 mm in diameter, while the males measure about 40 mm by 0.1 mm.

○ Adults produce microfilariae measuring 244 to 296 μm by 7.5 to 10 μm, which are sheathed and have nocturnal periodicity, except the South Pacific microfilariae which have the absence of marked periodicity.

○ The microfilariae migrate into lymph and blood channels moving actively through lymph and blood.

○ A mosquito ingests the microfilariae during a blood meal.

○ After ingestion, the microfilariae lose their sheaths and some of them work their way through the wall of the proventriculus and cardiac portion of the mosquitoes midgut and reach the thoracic muscles.

○ There the microfilariae develop into first-stage larvae and subsequently into third-stage infective larvae.

○ The third-stage infective larvae migrate through the hemocoel to the mosquitoes proboscis and can infect another human when the mosquito takes a blood meal.

Lab Diagnosis

○ **Thick blood smear:**

▪ The standard method for diagnosing active infection is the identification of microfilariae in a blood smear (multiple thin and thick blood smear) by microscopic examination.

▪ Blood collection should be done at night to coincide with the appearance of the microfilariae, and a thick smear should be made and stained with Giemsa or hematoxylin and eosin.

▪ Giemsa stain does not stain the microfilarial sheath adequately. Sheathed microfilariae often lose their sheath when drying on thick films. At least 2 thick smears and 2 thin smears must be prepared.

- For increased sensitivity, concentration techniques can be used.

○ **Thin blood smear:** Examination of a thin blood film for microfilariae should include low-power review of the entire film, not just the feathered edge.

○ **Membrane filtration method:**

- It is the concentration technique used to trap microfilariae on the polycarbonate filter after red blood cells are lysed.
- 1–2 mL intravenous blood filtered through 3μm pore size membrane filter and the filter paper may be examined directly on a microscope slide (filters are transparent when wet).

○ **DEC (Diethylcarbamazine) provocative test (2 mg/Kg):**

- It is somewhat impractical to obtain sample blood from a patient at late night.
- DEC provocation test is done to bring microfilariae in the periphery during day time.
- After consuming DEC, microfilariae enter into the peripheral blood in day time within 30–45 minutes.

○ **Wet mount:** Microfilariae are seen in microscopic mounts by their undulating motion displacing the RBCs side to side as they move.

○ Acridine orange microhematocrit tube technique is used for detection of microfilariae. After centrifugation, the parasites get concentrated in buffy coat and can be visualized through clear glass wall of tube. Acridine orange stains the DNA and morphological characters and nuclear patterns in tail sections. When examined under fluorescence microscope, species identification can be done.

○ **Knott concentration method:** After mixing 2 mL of blood with 10 mL of 2% solution in formalin, the mixture is allowed to stand for 10 minutes and then centrifuged at 200 g for 2 minutes. The sediment is examined for microfilariae

○ Adult worms can be seen in biopsied lymph node

○ Filarial antigen is detected in serum by enzyme immunoassays by using monoclonal antibodies.

○ Filarial antibodies can be detected by ELISA, IFA, IHA and RIA

○ PCR is available for *W. bancrofti* and *Brugia malayi*.

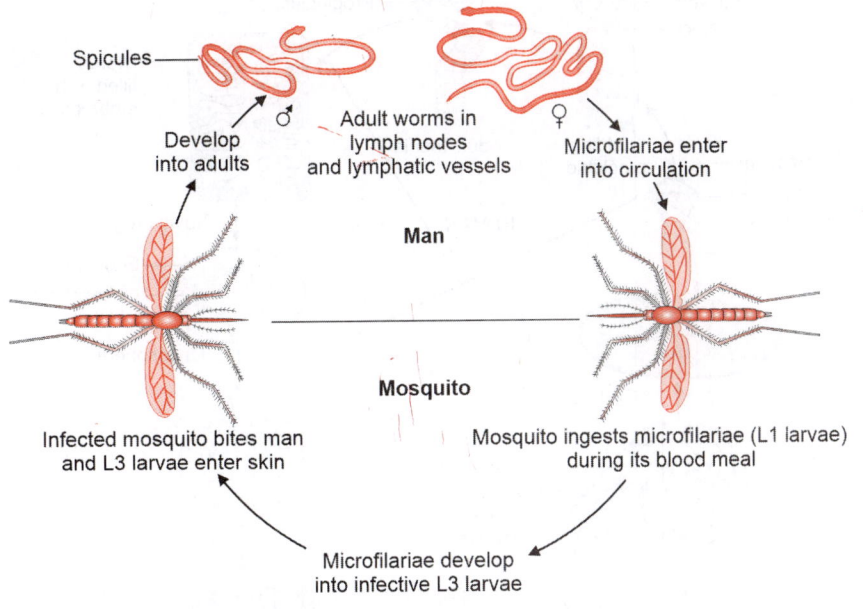

Fig. Life cycle of Wuchereria bancrofti

2. **Write short notes on :**

a. **Life Cycle of T. solium**

   (Ref: Arora Parasitology, 5th ed, pg. 131)

ANSWER

Life Cycle

The life-cycle of *Taenia solium* is complicated and digenetic, being completed in two hosts. The primary host is man and the secondary host is pig.

Fertilization

Self-fertilization takes place in Taenia. The eggs are fertilized in the oviduct and get surrounded with yolk and egg- shell in the ootype. The capsulated egg enters the uterus and is collected there. The uterus enlarges in size, gets branched and occupies the whole space. The eggs are very small in size measuring about 40 microns in diameter.

Cleavage

The division in the eggs start, while these are- still inside the uterus. The first cleavage is unequal so that a large vitelline cell and a small embryonic cell is formed. The embryonic cell undergone repeated divisions and a solid ball of cells, the morula is formed. The divisions are unequal so the morula consists of a few larger cells, the macromeres forming an outer or peripheral layer and inner mass of small cells or micromeres.

Hexacanth Larva

The micromeres develop into a hexacanth or oncosphere larva.

Infection to Secondary Host

The development of egg up to the formation of oncosphere takes place inside the uterus of gravid proglottid. The further development is not possible inside the host body. The gravid proglottids detach from the body of the parasite and come out along with the host feces. These infect the secondary host when pig feeds upon the contaminated feces.

Cysticercus or Hydatid Larva or Bladder Worm Stage

The numerous hexacanths are set free in the stomach, where the embryonic membranes of on chospheres is dissolved. These bore through the intestinal wall the help of hooks and enter the blood stream or lymph vessels. Travelling through the heart, these enter the muscles of various parts in the body. The usual site where the hexacanths gey encysted is the voluntary muscles of tongue, heart, liver and shoulder.

Infection of Final Host

Further development of the bladder worm takes place only inside the definitive host. Infection of man occurs when inadequately cooked pork infected with bladder worms is eaten. The cysticerci become active in the intestine. The scolex takes a firm hold of intestinal wall of the host. The bladder is thrown off and the neck starts budding off segments an adult tapeworm is formed.

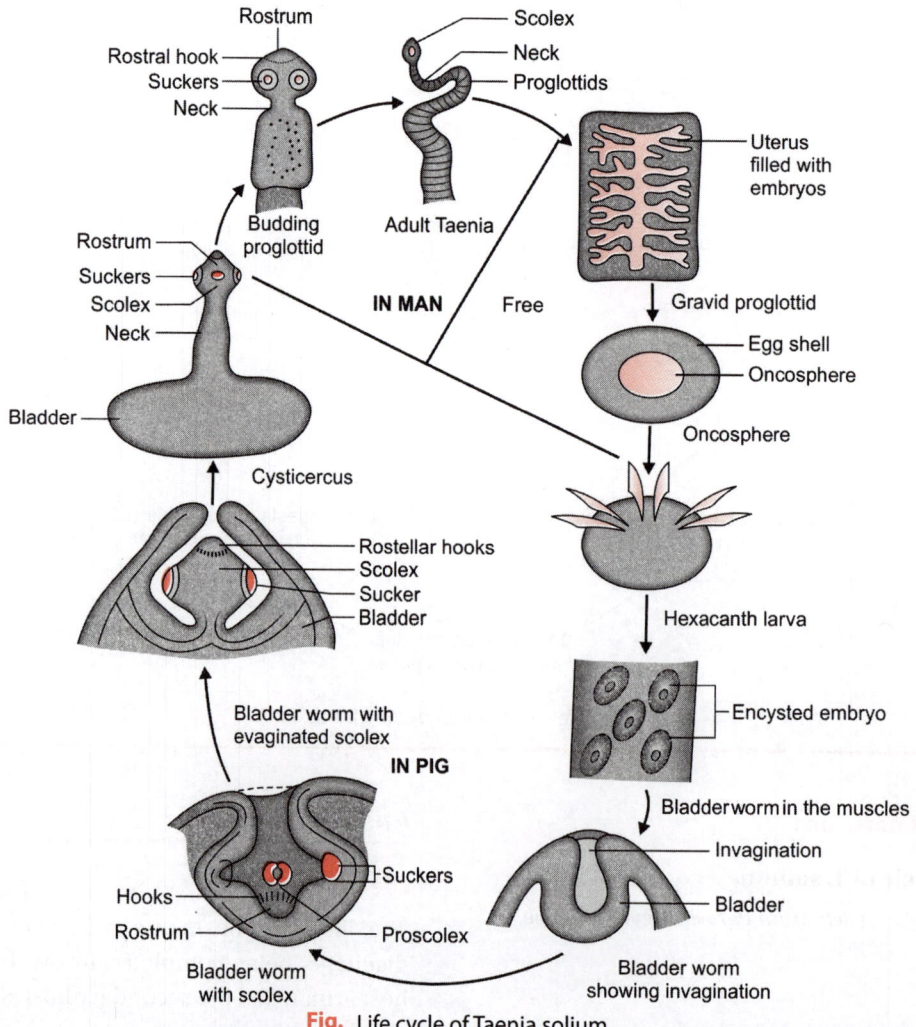

Fig. Life cycle of Taenia solium

b. **Visceral larva migrans**

(Ref: Arora Parasitology 5th ed. pg. 215)

ANSWER

Visceral Larva Migrans

○ Also known as systemic toxocariasis
○ It is a condition in humans caused by the migratory larvae of certain nematodes, humans being a dead end host.
○ Nematodes causing such zoonotic infections Toxocara canis, Toxocara cati, and Ascaris suum.
○ These nematodes can infect but not mature in humans and after migrating through the intestinal wall, travel with the blood stream to various organs where they cause inflammation and damage.
○ Affected organs can include the liver, heart (causing myocarditis) and the CNS (causing dysfunction, seizures, and coma).
○ A special variant is ocular larva migrans where usually T. canis larvae travel to the eye.
○ Other roundworms that are implicated in visceral larva migrans:
  ▪ Angiostrongylus cantonensis
  ▪ Gnathostoma spinigerum
  ▪ Anisakis simplex
  ▪ Baylisascaris procyonis
○ The larvae are attacked by phagocytic cells wherever they settle in the body
○ The primary phagocytic cells involved are eosinophils, histiocytes and giant cells that lead to the formation of granulomatous lesion and arrest the progress.

Predisposing Factors

○ Breeding of animals inside the house
○ Household pet that has not been treated for worms
○ Consumption of raw/unboiled milk
○ Ingestion of raw or undercooked meat infected with toxocara larva- the liver and other tissues act as host to the parasite.

Clinical Manifestation

The severity of symptoms may vary among the affected individuals. Some commonly reported signs and symptoms are:

○ Fever and headaches
○ Abdominal pain or discomfort
○ Coughing
○ Weakness or tiredness
○ Muscle pain
○ Hypereosinophilia, hepatomegaly, pneumonitis

○ Vision abnormalities
○ Confusion and memory-related problems

Diagnosis

○ Complete medical history and thorough physical examination
○ Blood test—to measure the level of eosinophils
○ Identification of larvae in autopsy or biopsy specimens and by IHA and IFA test

Complications

Depend on the location of the infecting roundworms in the body. It may include:

○ Damage to the infected organ resulting in organ failure
○ Convulsions (epilepsy)
○ Bowel dysfunction
○ Pneumonia(Infection of the lungs)

Treatment

○ Albendazole-Anti-parasitic drugs
○ If symptoms are severe/persistent- Surgical removal of the infection.

PART-II

3. **Enumerate the opportunistic fungal infections. Describe briefly the laboratory diagnosis of any one of them.**

(Ref: Ananthanarayan and Paniker's, 10th ed, pg. 615)

ANSWER

Opportunistic Fungal Infections

○ **Candidiasis:** Caused by *candida albicans*
○ **Aspergillosis:** Caused by species of *Aspergillus*
○ **Cryptococcosis:** Caused by *Cryptococcus*
○ **Zygomycosis/Mucormycosis:** Caused by *Mucor, Rhizopus, Absidia, Rhizomucor*
○ **Pencilliosis:** Caused by *Penicillium*

Laboratory Diagnosis of Candidiasis

○ **By microscopy and culture:**
  ▪ Candida can be detected in unstained wet preparations or Gram stained preparations of sample.
  ▪ In Gram stained smears, Candida appears as Gram-positive budding yeast cells (blastoconidia) and/ or pseudohyphae showing regular points of constriction.

- Demonstration of mycelial forms indicate colonization and tissue invasion.
  - ○ **Culture on SDA (Sabouraud dextrose agar):**
    - *Candida albicans* grows well on Sabouraud dextrose agar and most routinely used bacteriological media.
    - Cream colored pasty colonies usually appear after 24–48 hours of incubation at 25–37°C.
    - The colonies have a distinctive yeast smell and the budding cells can be easily seen by direct microscopy in stained or unstained preparations.
  - ○ In Blood agar, *Candida albicans* gives white, creamy colored colonies which can be mistaken for Staphylococcus spp.
  - ○ **Test for species identification:**
    - **Dalmau plate culture technique:** *C. albicans* forms chlamydospores on corn meal agar cultures at 20°C, which is highly characteristic of this strain.
    - **Reynolds-Braude phenomenon(Germ tube test):**
      - ♦ When incubated in human serum at 37°C, *C. albicans* produces germ tubes within 2 hours.
      - ♦ Specific for *Candida albicans*
      - ♦ No constriction at the origin differentiates it from pseudohyphae

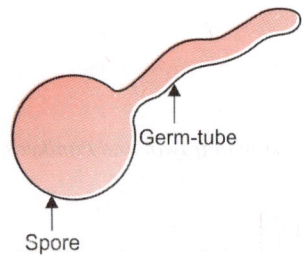

Fig. Germ tube test of *Candida albicans*

- **CHROM agar:** different species produces different colors that helps in the identification of different species
- **Growth at 45°C:** *C. albicans* grows well at 45°C and differentiated from *C. dubliniensis*
  - ○ *C. albicans* can be differentiated from other species also by sugar assimilation and fermentation tests.
  - ○ **Immunodiagnosis:**
    - **Antigen detection:** ELISA is performed for cytoplasmic and cell wall mannan antigen detection
    - **Antibody detection:** against cell wall antigen(mannan)
    - **Enzyme detection:** enolase, aspartate proteinase, etc. specific for Candida
    - **G test:** detection of α 1-3 glucan

- **Metabolites detection:** Detection of mannitol, arabinitol that is specific for *Candida*

---

4. **Write short notes on:**

a. **Rabies Vaccine**

(Ref: Ananthanarayan and Paniker, Textbook of Microbiology,10th ed, pg. 538-539)

ANSWER

Prophylaxis of Rabies

- ○ It is prevented by vaccination with a killed vaccine (HDCV, commercially called Imovax-Rabies) or treated with rabies immunoglobulin (RIG, commercially called Imogam-Rabies).
- ○ In India, tissue culture vaccine are used:
  - Human Diploid cell vaccine (HDC)
  - Purified chick embryo cell vaccine (PCEC)
  - Purified Vero Cell Vaccine
- ○ Vaccination schedule :
  - Pre-exposure Prophylaxis: 0, 7, 21 or 0, 28, 56; Booster after 1 year and then after 5 years
  - Post-exposure prophylaxis: 0, 3, 7, 14, 30 and optionally 90.

Pre-exposure Rabies Prophylaxis Regimen

- ○ **Intramuscular:**
  - One intramuscular dose is given on each of days 0, 7 and 21 or 28
  - **Site of injection:** Deltoid area of the arm for adults; anterolateral area of the thigh is recommended for children aged less than 2 years
- ○ **Intradermal:**
  - One intradermal injection of 0.1 mL is given on each of days 0, 7, and 21 or 28
- ○ Administration of booster dose if antibody titre is less than 0.5 IU/mL

Post Exposure Prophylaxis
Wound Treatment

- ○ Should be immediate
- ○ Is essential even if the person presents long after exposure
- ○ **Consists of:**
  - Immediate washing and flushing wound for 15 minutes with soap and water, or water alone
  - Disinfection with detergent, ethanol (700 mL/L), iodine (tincture or aqueous solution), or other substances with virucidal activity
  - Bleeding at any wound site indicates potentially severe exposure and must be infiltrated with either human or equine rabies immunoglobulin.

○ **IM regimen or Essen regimen:** Five doses (0.5 or 1 ml per dose) each on 0, 3,7,14 and 28 days and booster dose at 90 days. Day 0 is the date of first dose of vaccine.

○ **ID regimen:** 0.1 ml of vaccine given on days 0, 3, 7 and 28 on two sites per visit.

○ **Site of injection:** Deltoid region

○ **Other treatment include:**

■ Administration of antibiotics and tetanus prophylaxis

■ Administration of rabies immunoglobulin (RIG) to wounds classified as category III exposure, is of utmost importance in wound management.

■ Bites to the head, neck, face, hand and genitals are category III exposures

■ Infiltrate RIG into the depth of the wound and around the wound

■ RIG should be infiltrated around the wound as much as anatomically feasible

■ Remaining RIG should be injected at an intramuscular site distant from that of vaccine inoculation (e.g. into the anterior thigh)

Postexposure prophylaxis to previously vaccinated people:

○ Unknown titer or severe bite: 3 doses of vaccine at 0, 3, 7 days

○ Titer > 0.5 IU/ml – 2 doses, 0, 3 days

   b.   **Japanese encephalitis**

(Ref: Ananthanarayan and Paniker, Textbook of Microbiology,10th ed, pg. 527)

Answer

Introduction

○ It is single-stranded, RNA virus

○ It is the common and important cause of viral encephalitis in Asia

○ To differentiate it from encephalitis A in Japan, named as Japanese 'B' encephalitis

Pathogenesis

○ Vector in India—Culex vishnui

○ Tamil Nadu and Andhra Pradesh- endemic areas in India

Major vertebrate hosts: Domestic pigs (amplifying hosts); ardeid wading birds such as the black-crowned night heron (Nycticorax nycticorax), plumed egret (Egretta intermedia), domestic fowls; migratory birds, etc.

Reservoir host: Herons

Amplifier host:

○ Pigs

○ Human infection acts as dead end

Transmission Cycle

○ Numerous animals and birds are infected

○ Transmission cycles:

■ Pigs Culex pigs

■ Ardeid birds Culex Ardeid birds

Clinical Features

○ **Incubation period:** from 5-15 days

○ Exhibit subclinical infection- iceberg phenomena

○ Divided in to three stages:

■ Prodromal stage

■ Acute encephalitis stage

■ Late stage with neurological deficits and its sequelae.

○ Sudden onset of fever, headache and vomiting

○ After 1–6 days, convulsions, nuchal rigidity, altered sensorium and comma takes place

○ Fever: Continuous and high

○ Neurologic or psychiatric sequelae—50% survivors

○ Infection in pregnant female (I and IInd trimester)- may result in fetal death

Laboratory Diagnosis

○ Increased leucocyte count

○ Normal or raised sugar level with pleocytosis

○ Protein level in CSF is slightly raised

Vaccine

○ Live attenuated vaccine developed in China—JE Strain SA 14-14-2

○ Formalin inactivated mouse brain vaccine- Nakayama strain is used

○ **Licensed vaccine in India (for children of endemic areas):**

■ Inactivated Vero cell culture derived Kolar strain

■ Inactivated Vero cell culture derived SA-14- 14-2

PART-III

5. **Describe briefly the laboratory diagnosis of amoebic liver abscess.**

(Ref: Medical Parasitology, DR Arora and Brij Bala Arora, 5th ed, pg. 26)

Answer

Amoebic Liver Abscess

○ Amoebic liver abscess is an uncommon but potentially life-threatening complication of infection with the protozoan parasite Entamoeba histolytica

- Predominate in the age group of 20–60 years
- It has marked preference for right lobe of the liver. A section through the margins of liver abscess can be differentiated into 3 zones:
  - Necrotic center with thick pus and no amoebae
  - Intermediate zone of degenerated liver cells, a few red cells and occasionally trophozoites of *E. histolytica*
  - Outer zone of nearly normal hepatic tissues just being invaded by amoebae
- The center consists of viscous red brown (anchovy sauce appearance) or grey yellow fluid consisting of cytolysed liver cells, RBCs and WBCs

Laboratory Diagnosis of Amoebic Liver Abscess

- **Microscopic examination of stool:**
  - Intermittent shedding of amoebae so minimum three samples of stool are examined and demonstration of:
    - Trophozoites: Active infection
    - Quadrinucleated cysts: Represent carrier state
- **Stool culture:**
  - **Axenic culture:** Bacterial supplement , such as Diamond's medium is absent
  - **Polyxenic culture:**
    - Used in asymptomatic and chronic carriers with less number of cysts
    - Bacterial supplement present
    - Specificity—100% and sensitivity 50–70%
    - Culture media used:
      - Balamuth's medium, Nelson's medium
      - National Institute of Health media
      - Boeck and Drbohlav egg serum medium
- **Stool antigen detection(Copro-antigen):** ELISA or ICT for detection of lectin antigen. Usual presentation in stool is not seen but can be detected in serum, liver pus and saliva
- Detection of amoebic antigen in serum indicative of recent and active infection
- Detection of amoebic antibody in serum by ELISA, IHA, IFA but can not differentiate between recent and old infection because antibodies persistence even after the cure
- Exhibit charcot leyden crystal in stool and moderate leukocytosis
- **Zymodeme analysis:** For detection of isoenzyme marker like- hexokinase, malic enzyme, etc.
- Polymerase chain reaction—performed on amoebic liver pus
- **Ultrasonography of liver:** Demonstrate the site and extension of the abscess.

6. Write briefly on post exposure Prophylaxis in HIV infection.

(Ref: Ananthanarayan and Paniker, Textbook of Microbiology,10th ed, pg. 586)

ANSWER

Prophylaxis

Vaccine Research in HIV

- Modified whole virus has been tried
- Subunits based on envelope glycoprotein is under development
- Target cell protection by anti-CD4 antibody or genetically engineered CD4
- PEP – vaccine.

Strategy of Post Exposure Prophylaxis in HIV Infection

- **Assessment:**
  - Clinical assessment of exposure
  - Eligibility assessment for HIV post-exposure prophylaxis
  - HIV testing of exposed people and source if possible
  - Provision of first aid in case of broken skin or other wound
- **Counseling and Support**
  - Risk of HIV
  - Risks and benefits of HIV post-exposure prophylaxis
  - Side effects of treatment to be told
  - Enhanced adherence counseling if post-exposure prophylaxis to be prescribed
  - Specific support in case of sexual assault
- **Prescription**
  - Post-exposure prophylaxis should be initiated as early as possible following exposure
  - 28-day prescription of recommended age-appropriate ARV drugs
  - Drug information should be shared
- **Follow-up**
  - Assessment of underlying comorbidities and possible drug-drug interactions
  - HIV test at 3 months after exposure
  - Link to HIV treatment if possible
  - Provision of prevention intervention as appropriate

NACO guidelines for post exposure prophylaxis:

- **TLE Regimen:**
  - Single tablet consisting of- Tenofovir (TDF) 300 mg+ Lamivudine (3TC) 300 mg + Efavirenz (EFV) 600 mg once daily for 4 weeks
  - Ideally, therapy should be started within 2 hours of the exposure and definitely within 72 hours.
  - Indication: Health care workers exposed to HIV positive source.

Your Roll No. ....

Name of the Paper	:	**Microbiology Paper-I**
Name of the Course	:	**MBBS-2018**
Semester	:	**Annual**

Time: 3 Hours   **M.M.: 40**

INSTRUCTIONS

1. Write your Roll No. on the top immediately on receipt of this question paper
2. All questions are to be attempted
3. Answers to Parts I, II and III should be written in separate answer sheets provided
4. Attempt parts of a question in sequence

PART-I

1. List the different modes of transmission of genetic material in bacteria and describe any one method in detail.
                                                                                                                                         [5]

2. Write short notes on: [10]
   a. Agglutination
   b. Bacterial capsule.

PART-II

3. Enumerate the microorganisms causing meningitis. Describe the laboratory diagnosis of acute pyogenic meningitis.   [5]

4. Write briefly on: [10]
   a. Widal test
   b. Laboratory diagnosis of gas gangrene.

PART-III

5. Describe briefly the biomedical waste management in hospital settings.   [5]

6. Write the etiology of urinary tract infection (UTI). Describe the laboratory diagnosis of UTI.   [5]

PART-I

1. List the different modes of transmission of genetic material in bacteria and describe any one method in detail.

(Ref: Ananthanarayan and Paniker's, Textbook of Microbiology,10th ed, pg. 59)

ANSWER

Methods of Gene Transfer

○ Bacterial reproduction is by the asexual process of binary fission. With the exception of a de novo mutation, the resultant daughter cells are genetically identical to the parent cell. This lends itself to the question, "How then have bacteria undergone genetic variation resulting in the different virulence factors and antibiotic resistances?"

○ Three mechanisms have been observed to transfer novel genetic material into bacteria: Transformation, conjugation, and transduction.

▪ **Conjugation:** Transfer of genes between cells that are in physical contact with one another

▪ **Transduction:** Transfer of genes from one cell to another by a bacteriophage

▪ **Transformation:** Transfer of cell-free or "naked" DNA from one cell to another

○ Upon reception of the new genes, the genetic material must be stabilized either by reformation of a plasmid or by recombination. Linear DNA is always stabilized by homologous recombination.

○ Occasionally, a plasmid will be an episome and integrate into the bacterial chromosome by the process of site-specific recombination

Transformation

○ Transformation is the uptake of naked (free) DNA from the environment by competent cells.

○ Cells become competent (able to bind short pieces of DNA to the envelope and import them into the cell) under certain environmental conditions.

○ Some bacteria are capable of natural transformation (they are naturally competent): Haemophilus influenzae, Streptococcus pneumoniae, Bacillus species, and Neisseria species.

○ DNA (released from dead cells) is taken up. Newly introduced DNA is generally linear, homologous DNA; a similar type of cell but perhaps one that is genetically diverse.

○ The linear DNA is then stabilized by homologous recombination.

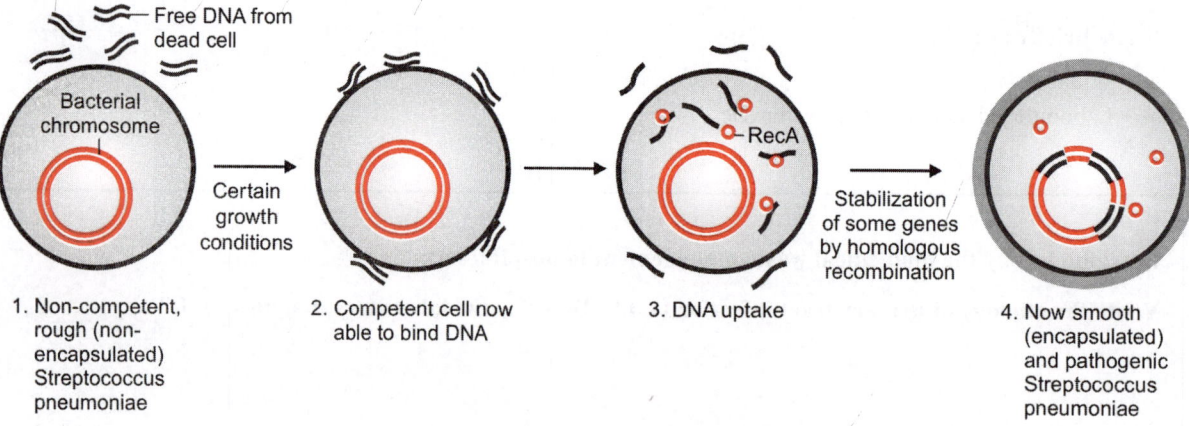

Fig. Transformation of a Non-encapsulated Streptococcus pneumoniae

Conjugation

○ Conjugation was the first extensively studied method of gene transfer

○ Conjugation requires donor cell-to-recipient cell contact and is mediated by sex pilus

○ Process occurs between two living cells

○ Requires mobilization of donor bacterium's chromosome/plasmid

○ Plasmid are genetic elements most frequently transferred by conjugation

Transduction

○ Phage mediated genetic recombination in bacteria i.e. phage is used to transfer DNA from one bacterium to another

○ **Transducing particle:** Bacterial nucleic acid in phage coat

- There are two broad categories of transduction
- **Generalized transduction:** Where virtually any genetic marker can be transferred
- **Specialized transduction:** Bacterial DNA who are adjacent to viral DNA in the prophage get transferred
- For artificial Genetic recombination purpose Temperate phage are preferred vehicle for gene transfer
- Transduction has been found to occur in a variety of bacterial populations including:
  - Escherichia coli
  - Pseudomonas spp
  - Salmonella spp
  - Staphylococcus spp.

2. Write short note on:

a. Agglutination

(Ref: Ananthanarayan and Paniker, Textbook of Microbiology, 10th ed, pg. 109)

ANSWER

Agglutination Tests

It is used to detect antibody union with large, particulate antigens.

- Rapid, slide identification of bacteria can occur by mixing a loopful of bacteria from the patient's culture with a battery of specific antibacterial antisera and noting which antiserum causes agglutination.
- Semi quantitative diagnostic test for bacterial diseases involves addition of the suspect bacterium (killed) to dilutions of the patient's serum. The highest dilution that results in visible agglutination is called the titer. A fourfold increase in titer is necessary for diagnosis due to low levels of "natural" antibodies occurring in the serum of most normal human beings.

Diagnostic Application of Agglutinations Tests

- **Slide agglutination**
  - It is used in blood grouping to determine qualitatively whether the donor's cells or serum possess antigens or antibodies that are reactive with the recipient's serum or cells.

- **Tube Agglutination**

  It is routinely used for

  - Typhoid fever (Widal test) Detects Ab against both H (Flagellar) and O (Somatic) Ag
  - Acute Brucellosis (Standard agglutination test)
  - **Coombs test or Antiglobulin test:**
    - Detects incomplete Rh antibodies.
    - Two variations of the Coombs test exist.
      - **Direct Coombs Test:** is designed to identify maternal anti-Rh antibodies that are already bound to infant RBCs or antibodies bound to RBCs in patients with autoimmune hemolytic anemia.

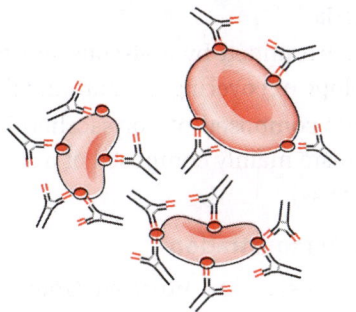 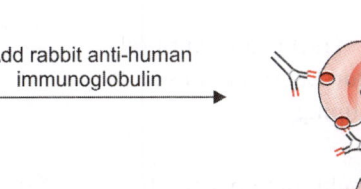 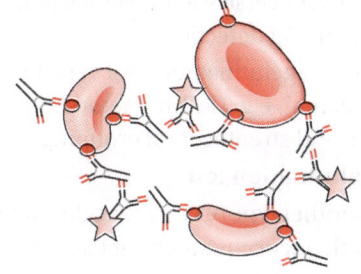

Baby's RhD+ cells already coated with mother's antibody to be used in the direct coombs test

Add rabbit anti-human immunoglobulin

Red cells agglutinated by the addition of rabbit anti-immunoglobulin serum

Fig. Direct Coombs test

- **Indirect Coombs test:** It is designed to identify Rh-negative mothers who are producing anti-Rh antibodies of the IgG isotype, which may be transferred across the placenta harming Rh-positive fetuses. The indirect Coombs is also used in the diagnosis of transfusion reactions.

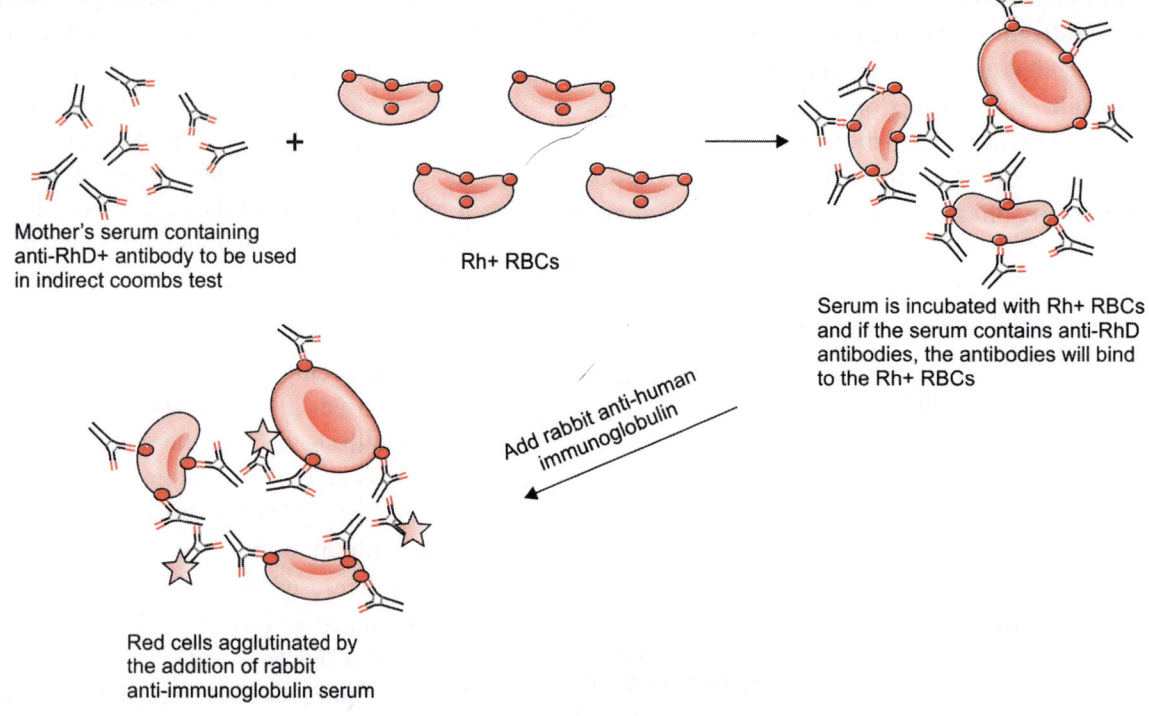

Mother's serum containing
anti-RhD+ antibody to be used
in indirect coombs test

Rh+ RBCs

Serum is incubated with Rh+ RBCs
and if the serum contains anti-RhD
antibodies, the antibodies will bind
to the Rh+ RBCs

Add rabbit anti-human immunoglobulin

Red cells agglutinated by
the addition of rabbit
anti-immunoglobulin serum

Fig. Indirect Coombs test

○ **Indirect or passive agglutination test:**

Antigen is coated on carriers such as Latex or RBCs to detect Antibody in serum. Examples:

- Indirect hemagglutination test (IHA)
- Latex agglutination Test (LAT) for antibody detection e.g. ASO

○ **Reverse passive agglutination test:**

Antibody is coated on carriers such as Latex or RBCs to detect Antigen in serum. Examples:

- RPHA (Reverse Passive Hemagglutination Assay), e.g. HBsAg detection
- Latex agglutination test (LAT) for antibody detection, e.g. CRP, RA actor, Capsular antigen in CSF and streptococcal grouping.

○ **Coagglutination test**

- It another type of Passive agglutination test, where Staphylococcus aureus act as carrier molecule.
- Some strains of S. aureus (Cowan 1strain) possess protein A on the surface, which has a property of binding to Fc portion of any IgG molecule (except IgG3) making the Fab portion free, which can agglutination with the corresponding antigen present in the clinical sample.

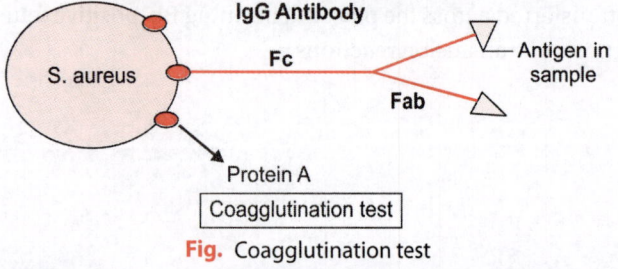

IgG Antibody

Fc

S. aureus

Fab

Antigen in sample

Protein A

Coagglutination test

Fig. Coagglutination test

b. Bacterial Capsule

(Ref: Ananthanarayan and Paniker's, Textbook of Microbiology, 10th ed, pg. 18)

ANSWER

Bacterial Capsule

○ A protective gelatinous covering present in certain bacteria

○ It is surrounded by a viscous substance forming a envelope or covering layer around the cell wall

○ Mainly composed of polysaccharide but in certain organism mainly composed of polypeptide(bacillus anthracis).

Capsule Demonstration

○ Ordinary stains are not used (Gram stain-low affinity for basic dyes)

○ **Use of India Ink:** Area occupied by the capsule in the cell are free of colloidal India ink particles

○ **Quellung reaction:** Use of specific antibody that causes swelling of the capsule. Example-Streptococcus pneumonia, Neisseria meningitides, Klebsiella, etc.

○ Serological methods

○ **Capsulated organisms are:**

Pneumococcus

Meningococcus

Bacillus anthracis

H. influenza

Yersinia
Cryptococcus (fungi)
Clostridium perfringens.

Functions

○ Protection from antibacterial agents like-lytic enzymes
○ Helps in bacterial adherence
○ Helps in laboratory diagnosis
○ Inhibition of phagocytosis
○ Bacterial typing and identification (by capsular antigen)

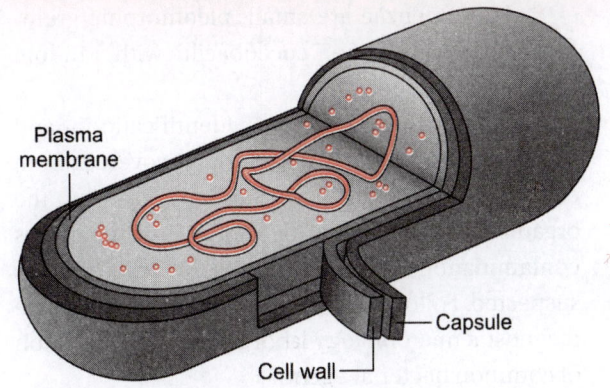

Mutation may result loss of capsule making the bacteria avirulent and also repeated subcultures in vitro may causes loss of capsules.

PART-II

3. **Enumerate the microorganisms causing meningitis. Describe the laboratory diagnosis of acute pyogenic meningitis.**

(Ref: Ananthanarayan and Paniker, Textbook of Microbiology, 10th ed, pg. 675-677)

ANSWER

Organisms Causing Meningitis

Bacteria	Fungi	Virus	Parasites
Adults: *Streptococcus pneumonia* *Neisseria meningitides* **Children:** *Streptococcus pneumonia* *Neisseria meningitides* *Haemophilus influenza*	*Candida albicans* *Cryptococcus neoformans* *Histoplasma capsulatum* *Aspergillus* species *Coccidioides immitis*	Enteroviruses (Polio, ECHO) Paramyxoviruses (Mumps, Measles) Adenoviruses Herpesviruses Arboviruses	Naegleria Entamoeba histolytica Toxoplasma gondii Acanthamoeba
Infants and Neonates: *E. coli* *Staphylococcus aureus* Group B streptococci (*Streptococcus agalactiae*) *Streptococcus pneumonia* *Listeria monocytogenes*			

Laboratory Diagnosis of Acute Pyogenic Meningitis

○ **CSF testing**
  ■ **CSF findings:**
    ♦ Increased CSF pressure (above 180 mm Hg)
    ♦ Turbid or frankly purulent CSF—due to pus accumulation in subarachnoid space
    ♦ Protein content: Markedly increased (more than 50 mg/dL)
    ♦ Polymorphonuclear leukocytosis (10-10000/μl)
    ♦ Glucose content: Decreased(below 40 mg/dL)
    ♦ **Oligoclonal band:** May be positive

○ **Bacteriologic examination:**
  ■ **CSF Gram staining:**
    ♦ If Cryptococcal meningitis is suspected, India ink preparation should be done
    ♦ N. meningitidis may occur intracellularly or extracellularly in PMN leukocytes and will appear as gram-negative, coffee-bean shaped diplococci.
    ♦ S. pneumoniae may occur intracellularly or extracellularly and will appear as gram-positive, lanceolate diplococci, sometimes occurring in short chains.

MICROBIOLOGY

♦ H. influenzae are small, pleomorphic gram-negative rods or coccobacilli with random arrangements

○ **Culture and Sensitivity:** Identification and susceptibility testing of bacteria recovered from cultures is routinely performed by growing the organisms in their specific culture media unless contamination during collection or processing is suspected. Following media are routinely used in the diagnostic microbiology laboratory for the isolation of common bacterial agents.

  ▪ **Chocolate agar:** On chocolate agar plate, H. influenzae appear as large colorless to gray, opaque colonies with no discoloration of the surrounding medium.

  ▪ **Blood Agar N. meningitidis on blood agar plate:**

    ♦ Overnight growth of N. meningitidis on blood agar plate appears as round, moist, glistening and convex colonies.

    ♦ S. pneumoniae appear as small grayish mucoid (watery) colonies with a greenish zone of alpha hemolysis surrounding them on the blood agar plate.

  ▪ **MacConkey Agar:** Antigen-antibody reactions

○ **Antigen testing:** Cryptococcal antigen latex agglutination test is preferred method in the suspected cases of Cryptococcal meningitis. Bacterial antigen testing on CSF is not recommended.

○ **Serology:**

  ▪ Serologic diagnosis is based on CSF to serum antibody index, 4-fold rise in acute to convalescent immunoglobulin G (IgG) titer, or a single positive immunoglobulin M (IgM).

  ▪ Submission of acute (3–10 days after onset of symptoms) and convalescent (2–3 weeks after acute) serum samples is recommended

  ▪ Mainly performed for S. pneumonia, H. influenza and N. meningitides

  ▪ **Detection of microbial antigen in urine:** Immunochromatography-based test for detection of S. pneumonia and latex agglutination-based test for detection of Cryptococcus neoformans.

○ **Detection of bacterial endotoxin:**

  ▪ **Limulus lysate test:** Detection of bacterial endotoxin

○ **Rapid Diagnostic Test:**

  ▪ Usually used for direct testing of CSF specimens

  ▪ Based on vertical flow immunochromatography principle.

4. Write short notes on:

  a. Widal test

(Ref: Ananthanarayan and Paniker, Textbook of Microbiology, 10th ed, pg. 302)

ANSWER

Widal Test

○ Widal Test is an agglutination test which detects the presence of serum agglutinins (H and O) in patients serum with typhoid and paratyphoid fever.

○ When facilities for culture are not available, the Widal test is the reliable test and can be of value in the diagnosis of typhoid fevers in endemic areas.

○ It was developed by Georges Ferdinand Widal in 1896.

○ The patient's serum is tested for O and H antibodies (agglutinins).

○ *Salmonella* antibody starts appearing in serum at the end of first week and rise sharply during the 3rd week of endemic fever.

○ In acute typhoid fever, O agglutinins can usually be detected 6–8 days after the onset of fever and H agglutinins after 10–12 days.

○ The main principle of Widal test is that if homologous antibody is present in patient's serum, it will react with respective antigen in the reagent and gives visible clumping on the test card and agglutination in the tube.

○ The antigens used in the test are "H" and "O" antigens of *Salmonella* typhi and "H" antigen of *S.* paratyphi.

○ The paratyphoid "O" antigen are not employed as they cross react with typhoid "O" antigen due to the sharing of factor 12.

Procedure

○ Patient serum serial dilution is prepared 1:40 to 1:320

○ Salmonella antigen in equal volume is added- by **Slide** method or as a **Tube** method

○ Two tubes used:

  ▪ Felix tube for O antigen

  ▪ Dreyer's tube for H antigen

○ Incubation of tubes for 12 hours or overnight

○ At zone of equivalence, agglutination takes place when antibodies meet antigens (lattice hypothesis)

○ O agglutination: exhibit disc-like pattern present at the bottom of the tube

○ H agglutination: Loose, cotton-woolly clumps

Interpretation

- Agglutination represent the highest dilution of the serum
- **Positive Widal test:**
  - "O" antigen titer is >1:160 demonstrate active infection
  - "H" antigen titer is >1:160, indicate past infection or in immunized persons
  - A increase in the titer fourfold (e.g., from 1:40 to 1:160) is diagnostic.

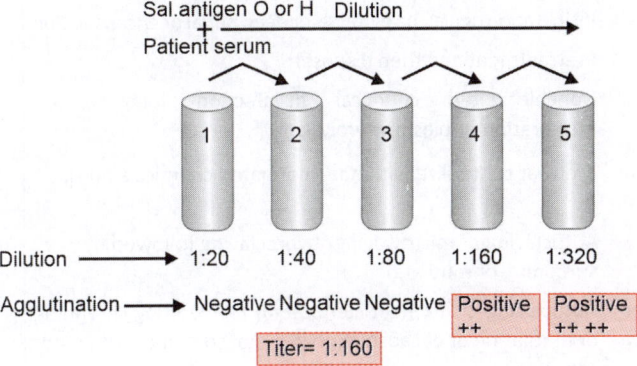

Fig. Widal test

- **O antigen:** Positive in acute stage and titer more than 1:160 and it appears early
- **H antigen:** Positive in the recovery stage and appears late
- **Vi antigen:** Indicate carrier stage.
- False positive test may be present in cross- reacting infections, like-malaria.

b. Laboratory diagnosis of gas gangrene

(Ref: Ananthanarayan and Paniker's, Textbook of Microbiology,10th ed, pg. 258)

ANSWER

Gas Gangrene

- Also known as Clostridial myositis, anaerobic myositis, etc.
- Gas gangrene is a bacterial infection that produces gas in tissues and this deadly form of gangrene usually is caused by *Clostridium perfringens* bacteria.

Laboratory Diagnosis of Gas Gangrene

- **Specimens:** Wound swab, discharge and affected tissue
- **Direct smear (Gram stained):** Shows brick-shaped large number of gram positive bacilli; spores are usually not seen- Diagnostic for *Cl perfringens*
- **Culture:** Specimen inoculated into cooked meat media as well as in a blood agar media and the latter is incubated anaerobically for 48–72 hours. In blood agar medium there is hemolysis around the colony.

- The bacterial culture is used for Nagler's reaction and biochemical tests.
- **Nagler's reaction:**
  - A test used for the detection of *Clostridium perfringens*
  - Serum or egg yolk agar is used for the reaction.
  - Colonies of *C. perfringens* grown in media consisting of 6% agar, 5% Fildes' peptic digest of sheep blood and 20% human serum with antitoxin present on the one – half of the plate revels no opacity around the colonies with the antitoxin because of alpha toxin neutralization while colonies present on the other half of the plate without antitoxin exhibits opacity round the colonies.
  - Thus, the presented lecithinase effect is called as "Nagler's reaction"
- **Biochemical reaction:** Glucose, lactose, maltose and sucrose fermentation in *Cl. perfringens* and production of gas and acid.

PART-III

5. Describe briefly the biomedical waste management in hospital settings.

(Ref: Ananthanarayan and Paniker, Textbook of Microbiology, 10th ed, pg. 657)

ANSWER

Biomedical Waste

- Biomedical waste means "any solid and/or liquid waste including its container and any intermediate product, which is generated during the diagnosis, treatment or immunization of human beings or animals".
- Biomedical waste poses hazard due to two principal reasons–the first is infectivity and the other, toxicity.

Classification

The World Health Organization (WHO) has classified medical wastes according to their weight, density and constituents into different categories. These are:

- **Infectious:** Material-containing pathogens in sufficient concentrations or quantities that, if exposed, can cause diseases. This includes waste from surgery and autopsies on patients with infectious diseases, sharps, disposable needles, syringes, saws, blades, broken glasses, nails or any other item that could cause a cut
- **Pathological:** Tissues, organs, body parts, human flesh, fetuses, blood and body fluids, drugs and chemicals that are returned from wards, spilled, outdated, contaminated, or are no longer required

○ **Radioactive:** Solids, liquids and gaseous waste contaminated with radioactive substances used in diagnosis and treatment of diseases like toxic goiter

○ **Others:** Waste from the offices, kitchens, rooms, including bed linen, utensils, paper, etc.

Table: Biomedical Waste categories

Color of the bag	Type of waste	Waste treatment
Yellow	Human anatomical waste	Incineration or plasma pyrolysis or deep burial
	Animal anatomical waste	Incineration or plasma pyrolysis or deep burial
	Soiled waste	Incineration or plasma pyrolysis or deep burial
	Expired or discarded medicines	Return back to the manufacturer or supplier for incineration at temperature >1200°C
	Chemical waste	Incineration or plasma pyrolysis or deep burial or encapsulation
	Chemical liquid waste	Pretreatment and then disposal
	Discarded linen, mattresses, beddings, contaminated with blood or body fluids	Nonchlorinated chemical disinfection followed by Incineration or plasma pyrolysis
	Microbiology, biotechnology and other clinical laboratory waste	Pretreat to sterilize with nonchlorinated chemicals on site
Red	Contaminated waste like plastic bag, bottles, pipes or containers	Autoclaving or microwaving/ hydroclaving followed by shredding or mutilation
White translucent	Waste sharps included needles, syringes with fixed needles, needles from needle tip cutter or burner, scalpels and blades	Autoclaving or dry heat sterilization followed by shredding or mutilation or encapsulation in metal container or cement concrete
Blue cardboard box with blue label	**Glassware:** Broken or discarded and contaminated glass including medicine vials and ampoules except those contaminated with cytotoxic wastes; metallic body implants	Disinfection with sodium hypochlorite treatment or autoclaving or microwaving or hydroclaving then sent for recycling

Salient Features of Biomedical Waste Management (Amendment) Rules, 2018

○ Bio-medical waste generators including hospitals, nursing homes, clinics, dispensaries, veterinary institutions, animal houses, pathological laboratories, blood banks, health care facilities, and clinical establishments will have to phase out chlorinated plastic bags (excluding blood bags) and gloves by March 27, 2019.

○ All healthcare facilities shall make available the annual report on its website within a period of two years from the date of publication of the Bio-Medical Waste Management (Amendment) Rules, 2018.

○ Operators of common biomedical waste treatment and disposal facilities shall establish bar coding and global positioning system for handling of bio-medical waste in accordance with guidelines issued by the Central Pollution Control Board by March 27, 2019.

○ The State Pollution Control Boards/ Pollution Control Committees have to compile, review and analyze the information received and send tis information to the Central Pollution Control Board in a new Form (Form IV A), which seeks detailed information regarding district-wise bio-medical waste generation, information on Health Care Facilities having captive treatment facilities, information on common bio-medical waste treatment and disposal facilities.

○ Every occupier, i.e. a person having administrative control over the institution and the premises generating biomedical waste shall pre-treat the laboratory waste, microbiological waste, blood samples, and blood bags through disinfection or sterilization on-site in the manner as prescribed by the World Health Organization (WHO) or guidelines on safe management of wastes from health care activities and WHO Blue Book 2014 and then sent to the Common biomedical waste treatment facility for final disposal.

6. **Write the etiology of Urinary Tract Infection (UTI). Describe the laboratory diagnosis of UTI.**

(Ref: Ananthanarayan and Paniker's, Textbook of Microbiology, 10th ed, pg. 678)

ANSWER

Etiology of Urinary Tract Infection

Bacteria	Fungi	Virus	Parasites
Gram positive cocci • *Staphylococcus aureus* • *Staphylococcus saprophyticus* **Gram negative cocci** • Neisseria gonorrhoea **Gram negative bacilli** • *Pseudomonas* • *E. coli* • *Proteus species* • *Klebsiella* **Others** • *Mycobacterium tuberculosis* • Salmonella species	*Candida albicans*	Adenovirus	*Enterobius vermicularis* Trichomonas vaginalis Schistosoma haematobium

Laboratory Diagnosis of Urinary Tract Infection

○ Diagnosis is done when significant bacteriuria is demonstrated using quantitative cultures developed by Kass. 100,000 bacteria per mL is considered significant count in a sample collected by voiding.

○ **Specimen:**
  ▪ For culture, a clean voided midstream sample of urine is cultured
  ▪ Suprapubic aspiration in infants
  ▪ From catheter: ideally it is not recommended; however, urine may be collected immediately after inserting the catheter.

○ **Culture:** Confirmatory test for UTI
  ▪ Media used are: MacConkey agar or CLED agar and blood agar

○ **Microscopic examination:**
  ▪ One bacilli/HPF in a gram-stained smear: indicative of UTI

○ **Griess nitrite test:** Normal urine does not contain nitrites. Presence of nitrites indicates nitrate-reducing bacteria

○ **Catalase test:** When hydrogen peroxide is added in urine sample and frothing develops, it indicates presence of catalase and hence, bacteriuria

○ **Triphenyl tetrazolium chloride:** A dye reduction test that signifies respiratory activity of growing bacteria

○ **Dip slide culture methods:** Agar coated slides are immersed in urine sample or can be exposed to stream of urine while the patient is voiding. These slides are incubated and the growth of the bacteria is estimated by either counting the colonies formed or the color change of indicators in the medium.

○ **Leukocyte esterase test**

MICROBIOLOGY

Your Roll No. ....

Name of the Paper	:	**Microbiology Paper-II**
Name of the Course	:	**MBBS-2018**
Semester	:	**Annual**

Time: 3 Hours   **M.M.: 40**

INSTRUCTIONS

1. Write your Roll No. on the top immediately on receipt of this question paper
2. All questions are to be attempted
3. Answers to Parts I, II and III should be written in separate answer sheets provided
4. Attempt parts of a question in sequence

PART-I

1. Describe briefly about the pathogenesis of visceral leishmaniasis and the lifecycle of Leishmania donovani.   [5]

2. Write short notes on: [10]
   a. Rapid diagnosis of malaria
   b. Life cycle of ascaris lumbricoides.

PART-II

3. Enumerate the methods of transmission of hepatitis B virus. Diagrammatically represent the serological markers in a patient of hepatitis B virus infection.   [5]

4. Write short notes on: [10]
   a. Define fungal dimorphism and give examples
   b. Laboratory diagnosis of candidiasis.

PART-III

5. List two each vector borne viral infections along with their vectors. Describe the laboratory diagnosis of any one of them.   [5]

6. Write briefly on Negri bodies.   [5]

PART-I

1. **Describe briefly about the pathogenesis of visceral leishmaniasis and the lifecycle of Leishmania donovani.**

(Ref: Medical Parasitology, DR Arora and Brij Bala Arora, 5th ed pg. 52-53)

ANSWER

Visceral Leishmaniasis

○ Also known as kala-azar, black fever or dum-dum fever

○ Caused by Leishmania donovani

○ Visceral leishmaniasis is most commonly transmitted through the bite of an infected female phlebotomine sand fly

○ Emerged as one of the most important opportunistic infection in HIV infected individuals

○ The most obvious sign of visceral leishmaniasis is the swelling/enlargement of the spleen.

Pathogenesis of Visceral Leishmaniasis

○ Incubation period: usually ranges from 3-6 months

○ Hematogenous spread of infection to reticuloendothelial system(spleen, bone marrow, lymph nodes, etc.)

○ Intracellular multiplication of amastigote results in granulomatous reaction leading to hyperplasia and hypertrophy of affected organs (like- spleen, liver, etc.)

○ Disease progression may results in suppression of bone marrow causing anemia, leucopenia/neutropenia. Lymphadenopathy and increased production of globulin leading to reversal of albumin: globulin ratio.

Lifecycle of Leishmania Donovani

○ **Two hosts are involved:**

■ Human and also dog (in some areas)—vertebrate host

■ Sandfly—invertebrate host

■ **Cycle in sandfly:**

♦ Sandfly carry the amastigotes form of the parasite and lodges in the midgut of the insect

♦ Amastigotes transformed in to promastigotes and multiplication occur resulting in huge number of parasites.

♦ Parasites reach pharynx and buccal cavity and block it with its infective blood meal between the 6th and 9th day

■ **Cycle in man:**

♦ Skin of the man is pricked by sandfly and promastigotes gain entry into the wound.

♦ Promastigotes are engulfed by fixed macrophages (present near by) and get converted into amastigotes within the cytoplasm of the host cell.

♦ Slow multiplication of amastigotes, more or less quiescent for weeks or months

♦ Parasitized macrophages enter into the blood stream and reaches to liver, spleen, bone marrow, etc.

♦ Entry and multiplication of amastigotes into the fixed macrophages (Kupffer's cells in the liver)

♦ Rupture of infected cell and liberation of parasites into the circulation

♦ Progressively, entire reticuloendothelial system is infected

♦ In blood stream, phagocytosis of free amastigotes by polymorphonuclear leucocytes and monocytes.

♦ Free amastigotes are taken up by the blood sucking insect during its blood meal and thus the cycle is repeated.

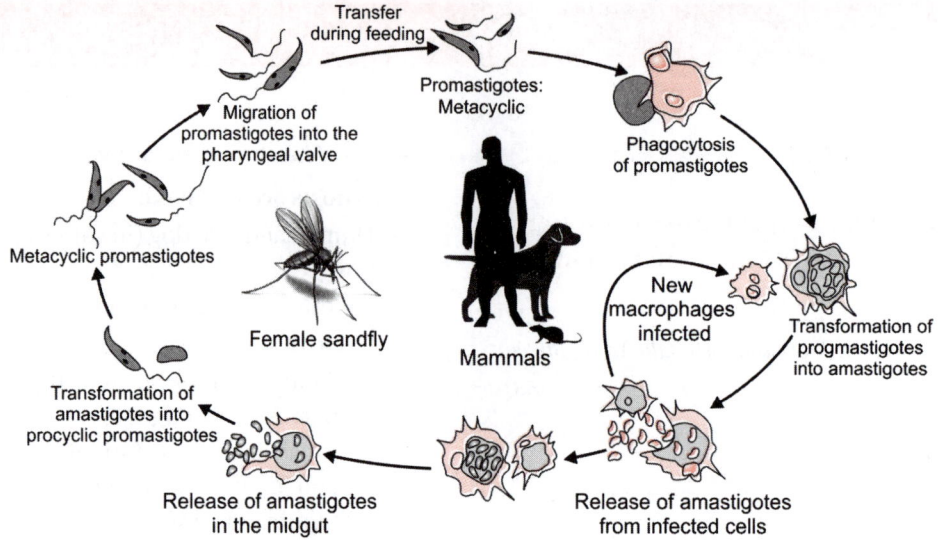

Fig. Life cycle of Leishmania donovani

2. Write short notes on:

a. Rapid diagnosis of malaria

(Ref: Medical Parasitology, DR Arora and Brij Bala Arora, 5th ed, pg. 82)

ANSWER

Rapid Diagnosis of Malaria

○ RDT is a device that can detect malaria antigen in a small amount of blood (5 μl) by immunochromatographic assay (colour change in an absorbing nitrocellulose strip) with monoclonal antibodies directed against the parasite antigen.

○ Depending on the target antigen, rapid tests that now exist may involve combinations of the following:

■ HRP-2 (Histidine Rich Protein-2) is a protein produced by the asexual stages and gametocytes of P. falciparum, expressed on the membrane of red blood cells (sensitivity: detects parasitemia of >40 parasites/μl). It often persists in patient's blood for weeks after successful treatment.

■ Plasmodium aldolase is an enzyme of the parasite glycolytic pathway expressed by all malaria species (pan malarial antigen- PMA).

■ Lactate dehydrogenase (LDH) is a glycolytic enzyme produced by asexual and sexual stages of parasites and released by infected red blood cells. (sensitivity: detects parasitemia of >100 parasites/μl)

Test Procedure

○ Consists of test strip (usually composed of nitrocellulose) is used

○ Blood is collected by finger prick method (2-50 μl)

○ Mixing of blood specimen in a separate test tube, or a sample pad with a buffer solution and if malaria antigen is present, formation of antigen- antibody complex takes place

○ Migration of antigen- antibody complex towards the detection line that contain capture antibodies

○ Washing buffer is used to remove the hemoglobin and to visualize the colored line on the strip

○ Presence of malarial antigen (P. falciparum or all Plasmodium spp.)—immobilization of labelled antigen-antibody complex at the lines containing capture antibodies and can be seen visually.

Advantages

○ The test donot require special equipment, electricity or training in microscopy

○ Easy to perform and interpret

○ Test can detect circulating antigens and thus may be used in the detection of deep seated (in the deep vascular compartment) infection caused by P.falciparum.

Disadvantages

○ No differentiation between *P. vivax*, P. ovale and P. malariae and not able to differentiate between pure P. falciparum infections and mixed infections

○ Costly procedure.

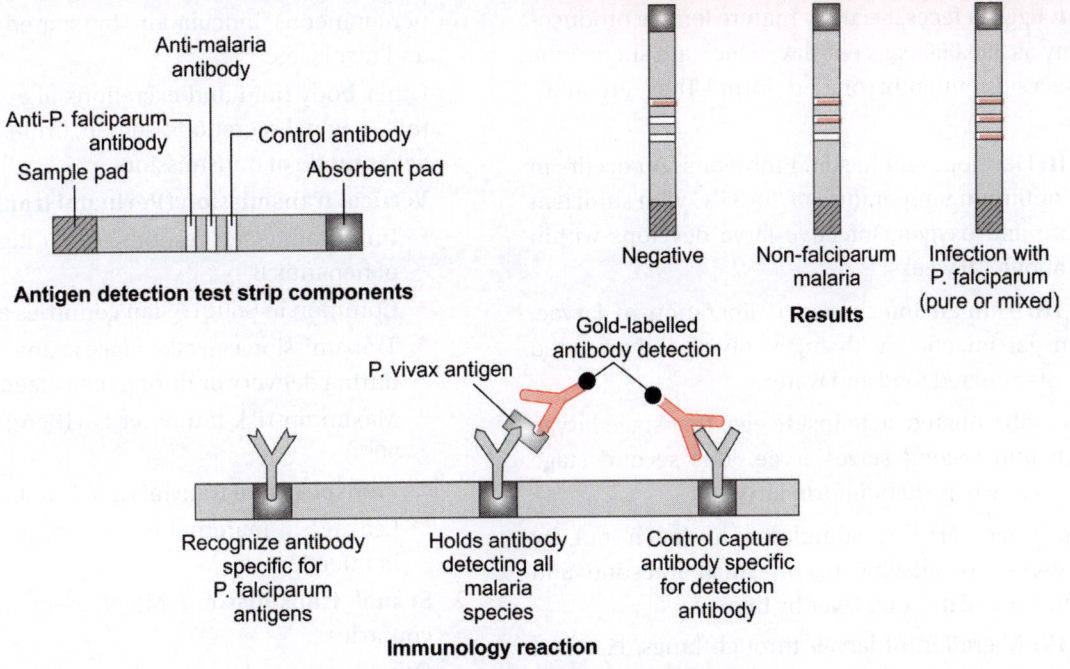

Fig. Procedure of rapid diagnostic test

b. **Life cycle of Ascaris lumbricoides**

(Ref: Medical Parasitology, DR Arora and Brij Bala Arora, 5th ed, pg. 195)

ANSWER

Introduction

Ascaris lumbricoides is an intestinal round worm. It is the largest intestinal nematode to infect humans.

Life Cycle

The life cycle of ascaris completes in single host—Human.

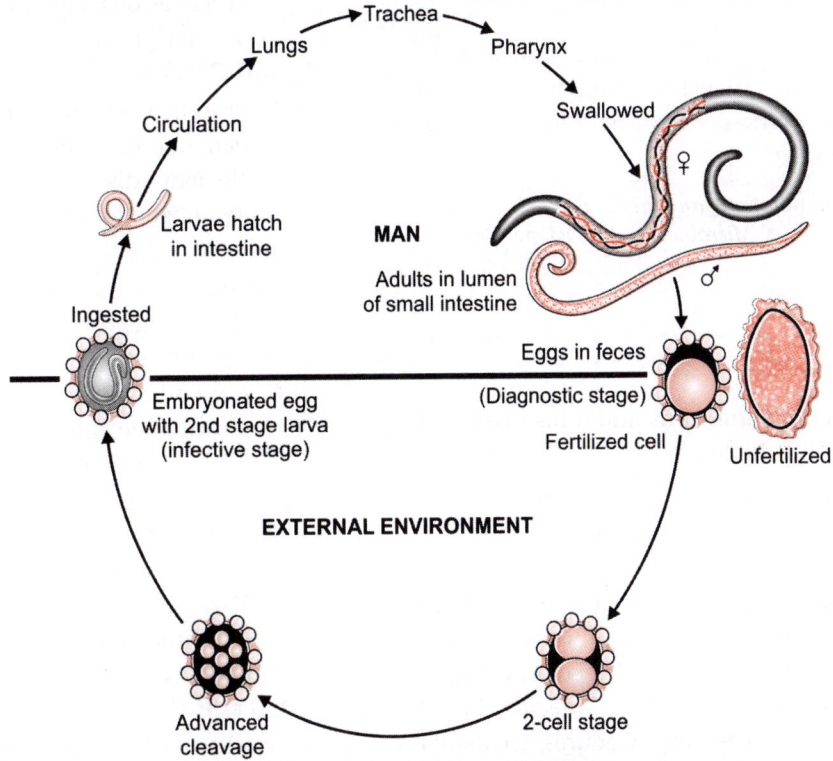

Fig. Life cycle of *ascaris lumbricoides*

Stage I: Eggs in feces. Sexually mature female produces as many as 200,000 eggs per day, which are shed along with feces in unembryonated form. They are non-infective.

Stage II: Development in soil. Embryonation occurs in soil as optimum temperature of 20–25°C with sufficient moisture and oxygen. Infective larva develops within egg in about 3-6 weeks.

Stage III: Human infection and liberation of larvae. Human get infection with ingestion of embryonated egg, contaminated food and water

Within embryonated state inside egg, first stage larvae develop into second stage larvae. This second stage larvae is known as rhabditiform larvae.

Second stage larva is stimulated to hatch out by the presence of alkaline pH in small intestine and solubilization of its outer layer by bile.

Stage IV: Migration of larvae through lungs. Hatched out larvae penetrates the intestinal wall and carried to liver through portal circulation

It then travels via blood to heart and to lungs by pulmonary circulation within 4–7 days of infection.

The larvae in lungs mold twice, enlarge and breaks into alveoli.

Stage V: Re-entry to stomach and small intestine. From alveoli, the larvae then pass up through bronchi and into trachea and then swallowed.

PART-II

3. **Enumerate the methods of transmission of hepatitis B virus. Diagrammatically represent the serological markers in a patient of hepatitis B virus infection.**

(Ref: Ananthanarayan and Paniker's, Textbook of Microbiology, 10th ed, pg. 550-551)

ANSWER

Transmission of Hepatitis B Virus

Hepatitis B is a blood borne virus and transmission of virus occur through multiple routes:

○ **Direct skin contact:** Mainly seen in children. Usually occur in infected open skin lesions like eczema, cuts, scratches, etc.

○ **Parenteral route:** Transmission of infected blood and blood products that occur through various modes – like, use of contaminated needles, syringes, skin prick, dialysis, transfusion, infected blood handling, surgical and dental procedures, accidental percutaneous inoculation by shared tooth brush and razors, etc.

○ Other body fluid and excretions like- saliva, breast milk, vaginal secretions, semen, urine, bile, etc. also act as mode of transmission

○ **Vertical transmission (Perinatal transmission):**
  ▪ Important factor responsible for high prevalence of hepatitis B
  ▪ Common in South Asian countries and China
  ▪ Transmission can take place at any age – in utero, during delivery or during breastfeeding
  ▪ Maximum risk if mother is HBeAg positive (60-90%)
  ▪ Transplacental transmission is not common
  ▪ Leakage of maternal blood into the baby results in infection

○ **Sexual transmission:** Mainly seen in developed countries

○ **Other routes:** Horizontal transmission (child to child), etc.

Serological Markers in a Patient of Hepatitis B Virus Infection

○ The surface antigen describes whether the patient is diseased or immune
  ▪ **HBsAg:**
    ♦ The surface antigen of the virus
    ♦ Having this antigen means the patient has the disease (chronic, acute, or asymptomatic carrier)
    ♦ Precedes onset of symptoms and elevation of liver enzymes
  ▪ **Anti-HBsAg:**
    ♦ Presence of this antibody indicates that patient is immune and/or cured
    ♦ No active disease present

○ The core antigen tells us how long the infection has been present
  ▪ **HBcAg:**
    ♦ The antigen of the core of the virus (HBsAg removed)
    ♦ Antibodies are not protective but yield information about the state of infection
    ♦ Positive antibodies seen during the "window period" (a period of active infection)
  ▪ **IgM anti-HBcAg:**
    ♦ New infection is present
    ♦ Most specific marker for diagnosis of acute HBV infection because it persists during the window period
  ▪ **IgG anti-HBcAg:**
    ♦ Old infection is present

○ The soluble component of the core antigen tells us how infective the patient is.

  ▪ **HBeAg:**
    ♦ A soluble component of the viral core
    ♦ Presence connotes high infectivity
  ▪ **Anti-HBeAg:**
    ♦ Presence connotes low infectivity

	Acute infection	Chronic carrier	Window period	Complete recovery	Immunized
HBs	+	+	–	–	–
Anti-HBs	–	–	–	+	+
Anti-HBc	+ (IgM)	+ (IgG)	+	+ (Ig)	–

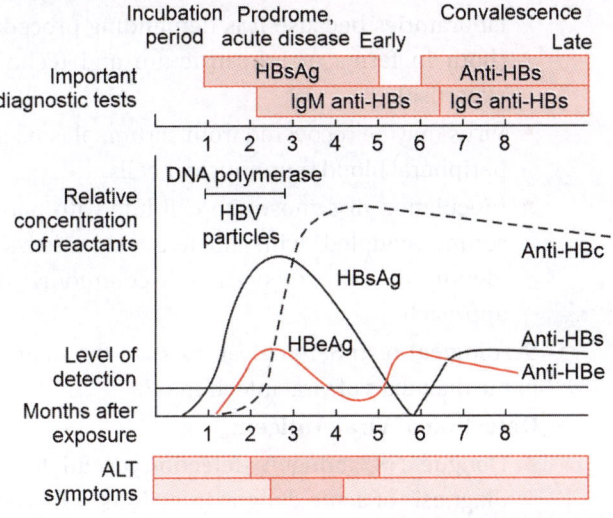

4. Write short notes on:

a. Define fungal dimorphism and give examples.
(Ref: Ananthanarayan and Paniker's, Textbook of Microbiology, 10th ed, pg. 609)

ANSWER

Fungal Dimorphism

○ Dimorphic means 2 morphological forms
○ Dimorphic fungi are the ones that grow as filamentous form in culture at 22–25°C and grow as yeast form in culture at 37°C
○ Most of the dimorphic fungi cause systemic mycoses and Sporothrix (one of the dimorphic fungus) causes subcutaneous mycoses.
○ **Common dimorphic fungi:**
  ▪ **Histoplasma capsulatum:** H. capsulatum is a dimorphic fungus that exists as a mold in soil and as a yeast in tissue. It causes histoplasmosis.
  ▪ **Blastomyces dermatitidis:** B. dermatitidis is a dimorphic fungus that exists as a mold in a soil and spherule in tissue. The yeast has a characteristic double refractive wall and a single broad based bud.
  ▪ **Paracoccidioides brasiliensis:** P. brasiliensis is a dimorphic fungus that exists as a mold in soil and yeasts in tissue. The yeast is thick walled and have multiple buds. It causes South American Blastomycosis.
  ▪ **Coccidioides immitis:** It is a dimorphic fungus that exists as a mold in soil and as a yeast in a tissue. It causes coccidioidomycosis.
  ▪ Among the subcutaneous mycoses, Sporothrix schenckii is a notable dimorphic fungus. It causes sporotrichosis.

Histoplasma Capsulatum

○ It is thermally dimorphic fungi that causes histoplasmosis
○ **Occur in two types:**
  ▪ Histoplasma capsulatum var. capsulatum-causes ubiquitous , classical histoplamosis
  ▪ Histoplasma capsulatum var. duboisii- causes African histoplasmosis
○ Commonly seen in USA and Africa
○ **Source of infection:** Soil, birds and rotting trees
○ Histoplasmosis is a pulmonary and hematogenous disease
○ It is often chronic and usually follows an asymptomatic primary infection
○ **Histoplasmosis has three main forms.**

1. Acute primary histoplasmosis is a syndrome with fever, cough, myalgias, chest pain, and malaise of varying severity. Acute pneumonia (evident on physical examination and chest X-ray) sometimes develops.

2. Chronic cavitary histoplasmosis is characterized by pulmonary lesions that are often apical and resemble cavitary TB. Manifestations are worsening cough and dyspnea, progressing eventually to disabling respiratory dysfunction. Dissemination does not occur.

3. Progressive disseminated histoplasmosis characteristically includes generalized involvement of the reticuloendothelial system, with hepatosplenomegaly, lymph-adenopathy, bone marrow involvement, and sometimes oral or GI ulcerations. The course is usually subacute or chronic, with only nonspecific, often subtle symptoms (e.g, fever, fatigue, weight loss, weakness, malaise); the condition of HIV-positive patients may inexplicably worsen

MICROBIOLOGY

○ **Laboratory diagnosis:**

▪ **Fungal culture:** Positive in 75% cases of Progressive disseminated histoplasmosis and chronic pulmonary histoplasmosis

▪ **Tissue specimen:** Exhibit yeast cell within phagocytic cells

▪ **At room temperature:** Spherical spores with tubercles (finger-like projections)- tuberculate spores

▪ **Serological diagnosis:** Latex agglutination, complement fixation and precipitation test

▪ **Skin test:** Done with Histoplasmin and more specific than serological test.

○ **Treatment:**

Table: Treatment of histoplasmosis

Type	Treatment
Chronic/Cavitary pulmonary	Itraconazole BD for at least 12 months
Acute pulmonary illness with diffuse infiltrates	Lipid amphotericin B ± glucocorticoids for 1-2 weeks Followed by Itraconazole for 12 weeks
Central nervous system involved	Lipid amphotericin B for 4-6 weeks followed by Itraconazole for 12 months
Progressive disseminated	Lipid amphotericin B for 1-2 weeks followed by Itraconazole for 12 weeks

b. **Laboratory diagnosis of candidiasis**

(Ref: Ananthanarayan and Paniker's, 10th ed, pg. 615)

ANSWER

For answer, refer 2019 paper-II, Q. 3, Pg. RP-165

PART-III

5. **List two each vector borne viral infections along with their vectors. Describe the laboratory diagnosis of any one of them.**

(Ref: Ananthanarayan and Paniker's, Textbook of Microbiology, 10th ed, pg. 529)

Vector Borne Viral Infections

Tick borne	Colorado tick fever, KFD, Crimean congo hemorrhagic fever
Rodent borne	Lassa fever, Hanta fever, Hemorrhagic fever with syndrome
Mosquito borne	Dengue, Chikungunya, JE, Yellow fever, Zika virus

Dengue Fever

○ Dengue fever is caused by dengue virus which is transmitted by Aedes aegypti

○ Also called as break bone fever

○ Manifests after an incubation period of 3–14 days

Laboratory Diagnosis

○ **Microscopy and Staining:** In this case, direct visualization of the virus in the sample (using electron microscopy or via fluorescent staining technique) is not done in diagnostic laboratories.

○ **Culture:**

▪ Virus isolation in cell culture is difficult and is not the commonly used method in diagnostic laboratories because it is demanding procedure (both in terms of infrastructure and technical expertise).

▪ Virus may be recovered from serum, plasma and peripheral blood mononuclear cells.

▪ Inoculation of a mosquito cell line with patient serum, coupled with nucleic acid assays to identify the recovered virus is commonly used approach.

○ **Serological test:** Serological tests are the mainstay in the diagnosis of viral infections.

○ **Detection of Viral Antigen:**

▪ Dengue NS1 antigen detection useful for the diagnosis of acute dengue infections. It has been detected in the serum of DENV infected patients as early as 1 day post onset of symptoms (DPO), and up to 18 DPO.

▪ NS1 ELISA based antigen assay is commercially available NS1 assay may also be useful for differential diagnostics between flaviviruses because of the specificity of the assay

○ Detection of Anti-dengue antibodies in serum or other body fluids by ELISA or other rapid tests.

○ Various methods (IgM/IgG ELISA, Hemagglutination Inhibition Test, or Rapid diagnostic kits) are available to detect Anti- Dengue Antibodies

○ **IgM detection:**

▪ Useful for the diagnosis of primary dengue infection and in distinguishing dengue from other flavi virus infections.

▪ IgM antibodies are detectable in 99% of patients by day 10 after onset of illness. IgM levels peak about two weeks after the onset of symptoms and then decline to undetectable levels over 2-3 months.

▪ **Sensitivity:** 65–75% sensitive in single acute serum sample.

○ **IgG detection:**
- Tests that detect IgG are useful in diagnosing secondary disease (IgG is the dominant immunoglobulin type in secondary infection).
- The test is complicated by cross-reactivity of IgG antibodies to heterologous flavivirus antigens (West Nile virus, tick-borne encephalitis virus, yellow fever virus, Zika virus).

○ **Molecular diagnosis:**
- Detection of viral RNA in plasma or serum or tissues using Nucleic Acid Amplification Tests (NAAT).
- RT-PCR based methods for rapid identification and serotyping of dengue virus in acute phase serum are available

6.   Write briefly on Negri bodies.

(Ref: Ananthanarayan and Paniker's, Textbook of Microbiology, 10th ed, pg. 538)

ANSWER

Negri Bodies
○ Eosinophilic intracytoplasmic inclusion bodies
○ Present in the brain cells of animals

○ **Demonstration of Negri bodies:**
- Zenker's fixative and 50% glycerol saline- for fixing brain tissue
- Seller's technique (methylene blue and basic fuchsin in methanol) is used for staining the impression smears of the brain
- Negri bodies present as purplish pink, oval or round intracytoplasmic structures with basophilic inner granules.

○ Size of Negri bodies approximately 3–27 μ
○ Common and abundant in cerebellum and hippocampus.

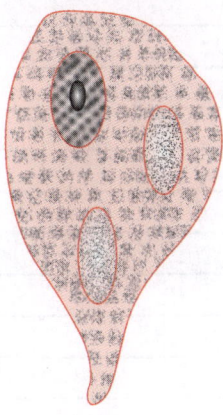

Fig. Negri body

Notes ✏️

Forensic Medicine & Toxicology

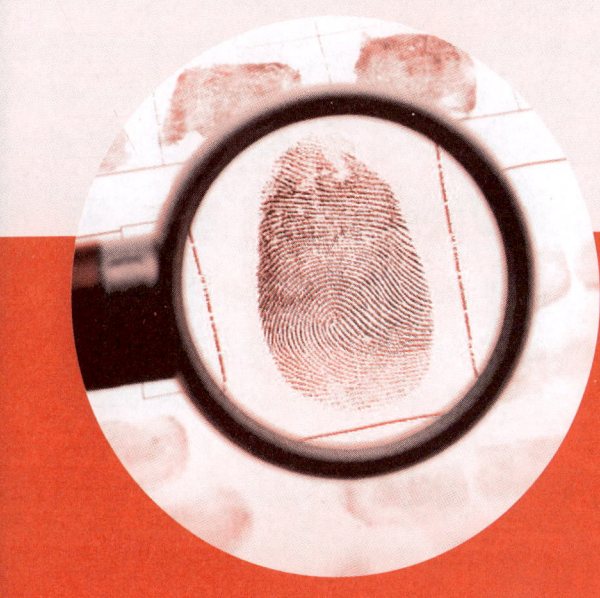

References Taken From:

○ *The Essentials of Forensic Medicine & Toxicology, KS Narayan Reddy & OP Murty, 34th edition*

○ *Parikh's Textbook of Medical Jurisprudence, Forensic Medicine and Toxicology, 8th edition*

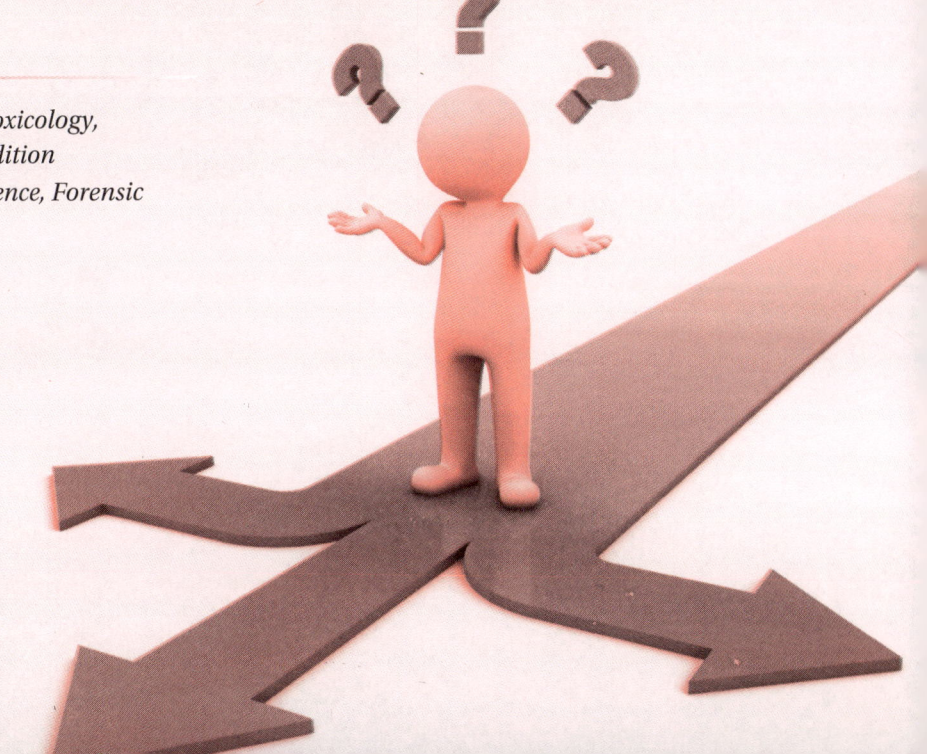

Your Roll No. ....

Name of the Paper	:	**Forensic Medicine & Toxicology**
Name of the Course	:	**MBBS-2019**
Semester	:	**Annual**

Time: 3 Hours   M.M.: 40

INSTRUCTIONS

1. Write your Roll No. on the top immediately on receipt of this question paper
2. All questions are to be attempted
3. Answers to Parts I, II and III should be written in separate answer sheets provided
4. Attempt parts of a question in sequence

PART-I

1. What are the findings, interpretation and medico-legal importance when it is stated that: [8]
   a. Red tears are present
   b. Person is showing motor cyclist's fracture
   c. Person is in suspended animation
   d. Person is an intersex.

2. Write short notes on: [6]
   a. Postmortem rigidity
   b. Somnambulism
   c. Delerium tremens.

PART-II

3. Classify poisons. Discuss clinical features, management and postmortem findings in acute organophosphate poisoning. What viscera shall you preserve in such cases?   [7]

4. Differentiate between: [6]
   a. Antemortem and postmortem blister
   b. Civil and criminal negligence
   c. Nulliparous and multiparous uterus.

PART-III

5. Describe the provisions under which pregnancy can be terminated as per provisions of MTP Act. Describe in detail the common methods of inducing criminal abortion in India.   [7]

6. Write short notes on: [6]
   a. Perjury
   b. Trench foot
   c. Latent prints.

PART-I

1. **What are the findings, interpretation and medico-legal importance when it is stated that:**

   a. **Red tears are present**
   (Ref: Parikh's Textbook of Medical Jurisprudence, Forensic Medicine and Toxicology, 8/e, pg. 649, Reddy, 34/e, pg. 485)

ANSWER

Red Tears are Present

Findings

Muscarine-like Effects

○ **Lacrimal glands:** Red tears or chromogenic tears shed from lacrimal glands owing to accumulation of porphyrin and Increased lacrimation

○ **Heart:** Slight bradycardia

○ **Pupils:** Slight miosis

○ **Ciliary body:** Blurring or dimness of vision

○ **Urinary bladder:** Frequency of micturition or Involuntary micturition

○ **Bronchial tree**
  ▪ Tightness in chest with prolonged wheezing expiration – suggestive of bronchospasm and increased secretion
  ▪ Discomfort or pain in chest
  ▪ Dyspnoea
  ▪ Cough
  ▪ Pulmonary oedema
  ▪ Froth at mouth and nose
  ▪ Cyanosis

○ **Gastrointestinal**
  ▪ Anorexia
  ▪ Nausea
  ▪ Vomiting
  ▪ Abdominal cramps
  ▪ Epigastric and substernal tightness
  ▪ Heartburn and eructation
  ▪ Diarrhoea
  ▪ Tenesmus
  ▪ Involuntary defaecation

○ **Sweat glands:** Increased sweating

○ **Salivary glands:** Increased salivation

Nicotine-like Effects

○ Striated muscle
  ▪ Easy fatigue
  ▪ Mild weakness
  ▪ Muscular fasciculations
  ▪ Cramps
  ▪ Generalised weakness of muscles of respiration with dyspnoea and cyanosis

○ Sympathetic ganglia
  ▪ Pallor
  ▪ Occasional elevation of blood pressure

CNS Effects

○ Irritability, apprehension and restlessness

○ Fine fibrillary tremors of hands, eye lids, face or tongue

○ Mental confusion progressing to stupor and muscular weakness with tremors and convulsions

○ Coma with absence of reflexes and depression of respiratory and circulatory centres

Interpretation

○ It is a case of Organophosphorus poisoning

Medicolegal Importance

○ Suicide – due to easy availability of pesticides, rodenticides and vermicides

○ Homicide – mixed with alcohol to mask the smell and can be used for homicidal purpose

○ Accidental – through contamination of edible things with these compounds

   b. **Person is showing motor cyclist's fracture**
   (Ref: Parikh's Textbook of Medical Jurisprudence, Forensic Medicine and Toxicology, 8/e, pg. 340, Reddy, 34/e, pg. 265)

ANSWER

Person is Showing Motor Cyclist's Fracture

Findings

○ Fracture of the skull with associated brain injury

○ Severe injuries as very little crushable material is there to absorb the impact and the driver or passenger is always thrown off

○ Primary injuries are usually open fractures of the tibia and fibula

○ Secondary injuries are usually fractures of the skull and cervical spine and also contusions of the brain

○ Head and neck injuries include skull fractures, contusions and lacerations of the brain, intracranial hemorrhages, ocular and orbital open lesions, facial fractures, cervical fractures and lesions of the spinal cord

Interpretation and Medicolegal Importance

- Such accidents are caused by turning in front of a vehicle from one side to another
- Most common cause of death is fracture of the skull with associated injury
- Multiple injuries produce a typical characteristic of fatal motor cycle accidents
- Submersion may result when moto cyclist attempts to cross a frozen lake and does not realizes that the ice is not thick enough to sustain the weight of the vehicle and its rider
- Crash helmets have reduced the rate of fatalities at low speeds but does not protect at high speeds

c. Person is in suspended animation

(Ref: Parikh's Textbook of Medical Jurisprudence, Forensic Medicine and Toxicology, 8/e, pg. 151, The Essentials of Forensic Medicine and Toxicology, K.S. Narayan Reddy 34/e, pg. 144)

ANSWER

Person is in Suspended Animation

Findings and Interpretation

- Condition in which signs of life i.e. vital functions of body (heart beat and respiration) are not found as they are at low pitch so cannot be detected by routine clinical examination
- Also known as apparent death as the person is not actually dead
- May persist for few seconds to several minutes after which the patient can be resuscitated successfully
- Metabolic rate is reduced in order to satisfy the individual cell requirement of oxygen through use of oxygen dissolved in body fluids

Medicolegal Importance

It is of two types

1. Voluntarily—yoga practitioners can pass into a trance, death like in character
2. Involuntary—lasts from few seconds to half an hour or more, may occur in apparently drowned, new born, after anesthesia, in cerebral concussion, electrocution, heat stroke, mesmeric trance, in prolonged illness such as typhoid fever, overdose by barbiturates or opiates, in deep shock

d. Person is an intersex

(Ref: Parikh's Textbook of Medical Jurisprudence, Forensic Medicine and Toxicology, 8/e, pg. 62, Reddy, 34/e, pg. 358)

ANSWER

Person is an Intersex

Findings and Interpretation

- **In gonadal agenesis**
  - Sexual organs i.e. testes or ovaries, have not developed
  - Chromatin negative
- **In gonadal dysgenesis**
  - In Klinefelter syndrome, a boy has:
    - Small testicles, firm consistency
    - Gynecomastia
    - Eunuchoidism: Long arms and legs, scanty pubic hair, scanty axillary hair, poor or no beard growth
    - Chromatin positive like female and sex chromosome pattern is XXY
- **In turner syndrome**
  - Sexual infantilism: Primary amenorrhea and consequent sterility
  - Short stature
  - Congenital abnormalities: Webbing of neck, cubitus valgus, coarctation of aorta, red green color blindness, renal abnormalities, osteoporosis
  - Lack of breast development with widely spaced nipples
  - Hypoplastic areolae
  - Scanty pubic hair
  - Infantile external genitalia, uterus and fallopian tubes
  - Streak ovaries with no ovarian follicles
  - Chromatin negative like a male and sex chromosome pattern is XO
- **True hermaphroditism**
  - External genitalia of both sexes
  - Internal genitalia have both ovaries and testes or ovotestes
  - Hypospadias
  - Cryptorchidism
  - Inguinal hernia
- **Pseudohermaphroditism**
  - External genitalia lack clear cut differentiation
  - Internal genitalia have only one sex

Medicolegal Importance

Complications pertain to:

- Marriage
- Inheritance
- Civil rights

2. Write short notes on:

a. Postmortem rigidity

(Ref: Parikh's Textbook of Medical Jurisprudence, Forensic Medicine and Toxicology, 8/e, pg. 157, Reddy, 34/e, pg. 151)

ANSWER

Postmortem Rigidity

Introduction

- In India, Postmortem Rigidity or Rigor mortis commences in 2-3 hours, takes around 12 hours to develop from head to foot, persists for another 12 hours, and takes around 12 hours to pass off thereby giving a rough estimate of time since death – Rule of 12
- Condition characterised by stiffening and shortening of muscles following the period of primary relaxation due to chemical changes involving structural proteins of muscle fibres indicating molecular death of its cells
- Also known as Cadaveric rigidity, reaction of muscle changes from slightly alkaline to distinctly acid due to local formation of lactic acid
- Persists until autolysis of myosin and actin filaments occurs as a part of putrefaction, when autolysis occurs, muscles become soft and secondary relaxation occurs
- It can be broken by mechanical force, therefore, when a limb is stiff due to rigidity, it is flexed forcibly at a joint, becomes flaccid and remains so after that – breaking of rigor mortis
- All voluntary and involuntary muscles are affected by rigor – appearing first in involuntary muscles and then in voluntary muscles
- Doesn't depend upon nerve supply and therefore, also develops in paralysed limbs
- **Tested by–**
  - Attempt to lift eyelids
  - Depress the jaw
  - Gently bend the neck and various other joints of body
- Rigidity passes off in the same order of appearance
- When erector pillae muscles of skin are affected, it presents a granular puckered appearance – cutis anserine, affecting mainly extremities

Sequence of Appearance of Postmortem Rigidity (or Rigor Mortis)

- In involuntary muscles, appears in heart within an hour after death
- In voluntary muscles
  - Muscles of eyelids in 3–4 hours

- Muscles of face in 4–5 hours
- Neck and trunk in 5–7 hours
- Muscles of upper extremities – 7–9 hours
- Muscles of legs – 9–11 hours
- Small muscles of fingers and toes in 11–12 hours

Medicolegal Importance

- Sign of death
- Helps in estimation of time since death
- Provides information about position of body at the time of death

Factors Affecting Postmortem Rigidity or Rigor Mortis

- **Age and condition of body –**
  - In children and old people, onset is earlier than adults
  - In strong muscular person, onset is late with prolonged duration
- **Mode of death**
  - In chronic diseases and convulsive disorders, onset is early and duration is short
  - In sudden death, onset is late with prolonged duration
  - In drowning, onset is early with prolonged duration
- **Surroundings**
  - Delayed by cold and accelerated by heat

b. Somnambulism

(Ref: Parikh's Textbook of Medical Jurisprudence, Forensic Medicine and Toxicology, 8/e, pg. 479, Reddy, 34/e, pg. 462)

ANSWER

Somnambulism

Introduction

- A state of dissociation arising in sleep which means walking in sleep usually occurring in children than adults

Clinical Picture

- Patient leaves the bed and makes way to study room or downstairs or may be out of house rarely injuring himself
- In this state, patient is not asleep but in a dissociated state of consciousness in which he may go through intense hallucinatory experience
- EEG studies do not show awake pattern
- Mental faculties are so concentrated at this stage that he can even solve a problem that he couldn't during waking period

Medicolegal Importance

- Patient may commit a theft or a murder in the state of dissociation
- This condition forms a good defence plea for criminal offences

c. Delirium Tremens

(Ref: Parikh's Textbook of Medical Jurisprudence, Forensic Medicine and Toxicology, 8/e, pg. 633, Reddy, 34/e, pg. 539)

ANSWER

Delirium Tremens

Findings

- Acute insanity
- Sleeplessness
- Marked tremors
- Excitement
- Fear
- Hallucinations: Visual and auditory
- Seeks escape from terrifying world by committing suicide

Interpretation

- State of excitement with hallucinations lasting 3–4 days

Medicolegal Importance

- Under section 84 IPC, person is not held responsible for his acts, if he lost consciousness to such an extent as would prevent him from knowing the nature of the act or distinguishing between right and wrong

PART-II

3. **Classify poisons. Discuss clinical features, management and postmortem findings in acute Organophosphate poisoning. What viscera shall you preserve in such cases?**

(Ref: Parikh's Textbook of Medical Jurisprudence, Forensic Medicine and Toxicology, 8/e, pg. 527, 649, Reddy, 34/e, pg. 467, 487)

ANSWER

Poisons

Introduction

- A substance which, when administered, inhaled or ingested is capable of acting deleteriously on the human body, therefore almost everything is a poison

Classification of Poisons

- **Corrosives**
  - Mineral acids—sulphuric acid, nitric acid, hydrochloric acid
  - Organic acids—oxalic acid, carbolic acid, acetic acid, salicylic acid
  - Vegetable acid—hydrocyanic acid
  - Concentrated alkalis—caustic soda, caustic potash and carbonates of ammonium, sodium and potassium
- **Irritants**
  - Inorganic
    - Non-metallic
      - Phosphorus
      - Chlorine
      - Bromine
      - Iodine
    - Metallic
      - Arsenic
      - Antimony
      - Mercury
      - Lead
      - Copper
      - Thallium
      - Zinc
      - Manganese
      - Barium
      - Radioactive substances
  - Organic
    - Vegetable poisons
      - Castor seeds
      - Croton
      - Abrus precatorius
      - Colocynth
      - Ergot
      - Capsicum
      - Semi carpus anacardium
      - Calotropis
      - Plumbago rosea
      - Plumbago zeylanica
    - Animal poisons
      - Cantharides
      - Snakes
      - Scorpions
      - Spiders
      - Poisonous insects
    - Mechanical
      - Coarsely powdered glass
      - Chopped hair
      - Dried sponge
      - Diamond dust

- ○ **Neurotics**
  - ▪ Cerebral—act on cerebrum
    - ◆ Somniferous
      - ▫ Opioids
    - ◆ Inebriant
      - ▫ Alcohol
      - ▫ Anaesthetics
      - ▫ Sedatives
      - ▫ Hypnotics
      - ▫ Fuels
      - ▫ Agrochemical compounds
    - ◆ Deliriant
      - ▫ Datura
      - ▫ Belladonna
      - ▫ Hyoscyamus
      - ▫ Cannabis indica
  - ▪ Spinal—act on spinal cord
    - ◆ Nux vomica and its alkaloids
    - ◆ Gelsemium
  - ▪ Peripheral – act on peripheral nerves
    - ◆ Curare
    - ◆ Conium
- ○ **Cardiac—act on heart**
  - ▪ Digitalis
  - ▪ Oleander
  - ▪ Aconite
  - ▪ Nicotine
- ○ **Asphyxiants—act on lungs**
  - ▪ Irrespirable gases
    - ◆ Carbon monoxide
    - ◆ Carbon dioxide
  - ▪ War gases
  - ▪ Sewer gas
- ○ **Miscellaneous**
  - ▪ Analgesics
  - ▪ Antipyretics
  - ▪ Antihistaminics
  - ▪ Tranquillizers
  - ▪ Antidepressants
  - ▪ Stimulants
  - ▪ Hallucinogens
  - ▪ Street drugs
  - ▪ Designer drugs

Organophosphate Poisoning

Clinical Picture of Organophosphate Poisoning

Toxic effects are of three types

1. **Muscarine-like effects—signs and symptoms are:**
   - ▪ Bronchial tree
     - ◆ Tightness in chest with prolonged wheezing expiration – suggestive of bronchospasm and increased secretion
     - ◆ Discomfort or pain in chest
     - ◆ Dyspnoea
     - ◆ Cough
     - ◆ Pulmonary oedema
     - ◆ Froth at mouth and nose
     - ◆ Cyanosis
   - ▪ Gastrointestinal
     - ◆ Anorexia
     - ◆ Nausea
     - ◆ Vomiting
     - ◆ Abdominal cramps
     - ◆ Epigastric and substernal tightness
     - ◆ Heartburn and eructation
     - ◆ Diarrhoea
     - ◆ Tenesmus
     - ◆ Involuntary defaecation
   - ▪ Sweat glands
     - ◆ Increased sweating
   - ▪ Salivary glands
     - ◆ Increased salivation
   - ▪ Lacrimal glands
     - ◆ Increased lacrimation
     - ◆ Tears can be red owing to porphyrin in lacrimal glands
   - ▪ Heart
     - ◆ Slight bradycardia
   - ▪ Pupils
     - ◆ Slight miosis
     - ◆ Ciliary body
     - ◆ Blurring or dimness of vision
   - ▪ Urinary bladder
     - ◆ Frequency of micturition
     - ◆ Involuntary micturition
2. **Nicotine-like effects**
   - ▪ Striated muscle
     - ◆ Easy fatigue
     - ◆ Mild weakness
     - ◆ Muscular fasciculations
     - ◆ Cramps
     - ◆ Generalised weakness of muscles of respiration with dyspnoea and cyanosis
   - ▪ Sympathetic ganglia
     - ◆ Pallor
     - ◆ Occasional elevation of blood pressure
3. **CNS effects**
   - ▪ Irritability, apprehension and restlessness
   - ▪ Fine fibrillary tremors of hands, eye lids, face or tongue
   - ▪ Mental confusion progressing to stupor and muscular weakness with tremors and convulsions
   - ▪ Coma with absence of reflexes and depression of respiratory and circulatory centres

Management

- ○ **Decontamination**
  - Physician and nurses should wear rubber gloves
  - Patient must be separated from the source of exposure and all clothes should be removed
  - Exposed areas should be washed with tap water and soap or some alkaline solution
  - In case of ingestion of poison, stomach should be washed with tap water
- ○ **Care of airway**
  - Foot end of the bed is raised to ensure drainage of respiratory muscles
  - Secretions should be aspirated and tracheostomy is required
  - Artificial respiration given, if required
  - Positive pressure oxygen should be given in case of pulmonary oedema
- ○ **Antidote**
  - Atropine blocks the peripheral actions of the excessive acetylcholine levels built up by the cholinesterase inhibitors
  - Dose – 2 mg every 15-30 minutes i.m. or i.v. till signs of atropinisation appear i.e. flushed face, dry mouth, dilated pupils, fast pulse and warm skin
- ○ **Cholinesterase reactivators**
  - Act by dephosphorylating the inactivated cholinesterase
  - Act as specific antidotes, used to supplement atropine therapy
  - Dose – 1-2 gm I.V. for adults and 25–50 mg/kg for children, as 5% solution in isotonic saline; repeated every 12 hours or if as required
- ○ **Other measures**
  - Diuretic and brisk saline purgative can be beneficial
  - Restlessness can be prevented by quick acting barbiturates or diazepam.

Postmortem Findings

- ○ **External**
  - Cyanosed face
  - Blood stained froth at nose and mouth
  - Kerosene-like smell can be perceived
- ○ **Internal**
  - Stomach contains greenish oily substances used as diluents
  - Kerosene-like or garlic smell is perceived
  - Blood stained contents of stomach
  - Congested mucosa
  - Submucous petechial haemorrhages are found

- Pulmonary oedema
- Capillary dilatation
- Petechial haemorrhages
- Hyperaemia of lungs, brain and other organs
- In delayed paralysis of extremities induced by parathion, malathion and other compounds - demyelination of ascending and descending spinal tracts with degeneration of motor horn cells

Medicolegal Importance

- ○ Suicide—due to easy availability of pesticides, rodenticides and vermicides
- ○ Homicide—mixed with alcohol to mask the smell and can be used for homicidal purpose
- ○ Accidental—through contamination of edible things with these compounds

Viscera to be Preserved in Case of Organophosphorus Poisoning

- ○ Stomach and its contents; wall of stomach should be preserved if the stomach is empty
- ○ Upper part of small intestine (around 30 cm in length) and its contents
- ○ Liver – 200-300 gm
- ○ Kidney – half of each kidney
- ○ Blood – 30 ml (minimum 10 ml)
- ○ Urine – 30 ml.

4. **Differentiate between:**

a. **Antemortem and postmortem blister**
(Ref: Parikh's Textbook of Medical Jurisprudence, Forensic Medicine and Toxicology, 8/e, pg. 354)

ANSWER

Antemortem and Postmortem Blister

Differentiating Characteristic	Antemortem blister	Postmortem blister
Line of redness	Seen	Not seen
Vesicles contain	Albuminous fluid and chlorides	Air
Infection	Present – Pus and sloughing	Nil
Healing	Occurs with granulation	Nil
Soot in upper respiratory tract	Seen	Not seen
Carboxyhemoglobin in blood	Not seen	Seen
Enzymes	Rise in enzymes	No such rise in enzymes is seen

FORENSIC MEDICINE & TOXICOLOGY

RP-195

b.   Civil and criminal negligence

(Ref: Parikh's Textbook of Medical Jurisprudence, Forensic Medicine and Toxicology, 8/e, pg. 37, Reddy, 34/e, pg. 41)

ANSWER

Civil and Criminal Negligence

Civil Negligence	Criminal negligence
Simply absence of required care and skill	Gross negligence, lack of attention and mismanagement
Arises when a patient or his relative sue the doctor for compensation of injury or when doctor brings a civil suit for realisation of his professional fees	Arises when patient gets seriously injured or dies due to criminal negligence or undue interference by doctor in treatment
Trial is done in civil court	Trial is done in criminal court
Strong evidence is needed	Guilt has to be proved apart from reasonable doubt
Litigation is between 2 parties	Litigation is between State and Doctor
Punishment is liability to pay compensation for damage done	Punishment is imprisonment with or without fine

c.   Nulliparous and multiparous uterus

(Ref: The Essentials of Forensic Medicine & Toxicology, KS Narayan Reddy, & OP Murty, 34/e, pg. 373)

ANSWER

Nulliparous and Multiparous Uterus

Characteristics	Nulliparous	Multiparous
Size	Small - 7 cm × 5 cm x 2 cm	Large - 10 cm × 6 cm x 2.5 cm
Weight	40 gm	80-100 gm
Ratio between body/cervix	Equal	2:1
Upper surface of fundus	Less convex and in line with broad ligament	More convex and at higher level than the line of broad ligament
External OS	Circular	Transverse slit
Internal OS	Circular, well defined	Ill defined
Uterine cavity	Triangular cavity and inner walls convex	Rounded cavity and inner walls concave
Arbor vitae	Present	Absent
Scar from placental attachment	Absent	Present

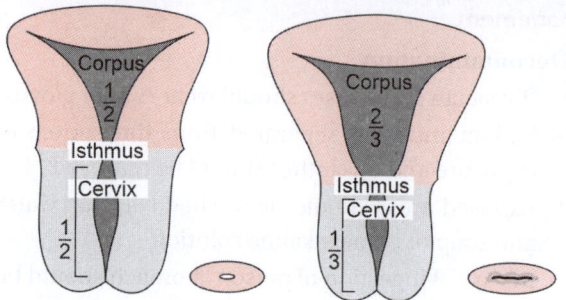

Nulliparous uterus
- Body & cervix same length
- Inner walls convex
- Triangular cavity
- Internal OS well defined
- External OS circular

Parous uterus
- Body twice the length of cervix
- Inner walls concave
- Rounded cavity
- Internal OS ill defined
- External OS transverse slit

PART-III

5.   **Describe the provisions under which Pregnancy can be terminated as per provisions of MTP Act. Describe in detail the common methods of inducing criminal abortion in India.**

(Ref: Parikh's Textbook of Medical Jurisprudence, Forensic Medicine and Toxicology, 8/e, pg. 430, Reddy, 34/e, pg. 374)

ANSWER

MTP Act, 1971 Medical Termination of Pregnancy Act, 1971

Medical Termination of Pregnancy Act, 1971 Legalises abortion on following grounds:

○ Therapeutic grounds – relate to conditions where continuation of pregnancy would risk
  - The life of pregnant woman
  - Grave injury to her physical or mental health
    - Organic heart disease with failure, active tuberculosis, severe diabetes
    - Hypertension complicated with cardiac or renal failure
    - Nephrotic syndrome
    - Pulmonary hypertension
    - Hepatocellular failure, acute hepatitis, acute pancreatitis
    - Toxaemia of pregnancy
    - Hydatidiform mole or acute hydramnios
    - Uterine haemorrhage or infected uterus after attempts at criminal abortion
    - Malignant neoplasms of breast or female genital tract
    - Repeated caesareans or irreducible prolapse of gravid uterus
    - Threatened insanity

- Eugenic grounds – conditions when there is substantial risk to the child, if born, will suffer from serious mental or physical abnormalities to be seriously handicapped
  - German measles, smallpox, chickenpox, viral hepatitis or other serious viral infections, if contracted within the first trimester of pregnancy
  - Exposure to X-rays and other radiation
  - When pregnant woman has received cytotoxic drugs, thalidomide, LSD etc.
  - When the parents have some inheritable mental condition or chromosomal abnormalities
- Humanitarian grounds
  - When pregnancy has been caused by rape, the anguish caused by such pregnancy is presumed to produce grave injury to her mental health
- Social grounds
  - Where pregnancy in a married woman is result of contraceptive failure
  - When the environment of pregnant woman, during the continuance of pregnancy and at the time when the child would be born and thereafter so far as is foreseeable would involve risk of injury to her health

Requirements for termination of pregnancy:

- In an emergency, any registered medical practitioner, irrespective of his experience or training in obstetrics and gynaecology can terminate pregnancy at any place, irrespective of its duration, if he is of opinion formed in good faith that the termination of such pregnancy is immediately necessary to save the life of the pregnant woman
- Except in an emergency, where duration of pregnancy does not exceed 12 weeks, a pregnancy can be terminated on the opinion of one registered medical practitioner and where the duration exceeds 12 weeks but is less than 20 weeks, opinion from 2 registered medical practitioners is necessary. It is essential that
  - Opinion must be formed in good faith
  - Registered medical practitioner must have specified experience or training in gynaecology and obstetrics
  - Such practitioner must have been registered with a certifying board for this purpose
  - Termination must be carried out in a hospital maintained by government or at a place approved by the government
  - Written consent of the woman only is essential
  - Consent of woman is not necessary
  - Written consent from her guardians in case where she is a minor or mentally defective

6. Write short notes on:

a. Perjury

(Ref: Parikh's Textbook of Medical Jurisprudence, Forensic Medicine and Toxicology, 8/e, pg. 10, Reddy, 34/e, pg. 13)

ANSWER

Perjury
Definition

- Giving wilful false or fabricated evidence or statement
- If a witness, after taking oath or making a solemn affirmation, wilfully makes a statement that he knows or believes to be false is guilty of the crime of Perjury under section 191 and section 192, IPC, 344, Cr PC.
- If the person's earlier statement regarding the facts on oath and subsequent statement on oath are opposed to each other, they cannot be reconciled
- Witness is liable to be prosecuted for perjury and his imprisonment may extend to 7 years under section 193, IPC

b. Trench foot

(Ref: Parikh's Textbook of Medical Jurisprudence, Forensic Medicine and Toxicology, 8/e, pg. 212, Reddy, 34/e, pg. 295)

ANSWER

Trench Foot
Introduction

- Type of cold injury to the foot resulting from sustained exposure to cold under moist conditions
- Typically experienced by soldiers during winter warfare, particularly in trenches

Symptoms and Signs

- Numbness of the affected feet, by erythema or cyanosis due to poor blood supply leading to necrosis of tissue.
- If the condition worsens, swelling of the feet may also occur.
- Advanced condition often involves blisters and open sores resulting in fungal infections; sometimes called tropical ulcer (jungle rot).
- If left untreated, usually results in gangrene, which may require amputation.
- If it is treated properly, complete recovery is normal, although it is marked by severe short-term pain when feeling returns.

Prevention

- By keeping the feet clean, warm, and dry

Treatment

- For gangrene, treatment is surgical debridement, and often includes amputation.
- Self-treatment can be done by changing socks two or three times a day and application of plenty of talcum powder.
- Whenever possible, shoes and socks should be taken off, the feet bathed for five minutes and patted dry, talcum powder applied, and feet elevated to let air get to them.

c. **Latent prints**

(Ref: The Essentials of Forensic Medicine & Toxicology, KS Narayan Reddy, & OP Murty, 34/e, pg. 83)

ANSWER

Latent Prints

Introduction

- It is a type pf fingerprint which is invisible or barely visible impression left on a smooth surface
- Also known as chance print

Development of Latent Prints

- Fingerprints may be taken from almost any surface with which the fingers come in contact, including certain fabrics and human skin
- Latent print may develop by dusting the area with colored powders to provide a contrast and its pattern is recorded by photography
- It may also be examined by oblique lighting
- Frequently used powder is grey powder (Chalk and mercury), but white powders (lead carbonate or French chalk) are used for dusting dark surfaces
- Fingerprints on paper, wood and fabrics are developed by treating them with 5% silver nitrate solution and then fixing them with sodium thiosulphate
- Fingerprints on paper can also be developed by exposing it to vapours of iodine or osmium tetroxide
- Electron autoradiography method uses a high energy beam of X-rays to irradiate the lead dust on fingermarks
- Scanning electron microscope visualizes latent fingerprints on metal and glass
- Using a continuous wave argon ion laser and observing through suitable filters, latent fingerprints show luminescence
- Even ten years old fingerprints can be developed

Your Roll No. ....

Name of the Paper : **Forensic Medicine & Toxicology**

Name of the Course : **MBBS-2018**

Semester : **Annual**

Time: 3 Hours   M.M.: 40

INSTRUCTIONS

1. Write your Roll No. on the top immediately on receipt of this question paper
2. All questions are to be attempted
3. Answers to Parts I, II and III should be written in separate answer sheets provided
4. Attempt parts of a question in sequence

PART-I

1. **What are the findings and medico-legal importance when it is stated that:**   [8]
   a. Female is having vaginismus
   b. Signature fracture is present over the skull
   c. Body is showing arborescent lines
   d. The boy is 12 years of age.

2. **Write short notes on:**   [6]
   a. Rule of nines
   b. Lochia
   c. Burtonian line.

PART-II

3. **Classify neurotic poisons. Discuss in detail signs, symptoms, management and post mortem findings in a case of death due to methyl alcohol poisoning.**   [7]

4. **Differentiate between:**   [6]
   a. Molecular and somatic death
   b. True and feigned insanity
   c. Male and female pelvis.

PART-III

5. **Define infanticide. Discuss in detail the post mortem findings of a live born foetus.**   [7]

6. **Write short notes on:**   [6]
   a. Vitriolage
   b. Atypical hanging
   c. Vicarious liability.

PART-I

1. **What are the findings and medico-legal importance when it is stated that**

   a. Female is having vaginismus

   (Ref: Parikh's Textbook of Medical Jurisprudence, Forensic Medicine and Toxicology, 8/e, pg. 385, Reddy, 34/e, pg. 360)

ANSWER

Female is Having Vaginismus

Findings

- Severe Involuntary pelvis muscle contraction
- Can be felt as varying constriction of the levator ani, right up to vaginal fornices
- Definite cramps like spasm of the adductor muscles
- Anticipation on attempted vaginal penetration

Interpretation

- Occurs due to fear, pain, disgust or apprehension for intercourse

Medicolegal importance: It may form grounds for:

- Nullity of marriage
- Divorce
- Adultery
- Legitimacy

   b. Signature fracture is present over the skull

   (Ref: Parikh's Textbook of Medical Jurisprudence, Forensic Medicine and Toxicology, 8/e, pg. 302)

ANSWER

Signature Fracture is Present Over the Skull

Findings

- Fractured bone is driven inward into skull cavity
- Outer table is pushed into the diploe, inner table is fractured erratically and to a larger extent and may be comminuted
- Resembles the shape of weapon used

Interpretation

- Caused by heavy weapon with a small striking surface for example, a hammer
- Shape of fracture indicates type of weapon used
- Differences in depth of various portions of depression suggests relative position of the assailant and victim when the blow was made
- Deepest part of the depression usually marks the most advanced part of the striking surface

Medicolegal Importance

- Given indication about the position of the victim and the assailant
- Suggests homicidal attack
- Indicates the kind of weapon used e.g. firearm, hammer, stone

   c. Body is showing arborescent lines

   (Ref: Parikh's Textbook of Medical Jurisprudence, Forensic Medicine and Toxicology, 8/e, pg. 371)

ANSWER

Arborescent Markings

Findings

- Superficial, thin, trivial lesions, involving only epidermal layer of skin (filigree burns or arborescent markings)
- Erythema with pattern like branches of tree
- Appears within minutes to hours of accident

Interpretation

- Indicate path taken by the discharge and disappears within a day or two if patient survives
- Caused due to natural electrical discharge from cloud to earth

Medicolegal Importance

- Depends on exclusion of any other cause of death
- History of thunderstorm in the vicinity
- Evidence of lightning such as damaged trees, dead cattle, appearance of various lesions on body such as filigree burns (arborescent markings), fractures, wounds, torn clothes, burns on body
- Death from lightning stoke are accidental

   d. The boy is 12 years of age

   (Ref: Parikh's Textbook of Medical Jurisprudence, Forensic Medicine and Toxicology, 8/e, pg. 63)

ANSWER

The Boy is 12 years of Age

Findings

- Teeth
  - Period of mixed dentition still persists
  - First bicuspid has erupted completely and second bicuspid has started erupting
  - Canines have started erupting
  - Second molars have not yet erupted
  - Space for last molar can not be seen

- Ossification of bones – as seen on X-ray studies
  - Lateral epicondyle of the humerus has not been united with trochlea and capitulum
  - Olecranon united with ulna
  - Pisiform already ossified
  - Heads of metacarpals and phalanges not yet fused

Interpretation

- Union of epiphysis in cartilaginous bones takes place earlier by 2 years in females than in males except in case of skull sutures where obliteration sets in little later and proceeds more slowly in female than in males
- The boy seems to be 12 years of age

Medicolegal Importance

- Criminal responsibility
  - Child under 12 years of age can not give valid consent to suffer harm which can occur from an act done in good faith and for its benefit eg. consent for operation
  - Person under 18 years of age cannot give valid consent whether express or implied to suffer any harm which may result from an act not intended to cause any grievous hurt eg. consent for wrestling
- Judicial punishment
  - Children (boys below 16 years and girls below 18 years of age), who have committed a crime, are tried by Juvenile court and if convicted, are entrusted to parents for special care or sent to correctional school with facilities for education, vocational training and rehabilitation
- Employment
  - Child below 14 years of age cannot be employed for any type of work
- Kidnapping
  - Kidnapping or abducting a minor, if boy is under 16 and girl is under 18 years is an offence

2. Write short notes on:

    a. Rule of Nines

    (Ref: Parikh's Textbook of Medical Jurisprudence, Forensic Medicine and Toxicology, 8/e, pg. 347, Reddy, 34/e, pg. 298)

ANSWER

Rule of Nines

Introduction

- In order to estimate the burnt surface area in an adult, rule of nines is used

Estimation of the Rule of Nines

- According to rule of nines,
  - 9% for head and each arm
  - 18% for front or back of trunk
  - 9% for front or back of each leg
  - 1% for perineum
- Thereby making 100% for the body
- Roughly, 1% of surface burn is equal to the area covered by the palm of the person

Diagrammatic Representation of the Rule of Nines

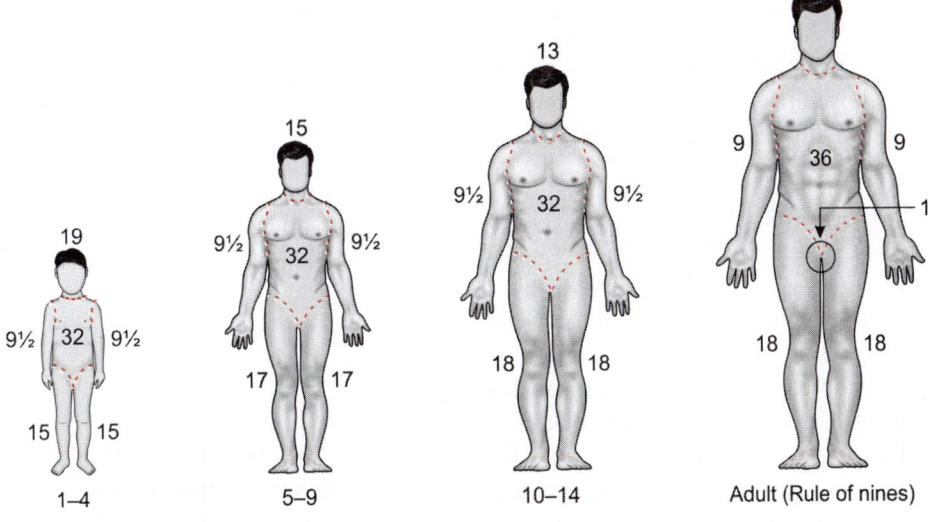

1–4   5–9   10–14   Adult (Rule of nines)

FORENSIC MEDICINE & TOXICOLOGY

b. **Lochia**

(Ref: Parikh's Textbook of Medical Jurisprudence, Forensic Medicine and Toxicology, 8/e, pg. 398, Reddy, 34/e, pg. 372)

ANSWER

Lochia

Definition

○ Vaginal discharge with peculiar sour odour after delivery

○ Contains red cells, leucocytes, decidual debris, vaginal epithelium, peptones and cholesterol crystals

○ Discharge in postpartum period which is part of healing process of uterus after child birth

○ Characteristic of full term delivery rather than premature birth

3 Stages of Lochia

○ Lochia rubra - Blood stained during first 3 days

○ Lochia serosa - Paler and serous for next 3 days

○ Lochia alba - Yellowish or greenish and then whitish for another 3 days, disappears after 15 days

Medicolegal Importance

○ Disappears within 10 days in strong, vigorous women or in multipara

○ Can indicate size of foetus and rapidity of the birth, from the extent of stretching and lacerations of parts

○ Sooner the woman is examined after delivery, more are the chances of getting useful information

c. **Burtonian line**

(Ref: Parikh's Textbook of Medical Jurisprudence, Forensic Medicine and Toxicology, 8/e, pg. 579, Reddy, 34/e, pg. 507)

ANSWER

Burtonian Line

Introduction

○ Stippled bluish black line on gums due to subepithelial deposition of lead sulphide granules on the gums at the junction with the teeth (not on the teeth)

○ It is seen in 50 – 70% cases of lead poisoning

○ Found on gums of carious or dirty teeth particularly on the upper jaw

○ Bluish black colour is owing to formation of lead sulphide due to the action of hydrogen sulphide released by microorganisms from decomposing protein food around carious teeth in the presence of circulating lead

○ Similar blue line can be found in cases of poisoning by copper, bismuth, mercury, iron or silver

3. **Classify neurotic poisons. Discuss in detail signs, Symptoms, management and post mortem findings in a case of death due to methyl alcohol poisoning.**

(Ref: Parikh's Textbook of Medical Jurisprudence, Forensic Medicine and Toxicology, 8/e, pg. 527, 640, Reddy, 34/e, pg. 467, 540)

ANSWER

Neurotic Poisons

Definition

○ Poisons which act mainly on nervous system

Classification

○ **Cerebral:** Act on cerebrum
  - Somniferous
    - Opioids
  - Inebriant
    - Alcohol
    - Anesthetics
    - Sedatives
    - Hypnotics
    - Fuels
    - Agrochemical compounds
  - Deliriant
    - Datura
    - Belladonna
    - Hyoscyamus
    - Cannabis indica

○ **Spinal:** Act on spinal cord
  - Nux vomica and its alkaloids
  - Gelsemium

○ **Peripheral:** Act on peripheral nerves
  - Curare
  - Conium

Methyl Alcohol poisoning

Clinical Picture

○ Symptoms usually get delayed but may appear within an hour

○ Headache

○ Nausea and vomiting

○ Dizziness

○ Pain in abdomen

○ Profound muscular weakness

○ Depressed cardiac action

○ Breath has spirit like odour

○ Dyspnoea

○ Cyanosis

○ Acidosis due to accumulation of acid metabolites

○ Effects in eyes—temporary blindness; optic nerve atrophy causing permanent blindness

○ Convulsions may occur

○ Intestinal contraction—small or large bowel or sometimes, both

○ Death due to respiratory failure

Fatal Dose

○ 60-240 ml in adults kills

○ 15 ml causes blindness

○ 1 ml/kg of denatured alcohol containing methyl alcohol in children causes serious symptoms

Fatal Period

○ Death may occur within 24 hours to 36 hours or 3-4 days

Management

○ Gastric lavage to prevent absorption with 5% solution of sodium bicarbonate in warm water

○ For acidosis, oral administration of sodium bicarbonate in a dose of 2 g in 250 mL of water every 2 hours is required to maintain neutral or slightly alkaline urine

○ In case, where oral therapy is not possible, 50 g of sodium bicarbonate dissolved in 1 litre of 5% dextrose solution can be given intravenously along with 10-15 units of insulin

○ Plasma bicarbonate level should be maintained at around 20 mEq/L

○ Intravenous administration of molar sodium lactate is beneficial

○ 50% ethyl alcohol in a dose of 0.75 to 1 mL/kg body weight should be given orally for 3-4 days to prevent methanol oxidation to formaldehyde and formic acid and helps in its excretion in urine and breath

○ Haemodialysis is indicated in – ocular findings, metabolic acidosis, renal failure and a blood methanol level above 50 mg%

○ Eyes should be covered to protect from strong light

○ Rest treatment is symptomatic

Postmortem Findings

○ Cyanosis is profound

○ Dark - fluid blood

○ Cerebral and pulmonary oedema can be observed

○ Inflamed gastrointestinal mucosa

○ Necrobiosis of liver

○ Kidneys show tubular degeneration

○ Viscera and postmortem blood should be preserved

Medicolegal Significance

○ Accidental poisoning may occur

○ Most commonly due to ingestion of liquor containing methyl alcohol by drinking cheap illicit liquor or accidently methanol getting into liquor

4. **Differentiate between:**

   a. **Molecular and Somatic death**
   (Ref: Parikh's Textbook of Medical Jurisprudence, Forensic Medicine and Toxicology, 8/e, pg. 147, Reddy, 34/e, pg. 128)

ANSWER

Molecular and Somatic Death

Molecular death	Somatic death
Tissues and cells survive for a varying period depending upon their oxygen requirements, When these individual tissues and cells die, it is termed as molecular death	Due to complete and irreversible cessation of vital functions of the brain, followed by cessation of the functions of heart and lungs
Not confused with suspended animation	May be confused with suspended animation
Muscles do not respond to electric stimuli	At this stage, muscles respond to electric stimuli
Organs can not be removed for transplantation at this stage	Organs can be removed for transplantation at this stage
It occurs after somatic death	It occurs before molecular death

   b. **True and feigned insanity**
   (Ref: Parikh's Textbook of Medical Jurisprudence, Forensic Medicine and Toxicology, 8/e, pg. 471, Reddy, 34/e, pg. 455)

ANSWER

True and Feigned Insanity

True insanity	False insanity
Gradual onset or rarely sudden but usually without any motive	Sudden onset and not without some motive
Predisposing or exciting cause may be present, e.g. family history of insanity, grief, sudden loss of money, etc.	No predisposing or exciting cause is usually present
Well-developed cases of insanity have a peculiar facial expression	Facial expression is generally normal even when the person pretends to be mad outright
The individual shows signs and symptoms of insanity irrespective of his conduct being observed or not	The individual pretends to be insane only when he is observed and there is total absence of symptoms when he is alone and unobserved

FORENSIC MEDICINE & TOXICOLOGY

Contd...

True insanity	False insanity
Signs and symptoms usually suggest a particular type of mental illness	Signs and symptoms are not uniform and do not suggest any particular type of mental illness
Can stand violent exertion for several hours or days without exhaustion, or sleep	Violent exertion leads to exhaustion, and sleep
Physical manifestations of true insanity, viz. dry, harsh skin, furred tongue, constipation, anorexia, and insomnia are present	Physical manifestations of true insanity, viz. dry, harsh skin, furred tongue, constipation, anorexia, and insomnia are not present
Not worried about being repeatedly examined	Dislike for repeated examination is obvious

c. Male and Female pelvis

(Ref: Parikh's Textbook of Medical Jurisprudence, Forensic Medicine and Toxicology, 8/e, pg. 82)

ANSWER

Male and Female Pelvis

Male pelvis	Female pelvis
Massive bony framework	Less massive bony framework
Inlet is Deep and narrow	Inlet is shallow and broad
Walls are not separated due to less expanded ilium	Walls are separated due to more expanded ilium
Anterior superior iliac spines are not separated widely	Anterior superior iliac spines are separated widely
V-shaped and narrow suprapubic arch, angle not more than 70°; distance between ischia is less	U-shaped and broad suprapubic arch, angle more than right angle, distance between ischia is more
Inverted ischial tuberosities	Everted ischial tuberosities
Obturator foramina is ovoid	Obturator foramina is triangular
Greater sciatic notch narrow, deep and less than a right angle	Greater sciatic notch broad, shallow and is almost a right angle
Wider and deeper acetabula	Narrow and shallow acetabula
Preauricular sulcus narrow, shallow and without marked edges	Preauricular sulcus broad, deep in a parous woman
Sacrum long and narrow, with five or more segments and well-marked promontory	Sacrum short and broad, with five segments and less marked promontory

PART-III

5. Define infanticide. Discuss in detail the post mortem findings of a live born foetus.

(Ref: Parikh's Textbook of Medical Jurisprudence, Forensic Medicine and Toxicology, 8/e, pg. 441, Reddy, 34/e, pg. 410)

ANSWER

Infanticide

Definition

- Unlawful destruction of a new born child, and is regarded as a murder in law
- Punishable under section 302 IPC, by death or transportation for life and also fine
- Differs from ordinary murder, as it is essential to prove that the child was born alive
- New born child means infant who is in first year of life
- Most commonly, infant is killed soon after birth
- Committed by
  - Unmarried women
  - Widows
  - Sometimes by married women also
  - In communities where dowry is prevalent, female infanticide is common
- Male infanticide is resorted to by prostitutes

Post Mortem Findings in Live Born Fetus

Live Born Fetus

- If a child exhibits signs of life such as crying, twitching of eyelids, movements of limbs, respirations and pulsations, after complete extrusion from the mother, though he may not have breathed or born completely

Signs of Live-birth

- In civil cases, proof of live birth is any sign of life after complete birth of the child seen by a witness such as a cry, movement of limb or body, contraction of muscle, movement or eye, pulsation of heart is felt etc.
- Vagitus uterinus – child may utter a cry in the uterus, Vagitus vaginalis – child may make a cry in vagina, which may be heard outside the delivery room and is due to rupture of membranes and air has gained entry to the uterus, and the infant has been aroused by asphyxia or some operative manipulation
- Muscles may twitch for certain time even after the body is dead as cellular life continues even after the death of the individual, hence it is not safe to believe that twitching of muscles is suggestive of life
- In criminal cases, signs of livebirth have to be determined by postmortem examination of the infant
- Internal examination may give strong, but not definite evidence of a livebirth

Degree of Maturity

○ In law, a foetus which has not attained the completion of the seventh month of intrauterine life is not viable unless excellent facilities for resuscitation are available

○ An immature infant weighs 2000 g or less at birth irrespective of the time of gestation

Viability

○ Stage of maturity at which a foetus with normal intrauterine development could maintain a separate existence after birth

○ Child is viable after 210 days or seven months if intrauterine life, and in some cases after 180 days or 6 months but in most of such cases the foetus is immature

Signs of Establishment of Respiration

○ **Shape of the chest:**
  ▪ Before respiration the chest is flat and its circumference is 1-2 cm less than the abdomen at the level of the umbilicus.
  ▪ Chest expands after respiration and becomes arched or drum shaped.

○ **The position of the diaphragm:**
  ▪ Abdomen should be opened before the thorax and the highest point of the diaphragm is observed which is located about the level of 4th or 5th rib if respiration has not taken place at the level of the 6th or 7th rib after breathing.
  ▪ It is influenced by decomposition gases.

○ **Lungs:**
  ▪ Breathing results in significant permanent changes in the lungs the extent of which is determined by the physical strength and period of respiration.

○ **Volume:**
  ▪ Non-respired lungs appear smaller being collapsed on to the hilum.
  ▪ Fully respired lungs fill the pleural cavities with the medial edges overlapping the mediastinum part of the pericardium.

○ **Margins:**
  ▪ The margins appear sharp before respiration and becomes round after respiration.
  ▪ Glistening bullae emerges along the margins.

○ **Consistency:**
  ▪ Dense, firm and non-crepitant lungs like liver before respiration.
  ▪ Become soft elastic, spongy and crepitant after respiration.

○ Colour and expansion of the air-vesicles:

▪ Uniformly reddish -brown or bluish red before respiration.
▪ Surface of the lobules is marked with shallow furrows
▪ Cut section appears uniform in colour and texture
▪ Distention of air cells with air after respiration and may be seen as polygon or angular areas on the surface of the lung giving it a fine mosaic appearance.

○ **Blood in the lung beds:**
  ▪ Amount of blood in the lung after respiration is around twice that in circulation before respiration.

○ **Weight:**
  ▪ **Static test or Fodere's test:**
    ◆ Lungs are ligated across their hila and separated.
    ◆ Average weight of both lungs before respiration varies between 30 g and 40 g and after respiration from 60 g to 66 g.
    ◆ Increase in weight is owing to increased blood flow.
  ▪ **Plocquet's test:**
    ◆ Blood flow in the lung bed is so increased after respiration that their weight is almost doubled from 1/70 of the body weight before respiration to 1/35 after respiration.
    ◆ Increase in weight is not constant and is not dependable sign of breathing

○ **Hydrostatic test**
  ▪ Hydrostatic test for live birth depends on changes in specific gravity of lungs due to respiration
  ▪ Specific gravity of non-respired lung is about 1050 i.e. heavier than water and that of a respired lung is about 950 i.e. lighter than water
  ▪ Non-respired lung sinks in water and respired lungs float
  ▪ If the test is positive – i.e. piece of lung floats in water then it means respiration has taken place
  ▪ **Findings:**
    ◆ Piece of lung floats in water – respiration has taken place
    ◆ If some pieces float while others sink that means feeble respiration
  ▪ **Medicolegal importance:**
    ◆ No value in forensic medicine as lungs of liveborn who has lived for few days may sink and lungs of still born may float
    ◆ Slightest degree of decomposition invalidates any interpretation of the floatation test
    ◆ Resuscitation attempts make evaluation of test difficult or even impossible

- ♦ Some expansion of air sacs of lungs in foetus does occur towards the end of pregnancy as a result of amniotic fluid moving in and out of bronchial tree
- ○ Changes in stomach and intestines
  - During respiration, air is swallowed into the stomach
  - After tying ligatures at each end of stomach and intestines, they are removed
  - If respiration has taken place, they will float otherwise they will sink
  - Also known as Breslau's second life test or stomach-bowel test
- ○ Changes in the middle ear
  - Also known as Wredin's test
  - Middle ear contains gelatinous embryonic connective tissue but no air, before birth
  - Sphincter at the pharyngeal end of eustachian tube relaxes with respiration and air replaces gelatinous substances in few hours to 5 weeks
  - After removing tegmen tympani, middle ear must be opened under water, a bubble of air will come out in case the test is positive

6. Write short notes on

a. Vitriolage

(Ref: Parikh's Textbook of Medical Jurisprudence, Forensic Medicine and Toxicology, 8/e, pg. 552, Reddy, 34/e, pg. 491)

ANSWER

Vitriolage

Definition

- ○ Throwing up of a corrosive on a person with spiteful intention, due to extreme dislike, jealousy or vengeance in order to seek revenge
- ○ Corrosive (not necessarily sulphuric acid) fluids are generally thrown on the face with intent of damaging vision or causing facial disfigurement causing grievous hurt
- ○ Most frequently used corrosive for this purpose is Sulphuric acid (oil of vitriol) and therefore called as Vitriolage
- ○ Sometimes Nitric acid and carbolic acids are also employed and use of caustic soda, caustic potash, iodine and marking nut juice has also seen

Effects

- ○ Severe chemical burns characterized by discoloration and staining of skin and clothing
- ○ Trickle marks

- ○ Absence of vesication and red line of demarcation
- ○ Presence of chemical substances in the stains

Treatment

- ○ Washing away of the corrosive immediately with large amount of water and soap or dilute solution of sodium or potassium bicarbonate
- ○ Then, a thick paste of magnesium oxide is applied
- ○ Raw surface can be covered with antibiotic ointment
- ○ If eyes are involved, they should be immediately washed with large amount of water followed by irrigation with 1% solution of sodium bicarbonate
- ○ Few drops of olive oil are instilled in the eyes
- ○ Eyedrops comprising antibiotics and steroids are beneficial

b. Atypical hanging

(Ref: Parikh's Textbook of Medical Jurisprudence, Forensic Medicine and Toxicology, 8/e, pg. 180, Reddy, 34/e, pg. 315)

ANSWER

Atypical Hanging

Introduction

- ○ Hanging is a form of asphyxia caused by suspension of the body by a ligature surrounding the neck, constricting force being the weight of the body
- ○ Atypical hanging – when the knot of ligature is anywhere else than on the occiput i. e on left or right or front of the neck

Cause of Death in Hanging

- ○ Asphyxia—owing to narrowing of laryngeal and tracheal lumina
- ○ Venous congestion—blockage of jugular veins
- ○ Combined venous congestion and asphyxia
- ○ Cerebral anemia—due to blockage of carotid artery
- ○ Reflex vagal inhibition causing sudden cardiac arrest
- ○ Fracture/dislocation of cervical vertebrae—observed in judicial hanging

Findings

External Appearance

- ○ Dribbling of saliva from corner of mouth opposite to the side on the knot due to pressure on salivary glands by the ligature
- ○ Neck is stretched due to upward pull of ligature and head is inclined to opposite side on knot
- ○ Pale face or congested and swollen with profuse petechiae in head and neck
- ○ Cyanosed hands and nail beds
- ○ Eyeballs prominent due to congestion
- ○ Tongue turgid or protruded and becomes dark brown or almost black

- Petechial haemorrhages on arms and legs
- Postmortem lividity seen on arms and legs and face and neck
- Ligature mark on the neck—above the level of thyroid cartilage between the larynx and chin

Internal Appearance

- Hyperaernia of the trachea and epiglottis
- Lymph nodes above or below the ligature mark present evidence of congestion and haemorrhage
- Frictional intimal tears of carotid arteries with sub-intimal haemorrhage
- Dissection of neck under the ligature mark exposes a dry and compressed white band of subcutaneous tissue with a few petechial haemorrhages into or around its substance and occasionally a few ecchymoses

Medicolegal Importance

- Whether death was due to hanging
- Whether it was suicidal, accidental or homicidal hanging

  c.   Vicarious Liability

  (Ref: Parikh's Textbook of Medical Jurisprudence, Forensic Medicine and Toxicology, 8/e, pg. 44, Reddy, 34/e, pg. 45)

ANSWER

Vicarious Liability

Definition

- Liability exists in spite of the absence of culpable conduct on the part of the master

- According to law, the master is held responsible for the negligent acts of his servants within the scope of his employment but in not so liable where he has employed an independent person to do something for him
- Hospital and nursing homes are liable for the negligent acts and omissions of their non-medical staff and full time junior medical staff but senior medical staff and honorary medical staff are in different position as there is not true relationship of a master and servant between them and managers of hospital
- Hospital management is held responsible for negligent acts of resident physicians and interns in training as they are considered employees while performing their normal duties
- Hospital management is not held responsible for negligent acts of senior medical staff, as they had employed well qualified and experienced staff
- Physician is held responsible for the acts of residents and interns carried out under his immediate direction and control
- Physicians and surgeons are not responsible for acts of qualified nurses unless such acts are carried out under their guidance
- Physician is held responsible under the doctrine of negligent choice, if he refers his patient to an incompetent or inappropriate doctor, otherwise he is not so responsible

Pathology

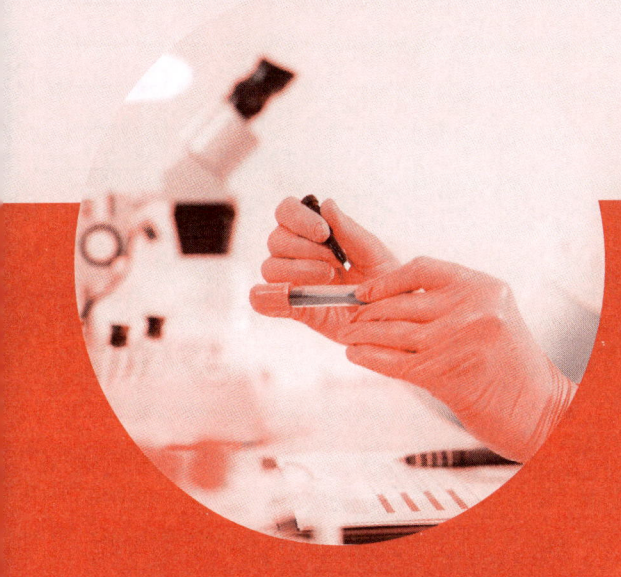

References Taken From:

- *Textbook of Pathology Harsh Mohan, 7th edition*
- *Robbins Pathologic Basis of Disease-South Asia edition*

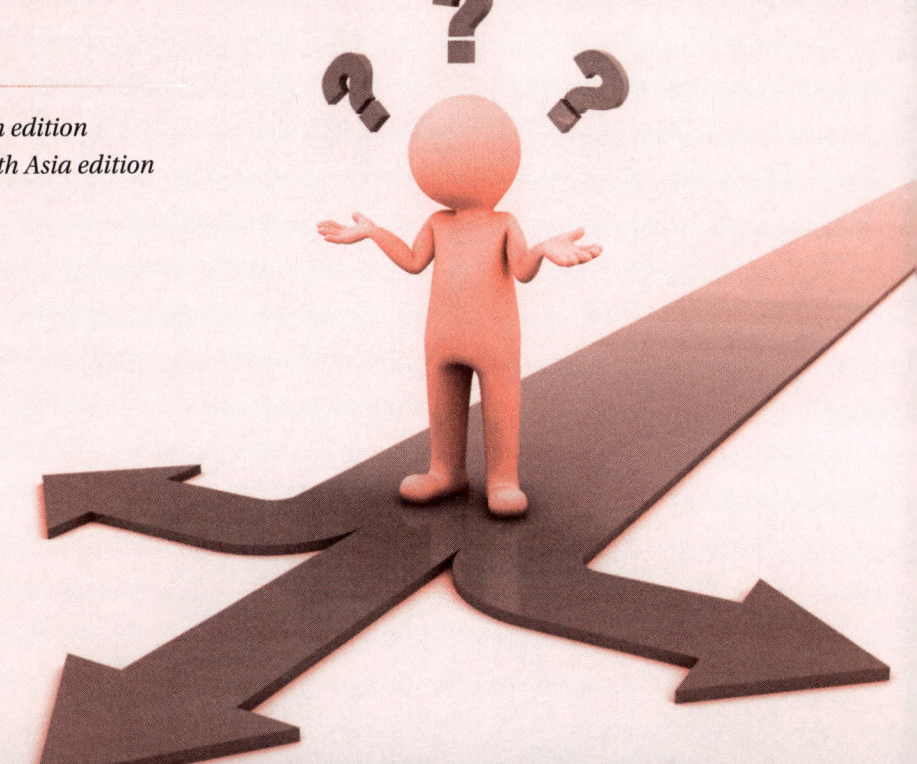

Your Roll No. ....

Name of the Paper	:	Pathology Paper-I
Name of the Course	:	MBBS-2017
Semester	:	Annual

Time: 3 Hours   M.M.: 40

INSTRUCTIONS

1. Write your Roll No. on the top immediately on receipt of this question paper
2. All questions are to be attempted
3. Answers to Parts I, II and III should be written in separate answer sheets provided
4. Attempt parts of a question in sequence

PART-I

1. **Differentiate between:**   [8]
   a. Laboratory findings in obstructive and hepatocellular jaundice
   b. Transudate and exudate
   c. Leukemoid reaction and chronic myeloid leukemia
   d. Primary and secondary amyloidosis

2. **Write briefly on:**   [6]
   a. Klinefelter syndrome
   b. Mechanisms of autoimmunity
   c. Chemical carcinogenesis

PART-II

3. **Write briefly on:**   [6]
   a. Causes of intravascular hemolysis and laboratory diagnosis of G6 PD deficiency
   b. Laboratory diagnosis of acute lymphoblastic leukemia

4. **Write briefly on:**   [6]
   a. Cause of thrombocytopenia and laboratory diagnosis of ITP
   b. Laboratory diagnosis of multiple myeloma

PART-III

5. **Write short note on:**   [8]
   a. Phagocytosis
   b. Complications of wound healing
   c. Tumor markers
   d. Acute radiation injury

6. **Write short notes on:**   [6]
   a. Transfusion reaction
   b. Activated partial thromboplastin time (aPTT)
   c. Hemolytic disease of newborn

PART-I

1. Differentiate between:

a. Laboratory findings in obstructive and hepatocellular jaundice

(Ref: Harsh Mohan, 7th ed. pg. 584, Robbins, SA ed. pg. 853)

ANSWER

Lab Findings in Obstructive and Hepatocellular Jaundice

Obstructive jaundice lab findings	Hepatocellular jaundice lab findings
• Conjugated bilirubin present in plasma	• Both conjugated and unconjugated bilirubin present
• Van den Bergh test is direct positive	• Van den Bergh test is biphasic
• Albumin decreases in later stages	• Decreased albumin
• Normal globulin	• Globulin increased
• A:G ratio normal usually	• A:G ratio decreased
• ALP/GGT markedly raised	• ALP/GGT slightly raised
• SGOP/AST slightly raised/ normal	• SGOP/AST markedly elevated
• SGPT/ALT slightly raised/ normal	• SGPT/ALT markedly raised
• Urobilinogen absent in complete obstruction	• Urobilinogen decreased
• Fat is markedly increased	• Fat is increased
• **Fecal stercobilinogen absent in complete obstruction**	• Fecal stercobilinogen reduced

b. Transudate and exudate

(Ref: THarsh Mohan, 7th ed. pg. 81, Robbins, SA ed. pg. 73)

ANSWER

Exudate and Transudate

Exudate	Transudate
• Associated with increased vascular permeability	• No change in endothelial permeability
• Protein content low (>3g/dL), high fibrinogen	• Protein content low (<3g/dL), low fibrinogen
• Specific gravity high(>1.015)	• Specific gravity is low(<1.015)
• LDH is high	• LDH low
• pH <7.3	• pH> 7.3

Exudate	Transudate
• Example- congestive heart failure, Uremia, myocardial infarction, or acute rheumatic fever.	• Example- malignancies, infections, Nephrotic syndrome or chronic liver disease

c. Leukemoid reaction and chronic myeloid leukemia

(Ref: Harsh Mohan, 7th ed. pg. 332, Robbins, SA ed. pg. 616)

ANSWER

Chronic Myeloid Reaction (CML) and Leukemoid Reaction

Features	CML	Leukemoid Reaction
• Etiology	• Clonal disorder	• Infections
• Total leucocyte count	• >50,000/cc	• <50,000/cc
• Immature cells	• Present, > 30%	• Present,< 5-10%
• Toxic granules	• Absent	• Present
• Dohle's bodies	• Absent	• Present
• Cytogenetics	• Presence of Philadelphia chromosome	• Absent
• Platelet	• Increased	• Normal or may be increased
• Splenomegaly	• Present	• Absent

d. Primary and secondary amyloidosis

(Ref: Harsh Mohan, 7th ed. pg. 71, Robbins, SA ed. pg. 258)

ANSWER

Primary and Secondary Amyloidosis

Primary amyloidosis	Secondary amyloidosis
• Common form of amyloidosis	• Less common as compared to primary amyloidosis
• Commonly affects skin, bowel, heart, skeletal muscle,etc.	• Solid visceral abdominal organs like- liver, kidney, spleen, adrenals, etc. affected
• Composed of light chain protein (AL)	• Composed of amyloid associated protein (AA)
• Commonly occurs in more than 40 yrs of age	• Can occur at any age including children
• Associated with plasma cell dyscrasias, like- multiple myeloma, B cell lymphomas, etc.	• Associated with chronic inflammation, like – infections, autoimmune diseases, cancers, etc.
• After treatment with permanganate, persistence of congophilia	• After treatment with permanganate, congophilia disappears.

2. **Write briefly on:**

    a. **Klinefelter syndrome**

ANSWER

Kinefelter Syndrome

(Ref: Textbook of Pathology, Harsh Mohan, 7th ed. pg. 253, Robbins, SA ed. pg. 185)

Introduction

- Male hypogonadism as a result of two or more X chromosome and one or more Y chromosome
- Sex chromosome trisomy

Pathogenesis

- Presence of extra (more than one) X or Y chromosome to a male karyotype give rise to abnormalities (both physical and cognitive)

Genetic Abnormality

- 47, XXY karyotype- classical type
- 46, XY/47, XXY, 47, XXY/48, XXXY- mosaic patterns

Clinical Features

- Most common in males
- Hypogonadism and infertility
- Long arms and legs
- "Eunuchoid body habitus" (long legs with increased length between soles and pubic bone)
- Sparse facial and axillary hair along with high pitched voice
- Gynecomastia and testicular atrophy
- Learning disability (IQ lower than normal)
- Increased risk of breast cancer, AML, deep vein thrombosis and pulmonary embolism
- Hormonal changes:
- Dysgenesis of seminiferous tubules → decreases inhibin B → Increases FSH.
- Abnormal Leydig cell function → decreases testosterone → Increases LH → Increases estrogen.

Treatment

- Testosterone supplementation (beginning of puberty)- for proper development of sexual characteristics, muscle bulk and bone structure.

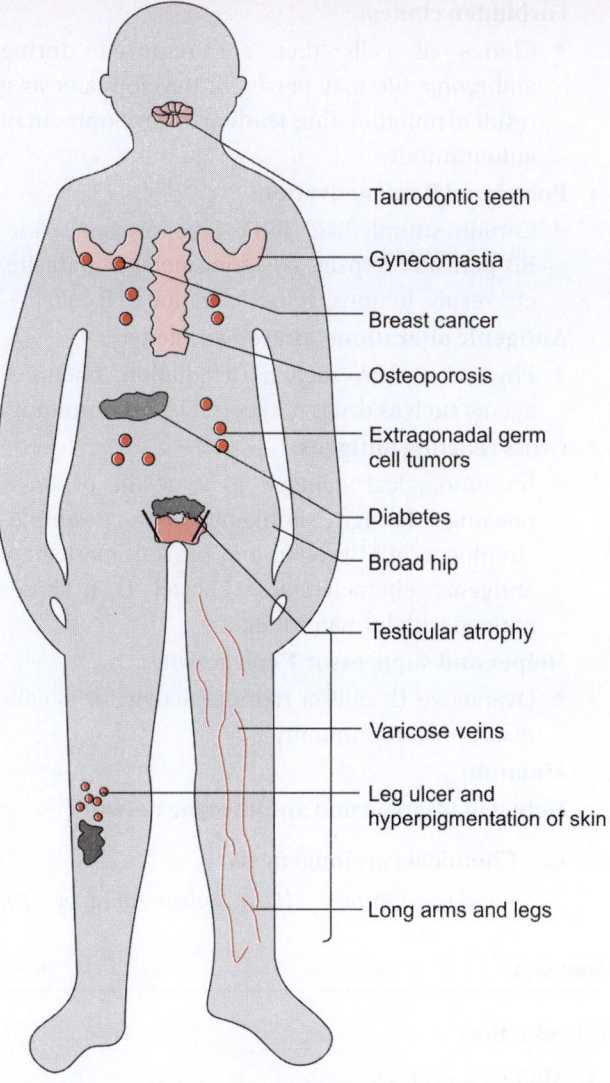

- Taurodontic teeth
- Gynecomastia
- Breast cancer
- Osteoporosis
- Extragonadal germ cell tumors
- Diabetes
- Broad hip
- Testicular atrophy
- Varicose veins
- Leg ulcer and hyperpigmentation of skin
- Long arms and legs

Fig. Klinefelter syndrome

b. **Mechanism of autoimmunity**

(Ref: Textbook of Microbiology, 5th/e, pg. 164, Robbins, SA ed. pg. 214)

ANSWER

Different Mechanism Responsible for Autoimmunity

- **Hidden or sequestered antigen:**
  - Certain self-antigen in embryonic life are present in close system and when exposed results in autoimmunity
  - **Examples:** Lens antigen of the eye, sperm antigen

- ○ **Forbidden clones:**
  - ▪ Clones of cells that are removed during embryonic life may persist or develop later as a result of mutation thus leading to development of autoimmunity
- ○ **Polyclonal B cell activation:**
  - ▪ Certain stimuli like- PPD, Lipopolysaccharide, EB parasite, trypsin, nystatin, malarial parasite, etc. results in nonspecific activation of B cells.
- ○ **Antigenic alterations/altered antigens:**
  - ▪ Physical agents, such as irradiation, chemical agents such as drugs may result in autoimmunity
- ○ **Cross reacting antigens:**
  - ▪ Immunological damage as a result of cross reacting foreign antigens. For example- streptococcal M protein and heart of man share antigenic characteristics, E. coli O14 shares antigen with human colon.
- ○ **Helper and suppressor T cell activity:**
  - ▪ Overactive Th cells or reduced activity of Ts cells results in autoimmunity
- ○ **Mutation**
- ○ **Defect in idiotype and antiidiotype network**

  c. **Chemical carcinogenesis**

  (Textbook of Patholoy, Harsh Mohan, 7th ed. pg. 210)

ANSWER

Introduction

- ○ Multistep process
- ○ Results due to mutation in the proto-oncogene and anti-oncogene

Stages of Chemical Carcinogenesis

Involve 3 stages

- ○ **Initiation:**
  - ▪ Induced by initiator chemical carcinogens
  - ▪ Causes permanent, irreversible damage
  - ▪ Not sufficient for tumor formation
- ○ **Promotion:**
  - ▪ Substances like phenols, artificial sweeteners, hormones, etc. act as promoters of carcinogenesis
  - ▪ No sudden change by promoters
  - ▪ No direct effect on DNA
  - ▪ Induced changes are reversible
  - ▪ Initiated cells may result in tumor
- ○ **Progression:**
  - ▪ Due to continuous formation of unstable chromosomes
  - ▪ Mutation due to genetic instability during promotion results in development of cells that inherit genetic and biochemical characteristics of malignancy

Chemical Carcinogens

- ○ **Direct-acting carcinogens:**
  - ▪ **Alkylating agents:** Anticancer drugs (cyclophosphamide, chlorambucil, etc.), epoxides, β-propiolactone
  - ▪ **Acylating agents:** Acetyl imidazole, dimethyl carbamyl chloride
- ○ **Indirect-acting carcinogens:**
  - ▪ Polycyclic aromatic hydrocarbons (in smoke, fossil fuel, tobacco, mineral oil, etc.): anthracenes, benzapyrene, etc.
  - ▪ **Aromatic amines, and azo dyes:** Benzidine, β-naphthylamine
  - ▪ **Naturally occurring products:** Betal nuts, actinomycin D, aflatoxin BI
  - ▪ **Miscellaneous:** Nitrosamines, nitrosamides, asbestos, arsenical compounds, etc.

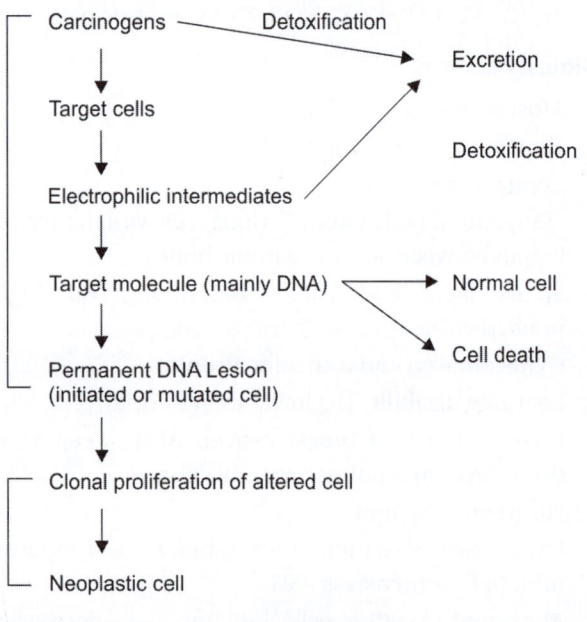

PART-II

3. **Write briefly on:**

   a. **Causes of intravascular hemolysis and laboratory diagnosis of G_6 PD deficiency**

   (Ref: Harsh Mohan, 7th ed. pg. 288, 293, Robbins, SA ed. pg. 631)

ANSWER

Causes of Intravascular Hemolysis

- ○ Lysis of red cells in the circulation and release of contents into the plasma
- ○ Marked increase in plasma hemoglobin

- Microangiopathic hemolytic anemia (sickle cell anemia, DIC, TTP)
- Autoimmune hemolytic anemia (AIHA)
- Thermal injury
- Mechanical trauma to red cells
- Paroxysmal nocturnal hemoglobinuria (PNH)
- G6PD deficiency
- Pregnancy induced hypertension (PIH)
- **Infections:** Malarial, bacterial, etc.

Laboratory diagnosis of G6 PD deficiency

Laboratory Findings

- **In normal phase:**
  - No anemia
  - Reduced red cell survival
- **In hemolytic phase:**
  - Intravascular hemolysis
  - Decreased hematocrit (25-30%)
  - Peripheral blood smear: Presence of -
    - Heinz bodies: dark inclusion within cells
    - Bite cells
    - Blister cells

Diagnosis: screening tests:

- **Indirect tests:**
  - Methemoglobin reduction test
  - Fluorescent screening test
  - Ascorbate cyanide screening test
- **Direct enzyme assay of red cell:**
  - In case of low enzyme level

b. **Laboratory diagnosis of acute lymphoblastic leukaemia**

(Ref: Harsh Mohan, 7th ed. pg. 353, Robbins, SA ed. pg. 590)

ANSWER

Introduction

- Malignancy of immature B (pre-B) or T(pre-T) cells
- Most common cancer of children (under 4 yrs of age)
- T-cell ALL can present as mediastinal mass (presenting as SVC-like syndrome).
- Associated with Down syndrome.

Laboratory Diagnosis

- **Complete blood count:**
  - Decreased hemoglobin
  - **Hematocrit:** Decreased
  - **Platelet count:** Reduced
  - **RBC count:** Decreased
  - **TLC:** Markedly increased
- **Peripheral blood smear:**
  - Marked leukocytosis (blast cells)

- High nucleo-cytoplasmic ratio with no cytoplasmic granularity
- Normocytic normochromic red cells
- Presence of smear cells"(degenerated leucocytes)

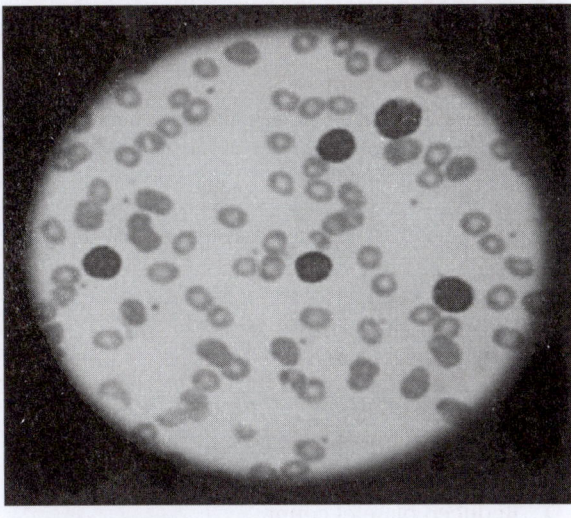

- **Bone marrow examination:**
  - **Bone marrow:** Hypercellular (mainly blast)
  - Decreased myeloid and erythroid precursors
  - Dyserythropoiesis
- **Cytochemistry:**
  - **PAS:** Positive
  - **MPO and Sudan black:** Negative
  - **Acid Phosphatase:** Focal positivity
- **Immunophenotyping:**
  - **Pre B cell:** CD19, CD10
  - **Pre T cell:** positive for CD1, CD2, CD3, CD5 and CD7
- **Cytogenetic analysis:**
  - Hyperploidy
  - Cytogenetic abnormality of (9; 22)
  - Philadelphia positive
- **Serum markers:**
  - **LDH:** Increased
  - **Uric acid:** Increased
  - **Phosphate:** Increased
  - **Calcium:** Decreased
- **Radiology:**
  - Leukemic lines in long bones

4. **Write briefly on:**

a. **Causes of thrombocytopenia and laboratory diagnosis of ITP**

(Ref: Harsh Mohan, 7th ed. pg. 310, Robbins, SA ed. pg. 657)

ANSWER

Introduction

- Thrombocytopenia is decreased blood platelet count (below 150,000/µl), i.e. below the lower limit of normal

Causes of Thrombocytopenia

Impaired/decreased platelet production	Increased platelet destruction and consumption	Splenic sequestration	Dilutional loss
Bone marrow failure, aplastic anemia, leukemia, myelofibrosis, marrow infiltrations	Idiopathic thrombocytopenic purpura, neonatal alloimmune thrombocytopenia, SLE,CLL, lymphoma,DIC, TTP, giant hemangiomas, sepsis	Hypersplenism- infection, inflammation, Red cell disorders, storage disease	Massive transfusion of blood
Drugs (quinine, sulfonamides, PAS) infection(CMV, Epstein barr virus, etc.)		Increase pooling in spleen	

Laboratory Diagnosis of ITP

- Large-sized platelets
- Reduced platelet count
- Reduced platelet life span
- Bone marrow findings: increased megakaryocytes with single non-lobulated nuclei and presence of cytoplasmic vacuoles along with decreased cytoplasmic granularity
- Presence of anti-platelet IgG antibody on platelet surface

b. Laboratory Diagnosis of Multiple Myeloma

(Ref: Harsh Mohan, 7th ed. pg. 363, Robbins, SA ed. pg. 600)

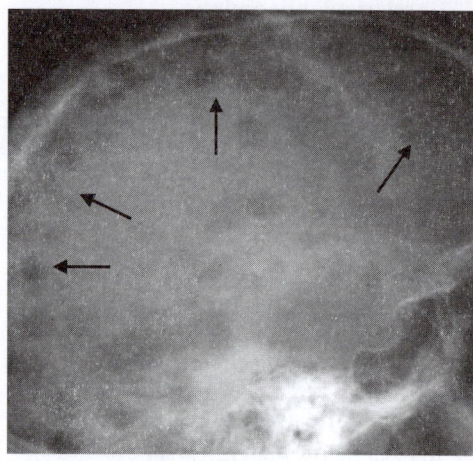

Fig. Lytic lesions

ANSWER

Introduction

- Clonal proliferation of malignant plasma cells with excessive production of monoclonal immunoglobulins (typically ineffective IgA or IgG) or immunoglobulin fragments (kappa/lambda light chains). MM primarily affects the elderly, peaking in the seventh decade. Risk factors include radiation, monoclonal gammopathy of undetermined significance (MGUS), and, possibly, petroleum products and pesticides.

History

- Seventy percent of MM patients present with bone pain or with a pathologic fracture (MM cells in filtrate bone marrow, where they activate osteoclasts, creating lytic lesions and weak bones). Anemia, hypercalcemia, and renal abnormalities are also seen.
- Patients are prone to infection (IgG and IgA produced by myeloma cells are monoclonal, thus making them ineffective) and have elevated monoclonal (M) proteins in the serum and/or urine

Diagnosis

- **Best initial test:** Serum protein electrophoresis showing IgG or IgA monoclonal spikes

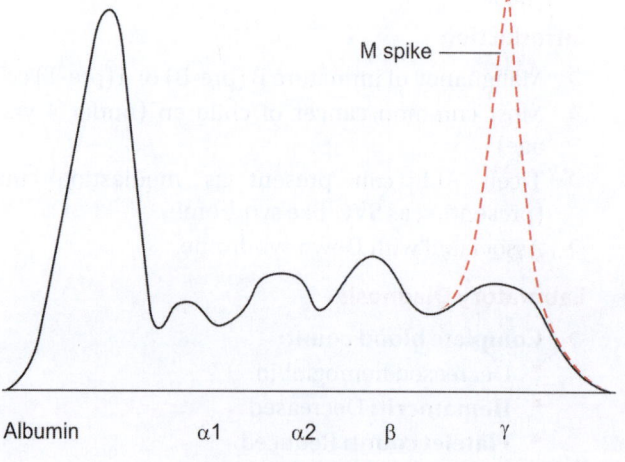

Fig. Monoclonal spikes

- **Most accurate test:** Bone marrow biopsy **showing > 10% monoclonal** CD138+ plasma cells.

- CBC with smear may show **Rouleaux** formation, Numerous plasma cells C with **"clock-face"** chromatin and intracytoplasmic inclusions containing immunoglobulin, whereas a urinalysis may show **Bence Jones protein** (paraprotein). **Total protein: albumin gap is often elevated.**

- M protein alone is insufficient for the diagnosis of MM, as MGUS, CLL, lymphoma, Waldenström macroglobulinemia, and amyloidosis can also ↑M protein.

- Patients should also be evaluated with a skeletal survey.

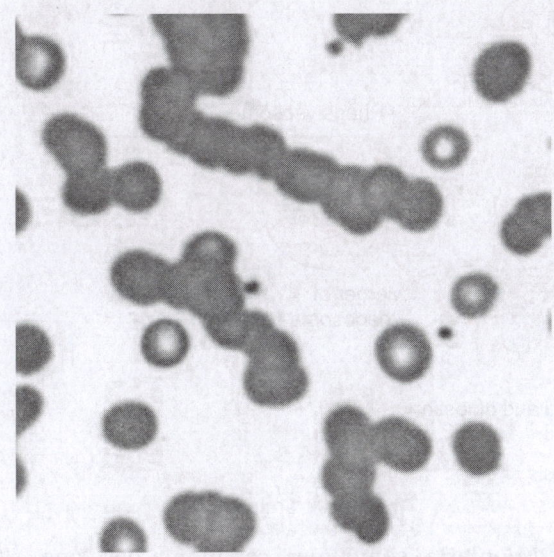

Fig. Rouleaux formation

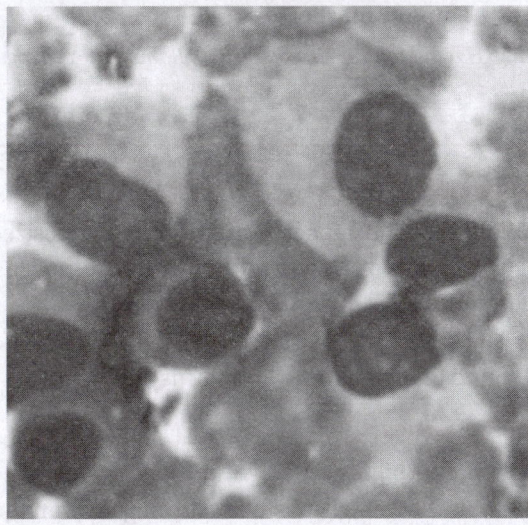

Fig. Numerous plasma cells

Treatment

- Young patients (< 70 years) can be treated with an autologous bone marrow transplant.

- Older patients are treated with melphalan (an oral alkylating agent) and prednisone.

PART-III

5. Write short note on:

a. **Phagocytosis**

(Ref: Harsh Mohan, 7th ed. pg. 120, Robbins, SA ed. pg. 9-10)

ANSWER

Introduction

- Defined as the process of ingestion or engulfment of solid particulate material by the cells

- Cells responsible for phagocytosis are called "phagocytes"

- Mainly, 2 types of phagocytes:
  - Polymorhonuclear leucocytes
  - Monocytes and macrophages

- **It involves three stages:**
  - Recognition and attachment
  - Engulfment
  - Killing and degradation

Recognition and Attachment

- Initiated by receptors expressed on the surface of leucocyte

- Mannose and scavenger receptors responsible for recognition of micro-organism

- **Opsonisation and Opsonins:** Process of coating of micro-organisms with specific proteins (opsonins) and the process is called opsonisation

- **Opsonins:** Fc portion of IgG(naturally occurring antibodies against bacteria), C3b (strongly chemotactic for attracting PMNs to bacteria), lectins (carbohydrate binding protein)

Engulfment

- Formation of cytoplasmic pseudopods and engulfment of opsonized particles

- Eventually, formation of phagocytic vacuoles or phagosome

- Fusion of lysosome of the cells and formation f phagolysosome

Killing and Degradation

- Mechanisms involved in killing and degradation as follows:
  - **Intracellular mechanism:** oxidative mechanism commonly involved in killing of micro-organism
    - **Oxidative bactericidal mechanism:**
      - Production of reactive oxygen metabolites (H_2O_2, HOCl, OH, O_2 etc.)
      - Bactericidal activity may be myeloperoxidase- dependent (present in azurophilic

PATHOLOGY

granules of neutrophils and monocytes) or myeloperoxidase-independent

- □ MPO- independent killing:

  $H_2O_2 \rightarrow OH'$ Presence of Fe Or O_2

- □ MPO-dependent killing

  $H_2O_2 \rightarrow HOCL + H_2O$ in presence of halides (cl', I', Br')

- **Non- Oxidative bactericidal mechanism:**
  - □ Certain granules like–lysosomal hydro-lase, lipases, proteases, etc.don't require oxygen for bacerticidal activity
- **Extracellular mechanism:**
  - ◆ Granules exerts its effect of proteolysis outside the cell.

- ◆ Immune- mediated lysis of micro-organism by cytolysis, antibody-mediated lysis and by cell-mediated cytotoxicity

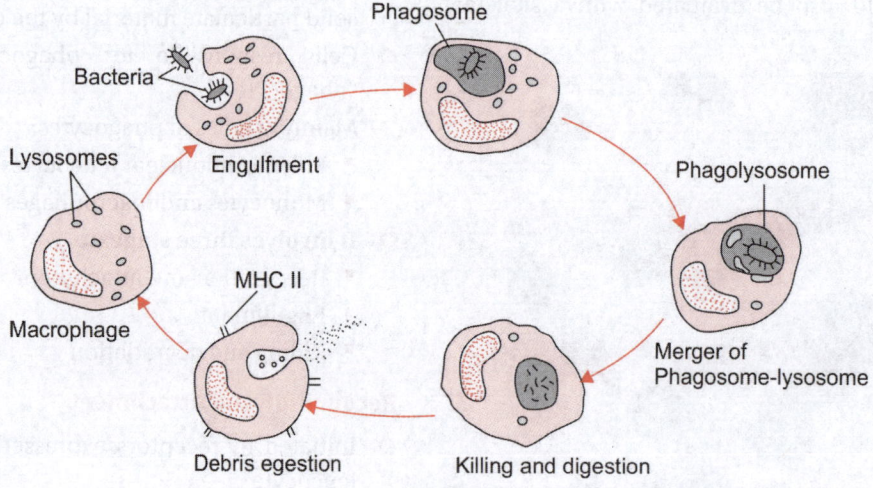

Fig. Phagocytosis

b. **Complications of wound healing**

(Ref: Harsh Mohan, 7th ed. pg. 159, Robbins, SA ed. pg. 109)

ANSWER

Complications of Wound Healing

- ○ **Hemorrhage:** Can be external or internal
- ○ **Infection:** As a result of bacteria that delays wound healing
- ○ **Deficient scar formation:** due to presence of inadequate granulation tissue
- ○ **Dehiscence:** stress on wound(coughing, vomiting, abdominal distension) resulting in separation of wound layers
- ○ **Implantation** cyst(epidermal cyst): Presence of epithelial cells after healing
- ○ **Pigmentation:** Hemosiderin may impart rust color to the healed wound
- ○ **Fistula**
- ○ **Hypertrophied scar and kleoid formation:** Formation of excessive collagen at the healing site result in keloid(claw-like) formation
- ○ **Contractures formation:** result in wound and surrounding tissue deformities

○ **Neoplasia:** sometimes, carcinoma develops at the site of scar formation, eg, Marjolin's ulcer

c. **Tumour markers**

(Ref: Harsh Mohan, 7th ed. pg. 229, Robbins, SA ed. pg. 337)

ANSWER

Introduction

- ○ Biological substances present in or synthesized by tumor itself or produced by host in response to a tumor
- ○ Usually proteins
- ○ Found in blood, urine or body tissues

Ideal Properties

- ○ Should be highly sensitive and specific
- ○ Should have high positive and negative predictive value
- ○ It should be able to differentiate between neoplastic and non-neoplastic disease
- ○ Should predict early recurrence and
- ○ Should have prognostic value
- ○ Clinically sensitive i.e., detectable at early stage of tumor
- ○ It should be easily assayable

Clinically Useful Tumor Markers

Alpha-fetoprotein (AFP)	Hepatoma, non-seminomatous testicular germ cell tumors, Yolk sac (endodermal sinus) tumor
Beta human chorionic gonadotropin (hCG)	Hydatidiform moles, Trophoblastic tumors, choriocarcinoma, Dysgerminoma
Calcitonin	Medullary carcinoma of the thyroid (alone and in MEN2A, MEN2B).
Carcinoembryonic antigen (CEA)	• **Major associations:** Colorectal and pancreatic cancers. • **Minor associations:** Gastric, breast, and medullary thyroid carcinomas.
CA-125	Malignant ovarian epithelial tumors
CA19-9	Malignant pancreatic adenocarcinoma
Placental Alkaline Phosphatase (ALP)	Seminoma, Metastases to bone or liver, Paget disease of bone
Prostate specific antigen (PSA)	Prostate cancer
Chromogranin	Neuroendocrine tumors
CA 15–3/CA 27–29	Breast cancer

d. Acute radiation injury

(Ref: Harsh Mohan, 7th ed. pg. 16, Robbins, SA ed. pg. 428)

ANSWER

Introduction

- Also known as "acute radiation syndrome"
- DNA damage by ionizing radiation
- Usually reversible (acute injuries)

Sign and Symptoms

- Depend on the degree or dose of radiation exposure
- Onset of symptoms depends on the dose of radiation

Phases

- Prodromal or initial
- Latent phase
- Manifest illness
- Recovery

Manifestations

- Hematopoietic syndrome
- Gastrointestinal syndrome
- Neurovascular syndrome

Hematopoietic Syndrome

- Nausea, vomiting, hemorrhage, weakness, neutropenic fever, sepsis etc.

Gastrointestinal Syndrome

- Loss of absorptive capacity
- Severe nausea, vomiting, fever, diarrhea, weakness
- Manifest illness phase - bloody diarrhea, anemia, cardiovascular collapse, shock, etc.

Neurovascular Syndrome

- Hypotension
- Loss of balance
- Confusion
- Respiratory distress
- Gross CNS sign, etc.

Low Doses

- Onset within 1 -6 hours, medium doses: onset within minutes, high doses: immediate onset of symptoms

Small Doses

- Nausea, vomiting, anorexia, diarrhea, fever, abdominal pain, low blood counts and bleeding.

Large Dose

- Headache, neurological symptoms, seizures, ataxia, severe fever and death.

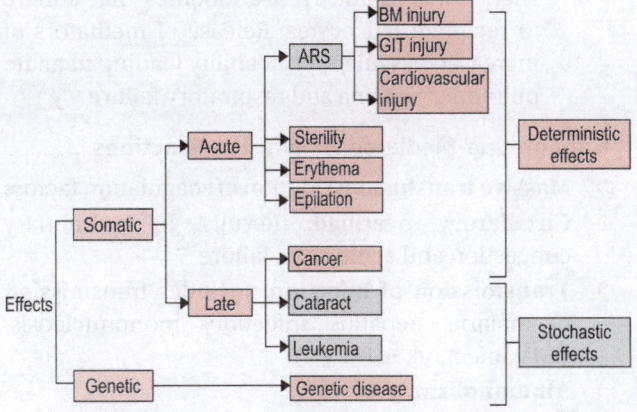

Fig. Human health effects of radiation exposure

Diagnosis

- History of radiation exposure
- Clinical symptoms.
- Blood test- to assess white blood cell count, especially if present with nausea and vomiting.

Treatment

- Blood transfusions—increase white blood cell count
- Antibiotics—to control infection
- Stem cell transplants

6. Write short notes on:

a. Transfusion reaction

(Ref: Textbook of Pathology, Harsh Mohan, 7th ed. pg. 318, Robbins, SA ed. pg. 665)

ANSWER

Two Types of Transfusion Reaction

- Immunological transfusion reaction
- Non- immunological transfusion reaction

Immune-Mediated Reaction

Are as follows:

- **Hemolytic transfusion reaction:**
  - Transfusion of mismatched blood due to ABO incompatibility
  - ABO isoagglutinins are responsible for most of the reactions
  - Severe intravascular hemolysis
  - Immune antibodies of the Rh system results in extravascular hemolysis
  - Delayed reactions results 1 to 4 weeks after the transfusion
  - Delayed reaction is less severe
  - Other reactions besides hemolytic transfusion reaction are: allergic reactions, graft-versus-host disease, anaphylactic shock, etc.
  - **Transfusion related acute lung injury (TRALI):** High levels of anti-HLA antibodies that adhere to recipient leucocytes. Release of mediators of increased vascular permeability leading to acute pulmonary edema and respiratory failure

Nonimmune-Mediated Transfusion Reactions

- **Massive transfusion:** Dilution of coagulation factors
- **Circulatory overload:** Results in pulmonary congestion and acute heart failure
- **Transmission of infection:** Includes transmission of malaria, hepatitis, infectious mononucleosis, CMV infection, AIDS, etc.
- **Air embolism**
- **Thrombophlebitis**
- **Transfusion hemosiderosis:** Occur after repeated transfusions, mainly in thalassaemia major, severe chronic refractory anemia

Lab Diagnosis of Acute Hemolytic Transfusion Reaction

- Increased serum LDH
- Decreased serum haptoglobin
- Serum indirect bilirubin level is increased
- Coomb's test for antibody detection

Lab Diagnosis of Allergic Transfusion Reaction

- **Serum IgA:** For screening test
- **Mast cell tryptase test:** Indicator of mast cell activation

Lab Diagnosis of Delayed Hemolytic Transfusion Reaction

- Increased LDH
- Increased bilirubin
- Decreased serum haptoglobin
- Reticulocytosis
- Direct antiglobulin test positive
- Prothombin time may be elevated (mainly in DIC)

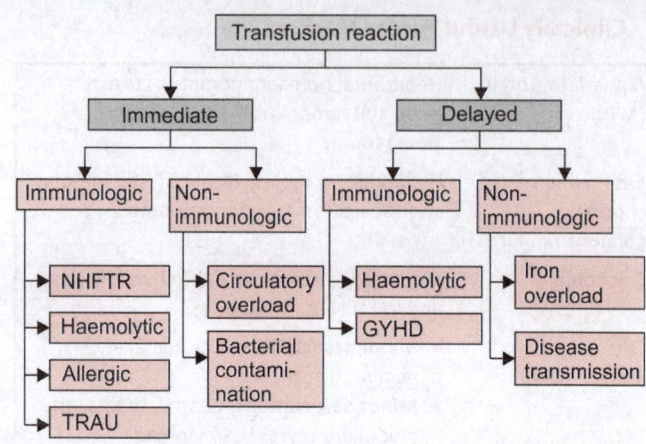

b. Activated partial thromboplastin time (aPTT)

(Ref: Textbook of Pathology, Harsh Mohan, 7th ed. pg. 307)

ANSWER

- It is the time taken in clotting of blood after addition of phospholipid (activator) along with calcium to it.
- Also known as "Kaolin Cephalin Clotting Time" or "Partial Thromboplastin Time with Kaolin"
- Screening test to assess the overall integrity of the intrinsic/common coagulation pathway
- Used in the assessment of heparin therapy
- **Method:** clotting time is observed after addition of three substances- phospholipid, calcium and a surface activator such as kaolin to the plasma
- Tissue factor III is not added to the mixture, thus termed "partial"

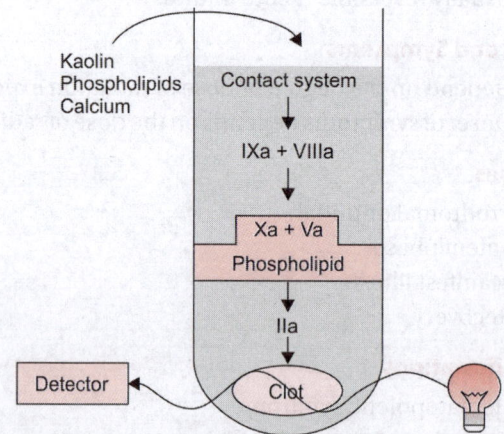

Fig. Kaolin cephalin clotting time

- **Normal value:** 30-40 seconds
- **Increased in:**
  - Heparin therapy
  - DIC
  - Hemophilia A and B
  - Vitamin K deficiency
  - Liver diseases
  - Oral anticoagulant therapy

c. Haemolytic disease of newborn

(Ref: Harsh Mohan, 7th ed. pg. 319, Robbins, SA ed. pg. 462)

ANSWER

Introduction

- Also known as "Erythroblastosis fetalis"
- Due to blood group incompatibility between mother and child
- As a result of passage of antibodies (IgG) from the mother across the placenta into the fetal circulation
- **Two forms:**
  - HDN due to Rh-D incompatibility
  - HDN due to ABO incompatibility
- **HDN due to Rh-D incompatibility:**
  - Causes severe form of HDN
  - Sensitisation of Rh- negative mother to Rh-positive blood results in Rh incompatibility
  - Usually, passage of Rh – positive red cells from Rh-positive fetus across the placenta into the circulation of Rh-negative mother.
- **HDN due to ABO incompatibility:**
  - Common than Rh incompatibility
  - Common in infants born to group O mothers, having anti-A and/or anti-B IgG antibodies.
  - Negative coomb's test
  - Less severe

Pathogenesis

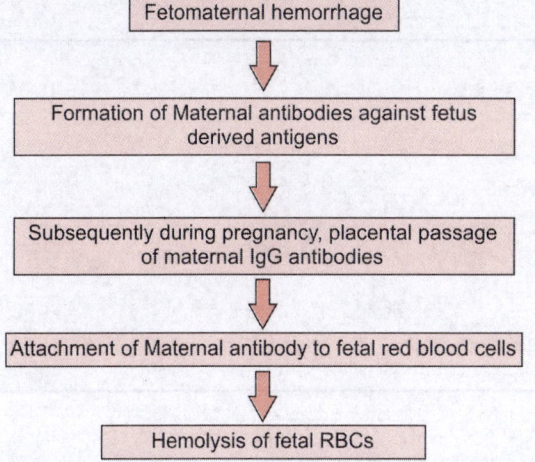

Clinical Features

- Anemia (main risk to fetus)
- Mild jaundice and anemia to hydrops fetalis
- Hepatosplenomegaly
- **Postnatal problems:**
  - Anemia
  - Coagulopathies
  - Edema (due to low serum albumin)
  - Pallor
  - Pulmonary hypertension
  - Kernicterus (due to hyperbilirubinemia)

Laboratory Findings

- **Cord blood:**
  - Reticulocytosis, increased serum bilirubin, positive direct Coomb's test (if cord blood Rh-D positive)
- **Mother's blood:**
  - Rh-D negative

Management

- **Treatment:**
  - **Maternal:** Intravenous immunoglobulin, plasma exchange
  - **Infant:** Exchange transfusion, intrauterine transfusion, phototherapy
- **Prevention:**
  - Rh immune globulin

Your Roll No. ....

Name of the Paper : **Pathology Paper-II**

Name of the Course : **MBBS-2017**

Semester : **Annual**

Time: 3 Hours   M.M.: 40

INSTRUCTIONS

1. Write your Roll No. on the top immediately on receipt of this question paper
2. All questions are to be attempted
3. Answers to Parts I, II and III should be written in separate answer sheets provided
4. Attempt parts of a question in sequence

PART-I

1. **Differentiate between:**   [8]
   a. Benign and malignant nephrosclerosis
   b. Vegetation of rheumatic and infective endocarditis
   c. Primary and secondary pulmonary tuberculosis
   d. Tubercular and typhoid ulcer of intestine

2. **Write briefly on:**   [6]
   a. Hashimoto thyroiditis
   b. Nodular sclerosis Hodgkin lymphoma
   c. Fibroadenoma breast

PART-II

3. **Write briefly on:**   [6]
   a. Osteogenic sarcoma
   b. Serological diagnosis of viral hepatitis

4. **Write briefly on:**   [6]
   a. Etiopathogenesis of cancer of uterine cervix
   b. Laboratory diagnosis of chronic renal failure

PART-III

5. **Write short note on:**   [8]
   a. Dysgerminoma
   b. Glioblastoma multiforme
   c. Advanced glycation end products
   d. Nutmeg liver

6. **Write short notes on:**   [6]
   a. Rapidly progressive glomerulonephritis
   b. Polyarteritis nodosa
   c. Asbestosis lung

PART I

1. Differentiate between:

a. Benign and Malignant Nephrosclerosis

(Ref: Harsh Mohan, 7th ed. pg. 677, Robbins, SA ed. pg. 938)

ANSWER

Benign and Malignant Nephrosclerosis

Benign nephrosclerosis	Malignant nephrosclerosis
• Occurs in Benign phase of hypertension	• Occurs in malignant phase of hypertension
• Most frequent form of renal disease	• Uncommon form
• Occurs in persons above 60 years of age due to increased severity of hypertension or diabetes mellitus	• Occurs in 5 % cases due to complication of pre-existing benign essential hypertension or in chronic renal diseases
• Gross appearance of kidneys – reduction in size and weight	• Gross appearance of kidneys – variable size
• Surface of kidney is finely granular and exhibits V-shaped areas of scarring	• Surface of kidney is oedematous, enlarged, have petechial hemorrhages and exhibits flea bitten kidney appearance
• Microscopic changes are Hyaline arteriosclerosis and intimal thickening	• Microscopic changes are Necrotising arteriolitis and Hyperplastic intimal sclerosis or onion skin proliferation
• Variation in blood pressure accompanied with headache, dizziness, palpitation and nervousness	• Malignant hypertension with headache and impaired vision
• Papilloedema is absent	• Papilloedema is present
• Proteinuria may or may not be present	• Proteinuria is present
• Renal failure is rare	• Renal failure occurs in 90% patients

b. Vegetations of Rheumatic and Infective endocarditis

(Ref: Harsh Mohan, 7th ed pg. 426, Robbins, SA ed. pg. 557, 559)

ANSWER

Vegetations of Rheumatic and Infective Endocarditis

Rheumatic endocarditis	Bacterial endocarditis
• Usually left sided valves (mitral valve) are affected	• Aortic and mitral valve get affected
• Vegetations present along the line of closure (on one side)	• Vegetations present on valve cusps (on one side)
• Grossly, multiple, translucent, firmly attached, vegetations that result in permanent valvular deformation	• Usually large, irregular, friable vegetations
• Microscopic picture shows fibrin along with platelets and no bacteria. endocardium exhibits edema, inflammatory cell infiltrate and proliferation of capillaries.	• Microscopically, composed of platelets and fibrin. deeper parts shows bacterial colonies along with granulation tissue present at the base

Jones Criteria

○ The Jones criteria are illustrated below. Diagnosis of rheumatic fever requires 2 major OR 1 major and 2 minor criteria, plus a preceding group A strep infection.

Table: WHO Criteria for Rheumatic Fever Based on Revised Jones Criteria

Major criteria	Minor criteria
• Carditis	• Fever
• Polyarthritis	• Polyarthralgia
• Chorea	• **Labs:** Elevated ESR or leukocyte count
• Erythema marginatum	• **ECG:** Prolonged P-R interval
• Subcutaneous nodules	

c Primary and secondary pulmonary tuberculosis

ANSWER

Primary and Secondary Pulmonary Tuberculosis

(Ref: Textbook of Pathology, Harsh Mohan, 7th ed. pg. 142, Robbins, SA ed. pg. 373)

Primary tuberculosis	Secondary tuberculosis
• Commonly occurs in children	• Commonly occurs in children and adults
• Affects exclusively lungs	• Affects lungs, lymph nodes, genitourinary tract, bones, meninges, brain, eyes, liver, spleen, intestine, skin etc

Primary tuberculosis	Secondary tuberculosis
• Lesions formed are Ghon's complex – consolidation found in lung, lymphatic vessels and hilar nodes lesions	• Lesions formed are tubercles, extensive caseation, miliary lesions, cavitation, fibrocaseous lesions, caseous pneumonia, pleurisy, effusion
• Healing is done by fibrosis and calcification but may get reactivated if immunity is weak	• Consolidation, parenchymal nodules, thickened pleura, amyloidosis, reactivation of healed lesion in weak immunity and AIDS

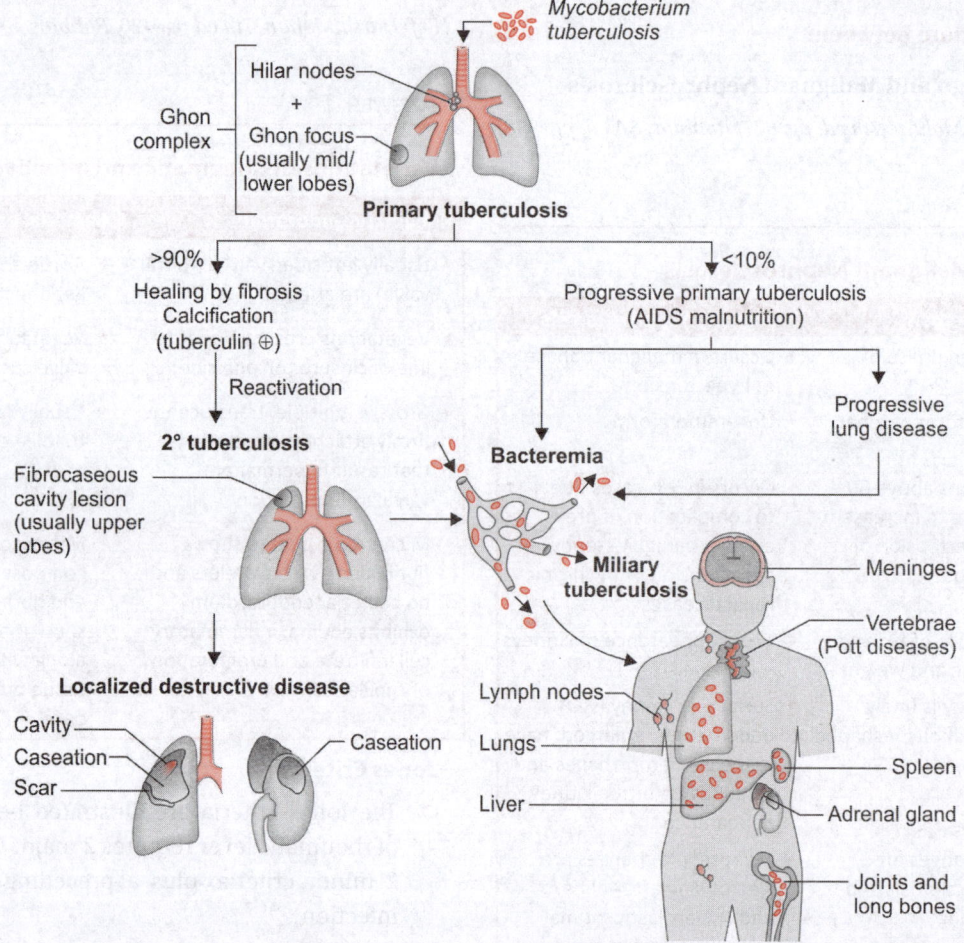

Fig. Primary and secondary tuberculosis

d. Tubercular and Typhoid ulcer of intestine

(Ref: Textbook of Pathology, Harsh Mohan, 7th ed. pg. 553)

ANSWER

Typhoid and Tubercular Ulcer of Intestine

Typhoid intestinal ulcer	Tubercular intestinal ulcer
• Caused by Salmonella typhii	• Caused by Mycobacterium tuberculosis
• Mostly located in terminal ileum in Payer's patch, or in jejunum and colon	• Can be located anywhere in small intestine, mostly in terminal ileum and caecum
• Occurs mainly in Payer's patch but may include lymphoid follicle	• Occurs mainly in lymphoid follicles, may involve Payer's patch

Typhoid intestinal ulcer	Tubercular intestinal ulcer
• Small ulcer with regular margins with absent caseous material, base is black due to sloughing of mucosa	• Large ulcer with irregular margins enclosing the gut with caseous material in the base of ulcers
• Microscopically, erythrophagocytosis, bacteria are present in macrophages, fibrosis is absent, perforation is common with bleeding	• Microscopically, typical caseous granuloma, AFB, epithelioid cells, giant cells with fibrosis on healing, perforation not present without bleeding

2. Write briefly on:

a. Hashimoto thyroiditis

(Ref: Harsh Mohan, 7th ed. pg. 795, Robbins, SA ed. pg. 1086)

ANSWER

Hashimoto Thyroiditis

Introduction

○ It is an autoimmune disease that attack the thyroid gland by a variety of cell and antibody mediated immune processes resulting in primary hypothyroidism

○ Results in thyroid failure due to autoimmune destruction of the thyroid gland

○ Also known as chronic lymphocytic thyroiditis

Etiology

Factors responsible are:

○ Hormones
○ Radiation exposure
○ Excessive iodine

Risk Factors

○ **Age:** Common in middle age
○ **Sex:** Females are more prone as compared to males
○ **Presence of other autoimmune disease:** Like type I diabetes, rheumatoid arthritis, etc.
○ Heredity

Pathogenesis

○ Autoimmune disease presents with reaction of immune system against thyroid antigens

○ Progressive loss of thyrocytes (thyroid epithelial cells) and replacement by infiltrate of mononuclear cells

○ Initial event- sensitization of thyroid antigens to autoreactive CD4+ T helper cells

○ **Steps involved are:**

▪ **CD8+ cytotoxic T cell mediated cell death:**
  ♦ Destruction of thyrocytes through- Perforin/granzyme exocytosis or involvement of CD95 (death receptor)
  ♦ **Cytokine–mediated cell death:** CD4+ T cells produces inflammatory cytokines with recruitment and activation of macrophages and damage to thyroid follicles

▪ **Binding of antithyroid antibodies:** antithyroidglobulin, antithyroid peroxidase, anti TSH receptor antibodies along with antibody dependent cell- mediated cytotoxicity

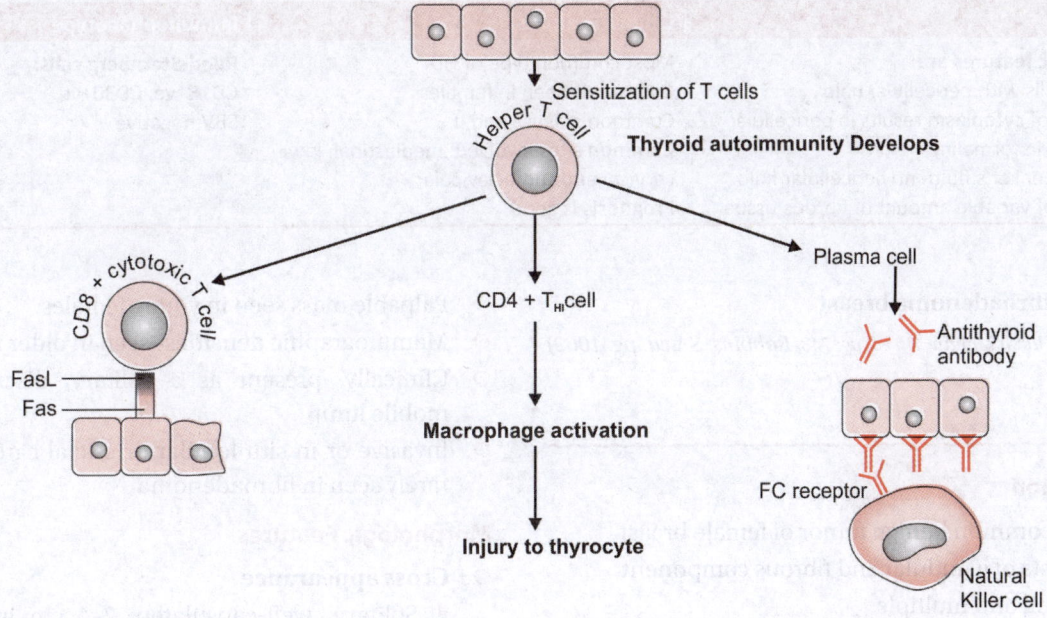

Clinical Features

○ Moderate enlargement of the thyroid gland
○ Painless, firm, diffuse and symmetrical

Morphology

- **Pathologically, two types:**
  - Classic form (common type)
  - Fibrosing variant
- **Classic form:** Presents with diffuse, firm, symmetric and rubbery enlargement of the gland
- **Fibrosing variant:** Gland is enlarged and firm along with surrounding tissue compression
- **Microscopically:**
  - Classic form exhibits lymphoid follicles with germinal centres and dense infiltration by lymphocytes, plasma cells, macrophages
  - Atrophic thyroid follicles, with decrease in number and no colloid
  - **Presence of Hurthle cells:** (Also known as oxyphilcells, oncocytes, Askanazy cells) follicular epithelial cells in degenerated form having abundant eosinophilic, granular cytoplasm and bizarre nuclei
  - Thickening of the fibrous septa dividing thyroid lobules

- Fibrosing variant consists of less extensive lymphoid infiltrate and fibrous and considerable amount of fibrous tissue replacing thyroid parenchyma

Diagnosis

- Decreased level of serum T3 and T4
- Increased TSH

b   Nodular sclerosis Hodgkin lymphoma

(Ref: Harsh Mohan, 7th ed. pg. 350, Robbins, SA ed. pg. 607)

ANSWER

Introduction

- Hodgkin's lymphoma arises in the lymph node (primarily)
- Bimodal incidence- between the age of 15–35 years and other after 5th decade of life
- **Diagnostic feature:** Presence of Reed-Sternberg cell

Features of Nodular Sclerosis Type of Hodgkin Lymphoma

Morphology	Clinical Features	Immunophenotype
Characteristic features are: • Lacunar cells with pericellular halo • Shrinkage of cytoplasm results in pericellular halo (fixed in formalin) • If fixed in Zenker's fluid- no pericellular halo • Presence of variable amount of fibrous tissue	Most common type of HD Commonly seen in females Common stages I and II Common sites involved: mediastinal, lower cervical and supraclavicular Prognosis is good	**Reed-Sternberg cells:** CD15+ve, CD30+ve EBV negative

c.   Fibroadenoma breast

(Ref: Harsh Mohan, 7th ed. pg. 748, Robbins, SA ed. pg. 1069)

ANSWER

Introduction

- Most common benign tumor of female breast
- Consists of glandular and fibrous component
- Bilateral and multiple
- Origin- may arise as a result of increase estrogen activity (may be absolute or relative)
- May be due to drug-induced

Clinical Features

- Occurs at any age of reproductive life, but usual presentation is between 15–30 years of age
- Usually upper quadrant of breast is involved

- Palpable mass seen in young females
- Mammographic densities- seen in older individuals
- Clinically, present as a solitary, discrete, freely mobile lump
- Invasive or in situ lobular or ductal carcinoma are rarely seen in fibroadenoma

Morphologic Features

- **Gross appearance**
  - Solitary, well-capsulated, 2–4 cm in diameter (small) mass
  - Usually upper quadrant of breast is involved
  - Giant fibroadenoma: Large size (up to 15 cm in diameter)
  - Cut surface is firm, slightly myxoid appearance, grey-white and shows slit-lke spaces formed as a result of compressed ducts

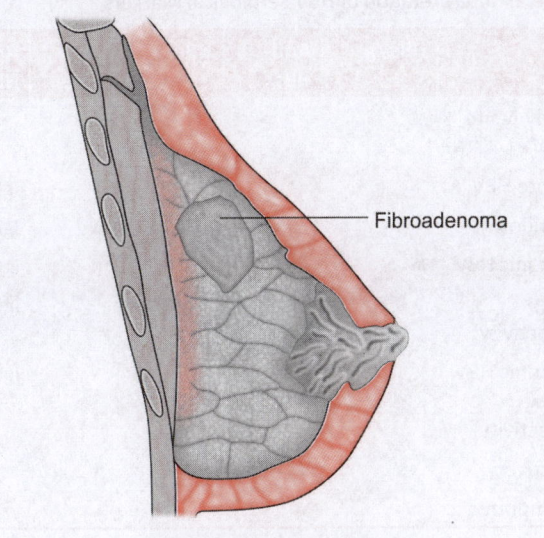

Fig. Fibroadenoma breast

○ **Microscopic findings:**

▪ Two types exist as a result of the arrangement pattern of ductal epithelium and fibrous stroma

Intracanalicular pattern:

♦ Compression of ducts by fibrous tissue into slit-like clefts lined by ductal epithelium or may present as cords of epithelial component with surrounding fibrous stroma

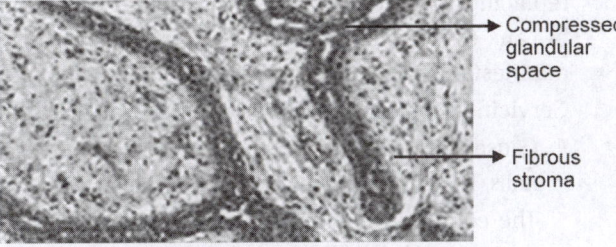

Compressed glandular space

Fibrous stroma

Fig. Intracanalicular pattern

▪ **Pericanalicular pattern:**

♦ Dilated or patent duct surrounded by fibrous stromal component

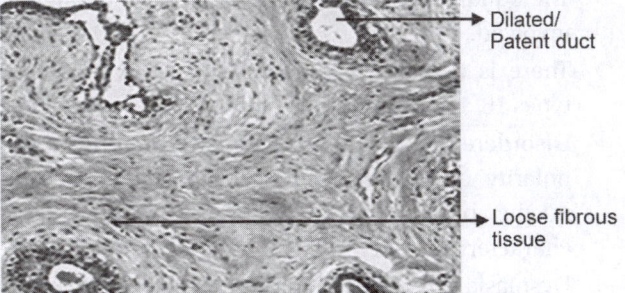

Dilated/ Patent duct

Loose fibrous tissue

Fig. Pericanalicular pattern

○ **Mammography:**

▪ Revels "popcorn" calcification

○ **Morphologic variants:**

▪ Tubular adenoma

▪ Lactating adenoma-seen in pregnancy or during lactation

▪ Juvenile fibroadenoma

PART II

3. **Write briefly on:**

a. **Osteogenic sarcoma**

(Ref: Harsh Mohan, pg. 832-835, Robbins, SA ed. pg. 1198)

ANSWER

Introduction

○ Common malignant bone tumor

○ Also known as osteosarcoma

○ Direct formation of osteoid or bone, or both from sarcoma cells

Types

Based on location, two types

○ Central osteosarcoma (medullary or classic)

○ Surface osteosarcoma (parosteal or periosteal)

Central Osteosarcoma (Medullary or Classic)

○ Common in males

○ Age- occurs between 10–20 years.

○ Sites commonly involved are-lower end of femur and upper end of tibia (approx. 60%), upper end of humerus, pelvis, etc.

○ Pain, swelling and tenderness of the affected part

○ **Pathogenesis:**

▪ Mutation in Rb gene, p53 and MDM2 (in primary)

▪ Pre-existing bone lesion like Paget's disease, fibrous dysplasia, etc. in secondary

○ **Radiographic features:**

▪ Sunburst appearance and presence of codman's triangle at the angle between the elevated periosteum and underlying surface of cortex

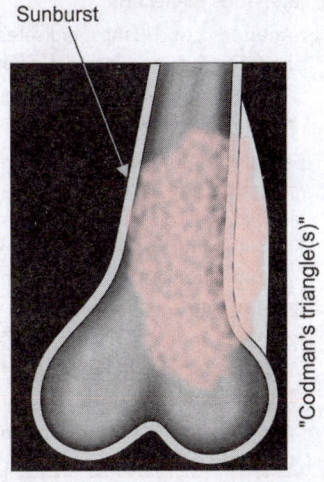

Sunburst

"Codman's triangle(s)"

PATHOLOGY

19

- ○ **Biochemical findings:**
  - Raised serum alkaline phosphatase level
  - Normal calcium and phosphorus level
- ○ **Histopathological findings:**
  - Composed of sarcoma cells that exhibits marked pleomorphism, polymorphism, hyperchromatism and atypical mitoses
  - Osteoid matrix and bone are also present in between the tumor cells
- ○ **Histologic variants:**
  - Small cell osteosarcoma
  - Telangiectataic osteosarcoma
  - Anaplastic osteosarcoma, etc.
- ○ **Prognosis:**
  - Poor

Surface Osteosarcoma

- ○ Common in older patients
- ○ **Common sites:** Lower end of femur and upper end of humerus
- ○ **Two variants:**
  - Parosteal osteosarcoma
  - Periosteal osteosarcoma
- ○ Microscopically, shows structural differentiation along with well-formed bony trabeculae
- ○ Better prognosis

b.　Serological diagnosis of viral hepatitis

(Ref: Textbook of Pathology, Harsh Mohan, 7th ed. pg. 590)

ANSWER

Table 1: Hepatitis serologic markers

Anti-HAV (IgM)	IgM antibody to HAV; best test to detect Acute hepatitis A.
Anti-HAV (IgG)	IgG antibody indicates prior HAV infection And/or prior vaccination; protects against Re-infection.
HBsAg	Antigen found on surface of HBV; indicates hepatitis B infection.
Anti-HBs	Antibody to HBsAg; indicates immunity to hepatitis B due to vaccination or recovery from infection.
HBcAg	Antigen associated with core of HBV.
Anti-HBc	Antibody to HBcAg; IgM = acute/recent infection; IgG = prior exposure or chronic infection. IgM anti-HBc may be the sole ⊕ marker of infection during window period.
HBeAg	Secreted by infected hepatocyte into circulation. Not part of mature HBV virion. Indicates active viral replication and therefore high transmissibility and poorer prognosis.
Anti-HBe	Antibody to HBeAg; indicates low transmissibility.

Table 2: Interpretation of HBV Serological Markers

	HBsAg	Anti-HBs	HBeAg	Anti-HBe	Anti-HBc
Early Acute HBV	√				
Acute HBV	√		√		IgM
Window				√	IgM
Chronic HBV	√		√		IgG
(High infectivity)	√				IgG
Chronic HBV (Low infectivity)				√	IgG
Recovery		√		√	
Immunized		√			

4.　Write briefly on:

a.　Etiopathogenesis of cancer of uterine cervix

(Ref: Harsh Mohan, 7th ed. pg. 715, Robbins, SA ed. pg. 1002)

ANSWER

Non-neoplastic Disorders

- ○ Erosion is characterized by columnar epithelium replacing squamous epithelium, grossly resulting in an erythematous area. Sometimes it is a manifestation of chronic cervicitis.
- ○ Cervicitis most often involves the endocervix.
  - Causes include staphylococci, enterococci, G. vaginalis, T. vaginalis, C. albicans, and C. trachomatis.
  - The condition is often asymptomatic. It may be manifested by cervical discharge.
- ○ Cervical polyps are inflammatory proliferations of cervical mucosa; they are not true neoplasms.

Dysplasia and Carcinoma in Situ

- ○ The squamocolumnar junction is most frequently involved.
- ○ There is a major association with HPV infection types 16, 18, 31, or 33.
- ○ Disordered epithelial growth manifested by loss of polarity and nuclear hyperchromasia, beginning at the basal layer and extending outward, is characteristic.
- ○ Dysplasia can progress through mild, moderate, and severe forms to carcinoma in situ and is classified as cervical intraepithelial neoplasia (CIN), with subtypes of CIN 1, CIN 2, or CIN 3, depending on the extent of epithelial involvement. CIN 3 (carcinoma in situ) is characterized by atypical changes extending through the entire thickness of the epithelium.

Invasive Carcinoma

- **General considerations**
  - The occurrence peaks in middle-aged women.
  - The cancer is most often squamous cell carcinoma; adenocarcinoma accounts for approximately 5% of cases.
  - Most frequently, the carcinoma arises from preexisting CIN at the squamocolumnar junction. It evolves through a series of increasing epithelial abnormalities proceeding from dysplasia to carcinoma in situ and then to invasive carcinoma.
  - Since the introduction of the Pap cytologic screening test, squamous cell carcinoma has exhibited a striking decrease in mortality.
- Epidemiologic factors (probable spread by sexual contact)
  - Early sexual activity and multiple sexual partners are associated with increased incidence.
  - Incidence is high in prostitutes, rare in celibates, and rare in some Jewish populations. The traditional belief that circumcision of male sexual partners exerts a protective effect has not been confirmed.
  - Incidence is increased in the economically deprived.
  - Cigarette smoking is also associated with increased incidence, but the relationship remains unclear.
- **Role of HPV**
  - Dysplastic cells frequently demonstrate koilocytosis (as in HPV-induced condyloma acuminatum).
  - HPV sequences are often integrated into genomes of dysplastic or malignant cervical epithelial cells; HPV types 16, 18, 31, and 33 are most common, as in most malignant genital squamous cell tumors, and are associated with more than 90% of cases. HPV viral proteins E6 and E7 bind and inactivate the gene products of p53 and Rb, respectively.

b   Laboratory diagnosis of chronic renal failure

(Ref: Harsh Mohan, 7th ed. pg. 592, Robbins, SA ed. pg. 898)

ANSWER

Laboratory Findings in Chronic Renal Failure
Introduction
- Progressive and irreversible deterioration of renal function owing to slow destruction of renal parenchyma leading to death

Etiopathogenesis
- All chronic nephropathies can result in CRF which are classified as
  - **Diseases causing glomerular pathology**
    - Primary glomerular pathology–chronic glomerulonephritis
    - Systemic glomerular pathology–systemic lupus erythematosus, serum sickness nephritis, diabetic nephropathy
  - **Diseases causing tubulointerstitial pathology**
    - Vascular causes–essential hypertension
    - Infectious causes–chronic pyelonephritis
    - Toxic causes–high intake of analgesics such as phenacetin, aspirin, acetaminophen
    - Obstructive causes–stones, blood clots, tumours, strictures, enlarged prostate

Laboratory Findings of CRF
- Elevated BUN and creatinine
- Decreased GFR
- Hyperkalaemia
- Hyponatremia
- Acidosis
- Hypocalcemia
- Hyperphosphatemia
- Elevated uric acid
- Hypoproteinemia
- Anaemia–normocytic, normochromic
- Increased serum cholesterol and triglyceride
- Hematuria and Proteinuria

PART III

5. **Write short notes on:**

   a. **Dysgerminoma**

   (Ref: Harsh Mohan, 7th ed. pg. 737, Robbins, SA ed. pg. 1030)

ANSWER

Introduction
- Dysgerminoma is a malignant ovarian tumor that is identical to testicular seminoma
- Common primitive germ cell tumor (malignant pure ovarian germ cell tumor)

Clinical Features
- **Age:** Between 15–30 years.
- Mass in the lower abdomen, abdominal enlargement
- Abdominal pain

○ Weight loss
○ Raised levels of hCG

Gross Appearance

○ Capsulated, solid mass of variable size
○ Cut section is lobulated with areas of necrosis and hemorrhage

Microscopic Features

○ Composed of large, uniform tumor cells with clear cytoplasm, vesicular nuclei and prominent nucleoli surrounded by connective tissue stroma with infiltration of lymphocytes

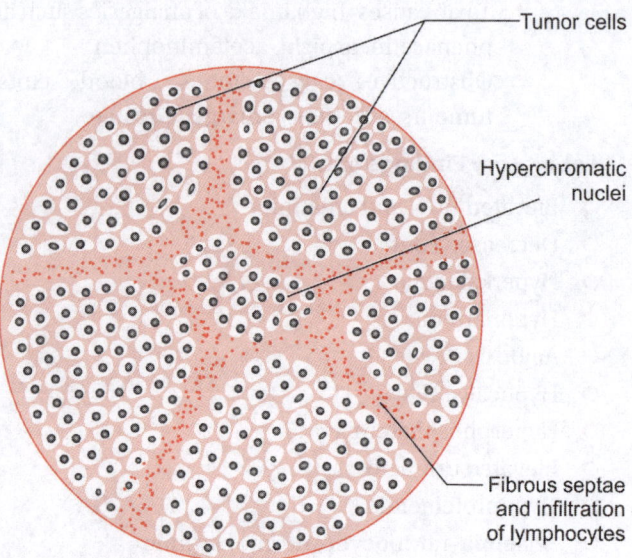

Behavior and Prognosis

○ Less aggressive, slow growing tumor
○ Hematogenous spread to liver, lungs, bones,etc.
○ Radiosensitive and chemosensitive
○ Prognosis is good

b.   Glioblastoma multiforme

(Ref: Textbook of Pathology, Harsh Mohan, 7th ed. pg. 879)

ANSWER

Introduction

○ Most aggressive form of astrocytoma
○ Due to neoplastic transformation of mature astrocytes
○ **Origin:** From embryonal cells

Clinical Features

○ Common in young patients
○ Frequently seen in males as compared to females

Symptoms occur depending on the location of the brain tumor, but commonly presents with

○ Persistent headache
○ Double or blurred vision
○ Vomiting
○ Loss of appetite
○ Changes in mood and personality
○ Changes in ability to think and learn
○ New onset of seizures
○ Gradual difficulty in speech

Morphology

○ **Gross appearance:**
  ▪ Variation in size and appearance depending on site
  ▪ Grey-white appearance to yellow and soft with hemorrhagic areas and necrosis
  ▪ Distorted surrounding brain tissue and infiltration by yellow tumor tissue
○ **Microscopic features:**
  ▪ Markedly anaplastic and cellular
  ▪ Tumor cells exhibit marked pleomorphism, mitoses and giant cells
  ▪ Marked endothelial proliferation- piled up vascular cells bulge into the vascular lumen (glomeruloid body)
  ▪ Areas of necrosis and highly malignant cells present along the edges of necrotic region giving pseudopalisading appearance

Diagnosis

○ **CT scan and MRI:** Assess the location of brain tumor
○ **Magnetic resonance spectroscopy (MRS):** To examine the tumors chemical profile
○ **PET scan:** Detection of tumor recurrence.

Grading

According to WHO, it is high grade (grade IV) astrocytoma

○ **Features:**
  ▪ Most malignant
  ▪ Rapid growth, aggressive
  ▪ Widely infiltrative
  ▪ Rapid recurrence
  ▪ Prone for necrosis

c.   Advanced glycation end products

ANSWER

Advanced Glycosylation end Products

Introduction

○ Non-enzymatic reaction between the amino group of both intracellular and extracellular protein with intracellular glucose-derived dicarbonyl precursors results in the formation of AGEs

○ Degree of glycosylation proportional to the blood sugar level

○ Hypglycemia accelerates the process of formation of AGEs

Properties

○ **Biological properties:**

- Monocyte emigratioan
- Increased vascular permeability, cellular proliferation and ECM preduction
- Monocytes and mesencymal cells binds to AGE receptors

○ **Chemical properties:**

- Resistance to proteolytic digestion of AGE
- Lipid oxidation
- Damage to nucleic acid
- Inactivation of nitric oxide
- Binding of these products to specific receptors, like RAGE present on the inflammatory cells results in certain vascular response:
  - ♦ Reactive oxygen species generation in endothelial cells
  - ♦ Procoagulant activity on macrophages and endothelial cells is increased
  - ♦ Extracellular matrix synthesis and increased proliferation of vasculsars smooth muscle Thus, results in compromised blood supply and functions of the organs

d. Nutmeg liver

(Ref: Harsh Mohan, 7th ed. pg. 91, Robbins, SA ed. pg. 116)

ANSWER

Nutmeg Liver

Introduction

○ Nutmeg liver is produced by chronic venous congestion of the liver due to right heart failure or occlusion of inferior vena cava and hepatic vein

Morphology

○ **Gross appearance:**

- Enlarged liver with tenderness and tense capsule

- Nutmeg appearance of cut surface owing to red and mottled appearance corresponding to congested center of lobules and fatty peripheral zone respectively

○ **Microscopic appearance:**

- Passive congestion can be seen in centrilobular zone which is farthest from blood supply and therefore the impact of hypoxia is observed mostly in centrilobular zone

---

6. Write short notes on:

a. Rapidly progressive glomerulonephritis

(Ref: Harsh Mohan, 7th ed. pg. 654, Robbins, SA ed. pg. 898)

ANSWER

Introduction

○ Also known as crescentic glomerulonephritis or extracapillary glomerulonephritis

○ Characterized by sudden/acute decrease in renal function causing acute renal failure within few weeks or months

Etiopathogenesis

Depending on the etiology and pathogenesis, RPGN is divided into 3 types:

○ **Type I RPGN (RPGN in systemic disease, Anti-GBM disease):**

- Good pasture syndrome is the classic example of anti-GBM disease
- Other systemic diseases like- SLE, vasculitis,etc. are also associated with the disease
- Linear deposits of IgG and C3.

○ **Type II RPGN (Immune-complex type):**

- Mainly post- infectious
- Granular deposits of IgG and C3 in glomerular capillary wall

○ **Type III RPGN (Pauci-immune RPGN):**

- Less or no glomerular deposit
- Includes Wegner's granulomatosis and polyarteritis nodosa
- Mainly ANCA positive (anti-neutophilcytoplasmic antibody)

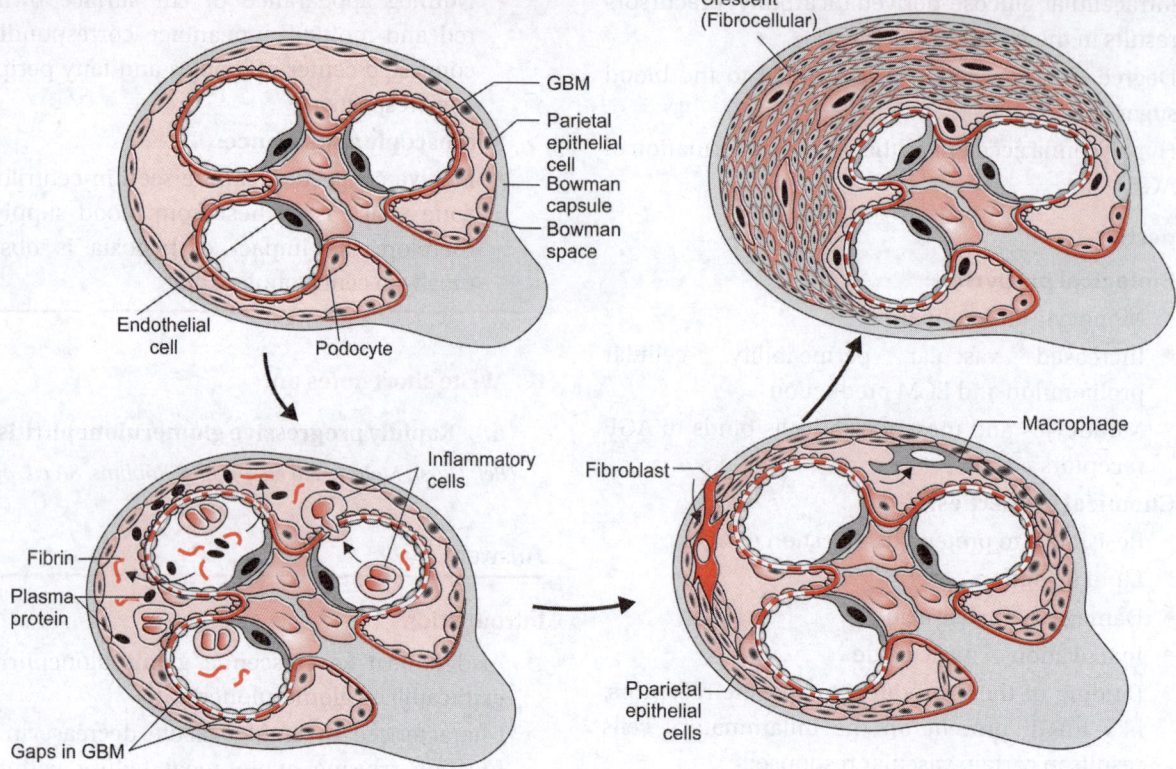

Microscopic Features

- Presence of "crescents" inside of Bowman's capsule
- Glomerular tufts exhibits increased cellularity
- Hyaline droplets along with casts, fibrin and red blood cells
- Infiltration of inflammatory cells, mainly lymphocytes and plasma cells in the interstitial tissue
- **Immunofluorescence:**
  Exhibits-
- In Goodpasture's syndrome-linear pattern of RPGN, consisting of IgG and C3 along the capillaries
    - **Type II RPGN:** granular pattern of post-infectious RPGN
    - **Type III RPGN:** Less or no deposits of immunoglobulin and C3
  b. **Polyarteritis nodosa**

(Ref: Harsh Mohan, 7th ed. pg. 383, Robbins, SA ed. pg. 509)

ANSWER

Polyarteritis Nodosa
Introduction

- Necrotising vasculitis of small and medium sized muscular arteries of multiple organs and tissues affecting mainly adult males

- Inflammation occurs in all the layers of vessel wall
- In descending order of frequency of involvement, commonly affected organs are kidneys, heart, liver, GIT, muscle, pancreas, testes, nervous system and skin

Clinical Features

- Fever
- Malaise
- Weakness
- Weight loss
- Renal symptoms—haematuria, albuminuria and renal failure
- Vascular lesions in alimentary tract—abdominal pain, melaena
- Peripheral neuritis
- Hypertension

Morphology

- Gross appearance
    - Lesions comprise sections of vessels at the bifurcations and branchings as tiny beaded nodules
- Microscopic appearance–3 stages of lesion evolution
    - Acute stage
        - Fibroid necrosis in the center of nodule surrounded by acute inflammatory response

- Periarteritis is seen with inflammatory infiltrate consisting mainly of neutrophils, eosinophils and mononuclear cells
- Thrombi can be seen at the lumen with aneurysm formation in the weakened wall
- **Healing stage**
  - Fibroblastic proliferation is found with firm nodularity
  - Inflammatory infiltrate comprises of lymphocytes, plasma cells and macrophages
- **Healed stage**
  - Thickening of arterial wall owing to dense fibrosis
  - Fragmented or lost internal elastic lamina
  - Haemosiderin laden macrophages and organised thrombus may be found

c. **Asbestosis lung**

(Ref: Harsh Mohan, 7th ed. pg. 437, Robbins, SA ed. pg. 690)

ANSWER

Introduction

- Prolonged exposure to asbestos dust results in lung asbestosis
- Characterized by interstitial fibrosis
- Common in workers engaged in fabrication of asbestos pipes, tiles, roofs, brake lining, etc. and mining

Etiopathogenesis

- Calcium, magnesium silicates, iron; chrysotile, amosite, crocidolite-responsible for fibrosis, asbestos body, thick alveolar walls and pleural plaques (rewrite).

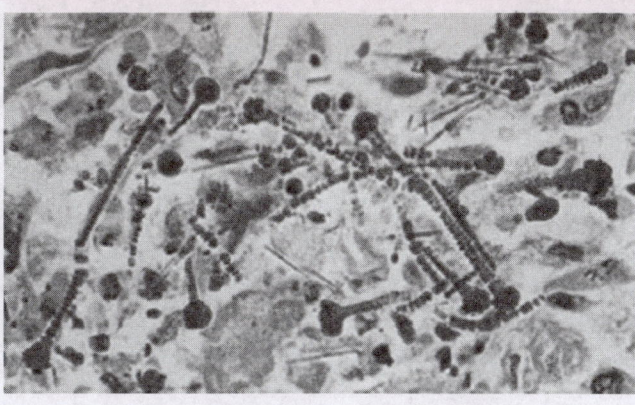

Fig. Ferruginous (asbestos) bodies. These asbestos fiber inclusions are coated with protein and iron and will appear blue when stained with Prussian blue

Clinical Features

- Slow growing illness
- Dyspnea
- Cough (dry or productive)
- In case of advanced disease- pulmonary hypertension, corpulmonale,etc.

Gross Features

- Pleural thickening
- Pulmonary fibrosis, esp. base of lungs and subpleural areas

Microscopic Features

- Interstitial fibrosis (non-specific)
- Asbestos bodies–asbestos fibers coated with hemosiderin and glycoprotein and dumb-bell shaped in appearance
- Enlarged airspaces- chances of emphysema

Name of the Paper : **Pathology Paper-I**

Name of the Course : **MBBS-2016**

Semester : **Annual**

Time: 3 Hours   M.M.: 40

INSTRUCTIONS

1. Write your Roll No. on the top immediately on receipt of this question paper
2. All questions are to be attempted
3. Answers to Parts I, II and III should be written in separate answer sheets provided
4. Attempt parts of a question in sequence

PART-I

1. **Differentiate between:**   [8]
   a. Iron deficiency anemia and beta thalassemia trait
   b. Necrosis and apoptosis
   c. Marasmus and Kwashiorkor
   d. Bleeding due to platelet defect and coagulation factor deficiency

2. **Write briefly on:**   [6]
   a. Pathogenesis of cardiac edema
   b. Free radical injury
   c. Spread of tumors

PART-II

3. **Write briefly on:**   [6]
   a. Septic shock
   b. Morphologic types of necrosis

4. **Write briefly on:**   [6]
   a. Laboratory features of folate deficiency anemia
   b. Factors predisposing to venous thrombosis

PART-III

5. **Write short notes on:**   [8]
   a. Coomb's test
   b. Turner syndrome
   c. Primary amyloidosis
   d. Ghon focus

6. **Write short notes on:**   [6]
   a. Mechanisms of apoptosis
   b. Role of p53 gene in neoplasia
   c. Factors affecting wound healing

PART -I

1. Differentiate between:

a. Iron deficiency anemia and beta thalassemia trait

(Ref. Harsh Mohan, 7th ed. pg. 286, 298, Robbins, SA ed. pg. 649, 639)

ANSWER

Iron deficiency Anemia and Beta Thalassemia Trait

Iron deficiency anemia	Beta- thalassemia trait
• Characterized by iron deficiency	• Characterized by deficiency of Hb chain
• Anemia is moderate	• Anemia is asymptomatic and mild
• RBC is decreased	• Raised RBC
• It is acquired deficiency	• Genetic in nature
• Serum iron and ferritin is reduced	• Normal serum iron and ferritin
• Increased TiBC	• Normal TiBC

b. Necrosis and apoptosis

(Ref: Harsh Mohan, 7th ed. pg. 31, Robbins, SA ed. pg. 41, 52)

ANSWER

Apoptosis and Necrosis

Apoptosis	Necrosis
• Programmed and coordinated cell death	• Cell death with degradation of tissue by hydrolytic enzymes
• Due to pathologic and physiologic processes	• Due to toxins, hypoxia
• Morphologic changes: shrinkage of cell, cytoplasmic blebs, chromatin condensation, apoptotic bodies and phagocytosis by macrophages, no inflammatory reaction	• Morphologic changes: death of adjacent cells, inflammatory reaction present, disruption of membrane along with nuclear disruption, phagocytosis of cell debris
• Intact lysosome	• Rupture lysosome
• Mechanism is genetically coordinated	• Due to ATP depletion, membrane damage, free radicals, etc.
• Electrophoresis shows step ladder pattern of DNA	• Diffuse DNA pattern on elctrophoresis

c. Marasmus and Kwashiorkor

(Ref: Harsh Mohan, 7th ed. pg. 240, Robbins, SA ed. pg. 433)

ANSWER

Marasmus and Kwashiorkor

Marasmus	Kwashirkor
• Characterized by the deficiency of protein and carbohydrate	• Protein deficiency is greater than carbohydrate deficiency
• Common between the age of 0–2 years	• Common in children < 5 years of age
• Weaning of children only on carbohydrate rich food and no protein absorption	• Weaning in early age without proper food
• Serum protein level may be normal or slightly decreased	• Marked decrease in serum protein level
• Severe mental retardation	• Less severe mental retardation
• No edema or hypoalbuminemia	• Presence of generalized or dependent edema
• Hepatomegaly is not present	• Hepatomegaly with fatty changes present
• Loose,dry and wrinkled skin	• Alternate bands of dark and pale hairs (flag sign), hair fall, loss of hair color, etc.
• Lymphoid atrophy is less	• Marked lymphoid atrophy

d. Bleeding due to platelet defect and coagulation factor deficiency

(Ref: Textbook of Pathology, Harsh Mohan, 7th ed. pg. 310, 333)

ANSWER

Bleeding due to Platelet Defect and Coagulation Factor Deficiency

Platelet defect	Coagulation factor deficiency
• Bleeding from superficial cut is present	• No bleeding from superficial cut
• On application of local pressure, bleeding does not stop quickly	• On application of local pressure, bleeding stops quickly
• Spontaneous bleeding common	• No usual spontaneous bleeding
• Hemarthrosis not present	• Hemarthrosis is characteristic
• Small and multiple ecchymosis	• Ecchymosis is large and solitary
• Bleeding after trauma is immediate, less and for short time	• Bleeding after trauma is delayed and persistent
• Presence of petechiae	• Petechiae is absent

PATHOLOGY

2. **Write briefly on:**

   a.   Pathogenesis of cardiac edema

   (Ref: Textbook of Pathology, Harsh Mohan, 7th ed. pg. 84)

ANSWER

Cardiac Edema Pathogenesis

○ Cardiac edema is dependent edema (influenced by gravity)

○ Hypovolaemia as a result of decreased cardiac output stimulates renin-angiotensin-aldosterone mechanism leading to sodium- water retention and edema

○ **Back pressure hypothesis:** Raised central venous pressure (as a result of heart failure) is mediated towards the venous end of the capillaries increasing the capillary hydrostatic pressure leading to transudation

○ **Forward pressure hypothesis:** Increase in capillary permeability in case of chronic hypoxia causes edema

○ In left heart failure- Pulmonary edema occurs as a result of venous congestion

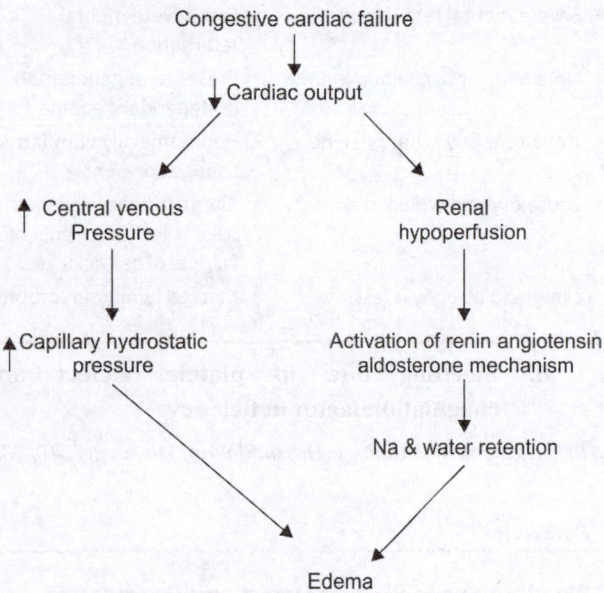

   b.   Free radical injury

   (Ref: Textbook of Pathology, Harsh Mohan, 7th ed. pg. 14-15)

ANSWER

Introduction

○ Highly reactive chemical species with a single unpaired electron in their outer orbit

○ They are reactive oxygen and nitrogen species

○ May damage the cell membrane and nucleic acids

○ Most common free radicals are hydrogen peroxide, hydroxyl radical and superoxide anion

Induction of Free Radicals

○ Enzymatic metabolism of chemicals and drugs. Example- CCl_4 to CCl_3

○ Radiation like- UV rays, X-rays

○ Oxidation-reduction reaction and formation of superoxide anion, hydrogen peroxide and hydroxyl ion

○ Transition metals like –iron, copper, etc. involved (Fenton reaction)

○ Nitric oxide produced from macrophages, endothelial cells, etc. and may be converted to peroxynitrite anion, NO_2, etc.

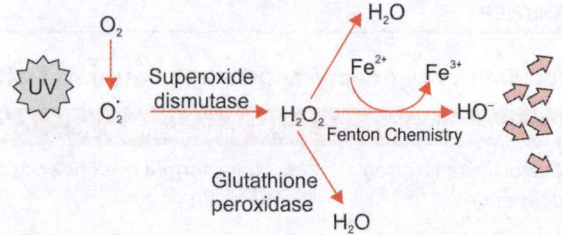

Effects

○ Mechanisms responsible for membrane damage caused by free radicals are as follows:

  ▪ **Protein oxidation:**
    ♦ Oxidation of amino acid residue side chain protein cross linkage, fragmentation of polypeptides results in cell destruction

  ▪ **Lipid peroxidation:**
    ♦ Oxygen–free radicals attack PUFA of membrane producing destructive PUFA radicals (lipid hydroperoxy and hypoperoxide radicals) and results in destruction and damage

  ▪ **DNA damage:**
    ♦ Results break in the single-strand of mito-chondrial and nuclear DNA causing cell injury

  ▪ **Damage of cytoskeleton:**
    ♦ Interference with cytoskeletal elements that results deletion in ATP

Conditions Associated with Free Radical Injury

○ Destruction of tumor cells

○ Ischemic reperfusion injury

○ Cellular ageing

○ Radiation injury

○ Microbial killing

○ Chemical carcinogenesis

○ Damage due to inflammation, etc.

   c.   Spread of tumors

   (Ref: Harsh Mohan, 7th ed. pg. 193-195, Robbins, SA ed. pg. 273)

ANSWER

Introduction

- Important feature of malignant tumor
- Invasion and destruction of adjoining tissues (direct spread)
- Dissemination to distant sites (metastasis)

Routes of Spread of Tumors

Direct Spread

- In benign tumors
- Circumscribed mass exhibiting expansion of the surrounding normal tissue
- No evidence of Infiltration, invasion and metastasis

Lymphatic Spread

- Common in carcinoma
- In sarcomas not usual path of spread
- Malignant cells/tumor cells involve the lymph nodes by "lymphatic permeation or in the form of "lymphatic emboli"
- **Regional nodal metastasis:** Involvement of regional lymph nodes. For example- breast carcinoma to axillary lymph nodes, from thyroid cancer to lateral cervical lymph nodes, etc.
- **Skip metastasis:** Sometimes, nearest lymph nodes may be by-passed because of venous-lymphatic anastomoses or due to obliteration of lymphatic channel.
- **Retrograde metastasis:** Lymph flow is disturbed due to obstruction of lymphatics and tumor cells spread against the flow of lymph. For example- metastasis of carcinoma prostate to the axillary lymph nodes, etc.
- **Virchow's lymph node:** Nodal metastasis from gallbladder, stomach or colon cancer to supraclavicular lymph node (preferably)

Hematogenous Spread

- Common route for sarcomas
- Common sites are liver, lungs, brain, bones, kidneys, adrenals, etc. for hematogenous spread
- Certain unfavourable sites that donot allow tumor metastasis are spleen, heart, skeletal muscle, etc.
- Appear as multiple, rounded nodules of varying size scattered throughout the organ
- **Examples:**
  - Tumours of bowel, spleen and pancreas have secondaries in liver because portal vein drain blood from these organs to liver
  - Pulmonary veins results in the spread of primary lung cancer but also provide route for metastatic growth in the lungs
  - **Retrograde spread:** Vertebral metastases in cancers of the thyroid and prostate

Uncommon Spread of Tumour

- **Transcoelomic spread:** Invasion of cancer cells through serosal wall and carried by coelomic fluid to a distant place. Peritoneal cavity is most commonly involved, pleural and pericardial cavities also involved.
  - **Examples:**
    - **Carcinoma of the bronchus and breast:** Spread to the pleura and pericardium
    - **Carcinoma of ovary:** Entire peritoneal cavity without infiltration of the underlying organs
    - **Stomach carcinoma:** Spread to both ovaries (Krukenberg tumor)
- **Spread through CSF:** Malignant tumors of the ependyma and leptomeninges
- **Spread along epithelial lined surfaces:** Through bronchus into alveoli, from kidney through uterus into lower urinary tract
- Implantation

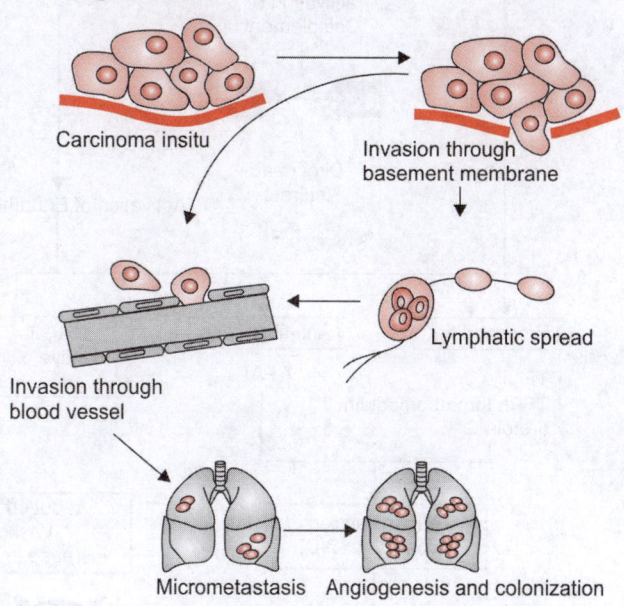

Carcinoma insitu

Invasion through basement membrane

Lymphatic spread

Invasion through blood vessel

Micrometastasis   Angiogenesis and colonization

PART-II

3. **Write briefly on:**

   a. **Septic shock**

   (Ref: Harsh Mohan, 7th ed. pg. 95, Robbins, SA ed. pg. 99)

ANSWER

Introduction

- Severe bacterial infection that results in hemostatic derangements, hemodynamic instability and malfunctioning of organ system

Etiology

- **Gram–negative bacteria (endotoxic shock):** Infection with E.coli (most common), Proteus, Klebsiella, Pseudomonas, Bacteroides

○ **Gram-positive bacteria (exotoxic shock):** Infection with streptococci, Pneumococci, Clostridia

○ **Viruses, Fungi, Parasites, etc.**

Source

○ **Endogenous:** Skin, Urinary tract, respiratory tract, GIT

○ **Exogenous:** Instruments, drapes, staff, imaging machines, etc.

Risk Factors

○ Malnutrition

○ Anemia

○ Malignancies

○ Major surgeries, trauma, extensive burn

○ Poor surgical technique, etc.

Pathogenesis

Consists of:

○ Macrophage-monocyte activation: results in liberation of free radicals and increased synthesis of nitric oxide resulting in vasodilatation and hypotension

○ Activation of inflammatory cascade, like-complement pathway, coagulation system, mast cells, kinin system

○ Results in vasodilatation and increased vascular permeability thus causing hyperdynamic circulation and inflammatory edema

○ Organ dysfunction as a result of hypotension and inadequate perfusion of cells and tissues

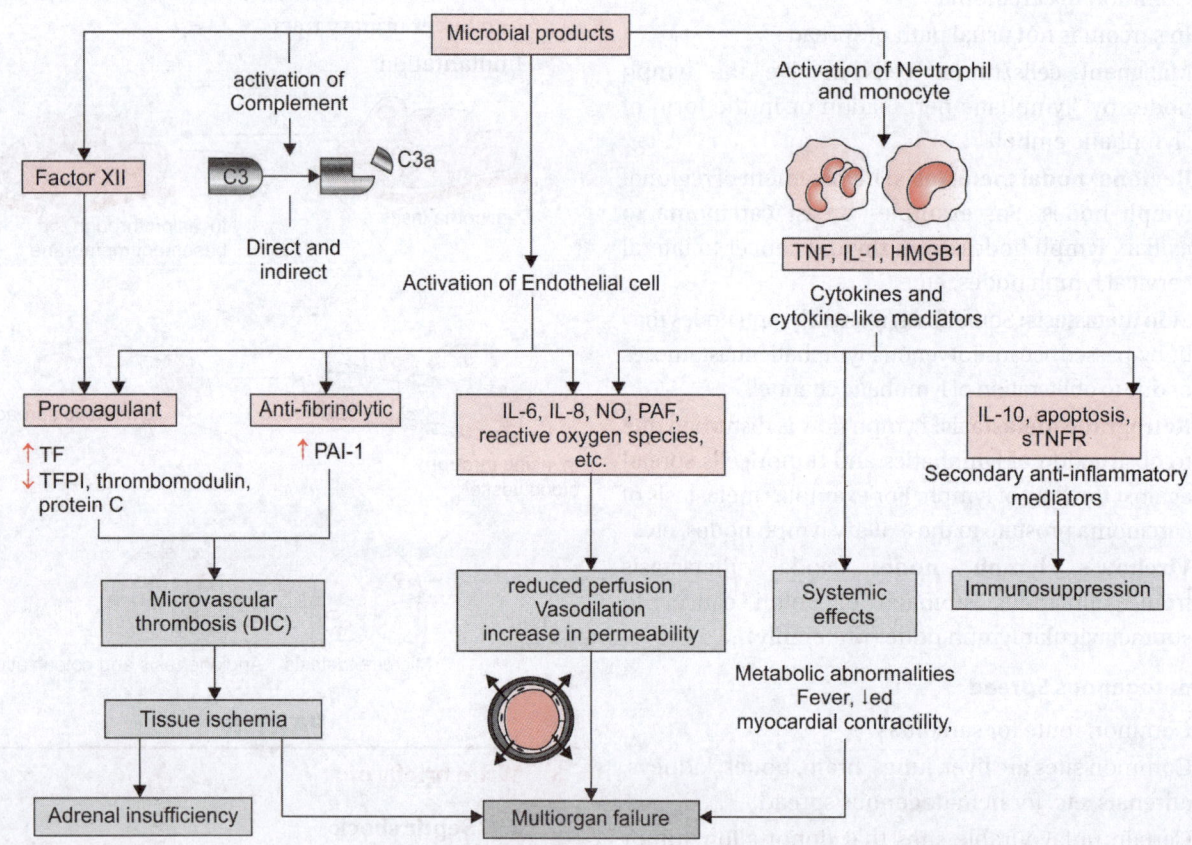

Clinical Features

○ Fever

○ Hypothermia

○ Hyperventilation

○ Confusion/disorientation

○ Tachypnoea

○ Tachycardia

○ Altered mental status

Treatment

○ Hemodynamic state to be improved

○ Tissue perfusion to be restored

○ Administration of oxygen and antibiotics(to combat infection)

○ Removal of septic focus

b. Morphologic types of necrosis

(Ref: Harsh Mohan, 7th ed. pg. 26, Robbins, SA ed. pg. 41)

ANSWER

Types of Necrosis

○ Depending on morphology, five types of necrosis:

  ▪ **Coagulative necrosis:**

- Most common type of necrosis occur as a result of focal irreversible injury (mainly ischemic necrosis)
- Commonly affected organs are- kidney, heart, spleen, etc.
- Microscopic appearance: loss of cytoplasmic and nuclear details but cellular outlines of the cells are retained

- **Caseous necrosis:**
  - Caseous means " cheese-like"
  - Common in tuberculosis, coccidiomycosis, etc.
  - Microscopic appearance: consist of necrosed, eosinophilic, granular material in the centre and peripherally surrounded by granulomatous inflammatory cells, mainly composed of epithelioid cells, giant cells and lymphocytes.

- **Fat necrosis:**
  - Commonly present in acute pancreatitis, breast, abdomen injury, etc.
  - Hydrolysis of fat cells results in release of free fatty acid and it combines with calcium thus forming calcium soaps (fat saponification)
  - **Microscopic appearance:** Cloudy appearance of necrosed cells with peripheral arrangement of inflammatory cell infiltrate. Calcium soaps in the form of basophilic, granular material is also evident

- **Liquefactive or colliquative necrosis:**
  - Loss of tissue architecture
  - Hydrolytic enzymes results in tissue degradation and formation of liquid viscous material
  - Example- CNS necrosis

- **Fibrinoid necrosis:**
  - Deposition of fibrin-like material and antigen-antibody complexes
  - Present in malignant hypertension, peptic ulcer, rheumatic fever, etc.
  - **Macroscopic features:** Deposition of hyaline-like material and debris of necrosed neutrophils

---

4. **Write briefly on:**

a. **Laboratory features of folate deficiency anemia**

(Ref: Harsh Mohan, 7th ed. pg. 282-283, Robbins, SA ed. pg. 648)

Laboratory Findings of Folate Deficiency Anemia

- The laboratory features are divided into:
  - **General laboratory findings:** Consist of CBC, bone marrow findings and biochemical test

- **Special/Specific test:** Consist of test that helps to differentiate whether the deficiency is due to vitamin B12 or folate

General Laboratory Findings

- **Complete blood count:**
  - **Hemoglobin:** Decreased
  - **Reticulocyte count:** May be reduced or normal
  - **MCV:** Increased (above 120 fl)
  - **MCHC:** Decreased/normal
  - **MCH:** Increased (above 50 pg)
  - **TLC:** May be decreased/normal
  - **Platelet:** Decreased (in case of moderate anemia)

- **Peripheral blood smear:**
  - Red cell macrocytosis
  - Marked anisocytosis, poikilocytosis
  - Macro-ovalocytes present
  - Hypersegmented neutrophils (more than 5 lobes) present
  - Presence of tear drop cells, and elongated red cells with inclusions like- basophilic stippling, Howell Jolly bodies and cabot's ring

- **Bone marrow findings:**
  - Hypercellular marrow
  - Decrease myeloid-erythroid ratio
  - Erythroid hyperplasia as a result of megaloblastic erythropoiesis
  - **Megaloblast:** Large, abnormal, nucleated erythroid precursor that exhibit less nuclear maturation than the development of cytoplasm. Large, sieve-like nuclei with open chromatin and in which nuclear maturation lags behind that of cytoplasmic maturation
  - Raised number and size of iron granules in erythroid precursor cells (positive for Prussian blue staining)
  - Band cells and giant form of metamyelocyte may also be present
  - Chromosomal abnormalities, like- chromosome breaks, centromere abnormalities, etc. may be present

Biochemical Findings

- Serum unconjugated bilirubin and LDH – increased
- Serum iron or ferritin- normal/raised

Special Test For Folate Deficiency

- Normal serum folate is 6–18 ng/mL
- Three tests are used to for the assessment of folate deficiency:
  - Urinary excretion of FIGLU
  - Serum folate assay
  - Red cell folate assay

Urinary Excretion of FIGLU

- In case of folate deficiency, urinary excretion of FIGLU is increased on oral intake of histidine

Serum Folate Assay

○ **Microbiological assay:**

▪ Presence of 5-methyl THF, a folic acid coenzyme is responsible for the activity of serum folate and also it is required for the growth of micro-organism, Lactobacillus casei

○ **Radioassay:**

▪ Pteroylglutamic acid or methyl-THF are used for radioassay

Red Cell Folate Assay

○ Reliable indicator of folate tissue stores than serum folate assay

○ Red cell folate values are reduced in megaloblastic anemia and in pernicious anemia

b. Factors predisposing to venous thrombosis

(Ref: Harsh Mohan, 7th ed. pg. 102, Robbins, SA ed. pg. 125)

ANSWER

Factors Responsible for Increased Risk of Venous Thrombosis

○ **Predisposing factors are:**

▪ Primary (hereditary)

▪ Secondary (acquired)

Primary Factors	Secondary Factors
Protein C and S deficiency:	**Clinical Conditions:**
• Autosomal dominant disorder with decreased protein C or S.	• Shock
	• Heart diseases, like- MI, CHF, cardiomyopathy, etc.
• Responsible for deep leg veins thrombosis	• Late pregnancy
Loss of Antithrombin III:	• Drugs like- oral contraceptives, anesthetic agents, etc.
• Autosomal dominant disorder	• Myeloproliferative disorders, dehydration, nephrotic syndrome,etc.
Factor V Leiden mutation:	
• Autosomal dominant disorder	• Vascular diseases- atherosclerosis, aneurysm, etc.
• Common cause of thrombophilia	• Trauma, fracture, burns, etc.
Coagulation factors:	**Risk Factors:**
• Raised level of coagulation factors- prothrombin and factor VIII may result in thrombosis	• Obesity
	• Bed-rest, if prolonged
	• Smoking
	• Elderly people
	Antiphospholipid antibody syndrome(APLA)
Fibrinolysis defect:	**Other factors:**
• Includes inherited disorders, like- plasminogen disorders	• Thrombocytopenia
	• Abortions
	• Transient ischemic attack, etc.

PART-III

5. Write short notes on:

a. Coomb's test

(Ref: Textbook of Pathology, Harsh Mohan, 7th ed. pg. 289)

ANSWER

Introduction

○ Also known as antiglobulin test

○ Discovered by Coombs et al.

Principle

○ During centifugation, Red cells sensitized with IgG or complement do not directly agglutinate

○ An additional antibody is required that reacts with Fc portion of the IgG antibody, or with the C3b or C3d component of complement for agglutination.

○ A "bridge"is formed between the antibodies or complement coating the red cells resulting in agglutination.

Methods

Two types:

○ **Direct Coomb's test:**

▪ Detection of incomplete antibodies coated on the surface of red cells (in vivo),like as in hemolytic disease of newborn

▪ **Indications:**

♦ Autoimmune hemolytic anemia

♦ Hemolytic disease of newborn

♦ Transfusion reactions

○ **Indirect Coomb's test:**

▪ Detection of incomplete antibodies in vitro (person's sera)

▪ **Indications:**

♦ In case of Rh positive child of a Rh negative mother and mother wants second conception

♦ In cross matching of blood for detection of incomplete antibodies in donar's serum

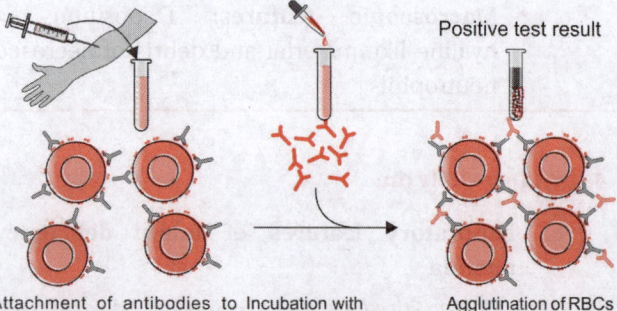

Attachment of antibodies to antigen on the surface of RBC

Incubation with antihuman antibodies (Coombs reagent)

Positive test result

Agglutination of RBCs

Fig. Direct coombs test

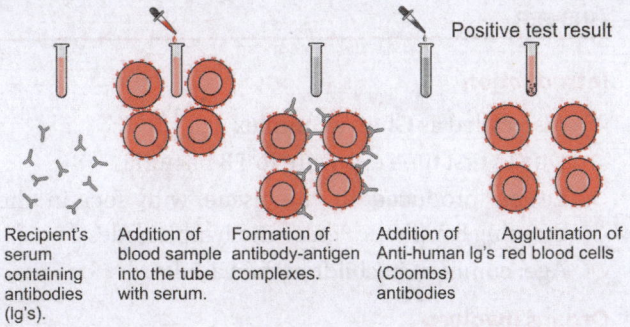

Fig. Indirect coombs test

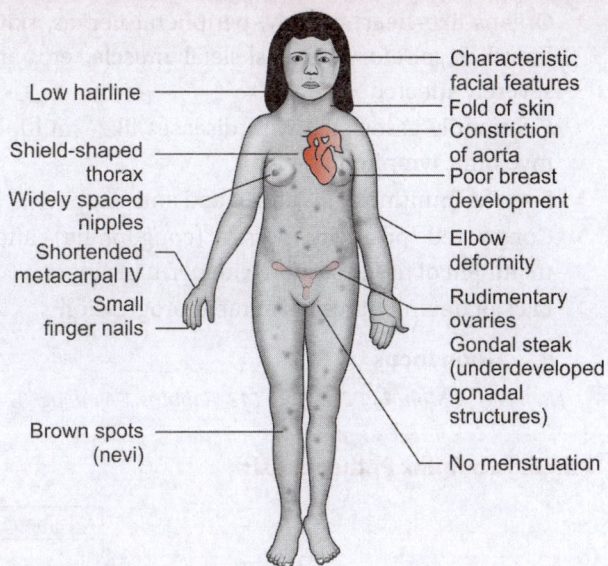

Fig. Turner syndrome

Interpretation

○ **Negative result:** No agglutination
○ **Positive result:** Seen in the following conditions-
  ▪ Hemolytic anemia
  ▪ Secondary to lymphomas
  ▪ Erythroblastosis fetalis (hemolytic disease of the newborn),
  ▪ Infectious mononucleosis,
  ▪ Systemic lupus erythematosus
  ▪ Idopathic
  ▪ Transfusion reaction, such as one due to improperly matched units of blood.
  ▪ Viral infections, Mycoplasma pneumonia,ETC.

b. Turner syndrome

(Ref: Harsh Mohan, 7th ed. pg. 253, Robbins, SA ed. pg. 166)

○ 4th metacarpal short
○ Pigmented nevi and cubitus valgus (increased carrying angle at the elbow)
○ Obesity, glucose intolerance, insulin resistance
○ Auto immune diseases
○ Mental status normal

c. Primary amyloidosis

(Ref: Harsh Mohan, 7th ed. pg. 71, Robbins, SA ed. pg. 258)

ANSWER

Introduction

○ Most common sex chromosome disorder
○ Seen in females
○ Monosomy (45, XO)

Genetic Abnormalities

○ **Classic type:** X chromosome missing in 57% (45, XO) (most common)
○ **Mosaic pattern:** 29% (45, XO/46, XX)
○ **Partial monosomy:** 14% cases

Clinical Features

○ **Cardiac abnormalities:** Coarctation of aorta and bicuspid aortic valve
○ Webbed neck and loose skin on the back of neck
○ Lower posterior hairline
○ Inadequate breast development
○ **Underdeveloped ovaries:** "Streak ovaries", infertility, amenorrhea
○ Broad chest and widely spaced nipples
○ Short stature and skeletal abnormalities(due to absence of copy of SHOX gene)

ANSWER

Introduction

○ Amyloid is a proteinaceous, pathological substance that is deposited between cells in various tissues and organs of the body
○ It is composed of—fibril material (95%) and P component along with other proteins
○ **Two types of amyloid proteins:**
  ▪ **Mutant proteins:** Unstable structurally, prone for aggregation and misfolding
  ▪ **Misfolded proteins:** Unstable and forms oligomers and fibrils

Primary Amyloidosis

○ A type of systemic(generalized) amyloidosis
○ Most common form of amyloidosis
○ Commonly seen in adults (more than 40 years of age)
○ Characterized by deposition of AL protein (light chain protein)mainly lambda chain than kappa
○ **Pathogenesis:** Stimulus/mutation→ proliferation of monoclonal B lymphocytes →no. of plasma cells increased→ light chain immunoglobulin→partial proteolysi) insoluble AL protein

○ Organs like–heart, kidney, peripheral nerves, skin, bowel, respiratory tract, skeletal muscle, etc. are severely affected

○ Commonly associated with diseases like- multiple myeloma, lymphomas, etc.

○ Specific immunostain- anti-λ and anti-kappa

○ Congo red positivity persist (congophilia) after treatment of tissue section with permanganate

○ Lack of treatment results in rapid progression

d. Ghon focus

(Ref: Harsh Mohan, 7th ed. pg. 142, Robbins, SA ed. pg. 374)

Primary complex Pathogenesis

ANSWER

Introduction

○ Also called as Ghon's complex

○ Due to first time exposure to TB bacteria

○ Lesion produced in the tissue with foci in the draining lymphatic vessel and lymph nodes

○ **Age:** common in children than adults

Organs Involved

○ Lungs and hilar lymph nodes- commonly involved

○ Other organs- tonsils, cervical lymph nodes, etc.

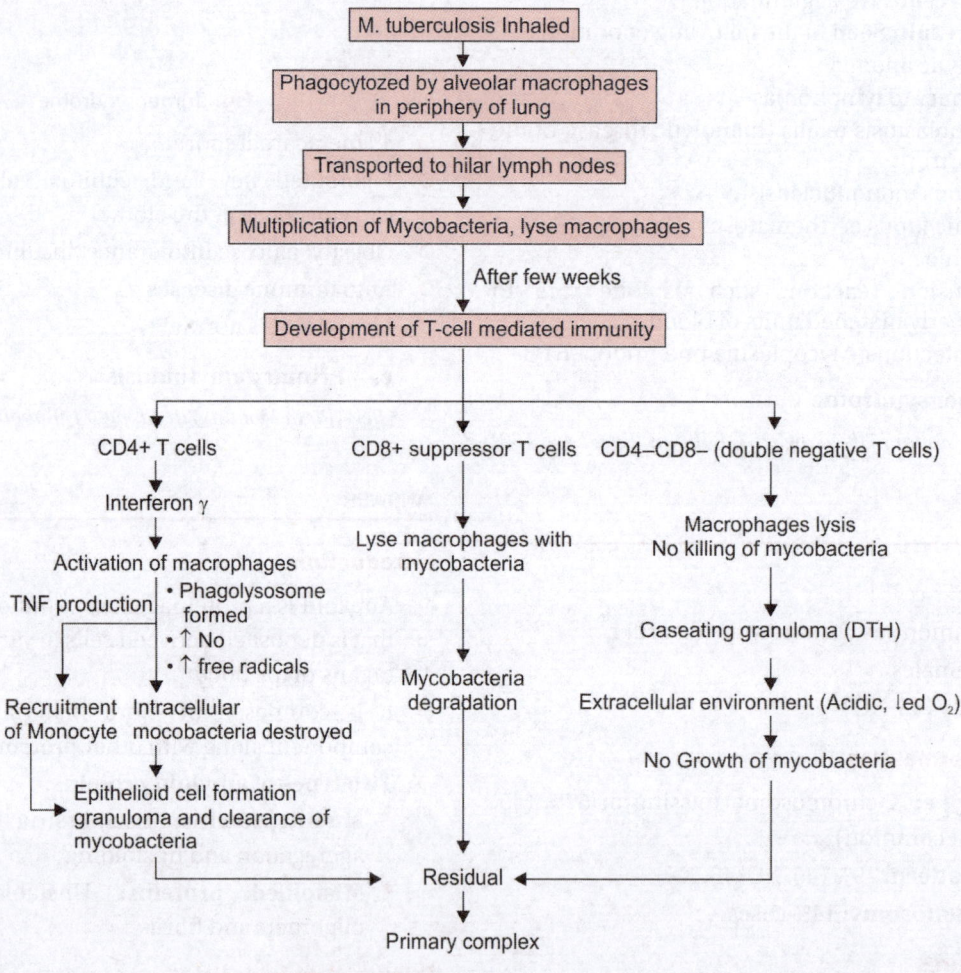

Flowchart: Primary complex Pathogenesis

Components

Three components:

○ **Pulmonary component:**
  ▪ Lesion in the lung is the primary focus or Ghon's focus
  ▪ 1–2 cm solitary area located more often in subpleural focus in the upper part of lower lobe

○ **Lymphatic vessel component:** Consist of
  ▪ Phagocytes with bacilli, miliary tubercles along the path of hilar lymph nodes

○ **Lymph node component**
  ▪ Enlarged matted, caseous lymph nodes (hilar and tracheobronchial lymph nodes)

Microscopic Findings

- Tuberculous granulomas with caseation necrosis in the center of the lesion

Fate of Primary Tuberculosis

- **Healing:**
  - Fibrosis and calcification
  - Bacilli may persist for life
  - Very small foci
- **Progressive primary tuberculosis:**
  - Spread to other areas of the same lung or opposite lung
- **Primary Miliary tuberculosis:**
  - Miliary spread to organs like lungs, liver, spleen, etc.
- **Progressive secondary tuberculosis:**
  - Reactivation of dormant primary complex

---

6. Write short notes on:

    a. **Mechanisms of apoptosis**

    (Ref: Harsh Mohan, 7th ed. pg. 29, Robbins, SA ed. pg. 52)

ANSWER

Introduction

- Means "falling off" or "droping off"
- Coordinated and internally programmed cell death
- Activation of intrinsic enzymes that lead to the degradation of cell's own DNA and proteins

Important Characteristics

- Membrane integrity preserved (no loss)
- No leakage of cellular contents
- Host reaction absent

Mechanism

- Two pathways- Mitochondrial pathway(intrinsic) and Death receptor pathway (extrinsic)
- Caspases activation

Mitochondrial (intrinsic) Pathway

- Major mechanism
- Due to increased mitochondrial permeability

- Damage to mitochondrial membrane and leakage of cytochrome C into cytoplasm leading to activation of caspase cascade

Death Receptor Initiated (Intrinsic) Pathway

- Death receptor activation on the cell membrane
- Death receptors: TNF-R1, Fas(CD95)
- Death receptors contain a cytoplasmic domain known as "death domain" required for delivering of apoptotic signals

Final Phase of Apoptosis

- Both of the mechanism results in activation of caspases
- **Mitochondrial pathway:** Activation of caspase-9
- **Death receptor pathway:** Activation of caspases-8 and 10
- Caspases results in activation of proteolytic actions leading to chromatin condensation, disruption of endoplasmic reticulum, mitochondrial damage and membrane permeability

Phagocytosis

- Membrane changes in dead apoptotic cells results in phagocytosis

Apoptosis

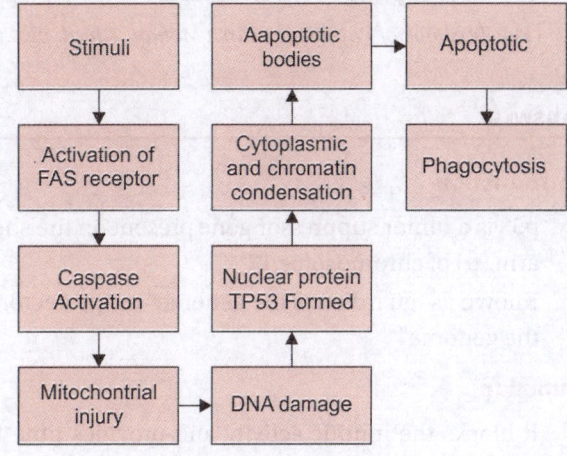

Fig. Steps of apoptosis

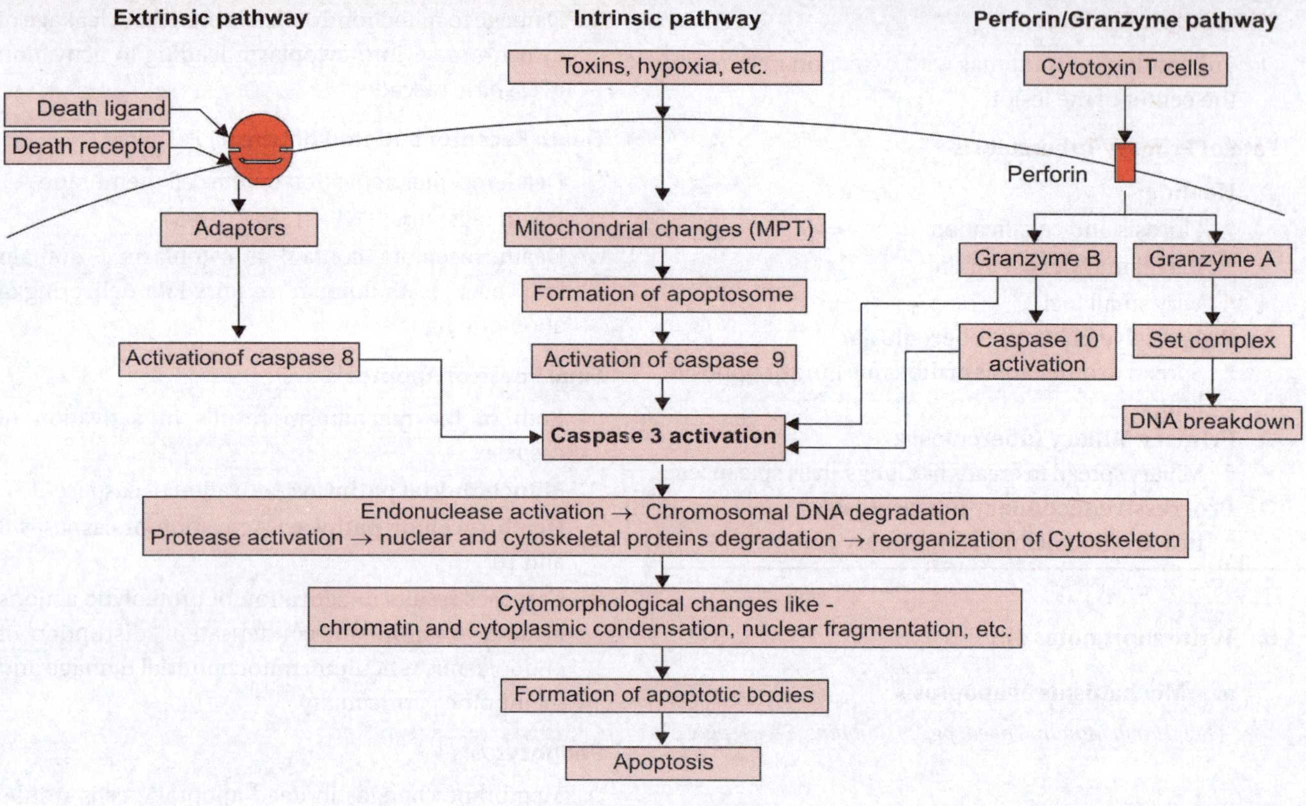

Extrinsic pathway
Intrinsic pathway
Perforin/Granzyme pathway
Toxins, hypoxia, etc.
Cytotoxin T cells
Death ligand
Death receptor
Perforin
Adaptors
Mitochondrial changes (MPT)
Granzyme B
Granzyme A
Formation of apoptosome
Activationof caspase 8
Activation of caspase 9
Caspase 10 activation
Set complex
DNA breakdown
Caspase 3 activation
Endonuclease activation → Chromosomal DNA degradation
Protease activation → nuclear and cytoskeletal proteins degradation → reorganization of Cytoskeleton
Cytomorphological changes like - chromatin and cytoplasmic condensation, nuclear fragmentation, etc.
Formation of apoptotic bodies
Apoptosis

Fig. Pathway of apoptosis

b. Role of p53 gene in neoplasia

(Ref: Textbook of Pathology, Harsh Mohan, 7th ed. pg. 206)

ANSWER

Introduction

- p53 is a tumor suppressor gene present on the short arm (p) of chromosome 17
- Known as "guardian of the genome" or "protector of the genome"

Function

- It blocks the mitotic activity and provides time for DNA repair thus inhibiting permanent mutational changes
- Promotes the apoptosis

Uses

- Helps in recognition of immune-phenotype of cancer cells
- To know the cancer origin
- Assess tumor behavior with tumor markers

Role in Neoplasia Development

- Normal cell- control cell proliferation and cell death and thus regulating cell growth
- Mutation in p53 results in-
  - Uncontrolled growth because mutated p53 acts as growth promoter
  - Most of the human cancers shows mutation in somatic cells gained as a result of homozygous loss of p53
  - Examples- breast cancer, cancer of head and neck, lung, etc.
  - Mutation of p53 gene is also evident in the progression of hyperplasia to invasive carcinoma along with carcinoma in situ

Stress signals like- inadequate metabolites, lack of growth factors, hypoxia, etc.
Stabilized and activated
Inactive functionally wild-type p53
Functionally active p53
Mutations
Cell death
Cell cycle arrest, repair of damaged DNA
Continuous proliferation, genomic instability and progression of tumor

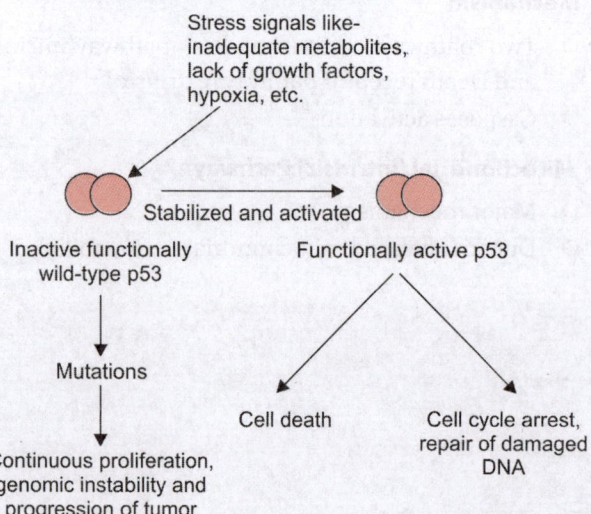

Fig. Role of p53 in development of neoplasia

c. **Factors affecting wound healing**

(Ref: Harsh Mohan, 7th ed. pg. 160, Robbins, SA ed. pg. 105)

ANSWER

Factors Affecting Wound Healing

○ **Local factors:**
- ▪ **Diminished blood supply:**
  - ♦ Decreases the rate of healing. For example–injuries in legs heals slowly whereas facial injuries heals faster
- ▪ **Location, size and type of wound:**
  - ♦ Responsible for the type of healing whether by- resolution or by organisation
- ▪ **Movement:**
  - ♦ Decreases the rate of healing
- ▪ Exposure to ionizing and ultraviolet radiation:
  - ♦ Ionising radiation delays healing whereas UV light enhances the healing process

- ▪ **Wound Infection:**
  - ♦ Decreases the healing process
- ▪ **Foreign bodies:**
  - ♦ Causes inflammatory reaction, infection and delays healing
○ **Systemic factors:**
- ▪ **Age:**
  - ♦ Healing is fast in young whereas slow rate of healing in older age group
- ▪ **Systemic infection:**
  - ♦ Decreases rate of healing
- ▪ **Nutrititional disorders:**
  - ♦ Nurtritional deficiencies like- vitamin A,C, Zinc, etc. delays wound healing
- ▪ **Diabetes:**
  - ♦ If uncontrolled, susceptible to infection with delayed wound healing
- ▪ **Hematologic defects:**
  - ♦ Bleeding disorders, neutropenia, etc. delays the healing

Name of the Paper : **Pathology Paper-II**

Name of the Course : **MBBS-2016**

Semester : **Annual**

Time: 3 Hours   M.M.: 40

INSTRUCTIONS

1. Write your Roll No. on the top immediately on receipt of this question paper
2. All questions are to be attempted
3. Answers to Parts I, II and III should be written in separate answer sheets provided
4. Attempt parts of a question in sequence

PART-I

1. **Differentiate between:**   [8]
   a. Syphillitic and aortic aneurysm
   b. Centriacinar and panacinar emphysema
   c. Crohn's disease and ulcerative colitis
   d. Conjugated and unconjugated hyperbilirubinemia

2. **Write briefly on:**   [6]
   a. Complications of atheromatous plaque
   b. Hodgkin lymphoma
   c. Pathogenesis of rheumatoid arthritis

PART-II

3. **Write briefly on:**   [6]
   a. Hydatidiform mole
   b. Minimal change glomerulonephritis

4. **Write briefly on:**   [6]
   a. Ulcerative lesions of small intestine
   b. Ewing sarcoma

PART-III

5. **Write short notes on:**   [8]
   a. Transitional cell carcinoma urinary bladder
   b. Sequelae of hepatitis B infection
   c. Astrocytoma
   d. Secondary pulmonary TB

6. **Write short notes on:**   [6]
   a. Teratoma
   b. Papillary thyroid carcinoma
   c. Renal changes in diabetes mellitus

PART I

1. **Differentiate between:**

    a. **Syphilitic and aortic aneurysm**

    (Ref: Harsh Mohan, 7th ed. pg. 386, Robbins, SA ed. pg. 501)

ANSWER

Syphilitic and Aortic Aneurysm

Syphilitic aneurysm	Aortic aneurysm
• Site of involvement is thoracic aorta	• Site of involvement is abdominal aorta
• Saccular in shape and around 3-5 cm in diameter	• Fusiform in shape and larger than 5-6 cm in diameter
• Healed syphilitic aortitis with adventitia showing fibrous thickening with endarteritis obliterans of vasa vasorum	• Atherosclerotic aneurysm wall loses its normal arterial structure
• Fibrous scar tissue may extend into media and intima	• Predominance of fibrous tissue in the media and adventitia with mild chronic inflammatory reaction
• Spirochetes may be found in syphilitic aneurysm, sometimes mural thrombus can be seen	• Intima and inner part of media exhibits remnants of atheromatous plaques and mural thrombus

• Effects include
  ▪ Rupture into pleural cavity, pericardial sac, trachea and oesophagus
  ▪ Compression on trachea causing dyspnoea, on oesophagus causing dysphagia, on recurrent laryngeal nerve leading to hoarseness, erosion of vertebrae, sternum and ribs
  ▪ Cardiac dysfunction
	• Effects include:
	  ▪ Rupture into peritoneum or into retroperitoneum leading to sudden and massive bleeding
	  ▪ Compression of ureter and erosion on vertebral bodies
	  ▪ Arterial occlusion

    b. **Centriacinar and Panacinar emphysema**

    (Ref: Harsh Mohan, 7th ed. pg. 461-62, Robbins, SA ed. pg. 675)

ANSWER

Panacinar and Centriacinar Emphysema

Panacinar Emphysema	Centriacinar Emphysema
• Central or proximal part of acinus is involved	• All portions of acinus are involved
• Associated with chronic bronchitis and coal miners' pneumoconiosis	• Associated with alpha1-antitrypsin in middle aged smokers
• Morphological changes, gross appearance – upper lobes of lungs are commonly affected	• Morphological changes, gross appearance – lower zone of lungs are commonly affected

    c. **Crohn disease and Ulcerative colitis**

    (Ref: Textbook of Pathology, Harsh Mohan, 7th ed. pg. 552)

ANSWER

Crohn Disease and Ulcerative Colitis

Characteristic	Crohn disease	Ulcerative colitis
Site of origin	Distal ileum, proximal colon	Rectum
Thickness of pathology	Transmural	Mucosa and submucosa only
Progression	Irregular (skip lesions)	Proximal, continuous from rectum; no skipped areas
Location	From mouth to anus	Involves colon and rectum; rarely extends to ileum
Change in bowel habits	Obstruction, abdominal pain	Bloody diarrhea
Classic lesions	Fistulas or abscesses, cobblestoning, string sign on barium radiographs	Pseudopolyps, lead-pipe colon on barium radiographs, toxic megacolon
Colon cancer risk	Slightly increased	Markedly increased
Surgery cures bowel disease?	No (can worsen it)	Yes (Proctocolectomy with ileoanal anastomosis)

Characteristic	Crohn disease	Ulcerative colitis

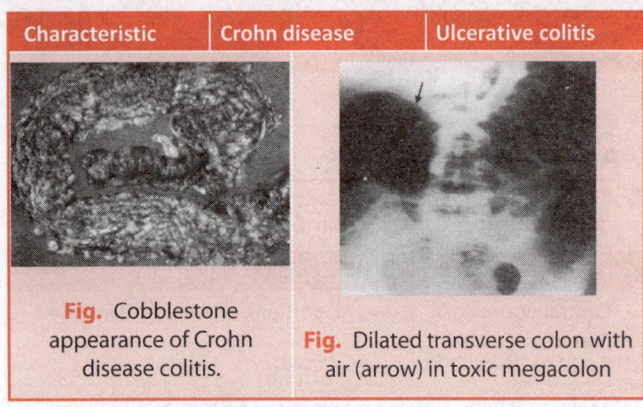

Fig. Cobblestone appearance of Crohn disease colitis.

Fig. Dilated transverse colon with air (arrow) in toxic megacolon

d. Conjugated and Unconjugated hyperbilirubinemia

(Ref: Textbook of Pathology, Harsh Mohan, 7th ed. pg. 582)'

ANSWER

Conjugated bilirubin	Unconjugated bilirubin
Normal serum level is decreased (less than 0.25 mg/dl)	Normal serum level is increased
Water solubility is present	Water solubility is not present
Alcohol solubility is not present	Alcohol solubility is present
Serum albumin binding is low	Serum albumin binding is high
Direct van der Bergh reaction	Indirect van der Bergh reaction
Excretion by kidneys is present	Excretion by kidneys is absent
Bilirubin albumin covalent complex is formed	Bilirubin albumin covalent complex is not formed
Brain tissue affinity is absent	Brain tissue affinity is present

2. Write briefly on:

a. Complications of atheromatous plaque

(Ref: Harsh Mohan, 7th ed. pg. 378, Robbins, SA ed. pg. 491)

ANSWER

Introduction

- Atherosclerotic lesion is known as atheromatous plaque
- Also known as "atheroma", fibrous plaque or "fibrofatty plaque"
- Abdominal aorta is most commonly affected with major involvement of iliac, femoral, carotid, coronary and cerebral arteries

Morphological Features

- **Gross appearance:**
  - Yellowish-white in colour
  - Small size(1–2 cm in diameter)
- Consists of white fibrous cap and a soft, yellow-white central core thus called as atheroma
- **Microscopic findings:**
  - Central soft core composed of lipids, cholesterol clefts, foam cells, fibrin and cellular debris
  - White fibrous cap composed of smooth muscle cells, dense connective tissue and extracellular matrix composed of proteoglycans and collagen
  - Cellular area present below the fibrous cap composed of foam cells, macrophages, lymphocytes and lipid containing smooth muscle cells

Complications

- **Calcification:**
  - Common in advanced atheromatous plaque mainly aorta and coronaries
  - Microscopic findings revels calcium salt deposition in the necrotic areas and lipid pool present deep into the thick intima
- **Thrombosis:**
  - Areas of endothelial damage and ulcerated plaque are the common sites
  - May get dislodged and lodges elsewhere in the circulation
  - May lodge into the arterial wall as mural thrombi
- **Ulceration:**
  - As a result of mechanical trauma
  - Release of lipid material and debris into the blood stream from emboli
  - Resulting in shallow, ragged ulcer with lipid debris in the base of the ulcer
- **Hemorrhage:**
  - Common complication in coronary arteries
  - Intimal hemorrhage in the atheromatous plaque due to blood in the vascular lumen or due to rupture of thin walled capillaries
- **Formation of aneurysm:**
  - Thinning and atrophy of media, fibrosis of adventitia results in weakening of the arterial wall thus aneurysmal dilatation

b. Hodgkin lymphoma

(Ref: Harsh Mohan, 7th ed. pg. 348, Robbins, SA ed. pg. 588)

ANSWER

Introduction

- Occurs in lymph nodes (commonly in cervical region)

Pathogenesis

- Transcription factor NF-κB activation – common in classical Hodgkin lymphoma
- Cytokines (IL-5, IL-10, M-CSF), chemokines (eg. eotaxin)and certain other factors (like – immunomodulatory factors) secreted by RS cells
- **Infections:** EBV, herpesvirus -6, HTLV-1 and II, etc.

Types

Subtype	Morphology	Immunophenotype	Ebv association	Clinical features
Mixed cellularity	Mononuclear cells	CD15+, CD30+;	70% EBV+ve	Common in India, stage III or IV; M>F; biphasic; prognosis is good
Lymphocyte rich	Mononuclear cells	CD15+, CD30+;	40% EBV+ve	Uncommon; M>F, prognosis is good
Lymphocyte depletion	Reticular variant	CD15+, CD30+;	90% EBV+ve	More common in males; HIV infected, not good prognosis
Nodular sclerosis	Lacunar cells, plasma cells and Fibrous strands	CD15+, CD30+;	Commonly EBV-ve	Common in World; M=F; usually stage I or II; mediastinal involvement is common, Good prognosis
Lymphocyte predominance	Lymphocytic and Histiocytic (popcorn cell)	CD20+, CD15-, C30-;	EBV-ve	Not common; young males with cervical or axillary lymph. nodes, prognosis is good

Morphology

- T lymphocytes surrounding RS cells in a rosette –like manner

Diagnosis

- **Reed-Sternberg cells:**
  - Binucleated or bilobed with two halves that appear as mirror image of each other
  - Nucleus shows large owl-eye nucleoli surrounded by a clear halo
- **Variants:**
  - **Lacunar cells:** Multilobed or folded nuclei surrounded by pale cytoplasm
  - **Mononuclear variant:** Round or oblong single nucleus
  - **Lymphocytic and histiocytic variant:** Popcorn appearance

Prognosis

- **Prognosis is poor if:**
  - Hemoglobin <10.5g/dL
  - Albumin<4.0 g/dL

Clinical Features

- **Lymphadenopathy:** Discrete, non-tender, rubbery lymph nodes
- Classical Pel Ebstein fever (cyclical pattern of fever, intermittent every alternate week)
- Fever
- Night sweats
- Unexplained weight loss (in advanced stage)
- Cutaneous allergy due to depressed cell-mediated immunity

- Sex-male
- Age- 45 years or more
- Stage – IV
- Lymphocytopenia
- Leucocytosis at or above 15000/mm³

c. **Pathogenesis of Rheumatoid arthritis**

(Ref: Harsh Mohan, 7th ed. pg. 843, Robbins, SA ed. pg. 1209)

ANSWER

Pathogenesis of Rheumatoid Arthritis

Introduction

- Chronic systemic inflammatory disorder which affects joints producing a non-suppurative proliferative synovitis which usually progresses to destruction of the articular cartilage and ankylosis of the joints and may involve tissues and organs such as skin, blood vessels, heart, lung and muscles
- Occurs in 30–40 years of age; females are more commonly affected

Etiopathogenesis

○ Genetic predisposition – HLA-DR4 or HLA-DR1
○ Autoimmunity–once inflammatory synovitis is triggered by exogenous factors, autoimmunity

(T cell mediate immunity) causes chronic destruction in RA
○ Infectious agents such as mycoplasma, EBV, CMV, rubella

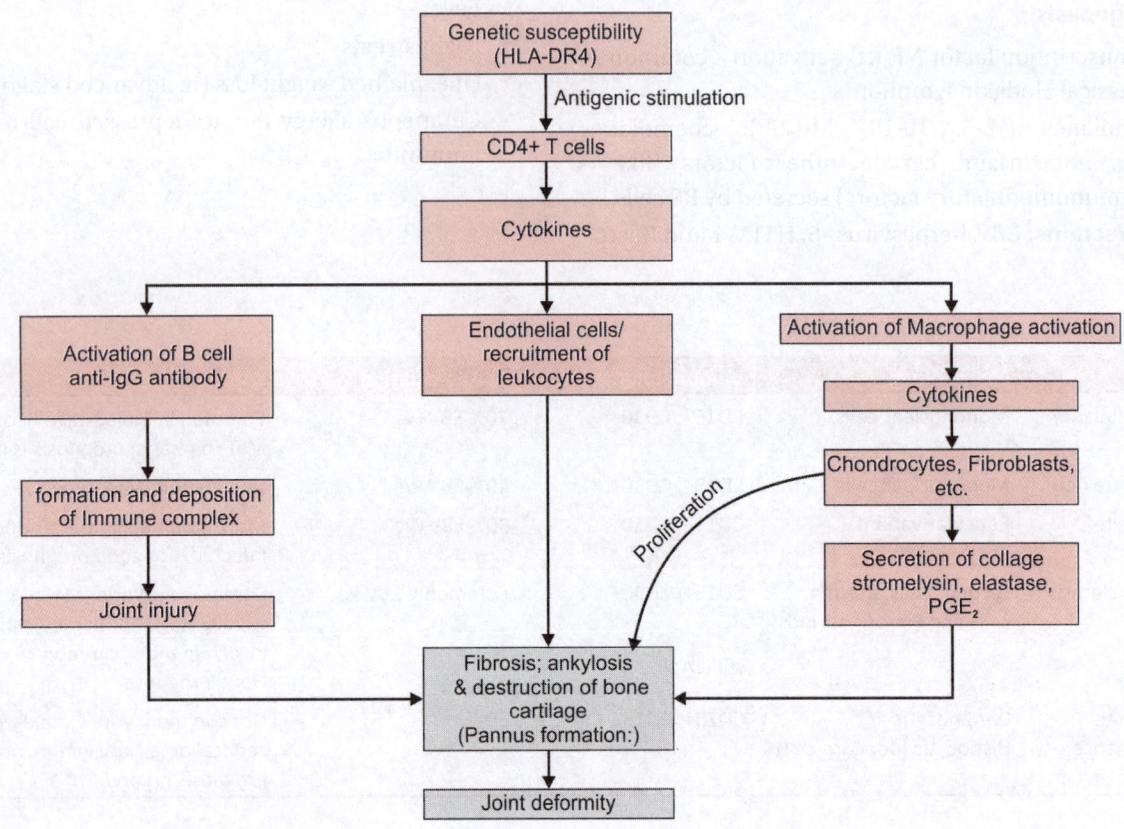

PART II

3. Write briefly on:

a. Hydatidiform mole

(Ref: Textbook of Pathology, Harsh Mohan, 7th ed. pg. 761)

ANSWER

Hydatidiform Mole

Introduction

○ Abnormal placenta with enlarged, hydropic and vesicular chorionic villi and variable trophoblastic proliferation
○ Appears after 4–5th month of pregnancy
○ Uterus is enlarged with presence of grape like vesicles
○ Symptoms are vaginal bleeding, with symptoms of toxaemia
○ HCG level in urine and plasma are increased
○ Survival rate – 2% develop choriocarcinoma

Types

○ Non-Invasive
  ▪ Partial mole
  ▪ Complete mole
○ Invasive

	Partial mole	Complete mole
Ploidy	Triploid	Diploid
Number of chromosomes	69, XXX; 69, XXY; 69, XYY	46 (All paternal) 46, XX; 46, XY
β-hCG	Elevated (+)	Elevated (+++)
Chorionic villi	Some are hydropic	All are hydropic
Trophoblast proliferation	Focal	Marked
Fetal tissue	Present	Absent
Invasive mole	2%	10%
Choriocarcinoma	Rare	2%
Components	2 sperm + 1 egg	Most commonly enucleated egg + single sperm egg + single sperm (subsequently duplicates paternal DNA)

b. **Minimal change glomerulonephritis**

(Ref: Harsh Mohan, 7th ed. pg. 656, Robbins, SA ed. pg. 917)

ANSWER

Minimal Change Glomerulonephritis

Introduction

○ Condition where nephrotic syndrome is associated with no evident change in glomeruli by light microscopy

○ Characteristic features are–absence of immune deposits but has an immunologic basis

Etiopathogenesis

○ Idiopathic

○ Cases associated with systemic diseases i.e. Hodgkin's disease, HIV infection and drug therapy such as NSAIDs, rifampicin, interferon-alpha

Morphology

○ **Gross appearance:** Kidneys are normal in size and shape

○ **Light microscopic appearance:**
  ▪ Glomeruli appear normal, slight increase in the mesangial matrix (minimal change lesion)
  ▪ Tubules–presence of fine lipid vacuolation and hyaline droplets in the cells of proximal convoluted tubules
  ▪ Interstitium–may have oedema
  ▪ Vessels–no noticeable change

○ **Electron microscopic appearance:**
  ▪ Diffuse effacement of foot processes of the visceral epithelial cells (podocytes)
  ▪ No electron dense deposits

○ **Immunofluorescence microscopic appearance:**
  ▪ No deposits of immunoglobulins or complement

Clinical Features

○ Prognosis is excellent – more than 90% cases respond rapidly to steroids

○ Renal function remains normal

○ No hypertension or hematuria

○ Selective proteinuria is found

---

4. **Write briefly on:**

  a. **Ulcerative lesions of small intestine**

ANSWER

Ulcerative Lesions of Small Intestine

Introduction

○ Small intestine includes duodenum, jejunum and ileum

○ Ulcerative lesions of small intestine includes:
  ▪ Peptic ulcer
  ▪ Ulcerative colitis
  ▪ Crohn's disease

Peptic Ulcer

○ Areas of degeneration and necrosis of GIT mucosa exposed to acid-peptic secretions

○ Can occur at any level of alimentary tract that is exposed to hydrochloric acid and pepsin

○ **Etiology**
  ▪ Psychological stress
  ▪ Physiological stress
    ◆ Shock
    ◆ Severe trauma
    ◆ Septicaemia
    ◆ Extensive burns
    ◆ Intracranial lesions
    ◆ Drug intake–aspirin, steroids, butazolidine, indomethacin
    ◆ H. Pylori
    ◆ Gastritis
    ◆ Dietary factors
    ◆ Psychological factors
    ◆ Hormonal factors
    ◆ Local irritants–e.g. alcohol, smoking, coffee

○ **Composed of 4 layers**
  ▪ Necrotic zone—base has thin layer of fibrinoid debris
  ▪ Superficial exudative zone—zone of neutrophil predominant infiltrate
  ▪ Granulation tissue zone—base has active granulation tissue with mononuclear leukocytes
  ▪ Zone of cicatrisation—zone of fibrous or collagenous scar

Ulcerative Colitis and Crohn's Disease

○ Extends into mucosa and submucosa

○ Mural thickening absent, serosal surface appears normal and strictures are not present

○ Has association with HLA-DR2, polymorphism in

IL-10 gene and abnormal T-cell response especially of Th2 cells

○ Involves rectum and extends proximally to include part of colon in continuous fashion—Pancolitis

○ Severe cases of pancolitis with mild mucosal inflammation of the distal ileum—backlash Ileitis in 10% cases

○ **Morphology of ulcerative colitis:**

- **Gross appearance:**

  ♦ Continuous involvement of rectum and colon without skipping any areas

  ♦ Mucosa exhibits non penetrating linear and superficial ulcers

  ♦ Inflammatory pseudopolyps are formed in intervening intact mucosa

  ♦ Thickening of muscle layer due to contraction thereby producing shortening and narrowing of affected colon with loss of normal haustral folds giving garden hose appearance

- **Microscopic appearance:**

  ♦ Crypt distortion, cryptitis, focal accumulation of neutrophils producing crypt abscesses

  ♦ Marked congestion, dilatation and haemorrhages from mucosal capillaries

  ♦ Superficial mucosal ulceration

  ♦ Reduced goblet cells

  ♦ Mucosal regeneration and mucodepletion of lining cells

  ♦ Epithelial cytologic atypia

○ **Morphology of Crohn's disease:**

- **Gross appearance**

  ♦ Multiple, well demarcated segmental bowel involvement with intervening uninvolved skip areas unlike ulcerative colitis

  ♦ Wall is thickened and hard, resembling a hose pipe

  ♦ Serosa studded with minute granulomas

  ♦ Narrow lumen of segment

  ♦ Serpiginous ulcers appear whereas intervening surviving mucosa is swollen with cobblestone appearance

- **Microscopic appearance:**

  ♦ Transmural inflammatory cell infiltrate

  ♦ Non-caseating sarcoid like granulomas

  ♦ Patchy ulceration of mucosa

  ♦ Widening of submucosa

  ♦ Increased fibrosis in all layers

b. Ewing Sarcoma

(Ref: Harsh Mohan, 7th ed. pg. 839, Robbins, SA ed. pg. 1203)

ANSWER

Ewing's Sarcoma

Introduction

○ Highly malignant small round cell tumour affecting patients of 5-20 years of age with preference for females

○ 3 types of Ewing's sarcoma are:

- Classic (skeletal) Ewing's sarcoma
- Soft tissue Ewing's sarcoma
- Primitive neuroectodermal tumour (PNET)

○ All 3 types are linked together by common neuroectodermal origin and by a common cytogenetic translocation abnormality t(11; 22) (q24; 12)

○ Skeletal Ewing's sarcoma begins in medullary canal of diaphysis or metaphysis

Clinical Features

○ Pain

○ Tenderness

○ Swelling of affected part

○ Fever

○ Leucocytosis

○ Raised ESR

Diagnosis

○ Radiographic examination shows predominantly osteolytic lesion with patchy subperiosteal reactive bone formation producing typical onion-skin appearance

Morphology

○ **Gross appearance:**

- Located in medullary cavity and affected diaphysis or metaphysis expands commonly extending to adjacent soft tissues

- Appearance of tumour tissue is grey-white, soft and friable

○ **Microscopic appearance:**

- Small round cell tumours involving other tumours such as PNET, neuroblastoma, embryonal rhabdomyosarcoma, lymphoma-leukaemias and metastatic small cell carcinoma

  ♦ Pattern–Fibrous septa divides the tumour into irregular lobules of closely packed tumour cells which are characteristically organised around capillaries forming pseudorosettes

  ♦ Tumour cells–Small, uniform tumour cells similar to lymphocytes and have indefinite cytoplasmic outlines, scanty cytoplasm and round nuclei having salt and pepper chromatin and recurrent mitoses

♦ Also known as round cell tumour or small blue cell tumour

♦ Cytoplasm contains glycogen which stains with periodic acid-Schiff (PAS) reaction

♦ Frequently expressed cell surface marker by tumour cells of ES/PNET group is CD99 which is a product of MIC-2 gene located on X and Y chromosome

PART III

5. Write short notes on:

a. Transitional cell carcinoma urinary bladder

(Ref: Textbook of Pathology, Harsh Mohan, 7th ed. pg. 687)

ANSWER

Transitional Cell Carcinoma Urinary Bladder

Introduction

○ Most of the tumours arise from transitional epithelial lining of bladder in continuity with that of renal, pelvis, ureters and major part of urethra

○ Out of all the cancers, bladder cancer comprises about 3%

○ More frequently affects men of 50 to 80 years of age group

Etiology

○ Cigarette smoking

○ Industrial exposure to substances like beta-naphthylamine and benzene

○ Schistosomiasis

○ Dietary factors–artificial sweeteners such as saccharin, coffee, caffeine and chronic alcoholism

○ Local lesions–ectopia vesicae, vesical diverticulum, leukoplakia etc

○ Drugs–immunosuppressive therapy with cyclophosphamide and patients having analgesic abuse nephropathy

○ Prior irradiation–for some pelvic cancers

Genetic Alterations

○ Fibroblast growth receptor 3, p53, RB gene and p21 gene

Clinical Symptoms

○ Painless hematuria

○ Frequency of micturition

○ Urgency of micturition

○ **Dysuria**

b. Sequelae of hepatitis B infection

(Ref: Textbook of Pathology, Harsh Mohan, 7th ed. pg. 591)

ANSWER

Clinical Features of Hepatitis B

○ Hepatitis B is an infectious disease caused by Hepatitis B virus

○ **In acute illness:**

▪ Incubation period from 30–180 days

▪ Clinically not apparent and usually mild

▪ Fever

▪ Anorexia

▪ Fatigue, jaundice

▪ **Phases:**

♦ **Viral replication phase (Phase 1):**

▫ Asymptomatic

▫ Demonstration of serological and enzyme markers

♦ **Prodromal phase (Phase 2):**

▫ Anorexia, nausea, vomiting, malaise, fatigue, urticaria, pruritus, taste alteration, etc.

♦ **Icteric phase (Phase 3):**

▫ Pale colored stools, dark urine, icterus, right upper quadrant pain and hepatomegaly

♦ **Convalescent phase (Phase 4):**

▫ Symptoms resolve

▫ Liver enzymes back to normal

○ **Chronic hepatitis B:**

▪ Persistent anorexia, weight loss and fatigue (suggestive of progression)

▪ Persistent hepatomegaly

○ **Extrahepatic findings:**

▪ Arthritis

▪ Arthralgia

▪ Glomerulonephritis

▪ Pleural effusion

▪ Pericarditis

▪ Generalized vasculitis

▪ Henoch-schonlein purpura, etc.

Sequelae of Hepatitis B: Infection

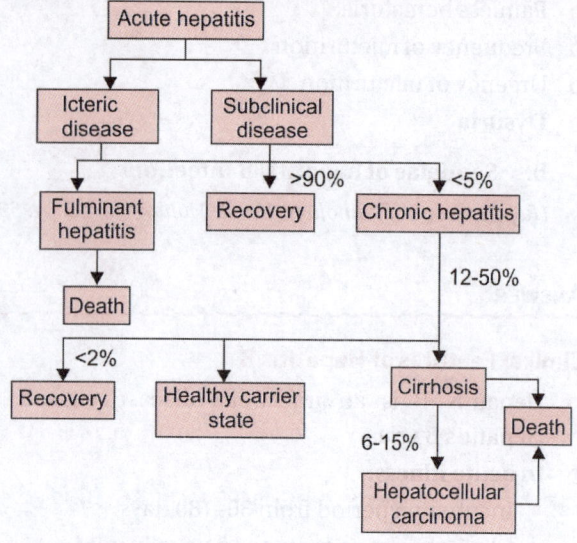

c. Astrocytoma

(Ref: Harsh Mohan, 7th ed. pg. 879, Robbins, SA ed. pg. 1306)

ANSWER

Astrocytoma

Introduction

○ Most frequent type of gliomas occurring in elderly age

○ Mostly found in cerebral hemispheres and rarely in spinal cord but in children and young adults, pilocytic astrocytomas appears in optic nerve, cerebellum and brainstem

○ Tends to progress from low grade to higher grades of anaplasia where low grade astrocytomas arise slowly and higher grades arise rapidly deteriorating patient's health

Classification

According to WHO

○ WHO Grade I–Diffuse astrocytoma

- Low grade tumour
- Prognosis is good
- Comprises of special histologic entities occurring in children
  - Juvenile pilocytic astrocytoma
    - Affects children and young adults in cerebellum, 3rd ventricle and optic nerve pathway
    - Grossly, cystic or solid and circumscribed
    - Microscopically, mainly composed of fusiform pilocytic astrocytes with unusually long, wavy fibrillary processes
  - **Pleomorphic xanthoastrocytoma**
    - Appears histologically pleomorphic and alarming
    - Satisfactory prognosis

○ **WHO Grade II (Well Differentiated)–Fibrillary astrocytoma**

- Most frequent type of glioma
- Occurs in 3rd -4th decade of life
- **Grossly**
  - Poorly defined
  - Grey-white appearance
  - Variable size
  - Distorts underlying tissue and merges with surrounding tissue
- **Histologically**
  - Composed of well differentiated astrocytes separated by variable amount of fibrillary background of astrocytic process
  - Depending on type of astrocytes, 3 subtypes are classified
    - Fibrillary
    - Protoplastic
    - Gemistocytic astrocytoma

○ **WHO Grade III (Anaplastic)**

- Arises from low grade astrocytoma
- **Grossly**
  - Indistinguishable from low grade astrocytoma
- **Histologically:**
  - Has characteristics of anaplasia such as hypercellularity, pleomorphism, nuclear hyperchromatism and mitoses
  - Proliferation of vascular endothelium

○ **WHO Grade IV (Glioblastoma Multiforme)**

- Originates by neoplastic transformation of mature astrocytes
- Most aggressive astrocytoma
- **Grossly:**
  - Multicolored appearance with few areas presenting grey white appearance whereas others are yellow and soft with foci of hemorrhages and necrosis
  - Distorted surrounding normal brain tissue with yellow tumour tissue infiltration
- **Histologically:**
  - Highly anaplastic and cellular appearance
  - Marked variation of cell types comprising of fusiform cells, small poorly differentiated round cells, pleomorphic cells and giant cells
  - Mitoses are common
  - Scanty glial fibrils
  - Presents areas of tumour necrosis around which tumour cells may form pseudo palisading
  - Noticeable microvascular endothelial proliferation

d. Secondary pulmonary TB

(Ref: Textbook of Pathology, Harsh Mohan, 7th ed. pg. 143)

ANSWER

Secondary pulmonary TB

Introduction

- Reinfection (exogenous source) or reactivation of silent primary tuberculosis focus (endogenous source)
- Occurs most frequently in lungs, other sites are lymph nodes, tonsils, pharynx, small intestine, skin
- Lesions begin as 1–2 cm apical area of consolidation of the lung which develops into a small area of central caseation necrosis and peripheral fibrosis
- Occurs due to lymphohematogenous spread of infection from primary complex to apex of affected lung where oxygen tension if high and favours growth of tubercle bacilli
- Microscopic appearance is characteristic of tuberculous granulomas with caseation necrosis
- Pattern of lesion is similar to that of primary tuberculosis – with involvement of hilar lymph nodes rather than cavitary apical lesions of the lung

Types of Secondary Pulmonary Tuberculosis:

- Fibrocaseous tuberculosis
- Tuberculous caseous pneumonia
- Military tuberculosis
- Tuberculous empyema

6. Write short notes on:

a. Teratoma

(Ref: Harsh Mohan, 7th ed. pg. 735-737, Robbins, SA ed. pg. 266)

ANSWER

Introduction

- Teratoma is composed of tissue elements derived from than one germ layer (endoderm, mesoderm and ectoderm)

Teratoma Testis

- Common in infants and children (approx.40%)
- May occur at any age group up to adult life
- Pure form – mainly in infants and chidren
- Usually raised hCG or AFP levels

Etiology

- Exact cause is not known, may be due to abnormal differentiation of the germ cells resulting in this condition

Clinical Features

- Testicular pain
- Testicular lump, feeling of heaviness in the scrotum
- Abdominal pain and swelling
- Blood in stool, urine
- Back pain
- Swelling of the legs
- Breast pain, mainly if accompanied by enlargement
- Trouble in breathing
- Anemia
- Changes in appetite
- Fatigue
- Frequent urination
- Paralysis

Morphology

Three types:

- Mature (difffferentiated) teratoma
- Immature teratoma
- Teratoma with malignant transformation

Gross Appearance

- Large, grey-white mass and involved testis is enlarged

Microscopic Features

- **Mature (differentiated) teratoma:**
  - Well-differentiated structures like smooth muscle, cartilage, mucus glands, epithelium(intestinal and respiratory), neural tissue present in an disorganized manner
  - Most common benign tumor
- **Immature teratoma:**
  - Composed of incompletely differentiated and primitive embryonic tissue with some mature components
  - Primitive tissue like poorly-formed cartilage, neural tissue, mesenchymal tissue,etc. are commonly present
- **Teratoma with malignant transformation**
  - Rare form of teratoma with malignant transformation of one or more tissue elements

Diagnosis

- Physical examination: for detection of in the testicles
- Biopsy
- Blood tests:
  - Complete blood cell count (CBC) blood test
  - Liver function blood test (LFT)
  - Serum tumor marker blood test to detect increases in human chorionic gonadotropin (hCG)
  - Alpha-fetoprotein (AFP) blood test

- Lactate dehydrogenase (LDH) blood test
- Testosterone levels blood test
- **Genetic analysis:** To assess mutations responsible for teratoma of testisis

Complications

- Retrograde ejaculation
- Excessive blood loss
- Infertility
- Metastasis and the loss of function of the organ

Teratoma Ovary

- Ovarian teratoma divided into 3 types:
  - Benign (mature) teratoma
  - Immature (malignant) teratoma
  - Specialized(monodermal) teratoma
- **Benign (mature) teratoma:**
  - Mostly benign and cystic
  - Common in young females
  - Develop from ectodermal differentiation of totipotent cells
  - **Morphological features:**
    - Unilocular cyst consisting of sebaceous secretion, hair masses along with areas of calcification and tooth structure
  - **Rokitansky protuberance:**
    - Inner lining of the cyst exhibiting prominence projecting from the wall towards the center of the cyst and contains tissue elements like- tooth, bone, cartilage, etc.
  - **Microscopic features:**
    - Lining of the cyst wall composed of stratified squamous epithelium and structures like sweat glands, sebaceous glands and hair follicles
- **Immature (malignant) teratoma:**
  - Occur in approx. 0.2% of all ovarian tumours(rare)
  - Common in young females and prepubertal adolescents
  - Commonly seen in under 20 yrs of age
  - **Microscopic features:**
    - Mostly composed of immature tissue
    - Immature tissue- may differentiate into cartilage, bone, neural tissue, etc
    - Immature neural tissue helps in determining the prognosis and histologic grading of tumor
- **Specialized(monodermal) teratoma:**
  - Rare entity
  - **Examples:** Struma ovarii and carcinoid tumor

b. **Papillary thyroid carcinoma**

(Ref: Textbook of Pathology, Harsh Mohan, 7th ed. pg. 802)

ANSWER

Introduction

- Most frequent type of thyroid carcinoma (75-85%)
- Affects people of all ages including children and young adults with predilection for advancing age
- More common in females (female/male ratio is 3:1)
- Characteristically slow growing tumour presenting as asymptomatic solitary nodule
- Prognosis is good
- 10 year survival rate is 80-95%

Morphology

- **Gross appearance:**
  - Ranging from small, multifocal nodules to 10 cm in diameter
  - Poorly delineated
  - Cut surface exhibits grey-white, hard and scar like tumour
  - Tumour may transform into a cyst into which numerous papillae project

Microscopic Appearance

- **Papillary pattern**
  - Composed of fibrovascular stalk and covered by single layer of tumour cells
  - Papillae are accompanied with follicles
- **Tumour cells**
  - Ground glass or optically clear appearance due to dispersed nuclear chromatin
  - Clear, oxyphilic cytoplasm
  - Apart from covering the papillae, tumour cells may form follicles and solid sheets
- **Invasion**
  - Invasion of capsule and intrathyroid lymphatics by tumour cells is seen but not of blood vessels
- **Psammoma bodies**
  - Half of papillary carcinomas exhibit typical small, concentric, calcified spherules in the stroma

c. **Renal changes in diabetes mellitus**

(Ref: Textbook of Pathology, Harsh Mohan, 7th ed. pg. 664)

ANSWER

Diabetic Nephropathy

Introduction

- Complication of diabetes mellitus – chronic kidney disease with renal failure results in death in more than 10% cases of diabetes
- More severe, development is early and more commonly in type I diabetes mellitus (30-40 % cases)

- Associated clinical syndromes are
  - Asymptomatic proteinuria
  - Nephrotic syndrome
  - Progressive renal failure
  - Hypertension
  - Cardiovascular disease

Morphology

- **Glomerular lesions**
  - **Capillary basement membrane thickening**
    - Most characteristic lesion
    - GBM thickening and mesangial widening
    - Tubular basement membrane thickening
  - **Diffuse mesangial sclerosis**
    - Most frequent change
    - Diffuse increase in mesangial matrix (PAS-positive)
    - Association with worsening renal function like proteinuria
  - **Nodular or intercapillary glomerulosclerosis or Kimmelstiel-Wilson disease**
    - Spherical, laminated, nodules of matrix at the periphery of glomerulus, which are PAS-positive
    - Capillary microaneurysms
    - Fibrin caps-accumulation of hyaline material in capillary loops
    - Capsular drops–hyaline material adherent to Bowman's capsules
- **Renal vascular lesions**
  - Arteriosclerosis–affects both afferent and efferent arteriole
  - Pyelonephritis, including necrotizing papillitis
  - Commences in interstitial tissue and extends to tubules, called as necrotizing papillitis

Name of the Paper	:	**Pathology Paper-I**
Name of the Course	:	**MBBS-2015**
Semester	:	**Annual**

Time: 3 Hours **M.M.: 40**

INSTRUCTIONS

1. Write your Roll No. on the top immediately on receipt of this question paper
2. All questions are to be attempted
3. Answers to Parts I, II and III should be written in separate answer sheets provided
4. Attempt parts of a question in sequence

PART-I

1. **Differentiate between:** [8]

   a. Normoblast and Megaloblast
   b. Benign and Malignant Tumors
   c. Lepromatous and Tuberculoid leprosy
   d. Granuloma and Granulation tissue

2. **Write briefly on:** [6]

   a. Mechanism of allograft rejection
   b. Lab diagnosis of neoplasia
   c. Role of cytochemistry in acute leukemia

PART-II

3. **Write briefly on.** [6]

   a. Laboratory diagnosis of disseminated intravascular coagulation (DIC)
   b. Laboratory diagnosis of Thalassemia

4. **Write briefly on:** [6]

   a. Cellular events in acute inflammation
   b. Pathogenesis of septic shock

PART-III

5. **Write short notes on:** [8]

   a. Prothrombin time
   b. Transfusion transmitted diseases
   c. Niemann Pick disease
   d. Tumour markers

6. **Write short notes on:** [6]

   a. Philadelphia chromosome
   b. Pathogenesis of amyloidosis
   c. Blood Components

PART I

1. Differentiate between:

a. Normoblast and Megaloblast

(Ref: Harsh Mohan, 7th ed. pg. 265, 283, Robbins, SA ed. pg. 632)

ANSWER

Normoblast and Megalobast

Normoblast	Megaloblast
Size is normal (78–100 fl)	Size larger than normal(>100 fl)
Seen in normal red cells	Formed in vitamin B12 and folic acid deficiency
Nucleus is small with clumped chromatin. Nucleoli is absent	Nucleus is three-fourth of the cell volume with "opened" chromatin. Nucleoli present (2-3 in number)
Cytoplasm is less basophilic	Cytoplasm is deeply basophilic

b. Benign and malignant tumors

(Ref: Harsh Mohan, 7th ed. pg. 186, Robbins, SA ed. pg. 267-275)

ANSWSER

Benign and Malignant Tumors

	Benign	Malignant
Gross	• Slow growing • Small size • Encapsulated or well-demarcated borders	• Rapid growth • Larger in size • Poorly demarcated • Necrosis and hemorrhage are commonly seen
Micro	• Expansile growth with well-circumscribed borders • Tend to be well differentiated • Noninvasive and never metastasize • Resemble the normal tissue counterpart from which they arise	• Vary from well to poorly (anaplastic) differentiated • Tumor cells vary in size and shape (pleomorphism) • Increased nuclear to cytoplasmic ratios • High mitotic activity with abnormal mitotic figures • Nuclear hyperchromasia and prominent nucleoli • Has potential to metastasize • Invasive growth pattern

c. Lepromatous and Tuberculoid leprosy

(Ref: Harsh Mohan, 7th ed. pg. 149, Robbins, SA ed. pg. 377-378)

ANSWER

Tuberculoid and Lepromatous Leprosy

Tuberculoid leprosy	Lepromatous leprosy
• Asymmetrical, macular, erythematous, hypopigmented may be single or few skin lesions	• Symmetrical, multiple, hypopigmented,, maculopapular skin lesion
• Lepromin test positive	• Negative lepromin test
• Immune response is good	• Immunity is suppressed
• Few lepra bacilli in granular or beaded form	• Lepra cells present with numerous lepra bacilli exhibiting "globi" or " cigarettes-in –pack" appearance
• Histopathologically, hard tubercle – similar to granulomas with no clear zone	• Histopathologically, lepra cells or Virchow cells in the dermis and separated from epidermis by a clear zone

d. Granuloma and Granulation tissue

(Ref: Harsh Mohan, 7th ed. pg. 135, 159, Robbins, SA ed. pg. 97, 98, 103)

ANSWER

Granulation Tissue and Granuloma

Granulation tissue	Granuloma
Composed of newly formed blood vessels (angiogenesis), proliferating fibroblasts and chronic inflammatory cells	Circumscribed, tiny lesion about 1 mm in diameter, composed predominantly of modified macrophages (epithelioid cells) and rimmed at periphery by lymphoid cells
Formed during healing and repair	Due to delayed hypersensitivity response
Giant cells absent	Langhans' type of giant cells with 20 or more nuclei arranged peripherally
Involvement of angiogenic and fibrogenic growth factors, like-VEGF, FGF, PDGF, etc.	Cytokines involved, like IL-1, IL-2
Remodelling (maturation and reorganization) of granulation tissue is evident	Remodeling not present

2. Write briefly on:

a. Mechanism of allograft rejection

(Ref: Harsh Mohan, 7th ed. pg. 170, Robbins, SA ed. pg. 231-33)

ANSWER

Introduction

○ Allograft rejection is directed against the antigen present on the graft

○ **Consist of two stages:**
  ▪ Recognition of antigen by the host lymphocytes
  ▪ Destruction of graft cells by cytotoxic T cells

○ Events that results in allograft rejection is known as "first-set of reaction"

○ **Histocompatibility antigen:** Set of membrane antigen expressed by individual cell and denotes immunological cell type of individual

Mechanism of Allograft Rejection

First-set Beaction

○ Demonstration of foreign cell MHC antigen -initial step

○ Activation of lymphatic T cells through graft antigen

○ Activated lymphocytes results in Tc, Th, and Td cells

○ Tc cells gain direct entry into the circulation

○ Td cells mobilization of phagocytic leucocytes

○ Tc cells responsible for the destruction of grafted tissue

Second-set Reaction

○ Rapid rejection of second graft within 3–5 days

○ As a result of rapid activation of Tc cells along with circulating complement fixing antibodies and NK cells, rapid destruction of blood vessels of the second graft occurs

○ Neutrophils, macrophages and Tc cells present in the circulation results in rapid and irreversible rejection of transplanted tissue.

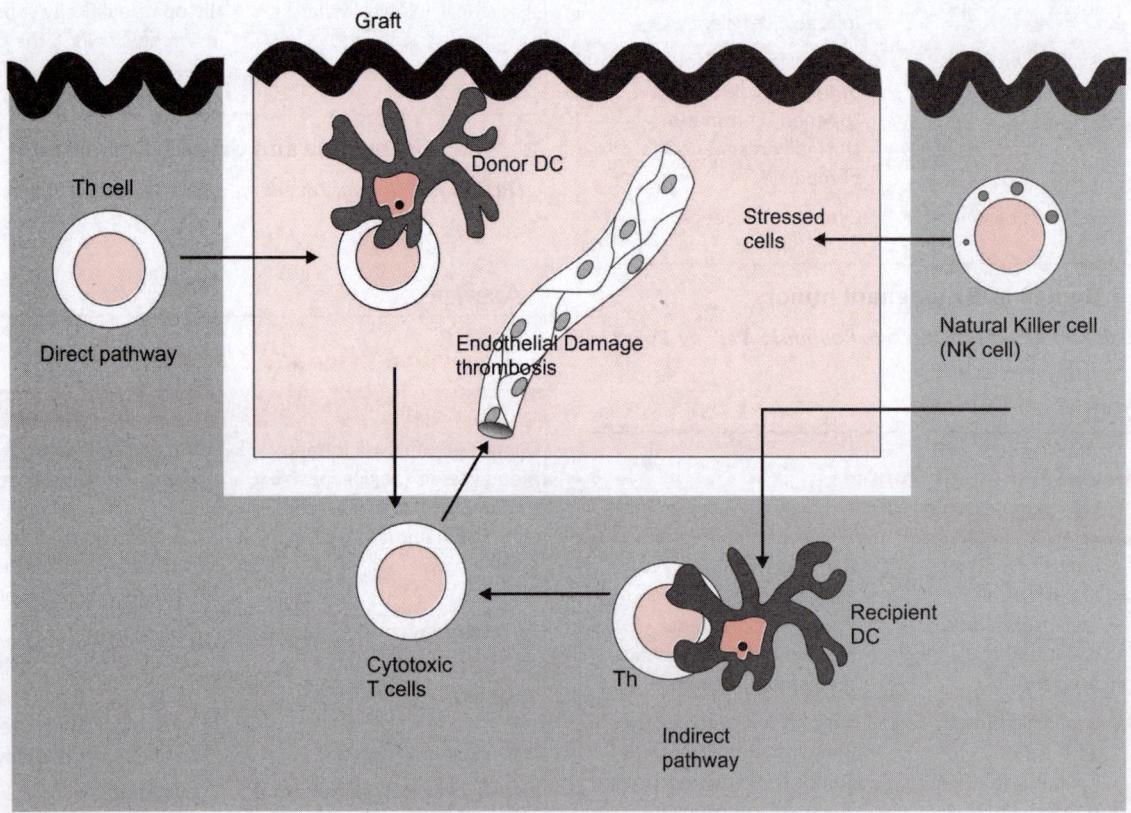

Fig. Mechanism of allograft rejection

    b. **Lab diagnosis of neoplasia**

(Ref: Textbook of Pathology, Harsh Mohan, 7th ed. pg. 226-230, Robbins, SA ed. pg. 337-338)

ANSWER

Different Methods used in the Diagnosis of Neoplasia

○ **Histologic methods:**
  ▪ Excisional/needle biopsy

- ◆ Microscopic examination of properly fixed and stained tissue
- ○ **Cytologic methods:**
  - ▪ FNAC
  - ▪ **Exfoliative cytology**
    - ◆ Used in the diagnosis of carcinoma cervix, stomach, bronchus
    - ◆ Cells are manually scraped/brushed off of a surface in the body or spontaneously shed by the body
- ○ **Immunohistochemistry:**
  - ▪ Specific antibodies are used
  - ▪ Helps in determining the site of origin of metastatic tumours
  - ▪ Helps in classification of undifferentiated malignant tumours
  - ▪ Identification of molecules with diagnostic and prognostic significance
  - ▪ Examples of certain tumours and their specific marker are given below

Tumor	Marker
• Sarcoma	• Vimentin
• Carcinoma (squamous cell carcinoma)	• Cytokeratin
• Neural tumours	• Neurofilament
• S-100	• Melanoma, Neuroendocrine tumour, Schwannoma
• HMB45	• Melanoma

- ○ **Histochemisty/Cytochemistry:**
  - ▪ Cytochemical stains (special stains) are used for the diagnosis, classification of tumor and also helps in identification of chemical composition of cells.
  - ▪ Examples-PAS stain–for basement membrane/collagen, alcian blue- for acid mucin, myeloperoxidase- for enzyme, etc.
- ○ **Electron microscopy:** for ultrastructural examination of tumor cell
- ○ **Molecular diagnosis:**
  - ▪ Polymerase chain Reaction
  - ▪ Array CGH(Comparative genomic hybridization)
  - ▪ Single nucleotide polymorphism array (SNP)
- ○ **Others:**
  - ▪ Flow cytometry:
    - ◆ Cell surface antigen identification
    - ◆ Analysis of DNA content
    - ◆ Used in bone marrow aspirates, blood cells, body fluids, etc.
  - ▪ In situ hybridization
  - ▪ Cell proliferation analysis
  - ▪ DNA microarray analysis of tumor

c. Role of cytochemistry in acute leukemia

(Ref: Textbook of Pathology, Harsh Mohan, 7th ed. pg. 226-230)

ANSWER

Introduction

- ○ **Two types of acute leukemia:** Acute lymphoblastic leukemia (ALL) and acute myeloid leukemia (AML).
- ○ Cytochemical stains are special stains that helps in differentiation of AML from ALL and in subclassification of AML.

A Use of Cytochemical Stains in Acute Leukemia

- ○ Special stains that helps in differentiation of AML from ALL and in subclassification of AML.
- ○ To identify the blast cells in acute leukemia as myeloid or non-myeloid
- ○ For identification of granulocytic and monocytic cells

Commonly used Cytochemical Stains

Cytochemical reaction	Stained cellular element	Indentified blasts
Myeloperoxidase (MPO)	Neutrophil primary granules	Myeloblasts strong positive; faint +ve monoblasts
Sudan Black B (SBB)	Phospholipids	Myeloblasts strong positive; faint +ve monoblasts
Specific esterase	Cellular enzyme	Strong positive myeloblasts
Nonspecific esterase (NSE)	Cellular enzyme	Strong positive monoblasts
Periodic acid-Schiff	Glycogen and related substances	Coarse or block-like positivity seen in lymphoblasts and pronormoblasts, usually myeloblasts negative but faint diffuse reaction may be seen occasionally

Cytochemistry of AML

FAB classification	Cytochemistry
M0	Myeloperoxidase negative in M0 myeloblast. Positive for myeloid cells containing granules and Auer rods
M1	Myeloperoxidase positive
M2	Strongly positive for myeloperoxidase
M3	Strongly positive for myeloperoxidase
M4	Positive(++)for myeloperoxidase and for non-specific esterase (+)
M5	Positive for non-specific estarase

FAB classification	Cytochemistry
M6	PAS and myeloperoxidase positive
M7	Positive for platelet peroxidase

Cytochemistry of ALL

FAB Classification	Cytochemistry
L1	May be positive or negative PAS or acid phosphatase
L2	PAS($\pm$) and acid phosphatase($\pm$)
L3	Both acid phosphatase and PAS negative

PART-II

3. Write briefly on:

a. Laboratory diagnosis of disseminated intravascular coagulation (DIC)

(Ref: Harsh Mohan, 7th ed. pg. 317, Robbins, SA ed. pg. 663-65)

ANSWER

Introduction

○ Acute, subacute or chronic thrombo-hemorrhagic disorder characterized by activation of coagulation pathway and formation of thrombi in the microcirculation of body

○ Also known as "defibrination syndrome" or "consumption coagulopathy"

Laboratory Diagnosis

○ **Hemogram:** Decreased platelet count

○ **Peripheral smear:** Schistocytes and fragmented red cells

○ **Coagulation test:** Prolonged thrombin time, prothrombin time, activated partial thromboplastin time

○ **Other investigation:**

○ Increased level of FDP (fibrin degraded product)

b. Laboratory diagnosis of Thalassemia

(Ref: Harsh Mohan, 7th ed. pg. 296, Robbins, SA ed. pg. 638-642)

ANSWER

Introduction

○ Thalassemia is genetically transmitted disorder characterized by decrease in globin chain synthesis

Types

○ α **Thalassemia** Reduction in α chain synthesis

○ β **Thalassemia:** Reduction in β chain synthesis

Laboratory Diagnosis

○ α Thalassemia

- ■ **Hb Bart's hydrops fetalis (Four α- gene deletion):**
  - ◆ **Anemia:** Severe(below 6 gm/dl)
  - ◆ Anisopoikilocytosis, microcytosis, basophilic stippling, target cells
  - ◆ **Reticulocyte count:** Increased
  - ◆ **Serum bilirubin:** Increased
  - ◆ **Hemoglobin electrophoresis:** 80–90% Hb-Bart's, small amount of Hg-H and Hb- Portland
- ■ **HbH disease (Three α- gene deletion):**
  - ◆ **Anemia:** Moderate
  - ◆ Severe microcytosis, basophilic stippling, target cells
  - ◆ Heinz bodies in mature red cells
  - ◆ **Hemoglobin electrophoresis:** 2–4% HbH and remaining HbA, HbA_2, HbF
- ■ α **Thalassemia trait: (Two α- gene deletion)**
  - ◆ **MCV, MCH, MCHC:** Slightly decreased
  - ◆ Microcytic and hypochromic red cell morphology
  - ◆ **Hemoglobin electrophoresis:** Hb-Bart's small amount in neonates and gradual disappearance in adults. HbA_2 slight reduction or normal

β- Thalassaemia

○ β-thalassaemia major

- ■ **CBC:**
  - ◆ Severe anemia (Hb: 3–6 gm/dL)
  - ◆ **MCH, MCV, MCHC:** Decreased
  - ◆ **Hematocrit:** Decreased (severely)
  - ◆ **WBC:** Raised (usually), shift of left of neutrophil series with presence of some myelocytes and metamyelocytes
- ■ **Peripheral blood smear:**
  - ◆ Severe microcytic hypochromic red cell
  - ◆ Marked anisopoikilocytosis
  - ◆ Target cells
  - ◆ Tear drop cells
  - ◆ Basophilic stippling
  - ◆ Cells with Cabot's ring
  - ◆ Pencil cells
  - ◆ Nucleated RBC's
- ■ **Hemoglobin electrophoresis:**
  - ◆ Increased HbF
  - ◆ Increased HbA_2
  - ◆ HbA–absent or sometimes present in variable amounts
- ■ **Bone marrow findings:**
  - ◆ Normoblastic erythroid hyperplasia
  - ◆ Intermediate and late normoblast predominant (smaller in size)

- Siderotic granules in the cytoplasm of normoblasts
    - Increased reticuloendothelial iron
  - **Biochemical findings:**
    - **Serum bilirubin (unconjugated):** Increased
    - **Serum iron:** Increased
    - **Urine urobilinogen:** Increased
    - **Serum ferritin:** Increased (300–3000 mg/dL)
  - **Osmotic fragility:** decreased
- β- thalassaemia minor(trait)
  - **CBC:**
    - Mild anemia
    - **Hematocrit:** Decreased
    - **MCV,MCH,MCHC:** Slightly decreased
  - **Peripheral blood smear:**
    - Abnormalities minor as compared to thalassaemia major
    - Hypochromic, microcytic RBC
    - Mild anisopoikilocytosis
    - Target cells (rare)
    - Basophilic stippling (occasional)
  - **Hemoglobin electrophoresis:**
    - **HbA$_2$:** Markedly increased
  - **Biochemical findings:**
    - **Serum bilirubin (unconjugated):** Normal/ slightly increased
  - **Osmotic fragility:** Decreased

---

4. **Write briefly on:**

   a. **Cellular events in acute inflammation**

   (Ref: Harsh Mohan, 7th ed. pg. 119, Robbins, SA ed. pg. 75-78)

ANSWER

Cellular Changes in Acute Inflammation

Extravasation or exudation of leucocytes: Movement and recruitment of leucocytes from vessels into the interstitial tissue(site of inflammation)

- **Lumen:**
  - **Margination and pavementing of neutrophils:** Due to stasis of blood flow, neutrophils move towards the periphery blood vessels
  - **Rolling and adhesion:** Neutrophils roll over the endothelial cells and adhere to the endothelial cells. Selectins, integrins molecules help in adhesion and rolling
- **Migration and diapedesis:**
  - Migration of leukocytes into extravascular space by piercing basement membrane in the presence of collagenase enzyme
  - **Molecules that are responsible:** Platelet endothelial cell adhesion molecule

- **Chemotaxis:**
  - Movement of leucocytes towards the site of injury in the presence of chemotactic agents
  - **Chemotactic agents include:**
    - **Exogenous:** Bacterial products
    - **Endogenous:** Complement system C5a, leukotrienes, cytokines
  - Production of arachidonic acid metabolites
  - Secretion of lysosomal enzyme

Phagocytosis

- Defined as the process of ingestion or engulfment of solid particulate material by the cells
- Cells responsible for phagocytosis are called "phagocytes"
- **Mainly, 2 types of phagocytes:**
  - Polymorhonuclear leucocytes
  - Monocytes and macrophages
- **It involves three stages:**
  - Recognition and attachment
  - Engulfment
  - Killing and degradation

Recognition and Attachment

- Initiated by receptors expressed on the surface of leucocyte
- Mannose and scavenger receptors responsible for recognition of micro-organism
- **Opsonisation and opsonins:** Process of coating of micro-organisms with specific proteins (opsonins) and the process is called opsonisation
- **Opsonins:** Fc portion of IgG (naturally occurring antibodies against bacteria), C3b (strongly chemotactic for attracting PMNs to bacteria), lectins (carbohydrate binding protein)

Engulfment

- Formation of cytoplasmic pseudopods and engulfment of opsonized particles
- Eventually, formation of phagocytic vacuoles or phagosome
- Fusion of lysosome of the cells and formation of phagolysosome

Killing and Degradation

- Mechanisms involved in killing and degradation as follows:
  - **Intracellular mechanism:** oxidative mechanism commonly involved in killing of micro-organism
    - **Oxidative bactericidal mechanism:**
      - Production of reactive oxygen metabolites (H_2O_2, HOCl, OH, O'_2 etc.)
      - Bactericidal activity may be myeloperoxidase- dependent (present in azurophilic

granules of neutrophils and monocytes) or myeloperoxidase-independent

- ◆ **Non- Oxidative bactericidal mechanism:**
  - ❑ Certain granules like–lysosomal hydrolase, lipases, proteases, etc.don't require oxygen for bacerticidal activity
- ▪ **Extracellular mechanism:**

- ◆ Granules exerts its effect of proteolysis outside the cell.
- ◆ Immune- mediated lysis of micro-organism by cytolysis, antibody-mediated lysis and by cell-mediated cytotoxicity

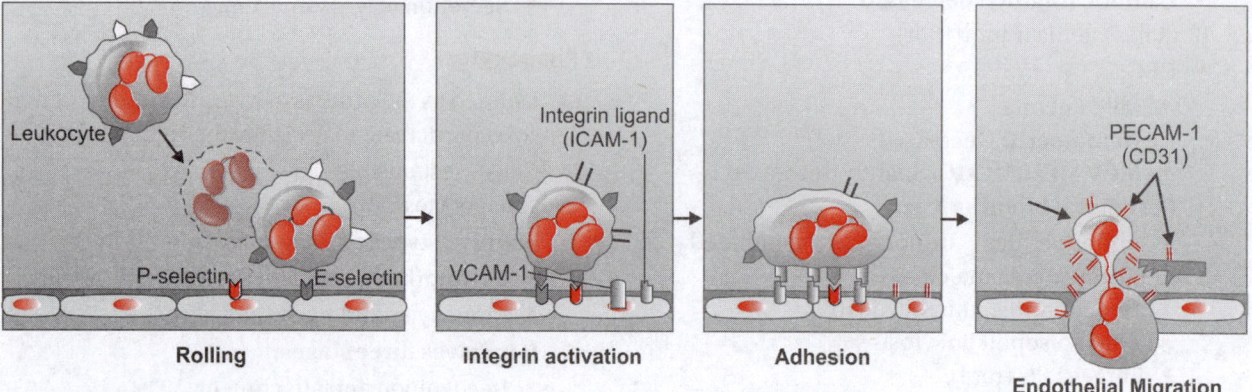

b   Pathogenesis of septic shock

(Ref: Harsh Mohan, 7th ed. pg. 96, Robbins, SA ed. pg. 131-133)

ANSWER

Introduction

- ○ Severe bacterial infection that results in hemostatic derangements, hemodynamic instability and malfunctioning of organ system

Pathogenesis

Consists of:

- ○ **Macrophage-monocyte activation:** Results in liberation of free radicals and increased synthesis of nitric oxide resulting in vasodilatation and hypotension
- ○ Activation of inflammatory cascade, like- complement pathway, coagulation system, mast cells, kinin system
- ○ Results in vasodilatation and increased vascular permeability thus causing hyperdynamic circulation and inflammatory edema
- ○ Organ dysfunction as a result of hypotension and inadequate perfusion of cells and tissues

   For diagrammatic presentation, refer to 2016 paper-I Q. 3 (a), Pg. 30

PART-III

5.   Write short notes on:

   a.   Prothrombin time

   (Ref: Harsh Mohan, 7th ed. pg. 308, Robbins, SA ed. pg. 119)

ANSWER

Introduction

- ○ Important screening test to assess coagulation
- ○ Blood coagulation test used for diagnosis of blood disorders
- ○ Helps in evaluation of total quantity of prothrombin in the blood

Prothrombin Time

- ○ Time taken by blood (plasma) to clot after addition of calcium and tissue thromboplastin to it
- ○ Measure defects of the extrinsic and common coagulation pathway
- ○ **Method:**
  - ▪ Tissue thromboplastin and calcium added to the blood (oxalated thus prothrombin not converted to thrombin)
  - ▪ Tissue thromboplastin activates prothombin and helps in blood coagulation
  - ▪ Use of calcium nullifies the effect of oxalate
  - ▪ Assessment of time taken by blood to clot after addition of tissue thromboplastin
- ○ **Normal prothrombin time:** 10-14 sec
- ○ **Causes for prolonged Prothrombin time:**
  - ▪ Liver disease (esp. obstructive liver disease)
  - ▪ Vitamin K deficiency
  - ▪ Disseminated intravascular coagulation
  - ▪ Oral anticoagulant drugs.

b.   Transfusion transmitted diseases

(Ref: Textbook of Pathology, Harsh Mohan, 7th ed. pg. 319)

ANSWER

Diseases Transmitted by Transfusion

- Cytomegalovirus infection (CMV)
- Hepatitis B virus
- Hepatitis C virus
- Malaria
- Syphilis
- HIV infection (AIDS)
- Parvo virus B-19 infection
- Bacterial infections
- Toxoplasmosis
- Leishmanisis

Cytomegalovirus Infection (CMV)

- CMV is a double–stranded, enveloped DNA herpes virus
- Post transfusion infection is mainly seen in immunocompromised patients
- **Indications:** Premature infants, HIV infection, bone marrow transplantation, etc.
- **Prevention:** Screening of blood components/ products and leukocyte free component transfusion

Hepatitis B Virus

- Transmission of HBV infection is through contaminated needles, syringes, needle-stick injury, intravenous and percutaneous drug abuse, transplacental, close postnatal contact, etc.
- **Three phases of acute HBV infection:** Preicteric phase, icteric phase and convalescent phase

Hepatitis C Virus

- Usually, parenteral route of transmission
- Less severe infection, short preicteric period, jaundice may be absent or mild
- **Clinical manifestation:** Acute hepatitis (approx. 80% cases), cirrhosis(10–20% cases)

Transfusion Associated HIV Infection

- Rapid progression of HIV infection related to transfusion
- **Mode of prevention:** Sterilization of blood components, safe transfusion, lab test and careful donar selection

Parvo Virus B19 Infection

- Parvo virus B19 is a nonlipid DNA virus
- Common disease
- Transmission through respiratory route (commonly)
- Mostly prevalent in donars of poor socioeconomic status, poor education level, poor living conditions, etc.

Malarial Infection

- Transfusion of malaria can take place through red blood cells, whole blood, platelets, cryoprecipitate, plasma, etc.

Transmission Associated Bacterial Infections

- Contamination of blood mainly occurs during collection and processing
- **Clinical features:** High fever, vomiting, headaches, chills, restlessness, etc. develops as result of bacterial infection
- Immunity of the patient, number of organism, type of antibiotic are the factors responsible for the severity of bacterial contamination

c.   **Niemann Pick disease**

(Ref: Harsh Mohan, 7th ed. pg. 258, Robbins, SA ed. pg. 152-153)

ANSWER

Introduction

- Autosomal recessive disorder that exhibits accumulation of cholesterol and sphingomyelin
- As a result of defect in acid sphingomyelinase
- Usually, liver, spleen, bone marrow, lungs and brain is involved

Types

Two types

- **Type A: Classic infantile form**
  - Common
  - Commonly seen in infancy (within first few months of life)
  - **Clinical features:**
    - Lymphadenopathy
    - Hepatosplenomegaly
    - CNS deterioration
    - Cherry-red spot in the eye (amaurosis)
    - Poor muscle tone
    - Feeding problems
- **Type B: Visceral juvenile form**
  - Appear in late childhood or adolescence
  - Impaired lung function
  - Mental retardation
  - Peripheral nerve problems
  - Delayed growth and short stature
  - High blood lipids
- **Type C: Subacute or juvenile form**
  - Abnormal posture of limbs, head, trunk, face
  - Seizures
  - Jaundice
  - Speech irregularity
  - Dementia
  - Sleep disorders, bipolar disorder, etc.
  - Sudden loss of muscle tone, etc.

Diagnosis

- **Type A and B:**
  - Measurement of ASM in white blood cell
  - DNA test (to determine the type)
- **Type C:**
  - DNA test
  - Biopsy of skin
- **Other test:**
  - Bone marrow examination
  - Liver biopsy, etc.

d. Tumour markers

(Ref: Textbook of Pathology, Harsh Mohan, 7th ed. pg. 229)

ANSWER

For answer, refer 2017 paper-I Q. No. 5 (c)

6. Write short notes on:

a. Philadelphia chromosome

(Ref: Harsh Mohan, 7th ed. pg. 335, Robbins, SA ed. pg. 317)

ANSWER

Introduction

- First tumor-specific chromosomal change discovered by Nowell and Hungerford in 1960
- Associated with CML (70-90% cases) and in certain cases of ALL

Chromosomal Abnormality

- Reciprocal translocation of chromosome 22 (parts of long arm) to the long arm of chromosome 9 (9;22)

- Fusion gene *bcr-abl* (oncogene) is formed on chromosome 22
- Expression of an enzyme with abnormal tyrosine kinase activity
- Abnormal gene products dysregulate the proliferation of hematopoietic stem cells.

Identification

- Fluorescent in situ hybridization (FISH)
- Reverse transcription Polymerase chain reaction (RT-PCR)

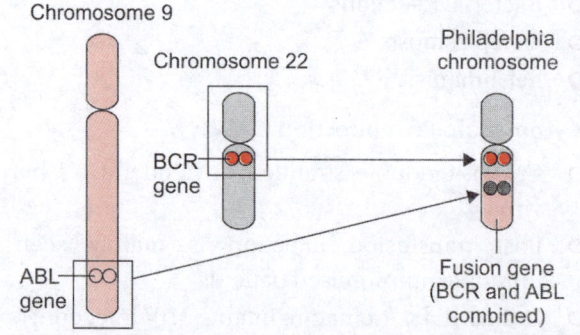

b. Pathogenesis of amyloidosis

(Ref: Harsh Mohan, 7th ed. pg. 69, Robbins, SA ed. pg. 258-262)

ANSWER

Mechanism Involved in Different Types of Amyloidosis

- Any stimulus result in deposition of amyloidgenic precursor protein
- Amyloid protein deposition or fibrillogenesis occur (AL in primary and SAA in secondary form)
- Partial degradation of fibrillar protein in macrophages or reticuloendothelial cells

- Fibrin stabilisation and protection from soublisation and degradation by non-fibrillar protein.

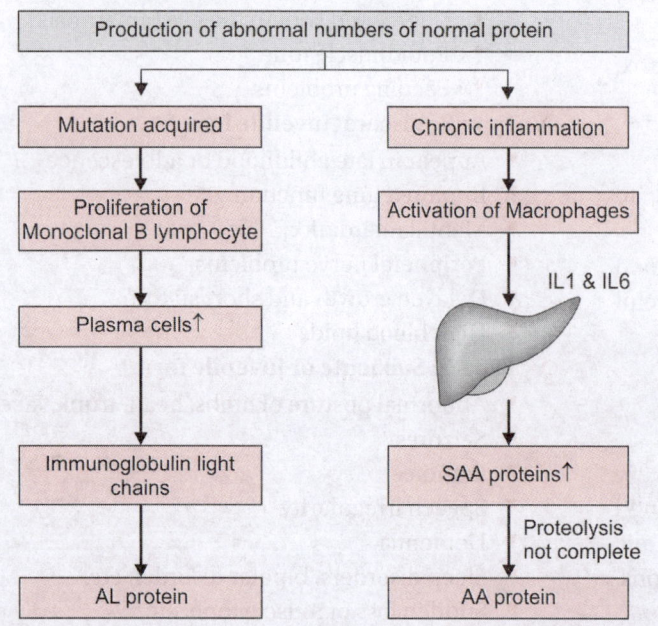

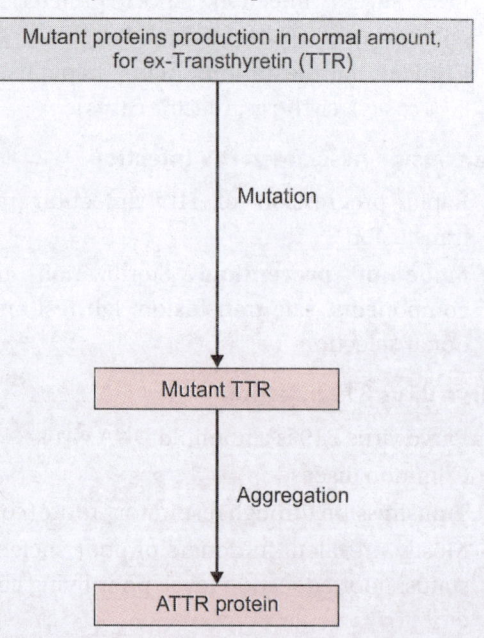

Fig. Amyloidosis pathogenesis

PATHOLOGY

c. Blood Components

(Ref: Textbook of Pathology, Harsh Mohan, 7th ed. pg. 319)

ANSWER

Blood Components

○ Whole blood is divided into components

○ **It mainly includes:**
  ▪ Packed RBC's
  ▪ Fresh frozen plasma
  ▪ Platelets
  ▪ Cryoprecipitate

○ **Procedure:**
  ▪ Whole blood centrifugation at low speed: packed RBC's and platelet-rich plasma(PRP)
  ▪ PRP centrifugation at high speed: random donar platelets and FFP
  ▪ FFP thawing and centrifugation: cryoprecipitate

Component	Uses
Packed RBC	To increase the oxygen carrying capacity of blood, anemia. 1 unit of packed RBC raise Hb by 1gm%
Platelets	Thrombocytopenia associated with hemorrhage.
Leukocyte reduced RBC's	In case of blood reaction by previous packed RBC's/WB
Fresh frozen plasma	Coagulation abnormality, TTP. Each unit of FFP raises coagulation factor by 2%
Cryoprecipitate	In fibrinogen deficiency, mild vonWillebrand's disease
Factor VIII concentrate	Hemophilia A
Albumin	Severe hypoproteinemia
Immune serum globulin	Hypogammaglobulinemia

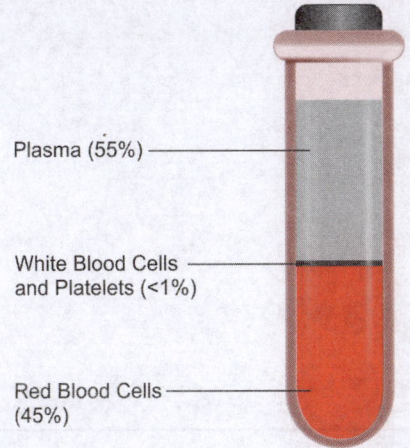

Plasma (55%)

White Blood Cells and Platelets (<1%)

Red Blood Cells (45%)

Your Roll No. ....

Name of the Paper : **Pathology Paper-II**

Name of the Course : **MBBS-2015**

Semester : **Annual**

Time: 3 Hours   M.M.: 40

INSTRUCTIONS

1. Write your Roll No. on the top immediately on receipt of this question paper
2. All questions are to be attempted
3. Answers to Parts I, II and III should be written in separate answer sheets provided
4. Attempt parts of a question in sequence

PART-I

1. **Differentiate between:**   [8]
    a. Transmural and subendocardial infarct
    b. Partial and Complete mole
    c. Panacinar and centriacinar emphysema
    d. Ulcerative colitis and Crohn's disease

2. **Write short notes on**   [6]
    a. Ewing's sarcoma
    b. Endometrial hyperplasia
    c. Papillary carcinoma thyroid

PART-II

3. **Write briefly on:**   [6]
    a. Rapidly progressive Glomerulonephritis
    b. Morphology and diagnosis of prostate cancer

4. **Write briefly on:**   [6]
    a. Etiopathogenesis and morphology of Hepatocellular carcinoma
    b. Etiopathogenesis and morphology of rheumatic heart disease

PART-III

5. **Write briefly on:**   [8]
    a. Amoebic colitis
    b. Morphological changes in chronic viral hepatitis
    c. Pheochromocytoma
    d. Diabetic nephropathy

6. **Write short note on:**   [6]
    a. Transitional cell carcinoma urinary bladder
    b. Pathogenesis and complication of acute pancreatitis
    c. Celiac disease

PART I

1. **Differentiate between:**

    a. **Transmural and subendocardial infarct**

    (Ref: Textbook of Pathology, Harsh Mohan, 7th ed. pg. 410)

ANSWER

Transmural and Subendocardial Infarct

Transmural infarct	Subendothelial infarct
• Commonly seen (95%)	• Less common
• Involves full thickness of ventricular wall and is solid	• Affects inner third to half of the myocardium
• Due to coronary stenosis (>75% cases)	• Due to hypoperfusion of myocardium
• Distribution to specific area of coronary supply	• Distribution is circumferential
• Coronary thrombosis is common	• Coronary thrombosis is rare
• Epicarditis is common	• No evidence of epicarditis

    b. **Partial and complete mole**

    (Ref: Textbook of Pathology, Harsh Mohan, 7th ed. pg. 741)

ANSWER

Partial and Complete Mole

	Partial Mole	Complete Mole
Ploidy	Triploid	Diploid
Number of chromosomes	69,XXX; 69,XXY; 69,XYY	46 (All paternal) 46,XX; 46,XY
β-hCG	Elevated (+)	Elevated (+++)
Chorionic villi	Some are hydropic	All are hydropic
Trophoblast proliferation	Focal	Marked
Fetal tissue	Present	Absent
Invasive mole	2%	10%
Choriocarcinoma	Rare	2%
Components	2 sperm + 1 egg	Most commonly enucleated egg + single sperm egg + single sperm (subsequently duplicates paternal DNA)

    c. **Panacinar and centriacinar emphysema**

    (Ref: Harsh Mohan, 7th ed. pg. 461, Robbins, SA ed. pg. 675)

ANSWER

For answer, refer 2016 paper-II Q. 1 (b), Pg. 39

    d. **Ulcerative colitis and Crohn's disease**

(Ref: Harsh Mohan, 7th ed. pg. 552, Robbins, SA ed. pg. 798-800)

ANSWER

For answer, refer 2016 paper-II Q. 1 (c), Pg. 39

2. **Write short notes on:**

    a. **Ewing's Sarcoma**

    (Ref: Harsh Mohan, 7th ed. pg. 839, Robbins, SA ed. pg. 1203)

ANSWER

For answer, refer 2016 paper-II Q. 4 (b), Pg. 44

    b. **Endometrial hyperplasia**

(Ref: Harsh Mohan, 7th ed. pg. 723, Robbins, SA ed. pg. 1012-13)

ANSWER

Endometrial Hyperplasia

Introduction

- Increased proliferation of glandular and stromal tissues
- Associated with prolonged, profuse and irregular uterine bleeding in women of menopausal age
- Results from prolonged oestrogenic stimulation unopposed with any progestational activity comprising conditions such as Stein-Leventhal syndrome, functioning granulosa-theca cell tumours, adrenocortical hyperfunction and prolonged administration of oestrogen
- Importance is owing to presence of cellular atypia which is closely associated to endometrial carcinoma

Classification

- **Simple hyperplasia without atypia (cystic glandular hyperplasia)**
  - Large and cystically dilated varying sized glands which are lined by atrophic epithelium
  - Scanty mitoses with no atypia
  - Sparsely cellular and oedematous stroma between glands
  - Minimal risk of adenocarcinoma

PATHOLOGY

○ **Complex hyperplasia without atypia (complex non-atypical hyperplasia)**

- Distinct proliferative pattern
- Increased number of glands varying in size and irregular in shape
- Glands are lined by multiple layers of tall columnar epithelial cells with large nuclei which have not lost basal polarity with no substantial atypia
- Crowding and complexity of glands without cellular atypia
- Dense, cellular and compact stroma
- 3% risk of developing adenocarcinoma

○ **Complex hyperplasia with atypia (complex atypical hyperplasia)**

- Presence of atypical cells in hyperplastic epithelium
- Extent of cellular atypia can be mild, moderate or severe
- Cytologic features–loss of polarity, large size, hyperchromatic nuclei, prominent nucleoli and altered nucleocytoplasmic ratio
- 20-25% cases progress to adenocarcinoma

c. **Papillary carcinoma thyroid**

(Ref: Textbook of Pathology, Harsh Mohan, 7th ed. pg. 802)

ANSWER

For answer, refer 2016 paper-II Q. 6 (b), Pg. 48

PART-II

3. **Write briefly on:**

a. **Rapidly progressive glomerulonephritis**

(Ref: Harsh Mohan, 7th ed. pg. 654, Robbins, SA ed. pg. 912-13)

ANSWER

Rapidly Progressive Glomerulonephritis

For answer, refer to 2017 paper II Q. 6 (a), Pg. 23

b. **Morphology and diagnosis of prostate cancer**

(Ref: Harsh Mohan, 7th ed. pg. 706, Robbins, SA ed. pg. 989-90)

ANSWER

Morphology and Diagnosis of Prostate Cancer

Introduction

○ Most common type of cancer in males affecting men above 50 years of age with increasing prevalence in increasing age

Classification

○ Latent carcinoma–small focus of carcinoma found during autopsy in men dying of other causes; 25–30% cases

○ Incidental carcinoma–15-20% prostatectomies done for BEP had incidental carcinoma of prostate

○ Occult carcinoma–patient had no symptoms but presents evidence of metastasis on clinical examination and investigation

○ Clinical carcinoma–identified by rectal examination and other investigations and confirmed by pathologic examination of biopsy of prostate

Morphology

○ **Gross appearance:**

- Enlarged, normal in size or smaller than normal prostate
- Located in posterior lobe of the peripheral zone
- Firm and fibrous prostate
- Cut surface is homogenous and consists of irregular yellowish areas

○ **Microscopic appearance:** 4 types are

- Adenocarcinoma–most frequent type (96%)
- Transitional cell carcinoma
- Squamous cell carcinoma
- Undifferentiated carcinoma

○ **Histologic characteristics of adenocarcinoma of prostate:**

- **Architectural disturbance**
  - Loss of intra-acinar papillary convolutions
  - Groups of acini are either closely packed in back to back organisation without intervening stroma or are randomly distributed
- **Stroma**
  - Malignant acini have no stroma between them
  - Tumour cells may penetrate and replace fibromuscular stroma
- **Gland pattern**
  - Small or medium sized glands, lined by single layer of cuboidal or low columnar cells
  - Cribriform or fenestrated glandular appearance of moderately differentiated tumours
  - Little or no glandular arrangement of poorly differentiated tumours but exhibit solid or trabecular pattern
- **Tumour cells**
  - Outer basal layer is lost
  - Clear, dark and eosinophilic cells
  - Clear cells have foamy cytoplasm, dark cells possess homogeneous basophilic cytoplasm and eosinophilic cells contain granular cytoplasm
  - Varying degree of anaplasia may be seen

- **Invasion**
  - Invasion of intra-prostatic perineural spaces
  - Lymphatic and vascular invasion may be present but difficult to be identified

Clinical Symptoms

- Urinary obstruction with dysuria
- Frequency of micturition
- Retention of urine
- Haematuria
- Pain in back due to skeletal metastases in 10 % cases

Diagnosis

- On digital rectal examination (DRE)—carcinoma is palpable as a hard and nodular gland fixed to the adjacent tissues
- **Serum tumour markers**
  - Prostatic acid phosphatase (PAP)—secreted by prostatic epithelium; elevated levels of PAP are found in prostatic cancer
  - Prostate-specific antigen (PSA)—identified by immunohistochemical method in the malignant prostatic epithelium and serum
- Transrectal ultrasound (TRUS)—guided core needle biopsy

---

4. **Write briefly on:**

a. **Etiopathogenesis and morphology of Hepatocellular carcinoma**

(Ref: Harsh Mohan, 7th ed. pg. 618, Robbins, SA ed. pg. 870-73)

ANSWER

Introduction

- Most frequent primary malignant tumour of liver, also called as Hepatoma
- **Incidence:** Noticeable geographic variation and is closely related two HBV and HCV in the region
- **Prevalence:** Less than 1% of all postmortem in US and Europe
- Male/female ratio is 4:1
- Most commonly occurs in 5th to 6th decades of life
- Supervenes cirrhosis in 70–80 % cases

Etiopathogenesis

- Relation to HBV infection—related to prolonged infection of HBV
  - Incidence of HBsAg-positive carriers is higher in HCC patients
  - In African and Asian patients, 95% cases of HCC have anti-HBc

- More direct evidence of integration of HBV-DNA genome is seen in the genome of tumour cells of HCC
- Relation to HCV infection–long standing HCV infection has developed as a major factor in the etiology of HCC, generally after more than 30 years of infection
  - Higher incidence of HCC was earlier recognized to endemic HBV infection in developed countries which has seen noticeable shift to HCV infection
  - 3 times higher risk of developing HCC in patients with anti-HCV and anti-HBc antibodies together
  - Prolonged HCV infection produces cirrhosis more frequently prior to development of HCC whereas HCC after HBV infection produces cirrhosis in half the cases and remaining have chronic hepatitis
  - HBV and HCV may synergistically produce HCC
- Relation to cirrhosis–all etiologic types of cirrhosis is associated with HCC but most commonly seen is post-necrotic cirrhosis
  - Liver cell dysplasia recognized by cellular enlargement, nuclear hyperchromatism and multinucleate cells is seen in 60% cirrhotic livers with HCC
- Relation to alcohol—4 times increase risk of HCC in alcoholics is seen
  - Alcohol may act as co-carcinogen with HBV or HCV infection, although alcohol does not seem to be hepatic carcinogen per se
- Mycotoxins—poorly stored wheat grains or groundnuts can be contaminated by mycotoxin, aflatoxin B1 produced by a mould Aspergillus flavus, in hot and humid weather which is responsible for higher incidence of HCC in some developing countries of Asia and Africa
- Chemical carcinogens—can induce liver cancer in experimental animals
  - Butter-yellow, safrole and nitrosamines commonly used as food additives
  - Bush trees containing pyrrolizidine, tannin acid
  - Pollutants such as pesticides and insecticides
- **Miscellaneous factors**
  - Haemochromatosis
  - Alpha -1-antitrypsin deficiency
  - Prolonged immunosuppressive therapy in renal transplant patients
  - Other types of viral hepatitis
  - Non–alcoholic steatohepatitis (NASH)
  - Tobacco smoking
  - Parasitic infestations such as clonorchiasis and schistosomiasis
  - Glycogen storage diseases

Pathogenesis

○ Depending on genetic mutations induced by one or more major etiologic factors which damage the DNA of hepatocytes leading to neoplastic transformation

  ▪ Inactivation of tumour suppressor oncogene p53 by HBV

  ▪ Binding of X-protein (HBxAg) generated from X-gene of HBV to p53

  ▪ Mutations of oncogenes such as KRAS

  ▪ Mutations in receptors for hepatocyte growth factors e.g. c-MYC, c-MET

  ▪ Activation of WNT and AKT pathways

Morphology

Gross Appearance

○ HCC may form one of the following 3 patterns of growth, in decreasing order of frequency

  ▪ Expanding type–most common; single, yellow-brown, large mass, most often in right lobe of liver with central necrosis, hemorrhage and occasional bile-staining

  ▪ Multifocal type–less common; multifocal multiple masses of 3-5 cm in diameter, dispersed throughout the liver

  ▪ Infiltrating type–rare; HCC forms diffusely infiltrating tumor mass

Microscopic Examination

○ Tumour cells resemble hepatocytes but vary with degree of infiltration, ranging from well-differentiated to highly anaplastic lesions

  ▪ Histologic patterns

    ♦ Trabecular or sinusoidal pattern–most frequent; trabeculae consist of 2-8 cell wide layers of tumour

    ♦ Pseudo glandular or acinar pattern–tumour cells are disposed around central cystic space

    ♦ Compact pattern–resembles trabecular pattern but tumour cells form large solid masses

    ♦ Scirrhous pattern–characterized by more abundant fibrous stroma

  ▪ Cytologic features

    ♦ Cells resemble hepatocytes having vesicular nuclei with prominent nuclei

    ♦ Cytoplasm is granular and eosinophilic but becomes increasingly basophilic with increasing malignancy

    ♦ Pleomorphism

    ♦ Bizarre giant cell formation

    ♦ Spindle shaped cells

    ♦ Tumour cells with clear cytoplasm

    ♦ Presence of bile within dilated canaliculi

    ♦ Intracytoplasmic Mallory's hyalin

b. Etiopathogenesis and morphology of rheumatic heart disease

(Ref: Harsh Mohan, 7th ed. pg. 418, Robbins, SA ed. pg. 557-559)

ANSWER

Introduction

○ Acute, systemic, post-streptococcal, non-suppurative inflammatory disease mainly affecting heart, joints, CNS, skin and subcutaneous tissues

○ Incidence – commonly affects children between 5–15 years of age group

○ Sex – both sexes are equally affected

Etiopathogenesis

○ **Environmental factors**

  ▪ History of infection of pharynx, upper respiratory tract 2–3 weeks prior to attack of RF

  ▪ Subsequent attacks of streptococcal infection

  ▪ Higher incidence of RF after epidemics of streptococcal infection of throat in children

  ▪ Administration of antibiotics resulting in low incidence

  ▪ Similar Cardiac lesions produced in experimental animals by induction of repeated infection with Beta-haemolytic streptococci of group A

  ▪ Socioeconomic status—poverty, inadequate nutrition, dense population

  ▪ Geographic distribution of disease

  ▪ Climatic conditions – higher in cold and damp regions such as near rivers and waterways

○ **Host factors**

  ▪ Clustering of disease in families

  ▪ Identical twins

  ▪ Persons with HLA class II alleles have strong association with RF

  ▪ Inherited susceptibility–first degree relatives of patients with RF and RHD

○ **Immunologic evidence**

  ▪ Patients with RF have elevated titres of antibodies to antigens of beta-haemolytic streptococci of group A such as anti-streptolysin O and S, anti-sterptokinase, anti-streptohyaluronidase and anti-DNAase B

  ▪ Cell wall polysaccharide of group A streptococcus forms antibodies which are reactive against cardiac valves

  ▪ Hyaluronate capsule of group A streptococcus is similar to human hyaluronate present in joint tissues which are the target of attack

  ▪ Membrane antigens of group A Streptococcus react with sarcolemma of smooth and cardiac muscle, dermal fibroblasts and neurons of caudate nucleus

Morphology

- **Cardiac lesions:** Pancarditis
  - Myocardium-Aschoff bodies or nodules–spheroidal or fusiform distinct tiny structures, 1-2 mm in size occurring in interstitium of heart in RF
  - **Endocardium**
    - Fibrinoid necrosis–within the cusps or tendinous cords
    - Verrucae–small vegetation of size 1–2 mm along the lines of closure
  - Pericarditis–associated with fibrinous or serofibrinous exudates—bread and butter pericarditis
- **Migratory polyarthritis**
  - Most frequently observed in adults
  - Large joints of the body are involved–one joint after the other (migratory)
  - Non-erosive arthritis–goes off suddenly without any residual deformability in the joints
- **Subcutaneous nodules**
  - Painless subcutaneous nodules on extensor surface of elbows, shin and occiput
- **Erythema marginatum**
  - Red macular rash appears in fair skinned people sparing the face
- **Syndenham's chorea**
  - Involuntary, purposeless movements associated with emotional liability of patient

PART III

5. Write briefly on:

a. Amoebic colitis

(Ref: Textbook of Pathology, Harsh Mohan, 7th ed. pg. 555)

ANSWER

Introduction
- Also known as amebiasis

Causative Organism
- Entamoeba histolytica

Clinical Features
- Present at any age, common in children
- Causative organism: entamoeba histolytica
- Spread through fecal-oral route
- Generalized involvement of large intestine or localized to cecum, ascending colon, sigmoid, rectum and appendix
- Abdominal pain
- Diarrhea (may be bloody)
- Fever, vomiting, weakness, unintentional weight loss
- **Ulcers:**
  - Discrete and flask-shaped ulcers with broad base and narrow neck along with normal mucosa
  - Size is pinhead to > 2.5 cm in diameter
  - Ulcer extends deep or may be superficial
  - No evidence of pseudopolyps

Morphology

Gross appearance: Lesion exhibits elevated mucosal surface advanced lesion exhibits flask -shaped ulcer with broad- base

Microscopic findings: Lesion consist of chronic inflammatory cell infiltrate composed of lymphocytes, plasma cells, macrophages, etc. trophozoites of Entamoeba present and usually present in the margins of the lesion

Differential Diagnosis
- Giardiasis-no bloody stool
- Ulcerative colitis-no abdominal pain
- Crohn's disease- barium enema studies help to rule out both ulcerative colitis and amebiasis
- Shigellosis-presence of high number of fecal leukocytes in the stool

Complications
- Perforation
- Hemorrhage
- Amoebic abscess or hepatitis
- Amoeboma formation

Diagnostic Tests
- **Stool test:** Presence of ameboid protozoan in the patient's stool
- **ELISA antigen tests**
- **Complete blood count:** Determination of the patient if become anemic due to bloody diarrhea
- **Metabolic profile:** To assess electrolyte status of the patient
- **Colonoscopy:** In case if stool test is negative for E. histolytica
- **Tissue samples:** Shows trophozoites and flask shaped ulcer (characteristic finding)

b. Morphological changes in chronic viral hepatitis

(Ref: Harsh Mohan, 7th ed. pg. 596, Robbins, SA ed. pg. 837)

ANSWER

Morphological Changes in Chronic Viral Hepatitis

Introduction

○ Ongoing or relapsing hepatic disease for more than 6 months with clinical symptoms along with biochemical, serologic, histopathologic sign of inflammation and necrosis

Causes

○ Most cases are result of infection with hepatotropic viruses – hepatitis B, hepatitis C and combined hepatitis B and D

○ **Non-viral causes are:**
  ▪ Wilson's disease
  ▪ Alpha1-antitrypsin deficiency
  ▪ Chronic alcoholism
  ▪ Drug-induced injury
  ▪ Autoimmune diseases

Morphology

○ **Piecemeal necrosis–periportal destruction of hepatocytes at the limiting plate**
  ▪ Necrosed hepatocytes at the limiting plate in periportal zone
  ▪ Interface hepatitis owing to expanded portal tract by infiltration of lymphocytes, plasma cells and macrophages
  ▪ Expanded portal tracts are frequently associated with proliferating bile ductules as a response to liver cell injury

○ **Portal tract lesions–varying degree of changes in portal tract**
  ▪ Inflammatory cell infiltration by lymphocytes, plasma cells and macrophages (triaditis)
  ▪ Proliferated bile ductules in expanded portal tracts
  ▪ Lymphoid aggregates or follicles with reactive germinal center and infiltration of inflammatory cells

○ **Intralobular lesions**
  ▪ Focal areas of necrosis and inflammation within hepatic parenchyma
  ▪ Scattered acidophilic bodies in lobule
  ▪ Kupffer cell hyperplasia
  ▪ Bridging necrosis in severe cases
  ▪ Regenerative changes in hepatocytes in persistent hepatocellular necrosis
  ▪ Moderate fatty change in chronic hepatitis C
  ▪ Scattered ground glass appearance of hepatocytes in chronic hepatitis B suggestive of HBsAg in cytoplasm in abundance

○ **Bridging fibrosis–onset of fibrosis is indicative of irreversible damage**
  ▪ Initially, periportal fibrosis at sites on interface hepatitis giving stellate-shaped appearance to portal tract
  ▪ Bridging fibrosis connecting portal tract to portal tract or portal tract to central vein traversing the lobule in progressive cases
  ▪ Dense collagenous septa destroying lobular architecture and forming nodules in end stage leading to postnecrotic cirrhosis

c.　Pheochromocytoma

(Ref: Harsh Mohan, 7th ed. pg. 790, Robbins, SA ed. pg. 1134-36)

ANSWER

Pheochromocytoma

Introduction

○ Tumour originating from pheochromocytes (i.e. chromaffin cells) of adrenal medulla

○ Characterised by dark brown black appearance of this tumour due to chromaffin oxidation of catecholamines

○ Occurs at any age, although common in 20-60 years of age

○ Frequently tumours are slow growing and benign but 10% of tumours can be malignant, invasive and metastasising

○ Commonly sporadic but 10 % are associated with familial syndromes of multiple endocrine neoplasia and are bilateral, medullary carcinoma of thyroid, hyperparathyroidism, pituitary adenoma, mucosal neuromas and von Recklinghausen's neurofibromatosis

Clinical Symptoms

Due to secretion of catecholamines – epinephrine and norepinephrine

○ Hypertension
○ Congestive heart failure
○ Myocardial infarction
○ Pulmonary oedema
○ Cerebral hemorrhages
○ Death

Diagnosis

○ 24-hour urinary catecholamines or their metabolites such as metanephrine and VMA

Morphology

○ **Gross appearance:**
  ▪ Soft, spherical, variable in size and weight, well demarcated from surrounding adrenal gland

- Cut surface of tumour is grey to dusky brown with haemorrhagic areas, necrosis, calcification and cystic change
- On immersion in dichromate fixative, tumour turns brown black due to oxidation of catecholamines

○ **Microscopic appearance:**

- Tumour cells are organised typically as well defined nests (zellballen pattern) separated by abundant fibrovascular stroma
- Other arrangements are as solid columns, sheets, trabeculae or clumps
- Large, polyhedral and pleomorphic tumour cells with abundant granular amphophilic or basophilic cytoplasm and vesicular nuclei
- Stain positively with neuroendocrine substances such as neuron-specific enolase (NSE) and chromogranin

d. Diabetic nephropathy

(Ref: Harsh Mohan, 7th ed. pg. 664, Robbins, SA ed. pg. 1119)

ANSWER

For answer, refer 2016 paper-II, Q. 6 (c), Pg. 48

6. **Write short notes on:**

a. Transitional cell carcinoma urinary bladder

(Ref: Textbook of Pathology, Harsh Mohan, 7th ed. pg. 687)

ANSWER

For answer, refer 2016 paper-II Q. 5 (a), Pg. 45

b. Pathogenesis and complication of acute pancreatitis

(Ref: Harsh Mohan, 7th ed. pg. 631, Robbins, SA ed. pg. 884-87)

ANSWER

Pathogenesis and Complication of Acute Pancreatitis

Introduction

○ It is an acute inflammation of the pancreas presents with acute abdomen

○ Severe form of the disease is acute hemorrhagic pancreatitis or acute pancreatic necrosis

Etiology

Mechanical	Cholelithiasis, trauma, iatrogenic injury
Metabolic	Alcoholism, hypercalcemia, hyperlipoproteinemia, certain drugs
Genetic	Cationic trypsinogen and trypsin inhibitor gene mutation

Mechanical	Cholelithiasis, trauma, iatrogenic injury
Vascular	Atheroembolism, shock, vasculitis
Infections	EBV, CMV and Mumps
Idiopathic pancreatitis	

Pathogenesis

○ Mechanism like–acinic cell damage, duct obstruction and blockage in exocytosis of pancreatic enzymes results in release and activation of following enzymes, like- protease, elastases, lipases and phospholipases that results in destructive effects on pancreas

Clinical Features

○ Common in adults between the age of 40 and 70 years.

○ Common in females than males

○ Acute severe pain in abdomen—involves upper left quadrant initially followed by generalized pain and may radiate to back

○ Nausea, vomiting

○ Tachycardia, hypotension,tachypnea followed by shock

Morphology

○ **Gross Appearance:**

- In early stage—swollen and edematous pancreas
- Grey—white pancreatic necrosis, chalky-whiye fat necrosis and blue-black hemorrhages seen
- In peritoneal cavity fat necrosis, blood stained ascetic fluid in the omentum, mesentery and peripancreatic tissue is seen

○ **Microscopic features:**

- Necrosis of pancreatic lobules, ducts, arteries and arterioles along with areas of hemorrhages and inflammatory cell infiltrate, mainly polymorphs

Laboratory Findings

○ **Radiological:** Ultrasound and CTscan

○ Increased neutrophil count

○ **Serum lipase:** More specific than serum amylase

○ **Serum amylase:** If value more than 4 times the normal value

○ **Urinary amylase:** Excreted in urine and increased level from 2nd day onwards

○ **Serum trypsin:** Specificity and sensitivity is highest for pancreatic injury

○ Hypocalcemia

Complications

○ Shock

○ Organ failure

- Acute respiratory distress syndrome
- Disseminated intravascular coagulation
- Renal failure
- Pancreatic abscess
- Chronic pancreatitis, etc.

    c. Celiac disease

(Ref: Harsh Mohan, 7th ed. pg. 557, Robbins, SA ed. pg. 782-83)

Answer

Celiac Disease

Introduction

- Type of malabsorption syndrome occurring in temperate climates
- Also known as coeliac sprue, non-tropical sprue, Gluten-sensitive enteropathy, Idiopathic Steatorrhoea)
- **Characteristics**
    - Substantial loss of villi in small intestine
    - Reduced absorptive surface area
- **Forms of celiac disease**
    - Childhood form–known as coeliac disease is found in infants and children
    - Adult form–known as idiopathic steatorrhoea is found in adolescents and early adult life

- Genetic abnormality leading to sensitivity to gluten and its derivative, gliadin (present in wheat, barley and rye) is seen
- Serum antibodies–IgA antigliadin and IgA antiendomysial are found
- Symptoms are relieved if gluten is removed from diet
- **Mucosal cell damage is caused due to**
    - Hypersensitivity reaction as found by gluten-stimulated antibodies
    - Toxic effect of gluten due to inherited enzyme deficiency in the mucosal cells

Morphology:

- Histologically, no difference can be seen in pathological findings in children and adults
- Variable degree of flattening of the mucosa, especially of the upper jejunum and duodenum and ileum to certain extent
- Cuboidal or low columnar type surface epithelial cells
- Partial villous atrophy is observed as replacement of normal villous pattern by convolutions or subtotal villous atrophy characterised by flat mucosal surface
- Increased number of plasma cells and lymphocytes seen in lamina propria

Sequela of Coeliac Sprue

- Incidence of intestinal carcinoma is higher

Your Roll No. ....

Name of the Paper	:	**Pathology Paper-I**
Name of the Course	:	**MBBS-2014**
Semester	:	**Annual**

Time: 3 Hours   **M.M.: 40**

INSTRUCTIONS

1. Write your Roll No. on the top immediately on receipt of this question paper
2. All questions are to be attempted
3. Answers to Parts I, II and III should be written in separate answer sheets provided
4. Attempt parts of a question in sequence

PART-I

1. **Differentiate between:**   [8]
    a. Dystrophic and metastatic calcification
    b. Leukemoid reaction and Chronic Myeloid leukemia
    c. Type II and Type III hypersensitivity reaction
    d. Intravascular and Extravascular Hemolysis

2. **Write briefly on:**   [6]
    a. Role of Arachidonic acid metabolites in acute inflammation
    b. Erythroblastosis fetalis
    c. Mode of spread of tumors

PART-II

3. **Write briefly on:**   [6]
    a. Causes and Laboratory diagnosis of disseminated intravascular coagulation
    b. Laboratory diagnosis of Multiple Myeloma

4. **Write briefly on:**   [6]
    a. DNA Oncogenic viruses
    b. Mechanism of Apoptosis

PART-III

5. **Write short notes on:**   [8]
    a. Erythrocyte Sedimentation Rate
    b. Stages of shock
    c. Hereditary spherocytosis
    d. Primary complex

6. **Write short notes on:**   [6]
    a. Pancytopenia
    b. Laboratory diagnosis in AIDS
    c. Fat embolism

PART-I

1. Differentiate between:

a. Dystrophic and Metastatic calcification

(Ref: Harsh Mohan, 7th ed. pg. 37, Robbins, SA ed. pg. 65-66)

ANSWER

Dystrophic and Metastatic Calcification

Dystrophic calcification	Metastatic calcification
• Deposition of calcium salts in dead and degenerated tissue	• Deposition of calcium salts in living/normal tissue
• Serum calcium level normal	• Elevated serum calcium level
• Can lead to organ dysfunction	• No usual clinical dysfunction of the organs evident
• Generally not reversible	• Can be reversed (depends upon correction of disorder)
• Due to infarcts, haematomas, necrosis, dead parasites, atheromas, certain tumours, cysts, etc.	• Due to Hyperparathyroidism, multiple myeloma, vitamin D related disorders, Milk-alkali syndrome, vitamin A toxicity, etc.

b. Leukemoid reaction and chronic myeloid leukemia

(Ref: Textbook of Pathology, Harsh Mohan, 7th ed. pg. 332)

ANSWER

Leukemoid Reaction and Chronic Myeloid Leukemia

For answer, refer to 2017 paper-I Q. 1 (c), Pg. 4

c. Type II and Type III hypersensitivity reaction

(Ref: Harsh Mohan, 7th ed. pg. 332, Robbins, SA ed. pg. 200)

ANSWER

Type II and Type III Hypersensitivity Reaction

Type II hypersensitivity reaction	Type III hypersensitivity reaction
• Antibody-mediated (cytotoxic) reaction	• Immune complex mediated (arthus)reaction
• Tissue-specific	• Not tissue-specific
• Neutrophils, non sensitized macrophages, B cells, NK cells, eosinophils are involved	• Leukocytes (neutrophils) and B cells are involved
• Requires 15-30 min for manifestation of hypersensitivity reaction	• Reaction manifestations appear within 6 hours

Type II hypersensitivity reaction	Type III hypersensitivity reaction
• Occurs as a result of exposure to foreign tissue/cells	• As result of persistent low grade infection, autoimmune process, environmental antigens, etc.
• Examples- transfusion reactions, ITP, Grave's disease, etc.	• Immune complex glomerulonephritis, SLE, rheumatoid arthritis, etc.

d. Intravascular and Extravascular Hemolysis

(Ref: Textbook of Pathology, Harsh Mohan, 7th ed. pg. 288)

ANSWER

Intravascular and Extravascular Hemolysis

Intravascular hemolysis	Extravascular hemolysis
• Hemolysis occurs in circulating blood vessels	• Occurs in organs like spleen, bone marrow, etc.
• Seen in G6PD deficiency	• Seen in thalassemia
• Serum bilirubin (unconjugated) increased	• Serum bilirubin (unconjugated) markedly increased
• Plasma hemoglobin present	• Plasma hemoglobin absent
• Reduced tissue iron	• Increased tissue iron
• Urine hemoglobin and hemosiderin present	• Urine hemoglobin and hemosiderin absent

2. Write briefly on:

a. Role of Arachidonic acid metabolites in acute inflammation

(Ref: Harsh Mohan, 7th ed. pg. 123, Robbins, SA ed. pg. 73)

ANSWER

Role of Arachidonic Acid Metabolites in Acute Inflammation

○ Also known as " eicosanoids"
○ Potent mediator of inflammation
○ 20-carbon polyunsaturated fatty acid
○ Form arachidonic acid metabolites by one of the following pathways:
  ▪ Cyclo-oxygenase pathway
  ▪ Lipo-oxygenase pathway
○ **Cyclo-oxygenase pathway:**
  ▪ Fatty acid enzyme that acts on activated arachidonic acid and results in three metabolites:
    ♦ Prostaglandins (PGD_2, PGE_2, PGF_2-α)
    ♦ Thtomboxane A_2 (TXA_2)
    ♦ Prostacyclin (PGI_2)

○ **Lipo-oxygenase pathway:**

- Present as enzyme in neutrophils acts on activated arachidonic acid and form hydroperoxy eicosatetraenoic acid which futher forms two metabolites:
  - ◆ Leukotrienes (LT)
  - ◆ Lipoxins (LX)

b. Erythroblastosis fetalis

(Ref: Harsh Mohan, 7th ed. pg. 319, Robbins, SA ed. pg. 462)

ANSWER

Introduction

○ Due to blood group incompatibility between mother and child

○ As a result of passage of antibodies (IgG) from the mother across the placenta into the fetal circulation

Two Forms

○ HDN due to Rh-D incompatibility

○ HDN due to ABO incompatibility

○ **HDN due to Rh-D incompatibility:**

- Causes severe form of HDN
- Sensitisation of Rh- negative mother to Rh-positive blood results in Rh incompatibility
- Usually, passage of Rh – positive red cells from Rh-positive fetus across the placenta into the circulation of Rh-negative mother.

○ **HDN due to ABO incompatibility:**

- Common than Rh incompatibility
- Common in infants born to group O mothers,having anti-A and/or anti-B IgG antibodies.
- Negative coomb's test
- Less severe

Pathogenesis

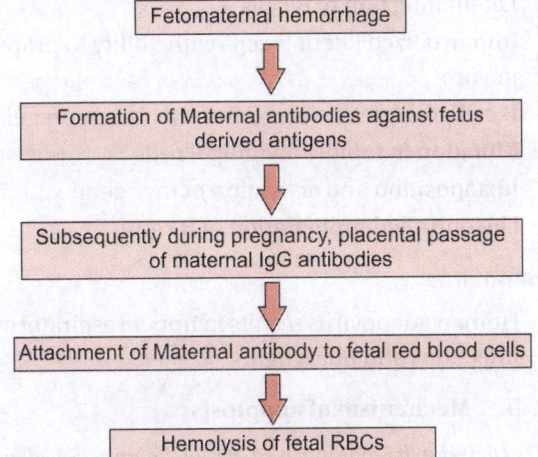

Fetomaternal hemorrhage

↓

Formation of Maternal antibodies against fetus derived antigens

↓

Subsequently during pregnancy, placental passage of maternal IgG antibodies

↓

Attachment of Maternal antibody to fetal red blood cells

↓

Hemolysis of fetal RBCs

Clinical Features

○ Anemia (main risk to fetus)

○ Mild jaundice and anemia to hydrops fetalis

○ Hepatosplenomegaly

○ **Postnatal problems:**

- Anemia
- Caogulopathies
- Edema (due to low serum albumin)
- Pallor
- Pulmonary hypertension
- Kernicterus (due to hyperbilirubinemia)

Laboratory Findings

○ **Cord blood:**

- Reticulocytosis, increased serum bilirubin, positive direct Coomb's test (if cord blood Rh-D positive)

○ **Mother's blood:**

- Rh-D negative

Management

○ **Treatment:**

- **Maternal:** Intravenous immunoglobulin, plasma exchange
- **Infant:** Exchange transfusion, intrauterine transfusion, phototherapy

○ **Prevention:**

- Rh immune globulin

c. Mode of spread of tumors

(Ref: Textbook of Pathology, Harsh Mohan, 7th ed. pg. 193-195)

ANSWER

Mode of Spread of Tumors

For answer, refer 2016 paper-I Q. 2 (c), Pg. 28

PART II

3. Write briefly on:

a. Causes and laboratory diagnosis of disseminated intravascular coagulation

(Ref: Harsh Mohan, 7th ed. pg. 315, Robbins, SA ed. pg. 663)

ANSWER

Introduction

○ Acute, subacute or chronic thrombo-hemorrhagic disorder characterized by activation of coagulation pathway and formation of thrombi in the microcirculation of body

○ Also known as "defibrination syndrome" or "consumption coagulopathy"

Etiology

○ Trauma and tissue injury
○ Infections, eg. certain viral infections, malaria, gram-negative bacilli, etc.
○ Vascular disorders, like hemangiomas
○ Innunologic disorders, like- GVHD, transplant rejection, etc.
○ Certain drugs, shock, ARDS, insect bite etc.

Laboratory Findings

○ **Hemogram:** Decreased platelet count
○ **Peripheral smear:** Schistocytes and fragmented red cells
○ **Coagulation test:** Prolonged thrombin time, prothrombin time, activated partial thromboplastin time
○ **Other investigation:**
○ Increased level of FDP(fibrin degraded product)

    b. Laboratory diagnosis of multiple myeloma

(Ref: Harsh Mohan, 7th ed. pg. 363, Robbins, SA ed. pg. 590)

ANSWER

For answer, refer 2017 paper-I Q. 4. (b), Pg. 8

---

4. Write briefly on:

    a. DNA oncogenic virus

(Ref: Textbook of Pathology, Harsh Mohan, 7th ed. pg. 217)

ANSWER

Introduction

○ Direct access and incorporation of the virus into genome of the host cell
○ **Five subtypes:**
    ■ Herpesvirus
    ■ Papovavirus
    ■ Adenovirus
    ■ Poxvirus
    ■ Hepadnavirus

Virus	Host	Neoplasm associated
Herpesvirus		
• Epstein-barr virus	Humans	Burkitt's lymphoma, nasopharyngeal carcinoma
• Human herpesvirus 8	Humans	Kaposi sarcoma
• Lucke's frog virus	Frog	Renal cell carcinoma

Virus	Host	Neoplasm associated
Poxvirus	Humans	Papilloma, molluscum contagiosum
Papovaviruses		
• Human papilloma virus	Humans	Cervical cancer, skin cancer, papillomas (warts) on skin, larynx, genital warts
• Papilloma viruses	Cotton tail rabbits	Papillomas
Hepadna virus		
• Hepatitis B virus	Human	Hepatocellular carcinoma
• Adenovirus	Hamster	Sarcoma

Mechanism of DNA Viral Oncogenesis

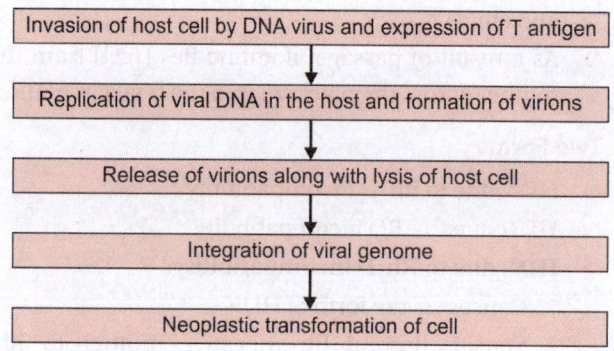

Invasion of host cell by DNA virus and expression of T antigen

↓

Replication of viral DNA in the host and formation of virions

↓

Release of virions along with lysis of host cell

↓

Integration of viral genome

↓

Neoplastic transformation of cell

Papilloma Virus

○ Replication in the layers of stratified squamous epithelium
○ Low risk HPV 1, 2, 4 and 7 involved in common viral warts
○ High risk HPVs are responsible for squamous cell carcinoma of anus, oral cavity, vagina, etc.

Epstein-Barr Virus

Responsible for:

○ Epithelial cells and B lymphocytes get infected via CD21
○ Latent infection of B cells
○ Immortalized latent B cells with ability to propagate in vitro
○ B cell proliferation and failure of immunoregulation
○ Mutation in rapidly dividing B cells
○ Juxtaposition and activation of myc gene
○ Uncontrolled proliferation of B cells

Adenovirus

○ Human adenovirus results in upper respiratory tract infections and pharyngitis

    b. Mechanism of apoptosis

(Ref: Harsh Mohan, 7th ed. pg. 29, Robbins, SA ed. pg. 52)

ANSWER

For answer, refer 2016 paper-I Q. 6. (a), Pg. 35

PART III

5. **Write short notes on:**

   a. **Erythrocyte sedimentation rate**

   (Ref: Harsh Mohan, 7th ed. pg. 270, Robbins, SA ed. pg. 99)

ANSWER

Introduction

○ It is the rate at which erythrocytes settle down when blood is (mixed with an anticoagulant) is allowed to stand in a vertical tube for one hour undisturbed.

○ Expressed in mm/hrs

○ Also known as "sed rate" or "Biernacki reaction"

○ Easy, inexpensive, non-specific widely used screening test

Normal Values

○ **Westergren method:**
   ▪ **Males:** 3 to 7 mm in 1hour
   ▪ **Females:** 5 to 9 mm in 1 hour

○ **Wintrobe method:**
   ▪ **Males:** 0 to 9 mm in 1hour
   ▪ **Females:** 0 to 15 mm in 1hour

Mechanism of Erythrocyte Sedimentation

○ **Stage I:**
   ▪ Aggregation of RBC and Rouleaux formation, for 10 minutes

○ **Stage II:**
   ▪ Last for 40 minutes, sinking of aggregates occurs

○ **Stage III:**
   ▪ Packing of aggregated cells at the bottom of tube, last for 10 minutes

Factors Affecting ESR

○ **Physiologic factors:**
   ▪ **Specific gravity of RBC:** increase in specific gravity, increases ESR.
   ▪ **Number of RBC:** Decrease in number of RBC, increases ESR. Usually seen in anemia. Increase in number of RBC, decrease ESR
   ▪ **Rouleaux formation:** Increases ESR
   ▪ **Size of RBC:** Increase in size of RBC, increases the ESR
   ▪ **RBC Count:** Decrease in RBC count, decreases the viscosity of blood, thus increasing the ESR.
   ▪ **Viscosity of blood:** Increased viscosity of blood, decreased ESR

▪ **Age:** Less in infants and children – more number of RBC's
▪ **Sex:** More in females than males
▪ **Pregnancy:** From 3rd month ESR increases upto 35 mm in 1 hour

○ **Laboratory factors:**
   ▪ **Temperature:** High temperature causes false high result due to reduced plasma viscosity
   ▪ **Time:** Test should be done within two hours of collection. Sample with EDTA should be used within six hours
   ▪ **Tube factor:** Longer tube-increase ESR
   ▪ **Anticoagulants:** Tri sodium citrate or K2EDTA should be used
   ▪ **Vibration:** Decrease in ESR
   ▪ **Position of tube:** Tube should be vertical. Angle of 3 degree from vertical—increase in ESR by ESR
   ▪ **Sunlight:** Direct sunlight increases ESR

Significance of ESR Determination

○ It helps in the confirmation of diagnosis as well as in prognosis.

○ It helps in the assessment of prognosis in certain conditions, like—Pulmonary tuberculosis, rheumatoid arthritis, temporal arteritis, etc.

   b. **Stages of Shock**

   (Ref: T Harsh Mohan, 7th ed. pg. 97, Robbins, SA ed. pg. 133)

ANSWER

Stages of Shock

○ **Compensated (initial, non-progressive, reversible) shock:**
   ▪ Activation of compensatory mechanism and perfusion of vital organs
   ▪ Compensatory mechanism are vasoconstriction, fluid conservation by kidney and adrenal medulla stimulation
   ▪ Result in tachycardia and cold clammy skin

○ **Progressive decompensated shock:**
   ▪ Normal compensatory mechanism not maintained
   ▪ Tissue hypoperfusion results in pulmonary hypoperfusion, tissue ischemia that leads to tachypnea, decreased cardiac output, mental confusion, decreased urinary output

○ **Irreversible decompensated shock:**
   ▪ Irreversible tissue injury multiple that results in increased vascular permeability, pulmonary hypoperfusion, progressive vasodilatation, etc.
   ▪ Effect multiple organs like–lungs (ARDS), brain (hypoxic encephalopathy), liver (necrosis), etc.

   c. **Hereditary spherocytosis**

   (Ref: Textbook of Pathology, Harsh Mohan, 7th ed. pg. 292)

Answer

Introduction

○ Characterized by intrinsic defect in the red blood cell membrane proteins leading to spherocytes

Inheritance Pattern

○ Autosomal dominant (75%), compound heterozygous (25%)

Structural Defect

○ Any defect in the membrane cytoskeleton protein (spectrin, actin, ankyrin, band-3, etc, most commonly ankyrin defect followed by band 3) results in loss of membrane fragments and reduced membrane stability

○ Reduced cell surface to volume ratio leads to spherocytic shape

Pathogenesis

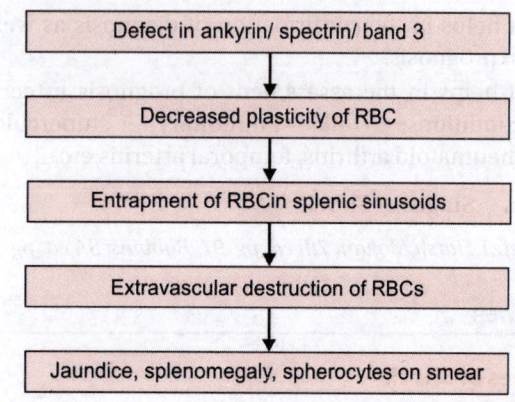

```
Defect in ankyrin/ spectrin/ band 3
            ↓
Decreased plasticity of RBC
            ↓
Entrapment of RBCin splenic sinusoids
            ↓
Extravascular destruction of RBCs
            ↓
Jaundice, splenomegaly, spherocytes on smear
```

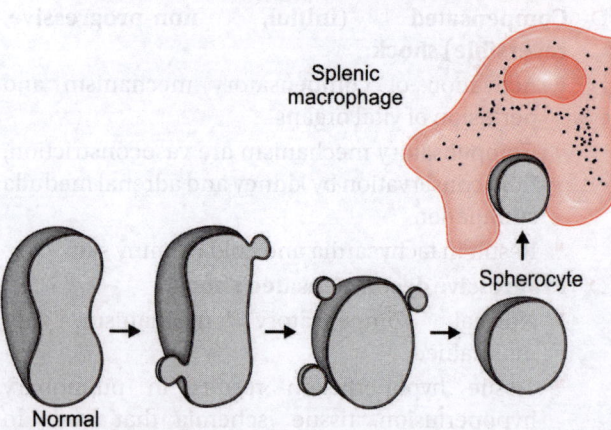

Splenic macrophage

Spherocyte

Normal

Clinical Features

○ Hemolytic anemia
○ Jaundice
○ Splenomegaly
○ Gallstones (pigment type)

Laboratory Findings

○ **Peripheral blood smear:** Anisocytosis microspherocytosis (lack of area of central pallor in dark appearing spherocytes)

○ **Bone marrow:** Erythroid hyperplasia
○ **Osmotic fragility test:** Increased fragility of RBC
○ **Direct Coombs' test:** Negative
○ Decreased MCV, increased MCHC, increased glycerol lysis test

Treatment

○ Splenectomy (anemia is corrected but spherocytes persist)

d. Primary Complex

(Ref: Textbook of Pathology, Harsh Mohan, 7th ed. pg. 142)

Answer

For answer, refer 2016 paper-I Q. 5. (d), Pg. 34

6. Write short notes on:

a. Pancytopenia

(Ref: Textbook of Pathology, Harsh Mohan, 7th ed. pg. 301)

Answer

Introduction

○ Clinico-hematological entity
○ Red blood cells, white blood cells and platelets are reduced in number, i.e. simultaneous presence of anemia, thrombocytopenia and leucopenia

Etiology

○ **Aplastic anemia:**
 ▪ Normocytic, normochromic anemia, Hb level decreased, decreased reticulocyte count
 ▪ **Leucopenia:** Absolute granulocyte count is low
 ▪ **Thrombocytopenia:** Reduced platelet count

○ **Paroxysmal nocturnal hemoglobinuria:**
 ▪ Chronic intravascular hemolysis
 ▪ Cells of myeloid progenitor lineage (red blood cells, white blood cells, platelets) is affected resulting in deficient haematopoiesis

○ Megaloblastic anemia
○ Hypersplenism
○ Myelodysplastic syndromes
○ Bone marrow infiltrations, like- osteopetrosis, myelofibrosis, storage diseases, haematologic malignancies, etc.

Clinical Features

○ Fever, fatigue, dizziness
○ Hepatomegaly, splenomegaly
○ Weight loss
○ Anorexia

- Night sweats
- Pallor, bleeding, lymphadenopathy, etc.

Diagnosis

- **Bone marrow examination:** Evaluation of abnormal infiltrate and its pattern of distribution, marrow architecture and focal bone marrow lesions

  b **Laboratory Diagnosis in AIDS**

(Ref: Harsh Mohan, 7th ed. pg. 57, Robbins, SA ed. pg. 243)

Answer

Tests Help in Establishment of Diagnosis in AIDS

- **Non-specific tests:**
  - **Total leucocyte and lymphocyte count:** Decreased (< 2000cu/mm)
  - Thrombocytopenia
  - **T cell subset assay:** Absolute CD4+ T cells is less than 200/µl, reverse T4: T8 ratio
  - Decrease in cell mediated immunity
  - Abnormalities on lymph node biopsy
  - Increased beta-2 microglobulin level
- **Specific tests:**
  - **Antigen detection:**
    - Viral antigen may be detectable in blood after about 2 weeks
    - First and foremost viral marker to appear in the blood is antigen p24
    - p24 capture ELISA assay is the method used
    - Highly increased free p24 Ag- stage of clinical disease
  - **Detection of antibody:**
    - Commonly used method
    - Appearance of IgM antibodies followed by IgM antibodies
    - **ELISA:**
      - Commonly used screening test
      - For early detection of infection- 4th generation ELISA can be used
      - Nowadays, p24 capture ELISA assay is used for screening
    - **Western blot test:**
      - Specific than ELISA
      - "Gold standard test"
  - **PCR:**
    - Sensitive test for demonstration of viral nucleic acid

- Qualitative PCR is used for diagnostic purpose
  - **Viral isolation:** for characterization of virus
- **Other tests:**
  - Oral fluid (saliva) HIV test
  - Urine test

c. **Fat Embolism**

(Ref: Harsh Mohan, 7th ed. pg. 107, Robbins, SA ed. pg. 128)

Answer

Introduction

- Obstruction of arterioles and capillaries by fat globules
- Occurs in individuals with severe skeletal injuries (90%)

Etiology

- Most commonly associated with fracture of long bones
- Trauma to soft tissue
- Pancreatitis
- Diabetes mellitus
- Extensive burn, etc.

Pathogenesis

- **Mechanical theory:**
  - Pulmonary or cerebral microvasculature by fat globules results in RBC and platelet aggregation and finally hypoxia of the organ/tissue
- **Biochemical injury:**
  - Free fatty acids formed from fat globules results in endothelial injury followed by platelet activation and recruitment of granulocytes producing free radicals, protease, eicosanoids thus resulting vascular damage

Clinical Features

- Pulmonary insufficiency
- Thrombocytopenia and anemia
- Neurological symptoms(restlessness, irritability, delirium and coma)
- Injury to endothelium

Laboratory Findings

- Anemia
- Thrombocytopenia
- Fat microglobulinemia
- Fat globules in urine

Your Roll No. ....

Name of the Paper : **Pathology Paper-II**

Name of the Course : **MBBS-2014**

Semester : **Annual**

Time: 3 Hours   M.M.: 40

INSTRUCTIONS

1. Write your Roll No. on the top immediately on receipt of this question paper
2. All questions are to be attempted
3. Answers to Parts I, II and III should be written in separate answer sheets provided
4. Attempt parts of a question in sequence

PART-I

1. **Differentiate between:**   [8]
   a. Benign and Malignant Gastric Ulcer
   b. Benign and Malignant Nephrosclerosis
   c. Lobar Pneumonia and bronchopneumonia
   d. Pre and post hepatic jaundice

2. **Write short notes on:**   [6]
   a. Multinodular goiter
   b. Osteogenic sarcoma
   c. Hyperplasia of prostate

PART-II

3. **Write briefly on:**   [6]
   a. Laboratory findings in chronic renal failure
   b. Etipathogensis and complications of atherosclerosis

4. **Write briefly on:**   [6]
   a. Laboratory diagnosis of Hepatitis B
   b. Laboratory diagnosis of Myocardial infarction

PART-III

5. **Write short notes on:**   [8]
   a. H. pylori and gastric diseases
   b. Nodular Sclerosis type of Hodgkin Lymphoma
   c. Astrocytoma
   d. Teratoma

6. **Write short notes on:**   [6]
   a. Choriocarcinoma
   b. Neuroblastoma
   c. Renal Stone

PART I

1. Differentiate between:

a. Benign and Malignant Gastric Ulcer

(Ref: Textbook of Pathology, Harsh Mohan, 7th ed. pg. 543)

ANSWER

Benign and Malignant Gastric Ulcer

Benign gastric ulcer	Malignant gastric ulcer
Common in younger age group	Frequent in older people
Frequently common in males	Less common in males
Commonly present at lesser curvature of pylorus and antrum	Present at greater curvature of antrum and pylorus
Grossly, it is small, regular in shape with radiating mucosal folds and ulcer bed is hemorrhagic	Grossly, large, irregular with interrupted mucosal folds and necrotic ulcer bed
Barium study revels punched out ulcer	Barium study shows irregular filling defect
Presents with normal to low acidity	Acidity may be normal or may present with achlorhtdria
Response to therapy is good	No response to medical therapy

b. Benign and Malignant Nephrosclerosis

(Ref: Textbook of Pathology, Harsh Mohan, 7th ed. pg. 677)

ANSWER

For answer, refer 2017 paper-II Q. 1 (a), Pg. 15

c. Lobar Pneumonia and Bronchopneumonia

(Ref: Harsh Mohan, 7th ed. pg. 454, Robbins, SA ed. pg. 702)

ANSWER

Lobar Pneumonia and Bronchopneumonia

Lobar Pneumonia	Bronchopneumonia
Part of a lobe of one or both lungs are affected	Terminal bronchioles extending into adjoining alveoli are affected
More frequent in adults	More frequent in infants and elderly people
Commonly affects healthy people	Commonly affects people with pre-existing diseases such as chronic debility, terminal illness, measles or flu

Lobar Pneumonia	Bronchopneumonia
Etiologic agents are Pneumococci, Klebsiella pneumoniae, Staphylococci, Streptococci	Etiologic agents are Staphylococci, Pseudomonas, Haemophilus influenzae
Pathology – stages of congestion (1-2days), early consolidation (2-4 days), late consolidation (4-8 days), resolution (1-3 weeks)	Pathology – patchy consolidation with central granularity, alveolar exudation, thickened septa
Diagnosis – neutrophilic leucocytosis, positive blood culture, X-ray exhibits consolidation	Diagnosis – neutrophilic leucocytosis, positive blood culture, X-ray exhibits mottled focal opacities
Prognosis is good, responds better to treatment	Prognosis is poor, variable response to treatment
Complications are pleural effusion, lung abscess, organisation	Complication are Bronchiectasis, pleural effusion, lung abscess

d. Pre and post hepatic jaundice

(Ref: Textbook of Pathology, Harsh Mohan, 7th ed. pg. 581)

ANSWER

Pre and Post Hepatic Jaundice

Pre-hepatic Jaundice	Post hepatic Jaundice
Due to hemolysis, excess amount of bilirubin is presented to liver – Haemolytic jaundice	Due to obstruction of bile flow, excretion is impaired
Unconjugated bilirubin is elevated	Conjugated bilirubin is elevated
Urobilinogen is increased	Urobilinogen is absent
Bile salts are absent	Bile salts are present
Liver function tests – clotting time, prothrombin time, plasma protein level, alkaline phosphatase level are normal	Clotting time, prothrombin time and alkaline phosphatase level are increased, plasma protein level is decreased

2. Write short notes on:

a. Multinodular goitre

(Ref: Harsh Mohan, 7th ed. pg. 798, Robbins, SA ed. pg. 1091)

ANSWER

Multinodular Goitre

Introduction

- Goitre is the enlargement of thyroid due to compensatory hyperplasia and hypertrophy of follicular epithelium caused by deficiency of thyroid hormone
- **Types of goitre**
  - Diffuse goitre also called as simple nontoxic goitre or colloid goitre
  - Nodular goitre also called as multinodular goitre or adenomatous goitre

Multinodular Goitre

- Considered as end stage of long standing diffuse goitre
- Symbolized by extreme degree of tumour like enlargement and typical nodularity
- Enlargement of thyroid gland results in cosmetic disfigurement, dysphagia and choking owing to compression of oesophagus and trachea

Etiology

- **Endemic goitre**
  - Lack of iodine in drinking water and food
  - Genetic factors
  - Goitrogens–substances interfering with synthesis of thyroid hormones, found in cabbage, cauliflower, turnips, cassava roots
- **Non-endemic or sporadic goitre**
  - Suboptimal iodine intake in conditions of higher demand such as puberty and pregnancy
  - Genetic factors
  - Dietary goitrogens
  - Hereditary defect in thyroid hormone synthesis and transport
  - Inborn errors of iodine metabolism
- **Other etiologic factors are**
  - Epithelial hyperplasia
  - Generation of new follicles
  - Irregular accumulation of colloid in follicles
  - Hemorrhages
  - Cystic change
  - Scarring
  - Calcification

Morphology

- **Gross appearance:**
  - Asymmetric and extreme enlargement of thyroid gland – weighing 100-500 g or more

- **5 important macroscopic features**
  - Nodularity with poor encapsulation
  - Fibrous scarring
  - Hemorrhages
  - Focal calcification
  - Cystic degeneration
- **Histologically:**
  - Partial or incomplete nodular encapsulation
  - Follicles vary from small to large and lined by flat to high epithelium
  - Areas of hemorrhages, haemosiderin-laden macrophages and cholesterol crystals
  - Fibrous scarring with foci of calcification
  - Micro-macrocystic change

  b. Osteogenic sarcoma

  (Ref: Harsh Mohan, 7th ed. pg. 832, Robbins, SA ed. pg. 902)

ANSWER

Osteogenic Sarcoma

For answer, refer 2017 paper-II Q. 3 (a), Pg. 19

  c. Hyperplasia of prostate

  (Ref: Textbook of Pathology, Harsh Mohan, 7th ed. pg. 705)

ANSWER

Introduction

- BPH is a part of natural aging process
- Characterized by hyperplasia of epithelial and stromal cells of prostate

Pathogenesis

- Increased epithelial cells and stromal component in the periurethral area
- **Responsible hormone:** Dihydrotestosterone (DHT)
- Production of growth factors due to action of DHT
- Growth factors induces proliferation of fibroblast and epithelial cells as well as decreased loss of epithelial cells
- Thus, epithelial and stromal cells increased resulting in enlarged prostate

Clinical Features

- Usually seen in older people (over 50 years of age)
- Due to urethra compression:
- Nocturia
- Painful micturition
- Increased frequency
- Dribbling or leaking after urination
- Decrease in urine stream

- Due to urine retention in the bladder:
  - Infection
  - Hypertrophy
  - Cystitis, etc.

Gross Appearance

- **Early nodules:** Usually composed of stromal cells but later epithelial cells predominate
- No true capsule but plane of cleavage present
- In glandular proliferation: consistency is soft and milky white prostatic fluid oozes out

Microscopic Features

- Composed of fibromuscular nodule to fibroepithe-lial nodulaes with dominant glandular tissue
- Glandular tissue composed of inner layer of columnar cells and outer layer of cuboidal or flattened epithelial cells
- Stromal component exhibits muscular and fibrous proliferation

Diagnosis

- Assessment of symptoms
- Digital rectal examination
- Ultrasonography-PV determination
- Urodynamic analysis
- Prostate specific antigen (PSA) measurement: prognostic marker for BPH

PART II

3. Write briefly on:

a. Laboratory findings in chronic renal failure

(Ref: Textbook of Pathology, Harsh Mohan, 7th ed. pg. 592)

ANSWER

Laboratory Findings in Chronic Renal Failure

For answer, refer 2017 paper-II Q. 4 (b), Pg. 21

b. Etiopathogenesis and complications of atherosclerosis

(Ref: Textbook of Pathology, Harsh Mohan, 7th ed. pg. 373)

ANSWER

Etiopathogenesis and Complications of Atherosclerosis

Etiology

Risk factors for Atherosclerosis

Modifiable risk factors	Non-modifiable risk factors	Other risk factors
Dyslipidaemia	Age – Increasing age	Infection (C. pneumoniae, Herpesvirus, CMV)
Hypertension	Sex – Males are commonly affected	Environmental influences
Diabetes mellitus	Family history	Obesity
Cigarette smoking	Genetic factors	Hormones – oestrogen deficiency, oral contraceptives
Physical inactivity	Stress	Alcohol consumption
Inflammation	Racial factors – Whites are more 5commonly affected than Blacks	Homocystinuria

Pathogenesis

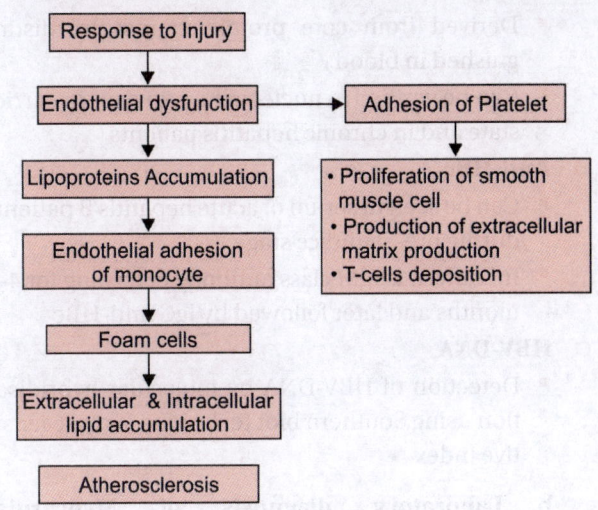

Complications

For answer, refer 2016 paper-II Q. 2 (a), Pg. 40

4. Write briefly on:

a. Laboratory diagnosis of Hepatitis B

(Ref: Harsh Mohan, 7th ed. pg. 592, Robbins, SA ed. pg. 831)

ANSWER

Laboratory Diagnosis of Hepatitis B

Laboratory diagnosis of Hepatitis B is done by Serological and viral markers:

○ **HBsAg**
  ▪ Appears early in blood after 6 weeks of infection
  ▪ Presence is suggestive of active HBV infection
  ▪ Disappears in 3–6 months
  ▪ If persists for more than 6 months – carrier state

○ **Anti-HBs**
  ▪ Appears late after 3 months of infection
  ▪ Response may be both IgM and IgG type

○ **HBeAg**
  ▪ Derived from core protein
  ▪ Present momentarily (3–6 weeks) during an attack
  ▪ If persists for more than 10 weeks suggests development of chronic liver disease and carrier state

○ **Anti-HBe**
  ▪ Appears after HBeAg disappears
  ▪ For resolution of infection during acute stage, seroconversion from HBeAg to anti-HBe is a prognostic sign

○ **HBcAg**
  ▪ Derived from core protein cannot be distinguished in blood
  ▪ Can be verified in nuclei of hepatocytes in carrier state and in chronic hepatitis patients

○ **Anti-HBc**
  ▪ Can be seen in serum of acute hepatitis B patients during pre- jaundice stage
  ▪ Initially, it is IgM class antibody persisting for 4-6 months and later followed by IgG anti-HBc

○ **HBV-DNA**
  ▪ Detection of HBV-DNA by molecular hybridisation using Southern blot technique is most sensitive index

  b. **Laboratory diagnosis of Myocardial Infarction**

  (Ref: Harsh Mohan, 7th ed. pg. 409, Robbins, SA ed. pg. 540)

Answer

Laboratory Diagnosis of Myocardial Infarction
Introduction

○ Life threatening condition resulting from coronary artery disease
○ Establishment of collateral circulation through anastomotic channels over a period of time may prevent myocardial damage
○ **Incidence:** Causes 10-25% of all deaths in developed countries
○ **Age:** Occurs at all ages, incidence being higher in old age
○ **Sex:** Males are more prone than females

Clinical Picture

○ Onset–sudden
○ Pain
○ Indigestion
○ Oliguria
○ Mild fever
○ Shock
○ Apprehension and anxiety
○ Acute pulmonary oedema

Diagnosis

○ **Electrocardiogram changes**–ST segment elevation, T wave inversion, appearance of wide deep Q waves
○ **Laboratory Findings:** Serum cardiac markers
  ▪ Creatinine phosphokinase (CK) and CK-MB–3 types are CK-MM (from skeletal muscle), CK-BB (from brain and lungs), CK-MB (from cardiac muscles and extracardiac tissue)
    ♦ Increased CK-MB is indicative of myocardial damage
    ♦ **Ratio of CK-MB2:** CK-MB1 above 4:1 is highly suggestive of acute MI after 4-6 hours of onset
    ♦ After 48 hours, it disappears from blood
  ▪ Lactate dehydrogenase (LDH)–2 isoforms–LDH 1 and LDH 2
    ♦ **Ratio of LDH 1:** LDH 2 more than 1 is suggestive of MI
    ♦ LDH levels rise after 24 hours, reach to peak in 3-6 days, returns to normal in around 14 days
  ▪ Cardiac-specific troponins (cTn)–2 types are cardiac troponin T (cTnT), cardiac troponin I (cTnI)
    ♦ cTnT and cTnI levels increase after myocardial injury
    ♦ cTnT remains elevated for 7-10 days and cTnI for 10-14 days
  ▪ Myoglobin–first cardiac marker to increase after MI, gets excreted rapidly in urine
    ♦ Returns to normal after 24 hours on MI

Complications

○ Arrhythmias
○ Cardiogenic shock
○ Rupture
○ Cardiac aneurysm
○ Congestive heart failure
○ Pericarditis
○ Postmyocardial infarction syndrome
○ Mural thrombosis and thromboembolism

PART III

5. Write short notes on:

a. H. Pylori and gastric diseases

(Ref: Textbook of Pathology, Harsh Mohan, 7th ed. pg. 531)

ANSWER

H. Pylori and Gastric Diseases

Introduction

- H. pylori is a spiral-shaped, gram-negative organism that has modified to flourish in acid
- It is common gastric pathogen which causes
  - Gastritis–Chronic Gastritis associated with H. Pylori occurs in 90% cases
    - Pylori display tropism for gastric epithelium
    - Not associated with intestinal metaplasia or duodenal epithelium
    - H. pylori are found within the stomach in the antrum (antral predominant gastritis or type B gastritis)
    - Intraepithelial neutrophils and subepithelial plasma are characteristic of H. pylori gastritis
  - Peptic ulcer disease – hyperplastic gastric polyps also called inflammatory polyps
  - Gastric adenocarcinoma
  - Low-grade gastric lymphoma

Virulence Factors of H. pylori

- Gram negative flagellated bacteria
- Flagella–permits motility of the bacteria in viscous mucus
- Urease–produces ammonia from endogenous urea-elevates local gastric pH and improves bacterial survival
- Adhesions–like BabA which enhances binding in people with blood group O
- Toxins–cytotoxin-associated gene A (CagA) and VacA

Diagnosis

- Gold standard–antral biopsy shows the bacilli, highlighted by Warthin-Starry silver stain
- Most specific investigation–culture of bacteria (done on Skirrow's medium)

b. Nodular sclerosis type Hodgkin Lymphoma

(Ref: Textbook of Pathology, Harsh Mohan, 7th ed. pg. 879)

ANSWER

Nodular Sclerosis Type Hodgkin Lymphoma

For answer, refer 2017 paper-II Q. 2 (b), Pg. 18

c. Astrocytoma

(Ref: Textbook of Pathology, Harsh Mohan, 7th ed. pg. 879)

ANSWER

Astrocytoma

For answer, refer 2016 paper-II, Q. 5 (c), Pg. 46

d. Teratoma

(Ref: Textbook of Pathology, Harsh Mohan, 7th ed. pg. 735-737)

ANSWER

Teratoma

For answer, refer to 2016 paper-II Q. 6 (a), Pg. 47

6. Write short notes on:

a. Choriocarcinoma

(Ref: Harsh Mohan, 7th ed. pg. 742, Robbins, SA ed. pg. 1041)

ANSWER

Choriocarcinoma

Introduction

- 2 types of choriocarcinoma are Gestational choriocarcinoma and non-gestational chorio-carcinoma
- Gestational choriocarcinoma is of placental origin and non-gestational choriocarcinoma is of ovarian origin
- Gestational choriocarcinoma is extremely malignant and extensively metastasising trophoblastic tumour, however, Non-gestational choriocarcinoma i.e. Ovarian choriocarcinoma is more malignant than placental choriocarcinoma
- **Incidence:** 50% cases occur after hydatidiform mole, 25% occur after spontaneous abortion, 20% occur after normal pregnancy and 5% occur after ectopic pregnancy

Clinical Picture

- Vaginal bleeding
- Patients present with metastases in brain or lungs

Diagnosis

○ Persistently high levels of Beta-hCG in plasma and urine

Morphology

○ Gross appearance:
  ▪ Haemorrhagic, soft and fleshy mass like appearance
  ▪ Can appear like a small, blood clot in the uterus
○ Microscopic appearance:
  ▪ Identifiable villi are absent
  ▪ Intermixed masses and columns of highly anaplastic and bizarre cytotrophoblast and syncytiotrophoblast cells
  ▪ Presence of hemorrhages and necrosis
  ▪ Infiltration of underlying myometrium and other structures, blood vessels and lymphatics

Treatment

○ Gestational choriocarcinoma gives good response with chemotherapy whereas non-gestational is resistant to chemotherapy with poor prognosis
○ Cure rate is 20-70 % 5-year survival rate with hysterectomy and chemotherapy
○ Total cure in localised tumours
○ Death is due to fatal hemorrhages in CNS or lungs or pulmonary insufficiency

b. Neuroblastoma

(Ref: Textbook of Pathology, Harsh Mohan, 7th ed. pg. 791)

ANSWER

Neuroblastoma

Introduction

○ Also known as sympathicoblastoma
○ Aggressive childhood malignancy
○ Origin- neural crest cells
○ Common in children less than 5 years of age
○ Sites-Adrenal medulla and paravertebral autonomic ganglia are commonly involved

Clinical Features

○ Common in children less than 5 years of age
○ Sites-Adrenal medulla, sympathetic chain, neck, thorax, retroperitoneum, etc are commonly involved
○ Fever
○ Weight loss
○ Abdominal distension and pain
○ Palpable abdominal mass
○ Bone pain or joint pain
○ Urinary retention
○ Neutologic deficits
○ Watery diarrhea, hypokalemia, flushing of skin-tumor produces kinins or prostaglandins
○ Metastatic spread to liver, lungs bones, etc.
○ Radiological finding: abdomen revels foci of calcification
○ Presence of vanillyl mandelic acid (VMA)and homovanillic acid(HVA)in 24 hour urine- diagnostic feature

Microscopic Findings

○ Tumor cells are round to oval in shape with hyperchromatic nuclei and arranged in the form of irregular sheets interspersed with fibrovascular stoma
○ Exhibits Homer-Wright's rosettes composed of cells that are radially arranged surrounding central core of fibrillar eosinophilic material

Diagnosis

○ Routine investigations
○ Bone marrow aspiration and biopsies
○ Vanillyl mandelic acid (VMA) and homovanillic acid(HVA) in 24 hour urine

Prognosis

○ Certain favorable prognostic features are:
  ▪ **Location of the tumor:** Extra-abdominal presents with favorable prognosis
  ▪ **Age of the child:** Less than 2 yrs is favorable
  ▪ Clinical stage I and stage II of tumor
  ▪ Histology of tumor-ganglionic or schwannian differentiation
  ▪ Genetic features, like – lack of amplification of N-MYC oncogene, absence of telomerase expression, etc.

c. Renal stones

(Ref: Textbook of Pathology, Harsh Mohan, 7th ed. pg. 672)

ANSWER

Renal Stones

Type of stone	Aetiology	Pathogenesis
• Calcium stones (75%)	• Hypercalciuria with or without hypercalcaemia; idiopathic	• Degree of supersaturation of ions in urine; alkaline pH of urine; increased excretion of oxalate and uric acid; reduced urinary volume
• Mixed struvite stones (15%)	• Urinary infection with urea-splitting organisms like Proteus	• Alkaline urinary pH produced by ammonia from splitting of urea by bacterially produced urease
• Uric acid stones (6%)	• Hyperuricosuria with or without hyperuricaemia as in primary and secondary gout	• Acidic urine (pH below 6) reduces the solubility of uric acid in urine and favours its precipitation
• Cystine stones (2%)	• Genetically-determined defect in cystine transport	• Cystinuria containing least soluble cystine precipitates as cystine crystals
• Other types (less than 2%)	• Inherited abnormalities of amino acid metabolism	• Xanthinuria

Name of the Paper	:	**Pathology Paper-I**
Name of the Course	:	**MBBS-2013**
Semester	:	**Annual**

Time: 3 Hours   **M.M.: 40**

INSTRUCTIONS

1. Write your Roll No. on the top immediately on receipt of this question paper
2. All questions are to be attempted
3. Answers to Parts I, II and III should be written in separate answer sheets provided
4. Attempt parts of a question in sequence

PART-I

1. **Differentiate between:**   [8]
   a. Myeloblast and Lymphoblast
   b. Necrosis and apoptosis
   c. Bleeding due to platelet defect and coagulation factor deficiency
   d. Lepromatous and Tuberculoid leprosy

2. **Write briefly on:**   [6]
   a. G6PD deficiency
   b. Type III hypersensitivity reaction
   c. Turner syndrome

PART-II

3. **Write briefly on:**   [6]
   a. Causes of microcytic hypochromic anemia and laboratory features of beta thalassemia major
   b. Viral carcinogenesis

4. **Write briefly on:**   [6]
   a. Laboratory diagnosis and prognostic factors in CML
   b. Pathogenesis of septic shock

PART-III

5. **Comment on:**   [8]
   a. Paraneoplastic syndrome
   b. Sickle cell anemia
   c. Fate of Thrombus
   d. Mechanism of immunodeficiency in HIV infection

6. **Write short notes on:**   [6]
   a. Acute hemolytic transfusion reaction
   b. Pathogenesis of DIC
   c. Graft vs Host disease

PART I

1. Differentiate between:

a. Myeloblast and Lymphoblast

(Ref: Textbook of Pathology, Harsh Mohan, 7th ed. pg. 326)

ANSWER

Myeloblast and Lymphoblast

Myeloblast	Lymphoblast
• Uniform and large in size	• Variable and small in size
• Granular cytoplasm	• Agranular cytoplasm
• Fine meshwork of nuclear chromatin	• Condensed and slightly clumped nuclear chromatin
• Fine nuclear membrane with indistinct nucleoli	• Dense nuclear membrane and prominent nucleoli
• Auer rods present (60-70% cases)	• Auer rods absent
• PAS negative	• PAS positive (75%)
• Myeloperoxidase positive	• Myeloperoxidase negative

b. Apoptosis and Necrosis

(Ref: Harsh Mohan, 7th ed. pg. 31, Robbins, SA ed. pg. 41, 52)

ANSWER

Apoptosis and Necrosis

Apoptosis	Necrosis
• Programmed and coordinated cell death	• Cell death with degradation of tissue by hydrolytic enzymes
• Due to pathologic and physiologic processes	• Due to toxins, hypoxia
• Morphologic changes: shrinkage of cell, cytoplasmic blebs, chromatin condensation, apoptotic bodies and phagocytosis by macrophages, no inflammatory reaction	• Morphologic changes: death of adjacent cells, inflammatory reaction present, disruption of membrane along with nuclear disruption, phagocytosis of cell debris
• Intact lysosome	• Rupture lysosome
• Mechanism is genetically coordinated	• Due to ATP depletion, membrane damage, free radicals, etc.
• Electrophoresis shows step ladder pattern of DNA	• Diffuse DNA pattern on elctrophoresis

c. Bleeding due to platelet defect and coagulation factor deficiency

ANSWER

For answer, refer 2016 paper-I Q. 1 (d), Pg. 27

d. Tuberculoid and Lepromatous Leprosy

ANSWER

For answer, refer 2015 paper-I Q. 1 (c), Pg. 51

2. Write briefly on:

a. G6PD Deficiency

(Ref: Harsh Mohan, 7th ed. pg. 293, Robbins, SA ed. pg. 634)

ANSWER

Introduction
- A genetic disorder .that occurs almost exclusively in males.

Pathogenesis
- A defect in glucose-6-phosphate dehydrogenase enzyme results in premature breakdown of red blood cells, thus, leading to hemolysis of red blood cells.

Genetics
- Mutation of G6PD gene

Epidemiology
- Inheritance of x -linked mutant gene, affecting males
- Females: Carrier

Clinical Features
- Hemolytic anemia- most common
- Paleness, fatigue, shortness of breath
- Dark urine, jaundice or yellowing of the skin and eyes, mainly in newborns
- Bacterial, viral infections or certain drugs may trigger hemolysis

$$\text{Glucose} \longrightarrow \text{Glucose-6-phosphate} \xrightarrow{\text{G6PD}} \text{6-Phosphogluconate}$$

$$\text{NADP+} \longrightarrow \text{NADPH}$$

No NADPH = No Glutathione
Oxidative stress = Hemolytic anemia

PATHOLOGY

Laboratory Findings

○ In normal phase:
  ▪ No anemia
  ▪ Reduced red cell survival

○ **In hemolytic phase:**
  ▪ Intravascular hemolysis
  ▪ Decreased hematocrit (25-30%)
  ▪ Peripheral blood smear: Presence of -
    ♦ Heinz bodies: dark inclusion within cells
    ♦ Bite cells
    ♦ Blister cells

Diagnosis

Screening tests-

○ **Indirect tests:**
  ▪ Methemoglobin reduction test
  ▪ Fluorescent screening test
  ▪ Ascorbate cyanide screening test

○ **Direct enzyme assay of red cell:**
  ▪ In case of low enzyme level

b. Type III Hypersensitivity reaction

(Ref: Harsh Mohan, 7th ed. pg. 60, Robbins, SA ed. pg. 200)

Answer

Introduction

○ Immune- complex mediated hypersensitivity reaction
○ Due to deposition of antigen-antibody complexes on tissues
○ Mediated by IgG, IgM antibodies
○ Onset of reaction approx. after 6 hours of the exposure

Etiology

○ Persistent low-grade infection
○ Environmental antigens (mainly exogenous)
○ Autoimmune process

Pathogenesis/Mechanism

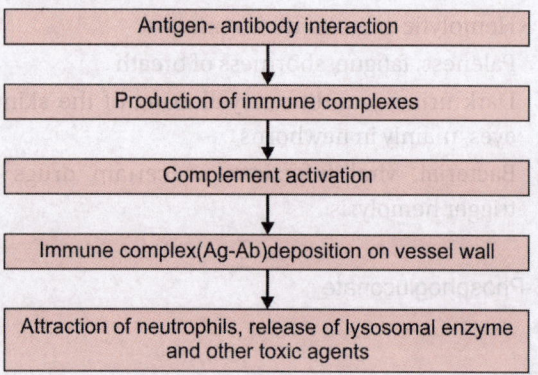

Examples

○ Systemic lupus eryhematosus
○ Subacute infective endocarditis
○ Hodgkin's disease
○ Arthus reaction (localized)
○ Rheumatoid arthritis
○ Glomerulonephritis (post-streptococcal)

c. Turner Syndrome

(Ref: Textbook of Pathology, Harsh Mohan, 7th ed. pg. 258)

Answer

For answer, refer 2016 paper-I Q. 5 (b), Pg. 33

PART II

3. **Write briefly on:**

  a. Causes of microcytic hypochromic anemia and laboratory features of beta thalassemia major

(Ref: Harsh Mohan, 7th ed. pg. 274, 300, Robbins, SA ed. pg. 638)

Answer

Causes of Microcytic Hypochromic Anemia

○ May be due to iron deficiency or other than ion deficieny, like- due to abnormal globin synthesis or due to abnormal heme or porphyrin synthesis
○ Decreased MCV,MCHC and MCH in microcytic hypochromic anem

Disorders of iron metabolism	Disorder of porphyrin and heme synthesis	Abnormal globin synthesis
• Iron deficiency anemia	• Sideroblastic anemia	• Thalassemia
• Atransferrinemia	• Lead poisoning	• HbC disease
• Anemia of chronic disease	• Vitamin B6 deficiency	• HbE trait and disease
	• Defective ALA synthetase activity	• Aluminium intoxication

Laboratory Features of Beta Thalassemia Major

○ **CBC:**
  ▪ Severe anemia (Hb:3-6 gm/dl)
  ▪ MCH, MCV, MCHC: decreased
  ▪ Hematocrit: decreased (severely)
  ▪ **WBC:** Raised (usually), shift of left of neutrophil series with presence of some myelocytes and metamyelocytes

- **Peripheral blood smear:**
  - Severe microcytic hypochromic red cell
  - Marked anisopoikilocytosis
  - Target cells
  - Tear drop cells
  - Basophilic stippling
  - Cells with Cabot's ring
  - Pencil cells
  - Nucleated RBC's
- **Hemoglobin electrophoresis:**
  - Increased HbF
  - Increased HbA_2
  - HbA – absent or sometimes present in variable amounts
- **Bone marrow findings:**
  - Normoblastic erythroid hyperplasia
  - Intermediate and late normoblast predominant (smaller in size)
  - Siderotic granules in the cytoplasm of normoblasts
  - Increased reticuloendothelial iron
- **Biochemical findings:**
  - Serum bilirubin(unconjugated): Increased
  - Serum iron: Increased
  - Urine urobilinogen: Increased
  - Serum ferritin: Increased (300–3000 mg/dl)
- **Osmotic fragility:** Decreased

b. Viral Carcinogenesis

(Ref: Textbook of Pathology, Harsh Mohan, 7th ed. pg. 216)

ANSWER

Introduction

- Viruses (DNA or RNA) results mutation in the target host cell

- High mutation rate associated with RNA virus

DNA Oncogenic Virus

- Human Papilloma virus
- Epstein-Barr virus
- Poxvirus
- Adenovirus, etc.

RNA Oncogenic Virus

- Human T cell lymphotropic virus
- Hepatitis C virus
- HCV
- Slow transforming virus

Oncogenesis by DNA Virus

- **Replication:**
  - Replication of DNA virus and formation of virions
- **Integration:**
  - Integration of viral DNA into the DNA of the host cell and expression of virus specific T antigen
  - Mutation and neoplastic transformation of the host cell

Oncogenesis by RNA Virus

- RNA virus consist of two identical strands of RNA and reverse transcriptase enzyme
- Reverse transcriptase acts as template in the synthesis of single strand of matching viral DNA followed by formation of double stranded viral DNA (provirus)
- Integration of provirus into the DNA of the host cell result in transformation of host cell into neoplastic cell
- Replication of the viral components followed by their assembly at the plasma membrane and released by budding

Virua	Mechanism	Associated Cancer
DNA Viruses		
EBV (Epstein-Bar virus)	Promotes polyclonal B-cell proliferation, which increases risk for (8:14) translocation	Burkitt's lymphoma, CNS lymphoma in AIDS, mixed cellularity Hodgkin's lymphoma, nasopharyngeal carcinoma
HHV-8 (human herpesvirus)	Acts via cytokines released from HIV and HSV	Kaposl's sarcoma in AIDS
HPV types 16 and 18, 31, 33 (human papillomavirus)	Type 16 (-50% of cancers); E6 gene product inhibits; TP53 suppressor gne Type 18 (-10% of cancers); E7 gene product inhibits; RB suppressor gene	Squamous cell carcinoma of vulva, vagina, cervix, anus (associated with and intercourse); larynx, oropharynx
RNA Viruses		
HCV	Produces postnecrotic cirrhosis	Hepatocellular carcinoma
HTLV-1 (human T-cell lymphotropic virus)	Activates TAX gene, stimulates polyclonal T-cell proliferation, inhibits TP53 suppressor gene	T-cell leukemia and lymphoma

PATHOLOGY

4. Write briefly on:

a. Laboratory Diagnosis and prognostic factors in CML

(Ref: Textbook of Pathology, Harsh Mohan, 7th ed. pg. 337, Robbins, SA ed. pg. 616)

ANSWER

Laboratory Diagnosis of CML

Laboratory Findings

- **Blood picture**
  - Normocytic normochromic anemia(moderate)
  - Marked leukocytosis (approx. 200, 000/μL or more)
  - Basophilia
  - Blast phase/blast crisis- ≥20%
- **Bone marrow examination:**
  - Hypercellular
  - Myeloid: erythroid ratio increased (myeloid cells predominate)
  - Increased, small dysplastic form of megakaryocytes
  - Sea blue histiocytes/pseudo-Gaucher cells
  - Reduced erythropoietic cells
  - Blasts less than 5%
- **Cytogenetics:**
  - Philadelphia chromosome present
- **Cytochemistry:**
  - LAP/NAP score reduced (helps to differentiate it from myeloid leukemoid reaction, in which LAP is elevated)
- **Other investigations:**
  - Hyperuricaemia
  - Raised serum B_{12} and vitamin B_{12} binding capacity

Prognostic Factors in CML

- **According to Sokal index:** based on chemotherapy treated patients
  - Circulating blast percentage
  - Platelet count
  - Size of spleen
  - Cytogenetic clonal evolution
- **According to Hassford system:** based on interferon alpha treated patients
  - Circulating blast percentage
  - Platelet count
  - Size of spleen
  - Eosinophils and basophil percentage

Adverse Prognostic Factors

- Spleen: Enlarged spleen
- Accelerated phase or blast phase
- Very high or very low platelet counts
- Increased number of basophils and eosinophils
- Age: 60 years or more
- Multiple chromosome changes
- Areas of bone damage

b Pathogenesis of septic shock

(Ref: Textbook of Pathology, Harsh Mohan, 7th ed. pg. 96)

ANSWER

For answer, refer 2016 paper-I Q. 3, Pg. 29 (a), 2015 paper-I Q. 4 (b), 56.

PART III

5. Comment on:

a. Paraneoplastic syndrome

(Ref: Harsh Mohan, 7th ed. pg. 225, Robbins, SA ed. pg. 330)

ANSWER

Introduction

- Group of disorders that develops in cancer bearing patients and that cannot be explained by direct or distant spread of tumor and nor by hormonal elaboration of the tumor(tissue of origin)
- Triggered by an altered immune system response
- Prevalent in middle-aged to older people
- Commonly seen in lung, ovarian, lymphatic, or breast cancer.

Clinical Features

- Difficulty in walking or swallowing
- Decrease muscle tone and fine motor coordination,
- Memory loss, sleep disturbances, dementia and seizures
- Loss of limb sensation and vertigo/dizziness.
- Commonly seen in patients with undiagnosed cancer, patients with active cancer, or those in remission.

Syndromes included in the PNS are as follows:

Syndrome	Form of cancer	Mechanism
Endocrine syndrome		
• Hypercalcaemia	Sq.cell car. of lung, kidney,breast, Adult T cell leukemia-lymphoma	Paratharmone like protein, vitamin D
• Cushing's syndrome	Small cell ca of lung, pancreas	ACTH or ACTH like substance
• Carcinoid syndrome	Bronchial carcinoid tumor, ca pancreas, stomach	Serotonin, bradykinin
• Polycythaemia	Kidney, liver	Erythropoietin
Neuromuscular syndrome		
• Myasthenia gravis	Thymoma	Immunologic
Hematologic syndromes		
• Thrombophlebitis	Pancreas, lungs. GIT	Hypercoagulability
• DIC	Adenocarcinoma, AML	Chronic thrombotic phenomenon
• Anemia	Thymoma	
Gastrointestinal syndromes		
• Malabsorption	Small bowel lymphoma	Hypoalbuminaemia
Renal syndrome		
• Nephrotic syndrome	Advanced cancer	Renal vein thrombosis
Cutaneous syndromes		
• Acanthosis nigricans	Gastric ca	Immunologic
• Exfoliative dermatitis	Lymphoma	
Osseous, joint and soft tissue		
• Hypertrophic osteoarthropath, clubbing of fingers	Bronchogenic carcinoma	

b. Sickle cell anemia

(Ref: Harsh Mohan, 7th ed. pg. 294, Robbins, SA ed. pg. 635)

ANSWER

Sickle Cell Anemia

○ Formation of HbS in the red cell with inheritance of abnormal gene from each parent.

Defect

○ **Genetic defect:** Single point mutation in 6th codon of β- globin

○ **Point mutation:** Replacement of glutamate residue with a valine residue

○ Polymerization of deoxygenated hemoglobin (HbS) results in sickle-shaped RBCs (sickling of RBC's)

Clinical Features

○ Vaso-occlusive crises/Acute painful crises: severe skeletal pain, hand-foot syndrome, chest syndrome

○ Hemolytic crises

○ Sequestration crises: sudden massive pooling of red cell in spleen with fall in Hb concentration

○ Aplastic crises

○ Stroke and retinopathy

○ Acute chest syndrome

○ Cardiomegaly

○ Aseptic necrosis, osteomyelitis-bones

○ Autosplenectomy

○ Renal cortical necrosis and hyposthenuria (inability to concentrate urine)

○ Chronic hemolysis: growth and development impaired

○ Pulmonary infections in lungs

○ Retinal hemorrhage, proliferative retinopathy

○ Septicemia and meningitis by pneumococci and H. influenzae

○ Erectile dysfunction

Lab Diagnosis

○ **CBC:**
  ▪ **Hemoglobin:** Moderate to severe anemia (6-9 g/dl)
  ▪ **Reticulocyte:** Increased

○ **Peripheral blood smear:**
  ▪ Sickle- shaped RBC's (elongated crescent-shaped)
  ▪ Target cells
  ▪ Howell- jolly bodies(feature of splenic atrophy)
  ▪ **Sickling test:** Use of sodium metabisulfite (reducing agent) induces sickling of RBC's (positive sickling test)

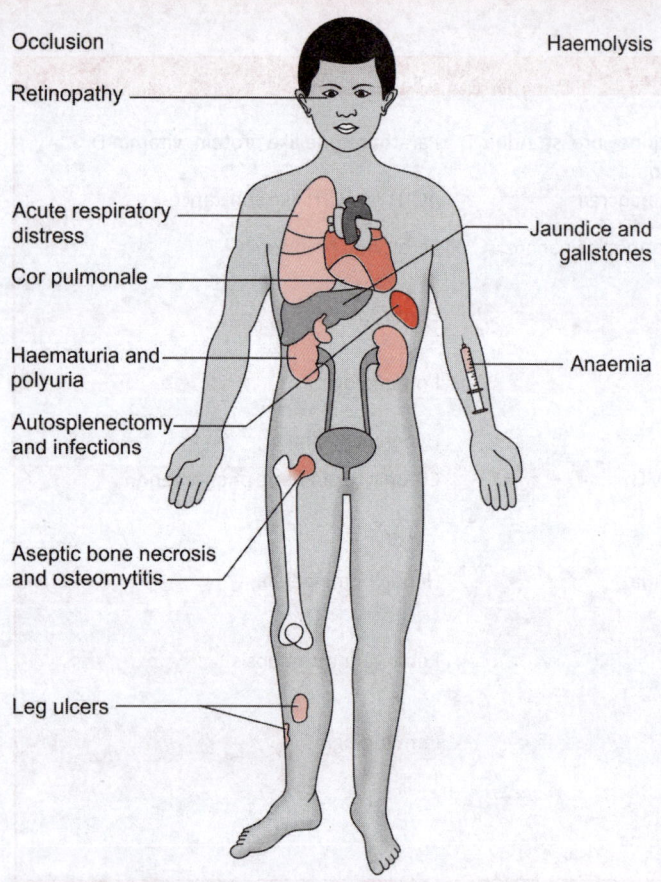

Occlusion

Retinopathy

Haemolysis

Acute respiratory distress

Cor pulmonale

Jaundice and gallstones

Haematuria and polyuria

Anaemia

Autosplenectomy and infections

Aseptic bone necrosis and osteomytitis

Leg ulcers

- **Hemoglobin electrophoresis:**
  - Decreased or absent HbA
  - Predominant HbS and 2–20% Hb
- **Solubility test:**
  - With reducing substance, eg. sodium dithionite, HbS polymerizes and produces turbid solution
- **Osmotic fragility test:**
  - Decreased fragility due to sickle shape
- **Prenatal Diagnosis:**
  - Analysis of fetal DNA
- **Biopsy :**
  - Spleen: Presence of Gamma gandy bodies
- **X-ray:**
  - Skull: "crew cut" appearance
  - Vertebrae: Fish mouth vertebra
- **High Performance Liquid Chromatography** (Hb-HPLC)

Radiological Findings: X-ray revels " cut –crew" appearance of skull and "fish mouth" vertebra

c. Fate of Thrombus

(Ref: Textbook of Pathology, Harsh Mohan, 7th ed. pg. 104)

ANSWER

Fate of Thrombus

Resolution

- Lysis and removal of thrombus by the fibrinolytic activity
- Effective in recently formed thrombus
- Older thrombus resistant to lysis due to extensive fibrin polymerization

Organization and Recanalization

- If thrombus is not removed, ingrowth of endothelial cells, smooth muscle cells, fibroblasts and formation of fibrin rich thrombus organization.
- New vascular channels may be formed re-establishing the blood flow

Propagation

- Obstruction of vessel due to accumulation of blood constituents resulting in large size of thrombus

Thromboembolism

- Thrombi may get dislodged and produce ill- effects at the site of thrombi

d. Mechanism of immunodeficiency in HIV infection

(Ref: Textbook of Pathology, Harsh Mohan, 7th ed. pg. 52)

ANSWER

Introduction

- Immunosuppression due to depletion of CD4+ T cells is responsible for HIV infection

Pathogenesis

- Events in the pathogenesis of infection are given below:
- Glycoprotein 120 (gp120) helps in the binding of virus to the CD4 receptor
- **Internalisation:**
  - HIV combines with CD4 receptor and CCR (chemokine coreceptor) and internalisation of gp41 glycoprotein of envelope in the CD4+ T cell membrane
- **Uncoating of the viral envelope and viral DNA formation:**
  - Reverse trancriptase forms single stranded DNA
  - Original RNA strand is degraded by ribonuclease H, and second strand of DNA is synthesized thus making double stranded DNA

- **Viral integration:**
  - The integrated HIV DNA is called " provirus"
- Viral DNA enters the host cell nucleus with the help of viral integrase enzyme
- Transcription of viral DNA into RNA along with production of multiple copies of RNA
- Destruction of CD4+ T cell followed by spread of infection to more CD4+ host cells

- Budding from the cell wall of the host cell and damage of the part of the cell membrane leading to death of the cell membrane of the host cell
- Other cells of the immune system like – circulating monocytes, macrophages, non- infected lymphoid cells, etc. are also get infected
- Thus, all the immunologic changes in the host results in immunosuppression rendering host to opportunistic infections.

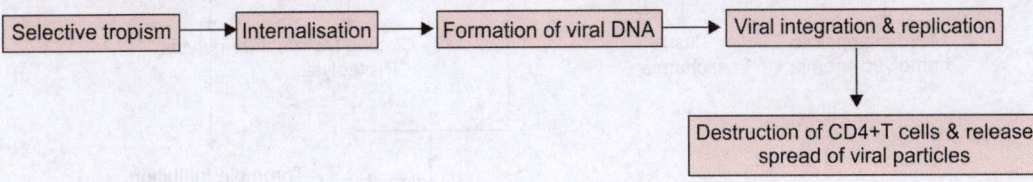

6. Write short notes on:

a. Acute Hemolytic Transfusion Reaction

(Ref: Harsh Mohan, 7th ed. pg. 318, Robbins, SA ed. pg. 665)

ANSWER

Introduction

- Transfusion of incompatible blood due to ABO incompatibility results in acute hemolytic reaction
- Occur within minutes and result in intravascular hemolysis

Mechanism

- Usually, ABO isoagglutinins are responsible for the reaction
- Antibodies present in the recipient plasma causes destruction of the transfused red cells

Clinical Features

- Fever, chills
- Hypotension
- Tachycardia, tachypnea
- Hemoglobinuria
- Flank pain

Laboratory Findings

- Serum indirect bilirubin: increased
- **Serum LDH:** Increased
- **Serum haptoglobin:** Reduced
- **Direct antiglobulin test:** For detection of antibody
- Re-cross matching of blood of both recipient and donar

b. Pathogenesis of DIC

(Ref: Harsh Mohan, 7th ed. pg. 315, Robbins, SA ed. pg. 663)

ANSWER

- Also known as "defibrination syndrome" or "consumption coagulopathy"

Pathogenesis

- **Activation of coagulation pathway:**
  - Release of tissue factor leading to activation of coagulation pathway
- **Thrombotic phase:**
  - Thrombi and emboli deposition throughout the microvasculature
- **Consumption phase:**
  - **Consumption of clotting factors and platelets**
- **Secondary fibrinolysis:**
  - Formation of fibrin degradation products(FDP'S)

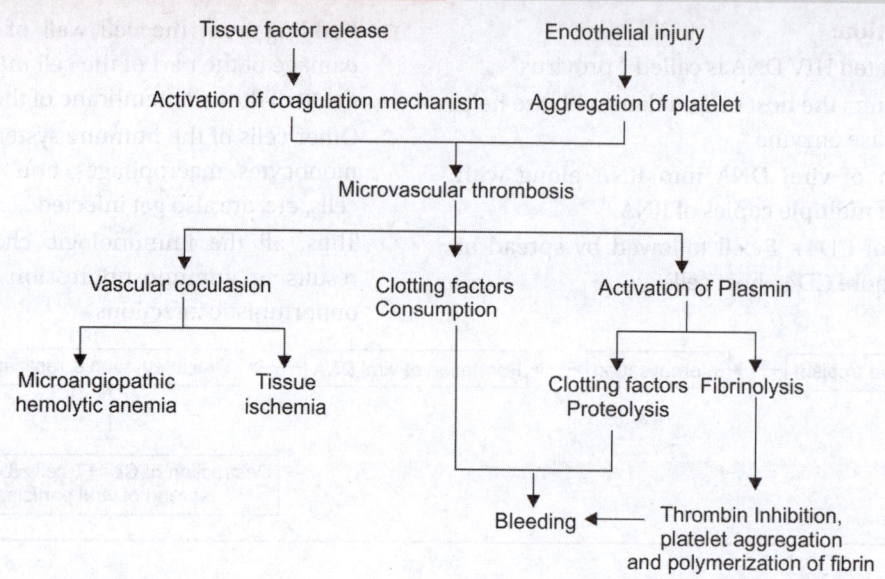

Tissue factor release   Endothelial injury

Activation of coagulation mechanism   Aggregation of platelet

Microvascular thrombosis

Vascular coculasion   Clotting factors Consumption   Activation of Plasmin

Microangiopathic hemolytic anemia   Tissue ischemia   Clotting factors Proteolysis Fibrinolysis

Bleeding ← Thrombin Inhibition, platelet aggregation and polymerization of fibrin

c. Graft versus Host Disease

(Ref: Harsh Mohan, 7th ed. pg. 50, Robbins, SA ed. pg. 802)

ANSWER

Introduction

○ A immune mediated disease

○ occurs when immunologically competent T cells or their precursors are transplanted into immunologically compromised recipient

Incidence 1–2 %

Pathophysiology

○ Immunologically competent T cells transplanted into immune- compromised host

○ Due to decreased immunity, host (recipient)cannot reject the graft

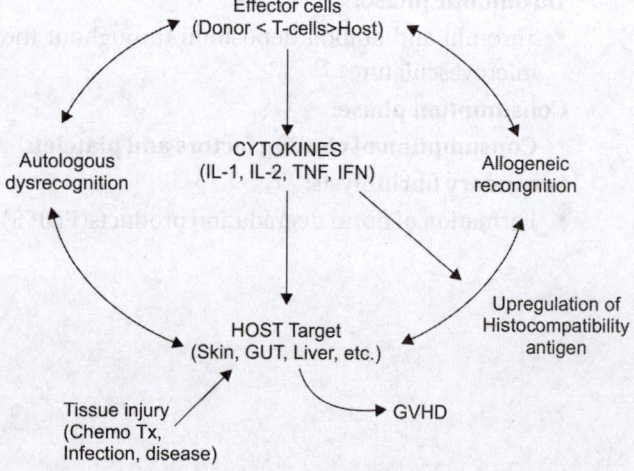

○ T cells consider host tissue as "foreign" and react against it

○ Results in activation of CD4 and CD8 T cells leading to inflammation and killing of host(recipient) cells.

Types

○ **Acute:**
  ▪ Appears within days to weeks of transplantation
  ▪ Dermatitis, hepatitis, enteritis- triad
  ▪ Infection by new organism or activation of silent infection(CMV causing pneumonia)
  ▪ Bloody diarrhea
  ▪ **Skin:** Pruritic and painful rash

○ **Chronic:**
  ▪ Jaundice
  ▪ Anorexia, dysphagia, esophageal stricture, abdominal cramps
  ▪ Restricted mobility of joints
  ▪ Wheeze, chronic cough, dyspnea
  ▪ Burning sensation of eyes, photophobia, keratoconjuctivitis sicca, corneal erosions,etc.
  ▪ Lichenoid lesions, contractures of skin
  ▪ Weakness, neuropathic pain

Investigations

○ Complete blood count

○ Liver function teasts

○ Barium swallow

○ Serum electrolyte

○ PFT, ABG

○ Biomarkers: IL8, TNF receptor 1, Hepatocyte growth factor, etc.

Your Roll No. ....

Name of the Paper	:	**Pathology Paper-II**
Name of the Course	:	**MBBS-2013**
Semester	:	**Annual**

Time: 3 Hours   **M.M.: 40**

INSTRUCTIONS

1. Write your Roll No. on the top immediately on receipt of this question paper
2. All questions are to be attempted
3. Answers to Parts I, II and III should be written in separate answer sheets provided
4. Attempt parts of a question in sequence

PART-I

1. **Differentiate between:** [8]
   a. Acute and subacute infective endocarditis
   b. Tuberculous and typhoid ulcer
   c. Nephritic and nephrotic syndrome
   d. Hepatitis A and Hepatitis B

2. **Write short notes on:** [6]
   a. Hashimoto's thyroiditis
   b. Giant cell tumor of bone
   c. Fibroadenoma

PART-II

3. **Write briefly on:** [6]
   a. Morphological features of rheumatic heart disease
   b. Wilms tumor

4. **Write briefly on:** [6]
   a. Obstructive uropathy
   b. Pathogenesis and complications of post infectious cirrhosis

PART-III

5. **Write briefly on:** [8]
   a. Glioblastoma multiforme
   b. Osteoporosis
   c. Bronchial asthma
   d. Seminoma

6. **Write briefly on:** [6]
   a. Coal workers' pneumoconiosis
   b. Risk factors in carcinoma cervix
   c. Pathology and complication of Amoebic colitis

PART I

1. **Differentiate between:**

   a. Acute and subacute infective endocarditis   *(Ref: Harsh Mohan, 7th ed. pg. 425, Robbins, SA ed. pg. 125)*

ANSWER

Acute and Subacute Infective Endocarditis

Acute infective endocarditis	Subacute infective endocarditis
• Caused by highly virulent bacteria such as Staphylococcus aureus, Beta-streptococci	• Caused by less virulent bacteria such as Streptococcus viridans
• Occurs in previously normal and healthy heart	• Occurs in previously diseased heart
• Duration of illness 2-6 weeks	• Duration of illness 6 weeks to few months
• Lesions produced are invasive, destructive and suppurative	• Lesions produced are not invasive or suppurative
• Clinical picture – symptoms of acute systemic infection	• Clinical picture – splenomegaly, clubbed fingers, petechiae

   b. Tuberculous and typhoid ulcer   *(Ref: Textbook of Pathology, Harsh Mohan, 7th ed. pg. 553)*

ANSWER

Tuberculous and Typhoid Ulcer

For answer, refer 2017, paper-II, Q. 1(d), Pg. 16

   c. Nephritic and Nephrotic syndrome   *(Ref: Harsh Mohan, 7th ed. pg. 649, Robbins, SA ed. pg. 913-914)*

ANSWER

Nephrotic and Nephritic Syndrome

Nephrotic syndrome	Nephritic syndrome
• Presents with mild edema	• Exhibits generalised peripheral edema
• Marked proteinuria present	• Mild proteinuria
• Presence of Hyperlipidemia evident	• Hyperlipidemia not present
• Hematuria/RBC cast not evident or mild in certain cases	• Heamaturia/RBC cast is evident
• Oligouria and uremia not present	• Presence of oligouria and uremia

   d. Hepatitis A and Hepatitis B   *(Ref: Harsh Mohan, 7th ed. pg. 591, Robbins, SA ed. pg. 831)*

ANSWER

Hepatitis A and Hepatitis B

Hepatitis A	Hepatitis B
• Causative agent is HAV	• Causative agent is HBV
• Spread is through faeco-oral route	• Spread is through contact or parenteral
• 15-45 days of incubation period	• Incubation period is from 30-180 days
• Non-enveloped RNA virus	• Enveloped DNA virus
• 27 nm in diameter	• 42 nm in diameter
• No role in development of hepatocellular carcinoma	• Responsible in the development of hepatocellular carcinoma
• Prognosis good	• Prognosis worsen as the age advances

2. Write short notes on:

a. Hashimoto's thyroiditis

(Ref: Textbook of Pathology, Harsh Mohan, 7th ed. pg. 795)

ANSWER

Hashimoto's Thyroiditis

Also refer 2017 paper-II Q. 2 (a), Pg. 16

Hashimoto's thyroiditis and Grave's disease

Hashimoto's thyroiditis	Grave's disease
• Most common cause of hypothyroidism	• Most common cause of hyperthyroidism
• Occurs at the age of 30-50 years and 10 times more common in females	• Occurs at the age of 30-40 years and 5 times more common in females

• Clinical triad consists of:
  ▪ Diffuse goitrous enlargement of thyroid
  ▪ Lymphocytic infiltration of thyroid gland
  ▪ Occurrence of thyroid autoantibodies
	• Clinical triad consists of:
	  ▪ Hyperthyroidism (thyrotoxicosis)
	  ▪ Diffuse thyroid enlargement
	  ▪ Ophthalmopathy

• Etiopathogenesis:
  ▪ HLA associated/genetic predisposition- familial occurrence in association with HLA-DR5, concordance in monozygotic twins is 40%
  ▪ Autoimmune association-associated with Graves' disease, SLE, rheumatoid arthritis
  ▪ Iodine intake – associated with high intake of iodine
	• Etiopathogenesis:
	  ▪ HLA associated/genetic predisposition – Familial occurrence in association with HLA-DR3, HLA-B8
	  ▪ Autoimmune disease association

• Morphology: gross appearance:
  ▪ Diffuse, symmetric, firm and rubbery enlargement of thyroid
  ▪ Cut section is fleshy with accentuation of normal lobulations, but shape of gland is intact
	• Morphology: gross appearance:
	  ▪ Diffuse, symmetric, smooth, soft enlarged gland with intact capsule
	  ▪ Cut section is soft, meaty resembling normal muscle

• Microscopic appearance:
  ▪ Extensive infiltration by lymphocytes, plasma cells, macrophages abd formation of lymphoid follicles with germinal center
  ▪ Reduced number and atrophied thyroid follicles, devoid of colloid
  ▪ Presence of Hurthle cells – epithelial cells of degenerated follicles having abundant eosinophilic and granular cytoplasm owing to large number of mitochondria and may contain large nuclei
  ▪ Fibrous thickening of septa
	• Microscopic appearance:
	  ▪ Follicular epithelial hyperplasia and hypertrophy-increased height of follicular lining cells and formation of papillary folding
	  ▪ Reduced colloid, light staining
	  ▪ Increased vascularity and lymphoid cells in stroma

• Lab finding:
  ▪ T3 and T4 decreased
  ▪ TSH increased
	• Lab finding:
	  ▪ T3 and T4 are increased
	  ▪ TSH decreased

b. Giant cell tumour of bone

(Ref: Harsh Mohan, 7th ed. pg. 837, Robbins, SA ed. pg. 1203)

ANSWER

Giant Cell Tumour of Bone

Introduction

- ○ Also known as osteoclastoma
- ○ Benign locally aggressive tumor
- ○ **Origin:** Fusion of stromal mononuclear cells
- ○ Molecular genetics: Expression of RANK (factor responsible for osteoclastic proliferation) in stromal

cells. RANK/RANKL signaling pathway may be responsible for formation of giant osteoclastic cells

Clinical Features

- ○ Common between 20-40 yrs. of age and no sex predilection
- ○ Common sites: lower end of femur and upper end of tibia, lower end of radius and upper end of fibula

Clinical Features

- ○ Pain usually on movement
- ○ Pathologic fracture and swelling
- ○ Arthritic symptoms (joints are involved)

Gross Appearance

○ Well-circumscribed, dark-tan and covered by a thin shell of subperiosteal bone

Microscopic Findings

○ Composed of osteoclast–like tumor giant cells scattered throughout the stroma

○ Stroma composed of sparse collagen fibers, spindle-shaped, plump, uniform mononuclear cells with areas of hemorrhage, macrophages and rich vascularity

Radiographic Findings

○ Appears as lobulated, large, osteolytic lesion usually solitary with "soap bubble" appearance

Prognosis

○ Recurrent and aggressive tumor

○ Mostly shows recurrence after curettage (40-60%)

○ Metastases to lungs is rare (approx. 4%)

c. Fibroadenoma

(Ref: Textbook of Pathology, Harsh Mohan, 7th ed. pg. 748)

ANSWER

Fibroadenoma

For answer, refer 2017 paper-II Q. 2 (c), Pg. 18

PART II

3. Write briefly on

a. Morphological features of Rheumatic Heart Disease

(Ref: Textbook of Pathology, Harsh Mohan, 7th ed. pg. 418)

ANSWER

For answer, refer 2015 paper-II Q. 4 (b), Pg. 64

b Wilms's tumour

(Ref: Harsh Mohan, 7th ed. pg. 683, Robbins, SA ed. pg. 479)

ANSWER

Wilms's tumour

Introduction

○ Also known as "Nephroblastoma"

○ Malignant tumor of kidney that occurs in childhood

○ Origin–from primitive renal tissue–both epithelial and mesenchymal components

Etiology

○ Mutation of WT1 gene (present at chromosome) 11p13 and mutation of WT2 gene increases chances of Wilms' tumor

Clinical Features

○ **Age:** Between 1 to 6 years. with equal incidence in males and females

○ Palpable abdominal mass

○ Hematuria, anemia

○ Pain, hypertension

○ Urethral obstruction as a result of compression

○ Anorexia, weight loss, dyspnea, etc.

○ **Associated syndromes:**

■ Denys-Drash syndrome

■ WAGR syndrome

■ Beckwith-Wiedemann syndrome

Morphological Appearance

○ Grossly, exhibits large, spheroidal, well circum-scribed tumor mass

○ cut section shows typical variegated appearance (soft, tan to grey color with foci of necrosis and hemorrhage)

○ **Microscopic Appearance:**

■ Consists of epithelial component, i.e. in the form of abortive tubules and glomerular structures and mesenchymal component, i.e. fibrous tissue, skeletal and smooth muscle, fat cells, etc.

■ Composed of small, spindle-shaped, anaplastic, sarcomatoid tumor cells

Prognosis

Improved prognosis and 5 year survival rate(80-90%) is due to:

○ Combination therapy of nephrectomy

○ Postoperative irradiation

○ Chemotherapy

4. Write briefly on:

a. Obstructive uropathy

(Ref: Harsh Mohan, 7th ed. pg. 672, Robbins, SA ed. pg. 950)

ANSWER

Obstructive Uropathy

Introduction

○ Urinary tract obstruction is frequent and important as it increases the susceptibility to infection and formation of stone

○ Can occur at any age and in either sex

Causes

- Intraluminal
  - Calculi
  - Tumours such as carcinoma of kidney and bladder
  - Blood clots
  - Sloughed renal papilla
  - Foreign body
- Intramural
  - Pelvi-ureteric junction(PUJ) obstruction
  - Vesicoureteric junction obstruction
  - Urethral stricture
  - Urethral valves
  - Inflammation such as phimosis, cystitis
  - Neuromuscular dysfunction
- Extramural
  - Gravid uterus
  - Retroperitoneal fibrosis
  - Tumours such as carcinoma of cervix, rectum, colon, caecum
  - Prostatic enlargement, prostatic carcinoma and prostatitis
  - Trauma

Types of Obstruction

- Unilateral
- Bilateral
- Partial
- Complete
- Sudden
- Insidious

Anatomic Sequelae of Obstruction

- Hydronephrosis
- Hydroureter
- Hypertrophy of bladder

b Pathogenesis and complications of post infectious cirrhosis

(Ref: Textbook of Pathology, Harsh Mohan, 7th ed. pg. 609)

ANSWER

Pathogenesis and Complications of Post Infectious Cirrhosis

Introduction

- Characterised by large and irregular nodules with broad bands of connective tissue and occurring most frequently after previous viral hepatitis

Etiology

- Viral hepatitis

- Drugs and chemical hepatotoxins
- Others–brucellosis, parasitic infestations, metabolic diseases such as Wilson's disease, advanced alcoholic liver disease
- Idiopathic

Morphology

- **Gross appearance:**
  - Liver is small (less than 1 kg) with distorted shape having irregular and coarse scars and variable size of nodules
  - Cut section exhibits scars and nodules (3 mm to few cm)
- **Microscopic appearance:**
  - Nodular pattern–lobular architecture of hepatic parenchyma is replaced by large nodules
  - Fibrous septa–dividing the variable sized nodules are usually thick
  - Necrosis, inflammation and bile duct proliferation–ordinary active liver cell necrosis; noticeable mononuclear inflammatory cell infiltrate forming follicles can be found in HCV chronic hepatitis; extensive proliferation of bile ductules derived from collapsed liver lobules
  - Hepatic parenchyma – liver cells are of variable size, regenerative nodules have multiple large nuclei

Clinical Features and Complications

- Portal hypertension and its effects–ascites, splenomegaly, development of collaterals (oesophageal varices, spider naevi)
- Progressive hepatic failure
- Development of hepatocellular carcinoma
- Chronic relapsing pancreatitis
- Steatorrhoea
- Gallstones
- Infections due to impaired phagocytic activity of reticuloendothelial system
- Haematologic derangements such as bleeding disorders, anemia
- Cardiovascular complications–atherosclerosis, myocardial infarction
- Musculoskeletal abnormalities such as digital clubbing, hypertropic osteoarthropathy and Dupuytren's contracture
- Endocrine disorders–gynaecomastia, testicular atrophy, impotence in men, amenorrhoea in women
- Hepatorenal syndrome – resulting in renal failure

PART III

5. Write short notes on:

a. Glioblastoma Multiforme

(Ref: Harsh Mohan, 7th ed. pg. 879, Robbins, SA ed. pg. 1187)

ANSWER

Glioblastoma Multiforme

For answer, refer 2017 Paper-II Q. 5 (b), Pg. 22

b. Osteoporosis

(Ref: Textbook of Pathology, Harsh Mohan, 7th ed. pg. 826)

ANSWER

Osteoporosis

Introduction

- Very common clinical syndrome of multiple bones presenting with quantitative reduction of bone tissue mass which is otherwise normal
- Leads to fragile skeleton linked with higher risk of fractures with pain and deformity
- Frequently seen in elderly and post-menopausal women

Diagnosis

- DEXA and SEXA scans (dual energy and single energy X-ray ansorptiometry)
- Quantitative CT
- Ultrasound

Pathogenesis

- Primary–
  - Results from osteopenia without any underlying disease or medication
  - Risk factors
    - Genetic factors–seen in Whites and Asians
    - Sex–Commonly seen in females
    - Reduced physical activity–old age
    - Deficiency of sex hormones–oestrogen deficiency in postmenopausal women and androgen deficiency in men
    - Combined deficiency of calcitonin and oestrogen
    - Hyperparathyroidism
    - Vitamin D deficiency
    - Local factors–stimulating osteoclastic resorption or slow bone osteoblastic bone formation
  - 2 Types are
    - Idiopathic–less common and is seen in young and juveniles

- Involutional–more common in postmenopausal women and elderly people
- Secondary–
  - Due to immobilisation, chronic anaemia, acromegaly, hepatic disease, hyperparathyroidism, hypogonadism, thyrotoxicosis and starvation
  - Effect of medication–hypercortisonism, anticonvulsants, large dose of heparin

Morphology

Grossly

- Immobilisation osteoporosis in restricted to affected limb
- Other forms have skeletal distribution
- Frequently seen fractures due to osteoporosis are – vertebral crush fracture, femoral neck fracture, wrist fracture
- Enlargement of medullary cavity
- Thinning of cortex

Histologically

- Active –
  - Increased bone resorption and formation i.e. enhanced turnover
  - Rise in number of osteoclasts with increased resorptive surface and increased quantity of osteoid with increased osteoblastic surfaces
- Inactive –
  - Minimal bone formation and diminished resorptive activity i.e. decreased turnover
  - Reduced number of osteoclasts with reduced resorptive surfaces and reduced amount of osteoid with reduced osteoblastic surface
  - Osteoid seams width appears reduced or normal

c. Bronchial asthma

(Ref: Harsh Mohan, 7th ed. pg. 463, Robbins, SA ed. pg. 679)

ANSWER

Bronchial Asthma

Introduction

- Increased airway sensitivity to various stimuli causes reversible bronchoconstriction of air passages along with inflammation and increased mucus secretion, generally due to immunological reaction, relieved spontaneously or by treatment
- Common and prevalent worldwide, occurs at all ages but approximately 10% cases develop before the age of 10 years
- Equally common in both sexes in adults, but in children, male-female ratio is 2:1

Clinical Symptoms

- Dyspnoea
- Wheezing
- Cough
- Severe and unremitting form which proves fatal is called as Status asthmaticus

Types: 2 types are Extrinsic (allergic, atopic) and Intrinsic (idiosyncratic, non-atopic) and a third type is Mixed type

Extrinsic asthma	Intrinsic asthma
Occurs in childhood	Occurs in adult
Family history is present	Family history is absent
Preceding allergic illness is present such as rhinitis, urticaria, eczema	Preceding allergic illness is absent
Allergens such as dust, pollens, danders are present	No such allergens are present
Not hypersensitive to any drug	Drug hypersensitivity is seen especially for aspirin
Serum IgE levels are raised	Serum IgE levels are normal
No association with chronic bronchitis or nasal polyps is observed	Association with chronic bronchitis or nasal polyps is found
Emphysema is not common	Emphysema is common

Pathogenesis

- Exaggerated TH2 response to normally harmless environmental antigens; type I hypersensitivity

Morphology

- Gross appearance:
  - Overdistended lungs due to over inflation
  - Cut section exhibits typical occlusion of bronchi and bronchioles by viscid mucus plugs
- Microscopic appearance:
  - Curschmann spirals–normal or degenerated respiratory epithelium forming twisted strips extrudes from mucus plugs
  - Charcot-Leyden crystals–sputum contains eosinophils and diamond shaped crystals derived from eosionophils
  - Creola bodies–ciliated columnar cells sloughed from bronchial mucosa
  - Thickening of basement membrane of bronchial epithelium
  - Submucosal oedema of bronchial wall and inflammatory infiltrate comprises of lymphocytes and plasma cells
  - Hypertrophied sub-mucosal glands and bronchial smooth muscle

d. Seminoma

(Ref: Textbook of Pathology, Harsh Mohan, 7th ed. pg. 697)

ANSWER

Seminoma

Introduction

- Most common malignant tumour of testis constituting 45% of all germ cell tumours
- 2 types are – classic seminoma and spermocytic seminoma
- Classic seminoma constitutes 95% of all seminomas
- Occurs in 4th decade of life and rare before puberty
- Most frequent in undescended testis
- Serum hCG levels are raised in 10% seminomas

Morphology

- **Gross appearance:**
  - Enlargement of testis upto 10 times but can maintain its normal shape as tumour does not invade tunica
  - Large tumour replaces the entire testis but small tumour is presented as a circumscribed mass in testis
  - Cut surface exhibits homogeneous and grey white lobulated appearance
- **Microscopic appearance:**
  - Tumour cells lie in sheets or columns forming lobules
  - Uniform in size and has clear cytoplasm with well-defined borders
  - Cytoplasm contains glycogen which stains positively with PAS reaction
  - Large, hyperchromatic and centrally located nuclei with 1-2 nucleoli
  - Around 10% seminomas show increased mitotic activity and aggressive behaviour and therefore categorised as anaplastic seminomas
  - Delicate fibrous tissue stroma dividing tumour into lobules
  - Typical lymphocytic infiltration suggests immunologic response of host to tumour

- Granulomatous reaction in stroma of around 20% tumours

Prognosis

Better than other germ cell tumours as tumour is highly radiosensitive

---

6. **Write briefly on:**

   a. **Coal workers' pneumoconiosis**

   (Ref: Textbook of Pathology, Harsh Mohan, 7th ed. pg. 468)

ANSWER

Coal Workers' Pneumoconiosis

Introduction

○ Most frequent type of pneumoconiosis and caused by inhalation of coal dust particles generally in coal miners engaged in handling soft bituminous coal for many years, around 20-30 years

Predisposing Factors

○ Old age of miners
○ Severity of coal dust burden engulfed by macrophages
○ Prolonged duration of exposure to coal dust
○ Concomitant tuberculosis
○ Additional role of silica dust

Morphology

○ **Gross appearance:**
  - Coal macules–small, black focal lesions of size less than 5 mm in diameter evenly distributed throughout the lung especially in the upper lobes, palpable macules are called nodules

- Dilated air spaces with little destruction of alveolar walls
- Black pigmentation on the pleural surface and regional lymph nodes

○ **Microscopic appearance:**
  - Coal macules comprises of aggregates of dust laden macrophages present in alveoli and bronchiolar and alveolar walls
  - Increase in the network of reticulin and collagen in coal macules
  - Distention of respiratory bronchioles and alveoli without any noticeable destruction of alveolar walls

Clinical Picture

○ Chronic cough with black expectoration
○ Radiological findings–nodularity in the lungs

   b. **Risk factors in carcinoma cervix**

   (Ref: Textbook of Pathology, Harsh Mohan, 7th ed. pg. 715)

ANSWER

Risk Factors in Carcinoma Cervix

For answer, refer 2017 paper-II Q. 4 (a), Pg. 20

   c. **Pathology and complications of Amoebic colitis**

   (Ref: Textbook of Pathology, Harsh Mohan, 7th ed. pg. 555)

ANSWER

Pathology and Complications of Amoebic Colitis

For answer, refer 2015 paper-II Q. 5 (a), Pg. 65

Your Roll No. ....

Name of the Paper	:	**Pathology Paper-I**
Name of the Course	:	**MBBS-2012**
Semester	:	**Annual**

Time: 3 Hours   **M.M.: 40**

INSTRUCTIONS

1. Write your Roll No. on the top immediately on receipt of this question paper
2. All questions are to be attempted
3. Answers to Parts I, II and III should be written in separate answer sheets provided
4. Attempt parts of a question in sequence

PART-I

1. **Differentiate between:**   [8]
   a. Leukemoid reaction and chronic myeloid leukemia
   b. Irreversible and reversible cell injury
   c. Primary and secondary amyloidosis
   d. Lymphatic and vascular spread of tumors

2. **Write briefly on:**   [6]
   a. Prothrombin time
   b. Role of human papilloma virus in neoplasia
   c. Fatty change liver

PART-II

3. **Write briefly on:**   [6]
   a. Hemophilia
   b. Gaucher's disease

4. **Write briefly on:**   [6]
   a. Enumerate the deficiency anemia seen in India. Give the blood, biochemical and bone marrow findings in iron deficiency anemia
   b. Pathogenesis of hypovolemic shock

PART-III

5. **Comment on:**   [8]
   a. Down's syndrome
   b. Types 1 hypersensitivity reaction
   c. Immune thrombocytopenia
   d. Role of interleukin's in acute inflammation

6. **Write short notes on:**   [6]
   a. Blood and urinary findings in nephrotic syndrome
   b. Cytochemistry, in acute leukemia
   c. Lab. Diagnosis of multiple myeloma

PART I

1. **Differentiate between:**

   a. **Leukemoid reaction and chronic myeloid leukemia**

ANSWER

Leukemoid Reaction and Chronic Myeloid Leukemia

For answer, refer 2017 paper-I Q. 1 (c), Pg. 4

   b. **Irreversible and reversible cell injury**

   (Ref: Harsh Mohan, 7th ed. pg. 12, Robbins, SA ed. pg. 40)

ANSWER

Irreversible cell injury	Reversible cell injury
On removal of injurious stimulus, induced structural and functional changes revert back to normal	On removal of injurious stimulus, induced structural and functional changes cannot revert back to normal
Calcification not present	Presence of dystrophic calcification
Lysosomal autophagy of organelles and no rupture	Lysosomal rupture and autolysis of cells
Swelling of Endoplasmic reticulum	Swelling and lysis of ER

   c. **Primary and secondary amyloidosis**

   (Ref: Harsh Mohan, 7th ed. pg. 71, Robbins, SA ed. pg. 256)

ANSWER

For answer, refer 2017 paper-I Q. 1 (d), Pg. 4

   d. **Lymphatic and vascular spread of tumors**

   (Ref: Textbook of Pathology, Harsh Mohan, 7th ed. pg. 192)

ANSWER

Lymphatic spread of tumors	Vascular spread of tumors
• Spread through lymph system	• Spread through blood circulation
• Common in carcinoma	• Common in sarcoma
• Growth of tumor cells in a continuous fashion(lymphatic permeation) or in the form of emboli	• Favored sites: lungs, liver, kidney, brain, bones, etc
• Regional lymph nodes results in regional nodal metastasis, eg. from breast carcinoma to axillary lymph nodes, from thyroid cancerto lateral cervical lymph nodes	• Invasion of wall of capillaries, veins and venules readily than arteries

2. **Write briefly on:**

   a. **Prothrombin time**

   (Ref: Textbook of Pathology, Harsh Mohan, 7th ed. pg. 308)

ANSWER

For answer 2015 paper-I Q. 5 (a), Pg. 56

   b. **Role of human papilloma virus in neoplasia**

   (Ref: Textbook of Pathology, Harsh Mohan, 7th ed. pg. 218)

ANSWER

Role of Papilloma Virus

- Human papilloma virus is the common etiologic agent in common skin warts or verruca vulgaris
- HPV 6 and 11 (low- risk) responsible for genital warts
- HPV 16,18,31, 33 and 45 (high- risk) responsible for invasive cervical cancer
- HPV 5 and 8 responsible for the causation of epidermodysplasia verruciformis

Role in Oncogenesis

- High risk HPV responsible for overexpression of viral proteins E6 and E7 with a high affinity for target host cells
- E6 and E7 viral proteins result in loss of p53 and Prb resulting in uncontrolled proliferation
- Activation of cyclin A and E and inactivation of CDKIs resulting in cell proliferation
- Viral proteins result in degradation of BAX (proapoptotic gene), resulting in inhibition of apoptosis
- Activation of telomerase thus immortalization of transformed target host cells

   c. **Fatty change liver**

   (Ref: Harsh Mohan, 7th ed. pg. 19, Robbins, SA ed. pg. 62)

ANSWER

Introduction

- Fatty change is the intracellular deposition of fat in the parenchymal cells
- Common in liver but also occur in heart, kidney, skeletal muscle, etc.

Types

On the basis of etiology and amount of deposition, it may be:

- Mild and reversible
- Severe and irreversible

Etiology

- Damage to liver cell: Conditions with liver cell injury are-
  - Alcoholic liver disease(common)
  - Protein calorie malnutrition
  - Starvation
  - Chronic illness, like tuberculosis
  - Hypoxia
  - Drugs, like steroids, methotrexate, etc.
- As a result of excess fat: conditions like-
  - Diabetes mellitus
  - Obesity
  - Congenital hyperlipidemia

Pathogenesis

Normal Fat Metabolism

- Free fatty acid from food or adipose tissue is esterified to triglycerides and changed into cholesterol, phospholipids and oxidized to ketone bodies.
- Secretion of triglycerides require lipid acceptor protein to form lipoprotein and released into the circulation as plasma lipoprotein.

In Fatty Liver

- Defect at any step from entry of free fatty acid to exit of lipoprotein may result in abnormal/excess accumulation of triglyceride resulting in fatty liver.
  - Increased FFA entry into liver- obesity, DM
  - Increased synthesis of FFA

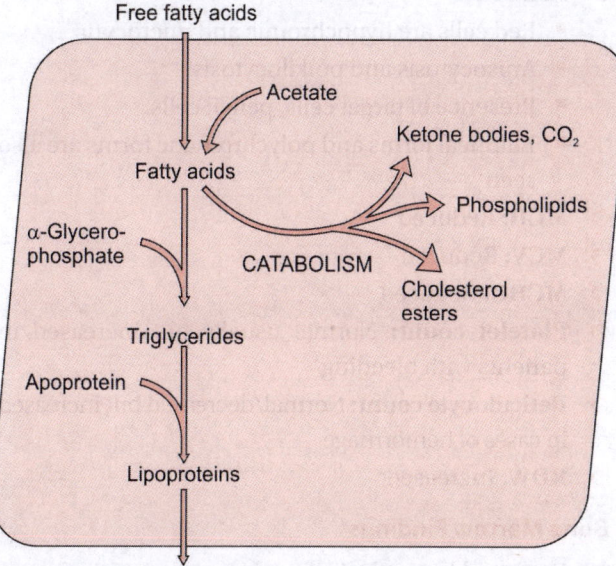

Fig. Pathogenesis of fatty liver

- Decreased fatty acid oxidation
- Decreased synthesis of lipid acceptor protein, thereby reduced formation of lipoprotein from triglycerides.

Gross Appearance

- Palcyellow enlarged liver
- Cytoplasmic vacuoles in the hepatocytes.

Microscopic Features

- Presence of cytoplasmic lipid laden vacuoles in the hepatocytes
- Cytoplasmic vacuoles may be microvesicular or macrovesicular
- Fat stains like – Sudan dye is used for demonstration of fat in the sections

PART II

3. Write briefly on:

a. Hemophilia

(Ref: Harsh Mohan, 7th ed. pg. 313-314, Robbins, SA ed. pg. 662-63)

ANSWER

Introduction

- A disorder of coagulation factor
- Common heredity coagulation disorders are – hemophilia A, hemophilia B and von Willebrand's factor

Hemophilia A

Pathogenesis

- Deficiency of factor VIII(anti-hemophilic factor) because of mutation in F8 gene
- Due to quantitative reduction of factor VIII (90%) cases and qualitative dysfunction of factor VIII(10%) cases
- Sex(X) recessive trait

Epidemiology

- Most of the clinical manifestation in males, females are carrier

Clinical Features

- Massive bleeding after trauma or injury (bleeding continues for hours to days)
- Painful, recurrent haemarthroses, hematomas commonly occur as a result of spontaneous hemorrhage

Laboratory Findings

- **Whole blood coagulation time:** Prolonged

- **Prothrombin time:** Normal
- **APTT or PTTK:** Prolonged
- **Confirmatory test:**
    - **Factor VIII assay:** Reduced plasma level or reduced function
    - **Cytogenetics:** Mutations in X chromosome, like- deletion, splicing defect, inversion, etc.

Treatment

- **Symptomatic cases:**
    - Factor VIII replacement therapy

Hemophilia B

- Due to deficiency of factor IX (Christmas factor or plasma thromboplastin component)
- Less common than hemophilia A
- **Treatment:**
    - Fresh frozen plasma infusion or plasma enriched with factor IX infusion (mainly in symptomatic cases)

b.   Gaucher's diseases

(Ref: Textbook of Pathology, Harsh Mohan, 7th ed. pg. 257)

ANSWER

Introduction

- An autosomal recessive disorder with deficiency of lysosomal enzyme, acid β-glucosidase (glucocer- ebrosidase).
- Lysosomal accumulation of ceramide-gluose (glu- cocerebrosidase) in pahagocytic cells and neurons (sometimes)

Clinical Features

- Based on neuronopathic involvement, classified into 3 tyes:
    - Type I/Classic form:
        - Most common type
        - Mainly seen in adults
        - Spleen, liver, lymph nodes,etc. are commonly involved
- **Type II:**
    - Infantile form
    - Progressively involved CNS
- **TYPE III:**
    - Juvenile form
    - Exhibits features of both type I and type II
- **Other Features:** bone pain, thrombocytopenia, pan- cytopenia, pathologic fracture, etc. are also evident

Microscopic Findings

- **Gaucher cells:** Enlarged macrophages

- **Cytoplasm:** Abundant, granular giving crumpled tissue paper appearance
- PAS, oil red O and Prussian – blue positive

Treatment

- For type I and type III:
    - Enzyme replacement therapy
    - Bone marrow transplantation

---

4.   Write briefly on:

a.   Enumerate the deficiency anemia seen in India. Give the blood, biochemical and bone marrow findings in iron deficiency anemia.

(Ref: Textbook of Pathology, Harsh Mohan, 7th ed. pg. 272)

ANSWER

Deficiency Anemia in India

- **Iron deficiency anemia:**
    - Most common form of anemia in the world
    - Occurs due to defective hemoglobin synthesis
- **Megaloblastic anemia:**
    - Due to vitamin B12 or folate deficiency
    - Other causes- drugs that interfere with DNA synthesis, acquired hematopoetic stem cell defect,etc

Blood, biochemical and bone marrow findings in iron deficiency anemia

Blood Picture

- **Hemoglobin:** Decreased
- **RBC count:** Decreased
- **Red cells:**
    - Red cells are hypochromic and microcytic
    - Anisocytosis and poikilocytosis
    - Presence of target cells, pencil cells
    - Elliptical forms and polychromatic forms are also seen
- **MCH:** Reduced
- **MCV:** Reduced
- **MCHC:** Reduced
- **Platelet count:** Normal usually but increased in patients with bleeding
- **Reticulocyte count:** Normal/decreased but increased in cases of hemorrhage
- **RDW:** Increased

Bone Marrow Findings

- Erythroid hyperplasia
- **Decreased myeloid:** Erythroid ratio

- Normoblastic erythropoiesis
- Micronormoblast predominant
- Iron stores: deficient, reduced sideroblast

Biochemical Findings

- **Serum iron:** Decreased
- **Serum ferritin:** decreased, reflecting poor iron stores in tissues
- **Total iron binding capacity:** Raised
- **Serum transferrin receptor protein:** Increased and indicates total red cell mass
- **Red cell protoporphyrin:** Decreased, due to insufficient iron supply

  b. Pathogenesis of hypovolemic shock

  (Ref: Harsh Mohan, 7th ed. pg. 95, Robbins, SA ed. pg. 131)

ANSWER

Introduction

- Inadequate circulating blood volume results in hypovolemic shock
- Also called as "haemorrhagic shock."
- Effects: Decreased cardiac output
- Decreased intracardiac pressure

Associated factors/Etiology

- Dehydration
- Hemorrhage (loss of red cell mass)
- Burns
- Acute pancreatitis
- Surgery
- Trauma

Types

Depending upon the amount of loss of blood volume, it is of 4 types:

- Compensated: ≤
- Mild: 1000-1500 ml
- Moderate : 1500-2000 ml
- Severe: > 2000 mL

Pathogenesis

Following three derangements results in shock:

- Decrease in effective circulatory blood volume
- Reduced supply of oxygen to tissues resulting in anoxia and cellular injury
- Release of inflammatory mediators and toxins in response to shock –induced cellular injury

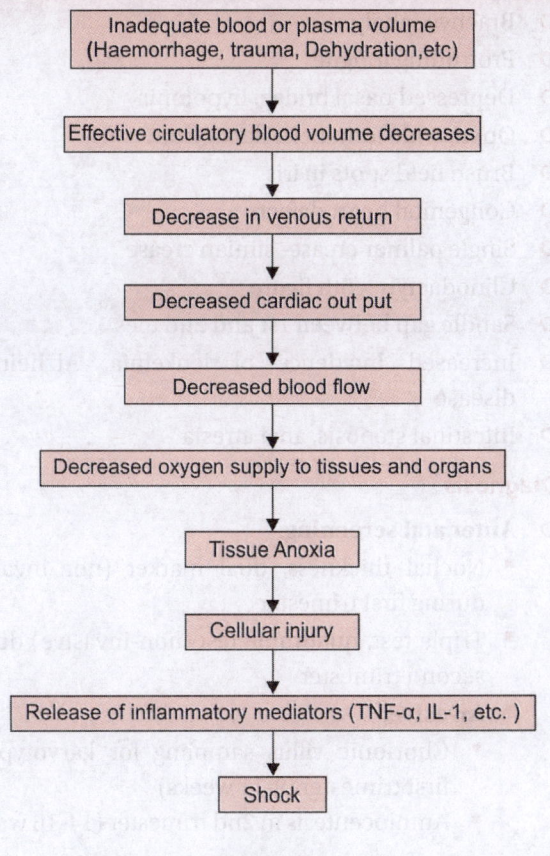

PART III

5. Comment on:

  a. Down's syndrome

  (Ref: Textbook of Pathology, Harsh Mohan, 7th ed. pg. 253)

ANSWER

Introduction

- Most common chromosomal abnormality
- Caused by maternal nondisjunction

Epidemiology

- Influenced with maternal age (increases with increasing maternal age)

Genetics

- Trisomy of the chromosome 21(most important and common)
- Least common- mosaic pattern (1-2%)

Clinical Features

- Mental Retardation
- Short stature

- Brachycephaly
- Protruding tongue
- Depressed nasal bridge, hypotonia
- Open, wide fontanele, flat occiput
- Brush field spots in iris
- Congenital heart defects
- Single palmar crease- simian crease
- Clinodactyly – 5th figure
- Sandle gap between 1st and 2nd toes
- Increased incidence of leukemia, Alzheimer's disease
- Intestinal stenosis, anal atresia

Diagnosis

- **Antenatal screening:**
  - Nuchal thickness, dual marker (non-invasive) during first trimester
  - Triple test, quadruple test (non-invasive) during second trimester
  - **Invasive:**
    - Chorionic villus sampling for karyotype in first trimester (9-11 weeks)
    - Amniocentesis in 2nd trimester (14-16 weeks)

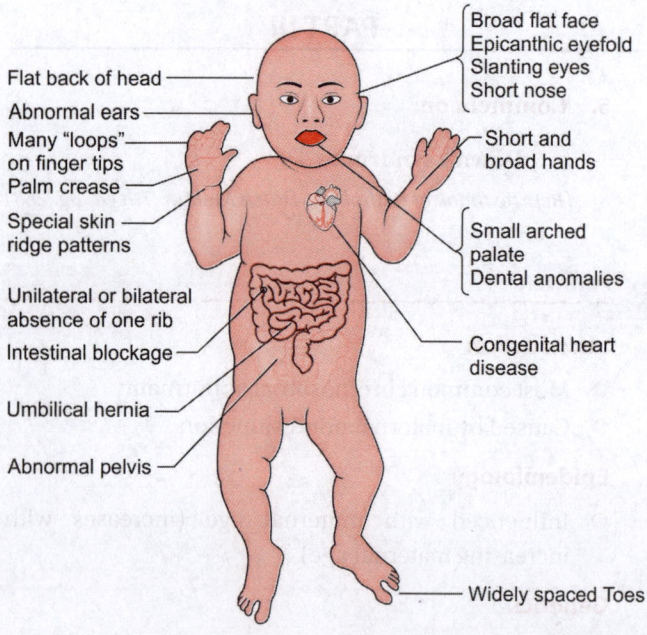

Flat back of head
Abnormal ears
Many "loops" on finger tips
Palm crease
Special skin ridge patterns
Unilateral or bilateral absence of one rib
Intestinal blockage
Umbilical hernia
Abnormal pelvis

Broad flat face
Epicanthic eyefold
Slanting eyes
Short nose
Short and broad hands
Small arched palate
Dental anomalies
Congenital heart disease
Widely spaced Toes

Fig. Down syndrome

b.   Type I Hypersensitivity reaction

(Ref: Harsh Mohan, 7th ed. pg. 58, Robbins, SA ed. pg. 200)

ANSWER

Introduction

- It is immediate type of "Atopic or Anaphylactic" hypersensitivity reaction

- Rapidly developing immunologic response in a previously sensitized individual

Etiology

- IgE antibodies mediated hypersensitivity reaction
- May be due to:
  - Viral infections
  - Environmental pollutants (allergen)
  - Genetic

Pathogenesis

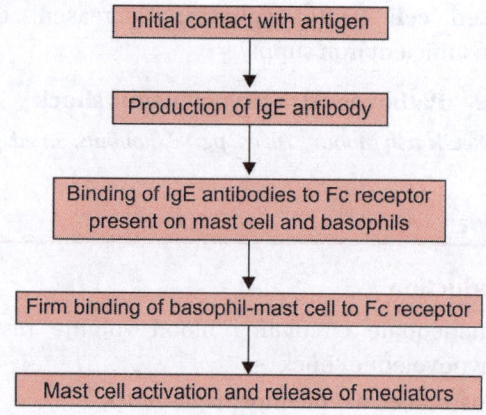

```
Initial contact with antigen
          ↓
Production of IgE antibody
          ↓
Binding of IgE antibodies to Fc receptor
present on mast cell and basophils
          ↓
Firm binding of basophil-mast cell to Fc receptor
          ↓
Mast cell activation and release of mediators
```

Mediators

- **Primary Mediators:**
  - Histamine
  - Adenosine
  - Eosinophil chemotactic factor
  - Proteases, etc.
- **Secondary Mediators:**
  - Leukotrienes B4, C4
  - Cytokines
  - Prostlandin

Examples

- Bronchial asthma
- Hay fever
- Food allergy
- Systemic anaphylaxis- administration of drugs, antisera, etc.

c.   **Immune thrombocytopenia**

(Ref: Textbook of Pathology, Harsh Mohan, 7th ed. pg. 311)

ANSWER

Introduction

- Characterized by immunological destruction of platelets resulting in severe thrombocytopenia

Types

Depending on duration of illness, two clinical forms-

- Acute ITP:
  - Self-limiting, sudden onset
  - Common in children with a history of viral infections (like-CMV, infectious mononucleosis, etc.)2-3 weeks before onset
- Chronic ITP:
  - Common in adults (mainly in females 20-40 years. of age)
  - Long-standing and develops slowly
  - Antiplatelet antibodies responsible in the pathogenesis of chronic ITP
  - Associated with remission and relapse

Clinical Features

- Mucosal bleeding– bleeding from gums, melaena, hematuria, nasal bleeding, etc, petechiae, bruising
- Splenomegaly and hepatomegly uncommon

Laboratory Diagnosis

- Large-sized platelets
- Reduced platelet count
- Reduced platelet life span
- Bone marrow findings: Increased megakaryocytes with single non- lobulated nuclei and presence of cytoplasmic vacuoles along with decreased cytoplasmic granularity
- Presence of anti-platelet IgG antibody on platelet surface

Treatment

- Corticosteroid therapy, immunosuppressive drugs, splenectomy
- Platelet transfusion(as palliative measure) - in case of severe hemorrhage

d. Role of Interleukin in acute inflammation

(Ref: Textbook of Pathology, Harsh Mohan, 7th ed. pg. 120)

ANSWER

Role of Interleukins

- Interleukins are cytokines and their role in acute inflammation as follows:
  - IL-1:
    - Elaboration mainly from monocytes/ macrophages, fibroblasts, B cells, endothelial cells and few epithelial cells
    - Responsible for:
      - Migration of neutrophils and macrophages
      - Expression of adhesion molecules
      - Production of acute phase protein
      - In fever and shock plays an imp role
  - IL-8:
    - Elaborated by T cells

- Targets are–neutrophils, basophils, T cells, monocytes/macrophages and endothelial cells
- Mainly responsible for:
  - Migration of neutrophils, macrophages and T cells
  - Release of histamine from basophils
  - Angiogenesis stimulation
- IL-6: Mainly responsible for:
  - T and B cell growth and differentiation
  - Acute phase protein production

6. Write short notes on:

a. Blood and Urinary Finding in nephrotic syndrome

(Ref: Textbook of Pathology, Harsh Mohan, 7th ed. pg. 648-649)

ANSWER

Introduction

- Nephrotic syndrome characterized by heavy proteinuria, hypoalbuminaemia, hyperlipidemia, edema, lipiduria and hypercoagulability

Blood and Urinary Findings

- Proteinuria:
  - Heavy proteinuria
  - More than 3 gm/day
- Lipiduria: Present (due to glomerular filtration barrier leakiness)
- Hyperlipidemia:
  - Present
  - Blood level of total lipids, cholesterol, triglycerides, LDL and VLDL increased
  - Reduced HDL levels
- Oligouria: Present in advanced cases
- Urine: Presence of frothy urine
- Cast: Presence of lipid cell cast cell
- Hypercoagulability: Present
  - Renal vein thrombosis
  - Pulmonary embolism
  - Arterial or venous thrombosis

b. Cytochemistry in acute leukemia

(Ref: Textbook of Pathology, Harsh Mohan, 7th ed. pg. 226–230)

ANSWER

For answer, refer 2015 paper-I Q. 2 (c), Pg. 53

c. Lab. Diagnosis of multiple myeloma

(Ref: Textbook of Pathology, Harsh Mohan, 7th ed. pg. 363)

ANSWER

For answer, refer 2017 paper-I Q. 4 (b), Pg. 8

Name of the Paper	:	**Pathology Paper-II**
Name of the Course	:	**MBBS-2012**
Semester	:	**Annual**

Time: 3 Hours   **M.M.: 40**

INSTRUCTIONS

1. Write your Roll No. on the top immediately on receipt of this question paper
2. All questions are to be attempted
3. Answers to Parts I, II and III should be written in separate answer sheets provided
4. Attempt parts of a question in sequence

PART-I

1. **Differentiate between:**   **[8]**
    a. Transmural and subendocardial infarct
    b. Partial and complete mole
    c. Papillary and medullary carcinoma of thyroid
    d. Hodgkin's disease–Nodular sclerosis and lymphocytic depletion type
2. **Write short notes on:**   **[6]**
    a. Radiological findings in bone tumors
    b. Astrocytoma
    c. Paget's disease of the breast

PART-II

3. **Write briefly on:**   **[6]**
    a. Morphological changes in Alzeheimer's disease
    b. Etiopathogenesis and morphology of hepatocellular carcinoma
4. **Write briefly on:**   **[6]**
    a. Role of H. Pylori in gastrointestinal disorders
    b. Laboratory findings in chronic renal failure

PART-III

5. **Write briefly on:**   **[8]**
    a. Minimal change disease
    b. Pleomorphic adenoma
    c. Barett's esophagus
    d. Cervical intra epithelial neoplasia
6. **Write briefly on:**   **[6]**
    a. Silicosis
    b. Hypersplenism
    c. Familial adenomatous polyposis coli

PART I

1. Differentiate between:

a. Transmural and subendocardial infarct

(Ref: Textbook of Pathology, Harsh Mohan, 7th ed. pg. 410)

ANSWER

Transmural and Subendocardial Infarct

For answer, refer 2015 paper-II Q. 1 (a), Pg. 61

ANSWER

b. Partial and complete mole

(Ref: Textbook of Pathology, Harsh Mohan, 7th ed. pg. 741)

ANSWER

Partial and Complete Mole

For answer, refer 2015 paper-II Q. 1 (b), Pg. 61

c. Papillary and medullary carcinoma of thyroid

(Ref: Textbook of Pathology, Harsh Mohan, 7th ed. pg. 802)

Papillary and Medullary Carcinoma of Thyroid

Papillary Carcinoma of Thyroid	Medullary Carcinoma of Thyroid
• Most common; occurs in 75-85% cases	• Less common; occurs in 5% cases
• Occurs in all ages	• Occurs in middle aged to old age
• Frequent in females than males; female/male ratio is 3:1	• Equally common among both males and females; female/male ratio is 1:1
• Gross appearance – small, multifocal	• Gross appearance – moderate size
• Relation to radiation is maximum	• Relation to radiation is absent
• Origin of cell is follicular	• Origin of cell is parafollicular
• RET gene over expression, NTRK gene rearrangement	• RET point mutation
• Pathognomonic microscopic features are nuclear features, papillary pattern	• Pathognomonic microscopic features are solid nests, amyloid stroma
• 10-year survival rate is 80-95%	• 10-year survival rate is 60-70%

d. Hodgkin's disease–Nodular sclerosis and lymphocytic depletion type

(Ref: Textbook of Pathology, Harsh Mohan, 7th ed. pg. 350)

ANSWER

Hodgkin's Disease– Nodular Sclerosis and Lymphocytic Depletion Type

Nodular Sclerosis Type Hodgkin's Disease	Lymphocytic Depletion Type Hodgkin's Disease
Most common type, occurs in 70% cases	Least common type, occurs in 1% cases
Microscopic features are lymphoid nodules, collagen bands	Microscopic features are scanty lymphocytes, atypical histiocytes and fibrosis
Reed-Sternberg cells are Frequent, lacunar type, CD15+, CD30+	Reed-Sternberg Cells are numerous, pleomorphic type, CD15+, CD30+
Prognosis is very good	Prognosis is poor

2. Write short notes on:

a. Radiological findings in bone tumors

(Ref: Textbook of Pathology, Harsh Mohan, 7th ed. pg. 831)

ANSWER

Radiological Findings in Bone Tumors

Introduction

- Tumours of bone and cartilage are not very common but clinically important as they are highly malignant
- Can be primary or metastatic
- Types–osseous and non-osseous

Diagnosis of Bone Tumour

- Clinical examination
- Pathological examination
- Radiological examination

Radiological Findings of Bone Tumours

Type of bone tumour	Radiological finding
• Osteoma	• Dense ivory like bony mass
• Osteoid osteoma	• Small radiolucent central focus or nidus surrounded by dense sclerotic bone
• Central Osteosarcoma	• Sunburst pattern owing to osteogenesis within the tumour and presence of Codman's triangle formed at the angle between the elevated periosteum and underlying surface of the cortex
• Surface osteosarcoma	• Dense bony mass attached to the outer cortex of the affected long bone
• Osteochondromas	• Exophytic lesions of long bones
• Enchondroma	• Radiolucent, lobulated tumour mass with spotty calcification
• Chondroblastoma	• Sharply circumscribed, lytic lesion with multiple small foci of calcification
• Chondromyxoid fibroma	• Abruptly outlined radiolucent area with foci of calcification and expansion of affected end of bone
• Chondrosarcoma	• Massively expansible and osteolytic growth with foci of calcification
• Osteoclastoma	• Giant cell tumour appears as large lobulated and osteolytic lesion at the end of and expanded long bone with soap bubble appearance
• Ewing's sarcoma	• Osteolytic lesion with patchy subperiosteal bone formation producing onion like appearance
• Chordoma	• Appearance of osteolytic lesion

b. Astrocytoma

(Ref: Textbook of Pathology, Harsh Mohan, 7th ed. 879)

ANSWER

For answer, refer 2016 paper-II, Q. 5 (c), Pg. 46

c. Paget's disease of the breast

(Ref: Textbook of Pathology, Harsh Mohan, 7th ed. pg. 755, Robbins, SA ed. pg. 1057)

ANSWER

Paget's Disease of the Breast

Introduction

- Eczematoid disease of nipple associated with invasive or non-invasive ductal carcinoma of breast
- In 50% cases nipple shows crusted, scaly and eczematoid lesion with palpable subareolar mass
- Most commonly, patients presenting with palpable mass have infiltrating duct carcinoma whereas patients with no palpable mass have intraductal carcinoma
- **Prognosis:** Favourable in ductal carcinoma with Paget's disease, less favourable in ductal carcinoma without Paget's disease

Pathogenesis

Two hypotheses have been explained

- Migration of tumour cells from underlying ductal carcinoma into lactiferous ducts and invasion into the epidermis producing skin lesions
- Represents a form of carcinoma in situ of the epidermis itself

Morphologic Features

- Grossly
  - Crusted, fissured and ulcerated skin of nipple and areola
  - Oozing of serosanguineous fluid from the erosions
- Histologically,
  - Presence of Paget's cells in the epidermis in small clusters or singly
  - Larger than epidermal cells, spherical having hyperchromatic nuclei with cytoplasmic halo
  - Underlying breast encloses invasive or non-invasive duct carcinoma presenting no obvious direct invasion of nipple skin

PART II

3. Write briefly on:

a. Morphological changes in Alzheimer's disease

(Ref: Harsh Mohan, 7th ed. pg. 876, Robbins, SA ed. pg. 1287)

ANSWER

Morphological Changes in Alzheimer's Disease

Introduction

- Most common type of degenerative disease
- Causes dementia in elderly
- Occurs usually after 5th decade of life

Causes

Exact cause is unknown

- Family history
- Deposition of A(beta) amyloid derived from amyloid precursor protein (APP) forming neuritic senile plaques and neurofibrillary tangles

Morphological Changes in Alzheimer's Disease

- Grossly,
  - Decreased weight of brain
  - Bilateral atrophy of brain
- Microscopically,
  - Senile neuritic plaque
    - Most noticeable lesion
    - Comprises of focal area with central core having A(beta)
  - Neurofibrillary tangle
    - Filamentous collection of neurofilaments and neurotubules within cytoplasm of neurons
  - Amyloid angiopathy
    - Deposition of amyloid in vessel wall same as deposited in amyloid core of plaque
  - Granulovacuolar degeneration
    - Presence of multiple, small intraneuronal cytoplasmic vacuoles, few of them contain one or more Hirano bodies (dark granules)

b. Etiopathogenesis and morphology of hepatocellular carcinoma

(Ref: Textbook of Pathology, Harsh Mohan, 7th ed. pg. 618)

ANSWER

For answer 2015 paper-II Q. 4(a), Pg. 63

4. Write briefly on:

a. Role of H. Pylori in gastrointestinal disorders

(Ref: Textbook of Pathology, Harsh Mohan, 7th ed. pg. 531)

ANSWER

Role of H. Pylori in Gastrointestinal Disorders

For answer, refer 2014 paper-II Q. 5 (a), Pg. 81

b. Laboratory Findings in Chronic Renal Failure

(Ref: Textbook of Pathology, Harsh Mohan, 7th ed. pg. 641)

ANSWER

For answer, refer 2017 paper-II Q.4 (b), Pg. 21

PART III

5. Write briefly on:

a. Minimal change disease

(Ref: Textbook of Pathology, Harsh Mohan, 7th ed. pg. 656)

ANSWER

For answer, refer 2016 paper-II, Q. 3 (b), Pg. 43

b. Pleomorphic adenoma

(Ref: Harsh Mohan, 7th ed. pg. 516, Robbins, SA ed. pg. 744)

ANSWER

Pleomorphic Adenoma

Introduction

- Most common benign tumor of the parotid gland
- Includes major (60-75%) and minor(approx. 50%) salivary glands (mixed tumor)

Clinical Features

- Common in 3rd- 4th decade of life
- Common in females
- Usually unilateral
- Painless, slow growing, solitary, nodular swelling
- Present below and in front of ear
- Dysphagia- deep lobe involvement
- Ear lobule raised
- Uvula and pharyngeal wall deviated towards midline
- Curtain sign- not movable above zygomatic bone

Gross Appearance

- Well-circumscribed, pseudoencapsulated, firm, swelling that is approx. 2-5 cm in diameter.

Microscopic Appearance:

○ Consists of epithelial component in the form of ducts, sheets, cords, acini and strands of ductal and myoepithelial cells

○ Columnar or cuboidal ductal cells whereas spindle-shaped or polygonal myoepithelial cells

○ Material present in the lumen of the duct like structures are PAS-positive

○ Mesenchymal component consist of myxoid, chondroid, and mucoid matrix in the form of pseudocartilage

○ Material present in the lumen of the duct like structures are PAS-positive

Investigations

○ FNAC- Diagnostic

○ CT scan and MRI

○ **Immunohistochemisty:** Immunoreactivity of epithelial component (cytokeratin, EMA, CEA) and of myoepithelial component (S-100, actin, vimentin) antibodies

Management

○ Parotidectomy- superficial (if only superficial lobe is involved)

○ Total conservative parotidectomy- (if both lobes are involved)

○ Enucleation- Avoided as a result of high recurrence

c.   Barrett's esophagus

(Ref: Harsh Mohan, 7th ed. pg. 523, Robbins, SA ed. pg. 757)

ANSWER

Barrett's Esophagus

Introduction

○ Characterized by replacement of distal stratified squamous epithelium of esophagus by columnar cells

○ Complication of severe form of GERD

Clinical Features

○ Age: 40-60 yrs.

○ Common in males as compared to females

○ Local ulceration

○ Bleeding

○ Heartburn, dysphasia

○ Hematemesis

○ Melena

○ Formation of stricture

Associated Conditions

○ Sliding hiatus hernia

○ Chronic gastric and duodenal ulcer

○ Nasogastric intubation

○ Surgical vagotomy

○ Delayed gastric empying, etc.

Pathogenesis

Lower part of esophagus shows ulceration and inflammation. As a result of adaptive response, differentiation of pluripotent stem cells into columnar cells that are resistant to acidity. These cells exhibits dysplasia(may be low grade or high grade) in low pH

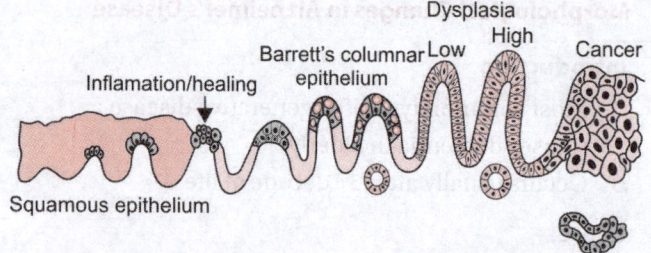

Morphological Findings

○ Endoscopy revels affected red and velvety mucosa along with hiatus hernia and Barret's ulcer (peptic ulcer at squamocolumnar junction)

○ **Microscopic Features:**

  ▪ Squamous epithelium revels intestinal metaplasia (metaplastic columnar cells with goblet cells) accompanied by high or low grade dysplasia

  ▪ Presence of fundic gastric glands or cardiac mucous glands accompanied by inflammatory cell infiltrate

d.   Cervical intra epithelial neoplasia

(Ref: Textbook of Pathology, Harsh Mohan, 7th ed. pg. 893)

ANSWER

Cervical Intra epithelial Neoplasia

Introduction

○ Also known as " cervical dysplasia"

○ A precancerous lesion that may progress to squamous cell carcinoma of cervix

Etiology/Risk Factors

○ Human papilloma virus infection(HPV)

○ Genital warts

○ Immunosuppression

○ Multiple sexual partners

○ Sexual activity in early age

○ Smoking

○ Use of oral contraceptives

○ Low socioeconomic strata

Pathology

Depending on the extent of dysplastic features (*pleomorphism, altered nucleocytoplasmic ratio, enlarged ir-*

regular nuclei, nuclear dyskeratosis, abnormal parabasal cells, etc.) within the epithelial layers, CIN is divided into mild, moderate, severe and carcinoma in situ.

- **CIN I (Mild dysplasia):**
  - Dysplasia present in the lower one-third of epithelium
  - Exhibits dysplastic features like– hyperchromatism, enlarged nucleus, coarse chromatin, etc.
- **CIN II (Moderate dysplasia):**
  - Dysplasia up to two-third of the epithelium
  - Dysplastic features like- hyperchromatism, loss of polarity, increased N:C ratio, abnormal mitoses, loss of maturation, etc.
- **CIN III (Severe dysplasia):**
  - Dysplastic cells present in 75-90% of epithelium

---

6. Write briefly on:

a. Silicosis

(Ref: Harsh Mohan, 7th ed. pg. 470, Robbins, SA ed. pg. 688)

ANSWER

Silicosis

Introduction

- Type of pneumoconiosis caused by prolonged inhalation of silica (silicon dioxide)
- Occurs in persons engaged in occupations which has exposure to siliceous rocks or sand and products manufactured from them such as
  - Miners (granite, sandstone, slate, coal, gold, tin and copper)
  - Quarry workers
  - Tunnellers
  - Sandblasters
  - Grinders
  - Ceramic workers
  - Foundry workers
  - Manufacture of abrasives containing silica

Clinical Picture

- Dyspnea
- Obstructive or restrictive pattern of disease may develop
- Complications such as
  - Pulmonary tuberculosis
  - Rheumatoid arthritis
  - Cor pulmonale

Pathogenesis

- Silica particles (0.5-5 microm) taken by macrophages as they reached alveoli and undergo necrosis

- New macrophages surround debris and repetitive cycle of phagocytosis and necrosis goes on
- Some silica-laden macrophages are carried to respiratory bronchioles, alveoli and in interstitial tissue
- While some are transported to subpleural and interlobar lymphatics and into regional lymph nodes
- Cellular aggregates containing silica are associated with lymphocytes, plasma cells, mast cells and fibroblasts
- Silica dust is fibrogenic, crystalline form is more fibrogenic than non-crystalline form
- Activation of T and B lymphocytes
- As silica is cytotoxic, it kills macrophages which surround it

Morphologic Features

- **Gross appearance:**
  - Chronic silicotic lung is embossed with well circumscribed, hard, fibrotic nodules – 1 to 5 mm in diameter which are dispersed throughout the lung parenchyma but more commonly located in upper regions of the lungs
  - Gross thickness and adherence of pleura to the chest wall
  - Ischemic necrosis and cavitation of lesions which may get complicated by tuberculosis and rheumatoid pneumoconiosis
- **Microscopic examination:**
  - Silicotic nodules in the region of respiratory bronchioles, adjacent alveoli, pulmonary arteries, in the pleura and the regional lymph nodes
  - They comprise of central hyalinized material with scanty cellularity and some amount of dust
  - Hyalinized center is encircled by concentric laminations of collagen which in turn is enclosed by more cellular connective tissue, dust filled macrophages and a few lymphocytes and plasma cells
  - Collagenous nodules present with cleft like spaces between the lamellae of collagen which on examination polariscopically may exhibit numerous birefringent particles of silica
  - Coalescence of adjacent nodules is seen in severe and progressive form of disease
  - Emphysema or hyperinflation of intervening lung parechyma

b. Hypersplenism

(Ref: Textbook of Pathology, Harsh Mohan, 7th ed. pg. 367)

ANSWER

Hypersplenism

- Characterized by excessive removal of erythrocytes, granulocytes or platelets from the circulation resulting in pancytopenia
- Due to increased sequestration of cells in the spleen or by antibody formation against respective blood cells
- Hypersplenism criteria:
  - Splenic destruction of cells in the peripheral blood
  - Splenomegaly
  - Normal or hyperplastic bone marrow cellularity

Splenomegaly

- Spleen enlargement is known as splenomegly
- May be mild, moderate or severe
- **Mild enlargement(up to 5cm):** Mainly seen in typhoid, acute malaria, SLE, bacterial endocarditis, etc.
- **Moderate enlargement (upto umbilicus):** present in lymphomas, cirrhosis, hepatitis, amyloidosis, etc.
- **Severe enlargement (below umbilicus):** present in CML, storage diseases, thalassaemia major, chronic malaria, etc.

Causes of Splenomegaly

Factors responsible for splenomegaly as follows:

- **Infective**
  - Bacterial:
    - Typhoid
    - Typhus
    - Tuberculosis
    - Septecaemia
    - Abscess
  - Viral:
    - Glandular fever (infectious mononucleosis)
  - Spirochaetal:
    - Syphillis
    - Leptospirosis
  - Protozoal:
    - Malaria.
  - Parasitic:
    - Hydatid cyst.
- **Inflammatory**
  - Rheumatoid arthritis
  - Sarcoidosis
  - Lupus
  - Amyloid
- **Neoplastic**
  - Leukemia
  - Lymphoma
  - Polycythemia vera
  - Myelofibrosis

- Hemolytic disease
  - Hereditary spherocytosis
  - Acquired hemolytic anemia
  - Thromocytopenic purpura
- **Storage Diseases**
  - Gaucher's disease
  - Niemann-Pick disease
- **Deficiency Diseases:**
  - Pernicious anemia
  - Severe iron deficiency anemia.
- **Splenic vein hypertension**
  - Cirrhosis
  - Splenic vein thrombosis
  - Portal vein thrombosis
- **Non-Parasitic cysts.**

c. **Familial adenomatous polyposis coli**

(Ref: Textbook of Pathology, Harsh Mohan, 7th ed. pg. 569)

ANSWER

Familial Adenomatous Polyposis Coli

Introduction

- Familial polyposis syndromes are group of disorders with multiple polyposis of the colon having autosomal dominant inheritance pattern which includes
  - Familial polyposis coli (adenomatosis)
  - Gardener's syndrome
  - Turcot's syndrome
  - Juvenile polyposis syndrome

Familial Polyposis Coli (Adenomatosis)

- Hereditary disease with presence of more than 100 neoplastic polyps (adenomas) on the mucosal surface of the colon
- Average number of neoplastic polyps are 1000
- Can be distinguished from multiple adenomas where number of adenomas does not exceed 100
- Occurs at 2nd -3rd decades of life
- Incidence–equally occurs in both sexes
- Has high malignant potential
- Colorectal cancer develops in 100% cases by 50 years of age if left untreated with colectomy

Causes

- Autosomal dominant transmission due to germline mutations in APC gene leading to occurrence of hundreds of adenomas progressing to invasive cancer

Morphologic Features

- Grossly and microscopically,
  - Commonest pattern of appearance is that of adenomatous polyps

Name of the Paper : **Pathology Paper-I**

Name of the Course : **MBBS-201I**

Semester : **Annual**

Time: 3 Hours   M.M.: 40

INSTRUCTIONS

1. Write your Roll No. on the top immediately on receipt of this question paper
2. All questions are to be attempted
3. Answers to Parts I, II and III should be written in separate answer sheets provided
4. Attempt parts of a question in sequence

PART-I

1. **Differentiate between:**   [8]
   a. Healing by primary and secondary intention
   b. Dysplasia and metaplasia
   c. Normoblast and megaloblast
   d. Granulation tissue and granuloma

2. **Write briefly on:**   [6]
   a. Pathogenesis of septic shock
   b. Chemical carcinogenesis
   c. Pancytopenia

PART-II

3. **Write briefly on:**   [6]
   a. Classification of Hemolytic anaemia and laboratory diagnosis of Beta-Thalassemia major
   b. Modes of spread of Tumours with suitable examples

4. **Write briefly on:**   [6]
   a. WHO classification of Acute Myelogenous Leukemia and laboratory diagnosis of Acute Promyelocytic Leukemia
   b. Immune Thrombocytopoenic Purpura (ITP)

PART-III

5. **Comment on:**   [8]
   a. CSF findings in acute pyogenic meningitis
   b. Reticulocyte
   c. Mechanisms of autoimmune disorder
   d. Turner Syndrome

6. **Comment on:**   [6]
   a. Von Willibrand disease
   b. Chemotaxis
   c. Pulmonary embolism

PART-I

1. Differentiate between:

a. Healing by primary and secondary intention

(Ref: Textbook of Pathology, Harsh Mohan, 7th ed. pg. 158)

ANSWER

Features	Healing by primary intention	Healing by secondary intention
• Tissue injury	• Limited to superficial layer of epithelium and connective tissue	• Extensive
• Site	• Clean, uninfected surgical incision	• Natural/ open wounds like abscess, inflammation etc.
• Scarring	• Less	• More
• Wound contraction	• Not present	• Present (characteristic of large surface wounds)
• Granulation tissue	• Formed but in less amount	• Formation in large amount

b. Dysplasia and metaplasia

(Ref: Harsh Mohan, 7th ed. pg. 41, Robbins, SA ed. pg. 270-71)

ANSWER

Metaplasia	Dysplasia
Change of one type of epithelial or mesenchymal cell to another type of adult epithelial or mesenchymal cell	Disordered cellular development
Epithelial and mesenchymal types	Only epithelial
Cellular development is mature	Disordered cellular development (loss of polarity, pleomorphism, mitosis, etc)
Bronchial mucosa, mesenchymal tissues like-cartilage, arteries, etc. are commonly affected	Bronchial mucosa, uterine cervix commonly affected

c. Normoblast and megaloblast

(Ref: Harsh Mohan, 7th ed. pg. 265–283, Robbins, SA ed. pg. 632)

ANSWER

For answer, refer 2015 paper-I Q. 1 (a), Pg. 51

d. Granulation tissue and Granuloma

(Ref: Harsh Mohan, 7th ed. pg. 135–159, Robbins, SA ed. pg. 99, 98, 103)

ANSWER

For answer, refer 2015 paper-I Q. 1 (d), Pg. 51

2. Write briefly on:

a. Pathogenesis of septic shock

(Ref: Harsh Mohan, 7th ed. pg. 96, Robbins, SA ed. pg. 131-133)

ANSWER

For answer, refer 2016 paper-I Q. 3 (a), Pg. 29 and 2015 paper-I Q. 4 (b), Pg. 56

b. Chemical carcinogenesis

(Ref: Textbook of Pathology, Harsh Mohan, 7th ed. pg. 210)

ANSWER

For answer, refer 2017 paper-I Q. 2 (c), Pg. 6

c. Pancytopenia

(Ref: Textbook of Pathology, Harsh Mohan, 7th ed. pg. 301)

ANSWER

For answer, refer 2014, paper-I Q. 6 (a), Pg. 74

PART-II

3. Write briefly on:

a. Classification of Hemolytic anemia and laboratory diagnosis of Beta-Thalassemia major

(Ref: Harsh Mohan, 7th ed. pg. 287–298, Robbins, SA ed. pg. 630, 638-641)

ANSWER

Classification of Hemolytic Anemia

Introduction

○ Hemolytic anemia due to increased red cell destruction either exrtravascular or intravascular

○ Generally classified into acquired hemolytic anemia (extracorpuscular) or hereditary hemolytic anemia (intracorpuscular)

Intracorpuscular Abnormalities

Hereditary

○ Red cell membrane disorders
  ▪ Spherocytosis, elliptocytosis,
  ▪ Lipid synthesis disorder
    Increase in membrane lecithin
○ Red cell enzyme deficiency:
  Pyruvate kinase, hexokinase
  G6PD, glutathione synthetase
○ Disorders of hemoglobin synthesis
  ▪ Deficient globin synthesis:
  ▪ Thalassemia syndrome
  ▪ Structural abnormality of globin chain (hemoglobinopathies):
  ▪ Sickle cell anemia

Extrinsic/extracorpuscular abnormalities Acquired

○ Antibodies mediated
  ▪ Isohemagglutinins
    ♦ Transfusion reaction
    ♦ Erythroblastosis fetalis
  ▪ Autoantiobodies
    ♦ Idiopathic, SLE, drug associated
    ♦ Malignant neoplasm
○ Mechanical trauma to red cells
  ▪ Microangiopathic hemolytic anemia (MAHA)
    ♦ Thrombotic thrombocytopenic purpura (TTP)
    ♦ DIC
  ▪ Cardiac traumatic hemolytic anemia
○ Infection
  Malarial, bacterial infection (Sepsis)
○ Chemical injury
  Lead poisoning
○ Sequestration in mononuclear phagocyte system
  Membrane defect: PNH
  Hypersplenism splenomegaly

Laboratory Diagnosis of Beta-thalassemia Major

β-thalassaemia Major

  ▪ **CBC:**
    ♦ Severe anemia (Hb: 3-6gm/dl)
    ♦ **MCH, MCV, MCHC:** decreased
    ♦ **Hematocrit:** decreased (severely)
    ♦ **WBC:** Raised (usually), shift of left of neutrophil series with presence of some myelocytes and metamyelocytes
  ▪ **Peripheral blood smear:**
    ♦ Severe microcytic hypochromic red cell

  ♦ Marked anisopoikilocytosis
  ♦ Target cells
  ♦ Tear drop cells
  ♦ Basophilic stippling
  ♦ Cells with Cabot's ring
  ♦ Pencil cells
  ♦ Nucleated RBC's
  ▪ **Hemoglobin electrophoresis:**
    ♦ Increased HbF
    ♦ Increased HbA_2
    ♦ HbA–absent or sometimes present in variable amounts
  ▪ **Bone marrow findings:**
    ♦ Normoblastic erythroid hyperplasia
    ♦ Intermediate and late normoblast predominant (smaller in size)
    ♦ Siderotic granules in the cytoplasm of normoblasts
    ♦ Increased reticuloendothelial iron
  ▪ **Biochemical findings:**
    ♦ **Serum bilirubin(unconjugated):** Increased
    ♦ **Serum iron:** Increased
    ♦ **Urine urobilinogen:** Increased
    ♦ **Serum ferritin:** Increased(300-3000 mg/dl)
  ▪ **Osmotic fragility:** Decreased

b. **Modes of spread of tumors with suitable examples**

(Ref: Textbook of Pathology, Harsh Mohan, 7th ed. pg. 193–195)

ANSWER

For answer, refer 2016 paper-I Q. 2 (c), Pg. 28

4. **Write briefly on:**

a. **WHO classification of Acute Myelogenous Leukemia and Laboratory Diagnosis of Acute promyelocytic leukaemia**

(Ref: Harsh Mohan, 7th ed. pg. 340, Robbins, SA ed. pg. 612-614)

ANSWER

WHO Classification of Acute Myelogenous Leukemia

○ **According to WHO:**
  ▪ Based on clinical, molecular and cytogenetic abnormalities AML is classified in to subtypes.
  ▪ Blasts count > 20% for diagnosis of AML

WHO Classification

○ AML with recurrent genetic abnormalities
  ▪ AML with t(8;21) (q22;q22)

- RUNX1-RUNX1T1
- AML with inv(16) (p13.1q22) or t916;16) (p13.1;p22); CBFB-MYH11
- Acute promyelocytic leukemia with t(15;17) (Q22;q12); PML-RARA
- AML with t(6.9)(q23;q34);DEK-NUP214
- AML(megakryoblastic) with t(1:22)(p13;q13); RBM15-MKL1
- Provisional AML with mutated CEBPA
○ AML with myelodysplasia-related changes
○ Therapy-related myeloid neoplasms
○ Acute myeloid leukemia, NOS
  - AML with minimal differentiation
  - AML without maturation
  - AML with maturation
  - Acute myelomonocytic leukemia
  - Acute myelomonocytic leukemia
  - Acute monoblastic and monocytic leukemia
  - Acute erythroid leukemia
  - Acute megakaryoblastic leukemia
  - Acute panmyelosis with myelofibrosis
  - Myeloid sarcoma
  - Myeloid proliferations related to Down syndrome
  - Transient abnormal myelopoiesis
  - Myeloid leukemia associated with Down syndrome
  - Blastic plasmacytoid dendritic cell neoplasm

Laboratory Diagnosis of Acute Promyelocytic Leukemia

Introduction

○ A subtype of acute myeloid leukemia
○ Classified as AML-M3 by FAB classification and acute promyelocytic leukemia with t(15;17) (q22;q12);PML-RARA in WHO classification

Laboratory Findings

○ **Bone Marrow examination:**
  - Abnormal promyelocytes (blasts may be <20%), packed with granules, numerous Auer rods (Hypergranular variant).
○ **Cytogenetics:**
  - APL with t(15;17)(q22;q12)
○ **Cytochemistry:**
  - MPO +++ positive
○ **Coagulation abnormality:** disseminated intravascular coagulation
○ **Anti-PML Immunofluorescent Antibody Test (POD Test):**
  - Rapidly performed, within 3-4 hours.
  - Cytogenetic and molecular testing is not required
  - Approx. 99% specific and sensitive.

b. **Immune Thrombocytopenic Purpura (ITP)**

(Ref: Textbook of Pathology, Harsh Mohan, 7th ed. pg. 311)

ANSWER

For answer, refer 2012 paper-I Q. 5 (c), Pg. 106

PART-III

5. **Comment on:**

a. **CSF findings in acute pyogenic meningitis**

(Ref: Harsh Mohan, 7th ed. pg. 867, Robbins, SA ed. pg. 1272)

ANSWER

Introduction

○ Acute pyogenic meningitis is acute infection of the pia-arachnoid and cerebrospinal fluid within the subarachnoid space.

CSF Findings

○ Increased CSF pressure (above 180 mm Hg)
○ Turbid or frankly purulent CSF- due to pus accumulation in subarachnoid space
○ Protein content: Markedly increased (more than 50 mg/dl)
○ Polymorphonuclear leukocytosis (10-10000/µl)
○ Glucose content: decreased(below 40 mg/dl)
○ Oligoclonal band: may be positive
○ Bacteriologic examination: Gram staining or culture of CSF shows causative organism .

b. **Reticulocyte**

(Ref: Textbook of Pathology, Harsh Mohan, 7th ed. pg. 265)

ANSWER

Reticulocyte

Introduction

○ Reticulocytes are newly formed RBC's released from bone marrow
○ Don't contain nuclei but can synthesize hemoglobin due to presence of ribosomal RNA
○ Normally present in the peripheral blood

Staining Characteristics

○ Can be stained with vital dyes like–new methylene blue, brilliant cresyl blue, Pure azure B–demonstrate deep blue reticulofilamentous material
○ Wright stain: polychromatophilic appearance of reticulocytes
○ **Normal range:**
  - 0.5-2.50 % (adults)
  - 2-6% (infants)

- **Estimation of Reticulocyte count:**
  - Reticulocyte maturation index/Immature reticulocyte fraction
  - Mean reticulocyte volume
  - Reticulocyte hemoglobin equivalent/ Reticulocyte hemoglobin concentration
- **Increased reticulocyte count:**
  - Intravascular hemolysis
  - Hemoglobinopathy
  - Autoimmune defect
  - Blood loss, metabolic defect, etc.
- **Decreased reticulocyte count:**
  - Iron deficiency
  - Marrow damage: infiltration, aplasia
  - Thalassemia
  - Sideroblastic anemia
  - Drug toxicity, etc.

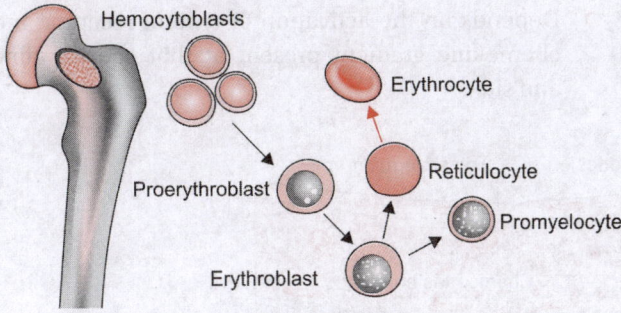

c. Mechanisms of autoimmune disorder

(Ref: Harsh Mohan, 7th ed. pg. 62, Robbins, SA ed. pg. 217)

ANSWER

Introduction

- Breakdown in the immune tolerance of the body causes "autoimmunity".

Factors Responsible for Autoimmunity/Autoimmune Diseases

- **Polyclonal lymphocytes activation:** Activation of CD4+ cells (stimulation of large number of T cells)
- **Activity of suppressor and helper T cells:** Decreased activity of suppressor T cell and increased activity of helper T cells leads to auto immunity
- Damage due to cross-reacting foreign antigens or due to cross-reacting antigens present on infection causing microorganism
- Release of sequestered or hidden antigens. For example- completely sequestered ocular antigen during development, if come in contact with systemic circulation act as foreign body and leads to immunologic response

- Certain genetic factors like increased expression of class II HLA antigens is also responsible autoimmunity.
- Certain infections mainly with viruses, (for example- EBV), bacteria(not common) may trigger the mechanism of autoimmunity

d. Turner Syndrome

(Ref: Harsh Mohan, 7th ed. pg. 253, Robbins, SA ed. pg. 166-167)

ANSWER

For answer, refer 2016 paper-I Q. 5 (b), Pg. 33

6. Comment on:

a. Von Willibrand disease

(Ref: Harsh Mohan, 7th ed. pg. 314, Robbins, SA ed. pg. 662, 665)

ANSWER

Introduction

- Most common hereditary coagulation disorder
- Result due to qualitative or quantitative defect in von Willebrand's factor (Vwf)
- Also known as "angiohemophilia", "pseudohemophilia"

Synthesis of Von Willebrand Factor (vWF)

- Endothelial ccells
  - Platelets
  - Megakarayocytes

Function of von Willebrand Factor (vWF)

- Adhesion of platelet to subendothelial collagen

Clinical Features

- Mucosal and cutaneous bleeding, GIT bleeding, etc.
- Hemarthroses, intramuscular hematoma

Types

Three types

- **Type I:**
  - Most common
  - Mild to moderate deficiency of vWF(approx. 50%)
- **Type II:**
  - Less common
  - Functional/qualitative defect in vWF
- **Type III:**
  - Most severe form
  - Inherited as Autosomal recessive trait

Laboratory Diagnosis

- Normal PT and TT

- Prolonged BT
- Prolonged apt
- Ristocetin (antibiotic), platelet aggregation test defective
- Decreased factor VIII activity
- **Serum electrophoresis:** vWF multimers reduced in type 1and 3

Treatment

- Desmopressin–sudden rise in vWF and factor VIII
- FFP (Fresh frozen plasma)

b.   Chemotaxis

(Ref: Harsh Mohan, 7th ed. pg. 120, Robbins, SA ed. pg. 77-78)

ANSWER

Introduction

- Process of migration of leukocytes after crossing several barriers like endothelium, basement membrane, etc. towards the site of injury is known as chemotaxis
- A chemotactic- factor mediated process.

Chemotactic Agents

- Cytokines (interleukins, mainly IL-8)
- Leukotriene B4
- Complement system components(C5a and C3a)
- Soluble bacterial products

Mechanism

- Chemotactic agents bind to specific receptors (seven–transmembrane G protein coupled receptor) present on the leukocyte cell surface.
- It results in induction of signals and thus, activation of second messenger
- As a result, migration of leukocytes towards inflammatory stimulus occur.
- During early stage of inflammation -predominance of neutrophils but in later stages replaced by monocytes and macrophages

Direction of Movement

- Depends on the activation of type of receptor and chemokine gradient present at that specific time and site

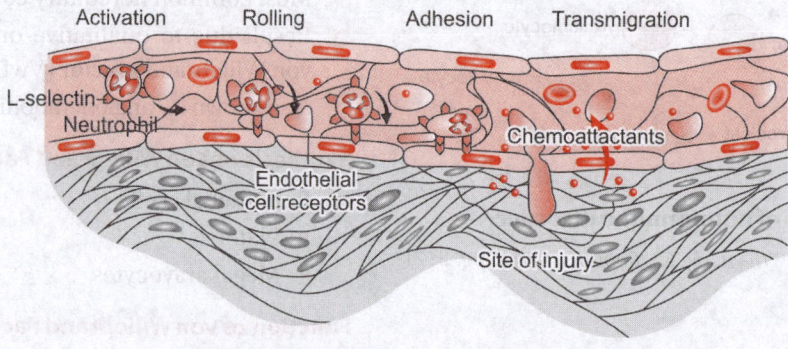

Fig. Chemotaxis mechanism

c.   Pulmonary embolism

(Ref: Harsh Mohan, 7th ed. pg. 106, Robbins, SA ed. pg. 127)

ANSWER

Introduction

- Most common and fatal form of thromboembolism resulting in occlusion of pulmonary artery and its branches
- Commonly seen in bed-ridden or hospitalized patients

Etiology

- Deep vein thrombosis (large vein of lower legs)- most common

- Thrombi in superficial veins of the legs, pelvis–less common

Pathogenesis

- Thrombus from its origin gets detached and is carried to right side of the heart through venous channel and enters into pulmonary circulation
- Large thrombus get lodged at the bifurcation of main pulmonary artery (saddle embolus) or may lodge in right ventricle or its outflow tract
- Multiple emboli lodges and occlude small pulmonary vessels
- Paradoxical emboli: passage of emboli through atrial or ventricular septal defects from right side to left side of the heart and thus enter into systemic circulation

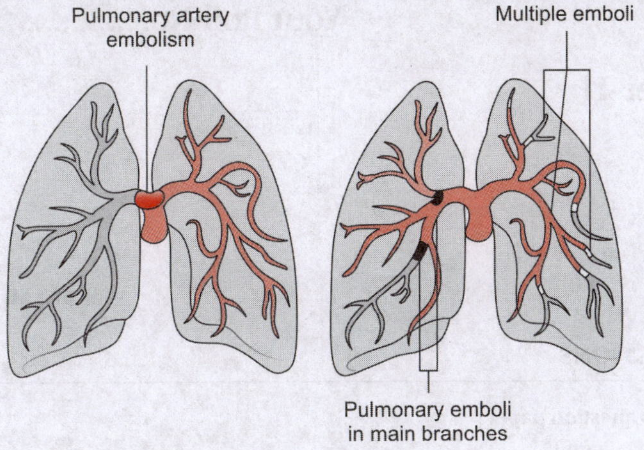

Pulmonary artery embolism

Multiple emboli

Pulmonary emboli in main branches

Consequences/Effects

○ Depends on–
- Size of the occluded vessel
- Number of emboli
- Cardiovascular status of patient

○ Consequences as follows-
- Sudden death
- Pulmonary infarction
- Acute cor pulmonale
- Pulmonary hemorrhage
- Pulmonary hypertension
- Chronic cor pulmonale and pulmonary aeteriosclerosis

Your Roll No. ....

Name of the Paper	:	Pathology Paper-II
Name of the Course	:	MBBS-2011
Semester	:	Annual

Time: 3 Hours   M.M.: 40

INSTRUCTIONS

1. Write your Roll No. on the top immediately on receipt of this question paper
2. All questions are to be attempted
3. Answers to Parts I, II and III should be written in separate answer sheets provided
4. Attempt parts of a question in sequence

PART-I

1. Differentiate between: [8]
   a. Benign and Malignant Gastric ulcer
   b. CSF findings in Viral and Tubercular meningitis
   c. Hepatitis A and Hepatitis B
   d. Amoebic and Ulcerative colitis

2. Write short notes on: [6]
   a. Primary Pulmonary Tuberculosis
   b. Multinodular Goitre
   c. Asbestosis Lung

PART-II

3. Write briefly on: [6]
   a. Etipopathogenesis of Colorectal Carcinoma
   b. Rapidly progressive Glomerulonephritis

4. Write briefly on: [6]
   a. Etiopathogenesis of Ischaemic Heart Disease
   b. Morphology of Alcoholic Liver Disease

PART-III

5. Write briefly on: [8]
   a. Advanced Glycosylation end products
   b. Chronic pyelonephritis
   c. Teratoma ovary
   d. Osteogenic sarcoma

6. Write briefly on: [6]
   a. Burkitt Lymphoma
   b. Fibrocystic disease of Breast
   c. Morphology and complications of Atheromatous plaque

PART-I

1. Differentiate between:

a. Benign and Malignant Gastric ulcer

(Ref: Textbook of Pathology, Harsh Mohan, 7th ed. pg. 543)

ANSWER

For answer, refer 2014 paper-II Q. 1 (a), Pg. 77

b CSF findings in Viral and Tubercular meningitis

(Ref: Textbook of Pathology, Harsh Mohan, 7th ed. pg. 868)

ANSWER

Viral meningitis	Tubercular meningitis
• Slightly turbid or clear appearance of CSF	• Appearance of CSF clear or slightly turbid but on standing, formation of fibrin web or coagulum is seen
• Protein content is slightly increased	• Increased protein content
• Normal glucose level	• Decreased glucose level
• Presence of 10-100 lymphocytes/μl	• Presence of 100-1000 lymphocytes/μl
• Increased CSF pressure(more than 250mm water)	• More than 300mm water of CSF pressure
• Causative organism not present	• Causative organism Tubercle bacilli present

c. Hepatitis A and Hepatitis B

(Ref: Harsh Mohan, 7th ed. pg. 591, Robbins, SA ed. pg. 831-833)

ANSWER

For answer, refer 2013 paper-II Q. 1 (d), Pg. 94

d. Amoebic and Ulcerative colitis

(Ref: Harsh Mohan, 7th ed. pg. 550–555, Robbins, SA ed. pg. 800, 801)

ANSWER

Amoebic colitis	Ulcerative colitis
• Common in children but can be seen at any age	• Peak incidence is between 20-25 years
• Flask shaped ulcer intervened with normal mucosa	• Ulcer with broad base and continuous lesion without normal mucosa in between
• No pseudopolyps	• Pseudopolyps present
• Extend deep upto muscularis propria or may be superficial	• Mainly superficial, limited to mucosa and submucosa
• Morphologically exhibits liquefactive necrosis with few inflammatory cells	• Morphologically revels crypt abscess along with infiltration of mononuclear leucocytes

2. Write short notes on:

a. Primary Pulmonary Tuberculosis

(Ref: Harsh Mohan, 7th ed. pg. 142, Robbins, SA ed. pg. 373)

ANSWER

For answer, refer 2016, paper-I Q. 5 (d), Pg. 34

b. Multinodular Goitre

(Ref: Harsh Mohan, 7th ed. pg. 48, Robbins, SA ed. pg. 1091-1092)

ANSWER

For answer, refer 2014 Paper-II Q. 2 (a), Pg. 77

c. Asbestosis Lung

(Ref: Harsh Mohan, 7th ed. pg. 437, Robbins, SA ed. pg. 690-692)

ANSWER

For answer, refer 2017 Paper-II Q. 6 (c), Pg. 25

PART II

3. Write briefly on:

a. Etiopathogenesis of Colorectal Carcinoma

(Ref: Harsh Mohan, 7th ed. pg. 570, Robbins, SA ed. pg. 448)

ANSWER

Introduction
- Colorectal carcinoma is the most common form of visceral carcinoma
- Affects caecum, colon and rectum

Etiology
- **Dietary Factors:**
  - Poor diet (high intake of refined carbohydrates, decreased intake of antioxidants, low fibers)
  - High intake of red meat (high cholesterol)

- ○ **Geographic Factors:**
  - ▪ Common in North Americans and North Europe than Asians, South Americans
- ○ **Adenoma-carcinoma sequence:**
  - ▪ Pre-existing adenoma is responsible for colonic adenocarcinoma
  - ▪ Certain factors that are responsible for increased risk of malignancy are:
    - ◆ **Size of adenomas:** Increased risk with large size adenoma
    - ◆ **Number of adenoma:** Familial polyposis coli syndrome
    - ◆ **Types:** Increased prevalence with more number of villous component
- ○ **Lynch syndrome (Hereditary non-polyposis colonic cancer):**
  - ▪ Autosomal dominant condition
  - ▪ In HNPCC, colorectal cancer is located at proximal colon commonly and shows better prognosis
  - ▪ Due to mutation in mismatch repair gene, human mutL homolog gene located on chromosome 2 and hMLH1 present on chromosome 3 causing DNA instability
- ○ **Other factors:**
  - ▪ Age- more than 50 yrs
  - ▪ Ulcerative colitis and chron's disease (more common in ulcerative colitis)

- ▪ Smoking
- ▪ Diabetes mellitus, acromegaly

Molecular Mechanism Involved in Colorectal Cancer

- ○ **Microsatellite instability pathway:**
  - ▪ **Responsible for only 10-15% cases of colonic cancer**
  - ▪ Mutation in DNA repair gene results in microsatellite instability and DNA repair genes that undergo mutation are TGF-β (mutation reesluts in uncontrolled proliferation of colonic epithelium) and BAX gene (defect causes loss of apoptosis and disregulation of growth)
- ○ **APC mutation/β- catenin mechanism:**
  - ▪ Mutation in oncogenes and antioncogenes results in chromosomal instability

Loss of APC gene located on long arm of chromosome 5 (5q)
↓
Mutation of K-RAS gene
↓
Loss of DCC gene located on long arm of chromosome 18 (18q)
↓
Loss of p53 gene on chromosome 17p

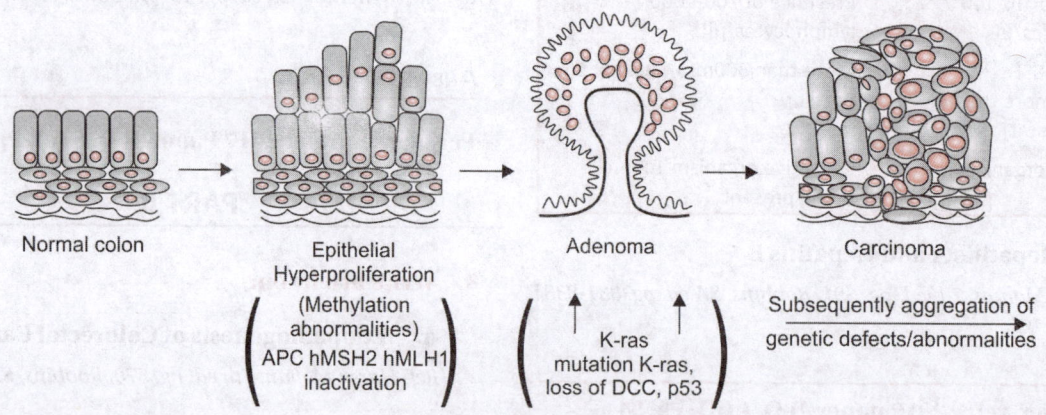

Fig. Mechanism involved in colorectal carcinoma

Normal colon → Epithelial Hyperproliferation (Methylation abnormalities) APC hMSH2 hMLH1 inactivation → Adenoma (K-ras mutation K-ras, loss of DCC, p53) → Carcinoma (Subsequently aggregation of genetic defects/abnormalities)

Clinical Features

- ○ **Location:**
  - ▪ Mostly rectum is involved (60% cases)
  - ▪ Sigmoid and descending colon (25%)
  - ▪ Caecum and ileocaecal valve (10%)
  - ▪ Asceding colon, splenic and hepatic flexures (5%)
  - ▪ Transverse colon is rarely involved

Right-sided growth of colorectal carcinoma	Left-sided growth of colorectal carcinoma
• Involves caecum and ascending colon	• Involves descending colon commonly
• Presents with weakness, fatigue, bleeding and iron deficiency anemia	• Melena, diarrhea, constipation, occult bleeding, change in bowel habits are present
• Grossly, exhibits large, cauliflower-like friable • mass that projects into lumen –"fungating polypoid carcinoma"	• Grossly, presents with "napkin-ring configuration- bowel wall encircled with fibrous tissue forming annular ring with central ulceration and slightly elevated margins
• Presents with good prognosis	• Prognosis is poor

○ **Difference between the right and left side growth is due to:**
- Contents present in ascending colon exhibits liquid nature that provides space for luminal growth on right side
- Contents present on left side presents with solid nature thus resulting growth into bowel wall

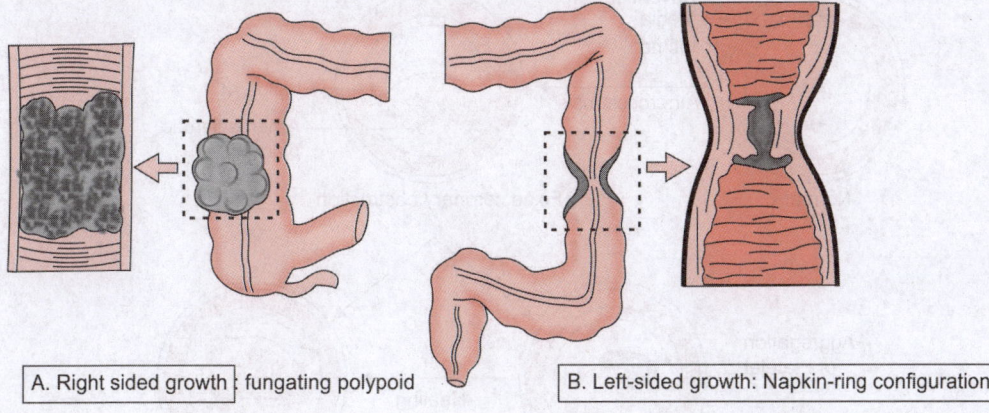

A. Right sided growth : fungating polypoid   B. Left-sided growth: Napkin-ring configuration

Microscopic Findings

○ Most of the colorectal cancers are adenocarcinomas (approx. 95%)

○ Undifferentiated carcinomas, signet ring cell carcinoma and adenosquamous carcinomas commonly seen in distal colon (approx. 5%)

○ Degree of differentiation may range from well- differentiated, to moderately differentiated and poorly differentiated

○ Secretion of mucin may be present

Complications

○ Obstruction
○ Hemorrhage
○ Secondry infection
○ Perforation

Diagnosis

○ Stool test- for occult blood
○ Proctoscopy
○ PR examination
○ CT scan and radiographic contrast studies
○ Tumor Marker- Estimation of CEA (100 % raised in metastatic colorectal cancer, 60-70% in advanced primary lesion)

Prognosis

○ Depends on-
- Metastases presence or absence

- Extent of involvement
- Location of tumor
- Histologic grade of the tumor

b. Rapidly progressive glomerulonephritis

(Ref: Harsh Mohan, 7th ed. pg. 654, Robbins, SA ed. pg. 912-913)

ANSWER

For answer, refer 2017 paper-II Q. 6 (a), Pg. 23

4. **Write briefly on:**

a. Etiopathogenesis of Ischemic Heart Disease

(Ref: Harsh Mohan, 7th ed. pg. 407, Robbins, SA ed. pg. 538, 539)

Introduction

○ IHD occur as a result of imbalance in between supply and demand of oxygenated blood in the heart

Etiopathogenesis

Mainly consists of-

○ **Coronary atherosclerosis:**
- Causes obstruction (90%)
- Most common cause of IHD
- Anterior descending branch of left descending artery (LAD) most commonly involved followed by RCA and CXA

- Commonly involved areas- bifurcation (at or near) of arteries, coronary ostia (approx. 3-4 cm away)
○ **Acute plaque changes:**
  - As a result of tachycardia, spasm, hypercholesterolemia, etc.
○ Platelet aggregation and spasm of coronary artery
○ Thrombosis of coronary artery: responsible for acute myocardial infarction
○ **Other causes:**
  - Embolism

- Vasospasm
- Arteritis
- Trauma
- Aneurysm
- Thrombotic disease, etc.

Pathogenesis

○ Reduced coronary blood as compared to myocardial demand as a result of atherosclerotic narrowing of coronary arteries, thrombosis, aggregation of platelets and vasospasm

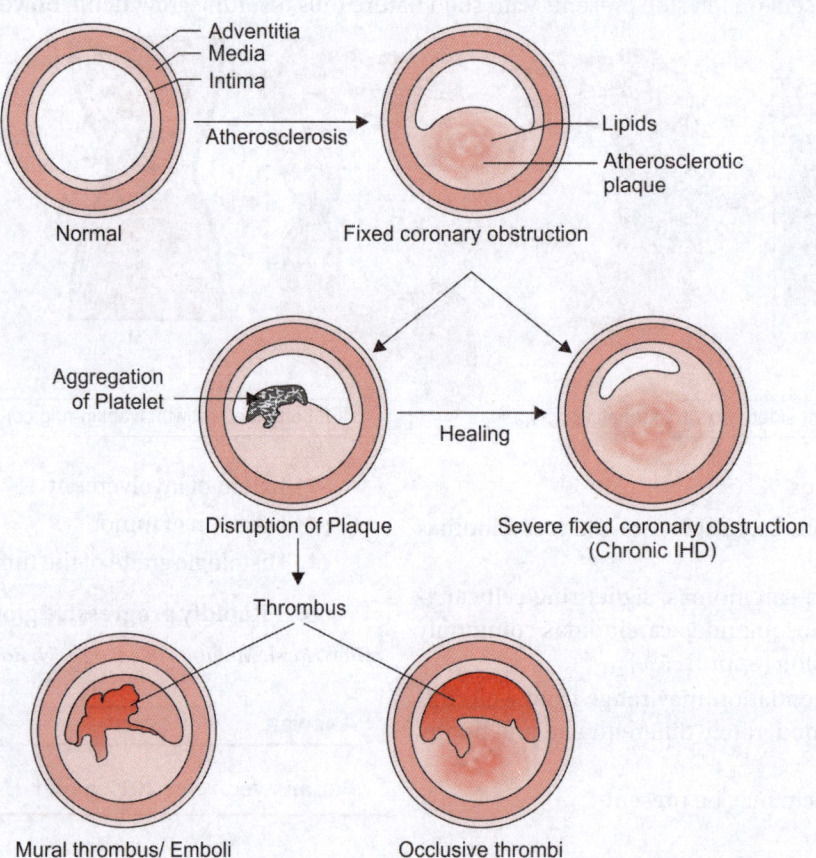

b. Morphology of Alcoholic Liver Disease

(Ref: Harsh Mohan, 7th ed. pg. 606, Robbins, SA ed. pg. 842-845)

ANSWER

Morphologic Features

Morphologically, it includes–alcoholic steatosis, alcoholic hepatitis, alcoholic cirrhosis

○ **Alcoholic steatosis:**
  - Grossly, liver is enlarged, yellow, firm with smooth capsule
  - **Microscopic findings:**
    ◆ Microvesicular and macrovesicular droplets of fat with peripheral displacement of nuclei

  ◆ Presence of fat cyst
  ◆ Lipogranulomas along with macrophages and giant cells may also present
○ **Alcoholic hepatitis:**
  - Develops as a of result of heavy drinking
  - **Microscopic findings:**
    ◆ Hepatocytes exhibit ballooning degeneration and necrosis
    ◆ Presence of Mallory bodies: swollen hepatocytes exhibits perinuclear intracytoplasmic eosinophilic inclusions
    ◆ Inflammatory cell infiltrate along with pericellular and perivenular fibrosis giving a chickenwire-like appearance also called as " creeping collagenosis"

- Alcoholic cirrhosis:
  - Most common form (60–70%)
  - Also known as Laennec's cirrhosis, portal cirrhosis, hobnail cirrhosis, micronodular cirrhosis, nutritional cirrhosis, etc.
  - **Gross Appearance:**
    - Micronodular cirrhosis with large, fatty liver
    - Tawny-yellow in color
    - Diffuse nodularity with very less variation in size giving hobnail appearance.
  - **Microscopic findings:**
    - Presence of micronodules with no central veins
    - Thick, dense fibrous septa dividing parenchyma into nodules
    - Fibrous tissue exhibit bile duct proliferation with scant inflammatory cell infiltrate
    - Cytoplasmic accumulation of hemosiderin is also evident

PART III

5. Write briefly on:

a. Advanced glycation end products

ANSWER

For answer, refer 2017 paper-II Q. 5 (c), Pg. 22

b. Chronic Pyelonephritis

(Ref: Textbook of Pathology, Harsh Mohan, 7th ed. pg. 669)

ANSWER

Introduction

- It is a chronic tubulointerstitial disorder
- Characterized by chronic tubular inflammation and scarring
- most common cause of end stage renal disease

Types

Based on etiology, two types-

- **Obstructive pyelonephritis:**
  - Urine outflow obstruction at different levels results in kidney infection
  - Can be bilateral (Urinary tract obstruction–posterior urethral valves) or unilateral (calculi and unilateral obstruction of ureter)
- **Reflux nephropathy:**
  - Reflux causes raised renal pelvis pressure followed by forceful accumulation of urine in the renal tubules thus resulting in damage to the kidney and scar formation

Clinical Features

- Slow onset
- Fever, loin pain, lumbar tenderness
- Dysuria, pyouria
- Bacteriuria
- Micturition frequency
- May show symptoms of hypertension and chronic renal failure

Gross Appearance

- Small and irregularly shrunken kidney
- U-shaped depression present on the cortical surface
- Dilatation of pelvis of the kidney and calyectasis

Microscopic Features

- Interstitial fibrosis along with chronic inflammatory cell infiltrate
- Atrophied and dilated tubules containing eosionphilic colloid cast (thyroidisationof tubules)
- Dilated renal pelvis and calyces
- Blood vessels are thick walled
- Glomeruli exhibits periglomerular fibrosis

c. Teratoma Ovary

(Ref: Harsh Mohan, 7th ed. pg. 735-737, Robbins, SA ed. pg. 1029)

ANSWER

Introduction

- Ovarian teratoma divided into 3 types:
  - Benign (mature) teratoma
  - Immature (malignant) teratoma
  - Specialized(monodermal) teratoma
- **Benign (mature) teratoma:**
  - Mostly benign and cystic
  - Common in young females
  - Develop from ectodermal differentiation of totipotent cells
  - **Morphological features:**
    - Unilocular cyst consisting of sebaceous secretion, hair masses along with areas of calcification and tooth structure
  - **Rokitansky protuberance:**
    - Inner lining of the cyst exhibiting prominence projecting from the wall towards the center of the cyst and contains tissue elements like-tooth, bone, cartilage, etc.
  - **Microscopic features:**
    - Lining of the cyst wall composed of stratified squamous epithelium and structures like sweat glands, sebaceous glands and hair follicles

○ **Immature (malignant) teratoma:**
  ▪ Occur in approx. 0.2% of all ovarian tumours (rare)
  ▪ Common in young females and prepubertal adolescents
  ▪ Commonly seen in under 20 yrs of age
  ▪ **Microscopic features:**
    ♦ Mostly composed of immature tissue
    ♦ Immature tissue- may differentiate into cartilage, bone, neural tissue, etc
    ♦ Immature neural tissue helps in determining the prognosis and histologic grading of tumor
○ **Specialized(monodermal) teratoma:**
  ▪ Rare entity
  ▪ **Examples**- struma ovarii and carcinoid tumor

  d. Osteogenic Sarcoma

(Ref: Harsh Mohan, 7th ed. pg. 832–835, Robbins, SA ed. pg. 1198-99)

ANSWER

For answer, refer 2017 paper-II Q. 3 (a), Pg. 19

6. Write briefly on:

  a. Burkitt Lymphoma

  (Ref: Harsh Mohan, 7th ed. pg. 357, Robbins, SA ed. pg. 597)

ANSWER

Introduction
○ High grade non- hodgkin's lymphoma
○ Rapidly progressive B cell tumor

Types
○ Non- endemic (sporadic) Burkitt lymphoma
○ Endemic (African) Burkitt lymphoma
○ HIV-associated aggressive lymphoma

Etioloy
○ EBV infection
○ Chromosomal translocation
○ Plasmodium falciparum infestation

Pathogenesis
○ Characterized by translocation of the c- myc gene on chromosome 8

Clinical Features
○ Common in children (mainly 4-8 yrs.) and young adults
○ Usually present at extranodal sites
○ Occur as mandibular mass- African type
○ Sporadic type- occur as abdominal mass involving peritoneum and ileocecal region

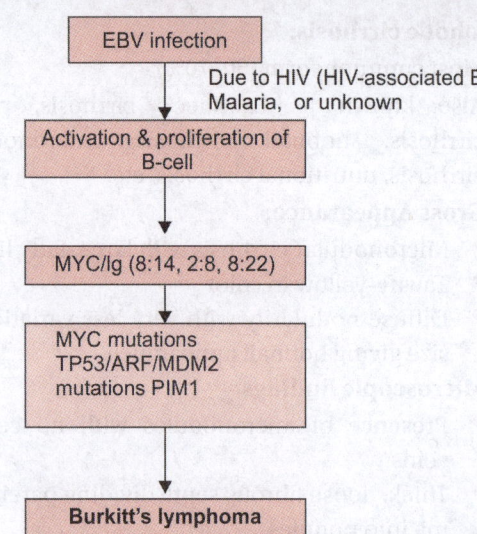

○ HIV-associated-common in bone marrow and lymph nodes
○ Nausea, vomiting, loss of appetite, GI bleeding, intestinal perforation, etc.

Microscopic Features
○ Tumor cells are intermediate in size with round, multiple nucleoli
○ Basophilic cytoplasm with lipid containing vacuoles
○ High mitotic rate and apoptotic death (presence of apoptotic cells)
○ Sheets of lymphocytes with interspersed macrophages containing tumor debris and surrounded by a clear space giving characteristic "starry sky" appearance

Investigations
○ **Cytology:**
  ▪ Cerebrospinal fluid, ascitic fluid, tumor aspirate are used for cytological analysis
○ **Radiology:**
  ▪ CT Scan
  ▪ Abdominal ultrasonography
○ **Others:**
  ▪ Serum electrolyte, urea, creatinine
  ▪ Serum LDH
  ▪ Serum uric acid, calcium, phosphate

  b. Fibrocystic Disease of Breast

  (Ref: Harsh Mohan, 7th ed. pg. 746, Robbins, SA ed. pg. 1048)

ANSWER

Introduction
○ Common benign condition of the breast that involves both epithelial and stromal component.
○ May be due to hormonal imbalance (increased estrogen and decreased progesterone)

Clinical Features

- **Incidence:** Common in 20-40 yrs of age, mainly in adult females
- Painful, tender swellings with defined edges
- Palpable lump
- Nipple discharge
- Calcification

Pathogenesis

Rupture of cyst → stromal tissue → inflammation and fibrosis → palpable, firm mass in the breast

Types

- Clinicopathologically divided into two types-
  - Nonproliferative changes (Simple fibrocystic change)
  - Proliferative changes (proliferative fibrocystic change)
- **Nonproliferative fibrocystic changes:**
  - Multiple and bilateral
  - Ranges from microcysts to 5-6 cm in diameter
  - Contains semi-transparent, turbid fluid giving brown to bluish color (blue-dome cyst)
  - **Microscopic Features:**
    - Formation of cyst with atrophied and flattened lining epithelium, apocrine metaplasia and increased fibrous stroma (fibrosis)
- **Proliferative fibrocystic changes:** Consists of
  - Epithelial hyperplasia:
    - Characterized by ductal hyperplasia and lobular hyperplasia
    - Ductal hyperplasia or epithelial hyperplasia may exhibit different grades of epithelial proliferations like – mild, moderate, severe
  - Sclerosing adenosis:
    - Charaacterized by benign proliferation of acini and intralobular fibrosis

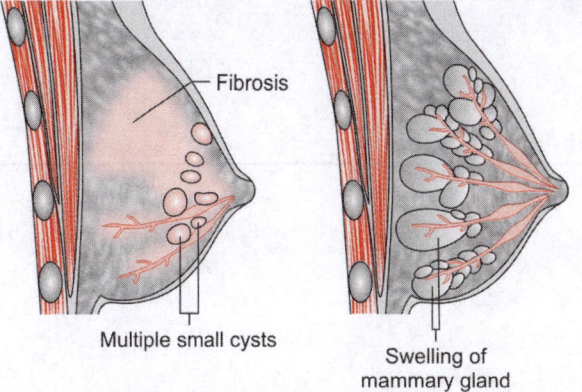

Fig. Fibrocystic breast changes

Multiple small cysts

Fibrosis

Swelling of mammary gland

c. **Morphology and complications of Atheromatous Plaque**

(Ref: Harsh Mohan, 7th ed. pg. 378, Robbins, SA ed. pg. 491)

ANSWER

Introduction

- Atherosclerotic lesion is known as atheromatous plaque
- Also known as "atheroma", fibrous plaque or "fibro-fatty plaque"
- Abdominal aorta is most commonly affected with major involvement of iliac, femoral, carotid, coronary and cerebral arteries

Morphological Features

- **Gross appearance:**
  - Yellowish-white in colour
  - small size(1-2 cm in diameter)
- Consists of white fibrous cap and a soft, yellow-white central core thus called as atheroma
- **Microscopic Findings:**
  - Central soft core composed of lipids, cholesterol clefts, foam cells, fibrin and cellular debris
  - White fibrous cap composed of smooth muscle cells, dense connective tissue and extracellular matrix composed of proteoglycans and collagen
  - Cellular area present below the fibrous cap composed of foam cells, macrophages, lymphocytes and lipid containing smooth muscle cells

Complications

- **Calcification:**
  - Common in advanced atheromatous plaque mainly aorta and coronaries
  - Microscopic findings revels calcium salt deposition in the necrotic areas and lipid pool present deep into the thick intima
- **Thrombosis:**
  - Areas of endothelial damage and ulcerated plaque are the common sites
  - May get dislodged and lodges elsewhere in the circulation
  - May lodge into the arterial wall as mural thrombi
- **Ulceration:**
  - As a result of mechanical trauma
  - Release of lipid material and debris into the blood stream from emboli
  - Resulting in shallow, ragged ulcer with lipid debris in the base of the ulcer
- **Hemorrhage:**
  - Common complication in coronary arteries
  - Intimal hemorrhage in the atheromatous plaque due to blood in the vascular lumen or due to rupture of thin walled capillaries
- **Formation of aneurysm:**
  - Thinning and atrophy of media, fibrosis of adventitia results in weakening of the arterial wall thus aneurysmal dilatation

PATHOLOGY

Name of the Paper : **Pathology Paper-I**

Name of the Course : **MBBS-2010**

Semester : **Annual**

Time: 3 Hours   M.M.: 40

INSTRUCTIONS

1. Write your Roll No. on the top immediately on receipt of this question paper
2. All questions are to be attempted
3. Answers to Parts I, II and III should be written in separate answer sheets provided
4. Attempt parts of a question in sequence

PART-I

1. **Differentiate between:**   [8]
   a. Transudate and exudate
   b. Apoptosis and necrosis
   c. Tuberculoid and lepromatous leprosy
   d. Hemophilia A and Von willebrand disease

2. **Comment briefly on**   [6]
   a. Special stains for amyloid
   b. Acute transplant rejection
   c. Hemolytic disease of newborn

PART-II

3. **Write briefly on:**   [6]
   a. Pathogenesis of renal edema
   b. Prognostic indicators of acute lymphoblastic leukemia

4. **Write briefly on:**   [6]
   a. Chemical carcinogenesis
   b. Laboratory diagnosis of CML

PART-III

5. **Write briefly on:**   [8]
   a. Phagocytosis
   b. Caisson's disease
   c. Primary complex
   d. Prothrombin time

6. **Write short notes on:**   [6]
   a. Bombay phenotype
   b. Kwashiorkor
   c. Clinicopathological features of sickle cell-anemia

PART-I

1. Differentiate between:

a. **Transudate and Exudate**

(Ref: Harsh Mohan, 7th ed. pg. 81, Robbins, SA ed. pg. 73)

ANSWER

Transudate and Exudate

For answer, refer 2017 paper-I, Q. 1 (b), Pg. 4

b. **Apoptosis and Necrosis**

(Ref: Harsh Mohan, 7th ed. pg. 31, Robbins, SA ed. pg. 15)

ANSWER

For answer, refer 2013 paper-I Q. 1 (b), Pg. 85

c. **Tuberculoid and Lepromatous Leprosy**

(Ref: Harsh Mohan, 7th ed. pg. 149, Robbins, SA ed. pg. 377-78)

ANSWER

For answer, refer 2015 paper-I Q. 1 (c), Pg. 51

d. **Hemophilia A and Von willebrand disease**

(Ref: Harsh Mohan, 7th ed. pg. 313–14, Robbins, SA ed. pg. 662-63)

ANSWER

Hemophilia A	Von willebrand disease
Deficiency of factor VIII	Qualitative or quantitative defect in von Willebrands's factor
X-linked recessive disorder	Inherited as an autosomal dominant trait
Defect in intrinsic pathway of coagulation	Defect in platelet aggregation and adhesion
Synthesis of factor VIII mainly in liver	Synthesis of vWF factor in endothelial cells, platelet cells and megakaryocytes
Bleeding time normal	Increased bleeding time
Petechiae absent	Petchiae present

2. Comment briefly on:

a. **Special stains for amyloid**

(Ref: Textbook of Pathology, Harsh Mohan, 7th ed. pg. 72)

ANSWER

Introduction

○ Pathological proteinaceous substance deposited between cells in various tissues and organs of the body in variety of diseases.

○ Consist of fibril material (95%) and remaining P component and other proteins

○ Categories of amyloid protein: Misfolded protein (production of abnormal amount of normal protein) and mutant protein (production of normal amount of mutant protein)

Stains for Amyloid

○ **Lugol's iodine:** Used on cut surface of a gross specimen or on frozen/paraffin section

○ **Hematoxylin and Eosin:** Appear as extracellular, homogeneous, structrueless eosinophilic hyaline material

Special Stains

○ **Congo red:** Pink red: Under ordinary light

Apple-green birefringence: under polarized light

○ **Metachromatic stain:** Methyl violet and crystal violet (rosaniline dye), rose-pink color to amyloid deposits

○ **Fluorescent stains:** Thioflavin T, fluorersces yellow under UV light

○ **Immunohistochemistry:** Most useful stain: anti AP stain

  ▪ For determination of biochemical type of amyloid: anti- AA, anti-lambda, anti-kappa, etc.

○ **Alcian blue:** impart blue color due to presence of glycosaminoglycans

○ **Periodic acid schiff (PAS):** Stains pink

○ **Other stains-** van Gieson, Immunoperoxidase, Toluidine blue

b **Acute Transplant Rejection**

(Ref: Textbook of Pathology, Harsh Mohan, 7th ed. pg. 49)

ANSWER

Introduction

○ Occur within a few days to few months of transplantation

○ Cellular or humoral mediated

○ Acute cellular rejection is common

Acute Cellular Rejection

○ Extensive infiltration of lymphocytes (mainly T cells), plasma cells (few) and PMNs (few)

○ Endothelialitis, tubulitis

○ Damage to blood vessels and necrosis of transplanted tissue

Acute Humoral Rejection

○ Also known as rejection vasculitis

○ Result of poor response to immunosuppressive therapy

○ Presence/deposition of C4d and inflammation of peritubular capillaries and glomeruli

○ Mononuclear cell infiltrate mainly of B lymphocytes and is less marked

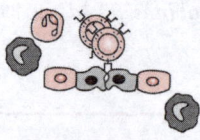
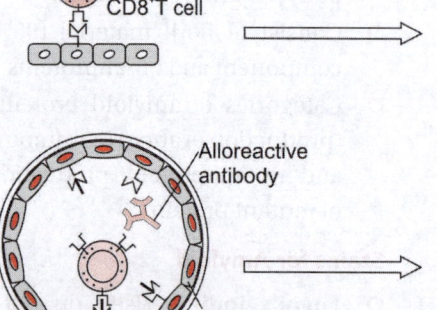
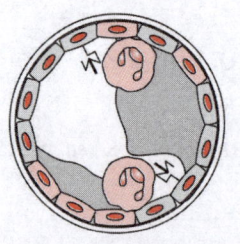

c. Hemolytic disease of newborn

(Ref: Textbook of Pathology, Harsh Mohan, 7th ed. pg. 319)

ANSWER

For answer, refer 2017 paper-I Q. 6 (c), Pg. 13

PART II

3. Write briefly on:

a. Pathogenesis of renal edema

(Ref: Textbook of Pathology, Harsh Mohan, 7th ed. pg. 84)

ANSWER

Introduction

○ Renal edema is characterized by heavy and persistent proteinuria resulting in reduced plasma oncotic pressure thus causing generalized edema

○ Present in nephrotic syndrome(nephrotic edema), nephritic syndrome(nephritic edema), acute tubular injury

Pathogenesis Due to -

○ **Intrinsic renal mechanism:**

▪ Severe hemorrhage (hypovolemia) results in renal ischemia that leads to reduced GFR and deceased excretion of sodium resulting in sodium retention

○ **Extra-renal mechanism:**

▪ Secretion of aldosterone by the renin-angiotensin – aldosterone system

▪ Increased tubular reabsorption of sodium and decreased excretion

○ **ADH mechanism:**

▪ Anti-diuretic harmone (ADH)influences the retention of sodium and water

▪ Increased sodium concentration in the plasma stimulates ADH release

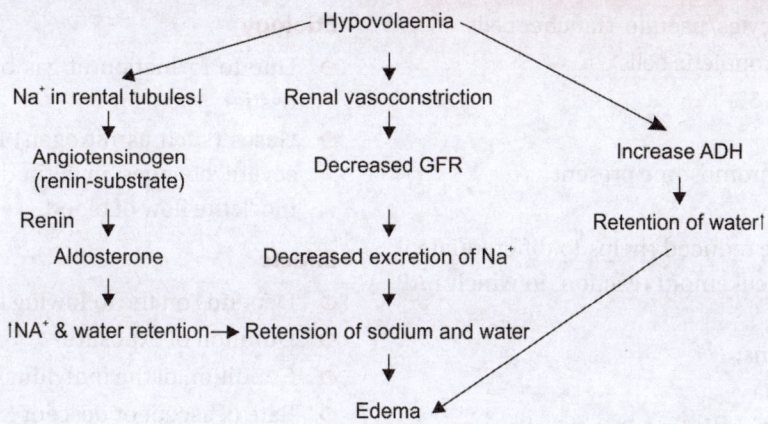

b. Prognostic indicator of acute lymphoblastic leukemia

(Ref: Harsh Mohan, 7th ed. pg. 353, Robbins, SA ed. pg. 590-93)

ANSWER

Introduction

- ○ Lymphoid malignancy of precursor series of B or T cells
- ○ Common in children under 4 years of age
- ○ According to FAB classification, it is of 3 types: L1(B/T cell childhood type), L2(adult T cell type) and L3(Burkitt type B cell)

Prognostic Factors

Factors	Favorable/good Prognosis	Unfavorable/poor Prognosis
Age	2-9 yrs.	Adult, < 1 yr, > 10 yr
Gender	Female	male
Race	white	black
CNS involvement	Absent	Present
Organomegaly(Lymph node, liver, spleen enlargement)	Absent	Present (massive)
Testicular involvement	Absent	Present
Ploidy	Hyperdiploidy	hypodiploidy
FAB	L1 Early pre-B cell ALL	L2-L3 Pre-B-cell ALL Mature B-cell
Hemoglobin	>10gm/dL	< 7gm/dL
WBC/μL	<10,000	>20,0000
Cytogenetic markers	t(12;21) trisomy 4,10,17	t(9;22), t(4;11)
Cytochemistry	PAS positive	PAS negative

4. Write briefly on:

a. Chemical Carcinogenesis

(Ref: Textbook of Pathology, Harsh Mohan, 7th ed. pg. 210)

ANSWER

For answer, refer 2017 paper-I Q. 2 (c), Pg. 6

b. Laboratory diagnosis of CML

(Ref: Harsh Mohan, 7th ed. pg. 335 Robbins, SA ed. pg. 617-18)

Introduction

- ○ A myeloproliferative disorder
- ○ Characterized by BCR-ABL gene and reciprocal translocation between chromosome 9 and 22

Epidemiology

- ○ Peak incidence: third and fourth decades of ife

Etiology

- ○ Radiation exposure, certain drugs, chemicals, RNA viruses, etc.

Clinical Features

- ○ Biphasic (sometimes triphasic)
- ○ Splenomegaly (massive)
- ○ Weakness, pallor, dyspnea, tachycardia (due to anemia)
- ○ Weight loss, anorexia, night sweats (due to hyper-metabolism)
- ○ Epistaxis, bruising, menorrhagia
- ○ Bone tenderness

Laboratory Findings

- ○ **Blood picture:**
  - ▪ Normocytic normochromic anemia (moderate)
  - ▪ Marked leukocytosis (approx. 200, 000/μL or more)
  - ▪ Basophilia
  - ▪ Blast phase/blast crisis- ≥20%
- ○ **Bone marrow examination:**
  - ▪ Hypercellular
  - ▪ **Myeloid:** Erythroid ratio increased (myeloid cells predominate)
  - ▪ Increased, small dysplastic form of megaryo-cytes

- Sea blue histiocytes/pseudo-Gaucher cells
- Reduced erythropoietic cells
- Blasts less than 5%
○ **Cytogenetics:**
  - Philadelphia chromosome present
○ **Cytochemistry:**
  - LAP/NAP score reduced (helps to differentiate it from myeloid leukemoid reaction, in which LAP is elevated)
○ **Other invstigations:**
  - Hyperuricaemia
  - Raised serum B_{12} and vitamin B_{12} binding capacity

Phases of CML

○ Accelerated phase:
  - 10-19% blast in blood or marrow
  - Basophilia ≥20%
  - Persistent thrombocytopenia and thrombocytosis
  - Increasing splenomegaly and WBC count
○ Blastic phase/blast crisis:
  - Blast cells > 20%
  - On bone marrow biopsy- clusters of blast cells
  - Anemia and thrombocytopenia
  - Generalized lymphadenopathy

Treatment

○ Imatinib oral therapy
○ Chemotherapy
○ Allogenic bone marrow (stem cell) transplantation
○ Interferon- alpha

PART III

5. Write briefly on:

a. Phagocytosis

(Ref: Harsh Mohan, 7th ed. pg. 120, Robbins, SA ed. pg. 9-10)

ANSWER

For answer, refer 2017 paper-I Q. 5 (a), Pg. 9

b. Caisson's Disease

(Ref: Textbook of Pathology, Harsh Mohan, 7th ed. pg. 108)

ANSWER

Introduction:

○ A specialized form of gas embolism
○ Also called as divers' palsy, aeroembolism, or decompression sickness
○ Common during deep sea diving or flying in a non-pressurized aircraft

Etiology

○ Due to formation of gas bubbles in the blood and tissue
○ Gases (such as nitrogen) form gas bubbles due to severe changes in altitude and air pressure and block the flow of blood

Effects

○ Depends on the following factors
○ Duration of exposure
○ Condition of the individual
○ Rate of ascent or descent
○ Depth or altitude reached

Clinical Effects

Two types:

○ **Acute form:**
○ Pain in joints, ligaments, tendons
○ Acute respiratory distress
○ Cerebral effects, like vertigo, coma,etc.
○ **Chronic Form:** Due to ischemic necrosis throughout the body
  - Neurological symptoms like paresthesia, paraplegia, etc.
  - Involvement of lung in the form of edema, amphysema, dyspnea, chest pain, non productive cough, etc.
  - Avascular necrosis of bone, eg. head of femur, tibia, etc.
  - Erythema, cyanosis, edema, itching of skin
  - Presence of lipid vacuoles in liver and pancreas

Diagnosis

○ Thorough medical history and physical examination
○ CT or MRI – for identification of bubbles

Treatment

○ 100% oxygen- initially
○ Hyperbaric oxygen therapy
○ Administration of fluids- reduce dehydration

c Primary Complex

(Ref: Textbook of Pathology, Harsh Mohan, 7th ed. pg. 142)

ANSWER

For answer, refer 2016, paper-I Q. 5 (d), Pg. 34 and 2014 paper-I Q. 5 (d), Pg. 74

d. Prothrombin Time

(Ref: Harsh Mohan, 7th ed. pg. 308, Robbins, SA ed. pg. 119)

ANSWER

For answer, refer 2015 paper-I Q. 5 (a), Pg. 56

6. Write short notes on:

a. Bombay Phenotype

(Ref: Textbook of Pathology, Harsh Mohan, 7th ed. pg. 318)

ANSWER

Introduction

- A rare condition observed by Dr. Bhende of Bombay in 1952.
- A blood group with absence of A, B and H antigens on red cells
- Anti A, anti-B and anti-H antibodies are present in serum
- Also known as Oh or (H/H) blood group

Properties

- Due to inheritance of two rare recessive h gene
- H antigen serve as a precursor in the formation of A and B antigen
- Deficiency/absence is known as H antigen deficient phenotype
- A,B,H non secretor(A, B or H substance not present in saliva
- Mode of inheritance is recessive
- A or B enzymes present in serum and red cells
- No A,B and H antigens: No agglutination with anti A, anti B or anti H lectin
- Serum grouping or reverse grouping is required for the detection of this group.

b. Kwashiorkor

(Ref: Textbook of Pathology, Harsh Mohan, 7th ed. pg. 240, Robbins, SA ed. pg. 433)

ANSWER

Introduction

- Deficiency of protein with sufficient calorie intake
- Also known as protein malnutrition, protein-calorie malnutrition or malignant malnutrition

Clinical Features

- Age: children between 6 months and 3 yrs of age
- Retardation of growth
- Early signs include, fatigue, irritability and lethargy
- Skeletal muscles are spared
- Loss of muscle mass
- Visceral protein compartment markedly reduced, thus sometimes life threatening

- **Hair changes:** Thin, dry, brittle, easily pluckable and sparse hair. "Flag sign" (alternate band of light and dark hair) evident.
- **Skin changes:** "Flaky paint" dermatosis
- **Edema:** Pitting edema (due to low albumin level)
- **Poor appetite:** Apathy, listlessness
- Large protuberant belly (pot belly)
- Hepatomegaly with fatty changes
- **Thymic and lymphoid atrophy:** Marked
- Severe infections with delayed recovery(reduced secretory IgA)
- Psychomotor changes

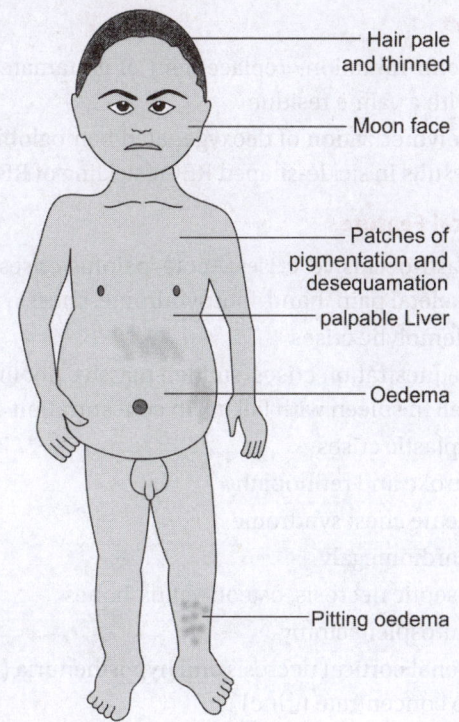

Labels:
- Hair pale and thinned
- Moon face
- Patches of pigmentation and desequamation
- palpable Liver
- Oedema
- Pitting oedema

Complications

- Anemia (low red blood cell count)
- Frequent infections
- Physical disability
- Poor wound healing
- Shock
- Skin pigmentation changes
- Fatty liver

Treatment

- Gradual increase in dietary protein
- Gradual increases in dietary calories from carbohydrates, sugars and fats
- Intravenous fluids to correct fluid and electrolyte imbalances
- Vitamin and mineral supplements to treat deficiencies
- Antibiotics to treat infections

PATHOLOGY

c. **Clinicopathological features of sickle cell anemia**

(Ref: Harsh Mohan, 7th ed. pg. 294, Robbins, SA ed. pg. 637-38)

ANSWER

Introduction

○ Sickle cell anemia is the most prevalent type of hemoglobinopathy

○ Present with hemoglobin S as the major component, small amount of hemoglobin A_2 and variable amount of hemoglobin F

Defect

○ Point mutation- replacement of glutamate residue with a valine residue

○ Polymerization of deoxygenated hemoglobin (HbS) results in sickle-shaped RBCs(sickling of RBC's)

Clinical Features

○ Vaso-occlusive crises/Acute painful crises: severe skeletal pain, hand-foot syndrome, chest syndrome

○ Hemolytic crises

○ Sequestration crises: sudden massive pooling of red cell in spleen with fall in Hb concentration

○ Aplastic crises

○ Stroke and retinopathy

○ Acute chest syndrome

○ Cardiomegaly

○ Aseptic necrosis, osteomyelitis-bones

○ Autosplenectomy

○ Renal cortical necrosis and hyposthenuria (inability to concentrate urine)

○ **Chronic hemolysis:** Growth and development impaired

○ Pulmonary infections in lungs

○ Retinal hemorrhage, proliferative retinopathy

○ Septicemia and meningitis by pneumococci and H. influenzae

○ Erectile dysfunction

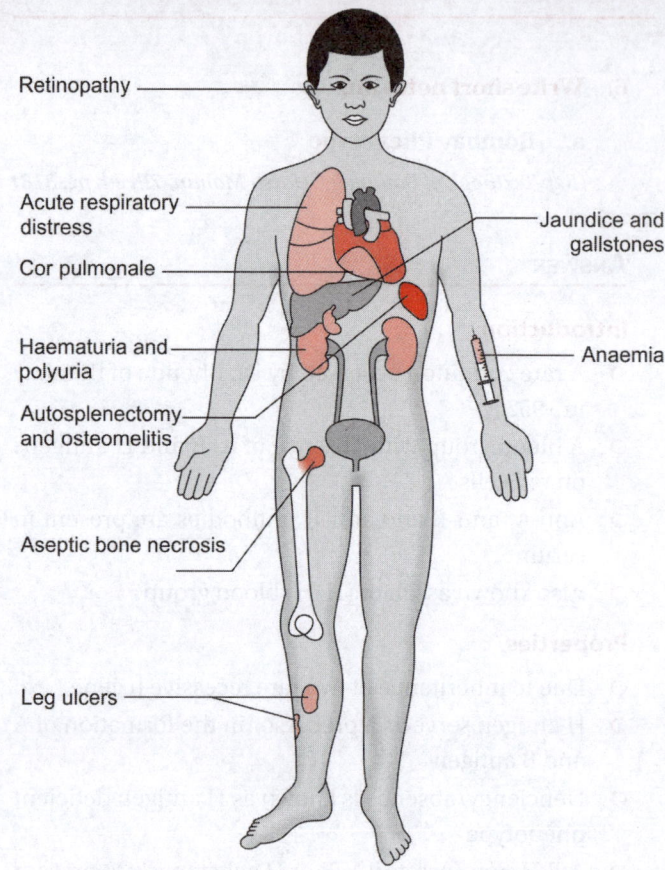

Retinopathy

Acute respiratory distress

Cor pulmonale

Jaundice and gallstones

Haematuria and polyuria

Anaemia

Autosplenectomy and osteomelitis

Aseptic bone necrosis

Leg ulcers

○ **Radiological Findings:** X-ray revels " cut –crew" appearance of skull and "fish mouth" vertebra

Laboratory Findings

○ Moderate to severe anemia (6-9g/dl)

○ **Peripheral blood smear:**
  ▪ Presence of sickle cells, target cells, Howell-Jolly bodies

○ **Sickling test**: Positive, using metabisulfite

○ **Serum electrophoresis:** Normal HbA absent, increased HbS(abnormal Hb)

○ **Osmotic fragility test:** Osmotic fragility decreased due to sickle shape of RBC's

Your Roll No. ....

Name of the Paper	:	**Pathology Paper-II**
Name of the Course	:	**MBBS-2010**
Semester	:	**Annual**

Time: 3 Hours   **M.M.: 40**

INSTRUCTIONS

1. Write your Roll No. on the top immediately on receipt of this question paper
2. All questions are to be attempted
3. Answers to Parts I, II and III should be written in separate answer sheets provided
4. Attempt parts of a question in sequence

PART-I

1. **Differentiate between:**   [8]
   a. Ulcerative colitis and crohn disease
   b. Alcoholic and Biliary Cirrhosis
   c. Partial and complete mole
   d. Ischemic and Nephrotoxic acute tubular necrosis

2. **Comment briefly on:**   [6]
   a. Hashimoto thyroiditis
   b. Meningioma
   c. Emphysema

PART-II

3. **Give pathogenesis of:**   [6]
   a. Ulcerative colitis
   b. Glomerulonephritis
   c. Apoptosis

4. **Short note on:**   [6]
   a. Carcinoma appendix
   b. Pleomorphic adenoma
   c. Benign Hypertrophy of Prostate
   d. Ghon Complex

PART-III

5. **Comment on:**   [6]
   a. Fibroadenoma breast
   b. Uroliathiasis
   c. Nodular sclerosis type of Hodgkin lymphoma

6. **Short note on:**   [8]
   a. Cushing syndrome   b. Retinoblastoma
   c. Dysgerminoma   d. Meningioma

PART-I

1. **Differentiate between:**

    a.   **Ulcerative colitis and crohn disease**   *(Ref: Harsh Mohan, 7th ed. pg. 552, Robbins, SA ed. pg. 798-801)*

ANSWER

For answer, refer 2016 paper-II Q. 1 (c), Pg. 39

    b.   **Alcoholic and Biliary Cirrhosis**   *(Ref: Harsh Mohan, 7th ed. pg. 604–609, Robbins, SA ed. pg. 827-28, 49)*

ANSWER

Alcoholic Cirrhosis	Biliary Cirrhosis
• Micronodular in appearance initially and in longstanding cases changes to mixed type (hobnail appearance)	• Chronic disorder presents with features (biochemical, morphological, clinical) of longstanding cholestasis of intrahepatic or extrahepatic origin
• Difficult to find the normal liver architecture	• Three types: Primary, secondary and primary sclerosing cholangitis • Primary: Cause is autoimmune, secondary: obstruction of extrahepatic bile duct, and primary sclerosing cholangitis may be associated with IBD
• Liver is fatty, enlarged, tan-yellow but later on becomes shrunken, and brown in color. Cut section exhibits, spheroidal nodules of fibrous seta	• Enlarged liver initially and greenish in appearance
• Initially fibrous septa are delicate, later on present with thick septa	• Pathologically, primary biliary cirrhosis revels cholangitis of intrahepatic bile ducts, secondary: stasis of bile in bile ducts and pyogenic cholangitis and fibrosing cholangitis with periductal fibrosis in primary sclerosing cholangitis
• Mallory body may be seen (not usual)	• Increased alkaline phosphatase and conjugated bilirubin with presence of autoantibodies in primary biliary cirrhosis, Increased alkaline phosphatase in secondary biliary cirrhosis and primary sclerosing cholangitis associated with hypergammaglobulinaemia and increased alkaline phosphatase and conjugated bilirubin

    c.   **Partial and complete mole**   *(Ref: Textbook of Pathology, Harsh Mohan, 7th ed. pg. 761)*

ANSWER

For answer, refer 2016 paper-II Q. 3 (a), Pg. 42

    d.   **Ischemic and Nephrotoxic acute tubular necrosis** *(Ref: Harsh Mohan, 7th ed. pg. 668, Robbins, SA ed. pg. 927-29)*

Ischemic acute tubular necrosis	Nephrotoxic acute tubular necrosis
• Renal ischemia is the causative factor	• As a result of toxic agents
• Causative agents are shock, hypotension, decreased renal perfusion	• Causative agents: drugs like gentamycin, poisons, contrast agents used in radiographs, organic solvents, etc.
• Affects straight segments of proximal tubules and ascending limbs of loop of Henle	• DCT and ascending loop of Henle may be affected
• Tubular injury and severe and persistent disturbance in blood flow responsible for the pathogenesis	• Occurs as a result of tubular injury

Ischemic acute tubular necrosis	Nephrotoxic acute tubular necrosis
• Morphologically, exhibits focal tubular necrosis and apoptosis along the nephron, BM rupture and tubular lumen occlusion by casts	Non specific acute tubular injury, for eg. in mercuric chloride poisoning large acidophilic inclusions in the injured cells
• Tubular necrosis is patchy, small areas are affected with large skip areas present in between	Extensive tubular necrosis with no skip areas

2. Comment briefly on:

a. Hashimoto thyroiditis

(Ref: Harsh Mohan, 7th ed. pg. 795, Robbins, SA ed. pg. 1086-88)

ANSWER

For answer, refer 2017 paper-II Q. 2 (a), Pg. 16

b. Meningioma

(Ref: Harsh Mohan, 7th ed. pg. 882, Robbins, SA ed. pg. 1314-15)

ANSWER

Introduction

- Slow growing benign tumor of adults
- Origin from the meningothelial cell of the arachnoid
- Molecular genetics: loss of chromosome 22q (NF2 gene)
- Positive for epithelial membrane antigens

Clinical Features

- Common in females as compared to males (3:2)
- Common sites involved are lateral cerebral convexities, midline along the falx cerebri, olfactory groove
- Less common sites are foramen magnum, cerebellopontine angle, cerebral ventricles and spinal cord
- Usually solitary
- May be present in patients with neurofibromatosis 2

Morphology

- **Gross appearance**
  - Present as masses in the well-defined dural base resulting in compression of underlying brain
  - Bosselated polypoid appearance
  - Hyperostosis of overlying bone
  - Cut surface is fibrous and firm with foci of calcification
- **Microscopic findings:** Five types-
  - **Fibrous (fibroblastic) meningioma:**
    - Parallel or interlacing bundles of tumor cells
    - Psammoma bodies and whorled pattern are less common
  - **Transitional (mixed) meningioma:**
    - Combination of syncytial and fibroblastic featues with whorled appearance of tumor

cells present around capillary sized blood vessel present in the centre
    - Psammoma bodies may be present at some places in whorls
  - **Meningotheliomatous (syncytial) meningioma:**
    - Resemblance to normal arachnoid cap cells
    - Solid masses of polygonal tumor cells with poorly defined cell membranes (called as syncytial appearance)
    - Granular cytoplasm with round to oval, central nuclei
  - **Angioblastic meningioma:**
    - Consist of two patterns-
      - Hemangioblastic pattern
      - Hemangiopericytic pattern
    - High recurrence rate
  - **Anaplastic (malignant) meningioma:**
    - Exhibits extraneural metastases, usually to lungs

Diagnosis

- Neurological, vision, and hearing tests
- Stereotactic neurosurgery/biopsy
- Imaging tests: Includes MRI, CT scan, cerebral angiogram

Factors Determining the Prognosis

- **Histology of tumor:**
  - Type of tumor, its grade and molecular features helps in determining treatment outcome
- **Patient's age:**
  - Younger the adult better is the prognosis
- **Extent of residual tumor:**
  - Removal of all the tumor- better prognosis
- **Location of tumor:**
  - Tumor can be formed in any part of CNS
  - Difficult removal if location is not easily accessible
- **Functional neurologic status:**
  - Neurologic status is assessed using Karnofsky Performance scale.
    A higher score-better prognosis
- **Metastatic spread:**
  - Rare spread to other parts of the body

c. Emphysema

(Ref: Harsh Mohan, 7th ed. pg. 459, Robbins, SA ed. pg. 675-678)

Answer

Introduction

- It is characterized as permanent abnormal dilatation of the airspaces present distal to the terminal bronchioles along with destruction of the walls of dilated air spaces without any fibrosis or little fibrosis

Etiology

- Air pollutants
- Tobacco smoke } most common
- Occupational exposure
- Infection
- Genetic and familial infuences

Pathogenesis

- Alveolar wall destruction due to deficiency of serum alpha-1- antitrypsin called as protease-antiprotease hypothesis
- Imbalance between protease and antiprotease activity results in elastolytic action
- **Protease:** Cellular protease, neutrophil elastase, matrix metalloproteinases, oxygen free radicals (inactivates alpha1 AT activity), macrophage elastase
- **Antiprotease:** alpha-1 antitrypsin (mainly in interstitium and blood), secretory leukoprotease inhibitor, alpha-1 microglobulin
- Lower zone is more commonly involved because extensive neutrophils are present in lower zone thus increased elastase activity

- Oxidants in smoke of cigarette decreases anti-elastase activity
- High elastse activity in smokers because of high (ten times more) phagocytes and neutrophils in present in the lungs

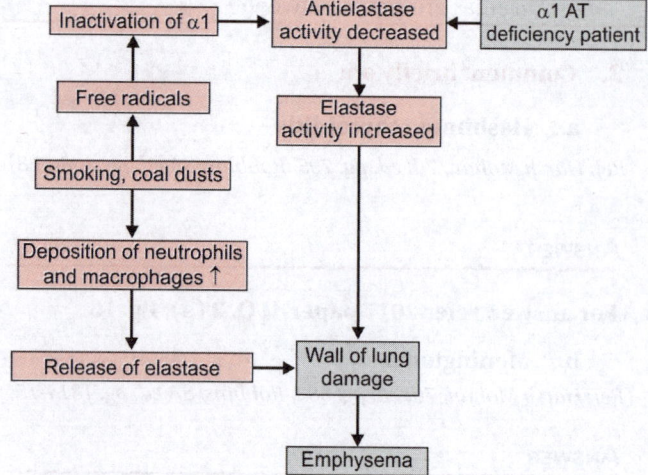

Clinical Features

Predominant emphysema presents with the following features-

- Severe exertional dyspnea
- Barrel-shaped chest with hyper resonance
- Use of accessory muscles of respiration producing discomfort
- Cough associated with scanty mucoid sputum
- Patient are known as "pink puffers" – tachypnoea and are well oxygenated
- Weight loss

Types

Centriacinar (Centrilobular emphysema)	Panacinar (Panlobular) emphysema	Paraseptal (distal acinar) emphysema	Irregular (Para-cicatricial) emphysema	Mixed (unclassified) emphysema
• Only central or proximal part of acini affected • Commonly present in heavy smokers • Upper lobe is commonly involved • Grossly, exhibits enlarged airspaces in the centre surrounded by a rim normal parenchyma in the same lobule	• Uniform enlargement of the acini • Associated with alpha 1 AT deficiency • Lower zone of the lungs is commonly involved	• Distal part of the acini is involved • Characterized by continuous, multiple and enlarged spaces forming cyst-like structures • Results in spontaneous pneuothorax in young adults • Commonly seen in upper part of lungs, adjacent to areas of fibrosis and atelectasis	• Irregularly involved acini • Most common form of emphysema	• More than one type of emphysema • No clear cut distinction between one type of emphysema and the other

Gross Appearance

- Pale, voluminous lungs with less blood
- Rounded edges
- Mild cases-dilatation of air spaces
- Advanced cases-subpleural bullae and blebs bulging from the surface of the lungs

Microscopic Features

- Destruction of alveolar septal wall
- Dilated air spaces
- Bullae and blebs if present–fibrosis and chronic inflammation of the walls

Diagnosis

○ Pulmonary function test
○ **Chest X-ray:** Hyperinflated lungs with small heart
○ **CT scan:** To assess the destruction of air spaces

PART-II

3. Give pathogenesis of:

a. **Ulcerative colitis**   *(Ref: Textbook of Pathology, Harsh Mohan, 7th ed. pg. 552, Robbins, SA ed. pg. 800)*

ANSWER

For answer, refer 2016 paper-II Q. 1 (c), Pg. 39

b **Glomerulonephritis**   *(Ref: Review of Neet/DNB Pattern Qs 2018, 1st ed. pg. 388, Robbins, SA ed. pg. 902-926)*

ANSWER

Table: Types of glomerular nephritis

Disease	Light microscopy	Fluorescence	Electron microscopy
Post streptococcal GN	Proliferation of endothelial and mesangial cells	Ig G, Ig M, C3 deposits in mesangium	
RPGN – I		Linear GBM deposits of Ig G and C3	
RPGN – II		Lumpy bumpy granular pattern of staining	
RPGN – III		No Ig or Complement deposits in GBM	
Membranous glomerulopathy	Diffuse capillary wall thickening	Granular Ig G, C3	Subepithelial deposits
Minimal change disease	Lipid deposit in tubules	Negative	Loss of foot process of podocytes
Focal segmental glomerulosclerosis	Focal and segmental sclerosis and hyalinosis	Focal – Ig M and C3	Loss of foot process of podocytes, Epithelial denudation
Membranoproliferative glomerulonephritis	Mesangial proliferation, BM thickening and splitting	Ig G + C3 and C1q + C4	Subendothelial deposits
Ig A nephropathy	Mesangial widening and proliferation	Mesangial deposition of Ig A, C3 and properdin	
Alport syndrome	Presence of foam cells in interstitial cells		Irregular foci of thickening and thinning in GBM with splitting and lamination of lamina densa (BASKET WEAVE appearance)
Good pasture syndrome	Focal necrosis, Intra-alveolar haemorrhage, Type II pneumocyte hypertrophy		Linear deposits of Ig along alveolar septa and GBM

c. **Apoptosis**

(Ref: Harsh Mohan, 7th ed. pg. 29, Robbins, SA ed. pg. 14-15)

ANSWER

For answer, refer 2016 paper-I Q. 6 (a), Pg. 35

4. Short note on:

a. **Carcinoma appendix**

(Ref: Robbins, SA ed. pg. 816)

ANSWER

Introduction

○ Appendix is a pouch-like tube attached to the cecum
○ It averages about 10 centimeters (about 4 inches) in length.
○ Considered part of the gastrointestinal (GI) tract.

Types

○ **Mucinous adenocarcinoma**:
  ▪ Second most common type of appendix cancer.

- Characterized by mucin production (responsible for spread of cancer to other parts of the body).
- Often identified after metastasis to the peritoneum (the lining of the abdominal cavity)
- **Adenocarcinoid tumors (Goblet cell carcinoids):**
  - Less common tumor.
  - Commonly seen in patients over the age of 50 yrs.
  - More aggressive than carcinoid tumors
  - Treatment similar to mucinous adenocarcinoma.
- **Intestinal-type adenocarcinoma:**
  - **Also known as colonic-type adenocarcinoma**
  - Accounts for approx. 10 percent of appendix tumors
  - Usually located near the base of the appendix
- **Signet-ring cell adenocarcinoma:**
  - Rare but aggressive type of appendix cancer
  - Commonly occur in the stomach or colon.
  - When develops in the appendix, causes appendicitis.
  - Called as signet-ring cell adenocarcinoma because cells has a signet ring inside it.

Risk Factors

- **Age:** Advancing age is the consistent risk factor
- **Gender:** Females are more prone for developing cancer
- **Medical history:** Patients with certain medical conditions like- Zollinger-Ellison syndrome, atrophic gastritis, etc.
- **Family history:** Patients with a family history of appendix cancer or multiple endocrine neoplasia type 1 (MEN1) syndrome have a higher risk
- Smokers are more prone to develop appendix cancer

Symptoms of Appendix Cancer

- Appendicitis – it is the most common symptom
- Acute Pain in the lower right side of the abdomen
- Bloating/increase in abdominal girth
- Changes in bowel function
- Ovarian mass
- Loss of appetite
- Appendicitis
- Indigestion
- Reflux
- Vomiting
- New hernias

Diagnosis

Depends on the following factors:

- Type of suspected cancer
- Signs and symptoms
- Age and medical condition
- Earlier medical test results

Tests used for Diagnosis

- Biopsy
- Magnetic resonance imaging
- Computed tomography scan
- Radionuclide scanning

Cancer Stage Grouping for Carcinomas of the Appendix

Stage	Features
Stage 0	Refers to cancer in situ. Found only in one place and has not spread (Tis, N0, M0)
Stage I	Spread of cancer to inner layers of appendix tissue but not to the regional lymph nodes (T1 or T2, N0, M0)
Stage IIA	Spread into the connective or fatty tissue next to the appendix but not spread to the regional lymph nodes or to other parts of the body (T3, N0, M0)
Stage IIB	Cancer grown through the lining of the appendix but not spread to the regional lymph nodes or to other parts of the body (T4a, N0, M0)
Stage IIC	Tumor grown into other organs, such as the colon or rectum, but has not spread to the regional lymph nodes or to other parts of the body (T4b, N0, M0)
Stage IIIA	Cancer spread to inner layers of appendix tissue and to 1 - 3 regional lymph nodes but not spread to other parts of the body (T1 or T2, N1, M0).
Stage IIIB	Cancer has grown into nearby tissue of the appendix or through the lining of the appendix and to 1 to 3 regional lymph nodes but has not spread to other areas of the body (T3 or T4, N1, M0).
Stage IIIC	Spread of tumor to four or more regional lymph nodes but not to other areas of the body (any T, N2, M0)
Stage IVA	Cancer that has spread to other areas in the abdomen but not to the regional lymph nodes; the cancer cells are well differentiated (any T, N0, M1a, G1)
Stage IVB	3 situations described: • Cancer spread to other areas in the abdomen but not to the regional lymph nodes; the cells are moderately or poorly differentiated (any T, N0, M1a, G2 or G3). • Cancer spread to other areas in the abdomen and to 1 to 3 regional lymph nodes; the cells may be any grade (any T, N1, M1a, any G). • Cancer spread to other areas in the abdomen and to 4 or more regional lymph nodes; the cells may be any grade (any T, N2, M1a, any G)
Stage IVC	Spread of cancer outside the abdominal area to distant parts of the body, such as the lungs (any T, any N, M1b, any G)
Recurrent	Cancer that come back after treatment are recurrent cancer, eg. carcinoid tumors and carcinomas

b.   Pleomorphic Adenoma

(Ref: Harsh Mohan, 7th ed. pg. 516, Robbins, SA ed. pg. 266-67)

ANSWER

For answer, refer 2012 paper-II Q. 5 (b), Pg. 111

c.   Benign Hypertrophy of Prostate

(Ref: Harsh Mohan, 7th ed. pg. 705, Robbins, SA ed. pg. 982-83)

ANSWER

For answer, refer 2014 paper-II Q. 2 (c), Pg. 78

d.   Ghon Complex

(Ref: Harsh Mohan, 7th ed. pg. 142, Robbins, SA ed. pg. 374-76)

ANSWER

For answer, refer 2016, paper-I Q. 5 (d), Pg. 47

Clinical Features

- Colicky pain (renal colic) is the clinical manifestation as the stone passes down along the ureter
- Hematuria
- May be asymptomatic

Types of Renal Stones

PART-III

5.   Comment on:

a.   Fibroadenoma Breast

(Ref: Harsh Mohan, 7th ed. pg. 748, Robbins, SA ed. pg. 1069)

ANSWER

For answer, refer 2017 paper-II Q. 2 (c), Pg. 18

b.   Uroliathiasis

(Ref: Harsh Mohan, 7th ed. pg. 672, Robbins, SA ed. pg. 951-52)

ANSWER

Introduction

- Urinary calculi formation at any level of the urinary tract
- Common in 2nd – 3rd decade of life

Type	Incidence	Etiology	Pathogenesis	Morphology
Calcium stone- made up of calcium oxalate (50%) or calcium phosphate (50%)or mixture of both	75%, M:F=2-3:1	Hypercalcemia, hyperoxalouria, hyperuricosuria, distal renal tubule acidosis, idiopathic, hypocitraturia, hyperparathyroidism	Alkaline pH of urine, less urinary volume, supersaturation of ions in urine	Small, hard along with granular surface, sharp-edged stones, dark brown in color Stones are radio-opaque
Uric acid Stones	5%, M:F= 3-4:1	Hyperuricosuria with or without hyperuricaemia (gout, dehydration, malignant tumors,etc.)	Decreased solubility of uric acid due to acidic urine	Stones are multiple, smooth, hard and yellowish-brown in color Stones are radiolucent
Mixed (struvite)stones, triple phosphate stones or infection induced stones - made up of magnesium-ammonium-calcium phosphate	10-15%, M:F=1:5	Urinary infection by Proteus (urease containing organism)	Alkaline urinary pH due to ammonia produced from urea (by urease)	Soft, irregular in shape and yellow-white or grey in color Staghorn stone- large, solitary stone present in renal pelvis
Cystine stones	1-2%, M:F= 1:1	Cystinuria as a result of genetic defect in the transport of cystine	Precipitation of cystine as cystine crystals	Multiple, Small, rounded and smooth, waxy and yellowish in color
Others	Approx.10%, M:F= (1:1)	Inherited abnormality of amino acid metabolism	Xanthinuria	Xanthine stones

Diagnosis

Includes physical examination and laboratory test

- Physical examination:
  - Tenderness of costovertebral angle
  - Painful testicles but appear normal
  - Constant movements of the body
  - Tachycardia
  - Hypertension
- Laboratory investigations
  - **Serum creatinine:** To evaluate renal function
  - **Dipstick test:** Demonstration of blood cells
  - 24 hour urine profile
  - Serum electrolyte
  - Complete blood count
- Imaging:
  - **Noncontrast abdominopelvic CT scan:** Mainly in case of acute renal colic
  - **Renal ultrasonography:** Renal stones, hydronephrosis but 30% stones are missed out
  - Plain abdominal radiograph (KUB)- 40% of stones are usually missed out
  - Urography (IVP)

Prognosis

- 80% - passes spontaneously
- Hospital intervention required- 20% cases due to:
  - Pain
  - Not able to retain enternal fluids
  - Proximal UTI
  - Inability to pass the stone

  c. **Nodular sclerosis type of Hodgkin lymphoma**

(Ref: Harsh Mohan, 7th ed. pg. 350, Robbins, SA ed. pg. 607-610)

ANSWER

For answer, refer 2017 paper-II Q. 2 (b), Pg. 18

---

6. **Short note on:**

    a. **Cushing syndrome**

(Ref: Harsh Mohan, 7th ed. pg. 832-835, Robbins, SA ed. pg. 1125)

ANSWER

Introduction

- Excessive secretion of glucocorticoids (cortisol) results in Cushing syndrome

Etiopathogenesis

Based on etiology, there are 4 major types of cushing syndrome

- **Adrenal Cushing's syndrome:**
  - Decreased ACTH level and increased glucocorticoid levels
  - Excessive secretion of cortisol due to cortical hyperplasia, carcinoma or cortical adenoma
- **Pituitary Cushing's syndrome:**
  - Bilateral adrenal cortical hyperplasia and raised ACTH levels
- **Iatrogenic Cushing's syndrome:**
  - Exogeneous glucocorticoids (administration of high doses of glucocorticoids)
  - Reduced ACTH level and increased glucocorticoid level
- **Ectopic Cushing's syndrome:**
  - ACTH is produced by no-endocrine tumors, e.g. small cell carcinoma of lung
  - Raised ACTH level and glucocorticoid level

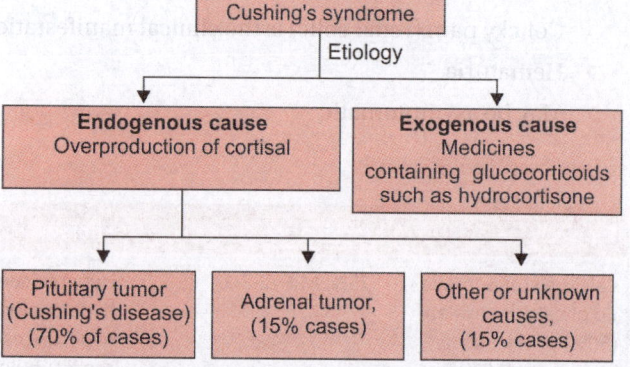

Clinical Features

- **Age:** 20–40 years
- **Incidence:** More in females as compared to males
- Central obesity
- Buffalo hump with moon facies
- Osteoporosis
- Wasting and thinning of skeletal muscles
- Weakness and fatigue
- Skin and subcutaneous tissue atrophy
- Striae on skin
- Hypertension
- Diabetes or impaired glucose tolerance
- Insomnia, depression, confusion
- Amenorrhoea, hirsutism, etc.

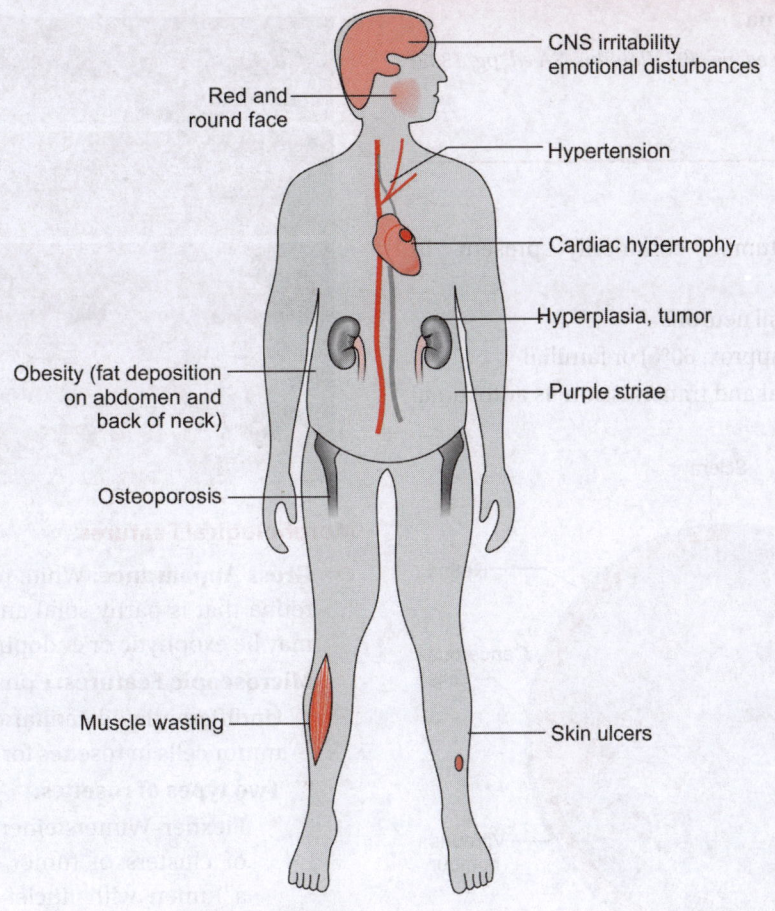

Fig. Symptoms of Cushing's syndrome

Diagnosis

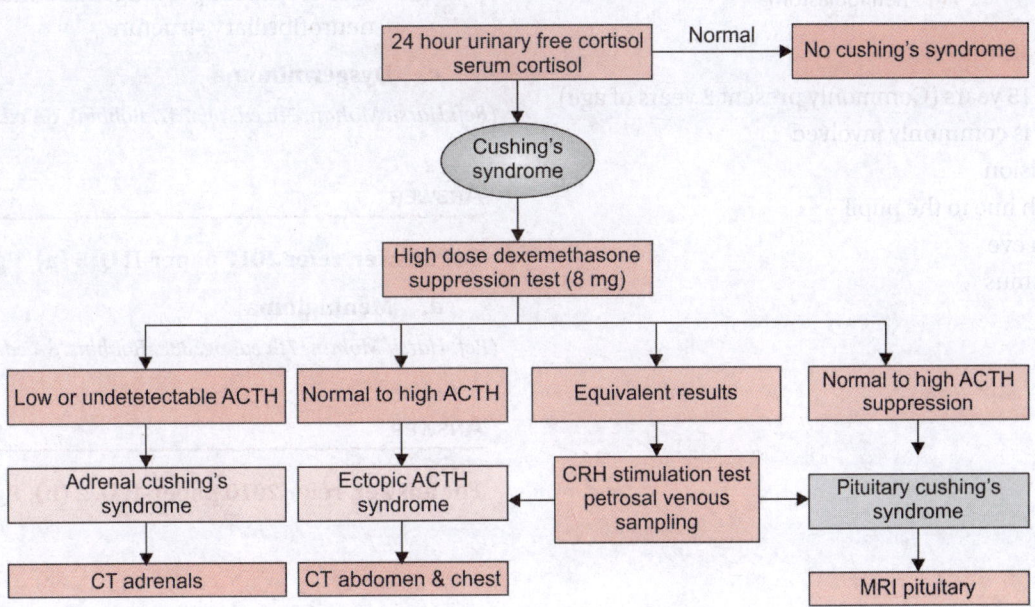

b. Retinoblastoma

(Ref: Harsh Mohan, 7th ed. pg. 493, Robbins, SA ed. pg. 1339)

ANSWER

Introduction

○ Malignant eye tumor commonly present in childhood
○ **Origin:** From retinal neurons
○ May be sporadic (approx. 60%) or familial
○ Familial- multifocal and transmission as autosomal dominant trait

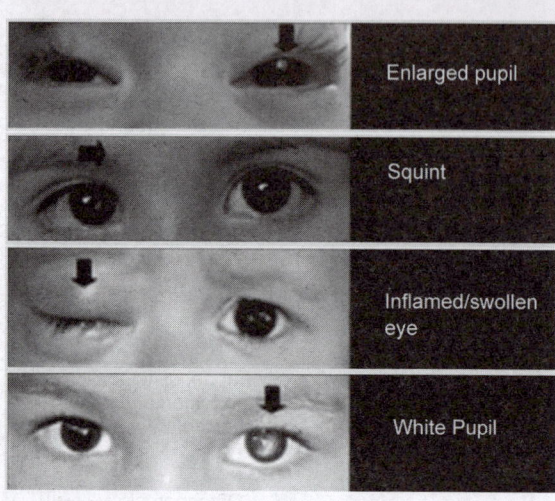

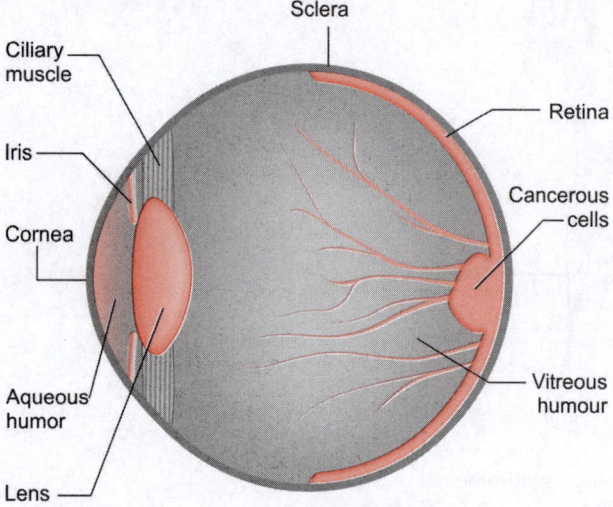

Fig. Retinoblastoma

Clinical Features

○ **Age:** < 15 years (Commonly present 2 years of age)
○ Retina is commonly involved
○ Poor vision
○ Whitish hue to the pupil
○ Pain in eye
○ Strabismus

Morphological Features

○ **Gross Appearance:** White nodular mass within the retina that is partly solid and partly necrotic and it may be exophytic or endophytic
○ **Microscopic Features:** Consists of –
  ▪ Undifferentiated retinal cells and differentiated tumor cells in rosettes form
  ▪ **Two types of rosettes:**
    ♦ Flexner–Wintersteiner rosette composed of clusters of tumor cells arranged around a lumen with nuclei placed away from the lumen
    ♦ Homer Wright rosette consist of tumor cells that are radially arranged around the central neurofibrillary structure

c. Dysgerminoma

(Ref: Harsh Mohan, 7th ed. pg. 737, Robbins, SA ed. pg. 1030-31)

ANSWER

For answer, refer 2017 paper-II Q. 5 (a), Pg. 21

d. Meningioma

(Ref: Harsh Mohan, 7th ed. pg. 882, Robbins, SA ed. pg. 1314-15)

ANSWER

For answer, refer 2010 paper-II Q. 2 (b), Pg. 139

Name of the Paper	:	**Pathology Paper-I**
Name of the Course	:	**MBBS-2009**
Semester	:	**Annual**

Time: 3 Hours   M.M.: 40

INSTRUCTIONS

1. Write your Roll No. on the top immediately on receipt of this question paper
2. All questions are to be attempted
3. Answers to Parts I, II and III should be written in separate answer sheets provided
4. Attempt parts of a question in sequence

PART-I

1. **Difference between in:**   [8]
   a. Myeloblast and Lymphoblast
   b. Healing by primary and secondary intention
   c. Antimortem and Postmortem clot
   d. Normoblast and megaloblast

2. **Write briefly on:**   [6]
   a. Septic shock
   b. Klinfelter syndrome
   c. Gaucher's disease

PART-II

3. **Write briefly on:**   [6]
   a. Pathogenesis of fatty change liver
   b. Complement system

4. **Write briefly on:**   [6]
   a. DIC
   b. Lab. Diagnosis of tuberculous meningitis

PART-III

5. **Short note on:**   [8]
   a. Opportunistic infections in AIDS
   b. Lab. Diagnosis of Beta-thalassemia
   c. Radiation injury
   d. Factors affecting ESR

6. **Write short notes on:**   [6]
   a. FAB classification of AML
   b. Mechanics of Apoptosis
   c. Etiopathogenesis of shock

PART-I

1. Differentiate between:

a. Myeloblast and Lymphoblast

(Ref: Textbook of Pathology, Harsh Mohan, 7th ed. pg. 326)

ANSWER

For answer, refer 2013 paper-I Q. 1 (a), Pg. 85

b. Healing by Primary and Secondary Intention

(Ref: Textbook of Pathology, Harsh Mohan, 7th ed. pg. 158)

ANSWER

For answer, refer 2011 paper-I Q. 1 (a), Pg. 116

c. Antemortem and Postmortem clot

(Ref: Harsh Mohan, 7th ed. pg. 104, Robbins, SA ed. pg. 125)

ANSWER

Antemortem clot	Postmortem clot
• Formed in response to normal hemostatic maintenance	• In dead persons due to settling down/sedimentation of blood compnents
• Strong adherence to vessel wall	• Weak attachment to vessel wall
• Grossly, it appears dry, granular, firm and friable	• Grossly, it is soft and rubbery
• Located anywhere in the body	• Seen in dependent part of the body kept after death

d. Normoblast and Megaloblast

(Ref: Harsh Mohan, 7th ed. pg. 265–283, Robbins, SA ed. pg. 816)

ANSWER

For answer, refer 2015 paper-I Q. 1 (a), Pg. 51

2. Write briefly on:

a. Septic shock

(Ref: Harsh Mohan, 7th ed. pg. 95, Robbins, SA ed. pg. 99-100, 131-33)

ANSWER

For answer, refer 2016 paper-I Q. 3 (a), Pg. 29

b. Klinefelter's syndrome

(Ref: Harsh Mohan, 7th ed. pg. 253, Robbins, SA ed. pg. 165-66)

ANSWER

For answer, refer 2017 paper-I Q. 2 (a), Pg. 5

c. Gaucher's disease

(Ref: Harsh Mohan, 7th ed. pg. 257, Robbins, SA ed. pg. 153-54)

ANSWER

For answer, refer 2012 paper-I Q. 3 (b), Pg. 104

PART II

3. Write briefly on:

a. Pathogenesis of fatty liver change

(Ref: Harsh Mohan, 7th ed. pg. 19, Robbins, SA ed. pg. 842-43)

ANSWER

For answer, refer 2012 paper-I Q. 2 (c), Pg. 102

b. Complement system

(Ref: Harsh Mohan, 7th ed. pg. 127, Robbins, SA ed. pg. 88-89)

ANSWER

Introduction

○ Complex set of 14 distinct serum proteins (nine components) that are involved in three separate pathways of activation.
○ Denoted by C followed by numbers and letters
○ A part of the innate immune system

Activation Mechanism

○ Classical pathway
○ Alternative or Properdin pathway
○ Lectin pathway (Mannose binding lectin pathway)

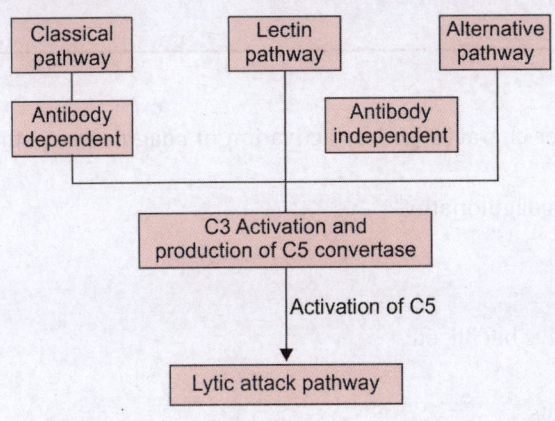

Classical Pathway

○ Pathway begins with the binding of antibody to cell surface and ends with lysis of cell

○ Three steps in this pathway: activation, amplification, and attack

○ Requires antibody for activation, either IgG or IgM, bound to cell surface antigen or as an antigen-antibody complex

○ C3 convertase and C4b2a formed

○ **Cleavage of C3 into two fragments:**

  ▪ **Larger C3b fragment:** Attachment to cell membrane and C4b2a

  ▪ **Small C3a fragment:** Has chemotactic and anaphylatoxic propeties

Alternative or Properdin Pathway

○ Part of innate immunity

○ Specific antibodies are not required for this pathway (antibody independent)

○ Four serum proteins- factor B, factor D, Properdin (P) and initiating factor (IF) involved in this pathway

○ Substances other than antigen-antibody complexes, like bacterial endotoxins, yeast cell wall, rabbit RBCs etc. are responsible for activation of alternative pathway

Lectin Pathway

○ Lectins are proteins that bind and recognize specific carbohydrate target

○ Not dependent on antibody for its activation

○ Activated by the binding of **mannose-binding lectin** (**MBL**) that results in activation of

MBL-associated serine proteases, **MASP-1** and **MASP-2**, which in turn activate **C4** and **C2**, and form the C3 convertase, **C4b2a.**

Functions of Complement

○ Opsonization and phagocytosis

○ Cell lysis

○ Chemotaxis

○ Activation of mast cells and basophils and enhancement of inflammation

○ Production of antibodies

○ Immune clearance

Complement deficiency and associated disease:

Complement deficiency	Associated disease
• C1, C2, C3 and C4 (early C components)	• Immune and rheumatic disorders
• C5, C6, C7 and C8 (late C components)	• Recurrent infections (Neisseria)
• C1q	• Combined immune deficiency state
• C1s	• Systemic lupus erythematosus
• C2	• Increased susceptibility to infections
• C3	• Severe pyogenic infections
• C5	• Recurrent infection of GI tract

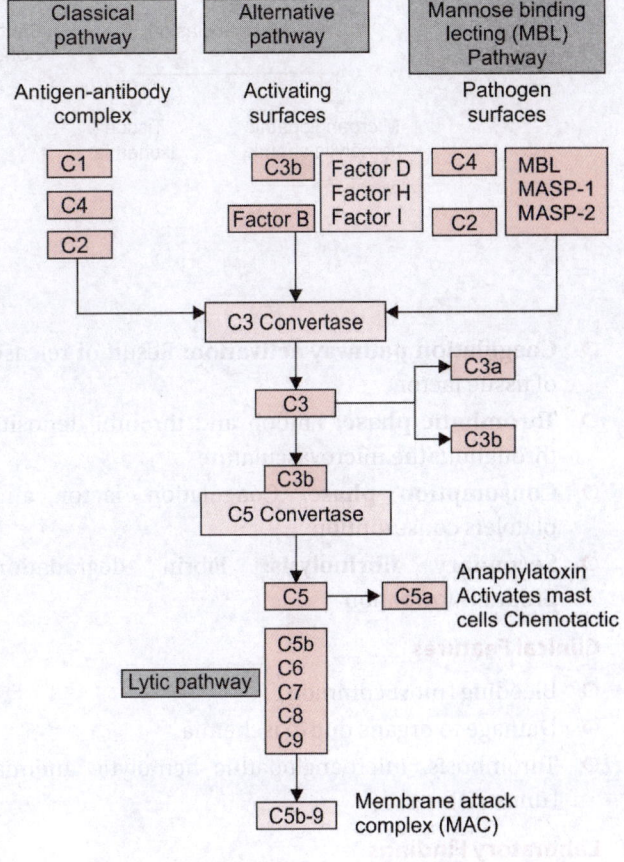

4. Write briefly on:

a. DIC (disseminated intravascular coagulation)

(Ref: Harsh Mohan, 7th ed. pg. 315, Robbins, SA ed. pg. 663-665)

ANSWER

Introduction

- Acute, subacute or chronic thrombo-hemorrhagic disorder characterized by activation of coagulation pathway and formation of thrombi in the microcirculation of body
- Also known as "defibrination syndrome" or "consumption coagulopathy"

Etiology

- Trauma and tissue injury
- Infections, eg. certain viral infections, malaria, gram-negative bacilli, etc.
- Vascular disorders, like hemangiomas
- Innunologic disorders, like- GVHD, transplant rejection, etc.
- Certain drugs, shock, ARDS, insect bite etc.

Pathogenesis

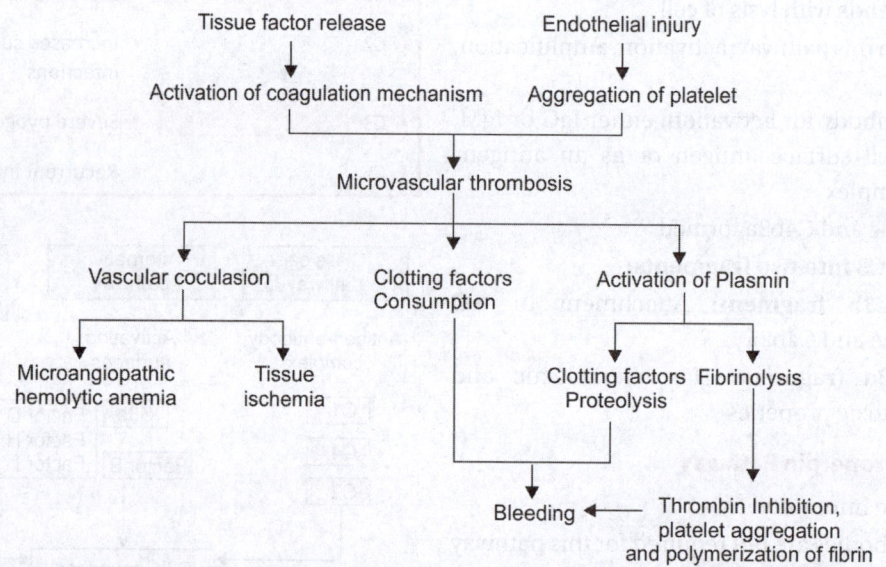

- **Coagulation pathway activation:** Result of release of tissue factor
- **Thrombotic phase:** Emboli and thrombi deposits throughout the microvasculature
- **Consumption phase:** Coagulation factor and platelets consumption
- **Secondary fibrinolysis:** Fibrin degradation products formation

Clinical Features

- Bleeding (most common)
- Damage to organs due to ischemia
- Thrombosis, microangiopathic hemolytic anemia (unusual)

Laboratory Findings

- **Hemogram:** Decreased platelet count
- **Peripheral smear:** Schistocytes and fragmented red cells
- **Coagulation test:** Prolonged thrombin time, prothrombin time, activated partial thromboplastin time

- **Other investigation:**
- Increased level of FDP (fibrin degraded product)

b.   Lab Diagnosis of Tuberculous Meningitis

(Ref: Textbook of Pathology, Harsh Mohan, 7th ed. pg. 867)

ANSWER

Introduction

- Meningitis is the inflammation of leptomeninges and CSF within the subarachnoid space.
- Tuberculous meningitis- a type of chronic meningitis
- Common in adults and children
- Hematogenous spread of infection

Laboratory Diagnosis

CSF findings are as follows-

- **Naked eye appearance**: Clear, slightly turbid and formation of fibrin coagulum/web on standing
- CSF pressure raised (above 300 mm water)

○ **Cells:**
  ▪ **RBC's:** normal
  ▪ **WBC:** 100-1000 lymphocytes/μl
○ **Protein:** Increased protein content
○ **Glucose:** Decreased concentration of glucose
○ **Bacteriology:** Presence of tubercle bacilli- Z N staining

PART III

5. **Short note on:**

   a. **Opportunistic infections in AIDS**

(Ref: Harsh Mohan, 7th ed. pg. 55, Robbins, SA ed. pg. 243-256)

ANSWER

Introduction

○ AIDS, caused by retrovirus, HIV-1 (usually common) or HIV-2
○ **Pathogenesis:** Depletion of CD4+ T cells resulting in immunosuppression
○ Affects multiple organs and involvement of multiple system

Opportunistic Infections

○ **Bacterial infections:**
  ▪ **Mycobacterium avium complex:**
    ◆ Common and associated with advanced stages of disease
  ▪ **M. tuberculosis:**
    ◆ Most common opportunistic infection
    ◆ Exhibits disseminated or extrapulmonary involvement
  ▪ **Salmonella:** causes recurrent septicemia
○ **Viral infections:**
  ▪ **Cytomegalovirus infection**
    ◆ CMV colitis, oesphagitis, pneumonia, encephalitis, etc.
  ▪ **Herpes simplex virus 1, 2 infection :**
    ◆ Mucocutaneous infections, like gingivostomatitis, recurrent fever blisters, visceral infections like, oesophagitis, keratitis, proctitis, etc.
  ▪ **Varicella zoster virus infection:**
    ◆ Vesicular or ulcerative lesion at any stage of HIV infection
  ▪ **Epstein-barr virus infection:**
    ◆ Causes oral hairy leukoplakia
  ▪ **Human herpes virus 6,8:**
    ◆ **HHV 8:** Kaposi sarcoma
    ◆ **HHV 6:** Cause of pneumonia in AIDS patients

○ **Fungal Infections:**
  ▪ **Candidiasis:**
    ◆ **Candida albicans:** Most common species causing fungal infection
    ◆ Mucocutaneous candidiasis—common
    ◆ Systemic candidiasis
  ▪ **Aspergillosis:**
    ◆ Fumigatus, A. niger, A. flavus are the important pathogens
    ◆ Causes allergic bronchopulmonary aspergillosis, intercavitary aspergilloma and invasive and disseminated disease with CNS involvement
  ▪ **Cryptococcosis:**
    ◆ **Life:** Threatening pathogen
    ◆ Meningitis, myocarditis associated with acute heart failure and pleural effusion
  ▪ **Histoplasmosis:**
    ◆ Hepatosplenomegaly, lymphadenopathy, gastrointestinal bleeding, endocarditis, erythema multiformae and oropharyngeal ulcers.
○ **Parasitic infections:**
  ▪ **Toxoplasmosis:**
    ◆ **Toxoplasma gondii:** Causes encephalitis and neurological deficits
    ◆ Seizures- common in toxoplasmosis
  ▪ **Cryptosporidiosis:**
    ◆ Results in life-threatening enteritis with persistent diarrhea and dehydration
  ▪ **Microsporidiosis:**
    ◆ Microsporidia- important cause of opportunistic infection
    ◆ Causes disseminated infections and liver, kidney, brain commonly involved organs

   b. **Lab Diagnosis of Beta – thalassemia**

(Ref: Harsh Mohan, 7th ed. pg. 300–301, Robbins, SA ed. pg. 638–641)

ANSWER

Introduction

○ Decreased rate of β chain synthesis that results in decreased formation of HbA in the red cells.
○ **Types:** Based on reduction in β chain synthesis, 3 types of β- thalassaemia:
○ β-thalassaemia major
○ β-thalassaemia intermedia
○ β-thalassaemia minor(trait)

Laboratory Diagnosis

○ β-thalassaemia major

- **CBC:**
  - Severe anemia (Hb: 3-6 gm/dL)
  - **MCH, MCV, MCHC:** Decresed
  - **Hematocrit:** Decreased (severely)
  - **WBC:** Raised (usually), shift of left of neutrophil series with presence of some myelocytes and metamyelocytes
- **Peripheral blood smear:**
  - Severe microcytic hypochromic red cell
  - Marked anisopoikilocytosis
  - Target cells
  - Tear drop cells
  - Basophilic stippling
  - Cells with Cabot's ring
  - Pencil cells
  - Nucleated RBC's
- **Hemoglobin electrophoresis:**
  - Increased HbF
  - Increased HbA$_2$
  - HbA – absent or sometimes present in variable amounts
- **Bone marrow findings:**
  - Normoblastic erythroid hyperplasia
  - Intermediate and late normoblast predominant (smaller in size)
  - Siderotic granules in the cytoplasm of normoblasts
  - Increased reticuloendothelial iron
- **Biochemical findings:**
  - **Serum bilirubin (unconjugated):** Increased
  - **Serum iron:** Increased
  - **Urine urobilinogen:** Increased
  - **Serum ferritin:** Increased (300-3000 mg/dL)
- **Osmotic fragility:** decreased
- β- thalassaemia minor(trait)
  - **CBC:**
    - Mild anemia
    - **Hematocrit:** Decreased
    - **MCV, MCH, MCHC:** Slightly decreased
  - **Peripheral blood smear:**
    - Abnormalities minor as compared to thalassaemia major
    - Hypochromic, microcytic RBC
    - Mild anisopoikilocytosis
    - Target cells (rare)
    - Basophilic stippling (occasional)
  - **Hemoglobin electrophoresis:**
    - **HbA$_2$:** Markedly increased
  - **Biochemical findings:**
    - **Serum bilirubin(unconjugated):** Normal/ slightly increased
  - **Osmotic fragility:** Decreased

c   **Radiation Injury**

(Ref: Textbook of Pathology, Harsh Mohan, 7th ed. pg. 16)

ANSWER

Introduction

- As a result of exposure to ionizing radiation, mainly X-Rays, alpha, beta and gamma rays, radioactive isotopes, protons, neutrons, etc.

Types

- Due to external irradiation
- Radioactive material contamination
- Radioactive material incorporation into body cells, tissues, or organs.

Determinants of the Biologic Effects of Radiation

- Cell proliferation
- Oxygen content of tissues
- Vascular damage
- Rate of delivery and field size of exposure.

Major Effects of Radiation Injury

- **Skin:** Erythema, edema, depigmentation (weeks to month), atrophy and cancer(months to years)
- **Gastrointestinal tract:** In early cases, mucosal injury and ulceration, later on, fibrosis
- **Blood and bone marrow:** Thrombocytopenia, granulocytopenia, anemia, lymphopenia
- **Lymph nodes:** Atrophy and fibrosis (in later cases)
- **Brain:** Destruction of neurons and glial cells (embryonic)
- **Gonads:** Atrophy and fibrosis of testes and ovaries

Acute Radiation Syndrome

- Also known as radiation poisoning, radiation sickness or radiation toxicity
- High amount of ionizing radiation results in combination of health effects which present within 24 hours of exposure

d.   **Factors affecting ESR**

(Ref: Harsh Mohan, 7th ed. pg. 270, Robbins, SA ed. pg. 99)

ANSWER

Introduction

- It is the rate at which erythrocytes settle down when blood is (mixed with an anticoagulant) is allowed to stand in a vertical tube for one hour undisturbed.
- Expressed in mm/hrs
- Also known as "sed rate" or "Biernacki reaction"
- Inexpensive widely used screening test

Normal Values

- **Westergren method:**
  - **Males:** 3 to 7 mm in 1 hour
  - **Females:** 5 to 9 mm in 1 hour
- **Wintrobe method:**
  - **Males:** 0 to 9 mm in 1 hour
  - **Females:** 0 to 15 mm in 1 hour

Factors Affecting ESR

- **Physiologic factors:**
  - **Specific gravity of RBC:** Increase in specific gravity, increases ESR.
  - **Number of RBC:** Decrease in number of RBC, increases ESR. usually seen in anemia. Increase in number of RBC, decrease ESR
  - **Rouleaux formation:** Increases ESR
  - **Size of RBC:** Increase in size of RBC, increases the ESR
  - **RBC count:** Decrease in RBC count, decreases the viscosity of blood,thus increasing the ESR.
  - **Viscosity of blood:** Increased viscosity of blood, decreased ESR
  - **Age:** Less in infants and children – more number of RBC's
  - **Sex:** More in females than males
  - **Pregnancy:** From 3rd month ESR increases upto 35 mm in 1 hour
- **Laboratory factors:**
  - **Temperature:** High temperature causes false high result due to reduced plasma viscosity
  - **Time:** Test should be done within two hours of collection. Sample with EDTA should be used within six hours
  - **Tube factor:** Longer tube- increase ESR

- **Anticoagulants:** Tri sodium citrate or K2EDTA should be used
- **Vibration:** Decrease in ESR
- **Position of tube:** Tube should be vertical. Angle of 3 degree from vertical – increase in ESR by ESR
- **Sunlight:** Direct sunlight increases ESR
- **Pathologic factors:**
  - Tuberculosis, hodgkin's disease, multiple myeloma, macrocytosis, chronic infective or inflammatory conditions: increased ESR
  - Polycythemia, leukocytosis, spherocytosis, congestive cardiac failure: decrease in ESR
- Temperature of body, obesity, medicines-like Aspirin, NSAIDs: No effect on ESR

---

6. **Write short notes on:**

a. **FAB Classification of AML**

(Ref: Textbook of Pathology, Harsh Mohan, 7th ed. pg. 34)

ANSWER

Introduction

- Neoplasm of myeloid cells
- Common in adults (50yrs median age)

Etiology

- Mutation resulting in inhibition of myeloid stem cell maturation

FAB (French American British) Classification

- Based on morphology and cytochemistry, divided into 7 subtypes

Fab class		Percent cases	Morphology	Cytochemistry
MO:	Minimally differentiated AML	2	Blasts lack definite cytologic and cytochemical features but have myeloid lineage antigens	Myeloperoxidase -
M1:	AML without maturation	20	Myeloblasts predominate; few if any granules or auer rods	Myeloperoxidase +
M2:	AML with maturation	30	Myeloblasts with promyelocytes predominate; Auer rods may be present	Myeloperoxidase +++
M3:	Acute promyelocytic leukaemia	5	Hypergranular promyelocytes; often with multiple auer rods per cell	Myeloperoxidase +++
M4:	Acue myelomonocytic leukaemia (Naegeli type)	30	Mature cells of both myeloid and monocytif series in peripheral blood; myeloid cells resemble M2	Myeloperoxidase++ Non-specific esterase+
M5:	Acute monocytic leukaemia (Schilling type)	10	Two subtypes: M5a shows poorly-differentiated monoblasts, M5b shows differentiated promonocytes and monocytes	Non-specific esterase ++
M6:	Acute erythroleukaemia (Di Guglielmo's) syndrome)	<5	Erythroblasts predominate (>50%) myeloblasts and promyeloytes also increased	Erythroblasts PAS+ Myeloblasts: myeloperoxidase+
M7:	Acute megakaryocytic leukaemia	<5	Pleomorphic undifferentiated blasts pedominatereat with antiplatelet antibodies	Platelet peroxidase+

b **Mechanism of apoptosis**

(Ref: Textbook of Pathology, Harsh Mohan, 7th ed. pg. 94)

ANSWER

For answer, refer 2014 paper-I Q. 4 (b), Pg. 72

c. **Etiopathogenesis of shock**

(Ref: Robbins, SA ed. pg. 131-134)

ANSWER

Introduction

○ A physiologic state characterized by systemic reduction in tissue perfusion resulting decreased oxygen supply to tissues

Etiology and Types of Shock

○ **Hypovolemic shock**
○ Dhydration, blood loss, burns, pancreatitis, peritonitis
○ **Septic shock:**
  ▪ **Gram negative bacteria, like:** E. coli, Proteus, Pseudomonas, Klebsiella, etc.
  ▪ **Gram positive bacteria, like:** Streptococci, Pneumococci,etc.
○ **Cardiogenic shock:**
  ▪ Obstruction of outflow, e.g. Pulmonary embolism, Ball valve thrombus, etc.
  ▪ Deficient filling, e.g. cardiac temponade
  ▪ Deficient empyting, e.g. myocardial infarction, cardiomyopathies, arrhythmias, etc.
○ **Traumatic shock:**
  ▪ Severe injuries, obstetrical trauma, etc.

○ **Neurogenic shock:**
  ▪ Severe head injury, accidental high spinal anesthesia, etc.
○ **Hypoadrenal shock:**
  ▪ Administration of high doses of glucocorticoids, secondary adrenal insufficiency (e.g. tuberculosis, metastatic disease, etc.)
○ **Anaphylactic shock:**
  ▪ Immediate hypersensitivity reaction

Pathogenesis

Following three derangements results in shock

○ Decrease in effective circulatory blood volume
○ Reduced supply of oxygen to tissues resulting in anoxia and cellular injury
○ Release of inflammatory mediators and toxins in response to shock–induced cellular injury

Effective circulatory blood volume decreases
↓
Decrease in venous return
↓
Decreased cardiac out put
↓
Decreased blood flow
↓
Decreased oxygen supply to tissues and organs
↓
Tissue Anoxia
↓
Cellular injury
↓
Release of inflammatory mediators (TNF-α, IL-1, etc.)
↓
Shocks

Your Roll No. ....

Name of the Paper	:	**Pathology Paper-II**
Name of the Course	:	**MBBS-2009**
Semester	:	**Annual**

Time: 3 Hours   M.M.: 40

INSTRUCTIONS

1. Write your Roll No. on the top immediately on receipt of this question paper
2. All questions are to be attempted
3. Answers to Parts I, II and III should be written in separate answer sheets provided
4. Attempt parts of a question in sequence

PART-I

1. **Differentiate between:**   [8]
   a. Etiopathogenesis of obstructive and hemolytic jaundice
   b. Pathology of Typhoid and tubercular intestinal ulcer
   c. Causes and sequalae of constrictive and fibrinous pericarditis
   d. Hashimoto's thyroiditis and grave's disease

2. **Comment briefly on:**   [6]
   a. Etiopathogenesis of chronic gastric ulcer
   b. Serological diagnosis of hepatitis C virus infection
   c. Etiopathogenesis and morphology of fibro congestive spleen

PART-II

3. **Write short notes on:**   [6]
   a. Membranous glomerulo nephritis
   b. Secondary pulmonary tuberculosis and its sequalae

4. **Write briefly on:**   [6]
   a. Colorectal carcinoma
   b. Bacterial endocarditis

PART-III

5. **Write briefly on:**   [8]
   a. Nephrosclerosis
   b. Panacinar emphysema
   c. Alcoholic cirrhosis
   d. Barret esophagus

6. **Write briefly on:**   [6]
   a. Cervical intraepithelial neoplasia
   b. Microscopic changes in renal cell carcinoma
   c. Metastasis of testicular tumors

PART I

1. Differentiate between

a. Etiopathogenesis of obstructive and haemolytic jaundice

(Ref: Harsh Mohan, 7th ed. pg. 581, Robbins, SA ed. pg. 894-95)

ANSWER

Etiopathogenesis of obstructive and haemolytic jaundice

For answer, refer 2014 paper-II Q. 1 (d), Pg. 77

b. Pathology of Typhoid and tubercular intestinal ulcer

(Ref: Textbook of Pathology, Harsh Mohan, 7th ed. pg. 553)

ANSWER

For answer, refer 2017 paper-II Q. 1 (d), Pg. 16

c. Causes and sequelae of constrictive and fibrinous pericarditis

(Ref: Harsh Mohan, 7th ed. pg. 437, Robbins, SA ed. pg. 573-75)

ANSWER

Causes and sequelae of constrictive and fibrinous pericarditis

Constrictive pericarditis	Fibrinous pericarditis
Chronic form of pericarditis	Acute form of pericarditis
Causes are: Uraemia, myocardial infarction, rheumatic fever, trauma such as in cardiac surgery, acute bacterial infections	Causes are: viral infection e.g. coxsackie A or B viruses, influenza virus, mumps virus, adenovirus and infectious mononucleosis; rheumatic fever, rheumatoid arthritis, systemic lupus erythematosus, involvement of pericardium by malignant tumour in the vicinity such as carcinoma lung, mesothelioma and mediastinal tumours, tuberculous pericarditis in early stage
Less common	More common
Pericardial space is obliterated due to the organization of the underlying pericardial lesion, producing dense fibrosis	Pericardial space is filled with thick mixture of serous fluid with fibrinous exudate
Fibrinous exudates may resolve without sequelae or may resolve without sequelae or undergo organization	Fibrotic scar may undergo calcification
As heart gets encased in a dense fibrotic or fibrocalcific scar, it limits diastolic expansion, thus inability of ventricular filing, decreased ventricular end diastolic volume, stroke volume and cardiac output	Generally, no functional compromise

d. Hashimoto's thyroiditis and Grave's disease

(Ref: Harsh Mohan, 7th ed. pg. 795, Robbins, SA ed. pg. 89, 1090, 1086-1088)

ANSWER

For answer, refer 2013 paper-II Q. 2 (a), Pg. 95

2. Comment briefly on:

a. Etiopathogenesis of chronic gastric ulcer

(Ref: Textbook of Pathology, Harsh Mohan, 7th ed. pg. 533)

ANSWER

Etiopathogenesis of chronic gastric ulcer

Introduction

○ Chronic, solitary lesion with size less than 4 cm located in any part of GIT that is exposed to acid and peptic juices

Etiology

○ Helicobacter Pylori gastritis
○ NSAIDs-induced mucosal injury
○ Acid-pepsin secretions
○ Gastritis
○ Other local irritants such as spicy foods, alcohol, cigarette smoking, unbuffered aspirin
○ Dietary factors–nutritional deficiencies such as in lower socioeconomic strata, South India
○ Psychological factors–stress, anxiety, fatigue, ulcer type personality

- Genetic factors-Blood group O is more prone to gastric ulcers
- Hormonal factors–such as elaboration of gastrin by islet-cell tumour in Zollinger-Ellison syndrome, endocrine secretions in hyperplasia and adenomas od parathyroid glands, adrenal cortex, anterior pituitary

Pathogenesis of Gastric Ulcer

- Depends on the impaired gastric mucosal defences against acid-pepsin secretions
- Increased serum gastrin levels followed by consumption of food in an atonic stomach results in hyperacidity
- Some patients have low to normal gastric acid levels, ulcer results in such patients due to gastritis, bile reflux, cigarette smoke
- Gastric mucus barrier is deranged in gastric ulcer which may be due to colonisation of gastric mucosa by H. Pylori in 75–80 % cases

b. Serological diagnosis of hepatitis C virus infection

(Ref: Textbook of Pathology, Harsh Mohan, 7th ed. pg. 590)

ANSWER

Serological diagnosis of hepatitis C virus infection

For answer, refer 2017 paper-II Q. 3 (b), Pg. 20

c. Etiopathogenesis and Morphology of fibro congestive spleen

(Ref: Harsh Mohan, 7th ed. pg. 367, Robbins, SA ed. pg. 833-835)

ANSWER

Etiopathogenesis and Morphology of fibro congestive spleen

Etiopathogenesis

For answer, refer 2012 paper-II Q. 6 (b), Pg. 113

Morphology

- **Gross appearance:**
  - Enlarged, heavy and firm spleen
  - Tense and thickened capsule
  - Cut surface is firm with prominent trabeculae
- **Microscopic appearance:**
  - Dilatation of sinusoids with prominent splenic cords
  - White pulp is atrophic with thickened travbeculae
  - Haemorrhages and Gamna-Gandy bodies are formed sue to long standing congestion leading

to fibrocongestive splenomegaly–termed as Banti's spleen

PART II

3. **Write short notes on:**

   a. **Membranous glomerulonephritis**

   (Ref: Harsh Mohan, 7th ed. pg. 656, Robbins, SA ed. pg. 915)

ANSWER

Membranous glomerulonephritis

Introduction

- Widespread thickening of glomerular capillary wall and most frequent cause of nephrotic syndrome in adults
- Around 85% cases are idiopathic whereas 15% cases are secondary to underlying condition such as SLE, malignancies, infections – hepatitis B and C, syphilis, malaria and drugs

Morphology

- Gross appearance:
  - Enlarged, pale and smooth kidneys
- Microscopic appearance:
  - Glomeruli
    - Diffuse thickening of glomerular capillary walls with all the glomeruli being affected uniformly
    - Duplication (formation) of new basement membrane occurs as deposits are incorporated into hugely thickened basement membrane
    - Changes are observed by silver impregnation stains (black) or by periodic acid-Schiff stain (pink)
  - Tubules
    - Renal tubules remain normal initially when lid vacuolation of proximal convoluted tubules is found
  - Interstitium
    - Exhibits fine fibrosis and sparse chronic inflammatory cells
  - Vessels
    - Not prominent in initial stage but later hypertensive changes of arterioles are seen
- Electron microscopy
  - Typical electron dense deposits are seen in subepithelial location
  - Basement membrane protrudes between deposits as spikes
- Immunofluorescence microscopy

- Shows granular deposits of immune complexes consisting of IgG associated with complement C3
- Secondary cases may observe relevant antigen such as hepatitis B or tumour antigen

Clinical Picture

○ Proteinuria
○ Microscopic haematuria
○ Hypertension
○ Impaired renal function
○ Progressive azotaemia
○ Progression to End stage renal disease
○ Renal vein thrombosis due to hypercoagulability

b. Secondary pulmonary tuberculosis and its sequelae

(Ref: Harsh Mohan, 7th ed. pg. 143, Robbins, SA ed. pg. 373-376)

ANSWER

For answer, refer 2016 paper-II, Q 5 (d), Pg. 47

4. Write briefly on:

a. Colorectal carcinoma

(Ref: Harsh Mohan, 7th ed. pg. 570, Robbins, SA ed. pg. 448)

ANSWER

Colorectal carcinoma

For answer, refer 2011 paper-II Q. 3 (a), Pg. 123

b. Bacterial endocarditis

(Ref: Harsh Mohan, 7th ed. pg. 426, Robbins, SA ed. pg. 559-61)

ANSWER

Bacterial endocarditis

For answer, refer 2017 paper-II, Q. 1 (b), Pg. 15

PART III

5. Write briefly on:

a. Nephrosclerosis

(Ref: Harsh Mohan, 7th ed. pg. 677, Robbins, SA ed. pg. 938-939)

ANSWER

Nephrosclerosis

For answer, refer 2017 paper-II Q. 1 (a), Pg. 15

b. Panacinar emphysema

(Ref: Harsh Mohan, 7th ed. pg. 461–462, Robbins, SA ed. pg. 675)

ANSWER

Panacinar emphysema

For answer, refer 2016 paper-II, Q. 1 (b), Pg. 39

c. Alcoholic cirrhosis

(Ref: Harsh Mohan, 7th ed. pg. 606, Robbins, SA ed. pg. 827)

ANSWER

Alcoholic cirrhosis

For answer, refer 2011 paper-II Q. 4 (b), 126

d. Barret oesophagus

(Ref: Harsh Mohan, 7th ed. pg. 523, Robbins, SA ed. pg. 757-58)

ANSWER

Barret oesophagus

For answer, refer 2012 paper-II Q. 5 (c), Pg. 112

6. Write briefly on:

a. Cervical intraepithelial neoplasia

(Ref: Harsh Mohan, 7th ed. pg. 893, Robbins, SA ed. pg. 1003-04)

ANSWER

Cervical intraepithelial neoplasia

For answer, refer 2012 paper-II Q. 5 (d), Pg. 112

b. Microscopic changes in renal cell carcinoma

(Ref: Harsh Mohan, 7th ed. pg. 682, Robbins, SA ed. pg. 953-955)

ANSWER

Microscopic changes in renal cell carcinoma

Microscopic Appearance of Renal Cell Carcinoma

○ Clear cell type (70%)
- Most frequent pattern
- Clear cytoplasm owing to removal of glycogen and lipid from cytoplasm during processing of tissues
- Various patterns of tumour cells – solid, trabecular, tubular, separated by delicate vasculature
- Well differentiated tumours

- **Papillary cell type (15%)**
  - Organisation of tumour cells in papillary pattern over fibrovascular stalks
  - Cuboidal cells with round small nuclei
  - Psammoma bodies may appear
- **Granular cell type (8%)**
  - Tumour cells possess acidophilic cytoplasm in abundance
  - More marked nuclear pleomorphism, hyperchromatism and cellular atypia
- **Chromophobe type (5%)**
  - Exhibits admixture of pale clear cells with perinuclear halo and acidophilic granular cells
  - Cytoplasm contains many vesicles
- **Sarcomatoid type (1.5%)**
  - Most anaplastic and poorly differentiated type
  - Characterised by whorls of atypical spindle tumour cells
- **Collecting duct type (0.5%)**
  - Rare form which occurs in medulla
  - Consists of a single layer of cuboidal tumour cells organised in tubular and papillary pattern

c. Metastasis of testicular tumours

(Ref: Textbook of Pathology, Harsh Mohan, 7th ed. pg. 694)

ANSWER

Metastasis of Testicular tumours

- Testicular tumours are developed from totipotent germ cells, hence forward and backward differentiation can be observed, however most of the tumours metastasise true
- Lymphatic spread is frequent in all types of testicular tumours
- Initially, retroperitoneal paraaortic nodes are involved, and then mediastinal and supraclavicular nodes
- Haematogenous spread mainly occurs in lung, it also involves liver, brain, bones
- Seminoma metastasizes principally through lymphatic, and later, hematogenous spread occurs
- Non-seminomatous germ cell tumours metastasise early and hematogenous route is mostly involved

Name of the Paper : **Pathology Paper-I**

Name of the Course : **MBBS-2008**

Semester : **Annual**

Time: 3 Hours **M.M.: 40**

INSTRUCTIONS

1. Write your Roll No. on the top immediately on receipt of this question paper
2. All questions are to be attempted
3. Answers to Parts I, II and III should be written in separate answer sheets provided
4. Attempt parts of a question in sequence

PART-I

1. **Differentiate between:** [8]
   a. Healing by primary and secondary intention
   b. Clonal deletion and Clonal anergy
   c. Metaplasia and Dysplasia
   d. CML and Leukemoid reaction

2. **Comment briefly on:** [6]
   a. Laboratory diagnosis of diabetes mellitus
   b. Down's syndrome
   c. Type III hypersensitivity reaction

PART-II

3. **Write briefly on:** [6]
   a. DNA virus in Neoplasia
   b. Modes of spread of Tumors with suitable examples

4. **Write briefly on:** [6]
   a. Indication of BM aspiration
   b. CML

PART-III

5. **Short notes on:** [8]
   a. Coomb's test
   b. Haemophilia
   c. Bombay Blood group
   d. Red infarct

6. **Short note on:** [6]
   a. Role of complement in inflammation
   b. G6PD deficiency
   c. Chemotaxis

PART-I

1. Differentiate between:

a. Healing by primary intention and secondary intention

(Ref: Textbook of Pathology, Harsh Mohan, 7th ed. pg. 158)

ANSWER

For answer, refer 2011 paper-I Q. 1 (a), Pg. 116

b   Clonal deletion and clonal energy

ANSWER

Clonal deletion	Clonal anergy
• Due to activation induced cell death	• Prolonged or irreversible functional inactivation of lymphocytes
• Antigen presented by cells bear B7 ligand (bind to CD28 of T cells)	• Do not bear CD 28 ligand
• Results in self tolerance	

c. Metaplasia and Dysplasia

(Ref: Textbook of Pathology, Harsh Mohan, 7th ed. pg. 39–41)

ANSWER

For answer, refer 2011 paper-I Q. 1 (b), Pg. 116

d. CML and leukemoid reaction

(Ref: Harsh Mohan, 7th ed. pg. 332, Robbins, SA ed. pg. 270-71)

ANSWER

For answer, refer 2017 paper-I Q. 1 (c), Pg. 4

2. Comment briefly on:

a. Laboratory diagnosis of diabetes mellitus

(Ref: Textbook of Pathology, Harsh Mohan, 7th ed. pg. 816)

ANSWER

Introduction

○ According to WHO, diabetes mellitus is defined as heterogeneous disorder characterized by common feature of chronic hyperglycemia with disturbance of carbohydrate, fat and protein metabolism.

○ **Types:** Type 1 DM (10%) and Type 2 DM (80%)– Based on etiology

Laboratory Diagnosis

○ Fundamental basis for diagnosis-Hyperglycemia

○ According to American Diabetes Association (2007), definite diagnostic criteria for diagnosis of diabetes is as follows:

Test[a]	Threshold	Qualifier
Hemoglobin A1c or	$\geq 6.5\%$	Lab NGSP-certified, standardized DCCT assay
Fasting glucose or	$\geq$ 126 mg/dL (7.0 mmol/L)	No caloric intake for at least 8 hours
2- hour glucose or	$\geq$ 200 mg/dL (11.1 mmol/L)	After 75 g of anhydrous glucose
Random glucose	$\geq$ 200 mg/dL (11.1 mmol/L)	Plus classic hyperglycemia symptoms or crisis
NGSP, National Glycohemoglobin Standardization Program; DCCT, Diabetes Control and Complications Trial [a] Results must be confirmed by repeated testing		

Investigations in the Diagnosis of Diabetes Mellitus

○ **Urine testing:** For the presence of glucose and ketones
  ▪ **Glucosuria:**
    ♦ Benedict's qualitative test
    ♦ **Dipstick method:** Specific for glucose
  ▪ **Ketonuria:** To assess the severity of diabetes
    ♦ Rothera's test
    ♦ Strip test

○ **Single blood sugar estimation:** Fasting plasma glucose value above 126 mg/dL ($\geq$ 7 mmol/L) is indicative of diabetes
  ▪ O-toluidine method
  ▪ Somogyi- Nelson method
  ▪ Glucose oxidase method

○ **Fasting glucose test screening:** Screening test for type 2 DM

○ **Oral glucose tolerance test:** Mainly done in patients with borderline fasting plasma glucose value (between 100–140 mg/dL)

○ **Other tests:**
  ▪ Glycosylated Hemoglobin
  ▪ Extended GTT

PATHOLOGY

- Glycated albumin
- Insulin assay
- Intravenous GTT
- C-peptide assay

b.   Down syndrome

(Ref: Textbook of Pathology, Harsh Mohan, 7th ed. pg. 253)

ANSWER

For answer, refer 2012 paper-I Q. 5 (a), Pg. 105

c.   Type III hypersensitivity reaction

(Ref: Textbook of Pathology, Harsh Mohan, 7th ed. pg. 60)

ANSWER

For answer, refer 2013 paper-I Q. 2 (b), Pg. 86

3.   Write briefly on:

a.   DNA virus in neoplasia

(Ref: Textbook of Pathology, Harsh Mohan, 7th ed. pg. 217)

ANSWER

For answer, refer 2014 paper-I Q. 4 (a), Pg. 72

b.   Mode of Spread of Tumors with suitable examples

(Ref: Textbook of Pathology, Harsh Mohan, 7th ed. pg. 193–195)

ANSWER

For answer, refer 2016 paper-I Q. 2 (c), Pg. 28 and 2014 paper-I Q. 2 (c), Pg. 71

4.   Write briefly on:

a.   Indication of BM aspiration

(Ref: Textbook of Pathology, Harsh Mohan, 7th ed. pg. 262)

ANSWER

Introduction

○ Bone marrow examination provides diagnostic help and confirmation of a suspected diagnosis
○ Short-bevelled, wide bore needle with a adjustable guard and stylet is used for aspiration (Salah bone marrow aspiration needle)

Site

○ Posterior iliac crest and sternum
○ In infants- head of tibia

Indications

○ **Myeloproliferative disorders:** Chronic myeloid leukemia, Polycythemia vera
○ **White cell disorders:** Neutropenia, suspected leukemias
○ **Red cell disorders:** Megaloblastic anemia
○ Pancytopenia
○ Myelodysplastic syndromes
○ **Storage diseases:** Niemann Pick's disease, Gaucher's disease
○ **Parasitic diseases:** Kala- azar, malaria, etc.
○ Granulomatous conditions
○ Unexplained liver, spleen or lymph nodes enlargement

b.   CML (Chronic myeloid leukemia)

(Ref: Textbook of Pathology, Harsh Mohan, 7th ed. pg. 335)

ANSWER

For answer, refer 2010 paper-I Q. 4 (b), Pg. 133

PART III

5.   Write short notes on:

a.   Coomb's test

(Ref: Textbook of Pathology, Harsh Mohan, 7th ed. pg. 289)

ANSWER

For answer, refer 2016 paper-I Q. 5 (a), Pg. 32

b.   Hemophilia

(Ref: Textbook of Pathology, Harsh Mohan, 7th ed. pg. 313)

ANSWER

For answer, refer 2012 paper-I Q. 3 (a), Pg. 103

c.   Bombay blood group

(Ref: Textbook of Pathology, Harsh Mohan, 7th ed. pg. 318)

ANSWER

For answer, refer 2010 paper-I Q. 6 (a), Pg. 135

d.   Red infarct

(Ref: Textbook of Pathology, Harsh Mohan, 7th ed. pg. 112)

ANSWER

Introduction

○ A localized area of necrosis developed as a result of obstruction in arterial blood supply or venous drainage to a particular tissue

Types of Infarcts

o **According to color:**
  ▪ Anemic/Pale
  ▪ Red/Hemorrhagic
o **Depending on their age:**
  ▪ Fresh/recent
  ▪ Old/healed
o **Depending on presence or absence of infection:**
  ▪ Septic
  ▪ Bland

Etiology

o Occlusion of arterial supply
o Venous obstruction

Commonly Affected Organs

o Usually, lung and gastrointestinal tract (spongy organs)
o Organs with dual blood supply(lungs)
o Previously congested organs
o Reperfused organs/tissues

Morphologic Changes

o Large red area, congested and may become firm later but never pale
o Hemorrhagic margins are not sharply defined
o Organs exhibits edema

Microscopic Feature

o Presence of coagulative necrosis of the affected organ- characteristic feature

---

6. Write short notes on:

  a. Role of complement in inflammation

  (Ref: Textbook of Pathology, Harsh Mohan, 7th ed. pg. 127)

ANSWER

Introduction

o Complement system helps in both innate and adaptive immunity
o All the three pathways (classical, alternative and lectin) leads to the formation of membrane attack complex (MAC) responsible for lysis of cells/organisms like bacteria

Role of Complement

Complement	Function
C5a, C3a, C4a (anaphylatoxins)	Increase vascular permeability and vasodilatation Degranulation of mast cells and release of histamines Activation of lipoxygenase pathway o arachidonic acid metabolism in monocytes and neutrophils
C5a	Chemotaxis, neutrophil activation
C3b, C4b	Opsonization and phagocytosis by macrophages and neutrophils
C3,C5	Activation of proteolytic enzymes like –plasmin, lysosomal enzymes from neutrophils present in the inflammatory exudate

  b. G6PD Deficiency

  (Ref: Textbook of Pathology, Harsh Mohan, 7th ed. pg. 293)

ANSWER

For answer, refer 2013 paper-I Q. 2 (a), Pg. 85

  c. Chemotaxis

  (Ref: Textbook of Pathology, Harsh Mohan, 7th ed. pg. 120)

ANSWER

For answer, refer 2011 paper-I Q. 6 (b), Pg. 120

Name of the Paper : **Pathology Paper-II**

Name of the Course : **MBBS-2008**

Semester : **Annual**

Time: 3 Hours M.M.: 40

INSTRUCTIONS

1. Write your Roll No. on the top immediately on receipt of this question paper
2. All questions are to be attempted
3. Answers to Parts I, II and III should be written in separate answer sheets provided
4. Attempt parts of a question in sequence

PART-I

1. **Differentiate between:** [8]
   a. Nephrotic and Nephritic Syndrome
   b. Benign and Malignant Gastric Ulcer
   c. Rheumatic and Bacterial Endocarditis
   d. Atheroma and Fatty Streak

2. **Comment briefly on:** [6]
   a. Prognostic factors in carcinoma breast
   b. Clinical features and sequelae of Hepatitis B
   c. Non-seminomatous germ cell tumours

PART-II

3. **Write a brief account of:** [6]
   a. Cushing syndrome
   b. Osteogenic sarcoma

4. **Write briefly on:** [6]
   a. Hypersplenism and causes of splenomegaly
   b. Cervical intra epithelial neoplasia

PART-III

5. **Write briefly on:** [8]
   a. Bronchogenic carcinoma
   b. Krukenberg tumour
   c. Barrett esophagus
   d. Wilms tumor

6. **Write short notes on:** [6]
   a. Complications of acute myocardial infarction
   b. Etiopathogenesis and complications of gall stones
   c. Neuroblastoma

PART-I

1. Differentiate between:

a. Nephrotic and nephritic syndrome

(Ref: Textbook of Pathology, Harsh Mohan, 7th ed. pg. 649)

ANSWER

For answer, refer 2013 paper-II, Q. 1 (c), Pg. 94

b. Benign and malignant gastric ulcer

(Ref: Textbook of Pathology, Harsh Mohan, 7th ed. pg. 543)

ANSWER

Benign gastric ulcer	Malignant gastric ulcer
• Commonly seen in younger age group	• Usually older age people are involved
• Present at lesser curvature of pylorus and antrum	• Present at greater curvature of pylorus and antrum
• Exhibits small size, smooth radiating folds and overhanging margins	• Large size with interrupted, nodular folds
• Hemorrhagic base of the ulcer	• Necrotic base
• Healing is within 8-10 weeks	• Healing is not

c. Rheumatic and bacterial endocarditis

(Ref: Textbook of Pathology, Harsh Mohan, 7th ed. pg. 426)

ANSWER

For answer, refer 2017 paper-II Q. 1 (b), Pg. 15

d. Atheroma and fatty streak

ANSWER

Atheroma	Fatty streak
• Large amount of extracellular lipid	• Mainly intracellular lipid accumulation
• Eccentric whitish-yellow raised lesion of 0.5 to 1.5 cm in diameter	• Flat, yellow multiple lesions with less than 1mm in diameter
• Mainly elastic, large and medium sized muscular arteries are involved	• Areas not affected by atherosclerosis are involved
• Mainly seen in older age group	• can be seen in children(may be < 1 year)

2. Comment briefly on:

a. Prognostic factors in carcinoma breast

(Ref: Textbook of Pathology, Harsh Mohan, 7th ed. pg. 758)

ANSWER

Prognostic factors for breast carcinoma

- **Major prognostic factors:**
  - **Size of tumor:**
    - If tumor size < 1 cm, then 10 years. Survival rate (90% cases) and in tumor size>2cm survival rate decreases to approx. 77%
  - **Lymph node metastasis:**
    - Involvement of axillary lymph node is the important prognostic factor.
    - 10 years. Survival rate (70–80%)-with no involvement
    - 1–3 positive nodes-survival rate 35–40%
    - Capsular invasion and huge metastatic deposits indicates poor prognosis
  - **Distant metastasis:**
    - Presence of distant metastasis indicates poor prognosis
  - **Invasive carcinoma versus in situ disease:**
    - Invasion through basement membrane and spread beyond ductal system in invasive carcinoma whereas in situ carcinoma is confined to ductal system. Thus, in situ carcinoma presents with better prognosis.
  - **Inflammatory carcinoma:**
    - Malignancy with redness, inflammation, thick skin indicates poor prognosis
  - **Locally advanced disease:**
    - Skeletal muscle and skin invasion revels poor prognosis
- **Minor prognostic factors:**
  - **Histologic grading:**
    - Histologic grading based on tubule formation, mitotic rate and nuclei regularity classified invasive carcinoma into three groups, i.e. (low grade, moderate and high grade)
  - **Histologic subtype:**
    - Tubular, colloid, medullary, papillary and lobular types of invasive carcinomas have better prognosis.

PATHOLOGY

Rate of proliferation:
  - High proliferative rate indicates poor prognosis
- High levels of estrogen and progesterone receptor in tumor indicates better prognosis
- Poor prognosis associated with lymphovascular invasion
- overexpression of HER2/neu associated with poor prognosis
- Abnormal DNA content in aneuploid tumor indicates poor prognosis
- Response of tumor to neoadjuvant therapy before surgery is an important prognostic factor

b.　Clinical Features and sequelae of hepatitis B

(Ref: Textbook of Pathology, Harsh Mohan, 7th ed. pg. 591)

ANSWER

For answer, refer 2016 paper-II Q. 5 (b), Pg. 45

c.　Non-seminomatous germ cell tumors

(Ref: Textbook of Pathology, Harsh Mohan, 7th ed. pg. 758)

ANSWER

Non-seminomatous Germ Cell Tumors

- A germ cell tumor of testis
- Small with loss of testicular contour
- Early metastasis mainly by hematogenous route
- Raised levels of hCG, AFP, LDH, etc.
- Resistant to radiation
- Aggressive tumor with poor prognosis

Types of Non-seminomatous Germ Cell Tumors

- **Embryonal carcinoma:**
  - Common in 25–25 years of age
  - Present as small, rounded, irregular mass
  - Raised levels of AFP or hCG or both
  - Grossly, shows invasion of tunica and epididymis
- **Choriocarcinoma:**
  - Rare tumor(1-2%)
  - Common in 2nd, 3rd decade of life
  - Distant metastasis- to lungs and brain
  - Increased levels of hCG
  - Histopathologically, consist of syncytiotrophoblastic cells and cytotrophoblastic cells
- **Yolk sac tumour:**
  - Common in infants and young children (up to the age of 4 years)
  - Increased AFP
  - Homogenous, non-encapsulated, mucinous appearance

- Microscopically, consist of flattened to cuboidal epithelial cells with clear vacuolated cytoplasm
- **Schiller:** Duval bodies present (perivascular structures)
- Presence of intracellular and extracellular PAS positive hyaline globules
- **Teratoma:**
  - Common in children and infants (approx. 40%)
  - In adults (approx. 5 %)
  - Raised AFP or hCG levels (20–25% cases)
  - **Types:**
    - Mature
      - Composed of well-differentiated structures like-cartilage, smooth muscles, etc. in a disorganized manner
    - **Immature**
      - Composed of primitive and incompletely differentiated tissue
    - **Teratoma with malignant transformation**
      - Rare form
      - Exhibits malignant changes
- **Mixed germ cell tumor**
  - Most common type of NSGCT
  - Teratoma and embryonal cell carcinoma is the most common combibation

PART-II

3.　Write a brief account of:

a.　Cushing syndrome

(Ref: Textbook of Pathology, Harsh Mohan, pg. 832-835)

ANSWER

For answer, refer 2010 paper-II Q. 6 (a), Pg. 144

b.　Osteogenic Sarcoma

(Ref: Textbook of Pathology, Harsh Mohan, 7th ed. pg. 832–835)

ANSWER

For answer, refer 2017 paper-II Q. 3 (a), Pg. 19

4.　Write briefly on:

a.　Hypersplenism and causes of splenomegaly

(Ref: Textbook of Pathology, Harsh Mohan, 7th ed. pg. 367)

ANSWER

For answer, refer 2012 paper-II Q. 6 (b), Pg. 113

b. **Cervical intra epithelial neoplasia**

(Ref: Textbook of Pathology, Harsh Mohan, 7th ed. pg. 893)

ANSWER

For answer, refer 2012 paper-II Q. 5 (d), Pg. 112

PART-III

5. **Write briefly on:**

   a. **Bronchogenic carcinoma**

   (Ref: Textbook of Pathology, Harsh Mohan, 7th ed. pg. 523)

ANSWER

Introduction

- Commonly known as "lung cancer"
- Characterized by carcinoma of the respiratory epithelium lining bronchi, bronchioles and alveoli
- Most common primary malignant tumor

Etiology

- Smoking (tobacco smoking) – most common
- Pollution
- Radiation exposure
- Dietary factors, like- vitamin A deficiency
- Occupational, example- workers exposed to asbestos, arsenic, nickel, beryllium, etc.

Clinical Features

- Common in middle age with peak incidence between 55–65 years of age
- **Local symptoms:** Cough, chest pain, dyspnea, hemoptysis
- Fever
- Pleural effusion
- Weight loss
- Painful bony lesion, paralysis of recurrent nerve, superior vena caval syndrome(as a result of metastasis)
- Paraneoplastic syndromes, like-polymyositis, peripheral neuropathy, calcitonin producing hypocalcaemia, etc.

Morphology

- **Two main types:**
  - Hilar type: involves main bronchus or its branches in the hilar part, chiefly right side
  - Peripheral type: single or multiple nodular tumor present in the lung periphery exhibiting pneumonia like consolidation of a large part of the lung

- **Microscopic findings:** Five main histologic subtypes
  - **Squamous cell carcinoma:**
    - Most common type
    - Common in males
    - Microscopically, exhibits keratinization or intercellular bridges
  - **Adenocarcinoma:**
    - Common in females
    - Categorized into preinvasive, minimally invasive and invasive adenocarcinoma
  - **Small cell carcinoma:**
    - **Two subtypes:**
      - **Pure small cell carcinoma:** Consists of small, round, oat-like cells arranged in the form of cords, ribbons forming pseudorosettes
      - **Combined small cell carcinoma:** Consist of a definite component of small cell carcinoma along with component of non-small lung carcinoma
  - **Large cell carcinoma:** Undifferentiated carcinomas and composed of tumor cells with large nuclei, abundant cytoplasm, prominent nucleoli and well defined borders
  - **Adenosquamous carcinoma:** Exhibit keratinization and glandular differentiation

Diagnosis

- Sputum examination (cytological)
- Radiological examination of the chest
- Bronchioalveolar lavage and bronchial washing

   b. **Krukenberg tumor**

   (Ref: Textbook of Pathology, Harsh Mohan, 7th ed. pg. 740)

ANSWER

Introduction

- It is a bilateral metastatic ovarian malignancy
- **Common primary sites for metastasis:**
  - Gastrointestinal tract (gastric carcinoma)
  - Other sites- breast, colon, appendix, etc.
- Metastasis-by transcoelomic spread

Clinical Features

- Common in 30–40 years of age
- Clinically, silent
- Abdominal pain or pelvic pain
- Ascites
- Bloating
- Vaginal bleeding or change in menstrual habits

Gross Appearance

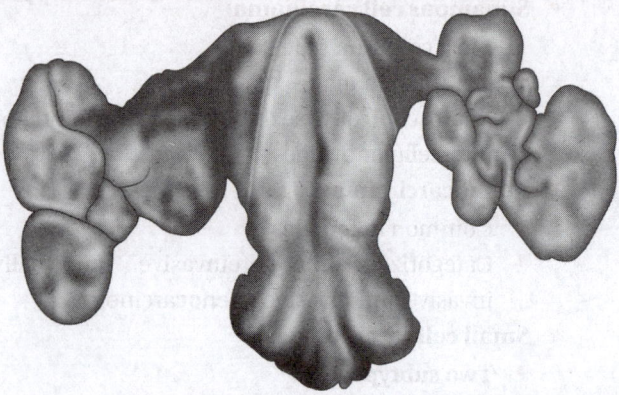

Fig. Krukenberg tumor

- Multinodular mass in both ovaries that are round to kidney shaped, firm, grey-white to yellow in color with areas of necrosis and hemorrhage

Microscopic Findings

- Presence of signet ring cells filled with mucin and proliferation of ovarian stromal cells

Diagnosis

- Confirmatory diagnosis based on –
  - Laparotomy
  - CT scan
  - Ovarian biopsy

   c. Barret oesophagus

(Ref: Textbook of Pathology, Harsh Mohan, 7th ed. pg. 523)

ANSWER

For answer, refer 2012 paper-II Q. 5 (c), Pg. 112

   d. Wilms' tumor

(Ref: Textbook of Pathology, Harsh Mohan, 7th ed. pg. 740)

ANSWER

For answer refer 2013 paper-II Q. 3 (b), Pg. 96

6. Write short notes on:

   a. Complications of acute myocardial infarction

(Ref: Textbook of Pathology, Harsh Mohan, 7th ed. pg. 415)

ANSWER

- **Important complications which may arise in case of acute myocardial infarction are:**
  - **Congestive heart failure:**
    - Right ventricular failure, LVF or both are common in patients of acute MI

- **Arrhythmias:**
  - Most common complication of acute MI
  - As a result of ischemic injury of the conduction system or may be due to raised lactate and free fatty acid concentration in the tissue fluid, etc.
  - **Includes:** Sinus bradycardia, sinus tachycardia, atrial fibrillation, premature systole, etc.
- **Cardiac aneurysm:**
  - Common in left ventricle
  - Results on impairment of heart function and responsible for mural thrombi
  - Present in healed infarcts
- **Thromboembolism:**
  - As a result of intracardiac thrombi and thrombosis in the leg veins (approx. 20-45% cases)
  - Thromboemboli as a result of prolonged bed rest causing venous thrombosis in the leg veins
  - Also results in occlusion of the renal, pulmonary, splenic, mesenteric, etc. arteries followed by infarcts
- **Rupture:**
  - Common in infarcted ventricular wall upto the pericardial cavity
  - Resuts in hemopericardium and tamponade
  - Incomplete rupture resulting in pseudoaneurysm
- **Pericarditis:**
  - Pericardial effusion along with fibrinous pericarditis
- **Postmyocardial infarction syndrome:**
  - Mainly occurs 1 to 6 weeks after the attack
  - Also called as " Dressler's syndrome"
  - Pneumonitis is common
  - Present mild symptoms and disappear within few weeks
- **Cardiogenic shock:**
  - Results in hypotension and also accompanied by oligouria, peripheral circulatory failure, etc.
- **Papillary muscle dysfunction**
- **Extension of infarct**
- **Formation of ventricular aneurysm**

   b. Etiopathogenesis and complications of gall stones

(Ref: Textbook of Pathology, Harsh Mohan, 7th ed. pg. 623-625)

ANSWER

Etiopathogenesis of Gall Stones

- **Gall stones consists of cholesterol, bile pigments and calcium salts**

Risk Factors

○ **For cholesterol stones:**

- Increased cholesterol content associated with advancing age
- Common in females and females on birth control pills (estrogen therapy)
- Obesity
- Low fiber content in diet
- Certain GI disorders like- Crohn's disease, ileal resection, etc.
- Mutation in CYP7A1 gene results in hypercholesterolemia and gall stones

○ **For pigment stones:**

- Hemolytic anemia
- Biliary infection
- Common in cirrhosis and hepatocellular disease
- Common in Asians

Pathogenesis

○ **Cholesterol stones:**

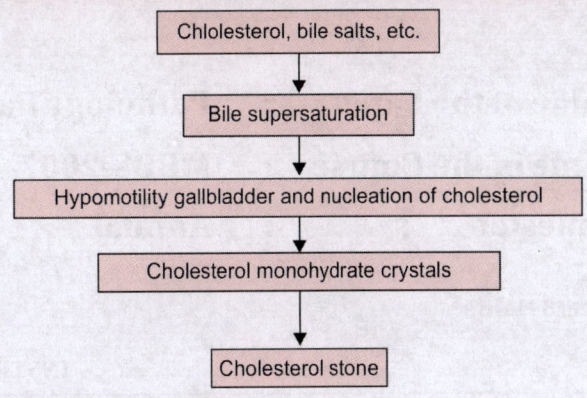

○ **Pigment stones:**

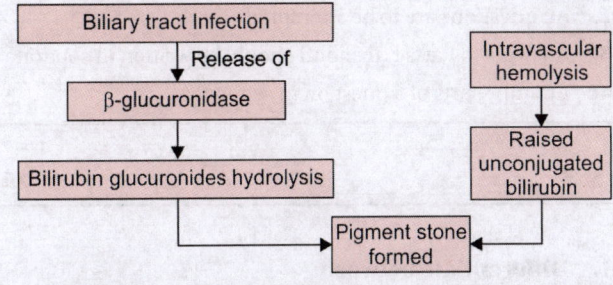

Complications of gall stones:

For answer, refer 2007 paper II Q. 5 (b), Pg. 179

    c. **Neuroblastoma**

(Ref: Textbook of Pathology, Harsh Mohan, 7th ed. pg. 791)

ANSWER

For answer, refer to 2014 paper-II Q. 6 (b), Pg. 82

Name of the Paper : **Pathology Paper-I**

Name of the Course : **MBBS-2007**

Semester : **Annual**

Time: 3 Hours **M.M.: 40**

INSTRUCTIONS

1. Write your Roll No. on the top immediately on receipt of this question paper
2. All questions are to be attempted
3. Answers to Parts I, II and III should be written in separate answer sheets provided
4. Attempt parts of a question in sequence

PART-I

1. **Differentiate between:** [8]
   a. Carcinoma and sarcoma
   b. Exudate and Transudate
   c. Dystrophic and metastatic calcification
   d. Bleeding in platelet and coagulation disorders

2. **Comment briefly on:** [6]
   a. Immune change in AIDS
   b. Pathogenesis of hypovolemic shock
   c. Mechanism of Transplant rejection

PART-II

3. **Write briefly on:** [6]
   a. Lab. Diagnosis of multiple myeloma
   b. Causes of intravascular hemolysis and lab. Diagnosis of sickle cell anaemia

4. **Write briefly on:** [6]
   a. Spread of tumors
   b. Mechanisms of auto immune diseases

PART-III

5. **Write briefly on:** [8]
   a. Mismatched blood transfusion and its. Lab diagnosis
   b. Philadelphia chromosome
   c. Prothrombin time
   d. Prognostic factors of ALL

6. **Write short note on:** [6]
   a. Pancytopenia
   b. Klinefelter's syndrome
   c. Lab. Diagnosis of chronic renal failure

PART-I

1. Differentiate between:

a. Carcinoma and Sarcoma

(Ref: Textbook of Pathology, Harsh Mohan, 7th ed. pg. 104)

ANSWER

Carcinoma	Sarcoma
• Malignant tumor of epithelial tissue origin	• Malignant tumor of mesenchymal origin (muscle, bone, cartilage, vascular, fibrous, fat tissue, etc.)
• Common	• Relatively rare
• Commonly seen in people over 50 years . of age	• Commonly seen in people below 50 yrs . of age
• Rate of growth is rapid	• Comparatively slow rate of growth
• Spread is initially by lymphatics	• Mainly haematogenous spread of tumor
• Prognosis comparatively better	• Poor prognosis
• Examples- Squamous cell carcinoma, adenocarcinoma, basal cell carcinoma, etc.	• Examples- Osteosarcoma, Liposarcoma, chondrosarcoma, etc.

b. Exudate and Transudate

(Ref: Textbook of Pathology, Harsh Mohan, 7th ed. pg. 81)

ANSWER

For answer, refer 2017 paper-I Q. 1 (b), Pg. 4

c. Dystrophic and Metastatic Calcification

(Ref: Textbook of Pathology, Harsh Mohan, 7th ed. pg. 37)

ANSWERS

For answer, refer 2014 paper-I Q. 1 (a), Pg. 70

d. Bleeding in platelet and coagulation disorders

(Ref: Textbook of Pathology, Harsh Mohan, 7th ed. pg. 310–333)

ANSWER

Platelet Disorder	Coagulation Disorder
• Bleeding from superficial cut is present	• No bleeding from superficial cut
• On application of local pressure, bleeding does not stop quickly	• On application of local pressure, bleeding stops quickly
• Spontaneous bleeding common	• No usual spontaneous bleeding
• Hemarthrosis not present	• Hemarthrosis is characteristic
• Small and multiple ecchymosis	• Ecchymosis is large and solitary
• Bleeding after trauma is immediate, less and for short time	• Bleeding after trauma is delayed and persistent
• Presence of petechiae	• Petechiae is absent

2. Comment briefly on:

a. Immune change in AIDS

(Ref: Textbook of Pathology, Harsh Mohan, 7th ed. pg. 54)

ANSWER

Introduction

○ Caused by an RNA virus (retrovirus)- human immunodeficiency virus

○ **Two types:** HIV-1 and HIV-2

○ Depletion of CD4+ T cells resulting in immunosuppression

○ Immunological changes due to HIV infection results in immunosuppression making the host susceptible to infections, tumors, etc.

Immune Changes in AIDS

○ **Depletion of CD4+T cells causes immunodeficiency:** major cause of depletion is apoptosis and other causes include induction of syncytium formation, alteration of membrane permeability, mitochondrial dysfunction, etc.

○ **Reversal of CD4:** CD8 cell ratio

○ **Loss of function of CD4+ T cells:** Due to functional defects in the immune system (binding of gp120 molecules to the surface of CD4+ T cells.)

○ **Cytokine dysregulation and coagulopathy in HIV infection:**

▪ Secretion of T-helper 1 (Th1) cytokines, such as Interleukin -2 and INF-gamma decreased.

▪ IL-1, IL-6, TNF-α is increased

▪ Reduced NK cells

- **Altered monocyte –macrophage response:**
  - Altered balance of Th1 and Th2 response
  - Decrease chemotaxis and phagocytosis
  - Decrease HLA II expression
- **Polyclonal B cell activation:**
  - Loss of control/signal for B cell function in vitro
  - Hypergammaglobulinemia and circulating immune complexes

b. Pathogenesis of Hypovolemic Shock

(Ref: Textbook of Pathology, Harsh Mohan, 7th ed. pg. 95-96)

ANSWER

For answer, refer 2012 paper-I Q. 4 (b), Pg. 105

c. Mechanism of transplant rejection

(Ref: Textbook of Pathology, Harsh Mohan, 7th ed. pg. 50)

ANSWER

Introduction

- The rejection reaction depends on the amount of genetic differences between donar and recipient in HLA system.
- The more is the genetic disparity (between donar and recipient), stronger and fast will be the rejection reaction.

Types of Graft

- Autografts
- Allografts
- Isografts
- Xenografts

Rejection Pathways

- **Cell mediated immune reactions:**
  - Responsible for rejection and are T cell mediated
  - In case of incompatibility, recipient lymphocytes sensitized with contact of HLA antigen of donar
  - Cytotoxic T cells (CD8+) as well as helper T cells (CD4+) are responsible for the destruction of graft.
- **Humoral immune reactions:**
  - Humoral antibodies play an important role in certain rejection reactions.
  - For example- preformed circulating antibodies (pre-sensitised recipient), or complement dependent cytotoxicity, antibody–dependent cell mediated cytotoxicity (ADCC) in non-sensitised individuals.

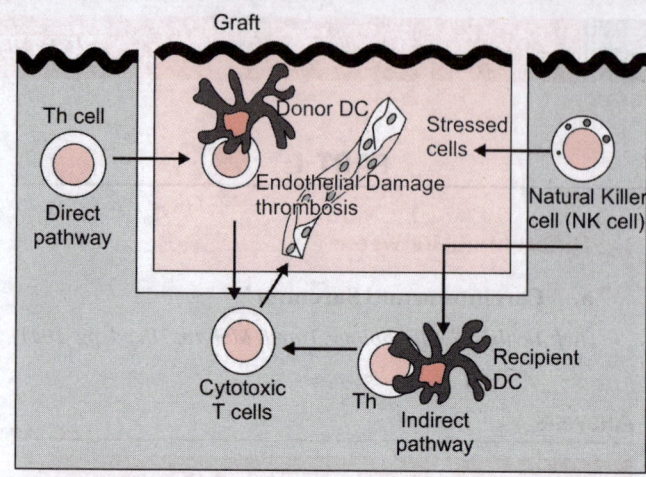

Types of Rejection Reactions

Three types of rejection reaction

- **Hyperacute:** Evident within minutes to hours
- **Acute:** Few days to a few months
- **Chronic:** Appear after repeated attacks of acute rejection or develop slowly

PART–II

3. Write briefly on:

a. Lab Diagnosis of Multiple Myeloma

(Ref: Textbook of Pathology, Harsh Mohan, 7th ed. pg. 363)

ANSWER

For answer, refer 2017 paper-I Q. 4 (b), Pg. 8

b. Causes of intravascular hemolysis and lab diagnosis of sickle cell anemia

(Ref: Textbook of Pathology, Harsh Mohan, 7th ed. pg. 296)

ANSWER

Intravascular Hemolysis

- Lysis of red cells in the circulation and release of contents into the plasma
- Marked increase in plasma hemoglobin

Causes

- Microangiopathic hemolytic anemia (sickle cell anemia, DIC, TTP)
- Autoimmune hemolytic anemia(AIHA)
- Thermal injury
- Mechanical trauma to red cells
- Paroxysmal nocturnal hemoglobinuria (PNH)
- G6PD deficiency

- Pregnancy induced hypertension (PIH)
- **Infections:** Malarial, bacterial, etc.

Sickle Cell Anemia

- Formation of HbS in the red cell with inheritance of abnormal gene from each parent.
- **Genetic defect:** Single point mutation in 6th codon of β- globin

Lab Diagnosis

- **CBC:**
  - **Hemoglobin:** Moderate to severe anemia (6–9 g/dL)
  - **Reticulocyte:** Increased
- **Peripheral blood smear:**
  - Sickle- shaped RBC's (elongated crescent-shaped)
  - Target cells
  - Howell- jolly bodies(feature of splenic atrophy)
  - **Sickling test:** Use of sodium metabisulfite (reducing agent) induces sickling of RBC's (positive sickling test)
- **Hemoglobin electrophoresis:**
  - Decreased or absent HbA
  - Predominant HbS and 2–20% Hb
- **Solubility test:**
  - With reducing substance, eg. sodium dithionite, HbS polymerizes and produces turbid solution
- **Osmotic fragility test:**
  - Decreased fragility due to sickle shape
- **Prenatal diagnosis:**
  - Analysis of fetal DNA
- **Biopsy:**
  - **Spleen:** Presence of gamma gandy bodies
- **X-ray:**
  - **Skull:** "Crew cut" appearance
  - **Vertebrae:** Fish mouth vertebra
- **High performance liquid chromatography** (Hb-HPLC)

---

4. **Write briefly on:**

    a. **Spread of tumors**

    (Ref: Textbook of Pathology, Harsh Mohan, 7th ed. pg. 193-195)

ANSWER

For answer, refer 2016 paper-I Q. 2 (c)

    b. **Mechanism of autoimmune diseases**

    (Ref: Textbook of Pathology, Harsh Mohan, 7th ed. pg. 62)

ANSWER

For answer, refer 2011 paper-I Q. 5 (c), Pg. 119

PART III

5. **Write briefly on:**

    a. **Mismatched Blood Transfusion and its Lab Diagnosis**

    (Ref: Textbook of Pathology, Harsh Mohan, 7th ed. pg. 318)

ANSWER

Introduction

- Transfer of blood or blood components from donar into the bloodstream of recipient is called as " blood transfusion"

Mismatched Blood Transfusion

- Due to ABO and Rh incompatibility.
- Adverse reactions that occur due to transfusion of mismatched blood
- Occur between recipient plasma and donar RBC's
- Mismatched blood transfusion leads to hemolytic reactions
- Severity of reaction depends upon the type of reaction, amount of blood transfused and general health of the patient

Immune Mediated Reaction

- **Hemolytic transfusion reaction:**
  - Transfusion of mismatched blood due to ABO incompatibility
  - ABO isoagglutinins are responsible for most of the reactions
  - Severe intravascular hemolysis
  - Immune antibodies of the Rh system results in extravascular hemolysis
  - Delayed reactions results 1 to 4 weeks after the transfusion
  - Delayed reaction is less severe
  - **Other reactions besides hemolytic transfusion reaction are:** Allergic reactions, graft-versus-host disease, anaphylactic shock, etc.
  - **Transfusion related acute lung injury (TRALI):** High levels of anti-HLA antibodies that adhere to recipient leucocytes. Release of mediators of increased vascular permeability leading to acute pulmonary edema and respiratory failure

Non-immune Transfusion Reactions

- **Massive Transfusion:** Dilution of coagulation factors

- **Circulatory overload:** Results in pulmonary congestion and acute heart failure
- **Transmission of infection:** includes transmission of malaria, hepatitis, infectious mononucleosis, CMV infection, AIDS, etc.
- **Air embolism**
- **Thrombophlebitis**
- **Transfusion hemosiderosis:** Occur after repeated transfusions, mainly in thalassaemia major, severe chronic refractory anemia

Lab Diagnosis of Acute Hemolytic Transfusion Reaction

- Increased serum LDH
- Decreased serum haptoglobin
- Serum indirect bilirubin level is increased
- Coomb's test for antibody detection

Lab Diagnosis of Allergic Transfusion Reaction

- **Serum IgA:** For screening test
- **Mast cell tryptase test:** Indicator of mast cell activation

Lab Diagnosis of Delayed Hemolytic Transfusion Reaction

- Increased LDH
- Increased bilirubin
- Decreased serum haptoglobin
- Reticulocytosis
- Direct antiglobulin test positive
- Prothombin time may be elevated (mainly in DIC)

b.   Philadelphia chromosome

(Ref: Textbook of Pathology, Harsh Mohan, 7th ed. pg. 335)

ANSWER

For answer, refer 2015 paper-I Q 6 (a), Pg. 58

c.   Prothrombin time

(Ref: Textbook of Pathology, Harsh Mohan, 7th ed. pg. 308)

ANSWER

For answer, refer 2015 paper-I Q. 5 (a), Pg. 56

d.   Prognostic Factors of ALL

(Ref: Textbook of Pathology, Harsh Mohan, 7th ed. pg. 354)

ANSWER

For answer, refer 2010 paper-I Q. 3 (b), Pg. 133

6.   **Write short notes on:**

a.   Pancytopenia

(Ref: Textbook of Pathology, Harsh Mohan, 7th ed. pg. 301)

ANSWER

For answer, refer 2014, Paper I Q. 6 (a), Pg. 74

b   Kinefelter's syndrome

(Ref: Textbook of Pathology, Harsh Mohan, 7th ed. pg. 253)

ANSWER

For answer, refer 2017 paper-I Q. 2 (a), Pg. 5

c.   Lab diagnosis of chronic renal failure

(Ref: Textbook of Pathology, Harsh Mohan, 7th ed. pg. 592)

ANSWER

For answer, refer 2017 paper-II 4 (b), Pg. 21

Name of the Paper	:	**Pathology Paper-II**
Name of the Course	:	**MBBS-2007**
Semester	:	**Annual**

Time: 3 Hours   **M.M.: 40**

INSTRUCTIONS

1. Write your Roll No. on the top immediately on receipt of this question paper
2. All questions are to be attempted
3. Answers to Parts I, II and III should be written in separate answer sheets provided
4. Attempt parts of a question in sequence

PART-I

1. **Differentiate between** [8]
   a. Transmural and sub-endocardial infarct
   b. Benign and malignant gastric ulcer
   c. Lab findings in obstructive and hepato-cellular jaundice
   d. Hapatitis B and hepatitis C infection

2. **Write briefly on** [6]
   a. Tubercular osteomyelitis
   b. Morphology and complication of atheromatous plaque
   c. Acute pancreatitis

PART-II

3. **Write briefly on:** [6]
   a. Giant cell tumor of bone
   b. Amoebic colitis

4. **Write briefly on:** [6]
   a. Glioblastoma multiforme
   b. Atherosclerosis

PART-III

5. **Write short notes on:** [8]
   a. Fibrocytic carcinoma of breast
   b. Complication of gall stones
   c. Teratoma testis
   d. Carcinoid

6. **Comment on:** [6]
   a. Advanced glycolysation end products
   b. Complication of bronchiectasis
   c. Hodgkin Lymphoma

PART-I

1. Diferentiate between:

a. Transmural and sub-endocardial infarct

(Ref: Textbook of Pathology, Harsh Mohan, 7th ed. pg. 410)

ANSWER

For answer, refer 2015 paper-II Q. 1 (a), Pg. 61

b. Benign and malignant gastric ulcer

(Ref: Textbook of Pathology, Harsh Mohan, 7th ed. pg. 543)

ANSWER

For answer, refer 2014 paper-II Q. 1 (a), Pg. 77

c. Lab findings in obstructive and hepato-cellular jaundice

(Ref: Textbook of Pathology, Harsh Mohan, 7th ed. pg. 584)

ANSWER

For answer, refer 2017 paper-I Q. 1 (a), Pg. 4

d. Hapatitis B and hepatitis C infection

(Ref: Textbook of Pathology, Harsh Mohan, 7th ed. pg. 591)

ANSWER

Hepatitis B infection	Hepatitis C infection
• Causative agent is HBV	• Causative agent is HCV
• **Genome:** DNA, ss/ds	• **Genome:** RNA,ss, linear and circular
• Incubation period is 30-180 days	• Incubation period is 20–90 days
• Double- shelled enveloped virus	• Enveloped virus
• **Antigen:** HBsAg, HBcAg, HBeAg, HBxAg	• **Antigen:** HCV RNA, C 100-3, C33c, NS5
• **Antibodies:** Anti-HBs, abti-HBc, anti-HBe	• **Antibodies:** Anti-HCV
• Severe occsionally	• Moderately severe
• Prognosis worsen with age	• Moderate prognosis

2. Write briefly on

a. Tubercular Osteomyelitis

(Ref: Textbook of Pathology, Harsh Mohan, 7th ed. pg. 824)

ANSWER

Introduction

○ Common condition seen in underdeveloped and developing countries of the world

Causative Agent

○ Tubercle bacilli, Mycobacterium tuberculosis

Spread

○ Hematogenous spread usually from lungs and direct or lymphatic spread from pulmonary or gastrointestinal tuberculosis

Age

○ Common in young adults and adolescents

Sites

○ Spine (Pott's disease, thoracic, lumbar) and bones of extremities are commonly involved
○ Joint spaces and intervertebral discs are also involved

Clinical Features

○ Onset of the disease is insidious
○ Localized tenderness present
○ Pain on motion
○ Weight loss, low grade fever and chills

Morphology

○ Lesion exhibits areas of bone destruction and caseous material along with multiple discharging sinus through the soft tissues and skin
○ Psoas abscess or lumbar cold abscess: Caseous material along with pus extend from the lumbar vertebrae to the sheaths of psoas muscle producing psoas abscess or lumbar cold abscess
○ Microscopically, consist of central areas of caseous necrosis surrounded by granulation tissue composed of Langhan's giant cells along with fragments of necrotic bone

Diagnosis

○ Acid Fast Bacilli detection in sputum or aspirated material
○ Culture of Mycobacterium (traditionally, LJ medium is used for 4-8 weeks)
○ Polymerase chain reaction

Complications

○ Kyphosis

- Scoliosis
- Tuberculous arthritis
- Ankylosis
- Neurologic deficit as aresult of compression of spinal cord
- Amyloidosis

b. Morphology and complications of atheromatous plaque

(Ref: Textbook of Pathology, Harsh Mohan, 7th ed. pg. 378)

ANSWER

For answer, refer 2011 paper-II Q. 6 (c), Pg. 129

c. Acute pancreatitis

(Ref: Textbook of Pathology, Harsh Mohan, 7th ed. pg. 631)

ANSWER

Introduction

- It is an acute inflammation of the pancreas presents with acute abdomen
- Severe form of the disease is acute hemorrhagic pancreatitis or acute pancreatic necrosis

Etiology

Mechanical	Cholelithiasis, trauma, iatrogenic injury
Metabolic	Alcoholism, hypercalcemia, hyperlipoproteinemia, certain drugs
Genetic	Cationic trypsinogen and trypsin inhibitor gene mutation
Vascular	Atheroembolism, shock, vasculitis
Infections	EBV, CMV and Mumps
Idiopathic pancreatitis	

Pathogenesis

- Mechanism like–acinic cell damage, duct obstruction and blockage in exocytosis of pancreatic enzymes results in release and activation of following enzymes, like- protease, elastases, lipases and phospholipases that results in destructive effects on pancreas

Clinical Features

- Common in adults between the age of 40 and 70 yrs.
- Common in females than males
- Acute severe pain in abdomen- involves upper left quadrant initially followed by generalized pain and may radiate to back
- Nausea, vomiting

- Tachycardia, hypotension,tachypnea followed by shock

Morphology

- **Gross appearance:**
  - In early stage- swollen and edematous pancreas
  - Grey-white pancreatic necrosis, chalky-whiye fat necrosis and blue-black hemorrhages seen
  - In Peritoneal cavity fat necrosis, blood stained ascetic fluid in the omentum, mesentery and peripancreatic tissue is seen
- **Microscopic features:**
  - Necrosis of pancreatic lobules, ducts, arteries and arterioles along with areas of hemorrhages and inflammatory cell infiltrate, mainly polymorphs

Laboratory Findings

- **Radiological:** Ultrasound and CT scan
- Increased neutrophil count
- **Serum lipase:** More specific than serum amylase
- **Serum amylase:** If value more than 4 times the normal value
- **Urinary amylase:** Excreted in urine and increased level from 2nd day onwards
- **Serum trypsin:** Specificity and sensitivity is highest for pancreatic injury
- Hypocalcemia

Complications

- Shock
- Organ failure
- Acute respiratory distress syndrome
- Disseminated intravascular coagulation
- Renal failure
- Pancreatic abscess
- Chronic pancreatitis, etc.

PART-II

3. Write briefly on:

a. Giant cell tumor of bone

(Ref: Textbook of Pathology, Harsh Mohan, 7th ed. pg. 837)

ANSWER

For answer refer 2013 paper-II Q. 2 (b), Pg. 95

b. Amoebic colitis

(Ref: Textbook of Pathology, Harsh Mohan, 7th ed. pg. 555)

ANSWER

For answer, refer 2015 paper-II Q. 5 (a), Pg. 65

PATHOLOGY

4. Write briefly on:

a. Glioblastoma multiforme

(Ref: Textbook of Pathology, Harsh Mohan, 7th ed. pg. 879)

ANSWER

For answer, refer 2017 Paper-II Q. 5 (b), Pg. 22

b. Atherosclerosis

(Ref: Textbook of Pathology, Harsh Mohan, 7th ed. pg. 373)

ANSWER

Introduction

○ Most common arterial disease
○ Fibrous plaque formed with lipid rich core in the tunica intima of arteries resulting in thickening and loss of elasticity of arterial walls

Risk Factors

Major risk factors		Additional risk factors
Modifiable	**Non-modifiable**	**Inflammation**
Hyperlipidemia	Stress	**Lifestyle factors:** Obesity, stress, physical inactivity, metabolic syndrome, atherogenic diet
Diabetes	Advancing age	Infections- CMV,Herpesvirus, etc.
Smoking (cigarette)	Gender: more in males	Increased level of homocysteine
Hypertension	Family history	Level of lipoprotein a
Inflammation	Genetic factors	Postmenopausal deficiency of estrogen
Physical inactivity		

Pathogenesis

○ **Stages that occur in the pathogenesis of atherosclerosis are:**
   ▪ Endothelial cell injury
   ▪ Leukocytes migration
   ▪ Migration of smooth muscle cell and proliferation
   ▪ Maturation of plaque

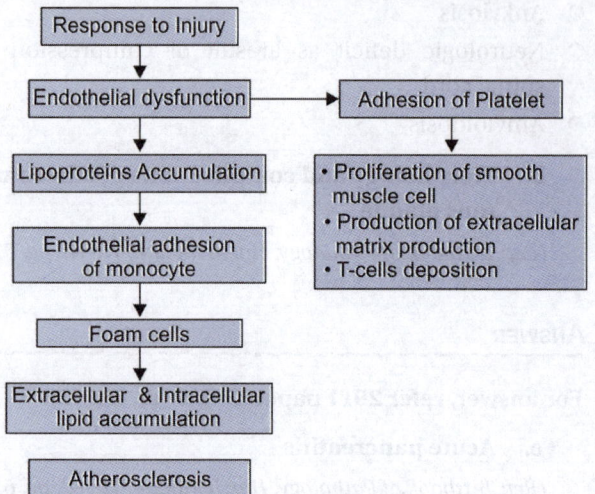

Clinical Features

○ Commonly involves arteries that supply heart, brain, kidney and lower extremities
○ **Clinical consequences are:**
   ▪ Cerebral infarction
   ▪ Myocardial infarction
   ▪ Lower limb peripheral vascular disease
   ▪ Ischemic bowel disease
   ▪ Renovascular hypertension

Morphology

○ **Fatty streaks and Dots:**
   ▪ Precursor lesions of atheromatous plaque
   ▪ Frequent in the aorta and other major arteries (common on the posterior wall)
   ▪ Microscopic Findings: composed of foam cells, lipid laden smooth muscle cells and few lymphoid cells
○ **Gelatinous Lesion:**
   ▪ Present in the intima of the aorta
   ▪ Circumscribed round or oval, grey elevations approx. 1cm in diameter
   ▪ Microscopic Findings: intima shows increased ground substance and thinned overlying epithelium

For Complications refer 2016 paper-II Q. 2 (a), Pg. 40

PART-III

5. Write short notes on:

a. Fibrocytic carcinoma of breast

(Ref: Textbook of Pathology, Harsh Mohan, 7th ed. pg. 751)

ANSWER

Fibrocystic breast carcinoma

- Common in left breast
- Upper outer quadrant of the breast is commonly involved

b. Complication of gall stones

ANSWER

Complications as follows:

- Origin usually from ductal epithelium
- Common types of breast carcinoma are :
  - Non-invasive (in situ)carcinoma
    - Lobular carcinoma in situ
    - Intraductal carcinoma
  - Invasive carcinoma
    - Infiltrative duct carcinoma-NOS
    - Tubular carcinoma
    - Invasive lobular carcinoma
    - Medullary carcinoma
    - Colloid carcinoma

(Ref: Textbook of Pathology, Harsh Mohan, 7th ed. pg. 625)

Cholecystitis	Mucocele and empyema	Choledocholithis	Biliary fistula	Pancreatits	Gallstone ileus	Gallbladder cancer
Biliary colic due to fatty meal, vomiting, fever, nausea and high serum bilirubin level	Gall bladder distension due to impacted stones in the neck of gall bladder	Gallstone in the common bile duct results in obstructive jaundice and pain Bacterialascendi-ng cholangitis results in fever	Fistula formed between one part of biliary system and bowel	Acute pancreatitis as a result of obstructive cholecystasis	Gallstone in the intestine may cause gallstone ileus	In cases with cholelithiasis, small risk of development of cancer

c. Teratoma testis

(Ref: Textbook of Pathology, Harsh Mohan, 7th ed. pg. 699)

ANSWER

Introduction

- Composed of tissue elements derived from than one germ layer (endoderm, mesoderm and ectoderm)
- Common in infants and children (approx.40%)
- May occur at any age group up to adult life
- Pure form – mainly in infants and chidren
- Usually raised hCG or AFP levels

Etiology

- Exact cause is not known, may be due to abnormal differentiation of the germ cells resulting in this condition

Clinical Features

- Testicular pain
- Testicular lump, feeling of heaviness in the scrotum
- Abdominal pain and swelling
- Blood in stool, urine
- Back pain
- Swelling of the legs

- Breast pain, mainly if accompanied by enlargement
- Trouble in breathing
- Anemia
- Changes in appetite
- Fatigue
- Frequent urination
- Paralysis

Morphology

Three types:

- Mature (diffferentiated) teratoma
- Immature teratoma
- Teratoma with malignant transformation

Gross Appearance

- Large, grey-white mass and involved testis is enlarged

Microscopic Features

- **Mature (differentiated) teratoma:**
  - Well-differentiated structures like smooth muscle, cartilage, mucus glands, epithelium(intestinal and respiratory), neural tissue present in an disorganized manner
  - Most common benign tumor

- ○ **Immature teratoma:**
  - ▪ Composed of incompletely differentiated and primitive embryonic tissue with some mature components
  - ▪ Primitive tissue like poorly-formed cartilage, neural tissue, mesenchymal tissue,etc. are commonly present
- ○ **Teratoma with malignant transformation**
  - ▪ Rare form of teratoma with malignant transformation of one or more tissue elements

Diagnosis

- ○ Physical examination: for detection of in the testicles
- ○ Biopsy
- ○ **Blood tests:**
  - ▪ Complete blood cell count (CBC) blood test
  - ▪ Liver function blood test (LFT)
  - ▪ Serum tumor marker blood test to detect increases in human chorionic gonadotropin (hCG)
  - ▪ Alpha-fetoprotein (AFP) blood test
  - ▪ Lactate dehydrogenase (LDH) blood test
  - ▪ Testosterone levels blood test
- ○ **Genetic analysis:** To assess mutations responsible for teratoma of testisis

Complications

- ○ Retrograde ejaculation
- ○ Excessive blood loss
- ○ Infertility
- ○ Metastasis and the loss of function of the organ

  d. Carcinoids

  (Ref: Textbook of Pathology, Harsh Mohan, 7th ed. pg. 559)

ANSWER

Introduction

- ○ Also known as argentaffinoma (tumors arising from endocrine cells)
- ○ Present at any age but peak incidence – 50 years
- ○ Contains argentaffin granules and non-argentaffin granules

Types

Based on the location of the tumor, divided into:

- ○ **Midgut carcinoids:**
  - ▪ Most common
  - ▪ Argentaffin positive
  - ▪ Involves terminal ileum and appendix
- ○ **Hindgut carcinoids:**
  - ▪ Involves rectum and colon
  - ▪ Occurrence (10–20%)

- ○ **Foregut carcinoids:**
  - ▪ Occurrence not frequent (10–20%)
  - ▪ Involves stomach, duodenum and esophagus
- ○ **Appediceal carcinoids:**
  - ▪ Common in 3rd- 4th decade of life
- ○ **Ileal carcinoids:**
  - ▪ Common in females with present commonly in 7th decade of life

Morphology

- ○ **Gross appearance:**
  - ▪ Small, submucosal elevations and overlying mucosa is ulcerated or intact
  - ▪ **Ileal and gastic carcinoids:** Often multiple
  - ▪ **Appendiceal carcinoids:** Solitary
- ○ **Microscopic appearance:**
  - ▪ Uniform appearance of tumor cells in the form of islands, strands, trabeculae or undifferentiated sheets
  - ▪ Infrequent mitoses
  - ▪ Scanty cytoplasm with round to oval stippled nucleus
  - ▪ Cellular atypisa is not common
  - ▪ Membrane bound granules with osmophilic centre, chromogranin A, neuron- specific enolase, synaptophysin may be present

Carcinoid Syndrome

- ○ Characterized by metastatic involvement of liver
- ○ Seen in approx. 1% of all carcinoid tumor
- ○ Consists of the following features:
  - ▪ Abdominal pain
  - ▪ Watery diarrhea
  - ▪ Dyspnoea due to bronchospasm
  - ▪ Right–sided heart failure

6. **Comment on:**

   a. **Advanced glycosylation end products**

ANSWER

For answer, refer 2017 paper-II Q. 5 (c), Pg. 22

   b. **Complication of bronchiectasis**

   (Ref: Textbook of Pathology, Harsh Mohan, 7th ed. pg. 465)

ANSWER

Introduction

- ○ Bronchiectasis is the chronic necrotizing infection of the bronchi and bronchioles that results in abnormal permanent dilatation of the airways

Complications

- ○ **Recurrent infection, breathing difficulty and increased sputum production:**
  - ■ Because lungs are not able to mobilize the secretions
- ○ **Pulmonary hypertension:**
  - ■ Constriction of the pulmonary arteries as a result of decreased oxygen supply results in raised pressure in the arteries
- ○ **Cor pulmonale:**
  - ■ Thickening of right ventricle
- ○ **Hemoptysis:**
- ○ **Heart failure and respiratory failure:**
  - ■ Cause of death in patients with bronchiectasis

- ○ Fibrosis of the bronchial and bronchiolar wall
- ○ Amyloidosis
- ○ Lung abscess
- ○ Peribronchiolar fibrosis
- ○ Metastatic brain abscess
- ○ Empyema of thorax

c. Hodgkin lymphoma

(Ref: Textbook of Pathology, Harsh Mohan, 7th ed. pg. 348)

ANSWER

For answer, refer 2016 paper-II Q. 2 (b), Pg. 40

Pharmacology

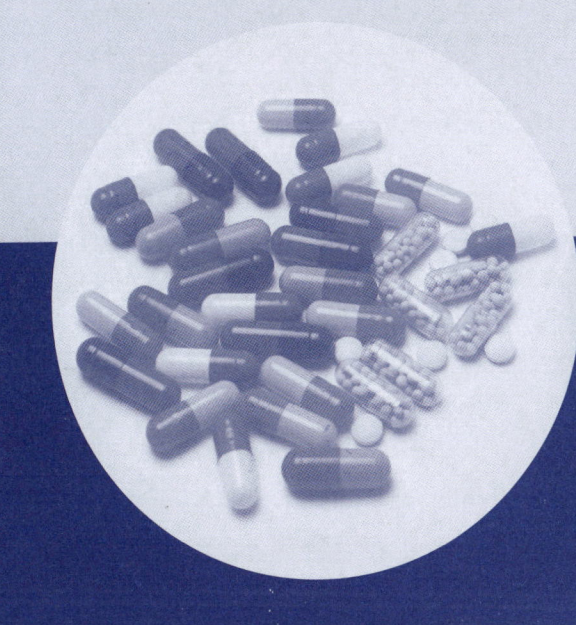

References Taken From:

○ *Essentials of Medical Pharmacology, KD Tripathi, 7th and 8th edition*

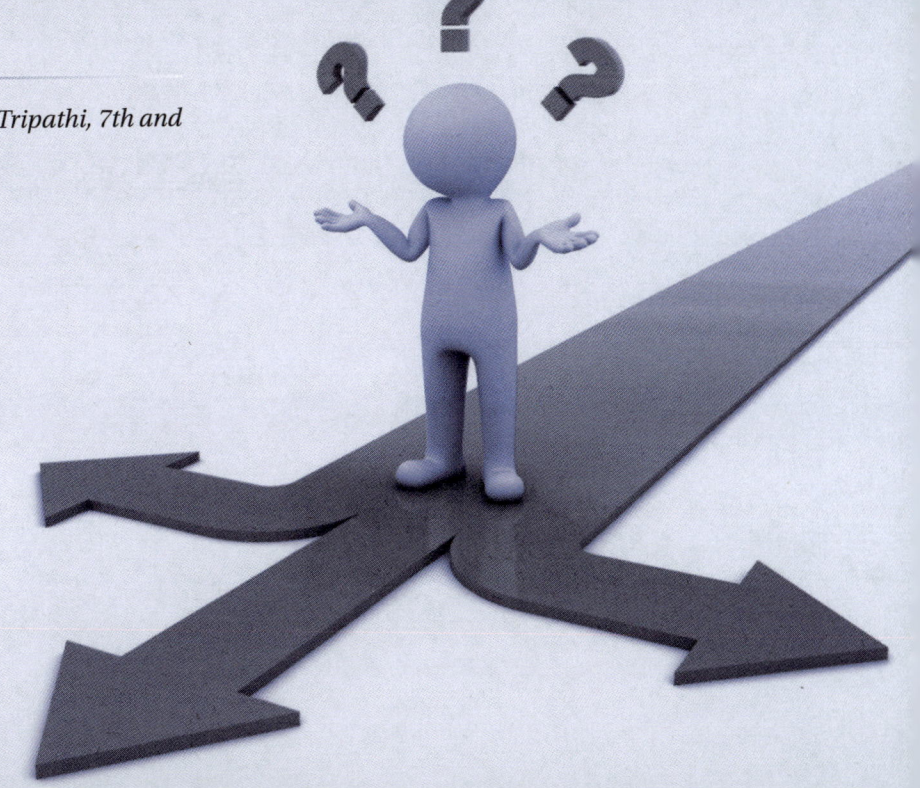

Your Roll No. ....

Name of the Paper : **Pharmacology Paper-I**

Name of the Course : **MBBS-2017**

Semester : **Annual**

Time: 3 Hours   M.M.: 40

INSTRUCTIONS

1. Write your Roll No. on the top immediately on receipt of this question paper
2. All questions are to be attempted
3. Answers to Parts I, II and III should be written in separate answer sheets provided
4. Attempt parts of a question in sequence

PART-I

1. **Explain Why?**   [8]
   a. Nitrates are effective in cyanide poisoning
   b. Some patient treated with succinylcholine suffer from apnoea
   c. Dopamine is administered in cardiogenic shock
   d. Lignocaine is combined with adrenaline for local anesthesia

2. **Enumerate antianginal drugs. Discuss the mechanism of action, therapeutic uses, precautions and adverse effects of nitroglycerine**   [6]

PART-II

3. **Write briefly on:**   [6]
   a. Spironolactone in heart failure
   b. Mannitol as a diuretic
   c. Dextromethorphan in cough
   d. Montelukast in bronchial asthma

4. **Discuss the drug treatment of:**   [6]
   a. Morphine poisoning
   b. Alcohol dependence

PART-III

5. **Discuss the therapeutic uses and adverse effects of:**   [6]
   a. Phenytoin
   b. Olanzapine

6. **Write short notes on:**   [6]
   a. Factors modifying drug bioavailability
   b. Generic drugs
   c. Clinical significance of enzyme induction

PART-I

1. Explain why?

a. Nitrates are effective in cyanide poisoning

(Ref: KD Tripathi, Essentials of Medical Pharmacology, 7th ed, 545, 8th ed, pg. 590)

ANSWER

Rationale for Nitrates being Effective in Cyanide Poisoning

- Nitrates on metabolism generate methemoglobin
- Methemoglobin exhibits great affinity for cyanide radical and leads to form cyanomethemoglobin and excreted out of body
- But, this may dissociate to release cyanide
- Hence, sodium thiosulfate is administered to generate Sodium thiocyanate; this is poorly dissociable and gets excreted in urine
- This also protects cytochrome and other oxidative enzymes from cyanide; including that which has complexed CN is reactivated
- The primary reason for using sodium nitrite is that it is a very weak vasodilator; even doses (>300 mg) are adequate to generate sufficient methaemoglobin that can be given intravenously without producing hypotension.

b. Some patient treated with succinylcholine suffer from apnoea

ANSWER

Rationale for Some Patients Suffering from Apnoea after Treatment with Succinylcholine

- **Mechanism of action:**
  - Acts on the nicotinic receptors of the muscles, stimulates them and eventually cause their relaxation
  - **This occurs in two steps:**
    - **Phase 1:** This is depolarizing phase; muscle fasciculations are caused while it is depolarizing the muscle fibers
    - **Phase 2:** This is desensitizing phase; sets in after adequate depolarization has occurred; the muscles no longer respond to ACh released by the nerve endings
- **Metabolism:** SCh undergoes rapid hydrolysis by plasma pseudocholinesterase to succinylmono-choline and afterwards succinic acid + choline

- But, there is possibility of genetically determined abnormality (that exhibit as low affinity for SCh), or pseudocholinesterase deficiency
- Not in heterozygous state; but in cases who are homozygous for the abnormal enzyme, prolonged phase II blockade occurs by SCh which results in muscle paralysis and apnea because SCh is a poor substrate for the more particular AChE located at the motor end plate
- Only mechanical ventilation can cater this prolonged apnea.

c. Dopamine is administered in cardiogenic shock

ANSWER

Dopamine

A dopaminergic (D1 and D2) as well as adrenergic α and β_1 (but not β_2) agonist

Mechanism of Action

- D1 receptors located in renal and mesenteric blood vessels are the most sensitive ones; dilatation of these vessels is caused even by small intravenous doses due to increase in intracellular cAMP
- Glomerular filtration rate is increased
- Exerting natriuretic effect (by D1 receptors) on PT cells
- Only large doses can cause vasoconstriction

Rationale for Using Dopamine in Cardiogenic Shock

- Due to its high sensitivity of D1 receptors on renal mesenteric vessels, there is resultant rise in BP and urine outflow
- Increase in cardiac output and systolic BP but less effect on diastolic BP
- Exerts no CNS effects as it does not penetrate blood-brain barrier
- **Dose:** 0.2–1 mg/min administered intravenously, BP and urine formation to be monitored so that to regulate doses given.

d. Lignocaine is combined with adrenaline for local anesthesia

ANSWER

Rationale to Combine Lignocaine with Adrenaline for Local Anesthesia

- Lignocaine is a short-acting local anaesthetic, that exhibits marked vasodilator and antiarrhythmic properties

○ Adrenaline is a sympathomimetic agent which causes activation of both α- and β-adrenoceptors

○ It is transient in its effect after parenteral administration since it gets rapidly metabolized

○ It is a vasoconstrictor and thus used to impede systemic absorption of infiltrated local anaesthetics

○ The addition of adrenaline 5 micrograms/ml (1:200,000) as a vasoconstrictor to local anaesthetic solutions slows down systemic absorption and extends the anaesthetic effect

○ In dental surgery, in which small volumes are injected, concentrations of 12.5 micrograms/ml (1:80,000) are commonly employed

○ **Note:** Adrenaline should not be used in ring block of digits or the penis or in other situations where there is a risk of local ischemia.

---

2. **Enumerate antianginal drugs. Discuss the mechanism of action, therapeutic uses, precautions and adverse effects of nitroglycerine**

(Ref: KD Tripathi, Essentials of Medical Pharmacology, 7th, ed, 8th ed, pg. 539-45)

ANSWER

Classification of Antianginal Drugs

Nitrates

○ **Short acting:** Glyceryl trinitrate (GTN, Nitroglycerine)

○ **Long acting:** Isosorbide dinitrate (it becomes short acting when given by sublingual route), Isosorbide mononitrate, Erythrityl tetranitrate, Pentaerythritol tetranitrate

β Blockers

○ Propranolol, Metoprolol, Atenolol and Others

Calcium Channel Blockers

○ **Phenyl alkylamine:** Verapamil

○ **Benzothiazepine:** Diltiazem

○ **Dihydropyridines:** Nifedipine, Felodipine, Amlodipine, Nitrendipine, Nimodipine, Lacidipine, Lercanidipine, Benidipine

Potassium Channel Opener

○ Nicorandil

Others

○ Dipyridamole, Trimetazidine, Ranolazine, Ivabradine, Oxyphedrine

Clinical Classification

○ **Those that are used to abort or terminate attack:** GTN, Isosorbide dinitrate (sublingually).

○ **Those that are used for chronic prophylaxis:** Rest of the drugs.

Nitroglycerine

○ **Mechanism of action:** The mechanism of action revolves around major action being direct nonspecific smooth muscle relaxation

Rapid denitration of organic nitrates enzymatically in the smooth muscle cell
↓
Release of the reactive free radical *nitric oxide (NO)*
↓
Activation of cytosolic guanylyl cyclase and leads to increased cGMP
↓ cGMP dependent protein kinase
Dephosphorylation of myosin light chain kinase
↓
Decreased availability of phosphorylated (active) MLCK which interferes with activation of myosin

Failure of myosin to interact with actin to cause contraction, thus relaxation occurs

Relaxation effect is also enhanced by elevated intracellular cGMP leading to decline in calcium ions entry

Nitrates causes generation of NO that activates cGMP production in platelets as well

Beneficial in unstable angina.

Therapeutic Uses

Nitroglycerine (NTG)

○ Nitroglycerine undergoes significant first pass metabolism by nitrate reductase and hence is not effective by oral route.

○ Sublingual Nitroglycerine is the drug of choice for treatment of an acute attack of stable and Prinzmetal (variant) angina, for which a buccal spray can also be used. To prevent an acute attack in case of expected stress, sublingual NTG should be taken five minutes before.

○ Sublingual Nitroglycerine is also drug of choice for treatment of pain associated with MI.

○ Buccal and transdermal route can be used for prophylaxis. Transdermal NTG is preferred for prophylaxis of nocturnal angina.

○ Intravenous nitroglycerine is used for treatment of pulmonary edema associated with acute CHF and for hypertensive emergency.

Isosorbide Dinitrate (IDN)

○ IDN also undergoes first pass metabolism but lesser than NTG. IDN is metabolized by denitration into IMN (Isosorbide mononitrate), the active form.

○ It is administered by sublingual route for an acute attack and by oral route for long term prophylaxis of angina.

○ By oral route it is also used along with hydrazine for treatment of chronic CHF.

Adverse Effects

○ Fullness in head and throbbing headache

○ Continued use results in tolerance

○ Lying down causes flushing, weakness, sweating; also causes palpitation, dizziness and fainting

○ **Methemoglobinemia:** Significant in severe anemia, this can further decrease O_2 carrying capacity of blood

○ Rarely, rashes, though relatively more common with pentaerythritol tetranitrate.

Precaution and Clinical Considerations

○ Tablets must not be stored in plastic container, instead use a tightly closed glass container so that the drug do not gets evaporated

○ While using sublingual route to terminate an attack, the tablet may be crushed under the teeth and then spread over buccal mucosa for absorption

○ The leftover may be swallowed or spit back when the anginal pain subsides

○ If using transdermal patch, then it is advised that the patch be taken off for 8 hours daily

○ If using a transmucosal dosage form, then to be stuck to the gums under the upper lip.

PART-II

3. **Write briefly on:**

   a.   Spironolactone in heart failure

   (Ref: KD Tripathi, Essentials of Medical Pharmacology, 7th ed, pg. 520-21, 8th ed, pg. 567-68)

ANSWER

○ **Spironolactone:** A potassium sparing diuretic

○ Diuretics form important modality of treatment in symptomatic CHF

○ Disease process is not influenced by diuretic therapy

○ Diuretics (high-ceiling) are used in CHF for following purposes:

   ■ Reduce circulating volume and ventricular efficiency is improved

   ■ Mobilize edema fluid and pulmonary congestion is relieved

○ **Rationale to use spironolactone in CHF:**

   ■ Despite providing symptom relief in CHF by regulating volume overload, resistance may develop in cases where furosemide is used; this can be overcome by use of spironolactone

   ■ Serum potassium concentration is improved, and thus counter the risk of hypokalemia and associated arrhythmic risk caused by non-potassium-sparing diuretics

   ■ The addition of spironolactone to standard therapy can reduce the risk of both morbidity and mortality in patients with severe heart failure.

   b.   Mannitol as a diuretic

ANSWER

○ **Mannitol:** An osmotic diuretic

○ **Osmotic diuretic:** Pharmacological inert substances that are filtered in the glomerulus but not reabsorbed by the nephron

○ **Mechanism of action**

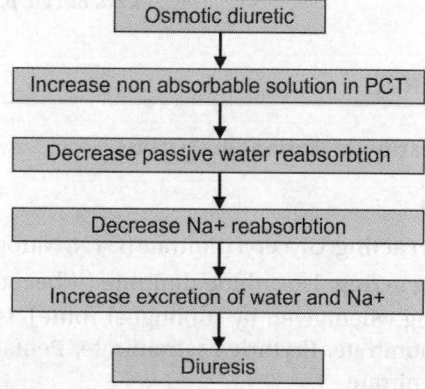

○ **Rationale for employing mannitol in cerebral edema:**

   ■ Never employed as natriuretic or for treating chronic edema

   ■ Employed in increased intracranial or intraocular tension (head injuries, stroke, acute congestive glaucoma, etc.)

   ■ It promotes water movement by osmotic action from CSF, brain parenchyma, and aqueous humour

   ■ Since it draws water out of the intracellular compartment, there is expansion of ECF volume, leading to reduction in edematous component

   ■ Although to increase urinary volume is the key action of mannitol, it also enhances excretion of all cations (Na_+, K_+, Ca_{2+}, Mg_{2+}) and anions (Cl^-, HCO_3^-, PO_{43}^-)

   ■ *Dose:* 1–1.5 g/kg is infused over 1 hour as 20% solution to momentarily raise osmolarity of plasma

- Employed before and after ocular/brain surgery so as to avoid acute upsurge in intraocular/ intracranial pressure
- **Note:** Mannitol is administered intravenously, as absorption is impeded via oral route.

c. Dextromethorphan in cough

(Ref: KD Tripathi, Essentials of Medical Pharmacology, 7th ed, pg. 220, 8th ed, pg. 239-40)

ANSWER

Dextromethorphan in Cough

○ Dextromethorphan is D isomer of opioid levomethorphan but is devoid of opioid agonistic effect.

○ Extensively used and safe antitussive agent that exhibits low affinity and also uncompetitive antagonism against NMDA receptors

○ Mucociliary function of the airway mucosa is not depressed

○ Used for suppression of nonproductive cough

○ **Note:** Though dextromethorphan is safe as well as effective in recommended dosage, it can cause euphoria at higher dosages. Thus cough formulations containing this drug has been used for abuse

○ It is not only associated with lesser side-effects but also is less effective than opioids and is an over the counter medication for mild cough. It can be combined with opioids if required.

○ Generally combined with various antihistamines, bronchodilators, mucolytics and other antitussives

○ **Dose:** Around 2 mg/kg PO has been suggested

○ The antitussive effects can stay for up to 5 hours.

○ Hallucinations and addiction are associated drawbacks.

Classification of antitussives

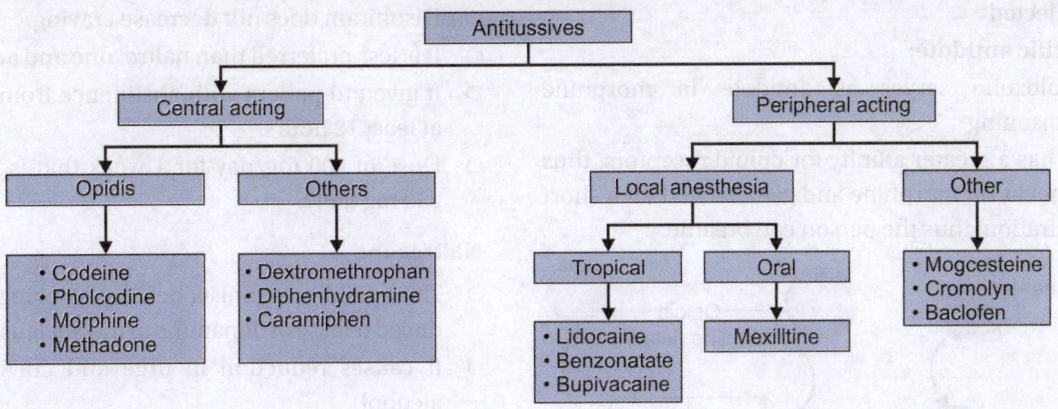

d. Montelukast in bronchial asthma

ANSWER

Leukotriene Antagonists

Montelukast and zafirlukast

Indications

○ Prophylactic therapy of mild-to-moderate asthma as alternatives to inhaled glucocorticoids

○ May be more acceptable in children

○ Additive effect with inhaled steroids in cases of severe asthma, may allow dose reduction of steroid and need for rescue b2 agonist inhalations

○ Not to be used for termination of asthmatic episodes

○ Modestly effective in aspirin-and exercise-induced asthma, but add no value in COPD

○ High safety profile; few side effects like headache and rashes, eosinophilia and neuropathy are

reported. Few cases of vasculitis with eosinophilia (Churg-Strauss syndrome) have been reported.

4. Discuss the drug treatment of:

a. Morphine poisoning

(Ref: KD Tripathi, Essentials of Medical Pharmacology, 7th ed, pg. 472, 8th ed, pg. 500-01)

ANSWER

Acute Morphine Poisoning

○ Acute poisoning with morphine and other opioids can occur with overdose of these drugs

○ This may be accidental or suicidal, or can also be observed in drug abusers

○ In humans, a dose of 250 mg is considered to be lethal dose

Clinical Manifestations of Morphine Poisoning

○ Stupor or coma
○ Flaccidity in muscles
○ Breathing gets shallower and occasional
○ Cyanosis, that presents as bluish discoloration of skin and mucus membranes
○ Pinpoint pupil
○ Fall in BP and condition of shock
○ Terminal stages presents pulmonary edema and demise due to respiratory failure

Treatment

○ **Respiratory support is mandatory:** Positive pressure respiration will also counteract pulmonary edema
○ **Maintenance of BP:** Intravenous fluids and vaso-constrictors
○ **Potassium permanganate:** Used for gastric lavage in order to remove the unabsorbed drug
   ▪ Lavage is advised even when morphine has been injected
○ **Specific antidote:**
   ▪ Naloxone serves as antidote in morphine poisoning
   ▪ It has a greater affinity for opioid receptors, thus knocks off morphine and get attached for a short duration; thus the person can breathe

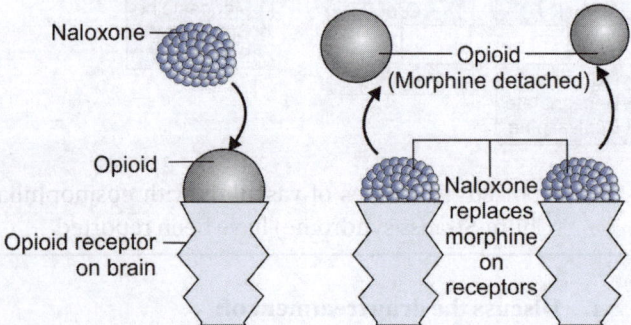

○ Doses recommended are 0.4–0.8 mg intravenously repeated every 2–3 minutes till respiration picks up and settles
○ Provides relief since it acts rapidly, and also does not exhibit any agonistic activity
○ Respiration is also not depressed per se
○ **Clinical key:** It has a short duration of action, thus should be repeated every 1 to 4 hours, as per the response of the patient.

   b.   **Alcohol dependence**

ANSWER

○ The FDA approved drugs for alcohol dependence one disulfiram, naltrexone and acamprosate.

Treatment of Alcohol Dependence

○ It can be based on two main objectives, including detoxification and rehabilitation
○ Drugs that are employed to prevent relapses and help in achieving complete abstinence can be classified as:
   ▪ **Aversion drugs:** Disulfiram
   ▪ **Opioid antagonists:** Naltrexone, Nalmefene
   ▪ **NMDA receptor antagonists:** Acamprosate
   ▪ **Supporting drugs:** Lithium, topiramate, carba-mazepine

Disulfiram

○ Disulfiram is an aversive agent which acts by inhibiting aldehyde dehydrogenase the enzyme for alcohol metabolism.
○ This leads to accumulation of acetaldehyde, toxic metabolite of alcohol which causes vomiting, flushing, hypotension, chest pain and other uncomfortable symptoms.
○ Disulfiram does not decrease craving.
○ It is less preferred than naltrexone and acamprosate.
○ It given to patient with abstinence from alcohol for at least 12 hours.
○ Dose of 500 mg/day for 1 week that is followed by 250 mg daily.

Naltrexone

○ The opioid antagonists help by blocking alcohol in-duced release of dopamine in the nucleus accumbens
○ It causes reduction in urge and craving towards alcohol
○ **Clinical key:** Disulfiram and naltrexone should not be combined as both are hepatotoxic

Acamprosate

○ This is an analog of GABA and acts as an agonist at GABA receptors as well as weak antagonist at the NMDA receptors
○ Reduces craving for alcohol in early abstinence phase and also decrease in voluntary alcohol consumption
○ **Note:** Can be given with disulfiram

Lithium

○ Oral lithium carbonate works by mood stabilizing activity and reduction in alcohol consumption.

Recent Advance

○ **Ondansetron:** Ondansetron is under trial for alcohol dependence to decrease craving.
○ **Nalmefene:** Nalmefene is under trial for alcohol dependence to decrease craving.

○ **Topiramate:** Topiramate is under trial for codependence on alcohol and smoking.

○ **Gabapentin, Vareniciline and Baclofen:** These are drug under trial to decrease craving in alcohol dependence.

PART-III

5. Discuss the therapeutic uses and adverse effects of:

a. Phenytoin

(Ref: KD Tripathi, Essentials of Medical Pharmacology, 7th ed, pg. 414, 8th ed, pg. 439-41)

ANSWER

Therapeutic Uses

○ **Generalized tonic-clonic, simple and complex partial seizures:** Useful in this type of seizures. Futile in absence seizures
  - **Dose:** 100 mg twice a day, maximum 400 mg/day; in children 5 to 8 mg/kg/day

○ **Status epilepticus:** Slow intravenous injection has been used many times; these days replaced by fosphenytoin

○ **Trigeminal neuralgia:** It is proven beneficial as second choice drug to carbamazepine

○ Limiting spread of seizure activity

Adverse Effects

○ Some adverse effects may appear at therapeutic concentrations *after* prolonged use while numerous side effects are seen at overdose or high plasma levels

○ **At therapeutic levels:**
  - **Gum hypertrophy:** Commonest seen (20% incidence); seen more in younger patients. Occurs due to overgrowth of gingival collagen fibres
  - Hirsutism, acne, coarsening of facial features forms the most problematic in young girls
  - Rashes and DLE can occur if the patient is hypersensitive to the drug
  - **Lymphadenopathy:** Increase in size of lymph nodes
  - **Megaloblastic anemia:** This drug causes turn down in folate absorption and also promotes its excretion
  - **Osteomalacia:** Metabolic activation of vitamin D is interfered with and also calcium absorption/metabolism is hampered
  - **Fetal hydantoin syndrome:** If administered during pregnancy, phenytoin can cause hypoplastic phalanges, cleft palate, hare lip, microcephaly, most probably caused by its arene oxide metabolite

○ **At high plasma levels (dose related toxicity):**
  - **Effects related to cerebellar and vestibular systems:** Ataxia, vertigo, diplopia, nystagmus, drowsiness, behavioral alterations, mental confusion, disorientation and rigidity
  - Epigastric pain, nausea and vomiting, can be minimized to a extent by taking the drug with meals
  - Local vascular injury by intravenous injection
  - Necrosis of the tissues if the solution extravasates
  - Intravenous administration also can cause fall in BP and cardiac arrhythmias, thus must to be administered under regular ECG monitoring.

b. Olanzapine

ANSWER

Olanzapine

Pharmacological Actions

○ Second generation antipsychotics; having weak D2 blocking but potent 5-HT2 antagonistic activity

○ Blockade of multiple monoaminergic (D2, 5-HT2, as well as muscarinic and H1 receptors

○ Minimal extrapyramidal side effects

○ Improvement in the impaired cognitive function in psychotics

○ Half-life is 24 to 30 hours

Therapeutic Uses

○ Serves broad spectrum efficacy in schizophrenia; both positive and negative symptoms appear to be benefitted

○ Used in monotherapy as well as mixed states of bipolar disorder

○ Adjunctive treatment of depression

○ Can also be employed to treat acute mania and anxiety

○ Relief in post-traumatic stress disorder and behavioral disturbances associated with dementia

Adverse Effects

○ Dry mouth and constipation due to potent antimuscarinic action

○ Causes weight gain

○ Increased chances of stroke in the elderly

○ Impairment of glucose tolerance or worsening diabetes; elevation of serum triglyceride

○ Drowsiness, dizziness, lightheadedness.

○ If has highest risk for EPS.

6. Write short notes on:

a. Factors modifying drug bioavailability

(Ref: KD Tripathi, Essentials of Medical Pharmacology, 8th ed, pg. 22)

Answer

Bioavailability

○ Defined as the rate at which and extent to which the active concentration of the drug is available at the site of action.

○ A measure of the fraction (F) of administered drug dose that will reaches the systemic circulation in the unchanged form

Factors Modifying Drug Absorption and its Bioavailability

○ **Physical properties of the drug itself:**
  ▪ Drugs in liquid forms are better absorbed than solids drug forms. Also, crystalloids are absorbed better than colloids

○ **Nature of the dosage forms**
  ▪ Bioavailability is 100% for intravenously given drugs; frequently lower after oral administration due to incomplete absorption of the drug and first pass metabolism
  ▪ Local binding of the drug may cause incomplete bioavailability in IM or SC routes
  ▪ Smaller particle size of the drug, for example, corticosteroids and antibiotics like chloramphenicol also enhances drug absorption

○ **Physiological factors**
  ▪ Weakly acidic drugs gets rapidly absorbed from stomach as they exist in an unionized form in the acidic medium
  ▪ Weakly basic drugs, like, pethidine and ephedrine are not absorbed until they reach the alkaline environment of the small intestine
  ▪ **Presence of other drugs and agents:** For example, vitamin C enhances oral iron absorption, while phytates retard that

○ **Disease states in patients**
  ▪ Drug absorption, bioavailability and first pass metabolism may be affected in conditions like thyrotoxicosis, liver cirrhosis, and biliary obstruction.

b. Generic drugs

Answer

Drug Nomenclature

○ **Can be of Three Types:** Chemical, generic, and trade/brand name

Generic Drugs/Generic Names of Drugs

○ Generic name is also known as non-proprietary name

○ These name are assigned by the United States Adopted Name Council, this is done only when the drug has been of potential therapeutic benefits

○ When a generic or non-proprietary name is included in official pharmacopoeia, it becomes an official name

○ **For examples**
  ▪ **Chemical name:** Acetyl salicylic acid
  ▪ **Generic name:** Aspirin
  ▪ **Brand name:** Ecospirin, Mejoral, etc.

c. Clinical significance of enzyme induction

(Ref: KD Tripathi, Essentials of Medical Pharmacology, 7th ed, pg. 26, 8th ed, pg. 33-4)

Answer

○ **Clinical Significance of Enzyme Induction:** Many drugs, insecticides and carcinogens interact with DNA and increase the synthesis of microsomal enzyme protein, especially cytochrome P_{450} and UGTs As a result rate of metabolism of inducing drug itself and/or other drugs is increased

○ Cytochrome P_{450} is microsomal enzyme protein

○ **Drugs Modulating Different Cytochrome P_{450} Enzyme Families:**
  ▪ **CYP3A isoenzymes:** Anticonvulsants (phenobarbitone, phenytoin, carbamazepine), rifampin, glucocorticoids
  ▪ **CYP2D6** by rifampin and **CYP2B1** by phenobarbitone
  ▪ **CYP2E1:** Isoniazid and chronic alcohol consumption
  ▪ **CYP1A isoenzymes:** Polycyclic hydrocarbons like 3-methylcholanthrene and benzopyrene found in cigarette smoke, charcoal broiled meat, omeprazole and industrial pollutants induce.
  ▪ Other important enzyme inducers: Phenylbutazone, griseofulvin, DDT

○ Induction includes microsomal enzymes both in liver and other organs

○ Also leads to an increase in the rate of metabolism by 2 to 4 fold
  ▪ **Drugs that are inactivated by metabolism:** Decreased intensity and/or duration of action, for example, contraception failure with oral contraceptives
  ▪ **Drugs that are activated by metabolism:** Increased intensity of action. This becomes very significant as acute paracetamol toxicity occurs due to one of its metabolitesv
  ▪ **Drug induces its own metabolism (autoinduction):** Tolerance, for example, carbamazepine
  ▪ Using an inducer intermittently interferes with dose adjustment of the other drug prescribed

on usual basis, for example, oral anticoagulants, antiepileptics, antihypertensive agents

○ **Metabolism of following drugs is considerably influenced by enzyme induction:** Phenytoin, tolbutamide, imipramine, warfarin, doxycycline, theophylline, griseofulvin, oral contraceptives, chloramphenicol, phenylbutazone.

Drugs Metabolized by CYP450 Enzymes

CYP450 Enzymes	Substrate Drugs
CYP1A2	Paracetamol Tacrine Theophylline Tamoxifen
CYP2B6	Cyclophosphamide Methadone Efavirenz Artemisinin
CYP2C9	Phenytoin Warfarin Glipizide Losartan

Contd...

CYP450 Enzymes	Substrate Drugs
CYP2C19	PPIs Clopidogrel is activated Propranolol
CYP2D6	Beta blockers except propranolol Drugs of psychiatry (TCA, SSRI, Antipsychotics)
CYP2E1	Enflurane Ethanol
CYP3A4	C : CCBs, Cyclosporine H : H mg CoA reductase inhibitors (Statins) A : Anti arrhythmics (Lidocaine, Mexiletine, Quinidine) R: Rapamycin L: Long acting benzodiazepines, e.g. diazepam I : Inhibitors of protease E : Erythromycin, Estrogen, Progesterone and its antagonist **Mifepristone**

Your Roll No. ....

Name of the Paper	:	**Pharmacology Paper-II**
Name of the Course	:	**MBBS-2017**
Semester	:	**Annual**

Time: 3 Hours   **M.M.: 40**

INSTRUCTIONS

1. Write your Roll No. on the top immediately on receipt of this question paper
2. All questions are to be attempted
3. Answers to Parts I, II and III should be written in separate answer sheets provided
4. Attempt parts of a question in sequence

PART-I

1. **Explain why?** [8]
   a. Alfacalcidol is preferred in renal rickets
   b. Azathioprine is given in combination with allopurinol
   c. Deferiprone is effective in acute iron poisoning
   d. Low molecular weight heparin is preferred over conventional heparin in the treatment of deep vein thrombosis

2. **Enumerate drugs used for treatment of diabetes mellitus. Discuss the mechanism of action, therapeutic uses and adverse effects of regular insulin.** [6]

PART-II

3. **Discuss the therapeutic status of:** [8]
   a. Misoprostol in pregnancy
   b. Bedaquiline in tuberculosis
   c. Ceftriaxone in typhoid fever
   d. Febuxostat in hyperuricemia

4. **Describe the drug treatment of:** [6]
   a. Urinary tract infection
   b. Chloroquine-resistant falciparum malaria

PART-III

5. **Discuss the therapeutic uses and adverse effects of:** [6]
   a. Methotrexate
   b. Dapsone

6. **Write short notes on:** [6]
   a. Anti-rabies vaccine
   b. Meropenem
   c. Post coital contraceptives

PART-I

1. Explain Why?

a. Alfacalcidol is preferred in renal rickets

(Ref: KD Tripathi, Essentials of Medical Pharmacology, 7th ed, pg. 342, 8th ed, pg.368)

ANSWER

Rationale to Prefer alfacalcidol in renal rickets

○ Prodrug rapidly hydroxylated in the liver to 1,25 (OH)2 D3 or calcitriol

○ Thus, it does not need hydroxylation at position 1 which is actually the limiting step in the synthesis of active form of vit D, occurring in the kidney

○ Hence, it is effective in renal rickets

○ Also indicated in conditions like vit D dependent rickets, vit D resistant rickets, hypoparathyroidism, etc. those conditions which require calcitriol

○ It gets metabolically activated in liver but not can be given to patients of severe liver disease

○ **Note:** Carefully watch out for hypercalcemia; prompt discontinuation of therapy for few days if that develops.

b. Azathioprine is given in combination with allopurinol

(Ref: KD Tripathi, Essentials of Medical Pharmacology, 7th ed, pg. 217, 8th ed, pg.228)

ANSWER

Rationale for Combining Azathioprine in Combination with Allopurinol

○ Allopurinol can be employed as *over producers* as well as *under excretors* of uric acid, mainly in more severe cases, with tophi or nephropathy

○ It is used for potentiating 6-mercaptopurine or azathioprine in chemotherapy of cancers and also in immunosuppressant therapy

○ When allopurinol is added to thiopurine (azathioprine and 6-MP) treatment in IBD patients that overproduce 6-MMP, there is reversal of metabolic shunting so that 6-MMP levels wanes and synthesis of the efficacious metabolite 6-TGN elevated

○ Also, combination azathioprine-allopurinol therapy is effective to reduce episodes of organ transplant rejection.

c. Deferiprone is effective in acute iron poisoning

ANSWER

Deferiprone

An iron chelator that is orally active.

Rationale to Use in Acute Iron Poisoning

○ Acute iron poisoning results in iron overload and also there is excessive iron in patients of liver cirrhosis

○ This overload can be cleared off by an iron chelator

○ Less effective than desferrioxamine that is parenterally administered

○ Due to expensive treatment and need of parenteral administration, the standard iron chelator deferoxamine not employed in many cases of acute and chronic iron poisoning

○ Also, treatment of transfusion siderosis in thalassemia patients has been simplified by defriprone

○ These patients have to be given repeated blood transfusions since extreme hemolysis happens, resulting in iron overload, and corrected by oral iron chelator, deferiprone.

d. Low molecular weight heparin is preferred over conventional heparin in the treatment of deep vein thrombosis

ANSWER

Low Molecular Weight (LMW) Heparin

○ Molecular weight 3,000–7,000

○ Selective inhibition of factor Xa with little effect on IIa

○ **LMW heparins are indicated in:**
  ▪ In high-risk cases for prophylaxis of deep vein thrombosis (DVT) and pulmonary embolism (surgery, stroke, etc.)
  ▪ Cases of established DVT
  ▪ Patients of unstable angina and myocardial infarction
  ▪ In patients undergoing dialysis for maintaining patency of cannulae and shunts

Rationale to Prefer LMW over Unfractionated Heparin

○ Less interference with hemostasis

○ Decreased frequency of thrombocytopenia

○ Provides better subcutaneous bioavailability (70–90%) matched to UFH (20–30%)

PHARMACOLOGY

○ Minimizing variability in response

○ Once daily subcutaneous administration due to long and consistent half-life

○ Dose calculation done based on body weight and no requirement of laboratory monitoring

○ LMW heparin affords less risk of osteoporosis after long term use

○ Lower incidence of hemorrhagic complications.

2. **Enumerate drugs used for treatment of diabetes mellitus. Discuss the mechanism of action, therapeutic uses and adverse effects of regular insulin**

(Ref: KD Tripathi, Essentials of Medical Pharmacology, 7th ed, pg. 296, 8th ed, pg.280, 285-304))

ANSWER

Diabetes Mellitus

A chronic, metabolic disorder characterized by the 3 Ps (polydipsia, polyuria, and polyphagia)

Classification of Drugs Used in Diabetes Mellitus

○ Enhance insulin secretion

- **Sulfonylureas:**
  - **First generation:** Tolbutamide
  - **Second generation:** Glibenclamide (Glyburide), glipizide, glimepiride, gliclazide
- **Meglitinide/phenylalanine analogues:** Repaglinide, Nateglinide
- **Glucagon-like peptide-1 (GLP-1) receptor agonists (injectable):** Exenatide, liraglutide
- **Dipeptidyl peptidase-4 (DPP-4) inhibitors:** Sitagliptin, vildagliptin, saxagliptin, alogliptin, linagliptin

○ Overcome insulin resistance

- **Biguanide:** Metformin
- **Thiazolidinediones:** Pioglitazone

○ Miscellaneous antidiabetic drugs

- **α-Glucosidase inhibitors:** Acarbose, miglitol, voglibose
- **Amylin analog:** Pramlintide
- **Dopamine-D2 receptor agonist:** Bromocriptine
- **Sodium-glucose cotransport-2 (SGLT-2) inhibitor:** Dapagliflozin

○ Insulin (Employed when OHAs fail to control blood glucose levels)

- **Rapid acting:** Insulin lispro, Insulin aspart, Insulin glulisine
- **Short acting:** Regular (soluble) insulin

- **Intermediate acting:** Insulin zinc suspension or lente, neutral protamine hagedorn (NPH) or isophane insulin
- **Long acting:** Insulin glargine, insulin detemir.

Mechanism of Action of Regular Insulin

Concentration of the injectable solution

↓

Self-aggregation of the insulin molecules to form hexamers around zinc ions

↓

Release of insulin monomers gradually by dilution after subcutaneous injection

↓

This results into slow absorption

↓

After 2–3 hours, peak action

↓

Continuation of action up to 6 to 8 hours

Therapeutic Uses

○ Better control on meal-time glycaemia and a lower incidence of late postprandial hypoglycaemia

○ Better marked reduction in HbA1c diabetes mellitus subjects

○ Must for type 1 diabetics

○ Employed in type 2 diabetes if not controlled by oral hypoglycemics, underweight patients and tide over surgery and pregnancy conditions

○ Used in diabetic ketoacidosis

○ Hyperosmolar coma (nonketotic hyperglycemic) coma in elderly type 2 patients

Adverse Effects of Regular Insulin

○ Subcutaneous administration just before a meal can often create a mismatch between insulin requirement and availability resulting in early postprandial hyperglycaemia and late postprandial hypoglycaemia

○ Not apt for a low constant basal level of action to be provided in the interdigestive period

○ It do not provide slow onset of action and prompt onset of action

○ **Note:** These shortcomings mandated developing and employing regular insulin analogs for better clinical outcomes.

PART-II

3. **Discuss the therapeutic status of:**

a. **Misoprostol in pregnancy**

ANSWER

Misoprostol in Pregnancy

○ It is prostaglandin E1 analog that has been used for medical abortion

○ It also has become an important drug in gynecologic practices since it possess uterotonic and cervical-ripening actions

○ Misoprostol is contraindicated in pregnancy as it exhibits abortifacient properties

○ **How it works for termination of pregnancy:**

- This causes contraction of smooth muscles of the uterus and leading to emptying of the uterus

- It can also cause softening the cervix and increases dilation for intrauterine procedures and facilitates expulsions

○ Also used in controlling postpartum haemorrhage

○ Used in MTP kits in association with mifepristone which acts by blocking progesterone receptors

○ Works best in the first 8 weeks of conception

○ It can be taken orally as well as vaginally.

○ Mifepristone (ru-486) is a partial agonist at progesterone receptors and hence act as antagonists in presence of progesterone. It also blocks glucocorticoid and androgen receptors.

○ It has high plasma protein binding and hence a long half-life.

○ Most common side effect is vaginal bleeding and other prostaglandins related side-effects like abdominal cramps and diarrhoea can be seen.

b. Bedaquiline in tuberculosis

ANSWER

Bedaquiline

○ Bedaquiline is a diarylquinoline which acts by inhibiting mycobacterial **ATP synthase**. It is a strong bactericidal and sterilizing drug that dramatically affects time to culture conversion in patients with MDR TB. It has been approved by FDA for treatment of MDR TB in 2012. In India it is currently available in 6 places under the conditional access program.

Pharmacokinetics

○ It has good oral absorption (oral route) and since food increases absorption, it should be taken with food.

○ It is highly distributed in to tissues as it is amphiphilic in nature and binds to tissue phospholipids following which it is slowly released and hence has an extended long half-life of 165 days (5.5 months).

The plasma half-life though is 24 hours. It is given at intermittent doses 200 mg three times a week followed by a two weeks of loading phase of 400 mg to avoid accumulation of drug in plasma and tissue.

○ It has a high plasma protein binding.

○ 75% of Bedaquiline is excreted unchanged by liver, whereas 25% is metabolized in liver by CYP3A4 in to active metabolites M2 and M3 which are less active than Bedaquiline.

○ It has a concentration-time dependent killing and the AUC decides its efficacy.

Contraindications

○ Bedaquiline can cause QT prolongation and hence is contraindicated in patients having prolonged QT interval (> 450 ms), cardiac arrhythmia and along with other drugs that can prolong QT. It is also contraindicated in patients with high risk of torsades like CHF, hypokalemia and family history of long QT syndrome.

○ It is contraindicated in age group less than 18 years of age.

○ It is also contraindicated in pregnancy and the female should be on non-hormonal contraceptives or has passed 2 years of post-menopausal period during drug therapy.

c. Ceftriaxone in typhoid fever

ANSWER

Third Generation Cephalosporins

○ Enhanced and highly augmented activity against gram-negative Enterobacteriaceae

○ Some few members cause inhibition of *Pseudomonas* as well

○ Less active on gram-positive cocci and anaerobes

○ **Cefotaxime:** Prototype of this group

- Exhibits potent action on both aerobic gram-negative and some gram-positive bacteria

- Inactive on anaerobes (particularly *Bact. fragilis*), *Staph. aureus* and *Ps. Aeruginosa*

- Valuable in meningitis caused by gram-negative bacilli, life-threatening resistant/hospital-acquired infections

- Beneficial in septicemias and infections in immunocompromised patients

- Potent alternative for typhoid fever, utilized for single dose therapy in PPNG urethritis

- Good penetration into CSF

○ **Ceftriaxone:** Distinctive feature its longer duration of action

- Highly effective extensively in serious infections including bacterial meningitis (particularly

PHARMACOLOGY

in children), multiresistant typhoid fever, complicated urinary tract infections

- In addition, inhibition of *B. fragilis* also.

○ **Cefixime:** Is the oral drug of choice for thyroid and is preferred in ambulatory medicine.

Mnemonics

Delhi: Cef**D**inir, Cef**D**inotren, cefo**D**oxime
P–Cefoperazone
M–Moxalactam, cef**T**izoxime, cef**T**azidime
Exam: Cefixime

d. Febuxostat in hyperuricemia

(Ref: KD Tripathi, Essentials of Medical Pharmacology, 7th ed, pg. 217, 8th ed, pg.235)

ANSWER

Febuxostat in Hyperuricemia

○ It is a nonpurine xanthine oxidase inhibitor

○ Almost equal or more effective than allopurinol to reduce blood uric acid level in patients with hyperuricemia and gout

○ An alternative drug to treat symptomatic gout only in individuals intolerant to allopurinol, or in those who are having any contraindications

○ Cover from NSAIDs/colchicine to be followed be provided for 1–2 months while initiating treatment with febuxostat

○ Cannot be given to patients with malignancy associated hyperuricaemia

○ Liver damage is the most important adverse effect; general ones being diarrhea, nausea and headache

○ Mercaptopurine, azathioprine and theophylline have adverse drug interactions; should not be given to patients consuming these drugs.

4. Describe the drug treatment of:

a. Urinary tract infection

(Ref: KD Tripathi, Essentials of Medical Pharmacology, 7th ed, pg. 708, 711, 8th ed, pg.759, 761-62)

ANSWER

Case	Treatment
Asymptomatic	In pregnant women, treatment for 3–7 days: **Before late 3rd trimester:** Amoxicillin or cephalexin or nitrofurantoin **Before third trimester:** Trimethoprim-sulfamethoxazole
Uncomplicated	Nitrofurantoin 100 mg BD for 5 days **Alternatively:** Fosfomycin 3g Or Trimethoprim-sulfamethoxazole 160/800 mg BD x 3 days*
Complicated UTI (also in uncomplicated pyelonephritis)	In case of mild/moderate illness, Oral therapy with ciprofloxacin 500 mg PO BD given for 5 to 14 days Or Trimethoprim-sulfamethoxazole 160/800 mg BD x 5 to 14 days In case of severe cases or pregnant, intravenous therapy with ceftriaxone 1 g IV qDay **Or Before the third trimester:** Trimethoprim-sulfamethoxazole or gentamicin or levofloxacin (not sued in pregnancy)

In uncomplicated cases, do not use amoxicillin empirically

○ Most acute uncomplicated urine tract infections respond promptly to cotrimoxazole

○ Courses of cotrimoxazole 3–10 days opined for lower as well as upper urinary tract infections

○ Ciprofloxacin used in complicated cases or cases with indwelling catheters/prostatitis, have been achieved.

b. Chloroquine resistance falciparum malaria

ANSWER

Treatment of Malaria

Vivax		Falciparum		Mixed Infection
Chloroquine 3 d + Primaquine 14 d	For all states	Artemether 3d + Lumefantrine 3d + Primaquine single dose on day 2	North East	Add primaquine for 14 days to falciparum regimen for North East

Vivax			Falciparum			Mixed Infection	
			Artesunate 3d + Sulfadoxine 3d + Pyrimethamine 3d +		Other state	Add primaquine for 14 days to falciparum regimen for other states	
d = days			Primaquine single dose on day 2				

Note: Primaquine is contraindicated in pregnant and infants.Part-III

5. Discuss the therapeutic uses and adverse effects of:

a. Methotrexate

(Ref: KD Tripathi, Essentials of Medical Pharmacology, 7th ed, pg. 210, 8th ed, pg.228)

ANSWER

Methotrexate

○ A dihydrofolate reductase inhibitor; exhibiting prominent immunosuppressant and anti-inflammatory property

Therapeutic Uses

○ It causes inhibition of cytokine production, chemotaxis and also cell-mediated immune reaction, thus beneficial in RA
○ Considered as DMARD of first choice
○ Used as standard treatment for most patients, that includes patients of juvenile RA
○ Predictable response that is sustained over long-term
○ Also forms one of the important drug in combination regimens of 2 or 3 DMARDs
○ Relatively rapid onset of symptom relief, thus ideal for initial treatment

Adverse Effects

○ Oral ulceration and gastric upset form major adverse effects of low dose regimen
○ Increased incidence of chest infection
○ It can cause dose dependent progressive liver damage
○ It can even depress bone marrow.

b. Dapsone

(Ref: KD Tripathi, Essentials of Medical Pharmacology, 7th ed, pg. 780, 8th ed, pg.831-32)

ANSWER

Dapsone

○ Diamino diphenyl sulfone

○ **Mechanism of action:** It leads to inhibition of incorporation of PABA into folic acid by the enzyme folate synthase
  ▪ PABA antagonizes the antibacterial activity of dapsone
  ▪ Leprostatic action at even very low concentrations

Therapeutic Uses

○ Multidrug treatment has find place in leprosy due to development of dapsone-resistance among *M. leprae*
○ There are two types of resistances: primary and secondary; one more important In addition to resistance, there is one more issue with dapsone use—"*persisters*" (drug sensitive bacilli which gets dormant, hide in some tissues and thus not affected by any drug)
○ Also employed in combination of pyrimethamine, as an alternative to sulfadoxine-pyrimethamine for treating *P. falciparum* and *Toxoplasma gondii* infections
○ Antifungal action against fungus *Pneumocystis jirovecii*
○ Can be employed for chloroquine-resistant malaria, toxoplasmosis and *P. jirovecii* infection

Adverse Effects

○ Mild hemolytic anemia
○ Nausea and anorexia occurs as gastric intolerance develops in the beginning
○ Headache and paraesthesias
○ Allergic rashes, phototoxicity
○ *Sulfone syndrome:* The reaction which develops 4–6 weeks after initiating dapsone treatment; it causes fever, malaise, enlargement of lymph nodes, desquamation of skin, and even jaundice and anemia.

6. Write short notes on:

a. Anti-rabies vaccine

(Ref: KD Tripathi, Essentials of Medical Pharmacology, 7th ed, pg. 922, 8th ed, pg.985-86)

PHARMACOLOGY

ANSWER

Anti-rabies Vaccine

There have been four rabies vaccines:

- **Antirabic vaccine carbolized (Semple vaccine):**
  - Also known as "Neural tissue vaccine"
  - Poorer efficiency, there was requirement for 14 daily painful large volume (2–5 ml) injections to be administered into the anterior abdominal wall

- **Purified chick embryo cell vaccine:**
  - Consists of Flury-LEP strain of rabies virus that are grown on chick fibroblasts and get deactivated by β-propiolactone
  - Pain at local site of injection, erythema, swelling and lymph node enlargement

- **Human diploid cell vaccine:**
  - Lyophilized inactivated rabies virus that are grown in human diploid cell culture
  - Redness and minor induration occurs that last for 1 to 2 days; in 10% cases
  - 1% cases have reported fever and arthralgia is reported in 1%
  - Approximately 100% effective

- **Purified vero cell rabies vaccine:**
  - Constitutes inactivated wistar rabies PM/WI38-1-503-3M strain
  - These are grown on vero continuous cell line
  - Therapy with intradermal route for all tissue culture rabies vaccines called the Thai regimen, recommended by the WHO since 1992, also been approved and notified by the Government of India in 2006
  - *Regimen:* 0.1 mL of PCEV or PVRV or 0.2 ml of HDCV is injected intradermally over deltoid of both arms
    - Given on days 0, 3 and 7 followed by one site injection on day 28 (or 30) and day 90, a total of 8 injections; no injection at day 14
    - 10–14 days are taken in the development of protective antibodies, simultaneous administration of rabies immunoglobulin recommended in category III bites.

b. Meropenem

(Ref: KD Tripathi, Essentials of Medical Pharmacology, 7th ed, pg. 731, 8th ed, pg.782)

ANSWER

Meropenem

- A newer carbapenem that do not get hydrolysed by renal peptidase
- No need to use with cilastatin like imipenem

- Active against both gram-positive and gram-negative bacteria; little more potent on gram-negative aerobes, particularly *Ps. aeruginosa* but less effective on gram-positive cocci
- Also acts against aerobes as well as anaerobes
- A reserve drug to treat serious nosocomial infections like septicaemia, febrile neutropenia, intraabdominal and pelvic infections, etc. that are caused by cephalosporin-resistant bacteria and diabetic foot
- To be combined with an aminoglycoside for treating *P.s. aeruginosa* infections
- Seizures are less common to occur.

c. Post coital contraceptives

ANSWER

Postcoital Contraception

- Postcoital contraception mandates emergency measures
  - **Emergency contraception:** Immediate measures instituted to prevent unwanted pregnancy in cases of unprotected sexual intercourse

Standard Regimen Used

- *Levonorgestrel* in a dose of 0.75 mg (twice with a gap of 12 hour), or single dose of 1.5 mg
  - Should be taken as soon as possible, but within 72 hour of unprotected sexual activity
  - Milder side effects, for example, headache, nausea, vomiting, and less pronounced than estrogen + progestin therapy
  - May result in delayed or disturbed menstrual cycles

- *Ulipristal* (recently approved)
  - It is a selective progesterone receptor modulator which is partial agonist at progesterone receptors and inhibits ovulation and implantation of fertilized ovum. It inhibits LH release and also inhibits LH induced follicular rupture in ovary.
  - This is also a well-tolerated method
  - It provides an extended window of protective action
  - Single dose of 30 mg single dose as soon as possible, within 120 hour of unprotected intercourse

- *Mifepristone*
  - Gideer
  - Is not FDA approved but can be used for emergency for 5 days.
  - Fewer side effects noted headache and abdominal pain
  - Single dose of 600 mg within 72 hour of unprotected sexual activity.
  - YUZPE regimen: Containing an estrogen as progesterone is less efficacious and hence not preferred.

Name of the Paper : **Pharmacology Paper-I**

Name of the Course : **MBBS-2016**

Semester : **Annual**

Time: 3 Hours   M.M.: 40

INSTRUCTIONS

1. Write your Roll No. on the top immediately on receipt of this question paper
2. All questions are to be attempted
3. Answers to Parts I, II and III should be written in separate answer sheets provided
4. Attempt parts of a question in sequence

PART-I

1. **Explain why?**   [8]
    a. In pharamacotherapeutics, children are not viewed as miniature adults
    b. Basic drugs are better absorbed in alkaline media and acidic drugs in acid media
    c. Spironolactone is especially useful in edema of cirrhosis of liver
    d. Adrenaline not noradrenaline, shows vasomotor reversal of Dale

2. **Explain by giving two examples how genetic factors can modify effect of a drug.**   [6]

PART-II

3. **Discuss the therapeutic status of:**   [8]
    a. Sodium nitroprusside in hypertensive emergencies
    b. Antihistamines in motion sickness
    c. Amyl nitrite in cyanide poisoning
    d. Dopaminergic agonists in parkinsonism

4. **Describe the drug treatment of:**   [6]
    a. Hypercalcaemia
    b. Anovulatory infertility

PART-III

5. **Discuss the therapeutic uses and adverse effects of:**   [6]
    a. Azithromycin
    b. Inhalational anaesthetic agents

6. **Write short notes on:**   [6]
    a. Drug dependence
    b. Therapeutic Index
    c. Intravenous anaesthetics

PART-I

1. Explain why?

a. In pharmacotherapeutics, children are not viewed as miniature adults

ANSWER

Rationale to Not Consider Children as Miniature Adults in Pharmacotherapeutics

- Children can neither be viewed nor treated as little adults as difference in size is not the only difference; there exist many other physiological and pathological variations as well
- Children have delicate skin and more prone to invasion, thus rendering them more susceptible to external pathogens
- Anatomic and physiological differences play important role to choose among routes of administration
- Oral bioavailability of drugs in pediatric and adult populations governed by factors such as gastric pH and emptying time, intestinal transit time, immature activity of bile and pancreatic fluid
- Drug distribution depends on membrane permeability, plasma protein binding and total body water, that exhibit major differences in children and adults
- Excretion of drugs also differ as determined by glomerular filtration (immature in children), renal tubular secretion and tubular reabsorption (at birth and their maturation determine excretion of drugs in the pediatric population).

b. Basic drugs are better absorbed in alkaline media and acidic drugs in acid media

ANSWER

Rationale for Better Absorption of Basic Drugs in Alkaline Medium and Acidic Drugs in Acidic Medium

- pH of the medium plays significant role in degree of ionization of drugs and their absorption
- Basic drugs are more ionized and less absorbed in acidic medium, whereas, they are nonionized (lipid soluble) and more absorbable in alkaline medium
- That is why, basic drugs best absorbed in intestine
- Weak acidic drugs will exist mainly in its unionized form (lipid soluble) in acidic medium and more readily absorbed into systemic circulation

- Hence, acidic drugs show better absorption in stomach.

c. Spironolactone is especially useful in edema of cirrhosis of liver

ANSWER

Rationale for Spironolactone being used in Edema due to Cirrhosis of Liver

- Proposed benefit of spironolactone therapy is through aldosterone antagonism
- It can be used to inhibit the **renin–angiotensin–aldosterone system (RAAS)** activation that occurs from administration of high-ceiling diuretics (e.g., furosemide) or some diseases that lead to congestion
- Employed for managing hepatic cirrhosis and resultant edema since it will inhibit ascites formation caused by excess aldosterone
- Thus, used in the management of fluid retention associated with noncardiac disease such as hepatic disease and nephrotic syndrome.

d. Adrenaline not noradrenaline, shows vasomotor reversal of Dale

(Ref: KD Tripathi, Essentials of Medical Pharmacology, 8th ed, pg. 138, 144)

ANSWER

Rationale for Adrenaline Showing Vasomotor Reversal of Dale

- A marked increase in both systolic as well as diastolic BP occurs due to rapid intravenous injection of adrenaline
- This occurs as alpha response predominates at high concentration and vasoconstriction in skeletal muscles also seen
- The mechanism involved is rapid uptake and distribution of Adr leads to reduced concentration around the receptor; low concentrations cannot act on α receptors but continued action on β2 receptors
- The α blockers (like ergotamine) block the pressor action of Adr, only producing vasodilatation and fall in BP due to β2 mediated vasodilatation
- This is known as *vasomotor reversal of Dale*
- On the contrary, noradrenaline acts on both alpha-1 and alpha-2 adrenergic receptors, no beta receptor action.

2. Explain by giving two examples how genetic factors can modify effect of a drug.

(Ref: KD Tripathi, Essentials of Medical Pharmacology, 7th ed, pg. 65, 8th ed, pg. 75-77)

ANSWER

Genetics Affecting Drug Action

○ Key factors of drug response, include transporters, metabolizing enzymes, ion channels, receptors with their couplers and effectors are controlled by genetics of each individual

○ Thus genetic makeup of races and individuals determine drug action

○ **Pharmacogenetics**: Study of genetic basis for variation in drug response

○ **Pharmacogenomics:** Defined as the use of genetic information to guide the choice of drug and dose on an individual basis

　▪ **Significance:**

　　♦ Aims to recognize individuals who are either more likely or less likely to respond to a drug, also including those who need altered dose of certain drugs

　　♦ Defining the genetic basis of an individual's profile of drug response and predicting most suited treatment option for the individual

○ Goal is "personalized medicine" on a wide scale

○ In case of most drugs, a constant variation with bell-shaped Gaussian frequency distribution is perceived

○ Examples of some specific genetic defects which may result into discontinuous variation in drug responses:

　▪ G-6PD deficiency is responsible for hemolysis with primaquine and other oxidizing drugs; this is X-linked monogenic trait more commonly seen in the Mediterranean, African and Southeast Asian races. Hemolysis is largely dose related. Severe hemolysis in homozygous deficient individuals of certain genotypes

　▪ Codeine fails to produce analgesia in CYP2D6 deficient, because this enzyme generates morphine from codeine

　▪ Mydriatics precipitate attack of angle closure glaucoma in individuals with narrow iridocorneal angle.

PART-II

3. Discuss the therapeutic status of:

　a. **Sodium nitroprusside in hypertensive emergencies**

(Ref: KD Tripathi, Essentials of Medical Pharmacology, 7th, ed, 8th ed, pg.568)

ANSWER

Sodium Nitroprusside in Hypertensive Emergencies
Sodium Nitroprusside

○ Nitroprusside is metabolized into nitric oxide, which causes dilation of both arteries and veins by cyclic GMP pathway as seen with nitrates.

○ It is also metabolized into cyanide, which is further metabolized in liver to thiocyanate. Thiocyanate can cause neuropsychiatric side-effects and hypothyroidism by inhibiting sodium iodide symporter in thyroid.

○ Nitroprusside is a **very short and fast acting** drug as the effect is seen within 30 seconds and terminates 3 minutes after infusion is stopped.

○ Currently it is a second line drug for treatment of hypertensive emergency. It can be used for treatment of CHF (associated pulmonary edema), MI (decreases myocardial oxygen demand) and to induce controlled hypotension in anaesthesia. In aortic dissection it is used along with beta blocker to prevent reflex tachycardia, which can worsen dissection.

　b. **Antihistamines in motion sickness**

(Ref: KD Tripathi, Essentials of Medical Pharmacology, 7th, ed, 8th ed, pg. 663-65)

ANSWER

Antihistamines in Motion Sickness

○ Few antihistaminics act as antiemetic based on anticholinergic, antihistaminic, weak antidopaminergic and sedative properties

○ Antiemetics with anticholinergic-antihistaminic property forms the preferred drugs for *motion sickness*

○ *Promethazine, dimenhydrinate, diphenhydramine:*

　▪ Provide protection to motion sickness for 4 to 6 hours

- Sedation and dryness of mouth occur
- Impede extrapyramidal side effects of metoclopramide, while enhancing its antiemetic activity
○ *Meclozine (Meclizine):*
- Less sedative and longer-acting
- Offers protection against sea sickness for around 24 hours
○ Cinnarizine:
- An antivertigo drug having antimotion sickness property.

c. Amyl nitrite in cyanide poisoning

(Ref: KD Tripathi, Essentials of Medical Pharmacology, 7th ed, pg. 545, 8th ed, pg. 544)

ANSWER

Amyl Nitrite in Cyanide Poisoning

○ Amyl nitrite is used as antidote for cyanide poisoning
○ Amyl nitrite and sodium nitrite antagonize cyanide toxicity in part by oxidizing hemoglobin to methemoglobin
○ Methaemoglobin generated by nitrates, which has high affinity for cyanide radical and leads to formation of cyanomethaemoglobin
○ Large doses (>300 mg) adequate to yield enough methaemoglobin can be intravenously injected without producing hypotension.

d. Dopaminergic agonists in Parkinsonism

ANSWER

Parkinsonism

Term used to describe the symptoms of tremors, slowness of movement, and muscle rigidity

Neurodegenerative Disorders

Parkinson's Disease

○ Parkinson's disease is caused by progressive depletion of dopaminergic neurons in corpus striatum.
○ Dopamine acts on D_2 (G_i) receptors in the corpus striatum and inhibits the action potential flow from cortex to spinal cord motor neurons. This has a physiological inhibitory effect on the movements.
○ In the absence of dopamine this inhibition is absent, and the movements are increased and leads to movement disorder called as Parkinson's disease.

Dopamine's Function in Striatum

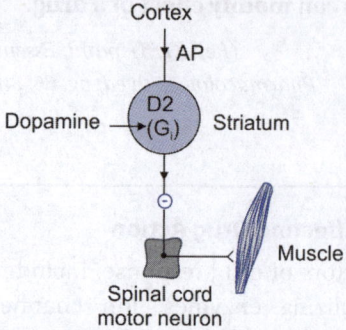

○ Thus, for treatment of PD either the level of dopamine can be restored or D_2 receptor can be stimulated (D_2 agonists). Dopamine level is restored by either giving a prodrug of dopamine i.e. levodopa or by inhibiting metabolism of dopamine by MAO and COMT inhibitors.

Mechanism of Action of Antiparkinsonian Drugs

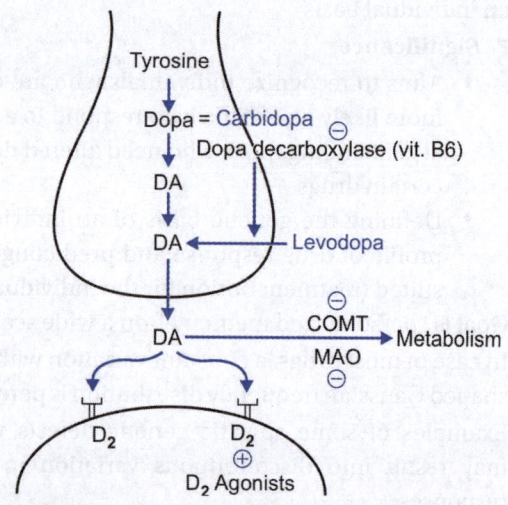

○ **Dose:** 0.25 mg thrice daily starting dose, titrated to a maximum of 4–8 mg thrice a day.

4. Describe the drug treatment of:

a. Hypercalcaemia

(Ref: KD Tripathi, Essentials of Medical Pharmacology, 7th ed, pg. 343, 8th ed, pg. 365-66)

ANSWER

Drug Treatment

○ **Bisphosphonates (BPNs):** Analogs of pyrophosphate
- Beneficial in metabolic bone diseases and hypercalcaemia
- Exhibit strong affinity for calcium phosphate and selective activity in calcified tissue

- Pamidronate (60–90 mg IV. over 2–4 hours) or zoledronate (4 mg IV over 15 min) are most effective drugs in treatment of **hypercalcemia of malignancy**, may be supplemented by IM calcitonin 6–12 hourly for 2 days
- Highly potent third generation BPN, zoledronate is indicated for hypercalcaemia
- Zoledronate is effective, faster acting than pamidronate and hence the drug of choice now

○ **Gallium nitrate:**
- A potent inhibitor of bone resorption
- Cause depression of ATP-dependent proton pump at the ruffled membrane of osteoclasts
- Employed in resistant cases of hypercalcaemia
- Administered by continuous intravenous infusion daily for 5 days

○ **Glucocorticoids:**
- Calcium excretion is enhanced and calcium absorption is reduced by giving high doses of prednisolone (and others)
- Adjuvant role in hypercalcaemia due to lymphoma, myeloma, leukaemia, carcinoma breast, etc.

b. **Anovulatory infertility**

ANSWER

Drug Treatment

○ **Clomiphene citrate:**
- Primarily used for infertility occurring due to failure of ovulation
- Dose is 50 mg OD for 5 days; initiated from 5th day of cycle
- Daily dose may be doubled for 2 to 3 cycles when treatment of 1–2 months fails to cause conception
- Acts as a pure estrogen antagonist
- Induction of gonadotropin secretion in females by hindering estrogenic feedback inhibition of pituitary
- Thus, increase in LH/FSH amount released at each secretory pulse, this causes ovaries to enlarge and if the ovaries are reactive to gonadotropin then, reovulation follows
- It can also modify endometrium and cervical mucus
- Menotropins or chorionic gonadotropin added to the therapy on the last 2 days of the course increases the success rate

Note: > 6 treatment cycles should not be tried.

○ **Gonadotropins:** When infertility is due to deficient production of Gns by pituitary

- Usually employed when ovulation cannot be induced by clomiphene or if anovulation is due to polycystic ovaries
- Ovulation occurs within the next 24–48 hours in about 75% cases, and conception can occur.

PART-III

5. Discuss the therapeutic uses and adverse effects of:

a. **Azithromycin**

ANSWER

Azithromycin

○ A macrolide-type antibiotic
○ Higher efficacy, better gastric tolerance, and convenient once daily dosing schedule
○ **Therapeutic uses:** First choice drugs for
- Legionnaires' pneumonia
- Chlamydia trachomatis
- Donovanosis caused by C. granulomatis
- Gonococcal urethritis
- Combating primarily respiratory diseases caused by Gram-positive pathogens and fastidious Gram-negative pathogens

○ **Adverse effect profile:**

Infections	• Candidiasis • Vaginal infection • Pneumonia • Fungal infection • Bacterial infection • Pharyngitis • Rhinitis • Oral candidiasis • Pseudomembranous colitis
Blood and lymphatic system disorders	• Leukopenia • Neutropenia • Eosinophilia • Thrombocytopenia • Haemolytic anemia
Immune system disorders	• Angioedema • Hypersensitivity
Metabolism and nutrition disorders	• Anorexia
Psychiatric disorders	• Nervousness • Insomnia
Nervous system disorders	• Headache • Dizziness • Somnolence • Dysgeusia • Paraesthesia

PHARMACOLOGY

b. Inhalational anaesthetic agents

ANSWER

Inhalational Anesthetic Agents

- **Classified as:**
  Gas
  - Nitrous oxide
  - Halothane
  - Isoflurane
  - Desflurane
  - Sevoflurane
  Volatile liquids
  - Ether

Techniques of Inhalation of Anesthetics

- **Open drop method:** Liquid anaesthetic poured over mask with gauze and inhalation of vapour with air. Ether is only drug to be administered like this

- **Through anaesthetic machines:** Reservoir bags, gas cylinders, specialized graduated vaporisers, flow meters, unidirectional valves, employed to deliver drug through face mask or endotracheal tube
  - Can be done by an open, closed, or semiclosed system

- **Therapeutic uses:**
  - **Nitrous oxide:** Nonirritating, but low potency anaesthetic
    - Recall of events during anesthesia may occur if maintenance on 70% N2O + 30% O2 along with muscle relaxants
    - Usually used as a carrier and adjuvant to other anaesthetic agents
  - **Halothane:** A volatile liquid with sweet odour, nonirritant and noninflammable
    - Rapid and pleasant induction
    - Affords precise control of concentration to be given
    - Relatively greater depression of respiration; breathing is shallow and rapid
    - Preferred for asthmatics
    - Used both for induction as well as maintenance in children
    - Used in maintenance anesthesia in adults after IV induction
  - **Desflurane:** Newer fluorinated congener of isoflurane
    - Used as an anaesthetic for outpatient surgery

- **Adverse Effects:**
  - Nephrotoxicity and hepatotoxicity
  - Cardiac arrhythmias
  - Postoperative nausea and vomiting
  - Neurotoxicity and respiratory depression and irritation
  - Malignant hyperthermia and postanesthesia agitation.

---

6. Write short notes on:

a. Drug dependence

ANSWER

Drug Dependence

A state in which use of drugs for personal satisfaction is rendered a higher priority than other basic requirements, often regardless of known risks to health

- **Related terminology and definitions describing different aspects of the problem:**
  - **Psychological dependence:** The individual believes that he/she can achieve optimal state of wellbeing only through the actions of the drug. The intensity of psychological dependence may vary from desire to craving.
  - **Physical dependence:** A changed physiological state produced when a drug is administered repeatedly, necessitating the sustained presence of the drug to maintain physiological equilibrium. Discontinuation of the drug results in withdrawal syndrome.
  - **Drug abuse:** Using a drug by self-medication in a manner and amount not in sync with the approved medical and social patterns in a given culture at a given time. There are two patterns: Continuous use or occasional use.
  - **Drug addiction:** A pattern of uncontrollable drug use characterized by irresistible involvement with the use of a drug.
  - **Drug habituation:** Less intensive involvement with the drug, the withdrawal will produce only mild discomfort.

b. Therapeutic Index

(Ref: KD Tripathi, Essentials of Medical Pharmacology, 7th ed, pg. 55, 8th ed, pg.65-66)

ANSWER

Therapeutic Index

- Safer drugs have higher TI values. Drugs with lower TI values frequently require monitoring.

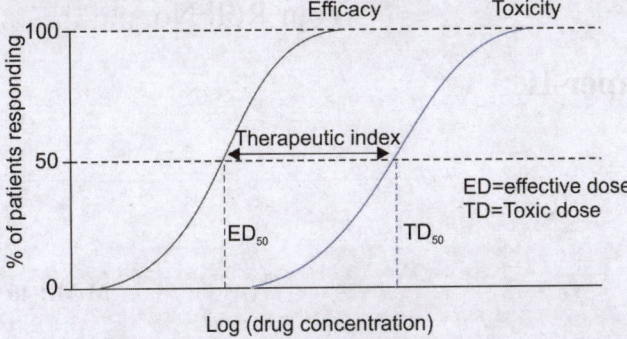

Intravenous Anesthetics

Drugs which when intravenously administered produce loss of consciousness in one arm-brain circulation time (around 11 s)

○ **Uses**
  - Usually employed for induction because exhibit rapid onset of action; maintenance usually done by an inhalational agent
  - Reduce the dose of maintenance anaesthetic
  - Serve as sole anesthetic when supplemented with analgesics and muscle relaxants

○ Examples include thiopentone sodium, propofol, etomidate

○ **Thiopentone sodium:**
  - Poor analgesic; so painful procedures not to be done unless an opioid or N_2O has been given
  - Cardiovascular collapse may occur if there are hypovolemia, shock or sepsis
  - Sometimes used for rapid control of convulsions
  - Facilitates verbal communication with psychiatric cases and employed in "narcoanalysis" in subanesthetic doses

○ **Propofol**: A fast-acting intravenous anesthetic
  - Used both for induction as well as maintenance
  - Occurrence of unconsciousness in 15–45 sec and remains for 5–10 minutes
  - Particularly suited for outpatient surgery
  - Preferred in asthmatics
  - Very low side effect profile.

○ Example: **W**arfarin, **T**heophylline, **D**igoxin, **L**ithium
  Mnemonics: **W**arning! **T**hese **D**rugs are **L**ethal!.

○ LD50 (lethal median dose) often replaces TD50 in animal studies.

○ The safety margin of a drug is determined by gap between the therapeutic effect and the adverse effect as determined by dose response curve; referred to as therapeutic index of that drug

○ Also known as therapeutic ratio; defined as ratio of drug dose needed to produce a toxic effect and the drug dose required to generate desired therapeutic response

○ **Significance:** The higher is the ratio, the greater is the relative safety of the drug

○ **Therapeutic index is calculated as:**

$$\text{Terapeutic index} = \frac{\text{Median lethal dose}}{\text{Median effective dose}}$$

○ Median effective dose: Dose that produces the specified pharmacological effect in 50% individuals

○ Median lethal dose: Dose that is sufficient to kill 50% of the recipients.

c.   Intravenous anaesthetics

(Ref: KD Tripathi, Essentials of Medical Pharmacology, 7th ed, pg. 381, 8th ed, pg. 408-12)

Name of the Paper : **Pharmacology Paper-II**

Name of the Course : **MBBS-2016**

Semester : **Annual**

Time: 3 Hours   M.M.: 40

INSTRUCTIONS

1. Write your Roll No. on the top immediately on receipt of this question paper
2. All questions are to be attempted
3. Answers to Parts I, II and III should be written in separate answer sheets provided
4. Attempt parts of a question in sequence

PART-I

1. **Explain why?**   [8]
   a. Corticosteroids should not be stopped abruptly
   b. Combination drug therapy is used in the treatment of tuberculosis
   c. Clopidogrel is used in cerebrovascular diseases
   d. Letrozole is used only in postmenopausal women suffering from carcinoma breast

2. Classify and enumerate antiemetic drugs. Discuss the mechanism of action, therapeutic uses and adverse effects of ondansetron.   [6]

PART-II

3. **Discuss the therapeutic status of:**   [8]
   a. Octreotide in the management of acromegaly
   b. Erythropoietin in anemia
   c. Cyclosporine in organ transplantation
   d. Linezolid in the treatment of community acquired pneumonia

4. **Describe the drug treatment of:**   [6]
   a. Paucibacillary leprosy
   b. Osteoporosis

PART-III

5. **Discuss the therapeutic uses and adverse effects of:**   [6]
   a. Oral contraceptives
   b. Insulin analogues

6. **Write short notes on:**   [6]
   a. Fibrinolytic agents
   b. Macrolide antibiotics
   c. Pentavalent vaccine

PART-I

1. Explain why?

a. Corticosteroids should not be stopped abruptly.

ANSWER

Rationale to Not Stop Corticosteroids Abruptly

○ Sudden cessation of corticosteroids result into withdrawal symptoms and signs
○ It may cause weakness, fatigue, decreased appetite, weight loss, nausea, vomiting, diarrhea, abdominal pain, mimicking many other medical problems
○ Tapering of the dose provides the adrenal glands time to return to their normal patterns of secretion
○ HPA axis may take more than 2 years for recovery
○ No tapering is needed if course has been of less than 1 week.

b. Combination drug therapy is used in the treatment of tuberculosis

ANSWER

Rationale to Use Combination of Antitubercular Drugs in Tuberculosis

○ **For preventing emergence of drug-resistant tuberculosis:**
   ▪ One most important step to ensure complete and effective treatment of tuberculosis is to prevent further emergence of drug-resistant tuberculosis
   ▪ Any inappropriate selection of antitubercular agent and monotherapy with any one drug has showed up risk of developing drug-resistant tuberculosis
   ▪ Drug resistance have been predominantly occurring due to multiple disruptions of treatment
   ▪ Also, if single dose preparations are given, patients are more likely to continue one drug and negligence towards others
   ▪ Use of fixed dose combinations of antitubercular agents results in limiting the risks of drug-resistant cases
○ Use of combinations also make prescription of drugs and management of drug supply simpler

○ **Overcoming limitations of treatment centers:**
   ▪ At times, drugs being out-of-stock in treatment facilities, may lead to continuation of some drugs, while new stocks of the others are awaited
   ▪ This epitomizes another possible source of monotherapy.

c. Clopidogrel is used in cerebrovascular diseases

(Ref: KD Tripathi, Essentials of Medical Pharmacology, 7th ed, pg. 630, 8th ed, pg. 678, 680)

ANSWER

Rationale to use Clopidogrel in Cerebrovascular Diseases

○ This drug exhibits ability of irreversible inhibition of platelet function and range of therapeutic efficacy
○ It is an oral antiplatelet agent used to inhibit platelet-initiated thrombosis in cerebrovascular disease
○ Leads to inhibition of adenosine diphosphate (ADP) receptor–mediated platelet activity
○ It is a prodrug and metabolized to an active metabolite through which it exerts its antiplatelet effect
○ It is more effective than aspirin alone and has been used concurrently with aspirin.

d. Letrozole is used only in postmenopausal women suffering from carcinoma breast

(Ref: KD Tripathi, Essentials of Medical Pharmacology, 7th ed, pg. 314, 8th ed, pg.339-40)

ANSWER

Rationale to Use Letrozole in Postmenopausal Women Suffering from Breast Cancer

○ An orally active nonsteroidal (type 2) compound which reversibly inhibits aromatization all over the body, (within the breast cancer cells, that lead to nearly total estrogen deprivation)
○ It is contraindicated in premenopausal women
○ A first line drug employed for adjuvant therapy after mastectomy in ER+ive postmenopausal women
○ It is recommended to be used as first line therapy in advanced breast carcinoma since it provides higher response rate as compared to tamoxifen
○ Should not be used alone in women with breast cancer who have preserved ovarian function

○ Should be only used in postmenopausal women, should be avoided in premenopausal women who have chemotherapy-induced amenorrhea with breast cancer since it may cause ovarian function to resume, this can cause failure or ineffective treatment.

2. **Classify and enumerate antiemetic drugs. Discuss the mechanism of action, therapeutic uses and adverse effects of ondansetron.**

(Ref: KD Tripathi, Essentials of Medical Pharmacology, 8th ed, pg. 710-13,716-17)

ANSWER

Classification of Antiemetics

○ **Anticholinergics:** Hyoscine, Dicyclomine

○ **H1 antihistaminics:** Promethazine, Diphenhydramine, Dimenhydrinate, Doxylamine, Meclozine (Meclizine), Cinnarizine

○ **Neuroleptics:** Chlorpromazine, (D2 blockers) Triflupromazine, Prochlorperazine, Haloperidol, etc.

○ **Prokinetic drugs:** Metoclopramide, Domperidone, Cisapride, Mosapride, Itopride

○ **5-HT3 antagonists:** Ondansetron, Granisetron, Palonosetron, Ramosetron

○ **NK1 receptor antagonists:** Aprepitant, Fosaprepitant

○ **Adjuvant antiemetics:** Dexamethasone, Benzodiazepines, Dronabinol, Nabilone.

Ondansetron

○ Developed to cater vomiting associated to chemotherapy/radiotherapy

○ **Mechanism of action:** Peripheral 5-HT3 receptor blockade on vagal afferents in GIT, including nucleus tractus solitarius (NTS) and chemoreceptor trigger zone (CTZ)

○ **Therapeutic profile in antiemesis:**

▪ Vomiting induced by cisplatin and other highly emetogenic drugs employed in cancer chemotherapy

▪ Also useful in postoperative nausea and vomiting; administered 4 h before surgery

▪ Used in cases of acute vomiting than delayed vomiting

▪ Effective in controlling vomiting which occurs as side effect of drugs or due to drug over dosage, uremia, neurological disorders and disorders of GI

▪ Poor efficacy in motion sickness

▪ Hyperemesis gravidarum (only given in pregnancy in unavoidable cases)

○ **Advantages over other antiemetics:** Does not produce dystonias or sedation

○ **Adverse effect profile:**

▪ Only common side effect is headache and dizziness

▪ Mild constipation

▪ Abdominal discomfort occurring in some patients

▪ Hypotension and bradycardia

▪ Chest pain may also occur

▪ Allergic reactions reported, particularly after intravenous injection.

PART-II

3. **Discuss the therapeutic status of:**

a. **Octreotide in the management of acromegaly**

(Ref: KD Tripathi, Essentials of Medical Pharmacology, 7th ed, 8th ed, pg. 238)

ANSWER

Octreotide in Acromegaly

○ This is a synthetic octapeptide surrogate of somatostatin

○ Potent in suppression of GH secretion and longer-acting, but weak inhibitor of insulin secretion

○ Thus employed for use in acromegaly

○ It helps in normalizing IGF-1 levels in 25 to 50% of patients with acromegaly

○ Also reduces the tumor size in about 25% of patients

○ Preferred over somatostatin for acromegaly and secretory diarrhoeas associated with carcinoid, AIDS, cancer chemotherapy or diabetes.

b. **Erythropoietin in anemia**

ANSWER

Erythropoietin

A sialoglycoprotein hormone; produced by peritubular cells of the kidney

How Erythropoietin Works?

○ Multiplying of colony forming cells of the erythroid series is stimulated

○ Formation of hemoglobin and maturation of erythroblast

○ Reticulocytes are released in the circulation

○ **Note:** Erythropoiesis is induced in a dose dependent manner, no impact on RBC lifespan

Erythropoietin in Anemia

○ Primarily indicated for anemia of chronic renal failure which occurs due to low levels of erythropoietin

○ Use of erythropoietin is considered only in symptomatic cases with Hb ≤ 8 g/dL

○ **Dose:** Subcutaneous or intravenous 25–100 U/kg thrice a week (max. 600 U/kg/week)

○ Hematocrit and hemoglobin is raised, need for transfusions is reduced

○ The treatment should be started with a low dose and then titrate upwards to maintain hematocrit between 30 and 36%, and Hb 10–11 g/dL

○ Cases where patients have low iron stores, concurrent parenteral/oral iron therapy may be needed for an optimal response.

c. Cyclosporine in organ transplantation

ANSWER

Cyclosporine

○ A highly selective immunosuppressant

○ Specific T-cell inhibitor which has strikingly increased success in organ transplantations

How it Works?

○ Target T cell signal transduction

○ Inhibit expression of IL-2

○ Inhibit IL-2 mediated T cell activation, proliferation, and differentiation

○ Arrest at G_0 or G_1 phase of lymphocytes

Used in Organ Transplants Patients Since

○ This compound preferentially suppresses cell-mediated immunity and prevents graft rejection

○ Most effective drug for use in renal, hepatic, cardiac, bone marrow and other transplantations

○ The recipient is yet left with sufficient immune activity to fight bacterial infection

○ **Added advantages:**
  ▪ No toxic effects on bone marrow and reticuloendothelial system
  ▪ Humoral immunity remains intact.

○ Effective therapy employs blood level monitoring as it is concentrated in WBCs and RBCs, metabolized in liver by CYP3A4 and excreted in bile.

d. Linezolid in the treatment of community acquired pneumonia

(Ref: KD Tripathi, Essentials of Medical Pharmacology, 7th ed, 8th ed, pg. 758)

ANSWER

Linezolid in Community Acquired Pneumonia

○ Belongs to oxazolidinone group, beneficial to treat resistant Gram-positive coccal (both aerobic and anaerobic) and bacillary infections

○ **Mechanism of action:** Mostly bacteriostatic; cidal activity exhibited against few streptococci, pneumococci, and *B. fragilis;* acts by inhibition of bacterial protein synthesis

○ Used in complicated or uncomplicated skin and soft tissue infections

○ Employed in nosocomial or community pneumonias or bacteremias

○ Used in drug-resistant Gram-positive infections, etc.

○ **Side Effect Profile:**
  ▪ Nausea and loose motions
  ▪ Disturbances in taste and mild pain abdomen
  ▪ Headache
  ▪ Rash and pruritus
  ▪ Oral/vaginal candidiasis
  ▪ Blood related effects, like anemia and thrombocytopenia may occur on prolonged use, etc.

4. Describe the drug treatment of:

a. Paucibacillary leprosy

(Ref: KD Tripathi, Essentials of Medical Pharmacology, 7th ed, pg. 783, 8th ed, pg. 835-36)

ANSWER

Leprosy has been Categorized by WHO into

○ *Paucibacillary leprosy (PBL):* Patient has few bacilli and is noninfectious

○ *Multibacillary leprosy (MBL):* Patient has large bacillary load and is infectious

Drug Treatment

○ Dapsone was used conventionally

○ 6-month two drug therapy has now been used for more than 25 years with very promising results

○ Follow-up for the subsequent 1 to 2 years should be done

○ Therapy can be extended for 12 months or longer till disease inactivity is achieved

○ Under standard multidrug therapy (MDT), the PBL cases treated with dapsone + rifampin for duration of 6 months

PHARMACOLOGY

○ **Multidrug therapy**
  - It helps achieve control on dapsone resistant strains of *M. leprae* and also to decrease the duration of treatment
  - It also prevents emergence of dapsone resistance
  - Offers quick symptom relief
  - Number of relapse cases also decline
  - The WHO expert group recommended continuing the treatment of PBL for 6 months
  - Resistance to rifampin was not developed when MDT was employed
  - Almost all *M. leprae* isolated from relapse cases showed full sensitivity to rifampin.

b. Osteoporosis

ANSWER

Osteoporosis

○ A condition in which bones become fragile, accompanied by an increased susceptibility to fracture

Drug Treatment

○ **Bisphosphonates:**
  - Most efficacious antiresorptive drug therapy
  - BPNs cause hastening of osteoclasts apoptosis
  - Osteoclasts differentiation is inhibited and interference with cytoskeleton
  - 2nd and 3rd generation BPNs (alendronate, risedronate) proven efficacious in osteoporosis in postmenopausal women
  - Also effective in osteoporosis cases due to age, idiopathic and steroid-induced in both genders
  - Bone mineral density is conserved and reduce the risk of vertebral and hip fractures significantly

○ **Raloxifene:**
  - Leads to preventing bone loss in postmenopausal women
  - Forms second line therapy in postmenopausal women for preventing and treating osteoporosis
  - Can be alternatively used in vertebral fractures for secondary prevention and treatment
  - Not approved for primary prevention fractures due to osteoporotic bone loss

○ **Calcium:**
  - Calcium and vitamin D_3 plays adjuvant role to drugs employed
  - Enhances benefits of raloxifene in prevention and treatment of osteoporosis
  - No reported effects in fracture prevention in healthy controls.

PART-III

5. Discuss the therapeutic uses and adverse effects of:

a. Oral contraceptives

(Ref: KD Tripathi, Essentials of Medical Pharmacology, 7th ed, pg. 321, 8th ed, pg.346-48)

ANSWER

Oral Contraceptives

Combined estrogen-progestin pills and even progestin-only pills are instituted in contraception

Therapeutic Uses

○ Used for reversible suppression of fertility and hence control unwanted births
○ Also employed in certain hormonal disorders, and polycystic ovarian disorder for regularizing menstrual cycles
○ Instituted as emergency postcoital contraception in certain preparations
○ Infrequently used to treat acne

Adverse Effects

○ **Nonserious side effects:** Frequent but disappear gradually
  - Nausea and vomiting: resembling morning sickness of pregnancy
  - Mild headache
  - Breakthrough bleeding (or spotting)
  - Disruption in cycle or prolonged amenorrhoea
  - Breast discomfort
○ **Late side effects:**
  - Weight gain and acne
  - Increased unwanted body hair
  - Pigmentation of cheeks, nose and forehead (referred as chloasma)
  - Mood swings and abdominal distention occasionally seen
○ **Serious complications**
  - *Leg vein thrombosis and pulmonary embolism:* Excessive risk gets normal shortly after stopping the OC
  - *Coronary and cerebral thrombosis* leading to *myocardial infarction or stroke*
  - *Genital carcinoma:* Animal studies have shown an increased incidence of vaginal, cervical, and breast cancers
  - Minor increase in breast cancer incidence among current OC users

- *Gallstones:* Estrogens cause an increased biliary cholesterol excretion; increased incidence of gallstones slightly.

  b. **Insulin analogues**

(Ref: KD Tripathi, Essentials of Medical Pharmacology, 7th ed, pg. 264, 8th ed, pg. 287-88)

ANSWER

Insulin Analogs

- Preparations made using recombinant DNA technology, with modified pharmacokinetics on subcutaneous injection, but similar pharmacodynamic effects
- Include following: Insulin lispro, Insulin aspart, Insulin glulisine, Insulin detemir, Insulin glargine

Therapeutic Uses

- Better control on meal-time glycaemia and a lower incidence of late postprandial hypoglycaemia
- Better marked reduction in HbA$_{1c}$ diabetes mellitus subjects
- Must for type 1 diabetics
- Employed in type 2 diabetes if not controlled by oral hypoglycemics, underweight patients and tide over surgery and pregnancy conditions
- Used in diabetic ketoacidosis
- Hyperosmolar coma (nonketotic hyperglycemic) coma in elderly type 2 patients

Adverse Effects

- **Hypoglycaemia:**
  - Most frequent and potentially serious reaction
  - May result due to inadvertent injection of large dose, missing a meal after injection or by carrying out vigorous exercise
  - Symptoms include sweating, anxiety, palpitation, tremor, dizziness, headache, behavioural changes, visual disturbances, hunger, fatigue, fall in BP
- Local reactions in form of swelling, erythema and stinging at times at the injected site
- Lipodystrophy at site of injection
- Allergy due to contaminating proteins
- Edema in some patients.

---

6. **Write short notes on:**

   a. **Fibrinolytic agents**

(Ref: KD Tripathi, Essentials of Medical Pharmacology, 7th ed, pg. 625, 8th ed, pg. 673-76)

ANSWER

Fibrinolytic Agents

- Drugs employed to lyse thrombi/clot to recanalize occluded blood vessels (mainly coronary artery)
- Therapeutic effect rather than prophylactic
- Activates the natural fibrinolytic system
- Important ones include streptokinase, alteplase (rt-PA), urokinase, etc.
- **Uses:**
  - **For MI:** An accelerated regimen of alteplase
    - Alternative first line approach to emergency percutaneous coronary intervention (PCI) with stent placement
    - Achievement of recanalization of thrombosed coronary artery
  - **For pulmonary embolism:** Dose of 100 mg IV infused over 2 hours
  - **For ischaemic stroke:** Dose of 0.9 mg/kg by IV infusion over 60 min
  - **Deep vein thrombosis:** Leads to decrease in pain and swelling
    - Chief use is preservation of venous valves and may be a reduced risk of pulmonary embolism
- All cases with STEMI are indicated for reperfusion therapy
- No consistent clinical value in non-STEMI cases
- Careful patient identification is important.

   b. **Macrolide antibiotics**

ANSWER

Macrolide-type Antibiotic

Include erythromycin, azithromycin, clarithromycin, etc.

- **How they work**
  - Irreversible binding to a site on the 50S subunit of the bacterial ribosome, thus blocking the translocation steps of protein synthesis
- Higher efficacy, better gastric tolerance, and convenient
- **Therapeutic uses:** First choice drugs for
  - Legionnaires' pneumonia
  - Chlamydia trachomatis
  - Donovanosis caused by C. granulomatis
  - Gonococcal urethritis
  - Combating primarily respiratory diseases caused by Gram-positive pathogens and fastidious Gram-negative pathogens

○ **Adverse effect profile:**

Infections	• Candidiasis • Vaginal infection • Pneumonia • Fungal infection • Bacterial infection • Pharyngitis • Rhinitis • Oral candidiasis • Pseudomembranous colitis
Blood and lymphatic system disorders	• Leukopenia • Neutropenia • Eosinophilia • Thrombocytopenia • Haemolytic anemia
Immune system disorders	• Angioedema • Hypersensitivity
Metabolism and nutrition disorders	• Anorexia
Psychiatric disorders	• Nervousness • Insomnia
Nervous system disorders	• Headache • Dizziness • Somnolence • Dysgeusia • Paraesthesia

c.   Pentavalent Vaccine

ANSWER

Pentavalent Vaccine

○ Constituted toxoids of tetanus and diphtheria along with pertussis vaccine, hepatitis B vaccine and *Haemophilus influenzae* type b (Hib) vaccine

○ Employed as alternative to triple antigen for primary immunization of infants

○ Offers protection against two extra common infections, and decreases the total number of injections received by the infants for protection against these five common infections

○ Currently, Government of India is also introducing it in a phased manner in the universal immunization programme employed in infants and children

○ Pentavalent vaccine will replace DPT 1, 2, 3 and Hep 1, 2, 3 doses

Note: Infants already started on DPT vaccination will continue and complete the schedule of DPT vaccine.

Your Roll No. ....

Name of the Paper	:	**Pharmacology Paper-I**
Name of the Course	:	**MBBS-2015**
Semester	:	**Annual**

Time: 3 Hours   M.M.: 40

INSTRUCTIONS

1. Write your Roll No. on the top immediately on receipt of this question paper
2. All questions are to be attempted
3. Answers to Parts I, II and III should be written in separate answer sheets provided
4. Attempt parts of a question in sequence

PART-I

1. **Explain why?** [8]
   a. Differences in bioavailability are of much greater concern with drugs that show a steep dose response relationship
   b. Thiazides should be use cautiously in patients on lithium therapy
   c. Pentazocine should be avoided in patients with morphine dependence
   d. Oxybutynin may be prescribed to patients with urological problems

2. **Classify and enumerate drugs modulating the Renin Angiotensin system, Discuss the mechanism of action, uses, adverse effects and contraindications of Enalapril.** [6]

PART-II

3. **Discuss the therapeutic status of:** [8]
   a. Vancomycin in bacterial infection
   b. Desmopressin in diabetes insipidus
   c. Latanoprost in glaucoma
   d. Trihexyphenidyl in Parkinsonism

4. **Discuss the drug treatment of:** [6]
   a. Grand mal epilepsy
   b. Status asthmaticus

PART-III

5. **Discuss the therapeutic uses and adverse effects of:** [6]
   a. Lignocaine
   b. Furosemide

6. **Write short notes on:** [6]
   a. Teratogenicity
   b. Centrally acting muscle relaxants
   c. Therapeutic applications of plasma half life

PART-I

1. Explain why?

a. Differences in bioavailability are of much greater concern with drugs that show a steep dose response relationship.

(Ref: KD Tripathi, Essentials of Medical Pharmacology, 8th ed, pg. 63-66)

ANSWER

Bioavailability

Defined as the rate at which and extent to which the active concentration of the drug is available at the site of action.

Dose Response Curve (DRC)

In general, an increase in dose results in increase in intensity of response, and the curve is a rectangular hyperbola

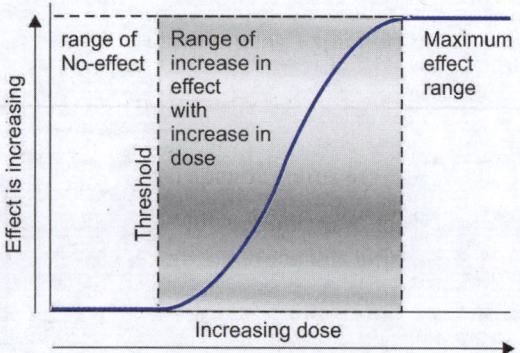

Fig. Dose-response curve

- ○ **DRC can be characterized by two parameters:**
  - Slope
  - Position
- ○ **Steep dose response:** Indicative of a drug that is rapidly and extensively absorbed and slowly eliminated.
- ○ Differences in bioavailability showing greater concern for such drugs—switching different brands for same drugs may lead to:
  - Therapeutic failure (decreased bioavailability)
  - Drug intoxication (increased bioavailability)
- ○ Examples: phenytoin, warfarin, etc.

b. Thiazides should be used cautiously in patients on lithium therapy.

ANSWER

Diuretics

- ○ Drugs that increase urine flow and induce urinary sodium loss.
- ○ Extensively used for therapy of hypertension, congestive heart failure, and edematous states.
- ○ Diuretics are typically classified as:
  - Thiazide diuretics (chlorothiazide, chlorthalidone, hydrochlorothiazide, indapamide, metolazone and polythiazide)
  - Loop diuretics (bumetanide, ethacrynic acid, furosemide, and torsemide)
  - Potassium-sparing agents (amiloride, eplerenone, spironolactone, and triamterene).
- ○ Mechanism of action for thiazides: Act on the early part of distal tubule and inhibit Na^+/Cl^- transport
- ○ Thiazides should be cautiously used in patients on lithium therapy since:
  - Thiazides (diuretic) cause enhanced reabsorption of lithium ions in proximal tubule
  - 24% reduction in the lithium clearance
  - Thus may cause lithium toxicity.

c. Pentazocine should be avoided in patients with morphine dependence.

ANSWER

Pentazocine

- ○ Pentazocine is a synthetic opioid with both agonist and antagonist activity against opiate receptors, thus categorized as mixed agonist-antagonist and partial agonist.
- ○ This drug is used in oral as well as parenteral forms as an analgesic for moderate-to-severe pain.
- ○ Morphine is the prototype opioid analgesic and a pure agonist (μ agonist as well). However, pentazocine works by agonizing κ-opioid receptors and antagonizing μ-opioid receptors.
- ○ Due to this opposite action on μ opioid receptors, any partial opioid agonist should not be administered in patients having pure opioid agonist as there is a risk of severe and abrupt withdrawal symptoms.

d. Oxybutynin may be prescribed to patients with urological problems.

ANSWER

Oxybutynin

○ Oxybutynin is a Tertiary Amine

○ **Mechanism of action and its therapeutic effect:**

  ▪ This drug is relatively vasicoselective anticholinergics and antimuscarinic.

  ▪ Oxybutynin and other antimuscarinic agents block muscarinic receptors and thus inhibit abnormal bladder contractions

  ▪ There is direct relaxant action on smooth muscles

  ▪ Oxybutynin may be thus prescribed in urological problems—urinary frequency, detrusor instability, urge incontinence.

---

2. **Classify and enumerate drugs modulating the Renin-Angiotensin system. Discuss the mechanism of action, uses, adverse effects and contraindications of Enalapril.**

(Ref: KD Tripathi, Essentials of Medical Pharmacology, 8th ed, pg. 530, 532)

ANSWER

Drugs Modulating Renin-angiotensin System ....

○ Sympathetic blockers

  ▪ Reduce release of renin

  ▪ Beta-blockers, central sympatholytics, adrenergic neuron blockers

○ Direct renin inhibitors

  ▪ Block release of renin

○ Angiotensin converting enzyme (ACE) inhibitors

  ▪ Inhibit formation of Ang II

○ Angiotensin receptor blockers

  ▪ Antagonize Ang II actions on the target cells

○ Aldosterone antagonists

  ▪ Block mineralocorticoid receptors

Enalapril (ACE inhibitor; a Prodrug)

Mechanism of Action

○ Overproduction of Ang I due to feedback increase in renin release

○ Conversion of Ang I to Ang II blocked

○ Diversion of Ang I to produce more Ang (1-7), having vasodilator property

○ Effect of vasodilation—BP lowering action

○ Decrease in total peripheral resistance—arterioles dilate and compliance of larger arteries increased

○ Fall in both systolic and diastolic BP.

Uses

○ **Hypertension:** ACE inhibitors now are the first line drugs used in hypertension. They have several benefits, e.g.

  ▪ No rebound hypertension on withdrawal

  ▪ No harmful effects on the lipid profile

  ▪ No postural hypotension and CNS effects

  ▪ Safe option for asthmatics, diabetics, etc.

○ **Congestive heart failure:** Enalapril reduces afterload as well as preload in CHF patients, thus symptomatic relief is attained in all grades of CHF.

○ **Myocardial infarction:** Enalapril should be administered within 24 hour of an attack and continued till 6 weeks (to many years).

○ **Diabetic nephropathy:** End-stage renal disease in type 1 or type 2 diabetics is prevented or delayed by this drug.

○ **Prophylaxis of subjects having high cardiovascular risk:** There is protective effect on myocardium as well as on vasculature.

○ **Scleroderma crisis:** Intense improvement has been noticed by administering enalapril (or other ACE inhibitors).

Adverse Effects

○ Hypotension

○ **Hyperkalemia:** More likely in cases of impaired renal function or patients having potassium sparing diuretics, beta blockers, or even NSAIDs

○ Urticaria and rashes

○ **Persistent and brassy cough:** This may occur in a subset of patients within 18 weeks

○ Reversible loss or alteration of taste (dysgeusia)

○ **Angioedema:** Swelling of mouth, nose, lips, pharynx may develop

○ Headache and dizziness

○ Nausea, vomiting, and upset bowel

○ **Acute renal failure (ARF):** ACE inhibitors can precipitate ARF in patients of bilateral renal artery stenosis

○ Hypoplasia of organs and growth retardation in foetus, if given in later half of pregnancy.

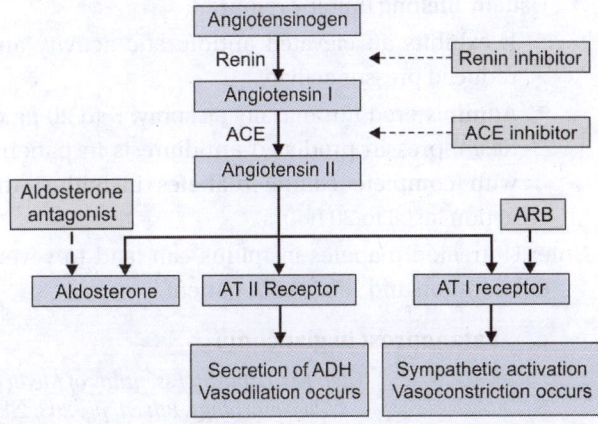

Contraindications

- **Pregnancy:** Enalapril is pregnancy category D. Some evidence suggests it will cause injury and death to a developing fetus
- Angioneurotic edema following other ACE inhibitors
- Bilateral renal artery stenosis: ARF may be precipitated
- Renal impairment
- Hyperkalemia.

PART-II

3. **Discuss the therapeutic status of:**

   a. **Propofol as an anesthetic agent**

   (Ref: KD Tripathi, Essentials of Medical Pharmacology, 8th ed, pg. 409-10)

ANSWER

Propofol

- Propofol is a fast acting intravenous anesthetic
- Used both for induction as well as maintenance
- Occurrence of unconsciousness in 15–45 sec and remains for 5–10 minutes
- Particularly suited for outpatient surgery
- Preferred in asthmatics
- Very low side effect profile:
  - Lacks airway irritancy
  - Less postoperative nausea and vomiting
  - No change or decrease in heart rate.

   b. **Desmopressin in diabetes insipidus**

   (Ref: KD Tripathi, Essentials of Medical Pharmacology, 8th ed, pg. 643-44)

ANSWER

- Selective V2 receptor agonist
- Indicated for neurogenic diabetes insipidus (DI)
- Not effective in nephrogenic DI
- Usually lifelong therapy required
  - It exhibits an elevated antidiuretic activity and reduced pressor activity
  - Administered intranasally as spray, 5 to 20 μg of desmopressin produced antidiuresis in patients with complete central diabetes insipidus; the action last 8 to 20 hours

Note: Untreated diabetes insipidus can lead to severe dehydration and seizures in patients.

   c. **Latanoprost in glaucoma**

   (Ref: KD Tripathi, Essentials of Medical Pharmacology, 8th ed, pg. 203, 206)

ANSWER

- PGF2α derivative
- Reduces intraocular tension 25–35%
- First choice drug for open angle glaucoma due to following reasons
  - Well sustained effect
  - Once daily application
  - No systemic side effects
- Can be used in normal pressure glaucoma also
- **Side effect profile:**
  - Pain and ocular irritation (common)
  - Blurring of vision, eyelashes darken and thicken, etc. (uncommon).

   d. **Trihexyphenidyl in Parkinsonism**

ANSWER

- Central anticholinergic action
- Works in patients of parkinsonism by reduction of the unbalanced cholinergic activity in the striatum
- Provide symptomatic relief, do not modify pathology of parkinsonism
- More beneficial in tremor than rigidity
- Least effect on hypokinesia
- May be used alone in mild cases or when levodopa is contraindicated
- Side effect profile:
  - Memory impairment
  - Organic confusional states
  - Blurring of vision
  - Often not tolerated by elderly.

4. **Discuss the drug treatment of:**

   a. **Grand mal epilepsy**

ANSWER

- **Alternative names:** Generalized tonic-clonic seizures (GTCS), major epilepsy, grand mal
- This is the commonest type
- An attack lasts 1–2 min
- **Drug treatment**
  - **First line:** Carbamazepine, Phenytoin
  - **Second line:** Valproate, phenobarbitone
  - **Add-on drugs:** Lamotrigine, gabapentin, topiramate, levetiracetam
- Initiate with a single drug, low dose is preferred
- Dose is increased gradually to maximum tolerated dose
- Substitute with another drug, if desired effect not achieved

○ If alternative drugs are to be instituted, combine drugs with different mechanisms of action

Tonic–Clonic Seizures

- **First-Line Agents**
  - Valproic acid
  - Lamotrigine
  - Topiramate
- **Alternative Agents**
  - Zonisamidet
  - Phenytoin
  - Carbamazepine
  - Oxcarbazepine
  - Phenobarbital
  - Primidone
  - Felbamte

b.   Status asthmaticus

ANSWER

Status Asthmaticus

○ Severe acute exacerbation of asthma

○ **Standard treatment in the emergency room:**
  - Oxygen by mask
  - Measurement of peak expiratory flow
  - Beta agonists (inhalation) to relax and open airways
  - Steroids such as prednisone (oral or intravenous)
  - Anticholinergic drugs (inhalation)

○ **Other medicines that can be administered in a patient with acute episode:**
  - Beta agonists, e.g., terbutaline (injection under skin)
  - Leukotriene modifiers, e.g., zafirlukast (oral)
  - Mg sulfate (intravenous)

○ Intubation or ventilation if needed.

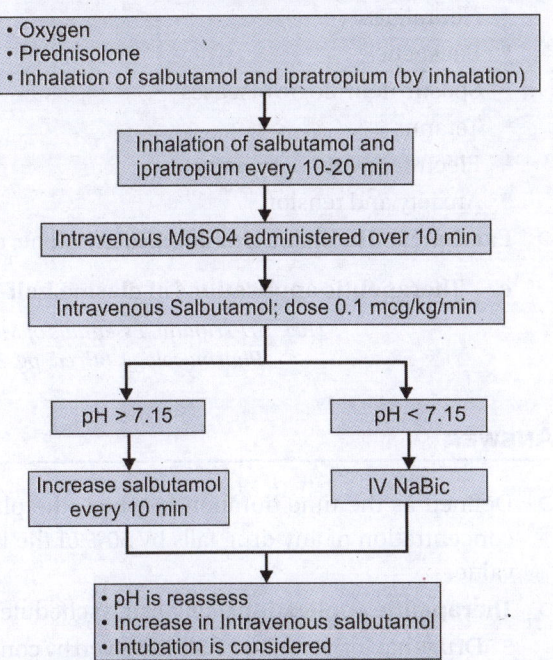

Fig. Treatment of status asthamaticus

PART-III

5. **Discuss the therapeutic uses and adverse effects of:**

   a.   **Lignocaine**

   (Ref: KD Tripathi, Essentials of Medical Pharmacology, 8th ed, pg. 392)

ANSWER

○ Most widely used local anesthetic

○ Categorized as intermediate potency and duration

○ **Therapeutic uses:**

  - **Surface application**
    ◆ This is produced by topical application to skin and mucous membranes
    ◆ It is widely used in the eye surgery and tonometry, intubation in pharynx and larynx, catheterization in urethra, stomatitis or painful ulcers in nose/ear.

  - **Nerve infiltration**
    ◆ This blocks sensory nerve endings in the area of operation as LA is infiltrated under the skin
    ◆ This is employed in minor procedures, e.g., incisions, excisions, herniorrhaphy, hydrocele, etc.

  - **Nerve block**
    ◆ The LA is injected around the nerve trunk or plexuses
    ◆ They are frequently used as in infraorbital, inferior alveolar, palatine nerve blocks in tooth extractions, ulnar, sciatic, femoral blocks.

  - **Regional block anesthesia**
    ◆ **Epidural:** Epidural injection can be made in thoracic, lumbar, or sacral regions acc. to desired area of anesthesia
    ◆ **Spinal:** The LA is injected in the subarachnoid space, below the lower end of spinal cord. It is employed in obstetric procedures, fracture setting, prostatectomy, etc.

○ **Adverse effects:**

  - Drowsiness
  - Mental clouding and dysphoria
  - Altered taste and tinnitus
  - Muscle twitching
  - Convulsions
  - Cardiac arrhythmias
  - Fall in BP, coma, and respiratory arrest.

   b.   **Furosemide**

   (Ref: KD Tripathi, Essentials of Medical Pharmacology, 8th ed, pg. 626-28)

ANSWER

Furosemide

○ Furosemide is a high ceiling diuretic

○ **Therapeutic uses:**

■ **Edema:** They can be used in cardiac, hepatic, or renal edema. They can be used in nephrotic and other forms of resistant edema.

■ **Acute pulmonary and cerebral edema:** Vasodilator action preceded the saluretic action, thus prompt relief is perceived in acute pulmonary edema. Osmotic diuretics are preferred in cerebral edema but furosemide can be given by intramuscular route.

■ Hypertension only when it is complicated by:

♦ Chronic renal failure

♦ Coexisting refractory congestive heart failure (CHF)

♦ Resistant to combination regimens containing a thiazide

♦ Marked fluid retention attributed to potent vasodilators

■ Symptomatic congestive heart failure

■ Forced diuresis: It can be used as an alternative to mannitol.

Adverse Effects

○ **Hypokalemia:** Manifestations are weakness, fatigue, muscle cramps. This is the most noteworthy problem.

○ **Dyslipidemia:** This results when furosemide is used as antihypertensive.

○ **Increased incidence of gout:** Long-term use may cause rise in blood urate and finally clinical gout.

○ **CNS and GIT effects:** Dizziness, paraesthesias, impotence in males, nausea, vomiting, diarrhea may occur.

○ **Hearing loss:** It can occur very rarely in few patients.

○ **Sudden cardiac death:** Episodes of torsades de pointes and ischemic ventricular fibrillation, etc.

6. Write short notes on:

a. Teratogenicity

(Ref: KD Tripathi, Essentials of Medical Pharmacology, 8th ed, pg. 99-101)

ANSWER

○ Defined as the capacity of a drug which grounds for foetal abnormalities when administered during pregnancy.

○ At following 3 stages, foetus can be affected by drugs:

■ Fertilization and implantation (conception–17 days)

■ Organogenesis (18–55 days)

■ Growth and development (≥ 56 days).

Proven Human Teratogens:	
Drug	**Abnormality**
Thalidomide	Phocomelia, multiple defects
Anti-neoplastic drugs	Multiple defects, foetal death
Androgens	Virilization, esophageal, cardiac defects
Progestins	Virilization of female foetus
Stilboestrol	Vaginal carcinoma
Tetracyclines	Discoloured teeth, bone defects
Warfarin	Nose, Eye, Hand defects, Growth retardation
Phenytoin	Cleft lip/palate, microcephaly, hypoplastic phalanges

b. Centrally acting muscle relaxants

ANSWER

○ Decrease muscle tone, no reduction in voluntary power

○ Orally given; parenteral at few times

○ **Indications:**

■ Overstretching of muscles

■ Ligament and tendon tearing

■ Rheumatic disorders, bursitis, etc.

■ Dislocation

■ Torticollis

■ Neuralgias

■ Backache

■ Spastic neurologic diseases

■ Tetanus

■ Electroconvulsive therapy

■ Anxiety and tension

○ **Examples:** Diazepam, tizanidine, dantrolene, etc.

c. Therapeutic applications of plasma half-life

(Ref: KD Tripathi, Essentials of Medical Pharmacology, 8th ed, pg. 39-40)

ANSWER

○ Defined as the time duration in which the plasma concentration of any drug falls by 50% of the initial value.

○ **Therapeutic applications:** on dosing schedules

■ Drugs having very short half-life given by constant intravenous infusion, e.g., dopamine

- Drugs having short half-life (30 min–2 hours) given at 6–8 hourly interval, e.g., cephalexin
- Drugs having medium half-life given at 12-hour interval

- Drugs having longer half-life, loading dose is followed by a maintenance dose, e.g., digoxin
○ Dose adjustments and change in intervals needed in renal/liver diseases
  - Due to alteration in half-life

Your Roll No. ....

Name of the Paper : **Pharmacology Paper-II**

Name of the Course : **MBBS-2015**

Semester : **Annual**

Time: 3 Hours   M.M.: 40

INSTRUCTIONS

1. Write your Roll No. on the top immediately on receipt of this question paper
2. All questions are to be attempted
3. Answers to Parts I, II and III should be written in separate answer sheets provided
4. Attempt parts of a question in sequence

PART-I

1. **Explain why?**   [8]
   a. Artemisinin derivatives are preferably prescribed in combination for treatment of malaria
   b. Low dose aspirin may be given in myocardial infarction (MI) and also post MI
   c. Live vaccines are contraindicated in immune compromised patients
   d. Dosing instructions in relation to food intake are extremely important while prescribing alendronate

2. **Classify and enumerate anti diabetic drugs. Discuss the mechanism of action, therapeutic uses, adverse effects and contraindications of metformin.**   [6]

PART-II

3. **Discuss the therapeutic status of:**   [8]
   a. Leflunomide in rheumatoid arthritis
   b. Fondaparinux in deep vein thrombosis
   c. Fluoroquinolones in tuberculosis
   d. Tamoxifen in breast cancer

4. **Discuss the drug treatment of**   [6]
   a. Typhoid fever
   b. Peptic ulcer

PART-III

5. **Discuss the therapeutic uses and adverse effects of:**   [6]
   a. Doxycycline
   b. Prednisolone

6. **Write short notes on:**   [6]
   a. Beta lactamase inhibitors
   b. Vitamin A preparations
   c. Penicillamine

PART-I

1. Explain why?

a. Artemisinin derivatives are preferably prescribed in combination for treatment of malaria

ANSWER

Artemisinin in Malaria

○ Active against *P. falciparum* resistant to all other antimalarial agents; also includes sensitive strains and other malarial species

○ **Mechanism of action:** In the erythrocytic schizogony cycle, acting on ring forms to early schizonts; exerts schizonticidal action

○ These drugs are also fatal to early stage malarial gametes but not mature ones; decreasing the population of gametes

○ Thus, disease transmission reduced but not totally interrupted

○ Primary liver forms or vivax hypnozoites are not killed

○ Their short acting action mandates monotherapy to be extended even after parasites disappear to prevent recrudescence

○ Can be totally prevented by combining 3 day artemisinin with a long-acting antimalarial drug

○ Examples include artesunate and artemether, etc.

b. Low dose aspirin may be given in myocardial infarction (MI) and also post MI

ANSWER

Aspirin

General use is to treat mild to moderate pain and reduce fever or inflammation

Rationale to Use in Myocardial Infarction (MI) as well as post-MI

○ Aspirin causes inhibition of platelet aggregation, thus lowering incidence of reinfarction

○ It also cause inhibition of thromboxane A2 synthesis in platelets at low doses

○ At a dose of 60–100 mg/day, incidence of myocardial infarction is reduced; thus now usually prescribed to postinfarct patients

○ At a dose of 100–150 mg/day for 12 weeks, reduces chances of "new onset" or "sudden worsening" angina to develop infarction

○ Not only reduces risk of transient ischemic attacks but also stroke incidence is reduced

○ Aspirin in low doses is adequate and selective in the long-term inhibition of TX-related platelet function in cases of post myocardial infarction.

c. Live vaccines are contraindicated in immune compromised patients

ANSWER

○ Inactive vaccines can be administered in accordance with the vaccination program to the immunocompromised patients, even though same levels of protective antibodies cannot be achieved in these cases when compared to healthy individuals

○ However, live vaccines (viral and bacterial) should not be administered during periods of immunosuppression

○ In conditions where drugs or diseases have strongly suppressed the immune system, the live vaccines would provide grounds for systemic infections to develop against vaccine strains

○ Therefore, live viral vaccines [for examples, polio, MMR (measles, mumps, rubella), varicella] and live bacterial vaccines (BCG) are contraindicated unless the patient is in the stage of remission

○ **Note:** Some live vaccines can only be administered in specific immune system disorders or when the benefit outweighs the risk.

d. Dosing instructions in relation to food intake are extremely important while prescribing alendronate

ANSWER

Alendronate

○ A potent 2nd generation amino-bisphosphonates, effective orally

○ Mainly used for prevention and treatment of osteoporosis both in males and females and also for Paget's disease

Rationale to Instruct Patient Adequately before Starting Therapy

○ Patient should be instructed to take the dose on empty stomach in the morning with a full glass of water

PHARMACOLOGY

○ Instruction should also be given to not lie down or take food for at least 30 minutes after the dose

○ These are important to prevent drug coming in contact with esophageal mucosa which can cause esophagitis

○ Also, calcium, iron, antacids, tea, coffee, even mineral water, fruit juice, interfere with absorption of alendronate

Note: NSAIDs cause accentuation of gastric irritation caused by alendronate.

2. Classify and enumerate anti diabetic drugs. Discuss the mechanism of action, therapeutic uses, adverse effects and contraindications of metformin

ANSWER

Oral Hypoglycemic Drugs (OHAs)

Drugs employed to lower blood glucose levels in blood when diet and exercise are not sufficient to maintain the recommended levels.

Pharmacology of Major OHAs

Drugs to treat type 2 diabetes	
Drugs which enhance action of insulin in peripheral tissues	Drugs which enhance endogenous secretion of insulin
• Thiazolidinediones • Metformin	• Sulfonylureas • Repaglinide, Netaglinide • GLP-1Analogues • DPP-IV inhibitors
Drugs that suppress endogenous production of glucose	Drugs which delay the carbohydrate absorption from GI Tract
• Metformin • Thiazolidinediones	• Alpha glucosidase inhibitors

OHA class	Pharmacological effects	Mechanism of action	Adverse effects
Sulfonylureas	• These drugs cause blood glucose lowering in normal subjects and in type 2 DM, but not in type 1 DM	• They exert their hypoglycemic effects by stimulating insulin secretion from the pancreatic β-cell • There is closure of ATP-sensitive K-channels in the β-cell plasma membrane • Thus initiate a chain of events resulting into insulin release	• Hypoglycemia • Nausea • Vomiting • Flatulence • Diarrhea or constipation • Mild headache and paresthesias • Hypersensitivity symptoms like rashes, purpura, transient leukopenia
Meglitinide analogues	• These are indicated only in those type 2 DM patients who suffer marked postprandial hyperglycemia, or supplementing metformin/long-acting insulin • These drugs are administered before each major meal to control postprandial glucose excursion	• Binding to sulfonylurea receptor leads to closure of ATP dependent K+ channels • Depolarization occurs → insulin release	• Mild headache • Dyspepsia • Arthralgia • Weight gain
GLP-1 receptor agonists	• GLP-1 based therapy is the most effective measure for preserving β cell function in type 2 diabetics	• Induces insulin release from pancreatic β cell • Inhibits release of glucagon • Suppresses appetite by activating specific GLP-1 receptors expressed on β and α cells, central and peripheral neurons, gastrointestinal mucosa, etc.	• Nausea and diarrhea infrequently • Weight loss • Hypoglycemia is rare with monotherapy, but can occur when combined with sulfonylureas/metformin.
DPP-4 inhibitors	• Mostly employed as adjuvant drugs in type 2 DM not well-controlled by metformin/insulin/sulfonylureas/pioglitazone	• Competitive and selective DPP-4 inhibitor • Boosts postprandial insulin release • Decreases glucagon secretion and lowers meal-time as well as fasting blood glucose in type 2 DM	• Nausea • Loose stools • Headache • Rashes • Allergic reactions and edema • Nasopharyngitis and cough

Contd...

OHA class	Pharmacological effects	Mechanism of action	Adverse effects
Biguanides	• Metformin is the first choice drug for all type 2 diabetics • Not effective in pancreatectomized animals and in type 1 DM	• Suppresses gluconeogenesis in liver and • Glucose output • Enhances insulin-mediated glucose uptake in peripheral tissues • Glycogen storage in skeletal muscle • Decreased lipogenesis in adipose tissue and enhanced fatty acid oxidation	• Frequent, but generally not serious • Abdominal pain • Anorexia • Bloating • Nausea • Metallic taste • Mild diarrhea and tiredness • Hypoglycemia in overdose. • Vit B12 deficiency • Lactic acidosis (not as pronounced as with phenformin which was banned in 2003)
Alpha-glucosidase inhibitors	• They may be used as an adjuvant to diet (with or without metformin/SU) in obese diabetics • Doses are taken at the start of each major meal.	• Reversibly inhibit α-glucosidases, which is the final enzyme for the digestion of carbohydrates in small intestine • It slows down and decreases digestion and absorption of polysaccharides • Postmeal glycemia declines without significant rise in insulin levels	• Flatulence, • Abdominal discomfort • Loose stool
Thiazolidinediones	• They are indicated in type 2 diabetics, but not in type 1 diabetics • Primarily used as supplement to SUs/metformin and in insulin resistance cases	• Act as selective agonists for the nuclear peroxisome proliferator-activated receptor γ which is expressed mostly in fat cells, but also in muscle and some other cells • Augments transcription of several insulin responsive genes • Entry of glucose into muscle and fat is improved. • Suppression of hepatic gluconeogenesis	• Greater fluid retention • Weight gain • Precipitation of CHF if using glitazones with insulin • Pioglitazone should not be used during pregnancy

Therapeutic Uses of Metformin

○ **Type 2 diabetes:** Employed in first choice treatment of type 2 diabetes cases

○ **Complications of type 2 diabetes:** Useful in preventing complications related to cardiovascular, ophthalmic, and renal complications in patients that are long-term cases of type 2 diabetes

○ **PCOS:** Also employed in treatment of polycystic ovarian syndrome

○ **Anti-cancer drug:** Metformin has demonstrated ability to slow tumor cells growth in vitro. This effect is also observed when metformin is used in combination with other anticancer treatments in breast cancer cells.

Contraindications of Metformin

○ If serum concentration of creatinine higher than 150 micromols/L (cutoff point for renal failure)

○ Periods when suspecting tissue hypoxia (MI, sepsis cases)

○ Use of intravenous contrast dye medium (3 days after iodine has been given)

○ Cases of alcohol abuse sufficient to cause acute hepatic toxicity

○ History of lactic acidosis.

PART-II

3. **Discuss the therapeutic status of:**

a. **Leflunomide in rheumatoid arthritis**

(Ref: KD Tripathi, Essentials of Medical Pharmacology, 8th ed, pg. 229)

ANSWER

Leflunomide in Rheumatoid Arthritis

○ An immunomodulator that impedes proliferation of stimulated lymphocytes in cases with active rheumatoid arthritis

○ It causes suppression of arthritic symptoms and retarding radiological progression of disease

○ Onset of benefit is fast and 4 weeks

○ An alternative to methotrexate or can be added to it, however, combined drug is more hepatotoxic

○ Combining it with sulfasalazine improves benefit

Mechanism of Action

○ Converted to active metabolite in the body that inhibits *dihydroorotate dehydrogenase* and pyrimidine synthesis in actively dividing cells

○ Depression of antibody production by B-cells

Adverse Effect Profile

○ Diarrhea and nausea

○ Headache

○ Rashes

○ Loss of hair

○ Thrombocytopenia and leukopenia

○ Increased risks of chest infection.

b.   Fondaparinux in deep vein thrombosis

(Ref: KD Tripathi, Essentials of Medical Pharmacology, 8th ed, pg. 672)

ANSWER

Fondaparinux in Deep Vein Thrombosis

○ An indirect thrombin inhibitor

○ Effective in the prevention of asymptomatic and symptomatic venous thromboembolic events in older acute medical patients

○ Less likely to result in thrombocytopenia as compared to even LMW heparins

○ Minimal risk of osteoporosis after continued use

Mechanism of Action

○ A specific sequence which binds with high affinity to AT III to selectively deactivate factor Xa without binding thrombin (factor IIa)

○ **Dose:** 5 mg (body weight <50 kg), 7.5 mg (50–100 kg), or 10 mg (>100 kg) subcutaneous once daily.

c.   Fluoroquinolones in tuberculosis

(Ref: KD Tripathi, Essentials of Medical Pharmacology, 8th ed, pg. 709)

ANSWER

Fluoroquinolones in Tuberculosis

○ These are quinolone antimicrobials having one or more fluorine substitutions

○ Employed in treating cases of tuberculosis primarily including resistance or intolerance to first-line antitubercular therapy

○ Successfully used in curing multidrug-resistant tuberculosis

○ Clinical trials have demonstrated that if used as first-line agents, even duration of therapy may be reduced to cure drug-sensitive TB

Mechanism of Action

○ **In Gram-negative bacteria:** Inhibition of the enzyme *bacterial DNA gyrase* (this enzyme is primarily active in gram negative bacteria

○ Binding to A subunit of this enzyme with high affinity

○ **In Gram-positive bacteria:** Inhibition of *topoisomerase IV*

○ Mammalian cells contain topoisomerase II instead of topoisomerase IV and DNA gyrase, hence confer low toxicity to host cells

d.   Tamoxifen in breast cancer

ANSWER

Tamoxifen

○ Selective estrogen receptor modulators

○ Acts in a tissue selective manner and exert estrogenic as well as antiestrogenic activities

Pharmacological Profile in Breast Cancer

○ Acts as potent estrogen antagonist in breast carcinoma cells, blood vessels and at some peripheral sites

○ Inhibition of human breast cancer cells and hot flushes

○ In early cases tamoxifen is given as postmastectomy adjuvant therapy

○ In advanced cases, instituted as constituent of palliative treatment

○ Higher response rates in ER-positive breast cancer cases

○ Approved for primary prophylaxis of breast cancer in high-risk women.

○ Single drug approved for primary as well as metastatic breast carcinoma in premenopausal patients

○ Effective in surgically treated cancer of male breast

Other Advantages

○ Reduction in total and LDL (bad) cholesterol

○ Stimulation of endometrial proliferation in postmenopausal women

○ Improvement in bone density in postmenopausal women.

4. **Discuss the drug treatment of:**

a. **Typhoid fever**

(Ref: KD Tripathi, Essentials of Medical Pharmacology, 7th ed, pg. 711, 8th ed, pg. 759-62)

ANSWER

Typhoid Fever

A bacterial infection caused by *S. typhi*, illness characterized by prolonged fever, headache, nausea, loss of appetite, and constipation, or sometimes diarrhea

Drug Treatment

○ **Ceftriaxone:** Most reliable and fast-acting bactericidal drug for enteric fever
  ▪ Active against practically all S. typhi isolates, including multidrug resistant ones
  ▪ **Dose**: Intravenous (4 g daily for 2 days followed by 2 g/day till 2 days after fever subsides; in children 75 mg/kg/day); costly therapy
  ▪ Usually 7 to 10 days treatment is needed
  ▪ Relapses and carrier stages are also prevented

○ **Fluoroquinolones:** Ciprofloxacin forms one of the first choice drugs in typhoid fever
  ▪ Number of nonresponsive resistant cases are reported
  ▪ Ceftriaxone (or cefotaxime/cefoperazone) are more commonly used
  ▪ **Dose:** Ciprofloxacin 750 mg twice daily for 10 days
  ▪ Quick defervescence; fever subsides in 4–5 days
  ▪ Less incidence of complications and relapse

○ **Chloramphenicol:**
  ▪ Infrequently used, only in cases of local strain sensitive to it and clinical experience supporting use
  ▪ **Dose:** Oral; 0.5 g 6 hourly until fever subsides, then 0.25 g 6 hourly for other 5 to 7 days

○ **Azithromycin:**
  ▪ Forms second-line alternative choice in MDR resistant typhoid cases
  ▪ **Dose:** 500 mg once daily for 7 days

○ **Cotrimoxazole:**
  ▪ Rarely used now
  ▪ In effect in cases of typhoid till plasmid mediated MDR spread among S. typhi

○ **Ampicillin/amoxicillin:**
  ▪ Cannot be taken as reliable therapy for typhoid since response rate is less and also late defervescence in responsive cases.

b. **Peptic ulcer**

ANSWER

Peptic Ulcer with *H. Pylori*

○ Gets attached to the surface epithelium
○ Maintains a neutral microenvironment around bacteria so as to protect against highly acidic gastric secretions
○ Around 90% cases of gastric and duodenal ulcers demonstrated positive test for *H. pylori*

Drug Treatment

○ *H. pylori* eradication therapy should be employed in all cases tested positive
○ H2 blockers and proton pump inhibitors (PPIs) form mainstay of treatment
○ Antibiotic therapy is mandatory, though no single antibiotic can be preferred as the organism develops resistance very rapidly
○ Antimicrobials used: Amoxicillin, Clarithromycin, tetracycline, and metronidazole/tinidazole
○ Combination regimens should include bismuth to be employed in case of double resistance to metronidazole and clarithromycin
○ H2 blockers/PPIs enhance efficacy antimicrobials active against *H. pylori* infections due to acid suppression
○ 1-week regimen may be sufficient; in some cases, high eradication rates with 2-week regimen
○ **Approved regimen:**
  ▪ Lansoprazole 30 mg + Amoxicillin 1000 mg + clarithromycin 500 mg, BD for 2 weeks
  ▪ Omeprazole 40 mg OD + Metronidazole 400 mg TDS + Amoxicillin 500 mg TDS
  ▪ For ulcers (> 10 mm in diameter) or presence of bleeding/perforation: Continue till complete healing
  ▪ In case of eradication failure: Quadruple therapy with CBS 120 mg QID + tetracycline 500 mg QID + metronidazole 400 mg TDS + omeprazole 20 mg BD.

PART-III

5. **Discuss the therapeutic uses and adverse effects of:**

a. **Doxycycline**

(Ref: KD Tripathi, Essentials of Medical Pharmacology, 7th ed, pg. 737, 8th ed, pg. 784, 786)

ANSWER

Therapeutic Uses of Doxycycline

- Often used when the nature and sensitivity of the infecting organism cannot be rationally estimated as empirical therapy
- Preferred in venereal diseases, for examples, 7-day treatment with doxycycline is effective in chlamydial nonspecific urethritis/endocervicitis; resolution of lymphogranuloma venereum in 2 to 3 weeks
- 3-week therapy in granuloma inguinale
- Duration of illness is reduced in atypical pneumonia
- Adjuvant value in cholera in limiting the duration of diarrhea
- Highly effective in brucellosis
- Highly efficacious in both bubonic and pneumonic plague

Adverse Effects

- Epigastric pain
- Nausea
- Vomiting and diarrhea on oral use
- Odynophagia and esophageal ulceration from capsules
- Thrombophlebitis of the injected vein
- **Phototoxicity:** A sunburn-like or other severe skin reaction on exposed parts
- **Teeth and bones:** Given between 3 months and 6 years of age disturb the crown of permanent anterior dentition
- **Superinfection:** Frequently responsible for superinfections since they cause more distinct suppression of the resident flora.

  b. Prednisolone

  (Ref: KD Tripathi, Essentials of Medical Pharmacology, 7th ed, pg. 288, 8th ed, pg. 313)

ANSWER

Therapeutic Uses

- Used to treat certain types of allergies, inflammatory conditions, and autoimmune disorders
- Some of conditions include rheumatoid arthritis, dermatitis, asthma, adrenocortical insufficiency, inflammation in the eyes, multiple sclerosis, etc.
- It can be used as oral dose, intravenously, as skin preparations, and eye drops
- Used for long-term treatment of asthma and to control severe exacerbations of asthmatic attack with inhaled steroids

Adverse Effects

Blood and lymphatic system disorders	Leukocytosis
Immune system disorders	Increased susceptibility and severity of infections with suppression of clinical symptoms and signs, opportunistic infections, recurrence of dormant tuberculosis
Endocrine disorders	Cushingoid facies, growth suppression in infancy, hirsutism, impaired carbohydrate tolerance with increased requirement for antidiabetic therapy, suppression of the hypothalamo-pituitary adrenal axis, and weight gain
Metabolism and nutrition disorders	Hypokalaemic alkalosis, potassium loss, sodium and water retention.
Psychiatric disorders	Marked euphoria leading to dependence; aggravation of epilepsy, behavioural disturbances, irritability, nervousness, anxiety, sleep disturbances, and cognitive dysfunction
Nervous system disorders	Intracranial pressure with papilloedema in children (pseudotumour cerebri) usually after treatment withdrawal
Eye disorders	Corneal or scleral thinning, scleral perforation, papilledema
Cardiac disorders	Risk of congestive heart failure in susceptible cases
Vascular disorders	Hypertension, thromboembolism
Gastrointestinal disorders	Abdominal distension, dyspepsia, nausea, increased appetite, oesophageal candidiasis, oesophageal ulceration, peptic ulceration with perforation and hemorrhage
Skin and subcutaneous tissue disorders	Acne, bruising, impaired healing, purple striae
Musculoskeletal and connective tissue disorders	Muscle weakness, wasting and loss of muscle mass.
Renal and urinary disorders	Nocturia, scleroderma renal crisis (frequency unknown).
General disorders and administration site conditions	Hypersensitivity including anaphylaxis, malaise.

6. **Write short notes on:**

   a. **Beta lactamase inhibitors**

   (Ref: KD Tripathi, Essentials of Medical Pharmacology, 7th ed, pg. 724, 8th ed, pg. 774-75)

ANSWER

β-lactamase Inhibitors

Inhibitors of this enzyme β-lactamase include clavulanic acid, sulbactam and tazobactam

- **Clavulanic acid:** It has a β-lactam ring, but no antibacterial action of its own
  - Inhibition of a wide variety (class II to class V) of β-lactamases produced by gram-positive as well as gram-negative bacteria
  - Known as "suicide" inhibitor, gets inactivated after binding to the enzyme
  - Addition of clavulanic acid re-established the action of amoxicillin against β-lactamase producing resistant *S. aureus, H. influenzae, N. gonorrhoeae, E. coli, Proteus,* etc.
  - Skin and soft tissue infections, intraabdominal and gynaecological sepsis
- **Sulbactam:** Semisynthetic β-lactamase inhibitor
  - Preferably given parenterally
  - Combined with ampicillin for use against β-lactamase producing resistant strains
  - Indicated in PPNG gonorrhea
  - Mixed aerobic-anaerobic infections, intraabdominal, gynecological, surgical and skin/soft tissue infections, especially those acquired in the hospital
- **Tazobactam:** Another β-lactamase inhibitor same as that of sulbactam
  - Combined with piperacillin for use in severe infections like peritonitis, pelvic/urinary/respiratory infections
  - Combined with ceftriaxone as well.

  b.   **Vitamin A preparations**

  (Ref: KD Tripathi, Essentials of Medical Pharmacology, 7th ed, pg. 910, 8th ed, pg. 968, 970)

ANSWER

Vitamin A Preparations

- Preformed vitamin A is present in the diet as retinyl or vitamin A esters
- Absorption is governed by factors that also determine lipid absorption
- Used for prophylaxis of vit A deficiency during pregnancy, breastfeeding, hepatobiliary diseases, and infancy

Retinoic Acid (Vit. A Acid)

- Exhibits vitamin A activity in epithelial tissues and also promoting growth
- Retinoic acid is however inactive in eye and reproductive organs

All-trans Retinoic Acid (Tretinoin)

- This is topically used
- Treatment of acne, psoriasis, ichthyosis

13-cis Retinoic Acid (Isotretinoin)

- Administered orally for acne
- Not stored but rapidly metabolized and excreted in bile and urine.

  c.   **Penicillamine**

  (Ref: KD Tripathi, Essentials of Medical Pharmacology, 8th ed, pg. 966)

ANSWER

Penicillamine

- Obtained as a degradation product of penicillin
- Exhibits strong copper chelating property and thus used for Wilson's disease
- Selective chelation of copper, mercury, lead and zinc

Indications

- **Wilson's disease (Hepatolenticular degeneration):** Occurs due to genetic deficiency of ceruloplasmin that results in high plasma concentration of free copper that gets deposited in liver, substantia nigra, basal ganglia of brain, and eventually local degeneration
  - Life-long therapy is needed to prevent disease progression
- **Copper/mercury poisoning:** Drug of choice for copper poisoning and alternatively used to dimercaprol/succimer for mercury poisoning
- **Chronic lead poisoning:** May be used as an adjuvant to $CaNa_2EDTA$
- **Cystinuria and cystine stones:** Promoting the excretion of cysteine and preventing its precipitation in the urinary tract
- **Scleroderma:** Employed in rheumatoid arthritis as disease modifying drug

Adverse Effects

- Various cutaneous reactions, itching and febrile episodes
- Prominent dermatological, renal, hematological and collagen tissue toxicities.

Your Roll No. ....

Name of the Paper : **Pharmacology Paper-I**

Name of the Course : **MBBS-2014**

Semester : **Annual**

Time: 3 Hours   M.M.: 40

INSTRUCTIONS

1. Write your Roll No. on the top immediately on receipt of this question paper
2. All questions are to be attempted
3. Answers to Parts I, II and III should be written in separate answer sheets provided
4. Attempt parts of a question in sequence

PART-I

1. **Explain why?**   [8]
   a. Tizanidine is effective in acute muscle spasm
   b. Pralidoxime is ineffective as an antidote to carbamate poisoning
   c. Furosemide is preferred drug for treatment of pulmonary edema anesthesia

2. **Classify antidepressant drugs. Discuss the mechanism of action, therapeutic uses and adverse effects of fluoxetine.**   [6]

PART-II

3. **Discuss the therapeutic status of:**   [8]
   a. Tamsulosin in benign hypertrophy of prostate
   b. Beta blockers in congestive heart failure
   c. Bimatoprost in open angle glaucoma
   d. Zafirlukast in bronchial asthma

4. **Discuss the drug treatment of:**   [6]
   a. Acute non-productive cough
   b. Petit mal epilepsy

PART-III

5. **Discuss the therapeutic uses and adverse effects of:**   [6]
   a. Spironolactone
   b. Methadone

6. **Write short notes on:**   [6]
   a. Clinical significance of plasma protein in binding of drugs
   b. Benzodiazepine-receptor agonists
   c. Bioequivalence of drugs

PART -I

1. Explain Why?

a. Tizanidine is effective in acute muscle spasm

ANSWER

Spasticity

A condition in which certain muscles are continuously contracted. This contraction can cause stiffness or tightness of the muscles and interfering with normal movement, speech, and gait.

- **How tizanidine works in spastic disorders?**
  - Central α_2 adrenergic agonist which inhibits release of excitatory amino acids in the spinal interneurons
  - Facilitation of the inhibitory transmitter glycine as well
  - Inhibition of polysynaptic reflexes which cause decrease in muscle tone and frequency of muscle spasms
- **Dose:** 2 mg TDS; max 24 mg/day
- **Indication:** Spasticity due to neurological disorders and in painful muscle spasms of spinal origin.
- **Side effect profile:**
  - Dry mouth
  - Drowsiness
  - Insomnia in night
  - Hallucinations
  - Dose-dependent elevation of liver enzymes.

b. Pralidoxime is ineffective as an antidote to carbamate poisoning

(Ref: KD Tripathi, Essentials of Medical Pharmacology, 7th ed, pg. 111, 8th ed, pg. 123)

ANSWER

Pralidoxime

An oxime; quaternary nitrogen which is positively charged and get attached to the anionic site of the enzyme.

Rationale to Pralidoxime being Ineffective as Antidote to Carbamate Poisoning

- In case of carbamate anti-ChEs (physostigmine, neostigmine, carbaryl, etc.), the anionic site of the enzyme is not free so as to offer attachment to oximes
- Contraindicated in carbamate poisoning since carbamylated enzyme is not reactivated, it also has weak anti-ChE activity of its own
- More prominent reactivation of skeletal muscle ChE than at autonomic sites and absolutely not in the CNS
- Used in organophosphate poisoning; secondary to that of atropine
- AChE inhibition due to carbamates is rapidly reversible
- Moreover, pralidoxime can reduce the protective effects of atropine in the treatment of one carbamate, carbaryl.

c. Furosemide is preferred drug for treatment of pulmonary edema anesthesia

ANSWER

Rationale to Prefer Furosemide in Treatment of Pulmonary Edema

- Furosemide is a loop diuretic; are indicated for patients with fluid overload
- Furosemide acts by reducing preload and hence provide relief in edema
- Should be withheld or judiciously employed in patients presenting with intravascular volume depletion
- **Mechanism of action:** It inhibits NaCl reabsorption in the thick ascending limb of the loop of Henle; and since a significant proportion of filtered NaCl is absorbed by the thick ascending limb of loop of Henle, thus diuretics acting at this location are highly efficacious
- No significant downstream compensatory reabsorption mechanisms seen; loop diuretics like furosemide are highly effective and are called high ceiling diuretics

2. Classify antidepressant drugs. Discuss the mechanism of action, therapeutic uses and adverse effects of fluoxetine.

ANSWER

Antidepressant Drugs

- Agents used to treat clinical depression, or other conditions, as characterized by manic or depressive effects; elevate mood; or prevent the mood disorders from recurring.

○ **Antidepressant drugs can be classified as:**
  ▪ **Reversible inhibitors of monoamine oxidase A (MAO-A):** Moclobemide, Clorgyline
  ▪ Tricyclic antidepressants (TCAs)
    ◆ Noradrenaline (NA) + serotonin (5-HT) reuptake inhibitors: Imipramine, amitriptyline, trimipramine, doxepin, dothiepin, clomipramine
    ◆ Predominantly noradrenaline (NA) reuptake inhibitors: Desipramine, nortriptyline, amoxapine, reboxetine
  ▪ **Selective serotonin reuptake inhibitors (SSRIs):** Fluoxetine, fluvoxamine, paroxetine, sertraline, citalopram, escitalopram, dapoxetine
  ▪ **Serotonin and noradrenaline reuptake inhibitors (SNRIs):** Venlafaxine, duloxetine
  ▪ **Atypical antidepressants:** Trazodone, mianserin, mirtazapine, bupropion, tianeptine, amineptine, atomoxetine.

Fluoxetine

○ First SSRI to be introduced
○ Longest acting SSRI.

Mechanism of Action

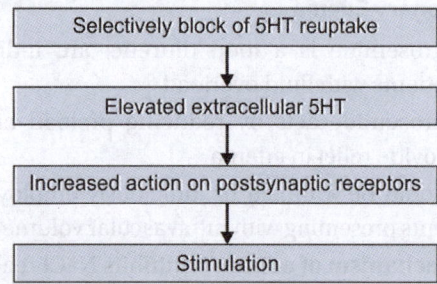

Selectively block of 5HT reuptake
↓
Elevated extracellular 5HT
↓
Increased action on postsynaptic receptors
↓
Stimulation

Therapeutic Uses

○ First line drugs in depression
○ Extensively used in anxiety and phobias, including social phobia
○ Obsessive-compulsive disorder (OCD) and related disorders
○ Panic disorder; eating disorders
○ Premenstrual dysphoric disorder, and post-traumatic stress disorder (PTSD).
○ Body dysmorphic disorder, compulsive buying, and kleptomania (an impulse control disorder that results in an irresistible, recurrent urge to steal, typically without regards to profit or need)
○ Can be used to cause delay in premature ejaculation.
○ Mood elevation and increased work capacity in few postmyocardial infarction and other chronic somatic illness patients.
○ Preferred for prophylaxis of recurrent depression.
○ **Note:** Approved to be used in children ≥7 years to treat depression and OCD, but should be given to children only when psychotherapy is unsuccessful.

Adverse Effects

○ Gastrointestinal (very prominent with almost all SSRIs)
  ▪ **Nausea:** This occurs due to stimulation of 5-HT₃ receptor stimulation, however, over time, tolerance gets developed.
  ▪ **Loose motions:** The blockade of 5-HT uptake in the gut and activation of 5-HT receptors on enteric plexus neurons can result in frequent loose motions.
  ▪ Gastric blood loss due to NSAIDs may be increased by fluoxetine (SSRIs).
○ Neurological
  ▪ Nervousness
  ▪ Sleeplessness
  ▪ Restlessness
  ▪ Anorexia
  ▪ Dyskinesia and headache
  ▪ **Note:** Administration of any serotonergic drug (e.g., MAOIs, tramadol, pethidine) in a patient receiving SSRIs can cause precipitation of "*Serotonin syndrome*" which manifests as agitation, restlessness, rigidity, hyperthermia, confusion, delirium, perspiring, twitchings, followed by convulsions.
○ **Cardiovascular:** Impairment of platelet function may result into increased incidence of epistaxis and ecchymosis
○ **Discontinuation reactions:** Paresthesias, bodyache, bowel upset, agitation and sleep disturbances in some patients.

PART-II

3. **Discuss the therapeutic status of:**

a. **Tamsulosin in benign hypertrophy of prostate**
    (Ref: KD Tripathi, Essentials of Medical Pharmacology, 7th ed, pg. 142, 8th ed, pg.156-57)

ANSWER

Benign Hypertrophy of Prostate (BHP)

○ Obstruction of urine due to BHP exhibits two types of components: static and dynamic.
○ Static due to increased size of prostate and dynamic is due to increased tone of neck of bladder or smooth muscles of prostate.

Tamsulosin in Benign Hypertrophy of Prostate

○ This drug is alpha-1 adrenergic blocker and it affects dynamic component by decreasing tone of prostatic/bladder neck muscles.

○ Blockade of a₁ adrenoceptors in bladder trigone, prostate and even prostatic urethra lead to relaxation in tone of smooth muscles, thus increasing flow rate of urine and more complete emptying of bladder BHP patients.

○ Irritative symptoms like urgency, frequency and nocturia are better relieved than voiding symptoms.

○ Size of prostate is not affected by tamsulosin.

○ May be used concurrently with finasteride.

○ **Note:** Problem of floppy iris has come across during cataract surgery.

b.   Beta blockers in congestive heart failure

ANSWER

Congestive Heart Failure (CHF)

A progressive chronic disease in which the heart becomes inefficient to pump sufficient blood and oxygen to meet the body requirements

β-adrenergic Blockers in CHF

○ Most useful in mild to moderate (NYHA class II, III) cases of dilated cardiomyopathy with systolic dysfunction

○ Not used in decompensated patients

○ **Mechanism of action:** Beta blocker therapy in patients with HFrEF is probably related to reduction of harmful effects of catecholamine stimulation including elevated heart rate, increased myocardial energy demands, adverse remodeling due to cardiac myocyte hypertrophy and death

○ Also affects interstitial fibrosis, impaired beta-adrenergic signaling, arrhythmia, and stimulation of other unfavorable systems, for example, renin-angiotensin-aldosterone axis

○ **Note:** To be stopped during acute heart failure episode.

c.   Bimatoprost in open angle glaucoma

ANSWER

Open Angle Glaucoma

A degenerative disease which affects patency of the trabecular meshwork and gradually lost past middle age

Bimatoprost in Open Angle Glaucoma

○ A prostaglandin analog

○ Increases uveoscleral outflow by increasing permeability of tissues in ciliary muscle or by acting on episcleral vessels

○ Current treatment approach starts with these drugs

○ Effect is well-sustained over long-term

○ Use: Reduces intraocular tension in normal pressure glaucoma also

○ Ocular hypotensive agent that works by increasing aqueous humor outflow

○ Indicated for the second-line treatment of open-angle glaucoma and ocular hypertension

○ Formulated as 0.03% ophthalmic solution

○ Provides an alternative treatment option for patients in whom beta-blockers are contraindicated.

d.   Zafirlukast in bronchial asthma

ANSWER

For answer, refer 2017 paper-I Q. 3 (d), Pg. 189

4.   Discuss the drug treatment of:
a.   Acute non-productive cough

ANSWER

Acute Nonproductive Cough

This type of cough has no useful function

Drug Treatment

○ Since no sputum is expelled during cough, drugs (mucolytics and expectorants) to clear airways not useful

○ Antitussives and cough suppressants are used

○ **Antitussives:**

▪ Drugs acting in the CNS to increase the threshold of cough centre or acting peripherally in the respiratory tract to reduce tussal impulses, or even both

▪ Aims at controlling rather than eliminating cough, used only for dry nonproductive cough or if cough is unduly tiring, disturbs sleep or if harmful (hernia, piles, cardiac disease, ocular surgery)

◆ **Codeine:**
  □ More selective for cough centre
  □ Regarded as the standard antitussive; cough is suppressed for about 6 h
  □ Constipation is major drawback
  □ Respiratory depression and drowsiness may occur at high doses

◆ **Ethylmorphine:**
  □ Closely related to codeine, antitussive and respiratory depressant properties are exhibited, less constipating effect

◆ **Noscapine:**
  □ Depresses cough but no narcotic, analgesic or dependence inducing properties

- Particularly useful in spasmodic cough
- Side effects occasionally seen in forms of headache and nausea
- Dextromethorphan
- *d*-isomer contains antitussive action while *l*-isomer possess analgesic action
- No depression of mucociliary function of the airway mucosa
- No constipating action

  ♦ **Antihistamines:**
  - First and second generations H1 antihistaminics are also included in the cough preparations.

b. Petit mal epilepsy

ANSWER

Petit Mal Epilepsy

○ Also known as absence seizures
○ More common in children than adults and can happen very frequently
○ Second most common type of seizure
○ Person becomes unconscious for a short time
○ May look blank and stare, or eyelids might flutter
○ During a typical absence seizure, the person becomes unresponsive for a few seconds

Drug Treatment

○ Ethosuximide is employed in *initial treatment* (less toxic than valproate and more effective than lamotrigine)
○ **Mechanism of action:** Antiepileptic effect is exerted by partial antagonism of T-type calcium channels of the thalamic neurons

↓

Decrease in burst firing of thalamocortical neurons

↓

Stabilizes the nerve activity in the brain

↓

Seizures are prevented

○ Alternatively, drugs of first choice are lamotrigine and valproate, particularly in case of generalized tonic-clonic seizures coexisting with absence seizures
○ Ethosuximide is not effective in latter case
○ It may result into drowsiness, dizziness, tiredness, headache, stomach upset, loss of appetite, nausea, vomiting, weight loss, diarrhea, or even loss of coordination as adverse effects

Note: *EEG gets normalized when complete control on seizure is achieved.*

PART-III

5. Discuss the therapeutic uses and adverse effects of:

a. Spironolactone

(Ref: KD Tripathi, Essentials of Medical Pharmacology, 7th ed, pg. 523, 8th ed, pg. 567-68)

ANSWER

Spironolactone

○ An aldosterone antagonist and a weak diuretic
○ Can benefit CHF by antagonizing direct and indirect effects of aldosterone in form of expansion of extracellular fluid volume and also increased cardiac preload

Therapeutic Uses

○ Edema particularly in case of cirrhotic and nephrotic syndrome
○ Add-on therapy to combination of ACE inhibitors and other drugs in moderate-to-severe CHF
○ Retarding disease progression, reduce episodes of decompensation and death due to heart failure as well as sudden cardiac deaths
○ Counteracting potassium loss due to loop diuretics, furosemide and thiazides
○ Restoring diuretic response to furosemide when refractoriness has developed
○ Primary hyperaldosteronism (Conn's syndrome)
○ Hypertension with thiazide

Adverse Effects

○ **Metabolic disorders:** Risk of hyperkalemia
○ **Frequently seen in male patients is gynecomastia:** Can be avoided by using eplerenone
○ **Nervous system disorders:** Ataxia, drowsiness, dizziness, headache and clumsiness
○ **Psychiatric conditions:** Lethargy, changes in libido, confusion
○ **Cardiac disorders:** Severe hyperkalemia may lead to paralysis, flaccid paraplegia and cardiac arrhythmias with subsequent cardiovascular collapse; can prove fatal in patients with impaired renal function
○ **Gastrointestinal disorders:** Gastritis, gastric bleeding, gastrointestinal disturbances, stomach cramps, diarrhoea, vomiting, nausea and ulceration frequently.

b. Methadone

(Ref: KD Tripathi, Essentials of Medical Pharmacology, 7th ed, pg. 476, 8th ed, pg.504)

ANSWER

Methadone

- Analgesic, respiratory depressant, antitussive, constipating and biliary activities similar to morphine
- Exhibits high oral: Parenteral activity ratio and firm binding to tissue proteins

Therapeutic Uses

- Primarily used as substitution therapy for opioid dependence
- Can also be used as an analgesic employed for the same conditions as morphine
- Occasionally used as antitussive

Adverse Effects

- **Short-term effects:**
  - Drowsiness, shallower and slower breathing
  - Dry eyes, nose and mouth
  - Fatigue
  - Decreased blood pressure
- **Long-term effects:**
  - Constipation
  - Sweating and itching
  - Nausea and vomiting
  - Vertigo very commonly
  - Edema of the lower extremities, etc.

---

6. **Write short notes on:**

   a. **Clinical significance of plasma protein in binding of drugs**

ANSWER

Binding to Plasma Proteins

- Greatly impacts drug efficacy, distribution, and disposition
- Common blood proteins to which the drugs bind to are human serum albumin, lipoprotein, glycoprotein, α, β, and γ globulins
- Binding of drug to plasma proteins affects drug's efficiency
- Less bound drug can more efficiently traverse cell membranes or diffuse, and also confers immediate start of action
- Bound drugs are pharmacologically inactive; and slowly dissociates
- Thus, highly protein bound drugs remain inside the body for a long period of time
- Bound drug is always is in equilibrium with the free drug.

b. **Benzodiazepine-receptor agonists**

ANSWER

Benzodiazepine-receptor Agonists

Highly potent anxiolytic benzodiazepine

Mechanism of Action

- Preferential action on midbrain ascending reticular formation and on limbic system
- Acts on primary medullary site of action to produce muscle relaxation and acts on cerebellum to produce ataxia
- These are not general depressants, however, exert relatively selective anxiolytic, hypnotic, muscle relaxant and anticonvulsant effects
- Some BZDs exhibit relatively selective antianxiety action
- REM phase of sleep is shortened, but more REM cycles may occur, so that effect on total REM sleep is less marked
- Clonazepam and diazepam exert more marked muscle relaxant property
- Diazepam and lorazepam are highly efficacious in short-term use in status-epilepticus
- Response to acute anxiety is better than chronic anxiety
- **Note:** If larger doses have been used, dose should be tapered gradually before withdrawing.

c. **Bioequivalence of drugs**

ANSWER

Bioequivalence

- Two drugs are considered bioequivalent if they are pharmaceutically equivalent, and if they have similar bioavailability, so that the efficacy and safety are principally the same
- If two medicines are bioequivalent there is no clinically significant difference in their bioavailability
- Bioequivalence is measured based on the relative bioavailability of the innovator medicine versus the generic medicine
- Determined by relating the ratio of the pharmacokinetic variables for innovator drug versus the generic medicine, wherein equality comes to be 1

Note: Drugs that are not listed as bioequivalent should not be substituted for each other.

Your Roll No. ....

Name of the Paper : **Pharmacology Paper-II**

Name of the Course : **MBBS-2014**

Semester : **Annual**

Time: 3 Hours   M.M.: 40

INSTRUCTIONS

1. Write your Roll No. on the top immediately on receipt of this question paper
2. All questions are to be attempted
3. Answers to Parts I, II and III should be written in separate answer sheets provided
4. Attempt parts of a question in sequence

PART-I

1. **Explain why?**   [8]

    a. Cancer chemotherapy is administered to patients in cycles
    b. Deferiprone may be administered to a patient of thalassemia
    c. N-acetylcysteine is given in paracetamol overdose
    d. Low molecular weight heparins are preferred over converntional heparin in the treatment of deep vein thrombosis

2. **Discuss inappropriate use of Antimicrobial agents. Write briefly the mechanisms for development of drug resistance and enumerate the strategies to prevent its development.**   [6]

PART-II

3. **Discuss the therapeutic status of:**   [8]

    a. Aromatase inhibitors in breast cancer
    b. Chloroquine in hepatic amoebiasis
    c. Sitagliptin in diabetes mellitus
    d. Corticosteroid in immunological condition

4. **Discuss the drug treatment of:**   [6]

    a. Thyrotoxic crisis
    b. Lepra reaction

PART-III

5. **Discuss the rational for the use of:**   [6]

    a. Methotrexate in rheumatoid arthritis
    b. Multidrug therapy in the treatment of tuberculosis

6. **Write short notes on:**   [6]

    a. Direct thrombin inhibitors
    b. Pentavalent vaccine

PART-I

1. Explain why?

a. Cancer chemotherapy is administered to patients in cycles

ANSWER

Intermittent Pulse Therapy

○ Use of drugs in intermittent schedules to attain selective toxicity has been called "pulsing" therapy

○ This type of intermittent chemotherapeutic regime employs maximum tolerated dose within a short administration period

○ Combination of 2–6 drugs given in intermittent pulses to achieve total cell-kill

Significance

○ Helps to attain goal of complete remission in cancer chemotherapy

Rationale to Use

○ Allows to schedule the administration of a drug at intervals so as to offer the normal cells a rest period for recovery before the cancer cells start multiplying back to baseline

○ Favors risk-benefit ratio

○ Intended for recovery of damaged normal host cells.

b. Deferiprone may be administered to a patient of thalassemia

(Ref: KD Tripathi, Essentials of Medical Pharmacology, 7th ed, pg. 908, 8th ed, pg. 967)

ANSWER

Defriprone

○ An iron chelator that is orally active

○ **Rationale to use in thalassemia:**
  ▪ Treatment of transfusion siderosis in thalassemia patients has been simplified by defriprone
  ▪ These patients have to be given repeated blood transfusions since extreme hemolysis happens
  ▪ This results in iron overload
  ▪ Thus, use of an iron chelator is mandated to clear this overload

○ Less effective than injected desferrioxamine

○ Also used in acute iron poisoning (less effective than desferrioxamine) and for iron load in patients of liver cirrhosis.

c. N-acetylcysteine is given in paracetamol overdose

ANSWER

Paracetamol Poisoning

Serious toxicity can occur with use of paracetamol if administered in large dose (>150 mg/kg or >10 g in adults).

○ Occurs particularly in small children as their hepatic glucuronide conjugating ability is low. Early manifestations include nausea, vomiting, pain abdomen and liver tenderness

○ Late manifestations include centrilobular hepatic necrosis after 12–18 hours; renal tubular necrosis may also occur

Treatment

○ **Supportive measures:**
  ▪ Gastric lavage or induction of vomiting should be done if the patient is brought at the start of symptoms
  ▪ Activated charcoal given orally or via tube prevents further absorption
  ▪ Other supportive measures, as required.

○ **Drug treatment:** This employs use of N-acetylcysteine
  ▪ **Rationale to use:** Replenishing glutathione stores in liver and prevention of binding of the noxious metabolite to other cellular constituents
  ▪ 150 mg/kg infusion intravenously over 15 minutes
  ▪ Same dose is followed IV over the next 20 hours
  ▪ May be orally administered as an alternative in a dose 75 mg/kg every 4–6 hours for 2–3 days
  ▪ Most effective when initiated within 8 hours of ingestion.

d. Low molecular weight heparins are preferred over conventional heparin in the treatment of deep vein thrombosis

ANSWER

For answer, refer 2017 paper-II Q. 1 (d), Pg. 195

2. **Discuss inappropriate use of Antimicrobial agents. Write briefly the mechanisms for development of drug resistance and enumerate the strategies to prevent its development**

(Ref: KD Tripathi, Essentials of Medical Pharmacology, 7th ed, pg. 691, 8th ed, pg. 745-49)

ANSWER

Inappropriate Antimicrobial Use

○ Defined as use of antimicrobial agent to which a pathogen is not maximally responding (is resistant); nonadherence to drug schedule or a delay or deferral in initializing appropriate treatment

○ One of the major issue that results due to inappropriate use of antimicrobials is drug resistance

○ Inappropriate use of antibiotics can lead to bacteria resistant to antibiotics in the community

Factors in Development of Drug Resistance

○ Regular use of broad-spectrum antimicrobial agents

○ Sustained use of antimicrobial agents

○ More frequent usage of invasive devices and procedures

○ Presence of patients who need prolonged hospitalization

Mechanisms of Development of Drug Resistance

○ **Mutation**
  ▪ A stable and inherited genetic change that may occur impulsively and randomly among microorganisms
  ▪ A few mutant cells are present in any sensitive microbe population that require high antimicrobial agent for their eradication
  ▪ They proliferate when the antimicrobials eliminate the sensitive cells
  ▪ Known as *vertical transfer* of resistance
  ▪ It may be single step, for example, Staphylococci to rifampin
  ▪ Multistep resistance; for example, resistance to erythromycin and tetracyclines by many organisms

○ **Gene transfer (infectious resistance)**
  ▪ The gene responsible for causing resistance is passed from one organism to the other
  ▪ Known as *horizontal transfer* of resistance
  ▪ Rapidly developed and spread
  ▪ This can develop through three modes: *conjugation, transduction and transformation*

Prevention of Drug Resistance

○ Only judicious use; no indiscriminate and insufficient or unduly prolonged use of antimicrobials: Minimizing the selection pressure and strains that are resistant will get less chance to preferentially spread

○ Choosing rapid-acting and selective (narrow-spectrum) antimicrobials in place of broad spectrum agents whenever possible

○ Employing multidrug combination of antimicrobials when continued prolonged therapy is needed, as in case of tuberculosis, etc.

○ Intensive treatment of infection caused by organisms infamous for developing resistance, for example, *Staph. aureus, E. coli*, etc.

PART-II

3. **Discuss the therapeutic status of:**

   a. **Aromatase inhibitors in breast cancer**

ANSWER

Aromatase inhibitors

○ Extensively used in breast cancer therapy

○ **Three generations:** Letrozole, Anastrozole and Exemestane

○ **Letrozole, Anastrozole:** Nonsteroidal agents, competitive inhibitors

○ **Exemestane:** Steroidal agent; irreversible inhibitor

○ **Mechanism of action:** Causes deprivation of estrogen in body by reversible inhibition of aromatization, including action on breast cancer cells

○ Orally administered regimen

Indications

○ Letrozole is employed as first line drug in early breast cancer cases for ER+ postmenopausal women post mastectomy

○ High response rate as compared to tamoxifen; forms first line drug in advanced cases of breast cancer

○ Also instituted as second line therapy if tamoxifen fails to bring the therapeutic outcome.

   b. **Chloroquine in hepatic amoebiasis**

(Ref: KD Tripathi, Essentials of Medical Pharmacology, 8th ed, pg. 875)

ANSWER

Chloroquine in Hepatic Amoebiasis

○ Exerts killing action on trophozoites of *E. histolytica*

- Highly concentrated in liver, hence, used in hepatic amoebiasis only
- Does not affect invasive dysentery and control on the luminal cycle since completely absorbed from the upper intestine and not so greatly concentrated in the intestinal wall to be effective
- Longer duration of treatment and frequent relapses
- For abolishing luminal cycle, a luminal amoebicide to be given with or after chloroquine
- **Dose:** 600 mg (base) for 2 days followed by 300 mg daily for 2 to 3 weeks
- Employed only when metronidazole fails to clear the infection or not tolerated

  Note: Resistance is not developed to choroquine by amoebae.

  c. **Sitagliptin in diabetes mellitus**

ANSWER

Sitagliptin in Diabetes Mellitus

- Competitive and selectiveDPP-4 inhibitor
- **Use:** Mostly employed as adjuvant drugs in type 2 DM not well-controlled by metformin/insulin/sulfonylureas/pioglitazone
- **Mechanism of action:** Works by inhibiting the DPP-4 enzyme which destroys GLP and GIP hormones, allowing both to function more effectively
- **Pharmacological Effects:**
  - Boosts postprandial insulin release
  - Decreases glucagon secretion and lowers meal-time as well as fasting blood glucose in type 2 DM
- **Adverse Effect Profile:**
  - Nausea
  - Loose stools
  - Headache
  - Rashes
  - Allergic reactions and edema
  - Nasopharyngitis and cough.

  d. **Corticosteriod in immunological condition**

  (Ref: KD Tripathi, Essentials of Medical Pharmacology, 7th ed, 8th ed, pg. 306)

ANSWER

Corticosteroids in Immunological Condition

- Impairment of immunological competence
- Suppression of all types of hypersensitization and allergic phenomena
- At therapeutic doses *in vivo,* no impairment of antibody production or complement function

- Suppression of leukocyte recruitment at the contact site with antigen and of inflammatory response to the immunological injury
- Used in organ transplantation cases and autoimmune diseases
- Greater suppression of cell mediated immunity in which T cells are primarily involved, for example, delayed hypersensitivity and graft rejection
- **Mechanism of action for effect in immunological condition:**
  - Inhibition of release of IL-1 from macrophages
  - Inhibition of production of IL-2 and action
  - Interruption of communication between cells that are involved in the immunological process by intrusive action in synthesis of or activities of lymphokines.

4. **Discuss the drug treatment of:**

   a. **Thyrotoxic crisis**

ANSWER

Thyroid Storm

Referred as thyrotoxic crisis; emergency condition arising due to decompensated hyperthyroidism

Drug Treatment

- **Nonselective β-blockers (e.g. propranolol):**
  - **Dose:** Intravenous 1–2 mg slowly; may be followed by 40–80 mg oral every 6 h
  - Provide dramatic relief in symptoms
  - Decreases peripheral conversion of T_4 to T_3
- **Propylthiouracil:**
  - Dose: Oral 200–300 mg 6 hourly
  - Synthesis of hormone and peripheral conversion of T_4 to T_3 both are reduced
- **Iopanoic acid:**
  - **Dose:** Oral 0.5–1 g once daily
  - Thyroid hormone release and peripheral conversion of T_4 to T_3 are inhibited
- **Corticosteroids:**
  - **Dose:** Hydrocortisone in a dose of 100 mg intravenously (8 hourly) followed by oral prednisolone
  - Adrenal insufficiency covered; peripheral conversion of T_4 to T_3 inhibited
- **Diltiazem:**
  - **Dose:** 60–120 mg BD oral; if propranolol fails to control tachycardia or if contraindicated
- Other measures include rehydration, anxiolytics, external cooling and proper antibiotic coverage.

PHARMACOLOGY

b. Lepra reaction

Lepra Reaction

- According to WHO, immunologically mediated episodes of acute or subacute inflammation known as reactions may occur during the course of leprosy, in up to 25% of patients with paucibacillary leprosy and as much as 40% with multibacillary leprosy
- It is an Arthus (Jarisch Herxheimer) type of reaction which occurs when killing of bacilli results into release of antigens
- Manifests as
  - Enlargement of existing lesions, redness, swelling and pain
  - New lesions may appear
  - Malaise and fever, etc.
- May be mild, severe or life-threatening, i.e. erythema nodosum leprosum (ENL)

Treatment

- **Prednisolone** in a dose of 40–60 mg/day is started immediately and continued till the reaction subsides in severe cases
- **Thalidomide**:
  - Can be used as an alternative to prednisolone as cytokines play an important role in generating symptoms in lepra reaction
  - Imparts anxiolytic, antiemetic with anti-inflammatory actions
  - Also has cytokine (TNFα, ILs, interferon) modulatory property. Thus, can be used as an alternative to prednisolone as cytokines play an important role in generating symptoms in lepra reaction
  - **Dose for ENL**: 100–300 mg once daily at bed time.
- **Clofazimine**:
  - Exerts leprostatic and anti-inflammatory actions
  - Dapsone-resistant *M. leprae* respond to clofazimine, after lag period of around 2 months
  - Also used in multidrug therapy of leprosy; due to its anti-inflammatory property, it is beneficial in lepra reaction.

PART-III

5. Discuss the rational for the use of:

a. Methotrexate in rheumatoid arthritis

(Ref: KD Tripathi, Essentials of Medical Pharmacology, 8th ed, pg. 228)

Methotrexate

A dihydrofolate reductase inhibitor; exhibiting prominent immunosuppressant and antiinflammatory property

Rationale to Use in Rheumatoid Arthritis (RA)

- It causes inhibition of cytokine production, chemotaxis and also cell-mediated immune reaction, thus beneficial in RA
- Considered as DMARD of first choice
- Used as standard treatment for most patients, that includes patients of juvenile RA
- Predictable response that is sustained over long-term
- Also forms one of the important drug in combination regimens of 2 or 3 DMARDs
- Oral ulceration and gastric upset form major adverse effects of low dose regimen
- Increased incidence of chest infection
- Relatively rapid onset of symptom relief, thus ideal for initial treatment.

b. Multidrug therapy in the treatment of tuberculosis

For answer, refer 2016 paper-II Q. 1 (b), Pg. 209

6. Write short notes on:

a. Direct thrombin inhibitors

(Ref: KD Tripathi, Essentials of Medical Pharmacology, 7th ed, pg. 620, 8th ed, pg. 666)

Direct Thrombin Inhibitors

Anticoagulant drugs that bind directly to thrombin and lead to its inactivation; no need to combine with and activate AT III

Lepirudin

- Firm binding to catalytic and substrate recognition sites of thrombin and their direct inhibition
- Indicated only in patients who exhibit risk of heparin induced thrombocytopenia
- Repeated/prolonged administration can result in prolonged anticoagulant effect and chances of anaphylaxis; irreversible

Bivalirudin

○ Slowly reversible action due to peptide bonds cleavage by thrombin itself

Argatroban

○ Reversible binding to the catalytic site of thrombin, but not to the substrate recognition site

○ Rapid and short-lasting antithrombin action.

b. **Pentavalent vaccine**

(Ref: KD Tripathi, Essentials of Medical Pharmacology, 8th ed, pg. 984)

ANSWER

For answer, refer 2016 paper-II Q. 6 (c), Pg. 214

Name of the Paper : **Pharmacology Paper-I**

Name of the Course : **MBBS-2013**

Semester : **Annual**

Time: 3 Hours M.M.: 40

INSTRUCTIONS

1. Write your Roll No. on the top immediately on receipt of this question paper
2. All questions are to be attempted
3. Answers to Parts I, II and III should be written in separate answer sheets provided
4. Attempt parts of a question in sequence

PART-I

1. **Explain why?** [8]
   a. Beta blockers are contraindicated in patients with variant angina
   b. Atracurium is preferred skeletal muscle relaxant in patients with altered hepatic and renal function
   c. Atropine is not preferred for treatment of chronic obstructive airway disease patients
   d. Nitrates are not given continuously in patients with stable angina

2. **Enumerate the depolarizing neuromuscular blockers. Write the mechanism of action, uses and adverse effects of succinylcholine.** [6]

PART-II

3. **Discuss the therapeutic status of:** [8]
   a. Aldosterone in Congestive heart Failure
   b. Losartan in hypertension
   c. Salbutamol in bronchial asthma
   d. Zolpidem in insomnia

4. **Discuss the drug treatment of:** [6]
   a. Glaucoma
   b. Myocardial infarction

PART-III

5. **Discuss the therapeutic uses and adverse effects of:** [6]
   a. Calcium channel blockers
   b. Anticholinergic drugs

6. **Write short notes on:** [6]
   a. Pharmacovigilance
   b. Inverse agonists
   c. Therapeutic drug monitoring

PART-I

1. Explain why?

a. Beta blockers are contraindicated in patients with variant angina

(Ref: KD Tripathi, Essentials of Medical Pharmacology, 8th ed, pg. 589)

ANSWER

Beta Blockers

Act by decreasing cardiac work and consumption of O_2

○ In angina pectoris, β-blockers have to be taken on a regular schedule, cannot be employed "as and when required" basis

○ Should be initiated nitrate ± CCB to counteract coronary vasospasm

○ **Contraindicated in patients with variant angina:**

  ▪ Considered first line therapy in patients with uncomplicated stable angina

  ▪ Decrease frequency and severity of attacks and increase in exercise tolerance in classical angina

  ▪ They cannot be used in variant angina as beta blockers are not direct vasodilators, thus not useful in vasospastic (variant) angina

  ▪ Instead variant angina is worsened due to unopposed β receptor mediated coronary constriction, which may worsen the coronary spasm.

b. Atracurium is preferred skeletal muscle relaxant in patients with altered hepatic and renal function

ANSWER

Atracurium

A bisquaternary competitive blocker that is four times less effective than pancuronium

○ Reversal is mostly not needed

○ **Preferred skeletal muscle relaxant in patients with altered hepatic and renal function:**

  ▪ The unique feature of atracurium is that it undergoes spontaneous degradation via a process known as Hofmann elimination as well as ester hydrolysis

  ▪ As a result, its duration of action is not altered by either renal or hepatic insufficiency

▪ Thus, it is the preferred muscle relaxant for liver/kidney disease patients as well as for neonates and the elderly

▪ Because of these properties, it rapidly gained favor for providing neuromuscular blockade in intensive care unit patients

▪ For this purpose, it is most commonly used by continuous infusion.

c. Atropine is not preferred for treatment of chronic obstructive airway disease patients

ANSWER

Bronchial Asthma, Asthmatic Bronchitis, COPD

○ Exhibits reflex vagal activity, thus causing bronchoconstriction and augmented secretion in chronic bronchitis and COPD, to a lesser extent in bronchial asthma

○ Impairment of mucociliary clearance

Antagonizing Muscarinic Effects of Drugs and Poisons

○ Atropine serves as the specific antidote for anti ChE and early mushroom poisoning

○ Used for myasthenia gravis, decurarization or cobra envenomation.

Side Effects of Atropine

○ Belladonna poisoning may result due to overdose or consumption of seeds and berries of belladonna/datura plant

○ **Dry mouth:** Causing difficulty in swallowing and talking

○ Dry, flushed and hot skin (especially over face and neck)

○ Fever, difficulty in micturition, decreased bowel sounds

○ **Skin:** A scarlet rash may appear

○ **Eye:** Pupil dilatation, photophobia, blurring of near vision, palpitation

○ Excitement, psychotic behaviour, ataxia, horrible visual hallucinations, delirium

○ Hypotension, weak and rapid pulse, cardiovascular collapse with respiratory depression.

Atropine not Preferred for Treatment of Chronic Obstructive Airway Disease

○ Some bronchodilation and reduction in secretions can be caused by atropine, this action is mediated by blocking of M3 receptors

PHARMACOLOGY

○ The efficacy of nonselective antimuscarinic drugs in treating chronic obstructive pulmonary disease is inadequate since blockade of M3 receptors on airway is opposed by blockade of autoinhibitory M2 receptors on postganglionic parasympathetic nerves by these drugs

○ Inhaled atropine lead to bronchodilatation, but systemic absorption via the lung results in unwanted adverse effects.

　　d.　**Nitrates are not given continuously in patients with stable angina**

ANSWER

Nitrates

Concurrently used with calcium channel blockers and may cut cardiac work and increase coronary perfusion

○ Particularly valuable in severe vasospastic angina, and cases when β–blockers are contraindicated

○ **Nitrates not given in patients with stable angina:**

　▪ In many patients with stable angina, continuous use of organic nitrates may lead to inducing tolerance and reduced therapeutic effect

　▪ This tolerance can be sidestepped by a nitrate-free interval each day, but threshold for episodes of angina may be lowered

　▪ Continuous treatment with organic nitrates also causes sympathetic activation, increase in oxidative stress, and induces endothelial dysfunction

　▪ Other undesirable effects of nitrates include flushing, headache, and postural hypotension.

2. **Enumerate the depolarizing neuromuscular blockers. Write the mechanism of action, uses and adverse effects of succinylcholine.**

ANSWER

Neuromuscular Blocking Agents

Nondepolarizing (Competitive) Blockers

○ **Long acting:** d-Tubocurarine, Pancuronium, Doxacurium, Pipecuronium

○ **Intermediate acting:** Vecuronium, Atracurium, Cisatracurium, Rocuronium, Rapacuronium

○ **Short acting:** Mivacurium

Depolarizing Blockers

○ Succinylcholine (SCh., Suxamethonium)

○ Decamethonium (C-10)

Directly Acting Agents

○ Dantrolene sodium

○ Quinine

Succinylcholine

○ **Mechanism of action:**

　▪ Acts on the nicotinic receptors of the muscles, stimulates them and eventually cause their relaxation

　▪ **This occurs in two steps:**

　　♦ **Phase 1:** This is depolarizing phase; muscle fasciculations are caused while it is depolarizing the muscle fibers

　　♦ **Phase 2:** This is desensitizing phase; sets in after adequate depolarization has occurred; the muscles no longer respond to ACh released by the nerve endings

○ **Therapeutic uses:**

　▪ Employed for brief procedures, for example, endotracheal intubation, laryngoscopy, esophagoscopy, and bronchoscopy

　▪ First-rate intubating state viz. relaxed jaw, vocal cords apart and immobile with no diaphragmatic movements is obtained

　▪ Used in reduction of fractures, dislocations, and for treating cases of laryngospasm

　▪ Employed in electroconvulsive treatment for preventing trauma

　▪ As adjuvant in anesthesia

○ **Adverse effects:**

　▪ Muscle fasciculations and soreness

　▪ Hyperkalemia: Potassium is released in blood during fasciculations

　▪ Changes in BP and HR and arrhythmias

　▪ Release of histamine: Precipitation of asthma by histamine releasing neuromuscular blockers.

　▪ Malignant hyperthermia: If used along halothane in general anesthesia

　▪ Risk of regurgitation and aspiration of gastric contents is increased in cases of GERD.

PART-II

3. **Discuss the therapeutic status of:**

　a.　**Aldosterone in congestive heart failure**

ANSWER

Aldosterone in congestive Heart failure

○ Aldosterone is a potent mineralocorticoid

○ It has a varied role in the pathogenesis of congestive heart failure

- It contributes to retention of salt and water
- Organ fibrosis is also promoted by this hormone
- It has a direct vascular effect aldosterone and may contribute to generalized vasoconstriction
- Increased plasma aldosterone levels can also cause depressed baroreflex sensitivity and related with increase in mortality severe heart failure patients

b. Losartan in Hypertension

(Ref: KD Tripathi, Essentials of Medical Pharmacology, 8th ed, pg. 506-07)

ANSWER

Losartan

Belongs to a class of drugs–angiotensin receptor blockers

- A competitive antagonist and inverse agonist
- No other receptor or ion channel is blocked, except thromboxane A_2 receptor
- **Losartan in hypertension:**
  - Acts as selective, competitive blocker of angiotensin II receptor type 1 and leads to a decrease in peripheral vascular resistance
  - It leads to fall in BP in hypertensive patients, lasting for 24 hours
  - No change in heart rate noticed
  - Peak plasma levels are obtained at 1 hour after oral ingestion
  - No significant effect on plasma lipid profile, carbohydrate tolerance, insulin sensitivity has been noted
  - Mild probenecid-like uricosuric action exhibited
  - In renal insufficiency, no adjustment in dose required
  - In hepatic dysfunction, dose to be reduced.

c. Salbutamol in Bronchial Asthma

(Ref: KD Tripathi, Essentials of Medical Pharmacology, 8th ed, pg. 252)

ANSWER

Salbutamol

Prototype drug of the group short-acting beta-2 receptor agonist

- Salbutamol in bronchial asthma:
  - Predominantly selective for beta-2 adrenergic receptors, and poorly selective for beta-1 receptors
  - *Mechanism of action:* Stimulation of beta 2 receptors stimulates formation of cAMP, thus relaxation of smooth muscles of airways, from trachea to the terminal bronchi

- Administered preferably by inhalation through a pressurized metered dose inhaler, nebulizers, and dry powder inhalers; as this is not only effective but also reduces systemic toxicity
- Bronchodilation starts within 1–5 minutes after inhalation
- It is used in terminating mild, moderate and severe acute asthmatic attacks
- Used in exercise induced asthma
- Also employed in mild intermittent asthma as needed basis
- Side effects include palpitations, restlessness, nervousness, throat irritation, at times angioedema, etc.
- **Note: While prescribing an inhaler, the patient must be taught synchronization of actuation of inhaler with inspiration or breathing to maximize drug delivery to lungs.**

d. Zolpidem in Insomnia

(Ref: KD Tripathi, Essentials of Medical Pharmacology, 8th ed, pg. 433-34)

ANSWER

Zolpidem

A selective BZD receptor agonist, but structurally non-BZD

- **Zolpidem in insomnia:**
  - Marked hypnotic effect
  - Shortens sleep latency, duration of sleep is prolonged in insomniacs
  - Indicated for short-term (1–2 weeks) use in sleep onset insomnia, also includes intermittent awakenings
  - Morning sedation or extension of reaction time can ensue if taken late at night
  - Few side effects reported; respiration not depressed even by large doses
  - One of the most commonly recommended hypnotics currently

Benefits

- Relative lack of effect on stages of sleep
- Residual daytime sedation is nominal
- When discontinued, no or very less rebound insomnia seen
- Doses to be reduced to half in elderly and patients of liver disease.

4. Discuss the drug treatment of:

a. Glaucoma

ANSWER

Open Angle Glaucoma

○ A degenerative disease which affects patency of the trabecular meshwork and gradually lost past middle age

○ Progressive increase in intraocular tension

Drug Treatment

○ **β-adrenergic blockers:**
- First line drugs till recently, replaced by PG F2α analogs
- Cause lowering of intraocular tension by reducing aqueous formation
- No effect on pupil size and tone of ciliary muscle or outflow facility
- Equally effective as miotics but less ocular side effects
- Mild and infrequent; stinging, eyes get red and dry, corneal hypoesthesia, allergic blepharoconjunctivitis, and blurring of vision
- *Note:* Absorbed through nasolacrimal duct; lethal bronchospasm conveyed in asthmatic and COPD patients

○ **α-edrenergic agonists:**
- Dipivefrine, Apraclonidine, Brimonidine, etc., used
- Dipivefrine, though better tolerated than adrenaline, leads to marked ocular burning and other side effects
- **Use of apraclonidine:** Short-term control of intraocular tension spikes after laser
- **Use of brimonidine:** Both short-term and long-term use in glaucoma; commonly used as add on therapy only

○ **Prostaglandin analogs:**
- Increases uveoscleral outflow by increasing permeability of tissues in ciliary muscle or by acting on episcleral vessels
- Current treatment approach starts with these drugs
- **Latanoprost:** Effect well-sustained over long-term
  - **Use:** Reduces intraocular tension in normal pressure glaucoma also
  - Due to better effectiveness and absence of systemic complications, forms the first choice drugs for open angle glaucoma cases despite side certain effects

○ **Carbonic anhydrase inhibitors**
- **Acetazolamide:** Dose of 0.25 g 6–12 hourly oral
  - **Use:** Supplement ocular hypotensive drugs for angle closure, before and after ocular surgery/laser therapy
  - Dorzolamide is also used

○ **Miotics**
- Now added only as the last option; due to several adverse effects.

b. Myocardial infarction

ANSWER

Myocardial Infarction

Drug treatment of Myocardial Infarction

○ **Pain relief:**
- Sublingual nitroglycerine in mild cases
- Slow intravenous infusion of morphine provides relief in severe pain
- Morphine may be repeated at an interval of 30 minutes, if needed

○ **Antiplatelet therapy:**
- Chewable aspirin 150-300 mg given as early diagnosis of MI made
- Aspirin is instituted at the time of acute myocardial infarction cases as well as regular schedule

○ **Inotropic drugs:**
- Drugs of choice are dopamine and dobutamine
- If they are unavailable, NA may be used

○ **Beta blockers:**
- These drugs may limit the size of infarct and early mortality is also reduced
- Contraindicated in cases of bronchospasm, absence of heart failure, and sympathetic overactivity
- Propranolol, metoprolol, and atenolol usually employed

○ **ACE Inhibitors:**
- Should be given within 24 h of onset of symptoms in all cases
- Left ventricular dysfunction is reduced and progression of CHF is slowed down

○ **Anticoagulants:**
- Heparin, particularly low molecular weight heparin is preferred
- Venous thrombosis and stroke is prevented

Other Important General Measures

○ Taking 100% Oxygen by face mask is very important alongwith rest and confining all movements

- Maintaining effective blood volume is very important; elevating lower limbs and thus increasing venous return to heart
- Thrombolytic therapy is most beneficial in patients with STEMI.
- Modification of cardiac risk factors including smoking, alcohol consumption, hypertension, obesity and diabetes mellitus, is very important after discharge and rehabilitation.

PART-III

5. **Discuss the therapeutic uses and adverse effects of:**

a. **Calcium channel blockers**

(Ref: KD Tripathi, Essentials of Medical Pharmacology, 8th ed, pg. 591-97)

ANSWER

Calcium Channel Blockers (CCBs)

Classified as:

- Verapamil—a *phenylalkylamine*
- Nifedipine—a *dihydropyridine* (DHPs)
- Diltiazem—a *benzothiazepine*
  - DHPs are the most potent CCBs

Therapeutic Uses

- *Angina pectoris:* Reduction in frequency and severity of both classical and variant angina
- *Myocardial infarction:* Used for evolution of myocardial infarction; also used for preventing further attacks
- *Hypertension:* Diltiazem, verapamil, and all DHPs are considered as first line drugs for hypertension
- *Cardiac arrhythmias:* Diltiazem and verapamil are very efficacious in PSVT and to control ventricular rate in case of supraventricular arrhythmias
- *Hypertrophic cardiomyopathy:* Verapamil plays salutary role due to negative inotropic action
- *Other uses:* Can be used to suppress nocturnal leg cramps (verapamil); alternatively used for premature labor; severity of Raynaud's episodes is reduced

Adverse Effects

- Frequent side effects are palpitation, flushing, and hypotension
- Ankle edema occurs very frequently
- Nervous system related adverse reactions include headache and drowsiness
- **Nausea:** Linked with peaks of drug level in blood; fractionated dose or using retard formulation can minimize this

- Post MI patients present higher mortality
- Increased difficulty in urine voiding in elderly males
- Lower esophageal sphincter relaxed—gastroesophageal reflux may get worsened.

b. **Anticholinergic drugs**

ANSWER

Therapeutic Uses

As Antisecretory

- Preanesthetic Medication
  - Administration of anticholinergics (atropine, hyoscine, glycopyrrolate) with ether made it mandatory to check increased salivary and tracheobronchial secretions as it was an irritant
  - With halothane etc., the need has decreased
  - Laryngospasm is also prevented by atropinic drugs. Also prevents vasovagal attack during anesthesia
- Peptic Ulcer
  - Decrease in gastric secretion by affecting fasting and neurogenic phase, but little effect on gastric phase, thus symptoms of peptic ulcers are relieved
- Pulmonary Embolism
  - Reduce pulmonary secretions induced reflexly by embolism
- For Checking Excessive Sweating or Salivation, for Example, Parkinsonism

As Antispasmodic

- **Intestinal and renal colic, abdominal cramps:**
  - If no mechanical obstruction exists, relief is provided
  - Atropine is less efficacious in biliary colic
- No use in infective diarrhea, can be helpful in nervous, functional and drug induced diarrhoea
- **Spastic constipation, irritable bowel syndrome:** Symptomatic relief is modest
- Providing relief in urinary urgency and frequency
- Partial suppression of gastritis, pylorospasm, gastric hypermotility, gastritis, and nervous dyspepsia

Bronchial Asthma, Asthmatic Bronchitis, COPD

- Exhibits reflex vagal activity, thus causing bronchoconstriction and augmented secretion in chronic bronchitis and COPD, to a lesser extent in bronchial asthma
- Impairment of mucociliary clearance

As Mydriatic and Cycloplegic

○ **Diagnostic use:**
  ▪ Mydriasis and cycloplegia both are required, for testing error of refraction
  ▪ Only mydriatic action needed to facilitate fundoscopy

○ Iritis, iridocyclitis, choroiditis, keratitis and corneal ulcer: Provides rest to the intraocular muscles and cuts down painful spasm

For Central Action

○ **Parkinsonism:** Used in mild cases or adjuvant to levodopa, as well as in drug induced extrapyramidal syndromes

○ **Motion sickness:** Hyoscine is most effective drug for motion sickness. Not useful in other types of vomiting

○ **Lie detector:** Hyoscine possess amnesic and depressant action

As Cardiac Vagolytic

○ Used in some cases of myocardial infarction and digitalis toxicity

Antagonizing Muscarinic Effects of Drugs and Poisons

○ Atropine serves as the specific antidote for anti ChE and early mushroom poisoning

○ Used for myasthenia gravis, decurarization or cobra envenomation.

Adverse Effects

○ Belladonna poisoning may result due to overdose or consumption of seeds and berries of belladonna/datura plant

○ **Dry mouth:** Causing difficulty in swallowing and talking

○ Dry, flushed and hot skin (especially over face and neck)

○ Fever, difficulty in micturition, decreased bowel sounds

○ **Skin:** A scarlet rash may appear

○ **Eye:** Pupil dilatation, photophobia, blurring of near vision, palpitation

○ Excitement, psychotic behaviour, ataxia, horrible visual hallucinations, delirium

○ Hypotension, weak and rapid pulse, cardiovascular collapse with respiratory depression.

---

6. **Write short notes on:**

   a. **Pharmacovigilance**

ANSWER

Pharmacovigilance

Defined in 2002 by the WHO as the "science and activities relating to the detection, assessment, understanding and prevention of adverse effects or any other drug related problems."

Benefits

▪ Information produced by pharmacovigilance is beneficial in educating doctors about adverse reactions of drugs

▪ Official regulation of drug use

▪ Reducing the risk of drug-related damage to the patient

○ Helps in assessing safety of medicines

Activities Involved

○ Postmarketing surveillance and ADR monitoring by other methods such as voluntary reporting by physicians

○ Medical record by computerized methods, prescription event monitoring, and some other cohort/case control studies

○ Data of adverse drug reactions disseminated through "drug alerts", advisories sent to doctors by pharmaceuticals and regulatory agencies, etc.

○ Labeling of medicines changed representing restrictions in use or statuary warnings, safeguards, by the regulatory decision making authority.

   b. **Inverse agonists**

(Ref: KD Tripathi, Essentials of Medical Pharmacology, 8th ed, pg .49)

ANSWER

Agonists

○ An agonist is an agent which stimulates a receptor to produce a pharmacological effect same as that of the physiological signal molecule

○ Contains both affinity and maximal intrinsic activity (IA = 1)

○ Examples include adrenaline, histamine, morphine

Inverse Agonist

○ An inverse agonist is an agent that stimulates a receptor to generate a pharmacological effect in the opposite direction to that of the agonist

○ Exhibits affinity, however, intrinsic activity presents a minus sign (IA between 0 and –1)

○ Examples include chlorpheniramine (on H1 histamine receptor)

○ **Simple example for easy understanding, if agonism of the receptor led to sedation, an inverse agonist might cause wakefulness.**

   c. **Therapeutic drug monitoring**

(Ref: KD Tripathi, Essentials of Medical Pharmacology, 8th ed, pg. 42)

ANSWER

Therapeutic Drug Monitoring (TDM)

Clinical practice of measuring specific drugs at selected intervals to sustain a constant concentration in bloodstream of patient, thereby optimizing individual dosage regimens

Particularly Used in the Following Conditions

○ Drugs with low safety margin, for example: Digoxin, anticonvulsants, antiarrhythmics, theophylline, aminoglycoside antibiotics, tricyclic antidepressants, lithium

○ Large individual variations, for example: Lithium, antidepressants

○ Potentially toxic drugs used if renal failure manifests, for example: Aminoglycoside antibiotics

○ Poisoning cases

○ Failure of response cases without any likely cause, for example: Antimicrobials

○ Patient compliance monitoring, for example: Psychopharmacological agents.

Name of the Paper : **Pharmacology Paper-II**

Name of the Course : **MBBS-2013**

Semester : **Annual**

Time: 3 Hours   M.M.: 40

INSTRUCTIONS

1. Write your Roll No. on the top immediately on receipt of this question paper
2. All questions are to be attempted
3. Answers to Parts I, II and III should be written in separate answer sheets provided
4. Attempt parts of a question in sequence

PART-I

1. **Explain why?**   [8]
   a. Primaquine is used for causal prophylaxis in malaria
   b. Heparin is effective for both in vitro and in vivo anticoagulation
   c. Tazobactum is combined with piperacillin for treatment of severe infections
   d. Patients need to be adequately instructed before starting therapy with alendronate

2. **Enumerate selective estrogen receptor modulators (SERMs). Write briefly the mechanism of action in correlation with their therapeutic uses.**   [6]

PART-II

3. **Discuss the therapeutic status of:**   [8]
   a. Metronidazole in amoebiasis
   b. Tamoxifen in breast cancer
   c. Sumatriptan in migraine
   d. Allopurinol in chronic gout

4. **Discuss the drug treatment of:**   [6]
   a. Osteoporosis
   b. H. pylori infection

PART-III

5. **Write short notes on:**   [6]
   a. Postantibiotic effect
   b. HAART
   c. Linezolid

6. **Explain the rationale for the use of:**   [6]
   a. Mifepristone in termination of first trimester pregnancy
   b. Liposomal Amphotericin B in Leishmaniasis
   c. Clofazimine in lepra reaction

PART-I

1. **Explain why?**

   a. **Primaquine is used for causal prophylaxis in malaria**

   (Ref: KD Tripathi, Essentials of Medical Pharmacology, 8th ed, pg. 875)

ANSWER

Primaquine

- A poor erythrocytic schizontocide
- Exhibits weaker action on *P. vivax*, but no response on blood forms of *P. falciparum*

Rationale to Use Primaquine for Causal Prophylaxis in Malaria

- Causal prophylaxis refers to targeting the pre-erythrocytic phase which occurs in liver, since this is the root *cause* of malarial infection and the clinical attacks
- Primaquine used as causal prophylactic for all the malarial species
- It exerts an extensive effect on both primary and secondary hepatic phases of the malarial parasite, hence target pre-erythrocytic phase
- Also, extremely active against gametocytes and hypnozoites
- Marked and better activity against the pre-erythrocytic stage of *P. falciparum* than *P. vivax*
- **Note:** Cannot be used in masses due to its toxic potential.

   b. **Heparin is effective for both** *in vitro* **and** *in vivo* **anticoagulation**

   (Ref: KD Tripathi, Essentials of Medical Pharmacology, 8th ed, pg. 663-64)

ANSWER

Heparin

- A powerful and promptly acting anticoagulant to be administered by intravenous or deep subcutaneous routes
- Effective both in vivo and in vitro anticoagulation

Rationale to Heparin Use for Both *in vivo* **and** *in vitro* **Anticoagulation**

- Chief reason is that it inhibits reactions that lead to the blood clotting and formation of fibrin clots both in vivo and in vitro
- Indirect action by activation of plasma antithrombin III

↓

Binding of heparin-AT III complex to clotting factors of the intrinsic and common pathways

↓

Inhibition of factor Xa and thrombin (IIa) mediated conversion of fibrinogen to fibrin

- Common pathway is affected by higher concentrations
- Selective interference with intrinsic pathway at lower concentrations.

   c. **Tazobactum is combined with piperacillin for treatment of severe infections**

   (Ref: KD Tripathi, Essentials of Medical Pharmacology, 8th ed, pg. 775)

ANSWER

Tazobactam

- A β-lactamase inhibitor which is similar to sulbactam
- Pharmacokinetics of tazobactum get matched with piperacillin

Rationale to Combine with Piperacillin

- Been combined with tazobactum to be used in case of severe infections like peritonitis, pelvic/urinary/respiratory infections caused due to β-lactamase producing bacilli
- Piperacillin is combined with tazobactum, β-lactamase inhibitor, in ratio of 8:1 for intravenous preparation
- Since piperacillin is susceptible to hydrolysis by β-lactamase, these days manufactured with tazobactam
- The combination of Piperacillin-tazobactam not approved by FDA to be employed use in infants aging less than 2 months
- Can be considered for neonates with proven bacterial infections, particularly those infected with difficult to treat polymicrobial sepsis or infections due to P. aeruginosa or K. pneumoniae
- **Dose:** 0.5 g combined with piperacillin 4 g injected intravenously over 30 minutes 8 hourly.

d.   **Patients need to be adequately instructed before starting therapy with Alendronate**

(Ref: KD Tripathi, Essentials of Medical Pharmacology, 8th ed, pg. 369)

ANSWER

For answer, refer 2015 paper-II Q. 1 (d), Pg. 223

---

2.   **Enumerate Selective estrogen receptor modulators (SERMs). Write briefly the mechanism of action in correlation with their therapeutic uses.**

(Ref: KD Tripathi, Essentials of Medical Pharmacology, 8th ed, pg. 337-39)

ANSWER

Selective Estrogen Receptor Modulators

Drugs that exhibit both estrogenic and antiestrogenic actions in a tissue selective manner

Mechanism of Action Correlating with the Therapeutic Uses

- Reflect anitestrogenic action; acting as potent estrogen antagonist in carcinoma cells of breast, blood vessels and at some peripheral sites
- Acting as partial agonist in uterus, bone, liver and pituitary
- Weaker estrogen agonistic action that manifests as stimulating endometrial proliferation, dropping of gonadotropin and prolactin levels in postmenopausal women
- Estrogenic action leads to a decrease in total and LDL cholesterol with no change in levels of HDL and triglyceride level
- Acting as estrogen HRT, it increases the risk of deep vein thrombosis by 2 to 3 times
- Till aromatase inhibitors, SERMs been treated as standard hormonal treatment of breast cancer in both pre- and postmenopausal women
- Given in early cases of postmastectomy adjuvant therapy, whereas in advanced cases, it is a component of palliative treatment
- Tamoxifen is the only drug approved for both primary and metastatic breast carcinoma in premenopausal women
- Also effective in cases of surgically treated cancer of male breast
- Also used as primary prophylaxis of breast cancer in high-risk women
- Due to antiresorptive effect and changes in lipid profile, leads to improved in bone mass
- May be used as alternative to clomiphene in male infertility
- Raloxifene is a different SERM; has a different pattern of action than tamoxifen
- Acts as an estrogen partial agonist in bone and CVS, but an antagonist in endometrium and breast
- It reduces the risk of vertebral fracture to half, however, long bones not included
- Provides protection against ER-positive breast cancer
- Acts as second line drug for prevention and treatment of osteoporosis in postmenopausal women
- Enhancing benefits by Ca_{2+} and vit D supplements.

PART-II

3.   **Discuss the therapeutic status of:**

a.   **Metronidazole in amoebiasis**

ANSWER

Metronidazole

- Broad-spectrum; cidal action against anaerobic protozoa and *Giardia lamblia*
- A highly active amoebicide

Mechanism of Action

Nitro group of the drug reduced by certain redox proteins functioning only in anaerobic microbes to a highly reactive nitro radical, exerting cytotoxicity

Therapeutic Profile in Amoebic Hepatitis

- First line drug employed in all forms of amoebic infection
- Hepatic amoebiasis responds promptly to metronidazole 800 mg 8-hourly for 5 days
- Effective in complete eradication of trophozoites from the liver (essential to avoid relapses)
- In patients where metronidazole is contraindicated or patient is unresponsive, dehydroemetine to be used
- Large abscesses may need to be aspirated.

b.   **Tamoxifen in breast cancer**

ANSWER

For answer, refer 2015 paper-II Q. 3 (d), Pg. 226

c.   **Sumatriptan in migraine**

ANSWER

Sumatriptan

- A selective 5-HT$_{1D/1B}$ agonist
- Most effective treatment of acute migraine attacks

Mechanism of Action

- Constriction of dilated cerebral blood vessels
- Especially the arteriovenous shunts in the carotid artery, which express 5-HT$_{1D/1B}$ receptors
- Resulting into diversion of blood flow away from brain parenchyma
- Also reduces 5-HT release at these blood vessels
- May cause inhibition of release of inflammatory neuropeptide around the affected vessels as well as extravasation of plasma proteins across dural vessels.
- Complete/significant relief is obtained within 2–3 hours in about three-fourths of patients
- Recurrence of headache noted in 20–40% of patients within 24 hours
- Advantage: Suppression of nausea and vomiting of migraine (unlike ergotamine accentuating these symptoms)

  Note: Restrict use of sumatriptan (or other triptans) to treatment of acute attacks of moderate to severe migraine which is not responding to analgesics or their combinations

Side Effect Profile

- Short lasting, but dose related side effects
  - Tightness in head and chest
  - Feeling of heat and other paresthesias in limbs
  - Weakness and dizziness

Contraindications

- Ischemic heart disease
- Hypertension
- Epilepsy
- Hepatic or renal impairment
- Pregnant women.

  d. Allopurinol in chronic gout

ANSWER

Chronic Gout

Pain and discomfort may be retained even in between sudden exacerbations or acute attack

Allopurinol in Chronic Gout

- A hypoxanthine analogue; competitively inhibits xanthine oxidase

- Preferred and standard therapy in chronic gout
- It is also used for hyperuricemic condition like tumor lysis syndrome, Lesch-Nyhan syndrome, and in post-transplant patients
- Its major metabolite, alloxanthine (oxypurine), is a noncompetitive inhibitor
- Alloxanthine is primarily responsible for uric acid synthesis inhibition in vivo
- While during administration, levels of uric acid are reduced and that of hypoxanthine and xanthine is slightly increased
  - Excretion of all three oxipurines in place of uric acid alone
  - Can be employed in both over-producers and under-excretors of uric acid
  - Thus, results in decreased uric acid levels in blood as well as urine
  - Due to raised levels of xanthine and hypoxanthine, feedback inhibition of de novo synthesis of purine and reuse of metabolically derived purine
- **Note:** Copious fluid intake is encouraged during allopurinol therapy.

4. Discuss the drug treatment of:

  a. Osteoporosis

ANSWER

For answer, refer 2016 paper-II Q. 4 (b), Pg. 212

  b. H. Pylori infection

ANSWER

For answer, refer 2015 paper-II Q. 4 (b), Pg. 227

PART-III

5. Write short notes on:

  a. Postantibiotic effect

ANSWER

Postantibiotic Effect (PAE)

- Term used to describe suppression of bacterial growth that persists after brief exposure of organisms to antimicrobials
- May pose a clinical effect on dose regimen of antimicrobials

- Aminoglycosides like gentamicin, fluoroquinolones like ofloxacin, and rifampin exhibit long and dose-dependent PAE
- When an organism is kept in an antibiotic free medium, multiplication begins again after a lag period which be determined by the organism as well as the antiomicrobial
- This lag interval in resumption of growth referred as "postantibiotic effect"
- This is the time needed to reachieve the logarithmic growth
- Usually calculated from the time needed to achieve a rise of tenfold in bacterial count in the culture for antibiotic exposed and unexposed tubes.

b. HAART

ANSWER

HAART in HIV

Stands for "highly active antiretroviral therapy"

- Antiretroviral therapy (ART) for AIDS is still evolving
- Better understanding of the biology of HIV infection and accessibility of various potent drugs has commanded HAART with combination of 3 or more drugs whenever indicated; monotherapy is contraindicated.
- It has been realized that even with HAART, few may survive within the resting CD4 lymphocytes and invariably cause relapse when treatment is discontinued despite no detectable viraemia and normal CD4 cell count for years
- HIV has very high rate of mutation; conferring resistance to one or the other antiretroviral drugs
- **Drug regimens:** It should always be HAART with at least three anti-HIV drugs
- Treatment with three drugs is considered optimal in treatment-naive patients
- Adding a fourth drug may be tried in failed patients only

NACO's Principles for Selecting First Line Regimens for Untreated Patients

- All regimens should have 2 NRTI+1NNRTI.
- Contain lamivudine in all regimens
- The other NRTI can be zidovudine or stavudine
- Choose one NNRTI from nevirapine or efavirenz
- Choose efavirenz in patients with hepatic dysfunction and in those concomitantly receiving rifampin. Efavirenz not to be used in pregnant women or likely to get pregnant.

c. Linezolid

ANSWER

Linezolid

Belongs to oxazolidinone group, beneficial to treat resistant Gram-positive coccal (both aerobic and anaerobic) and bacillary infections

- **Mechanism of action:** Mostly bacteriostatic; cidal activity exhibited against few streptococci, pneumococci, and *B. fragilis;* acts by inhibition of bacterial protein synthesis
- **Indications:**
  - Complicated or uncomplicated skin and soft tissue infections
  - Nosocomial or community pneumonias or bacteremias
  - Drug-resistant Gram-positive infections, etc.
- **Side Effect Profile**
  - Nausea and loose motions
  - Disturbances in taste and mild pain abdomen
  - Headache
  - Rash and pruritus
  - Oral/vaginal candidiasis
  - Blood related effects, like anemia and thrombocytopenia may occur on prolonged use, etc.

6. **Explain the rationale for the use of:**

a. **Mifepristone in termination of first trimester pregnancy**

(Ref: KD Tripathi, Essentials of Medical Pharmacology, 8th ed, pg. 345-46)

ANSWER

Mifepristone

- Possess antiprogestin action, when given during the follicular phase, leads to attenuation of the midcycle gonadotropin surge from pituitary which causes slowing of follicular development and delay/failure of ovulation
- A partial agonist and competitive antagonist at both A and B forms of PR

Rationale to Use in Terminating Pregnancy in First Trimester

- Progesterone acts on the endometrium to retain the lining for receiving and nourishing fertilized egg
- Acts on preventing secretory changes done by progesterone on uterus when given during the luteal phase
- It also blocks support of progesterone to the endometrium

○ It also stimulates uterine contractions

○ Sensitizing myometrium to PGs and menstrual bleeding is induced

○ To aid in terminating pregnancy, even if implantation occurs, blocking of decidualization and conceptus gets dislodged

○ Failing to production hCG, secondary luteolysis also occurs–decreasing endogenous progesterone secretion and softening of cervix

○ All these effects together lead to abortion.

b. Liposomal Amphotericin B in Leishmaniasis

(Ref: KD Tripathi, Essentials of Medical Pharmacology, 8th ed, pg. 839-40)

ANSWER

Liposomal Amphotericin B

It is one of the preparations of antifungal antibiotic

Rationale to Use Liposomal Amphotericin B in Leishmaniasis

○ It is used since leishmania is susceptible to this antibiotic; that has high affinity for ergosterol and acts by binding to it

○ Particularly suited for leishmaniasis because it delivers the drug inside the reticuloendothelial cells in spleen and liver where

○ the amastigotes live

○ AMB presently is the drug exhibiting highest cure rate in kala-azar

○ As per WHO, recommended as having higher preference over miltefosine

○ AMB forms the drug of choice in pregnant women and lactating women, but it is very expensive

○ Also beneficial in mucocutaneous leishmaniasis.

c. Clofazimine in lepra reaction

(Ref: KD Tripathi, Essentials of Medical Pharmacology, 8th ed, pg. 827)

ANSWER

Lepra Reaction

○ It is a Arthus (Jarisch Herxheimer) type of reaction which occurs when killing of bacilli results into release of antigens

○ Manifests as

- Enlargement of existing lesions, redness, swelling and pain

- New lesions may appear

- Malaise and fever, etc.

Rationale to Use Clofazimine in Lepra Reaction

○ Exerts leprostatic and anti-inflammatory actions

○ Antileprotic action of clofazimine exerted due to:

- Interfering with template function of DNA in *M.leprae*

- Changes in structure of membrane and its transport function

- Disrupting of mitochondrial electron transport chain

○ Dapsone-resistant *M. leprae* respond to clofazimine, after lag period of around 2 months

○ Also used in multidrug therapy of leprosy; due to its antiinflammatory property, it is beneficial in lepra reaction.

Your Roll No. ....

Name of the Paper : **Pharmacology Paper-I**

Name of the Course : **MBBS-2012**

Semester : **Annual**

Time: 3 Hours   M.M.: 40

INSTRUCTIONS

1. Write your Roll No. on the top immediately on receipt of this question paper
2. All questions are to be attempted
3. Answers to Parts I, II and III should be written in separate answer sheets provided
4. Attempt parts of a question in sequence

PART-I

1. **Explain why?**   [8]
    a. Beta blockers should not be stopped suddenly in a patient of angina pectoris
    b. Parenteral route of drug administration is not preferred for routine use
    c. Lorazepam is preferred over diazepam for treatment of status epilepticus
    d. Bupivacaine is preferred for epidural anesthesia during labour

2. **Enumerate opioid analgesics. Write the mechanism of action, uses and contraindications of morphine.**   [6]

PART-II

3. **Discuss the therapeutic status of:**   [8]
    a. Digoxin in congestive heart failure
    b. Pilocarpine in glaucoma
    c. Ethosuximide in epilepsy
    d. Amiodarone in arrhythmias

4. **Discuss the drug treatment of:**   [6]
    a. Severe bronchial asthma
    b. Insomnia

PART-III

5. **Discuss the therapeutic uses and adverse effects of:**   [6]
    a. High ceiling diuretics
    b. Angiotensin converting enzyme inhibitors

6. **Write short notes on:**   [6]
    a. Pharmacogenomics
    b. Essential drugs concept
    c. Factors modifying drug action

PART-I

1. **Explain why?**

   a. **Beta blockers should not be stopped suddenly in a patient of angina pectoris**

   (Ref: KD Tripathi, Essentials of Medical Pharmacology, 8th ed, pg. 597-98)

ANSWER

Beta Blockers

- Beta blockers lowers myocardial oxygen demand by reducing heart rate and blood pressure and reducing myocardial contractility
- Beta blockers exert their therapeutic effects in angina pectoris due to inhibition of beta1 receptor mediated stimulation of heart rate and myocardial contractility, which results in an enhanced oxygen supply-demand balance in the myocardium

Rationale Not to Suddenly Stop Use of Beta Blockers in a Patient of Angina Pectoris

- On abrupt discontinuation, there is a possibility of rebound effect and also a risk of precipitating arrhythmias, worsening angina, or even causing myocardial infarction
- Patients with ischemic heart disease may have exacerbation of angina or acute ischemic events
- Known as beta blocker withdrawal syndrome.

   b. **Parenteral route of drug administration is not preferred for routine use**

   (Ref: KD Tripathi, Essentials of Medical Pharmacology, 8th ed, pg. 13-14)

ANSWER

Parenteral Route of Drug Administration

- Parenteral route refers to administration of a drug by injection that takes the drug directly into the tissue fluid or blood without crossing the enteral mucosa
- Action is faster and surer

Rationale to Not Use Parenteral Route of Drug Administration Routinely

- The drug preparation has to be sterilized and is expensive
- Invasive and painful technique

- Other person is needed at most times (inulin may be self-injected)
- Possibilities of local tissue injury.

   c. **Lorazepam is preferred over diazepam for treatment of status epilepticus**

   (Ref: KD Tripathi, Essentials of Medical Pharmacology, 8th ed, pg. 428)

ANSWER

Lorazepam

- **Rationale to prefer lorazepam over diazepam for treatment of status epilepticus:**
  - Lorazepam is considered the benzodiazepine of choice for the initial treatment of seizures in view of its pharmacokinetic and safety profile
  - Better than intravenous diazepam or phenytoin for instantaneous control of status epilepticus
  - Exhibits more sustained action than that of diazepam
  - Better than diazepam in status epilepticus since it exhibits local thrombophlebitic complications
  - **Doses**: Initial dose should be 4 to 10 mg intravenously.

   d. **Bupivacaine is preferred for epidural anesthesia during labor**

   (Ref: KD Tripathi, Essentials of Medical Pharmacology, 8th ed, pg. 389)

ANSWER

Epidural Anesthesia

- LA injected acts primarily on nerve roots (both in the epidural and subarachnoid spaces to which it diffuses)
- Categorized into three categories based on the site of injection: thoracic, lumbar, and caudal
- More difficult than spinal anesthesia and larger drug volumes needed

Rationale to Prefer Bupivacaine during Labor

- Onset of anesthetic action is slower and duration of anesthesia is longer with bupivacaine
- This action can further be prolonged by adding adrenaline
- 0.25% bupivacaine helps to attain greatest separation between sensory and motor block

○ Particularly beneficial for obstetric purposes (participation in labor without feeling pain)
○ Also valuable for postoperative pain relief.

2. Enumerate opioid analgesics. Write the mechanism of action, uses and contraindications of morphine

ANSWER

Opioids

A broad group of pain-relieving drugs that work by interacting with opioid receptors in the body.

Classification of Opioids

○ **Natural opium alkaloids:** Morphine, Codeine
○ **Semisynthetic opiates:** Diacetylmorphine (Heroin), Pholcodine, Ethylmorphine
○ **Synthetic opioids:** Pethidine (Meperidine), Fentanyl, Methadone, Dextropropoxyphene, Tramadol

Note: Many opioids like, Hydromorphone, Oxymorphone, Hydrocodone, Oxycodone, Levorphanol, Dextromoramide, Dipipanone, Alfentanil, Sufentanil, Remifentanil, etc., are either not available or not used in India.

Mode of Action

○ **CNS:**
  ▪ Primarily interacts with the μ opioid receptor and imparts site specific depressant and stimulant actions in the CNS
  ▪ **Analgesia:**
    ♦ Better relief in nociceptive pain (due to stimulation of peripheral pain receptors) than neurotic pain (as in trigeminal neuralgia) which may occur due to inflammation or any damage to neural tissues or structures.
    ♦ Apprehension, fear, autonomic effects related to pain are also reduced suppression of pain perception
    ♦ Analgesic effect constitutes both spinal and supraspinal components
    ♦ 5-HT, NA, GABAergic, etc., neuronal systems seem to be involved in the action
  ▪ **Sedation:**
    ♦ Drowsiness and indifference to surroundings and one's own body
    ♦ No motor incoordination, ataxia, or excitement
  ▪ **Mood and subjective effects:**
    ♦ Loss of apprehension

♦ Lack of initiative
♦ Inability to concentrate

▪ **Respiratory center:** Depressant action on respiratory center dose dependently; this leads to decline in rate and tidal volume
▪ **Cough center:** Depressant action on cough center
▪ **Vasomotor center:** Depressed at high doses and results in a fall in BP
▪ **Temperature regulating center:** Hypothermia may occur
▪ **CTZ:** Sensitization of the CTZ to vestibular and other impulses; nausea and vomiting appear as side effcts
▪ **Edinger Westphal nucleus** of III nerve: Stimulant action leading to miosis. Intraocular tension is also reduced.
▪ **Vagal center:** Stimulant action, resulting in bradycardia.
▪ **Certain cortical areas and hippocampal cells:** Stimulant action; rigidity and immobility of muscles on exposure to high doses

○ **CVS:**
  ▪ Vasodilatation is caused due to: release of histamine release; depression of vasomotor center; decreased tone of blood vessels
  ▪ Decrease in peripheral resistance causes reduction in cardiac work; this is responsible for anti-ischemic effect of morphine
  ▪ Rise in intracranial tension

○ **Neuroendocrine:**
  ▪ Decreased hypothalamic influence on pituitary
    ♦ ↓FSH, LH, ACTH, sex hormones and cortisol (loss of libido, impotence and infertility in heavy abusers)
    ♦ ↑Prolactin and GH

○ **GIT:**
  ▪ Increase in tone and segmentation but decreased propulsive movements
  ▪ Spasmodic action on pyloric, ileocecal and anal sphincters
  ▪ Reduction in GI secretions
  ▪ Constipating effect

○ **Other Smooth Muscles:**
  ▪ **Urinary bladder:** Increase in tone of detrusor and sphincter muscle, results in urinary urgency and difficult micturition
  ▪ **Bronchi:** As morphine induce release of histamine, can cause bronchoconstriction.

Indications of Morphine

○ Relief of moderate to severe pain in both acute and chronic conditions

- Preoperative sedation and facilitation of induction of anesthesia
- Long-term treatment of terminally ill patients
- Acute pulmonary edema
- Obstetrical analgesia
- Antitussive in cough mixtures (preferentially codeine)
- MI related pain

Contraindications of Morphine

- Two extremes of age, infants and the elderly due to the respiratory depressant action of morphine
- **Patients with respiratory insufficiency (emphysema, pulmonary fibrosis, etc.):** Sudden deaths have been reported
- **Bronchial asthma:** An attack can be precipitated by its histamine releasing effect
- **Head injuries:** As mentioned earlier, retaining CO_2, it increases intracranial tension adding to that already caused by injury. Vomiting, miosis and altered mentation caused by morphine will restrict with assessment of improvement
- **Hypotensive states and hypovolemic cases:** Fall in BP may be exaggerated
- **Abdominal pain cases when diagnosis has not been established:** Biliary colic; inflamed appendix may even rupture
- **Elderly male:** Increased instances of urinary retention are reported
- Patients of hypothyroidism, liver and kidney disease, who may show high sensitivity to use of morphine.

PART-II

---

3. **Discuss the therapeutic status of:**

   a. **Digoxin in congestive heart failure**

   (Ref: KD Tripathi, Essentials of Medical Pharmacology, 8th ed, pg.129, 512, 517, 556)

ANSWER

Digoxin

- A cardiac glycoside with positive inotropic characteristics
- Suppresses the neurohormonal activation, thus very useful in chronic heart failure (systolic) patients
- Employed for long-term therapy

Mechanism of Action

Inhibits the Na-K adenosine triphosphatase (ATPase) pump at the cellular level

↓

Prevents Na-transport intracellularly to the extracellular space

↓

Effect on activity of Na-Ca

↓

Increased intracellular level of Ca, resulting in the inotropic effect of the drug.

Digoxin in CHF

- Systolic (ventricles are dilated, so adequate wall tension is not developed to eject sufficient quantity of blood) or diastolic dysfunction (ventricular filling is impaired, resulting in low cardiac output)
- Digoxin has properties to directly improve myocardial contractility as well as electrophysiological properties
- Moreover, it has vagomimetic action and alters sympathetic activity
- The filling pressure is increased and tissue perfusion demands are also fulfilled
- Thus, provides symptomatic relief in heart failure precipitated due to systolic dysfunction by reversing low ionotropic state of heart tissue.

   b. **Pilocarpine in glaucoma**

   (Ref: KD Tripathi, Essentials of Medical Pharmacology, 8th ed, pg. 108-09)

ANSWER

Pilocarpine in Glaucoma

- Acts as miotics
- Increase the tone of ciliary muscle and sphincter pupillae which pull on
- This improves alignment of the trabeculae, thus increased outflow facility, eventually fall in intraocular tension in case of open angle glaucoma
- Action is rapid and short lasting
- Effective in aphakic glaucoma
- Pilocarpine (with other drugs) is employed in angle closure glaucoma also
- Used to reverse the influence of mydriatics after refraction testing
- Helps in preventing formation of adhesions between iris and lens or iris and cornea, and even to break those which have formed due to iritis, corneal ulcer, etc.— alternated with a mydriatic.

   c. **Ethosuximide in epilepsy**

ANSWER

For answer, refer 2014 paper-I Q. 4 (b), Pg. 234

d. Amiodarone in arrhythmias

(Ref: KD Tripathi, Essentials of Medical Pharmacology, 8th ed, pg. 573)

ANSWER

Amiodarone in Arrhythmias

- Efficacious in a wide range of ventricular and supraventricular arrhythmias that includes PSVT, nodal and ventricular tachycardia, atrial fibrillation, etc.
- Most significant indications include resistant VT and recurrent VF
- Intravenous injection can rapidly terminate ventricular (VT and VF) and supraventricular arrhythmias
- Also employed to maintain sinus rhythm in AF after failure of other drugs
- Also suited for chronic prophylactic therapy since it has long duration of action
- In addition, long term use reduces sudden cardiac death
- Organ toxicity (pulmonary alveolitis and fibrosis, goiter, photosensitization, etc.) is caused; but its high and broad spectrum efficacy and relatively low proarrhythmic potential makes it among drugs most commonly employed in arrhythmias.

4. Discuss the drug treatment of:

a. Severe bronchial asthma

ANSWER

Status Asthmaticus

- Severe acute exacerbation of asthma
- Standard treatment in the emergency room:
  - Oxygen by mask
  - Measurement of peak expiratory flow
  - Beta agonists (inhalation) to relax and open airways
  - Steroids such as prednisone (oral or intravenous)
  - Anticholinergic drugs (inhalation)
- Other medicines that can be administered in a patient with acute episode:
  - Beta agonists, e.g., terbutaline (injection under skin)
  - Leukotriene modifiers, e.g., zafirlukast (oral)
  - Mg sulfate (intravenous)
- Intubation or ventilation if needed.

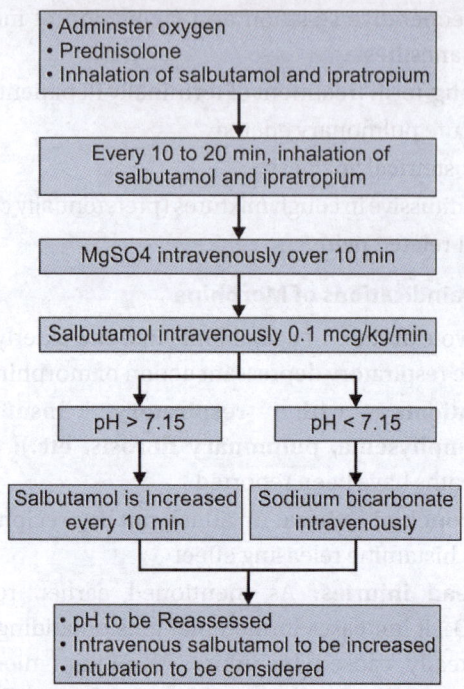

b. Insomnia

(Ref: KD Tripathi, Essentials of Medical Pharmacology, 8th ed, pg. 424)

ANSWER

Insomnia

Difficulty in falling asleep or staying asleep, even when a person has the chance to do so

Drug Treatment of Different Types of Insomnia

- Chronic insomnia (sleeplessness > 3 weeks)
  - Use of hypnotics in this is not well advocated
  - Obstructive sleep apnea patients exhibit poor sleep and feel sleepy during the day
  - However, all hypnotics worsen sleep apnoea and thus contraindicated
  - Use of a hypnotic intermittently, for example once in every 3 days may be tried
  - Slowly eliminated drugs preferred since rebound insomnia and withdrawal symptoms are very less marked
- Short-term insomnia (sleeplessness 3 to 21 days)
  - General causes include emotional problem (occupational stress, etc.) and physical illness|
  - Usually a hypnotic, without residual effects to be chosen
  - In elderly, short acting drugs are preferred
  - Use of hypnotic intermittently for 2 to 3 weeks
- Transient insomnia (sleeplessness 1 to 3 days)
  - It may be due to changes in the sleep circumstances, for examples, overnight train journey,

new place, unusual pattern of work, shift workers, intercontinental travel–jetlag, etc.

- A hypnotic that is rapidly eliminated or one with prominent distribution is preferred to escape residual effects the next morning.

PART-III

5. Discuss the therapeutic uses and adverse effects of:

a. High ceiling diuretics

ANSWER

For answer, refer 2015 paper-I 5 (b) (Furosemide), Pg. 219

b. Angiotensin converting enzyme inhibitors

(Ref: KD Tripathi, Essentials of Medical Pharmacology, 8th ed, pg. 530-35)

ANSWER

Therapeutic Uses

- **Treatment of hypertension:** All grades of essential and renovascular hypertension
- **Treatment of heart failure:** Along with non-potassium-sparing diuretics and, where appropriate digitalis
- **Prevention of symptomatic heart failure:** In asymptomatic patients with left ventricular dysfunction, retarding development of symptomatic heart failure, and also reduces hospitalization for heart failure

Adverse Effects

- **Gastrointestinal disorders:** Very common is nausea, commonly seen other adverse effects are diarrhoea, abdominal pain, alteration in taste
- **Blood and the lymphatic system disorders:** Anemia (uncommon; including aplastic and hemolytic); rarely seen are neutropenia, decreased hemoglobin, decreased hematocrit, thrombocytopenia, agranulocytosis
- **Nervous system and psychiatric disorders:** Headache and depression are common; uncommonly confusion, somnolence, insomnia, paresthaesia, vertigo
- **Eye disorders:** Very commonly occurring is blurred vision
- **Cardiac and vascular disorders:** Dizziness very commonly occurs; common: hypotension (including orthostatic hypotension), syncope, chest pain

- **Respiratory disorders:** Cough and dyspnea, sore throat and hoarseness uncommonly seen
- **Skin:** Rash, hypersensitivity/angioneurotic edema
- **General:** Fatigue.

6. Write short notes on:

a. Pharmacogenomics

(Ref: KD Tripathi, Essentials of Medical Pharmacology, 8th ed, pg. 75)

ANSWER

Pharmacogenomics

Defined as the use of genetic information to guide the choice of drug and dose on an individual basis

- **Significance:**
  - Aims to recognize individuals who are either more likely or less likely to respond to a drug, also including those who need altered dose of certain drugs
  - Defining the genetic basis of an individual's profile of drug response and predicting most suited treatment option for the individual
- Goal is "personalized medicine" on a wide scale
- In case of most drugs, a constant variation with bell-shaped Gaussian frequency distribution is perceived
- **Examples of some specific genetic defects which may result into discontinuous variation in drug responses:**
  - G-6PD deficiency is responsible for hemolysis with primaquine and other oxidizing drugs; more commonly seen in the Mediterranean, African and Southeast Asian races
  - Severe toxicity of 5-fluorouracil occurring in patients with dihydropyrimidine dehydrogenase (DPD) deficiency, etc.

b. Essential drugs concept

(Ref: KD Tripathi, Essentials of Medical Pharmacology, 8th ed, pg. 6)

ANSWER

Essential Drugs

- As per WHO, "those that satisfy the priority healthcare needs of the population. They are selected with due regard to public health relevance, evidence on efficacy and safety, and comparative cost effectiveness

○ These drugs are intended to be accessible within any functioning health systems setting at all times and in sufficient amounts, in appropriate dosage forms, with assured quality and adequate information, and at an affordable cost that can be easily paid by the individual and community

Significance

○ Improved availability of medicines, cost saving and optimum utilization of drugs

○ WHO criteria for guiding selection of an essential medicine.

 ▪ Adequate data on its efficacy and safety should be available from clinical studies

 ▪ It should be available in a form in which quality, including bioavailability, and stability on storage can be assured

 ▪ Its choice should depend upon pattern of prevalent diseases; availability of facilities and trained personnel; financial resources; genetic, demographic and environmental factors

 ▪ In case of two or more similar medicines, choice should be made on the basis of their relative efficacy, safety, quality, price and availability. Cost-benefit ratio should be a major consideration

 ▪ Choice may also be influenced by comparative pharmacokinetic properties and local facilities for manufacture and storage

 ▪ Most essential medicines should be single compounds

 ▪ Selection of essential medicines should be a continuous process which should take into account the changing priorities for public health action, epidemiological conditions as well as availability of better medicines/formulations and progress in pharmacological knowledge

 ▪ Recently, it has been emphasized to select essential medicines based on rationally developed treatment guidelines

○ A *National Essential Drugs List* has been provided by India in 1996 and revised in 2011 with the title "*National List of Essential Medicines*," including 348 medicines.

 c. Factors modifying drug action

Answer

Factors Modifying Drug Action

Physiological Factors

○ **Age**

 ▪ In children and neonates, there is ↓ gastric acid secretion, ↓ liver microsomal enzymes (glucuronyl transferase), ↓ plasma protein binding, ↓ GFR and tubular secretion, which affects drug action

 ▪ In elderly, there is ↓ kidney function, so gentamycin, digoxin, penicillins are contraindicated

○ **Sex**

 ▪ Testosterone increases the rate of biotransformation of drugs

 ▪ Decreased metabolism of some drugs in female (Diazepam)

○ **Pregnancy**

 ▪ Lipophilic drugs cross placental barrier & slowly excreted.

○ Body weight

○ Lactation

○ Food

 ▪ For example, presence of gastric juices or even food particles may interfere with drug absorption, in some cases.

Pathological Factors

○ Diseases may cause individual variation in drug response

○ Impaired liver microsomal enzymes- ↓ Diazepam-rifampicin-theophylline

Genetic Factors

Existence in a population of two or more phenotype with respect to the drug effect. For example, acetylation enzymes deficiency

Environmental Factors

Smokers metabolize drugs more rapidly than nonsmokers

Interaction with Other Drugs

Defined as condition in which a substance (usually another drug) affects the activity of a drug when both are administered together; may be additive as well as negative

○ Combination of amoxicillin with clavulanic acid inhibits species like, *B. fragilis* and *Branhamella catarrhalis*, that do not respond to amoxicillin given alone; also improved tolerance

○ Oral contraceptive failure can occur in patients treated with antitubercular chemotherapy.

Your Roll No. ....

Name of the Paper	:	**Pharmacology Paper-II**
Name of the Course	:	**MBBS-2012**
Semester	:	**Annual**

Time: 3 Hours   M.M.: 40

INSTRUCTIONS

1. Write your Roll No. on the top immediately on receipt of this question paper
2. All questions are to be attempted
3. Answers to Parts I, II and III should be written in separate answer sheets provided
4. Attempt parts of a question in sequence

PART-I

1. **Explain why?**   [8]
    a. Tetracyclines should not be administered to children
    b. Low dose of ritonavir is combined with other protease inhibitors like indinavir, saquinavir
    c. Toxicity of methotrexate cannot be overcome by folic acid
    d. Antimotility drug diphenoxylate is combined with atropine

2. **Classify corticosteroids. Discuss the mechanism of action, therapeutic uses and adverse effects of prednisolone.**   [6]

PART-II

3. **Discuss the therapeutic status of:**   [8]
    a. Metformin in diabetes
    b. Mefloquine in malaria
    c. Amphotericin B in fungal infections

4. **Describe the drug treatment of:**   [6]
    a. Diabetic ketoacidosis
    b. Osteoporosis

PART-III

5. **Write short notes on:**   [6]
    a. Desferrioxamine
    b. Tocolytic agents
    c. Radioactive iodine

6. **Explain the rationale for the use of:**   [6]
    a. Ondansetron in chemotherapy induced vomiting
    b. Estrogen in combination with progesterone as HRT in post-menopausal women
    c. Fixed dose combination of trimethoprim and sulfamethoxazole
    d. Indomethacin for closure of patent ductus arteriosus at birth

PART-I

1. **Explain why?**

   a. **Tetracyclines should not be administered to children**

   (Ref: KD Tripathi, Essentials of Medical Pharmacology, 7th ed, pg. 736, 8th ed, pg. 784-7

ANSWER

Tetracyclines

Primarily bacteriostatic; works by inhibiting protein synthesis.

Rationale to Not Administer Tetracycline in Children

○ Tetracyclines exhibit chelating property; thus gets chelated to calcium present in developing teeth and bones

○ Resultant calcium-tetracycline chelate deposit in developing teeth and bone

○ This would affect deciduous teeth and cause ill-formed, brown discoloration of teeth, increased susceptibility to caries if given during midpregnancy to 5 months of extrauterine life

○ Crowns of permanent anterior dentition are affected if administered between 3 months and 6 years of age

○ Temporary suppression of bone growth can occur if administered during late pregnancy or childhood

○ Prolonged use can result in height reduction and deformities.

   b. **Low dose of ritonavir is combined with other protease inhibitors like indinavir, saquinavir**

   (Ref: KD Tripathi, Essentials of Medical Pharmacology, 7th ed, pg. 810, 8th ed, pg.865)

ANSWER

Ritonavir

○ An HIV protease inhibitor that works by hindering with the reproductive cycle of HIV

   ▪ Also cause inhibition of cytochrome P-450 CYP3A

   ▪ It is a cytochrome P450 3A inhibitor and a potent protease inhibitor

Rationale to Combine Low Dose Ritonavir with Other PIs like Indinavir and Saquinavir

○ Usually employed in a low dose (dose of 100 mg twice daily) so as to boost other PIs including indinavir and saquinavir

○ Though it can be used alone as antiretroviral drug in a dose of 600 mg twice daily

○ Prominent drug interactions, and adverse effects such as nausea, diarrhea, paresthesias, fatigue and lipid abnormalities.

   c. **Toxicity of methotrexate cannot be overcome by folic acid**

   (Ref: KD Tripathi, Essentials of Medical Pharmacology, 7th ed, pg. 611, 8th ed, pg. 657)

ANSWER

Methotrexate

○ Used for treatment of rheumatoid arthritis and leukemia; also acts as teratogen that causes severe abnormalities on developing fetuses

○ Methotrexate is a competitive inhibitor of dihydrofolate reductase, which is the enzyme used to make folic acid

○ Thus, hypothesized that an increase in FA will overcome the inhibitory effects of methotrexate

Rationale to Not Use Folic Acid in Methotrexate Toxicity

○ Folinic acid is an active coenzyme form which does not require to be reduced by DHFRase before it can act

○ Methotrexate acts as a DHFRase inhibitor

○ Thus, antagonized by folinic acid but not counteracted by folic acid

○ This is the reason exogenous FA cannot be used as a mechanism to overcome the teratogenic effects of methotrexate.

   d. **Antimotility drug diphenoxylate is combined with atropine**

   (Ref: KD Tripathi, Essentials of Medical Pharmacology, 8th ed, pg. . 686)

ANSWER

Diphenoxylate

- Synthetic opioid, chemically related to pethidine; used particularly as constipating agent
- Action is similar to codeine
- **Dose:** Diphenoxylate (2.5 mg) + atropine (0.025 mg)

Rationale to Combine with Atropine

- This drug is systemically absorbed and crosses blood-brain barrier, thus CNS effects occur
- Atropine is combined in subpharmacological dose to discourage abuse by use of several tablets
- Caution to be exercised as overdose will result in disturbing atropinic side effects
- Response is more variable in children, thus contraindicated below 6 years of age
- **Note:** Due to these adverse effects, loperamide greatly superseded it.

---

2. **Classify corticosteroids. Discuss the mechanism of action, therapeutic uses and adverse effects of prednisolone.**

(Ref: KD Tripathi, Essentials of Medical Pharmacology, 7th ed, pg. 288, 8th ed, pg.306)

ANSWER

Classification of Corticosteroids

- **Functional classification:**
  - **Glucocorticoids:** Regulate carbohydrates, lipids, and proteins metabolism, e.g., hydrocortisone
  - **Mineralocorticoids:** Control electrolytes and water balance, e.g., aldosterone
- **Based on duration of action:**
  - **Short-acting:** Hydrocortisone, cortisone, fludrocortisone
  - **Intermediate-acting:** Methyl-prednisolone, prednisolone, triamcinolone
  - **Long-acting:** Betamethasone, dexamethasone.

Pharmacological Actions of Glucocorticoids

- **Carbohydrate and protein metabolism:**
  - Promoting gluconeogenesis and glycogen deposition (in liver)
  - Inhibition of peripheral glucose utilization by tissues
  - Increased release of glucose from liver
  - Breakdown of proteins and mobilization of amino acids, thus can cause muscle wasting, etc.

- **Fat metabolism:**
  - Promote lipolysis due to glucagon, growth hormone, adrenaline, and thyroxine
  - Redistribution of fat in body: fats lost by extremities gets deposited over face, neck and shoulder
  - Characteristic feature producing "moon face", "buffalo hump", and "fish mouth"
- **Calcium metabolism:**
  - Inhibition of intestinal absorption
  - Enhancement of renal excretion of calcium
- **Water excretion:**
  - Enhancement of secretory activity of renal tubules
- **Cardiovascular system:**
  - Maintain tone of arterioles and contractility of myocardium
  - Restriction of capillary permeability, etc.
- **Skeletal muscles:**
  - Excessive action of mineralocorticoid leads to hypokalemia, and eventually weakness
  - Excessive action of glucocorticoid cause wasting of muscles and myopathy, leading to weakness
- **Central nervous system:**
  - Mild euphoria when administered with pharmacological doses
  - Level of sensory perception and neurons excitability maintained
- **Stomach:**
  - Increase in secretion of gastric acid and pepsin
- **Lymphoid tissue and blood cells:**
  - Increase in the number of RBCs, neutrophils, and platelets
  - Lymphocytes, eosinophils and basophils are decreased
- **Inflammatory responses:**
  - Suppression of inflammation
  - **All stages of inflammation:** Raised capillary permeability, exudation, etc. all are tempered
- **Immunological and allergic responses:**

Allergies and hypersensitivity reactions are subdued

Indications Learn Pneumonic: (CORTICOSTE)

- **C:** Collagen disorders
- **O:** Osteoarthritis
- **R:** Rheumatoid arthritis
- **T:** Thyroid storm
- **I:** Intestinal disease (Ulcerative colitis, Crohn's disease)
- **C:** Cerebral edema
- **O:** Organ transplantation

- **S:** Skin disorders and allergic reactions
- **T:** Testing functioning of adrenal pituitary axis
- **E:** Eye diseases
- **R:** Rheumatic fever
- **O:** Other lung diseases, bronchial asthma
- **I:** Inflammatory and infective diseases; and immunosuppression
- **D:** Dermatitis (Atopic)
- **S:** Septic shock

Side Effects

- Central obesity, supraclavicular hump, characteristic rounded face and narrow mouth (Cushing's habitus)
- Purple striae on thighs and lower abdomen
- Skin becomes fragile
- Weakness in muscles
- Hyperglycemia
- **Hirsutism:** Unwanted growth of coarse hairs in women (male pattern)

- Wound healing is deferred
- Osteoporosis in vertebrae and other flat spongy bones
- Bleeding and perforation of peptic ulcers may occur
- Children may exhibit growth retardation when given for long periods
- Glaucoma may also develop, etc.

Therapeutic Uses

- Used to treat certain types of allergies, inflammatory conditions, and autoimmune disorders
- Some of conditions include rheumatoid arthritis, dermatitis, asthma, adrenocortical insufficiency, inflammation in the eyes, multiple sclerosis, etc.
- It can be used as oral dose, intravenously, as skin preparations, and eye drops
- Used for long-term treatment of asthma and to control severe exacerbations of asthmatic attack with inhaled steroids

Adverse Effects

• Blood and lymphatic system disorders	• Leukocytosis
• Immune system disorders	• Increased susceptibility and severity of infections with suppression of clinical symptoms and signs, opportunistic infections, recurrence of dormant tuberculosis
• Endocrine disorders	• Cushingoid facies, growth suppression in infancy, hirsutism, impaired carbohydrate tolerance with increased requirement for antidiabetic therapy, suppression of the hypothalamo-pituitary adrenal axis, and weight gain
• Metabolism and nutrition disorders	• Hypokalaemic alkalosis, potassium loss, sodium and water retention.
• Psychiatric disorders	• Marked euphoria leading to dependence; aggravation of epilepsy, behavioural disturbances, irritability, nervousness, anxiety, sleep disturbances, and cognitive dysfunction
• Nervous system disorders	• Intracranial pressure with papilloedema in children (pseudotumour cerebri) usually after treatment withdrawal
• Eye disorders	• Corneal or scleral thinning, scleral perforation, papilledema
• Cardiac disorders	• Risk of congestive heart failure in susceptible cases
• Vascular disorders	• Hypertension, thromboembolism
• Gastrointestinal disorders	• Abdominal distension, dyspepsia, nausea, increased appetite, oesophageal candidiasis, oesophageal ulceration, peptic ulceration with perforation and hemorrhage
• Skin and subcutaneous tissue disorders	• Acne, bruising, impaired healing, purple striae
• Musculoskeletal and connective tissue disorders	• Muscle weakness, wasting and loss of muscle mass.
• Renal and urinary disorders	• Nocturia, scleroderma renal crisis (frequency unknown).
• General disorders and administration site conditions	• Hypersensitivity including anaphylaxis, malaise.

PART-II

3. **Discuss the therapeutic status of:**

   a. **Metformin in diabetes**

ANSWER

For answer, refer 2015 paper-II, Q. 2, Pg. 224

   b. **Mefloquine in malaria**

(Ref: KD Tripathi, Essentials of Medical Pharmacology, 7th ed, pg. 824, 8th ed, pg. 876)

ANSWER

Mefloquine in Malaria

○ Effective against CQ-sensitive as well as resistant plasmodia

○ Fever can be controlled by a single dose (15 mg/kg) and circulating parasites in infections caused by *P. falciparum* or *P. vivax* in partially immune as well as nonimmune individuals eliminated

○ Does not exhibit gametocidal activity, even vivax hypnozoites are not killed

○ Subsequently, relapses occur in vivax malaria

○ Also acts as efficacious suppressive prophylactic for multiresistant *P. falciparum* and other types of malaria

○ Effective drug for multiresistant *P. falciparum*

○ Employed in prophylaxis of malaria among travellers to areas with multidrug resistance

○ **Mechanism of Action**
   ▪ It induces morphological changes produced in the intraerythrocytic parasite behaves like quinine and CQ induced changes
   ▪ It also get accumulated in infected RBCs, binds to heme and this complex damages membranes of the parasite

○ **Adverse Effect Profile**
   ▪ Bitter taste
   ▪ Dizziness
   ▪ Nausea, vomiting, and diarrhoea
   ▪ Abdominal pain, sinus bradycardia and Q-T prolongation

○ Safe in pregnancy, but should be avoided in first trimester unless completely essential

   Note: To be taken with plenty of water after meals.

   c. **Amphotericin B in fungal infections**

(Ref: KD Tripathi, Essentials of Medical Pharmacology, 8th ed, pg. 839

ANSWER

Amphotericin B in Fungal Infections

○ High affinity for ergosterol present in fungal cell membrane exerted by polyenes, thus exerting antifungal activity

○ Cholesterol that is present in host cell membranes, closely resembles ergosterol and so polyenes bind to it as well with somewhat lesser affinity

○ Do not affect bacteria as they do not have sterol

○ Active against extensive range of yeasts and fungi, including *Candida albicans, Histoplasma capsulatum, Cryptococcus neoformans, Blastomyces dermatitidis, Coccidioides immitis, Torulopsis, Rhodotorula, Aspergillus, Sporothrix,* etc.

○ Acts as fungicidal at high and static at low levels

○ Also active on various species of *Leishmania*, a protozoan

○ Administered orally for intestinal candidiasis without systemic toxicity

○ Extensive distribution in the body, but poor penetration in CSF

○ Given orally (50–100 mg QID) for intestinal moniliasis; also employed topically in vaginitis, otomycosis, etc.

4. **Describe the drug treatment of:**

   a. **Diabetic ketoacidosis**

(Ref: KD Tripathi, Essentials of Medical Pharmacology, 7th ed, pg. 267, 8th ed, pg. 290)

ANSWER

Diabetic Ketoacidosis

○ Acute major complication of diabetes, frequently occurring in type 1 diabetics, but infrequent in type 2 diabetics

○ Most common precipitating reason is infection; others include trauma, stroke, pancreatitis, stressful conditions and insufficient doses of insulin

○ Cardinal biochemical features of diabetic ketoacidosis are mentioned below:

Cardinal biochemical features	
• Plasma glucose	• >250 mg/dL
• Arterial pH	• <7.30
• Serum bicarbonate level	• <15 mEq/L
• Hyperketonemia	• >3 mmol/L
• Ketonuria	• >2+on std urine sticks

Drug Treatment

- **Insulin:**
  - Regular insulin employed to promptly rectify the metabolic abnormalities
  - Decline in blood glucose level by 10% per hour can be considered suitable response
  - Infusion is maintained until the patient gets fully conscious and routine therapy with subcutaneous insulin is set up
- **Intravenous fluids**
  - Vital for correcting dehydration
  - Normal saline intravenously infused
  - Once BP and heart rate stabilize, satisfactory renal perfusion is assured, change over to ½N saline
  - Glucose is also required for restoring the depleted hepatic glycogen
- **KCl**
  - During DKA, serum K+ is generally normal due to exchange with intracellular stores
  - Ketosis subsides after insulin therapy is instituted, but dangerous hypokalemia can precipitate
- **Sodium bicarbonate**
  - Routinely needed; acidosis subsides as control on ketosis is achieved
  - Bicarbonate infusion is continued gradually till blood pH rises above 7.2
- **Phosphate**
  - When serum phosphate is in the low normal range, infusion of 5–10 m mol/hr of sod./pot. Phosphate
- **Antibiotics**
  - Supportive measures and management of precipitating cause must be employed simultaneously.

  b. **Osteoporosis**

ANSWER

For answer, refer 2016 paper-II Q. 4 (b), Pg. 212

PART-III

5. **Write short notes on:**

   a. **Desferrioxamine**

   (Ref: KD Tripathi, Essentials of Medical Pharmacology, 7th ed, pg. 907, 8th ed, pg. 966)

ANSWER

Desferrioxamine

- Yielded from removal of iron from the iron complex ferrioxamine
- Exhibits very high affinity for iron; 1g able to chelate 85 mg of elemental iron
- Removes loosely bound iron and also from hemosiderin and ferritin
- Iron from hemoglobin or cytochrome is spared
- It also has property to show low affinity for calcium
- **Therapeutic uses:**
  - **Acute iron poisoning:** Life-saving in most children; forms most important indication
  - **Transfusion siderosis:** This occurs in thalassemia patients due to receiving repeated blood transfusion and leading to iron overload
- Desferrioxamine 0.5–1 g/day intramuscular helps in excreting the chronic iron overload
- **Adverse effect profile**
  - Fall in BP
  - Flushing
  - Abdominal pain and loose stools
  - Itching
  - Urticaria and rashes
  - Changes in lens and retina on repeated use.

   b. **Tocolytic agents**

ANSWER

Tocolytic Agents

- Drugs which reduce uterine motility
- Employed to delay or postpone labor, stop threatened abortion, and in dysmenorrhea

Examples Include:

- **Adrenergic agonists**
  - *Ritodrine*, exerts prominent uterine relaxant action
  - Permitted to subdue premature labour and to delay delivery in case of conditions like some exigency or acute fetal distress
  - Treatment beyond 48 hours is not recommended
- **Calcium channel blockers**
  - Since Ca_{2+} ions influx plays an important role in uterine contractions, Ca^{2+} channel blockers decrease myometrium tone and oppose contractions
  - At times, apprehension of fetal hypoxia due to reduced placental perfusion
- **Oxytocin antagonist**
  - Example include atosiban, peptide analog of oxytocin
  - Cause suppression of premature uterine contractions and postpone preterm delivery
- **Magnesium sulfate**
  - Acts as a tocolytic by contending with Ca^{2+} for entry into myometrium via both voltage sensitive as well as ligand gated Ca^{2+} channels

○ **Miscellaneous drugs**

- Ethyl alcohol, nitrates, indomethacin, progesterone, general anesthetics
- Halothane, effective uterine relaxant used as the anesthetic when external or internal version is attempted.

c. **Radioactive Iodine**

(Ref: KD Tripathi, Essentials of Medical Pharmacology, 8th ed, pg. 277)

ANSWER

Radioactive Iodine

○ 127I is the stable isotope of iodine

○ X-rays as well as β particles emitted by 131I

○ X-rays used in tracer studies by traversing the tissues and can be monitored by a counter, while the latter are used for their damaging effect on thyroid cells

○ Administered as sodium salt of 131I dissolved in water and to be taken orally

Uses

○ Used as diagnostic 25 to 100 μ curie; counting done at intervals

○ Therapeutic use in *hyperthyroidism* due to Graves' disease or toxic nodular goiter. Around 20 to 40% patients need one or more repeated doses

○ Used as palliative therapy after thyroidectomy in cases of metastatic carcinoma of thyroid

Merits

○ Simple, cost-effective, and convenient line of treatment

○ No surgical risk, no scar or damage to parathyroid glands/recurrent laryngeal nerves

○ Permanent cure once control on hyperthyroidism

Demerits

○ Hypothyroidism may be observed in about 5 to 10% patients of Graves' disease

○ Long latent period of response

○ Fetal thyroid will be destroyed leading to cretinism, thus contraindicated during pregnancy

○ Not suited for young patients.

6. **Explain the rationale for the use of:**

a. **Ondansetron in chemotherapy induced vomiting**

https://www.sciencedirect.com/topics/neuroscience/chemotherapy-induced-nausea-and-vomiting

ANSWER

Ondansetron

○ Developed to cater vomiting associated to chemotherapy/radiotherapy

- Used in Vomiting induced by cisplatin and other highly emetogenic drugs employed in cancer chemotherapy
- Also useful in postoperative nausea and vomiting; administered 4 h before surgery
- Used in cases of acute vomiting than delayed vomiting

○ **Mechanism of action:** Peripheral 5-HT3 receptor blockade on vagal afferents in GIT, including nucleus tractus solitarius (NTS) and chemoreceptor trigger zone (CTZ)

○ Vomiting induced by cisplatin and other highly emetogenic drugs employed in cancer chemotherapy

Rationale to use Ondansetron in Chemotherapy Induced Vomiting

○ Nausea mediated through the autonomic nervous system and vomiting mediated by stimulating vomiting center that receives input from neuronal pathways including CTZ, peripheral stimuli from the GI tract, cortical pathways, vestibular labyrinthine apparatus of the inner ear

○ Neurotransmitters include muscarinic, dopamine (D2), serotonin (5-HT3), neurokinin-1 (NK-1), histamine (H1)

○ Emesis results due to release of neurotransmitters (including serotonin) from intestinal enterochromaffin cells

○ Ondansetron acts as effective antiemetic agent due to providing control of vomiting by blocking neurochemical 5-HT3 receptor and thus inhibiting stimulation of the CTZ

○ **Dose:** 0.15 mg/kg q8h to max. of 8 mg.

b. **Estrogen in combination with progesterone as HRT in postmenopausal women**

(Ref: KD Tripathi, Essentials of Medical Pharmacology, 8th ed, pg. 334-36)

ANSWER

Introduction

Cessation of ovarian function at menopause leads to several physical, psychological and emotional consequences in postmenopausal women

Rationale to Use Estrogen in Combination with Progesterone as HRT

- Estrogen in combination with progestin employed in HRT (also known as menopausal hormone therapy) is highly effective in suppressing the perimenopausal syndrome of vasomotor instability and psychological disturbances

- Also provides prevention against atrophic changes and osteoporosis

- Also, estrogen seize genital and dermal atrophic changes

- Promote resolution of vulval and urinary problems

- Estrogen alone to be used in hysterectomised women and if a progestin is not tolerated or contraindicated.

c. Fixed dose combination of trimethoprim and sulfamethoxazole

ANSWER

Rationale to Combine Trimethoprim and Sulfamethoxazole

- Fixed dose combination of trimethoprim and sulfamethoxazole; referred as *cotrimoxazole*

- **Trimethoprim:** A diaminopyrimidine (associated to pyrimethamine) which selectively inhibits bacterial dihydrofolate reductase (DHFRase)

- Both sulfonamide and trimethoprim are bacteriostatic when used alone, but the combination acts cidal against many organisms

- Maximum synergism noticed in cases when even if an organism is moderately resistant to any one component, the action of the other (exhibiting sensitivity) may be enhanced

- Both have approximately the same half-life (~10 hour)

- Increased antibacterial spectra of the combination when compared to trimethoprim and sulfonamides independently

- Further organisms covered by the combination are— *Salmonella typhi, Serratia, Klebsiella, Enterobacter, E. coli, H. influenza, Yersinia enterocolitica, Pneumocystis jiroveci,* and many sulfonamide-resistant strains of *Staph. aureus,* etc.

- Resistance to the combination is slow as matched to either drug use alone.

d. Indomethacin for closure of patent ductus arteriosus at birth

ANSWER

Introduction

Pharmacological closure by indomethacin is customary if symptoms of PDA are not controlled adequately with fluid restriction and diuretics

Rationale to Use Indomethacin for Closure of Patent Ductus Arteriosus

- Prostaglandins are synthesized in the body when arachidonic acid is freed from lipid storage by phospholipase A_2

- Prostaglandins play a crucial role in the pathophysiology of PDA

- That is why inhibition of the production of these vasoactive substances forms mainstay of pharmacologic approaches

- Indomethacin is a prostaglandin inhibitor (holds true for ibuprofen also)

- It can enter the COX hydrophobic channel, competes with arachidonic acid for binding to the catalytic site, and hindering prostaglandin production

- Thus, helps achieve desired patency of ductus arteriosus and thus used in prophylaxis and treatment of PDA (by its closure).

Your Roll No. ....

Name of the Paper	:	**Pharmacology Paper-I**
Name of the Course	:	**MBBS-2011**
Semester	:	**Annual**

Time: 3 Hours   M.M.: 40

INSTRUCTIONS

1. Write your Roll No. on the top immediately on receipt of this question paper
2. All questions are to be attempted
3. Answers to Parts I, II and III should be written in separate answer sheets provided
4. Attempt parts of a question in sequence

PART-I

1. **Explain why?**   [8]

   a. Inhaled beclomethasone in not a broncho dilator but is used for the treatment of bronchial asthma

   b. Dopamine and not adrenaline is preferred for treatment of cardiogenic shock

   c. Pseudoephedrine and not ephedrine is used as a nasal decongestant

   d. Carvedilol is used in the treatment of hypertension

2. **Enumerate anti cholinergic drugs. Discuss their uses giving specific example. Write the adverse effects of atropine.**   [6]

PART-II

3. **Discuss the therapeutic status of:**   [8]

   a. Fenofibrate in the treatment of hypercholesterolemia

   b. Acetylcysteine in paracetamol poisoning

   c. Alprazolam in anxiety disorder

   d. Olanzapine in schizophrenia

4. **Discuss the drug treatment of:**   [6]

   a. Congestive cardiac failure

   b. Generalized tonic-clonic-seizures

PART-III

5. **Discuss the therapeutic uses and adverse effects of:**   [6]

   a. Enalapril

   b. Physostigmine

6. **Write short notes on:**   [6]

   a. Dissociative anesthesia

   b. Agonist and inverse agonist

   c. Fixed dose drug combination

PART-I

1. Explain why?

a. Inhaled beclomethasone in not a bronchodilator but is used for the treatment of Bronchial asthma

(Ref: KD Tripathi, Essentials of Medical Pharmacology, 7th ed, pg. 230, 8th ed, pg.250)

ANSWER

Inhaled Beclomethasone

- Glucocorticoids having high topical but low systemic actions
- Low systemic activity is due to poor absorption as well as prominent first pass metabolism

Rationale to Use in Treatment of Bronchial Asthma despite being a Bronchodilator

- Inhaled beclomethasone (steroids) cause suppression of bronchial inflammation
- Thus they increase peak expiratory flow rate, and chances of acute episodic asthma is reduced
- Airways inflammation is seen even in early mild disease as well, and there is start of bronchial remodelling
- This makes it significant to use inhaled beclomethasone to reduce this inflammation
- Since it do not cause any bronchodilation, not used in an acute attack or status asthmaticus
- Patients who are on oral steroid and need to be switched, inhaled steroid are given before additionally for 1 to 2 weeks before tapering doses of oral steroid to prevent withdrawal symptoms
- Currently inhaled steroids are not considered cases with mild and episodic asthma.

b. Dopamine and not adrenaline is preferred for treatment of Cardiogenic shock

(Ref: KD Tripathi, Essentials of Medical Pharmacology, 8th ed, pg. 146)

ANSWER

Dopamine

A dopaminergic (D1 and D2) as well as adrenergic α and b_1 (but not b_2) agonist

Mechanism of Action

- D1 receptors located in renal and mesenteric blood vessels are the most sensitive ones; dilatation of these vessels is caused even by small intravenous doses due to increase in intracellular cAMP
- Glomerular filtration rate is increased
- Exerting natriuretic effect (by D1 receptors) on PT cells
- Only large doses can cause vasoconstriction

Rationale for Using Dopamine but Not Adrenaline in Cardiogenic Shock

- *Due to its high sensitivity of D1 receptors on renal mesenteric vessels, there is resultant rise in BP and urine outflow*
- Increase in cardiac output and systolic BP but less effect on diastolic BP
- Exerts no CNS effects as it does not penetrate blood-brain barrier
- *Adrenaline is a sympathomimetic drug*
- The main *drawback* of the sympathomimetic drugs in cardiogenic shock is *that they produce extensive peripheral vasoconstriction*
- This is why, dopamine is preferred but not adrenaline.

c. Pseudoephedrine and not ephedrine is used as a nasal decongestant

(Ref: KD Tripathi, Essentials of Medical Pharmacology, 8th ed, pg. 134, 149

ANSWER

Rationale to Use Pseudoephedrine but Not Ephedrine as Nasal Decongestant

- Ephedrine mainly acts indirectly but exerts some direct action also on alpha and beta receptors
- Thus causing increased heart rate and BP, on repeated injections produce tachyphylaxis
- Also causes bronchodilation but less efficacious than epinephrine
- It also lacks selectivity, and efficacy is low
- Pseudoephedrine is a stereoisomer of ephedrine
- It particularly produces vasoconstriction in mucosae and skin, but a poor bronchodilator
- Because of this, it is taken orally as a decongestant which affects upper respiratory tract, nose and Eustachian tubes

○ Thus, symptomatic relief is provided in common cold, allergic rhinitis, blocked eustachian tubes and infection of upper respiratory tract after combining with antihistaminics, mucolytics, antitussives, etc.

○ Instead, ephedrine has been employed in mild chronic bronchial asthma.

d. Carvedilol is used in the treatment of hypertension

(Ref: KD Tripathi, Essentials of Medical Pharmacology, 7th ed, pg. 151, 8th ed, pg. 165)

ANSWER

Carvedilol

A $\beta_1 + \beta_2 + \alpha_1$ adrenoceptor blocker

Mechanism of Action

Vasodilatation is produced due to α_1 blockade, also including calcium channel blockade, and has antioxidant property

Rationale to Use in Treating Hypertension

○ Vasodilatation is caused, hence helps lowering blood pressure

○ It is a mild antihypertensive

○ All drugs, irrespective of related properties, have nearly equal effect

○ Considered as first choice drugs because of good patient acceptability and cardioprotective potential

○ It plays a protective role in CHF.

---

2. **Enumerate anti cholinergic drugs. Discuss their uses giving specific example. Write the adverse effects of atropine.**

ANSWER

Classification of Anticholinergic Drugs

(Ref: KD Tripathi, Essentials of Medical Pharmacology, 7th ed, pg. 113, 118, 8th ed, pg. 124-132)

○ *Natural alkaloids* Atropine, Hyoscine (Scopolamine)

○ *Semisynthetic derivatives* Homatropine, Atropine methonitrate, Hyoscine butylbromide, Ipratropium bromide, Tiotropium bromide

○ *Synthetic compounds*
- *Mydriatics:* Cyclopentolate, Tropicamide
- *Antisecretory-antispasmodics*:
  - *Quaternary compounds:* Propantheline, Oxyphenonium, Clidinium, Pipenzolate methylbromide, Isopropamide, Glycopyrrolate

- *Tertiary amines:* Dicyclomine, Valethamate, Pirenzepine
- *Vasicoselective:* Oxybutynin, Flavoxate, Tolterodine
- *Antiparkinsonian:* Trihexyphenidyl (Benzhexol), Procyclidine, Biperiden.

○ **Note:** Many drugs of other classes, including, tricyclic antidepressants, phenothiazines, antihistamines and disopyramide exhibit significant antimuscarinic actions

Therapeutic Uses

As Antisecretory

Preanesthetic Medication

○ Administration of anticholinergics (atropine, hyoscine, glycopyrrolate) with ether made it mandatory to check increased salivary and tracheobronchial secretions as it was an irritant

○ With halothane etc., the need has decreased

○ Laryngospasm is also prevented by atropinic drugs. Also prevents vasovagal attack during anesthesia

Peptic Ulcer

○ Decrease in gastric secretion by affecting fasting and neurogenic phase, but little effect on gastric phase, thus symptoms of peptic ulcers are relieved

Pulmonary Embolism

○ Reduce pulmonary secretions induced reflexly by embolism

For Checking Excessive Sweating or Salivation,

For example, parkinsonism

As Antispasmodic

○ **Intestinal and renal colic, abdominal cramps:**
- If no mechanical obstruction exists, relief is provided
- Atropine is less efficacious in biliary colic

○ No use in infective diarrhea, can be helpful in nervous, functional and drug induced diarrhoea

○ **Spastic constipation, irritable bowel syndrome:** Symptomatic relief is modest

○ Providing relief in urinary urgency and frequency

○ Partial suppression of gastritis, pylorospasm, gastric hypermotility, gastritis, and nervous dyspepsia

As Mydriatic and Cycloplegic

○ **Diagnostic use:**
- Mydriasis and cycloplegia both are required, for testing error of refraction
- Only mydriatic action needed to facilitate fundoscopy

- **Iritis, iridocyclitis, choroiditis, keratitis and corneal ulcer:** Provides rest to the intraocular muscles and cuts down painful spasm

For Central Action

- **Parkinsonism:** Used in mild cases or adjuvant to levodopa, as well as in drug induced extrapyramidal syndromes
- **Motion sickness:** Hyoscine is most effective drug for motion sickness. Not useful in other types of vomiting
- **Lie detector:** Hyoscine possess amnesic and depressant action

As Cardiac Vagolytic

- Used in some cases of myocardial infarction and digitalis toxicity

PART-II

3. Discuss the therapeutic status of:

a. Fenofibrate in the treatment of hypercholesterolemia

(Ref: KD Tripathi, Essentials of Medical Pharmacology, 7th ed, pg. 639, 8th ed, pg. 685)

ANSWER

Fenofibrate

A PPAR-alpha agonist; second generation prodrug fibric acid derivative

- Indicated for the treatment of hypertriglyceridemia and mixed dyslipidemia
- Approved for the treatment of hypercholesterolemia, lipid abnormalities commonly observed in patients at high risk of cardiovascular disease, including Type 2 diabetes and/or metabolic syndromes
- Possess superior HDL–CH raising and superior LDL-CH lowering action than other fibrates
- Considered apt as an adjunctive drug in patients with raised LDL-CH levels in addition to increased triglyceride levels
- There is no increase in LDL-CH in patients with high triglycerides concentrations
- Most suitable fibrate to be used in combination to statin
- **Side effect profile:**
  - Myalgia (Pain in muscles)
  - Hepatitis and rashes
  - Rarely seen are cholelithiasis and rhabdomyolysis
- **Dose recommended:** 200 mg once daily with meals.

b. Acetylcysteine in paracetamol poisoning

ANSWER

For answer, refer 2014 Paper-II Q. No. 1(c), Pg 237

c. Alprazolam in anxiety disorder

(Ref: KD Tripathi, Essentials of Medical Pharmacology, 8th ed, pg. 494)

ANSWER

Alprazolam

Highly potent anxiolytic benzodiazepine

- Additionally, some mood elevation is also part of action spectrum in mild depression
- Particular indication is anxiety associated with depression
- Panic disorders along with severe anxiety also show good response
- Withdrawal symptoms may manifest more when discontinued than other BZDs
- Like other benzodiazepines, to be used in the least possible dose
- Response to acute anxiety is better than chronic anxiety
- If larger doses have been used, dose should be tapered gradually before withdrawing
- Generally, 1/2 to 2/3 of daily dose is given at bed time, rest is divided in 2 to 3 doses given at daytime

d. Olanzapine in schizophrenia

ANSWER

For answer, refer 2017 paper-I Q. 5 (b), Pg 191

4. Discuss the drug treatment of:

a. Congestive cardiac failure

(Ref: KD Tripathi, Essentials of Medical Pharmacology, 8th ed, pg. 561-68)

ANSWER

Goals of Drug Treatment in CHF and Drugs Employed

- To provide relief of congestive/low output symptoms and restore cardiac performance
  - *Inotropic drugs*—Digoxin, dobutamine/dopamine, amrinone/milrinone
  - *Diuretics*—Furosemide, thiazides
  - *RAS inhibitors*—ACE inhibitors/ARBs

- *Vasodilators*—hydralazine, nitrate, nitroprusside
- β *blocker*—Metoprolol, bisoprolol, carvedilol, Nebivolol

○ To allow arrest/reversal of disease progression and prolong survival
- *ACE inhibitors/ARBs*, β *blockers*
- *Aldosterone antagonist*—Spironolactone, eplerenone

Rest and Salt Restriction are Significant Nonpharmacological Measures

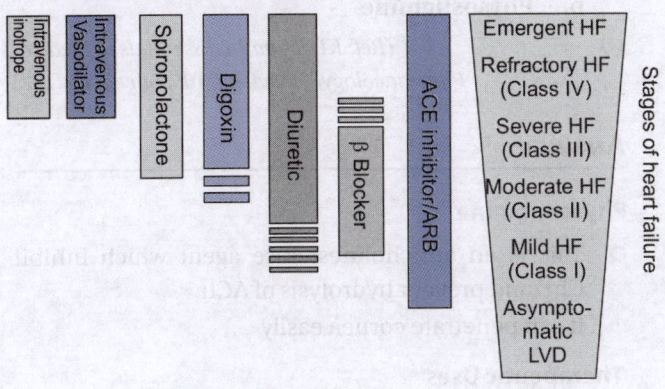

Fig. Drugs used in heart failure

Diuretics

○ Used to treat most symptomatic cases of CHF
○ High-ceiling diuretic are preferred, later metola-zone/spironolactone added to counter resistance if develops
○ Disease progression not affected, but symptoms improve
○ In mild heart failure: ACE inhibitors/ARBs ± β blockers to provide survival benefit, + Diuretics for symptom relief

Renin-angiotensin System (RAS) Inhibitors

○ These include ACE inhibitors and ARBs which form sheet anchor in CHF
○ They cause vasodilatation, retard/prevent ventricular hypertrophy, myocardial cell apoptosis, fibrosis, remodelling, etc. thus disease modifying advantages as well as symptom relief
○ Mild to severe cases and asymptomatic systolic dysfunction are all benefited

Vasodilators

○ *Nitrates* helps by reducing ventricular end-diastolic pressure and volume (preload reduction)
○ Affords rapid symptom relief in acute left ventricular failure
○ Employed in increased central venous pressure and dilated cardiomyopathy

○ *Hydralazine* works by dilation of resistance vessels and reduction of aortic impedance (afterload reduction)
○ When given alone, both hydralazine or nitrate not proven beneficial in the treatment of chronic heart failure; however, supplement each other when combined

β-adrenergic Blockers

○ Most useful in mild to moderate (NYHA class II, III) cases of dilated cardiomyopathy with systolic dysfunction
○ Not used in decompensated patients
○ **Note:** To be stopped during acute heart failure episode

Aldosterone Antagonist (Include Spironolactone, Eplerenone)

○ Indicated in moderate-to-severe CHF as add-on to ACE inhibitors + other drugs
○ Disease progression is retarded

Sympathomimetic Inotropic Drugs

○ **Dobutamine:** Preferred drug given intravenously in acute heart failure accompanied by myocardial infarction; in cardiac surgery
○ **Dopamine:** Preferred in cardiogenic shock due to MI and other causes
○ Not employed in long-term treatment as tolerance develops.

b. **Generalized tonic-clonic-seizures**

(Ref: KD Tripathi, Essentials of Medical Pharmacology, 8th ed, pg. 451)

ANSWER

Generalized Tonic-clonic Seizures (GTCS)

○ **Alternative names:** Major epilepsy, grand mal epilepsy
○ This is the most common type
○ An attack lasts 1–2 minutes

Drug Treatment

- **First line:** Carbamazepine, phenytoin
- **Second line:** Valproate, phenobarbitone
- **Add-on drugs:** Lamotrigine, gabapentin, topiramate, levetiracetam

○ Initiate with a single drug, low dose is preferred
○ Dose is increased gradually to maximum tolerated dose
○ Substitute with another drug, if desired effect not achieved

○ If alternative drugs are to be instituted, combine drugs with different mechanisms of action

Tonic–Clonic Seizures
• **First-Line agents**
▪ Valproic acid
▪ Lamotrigine
▪ Topiramate
• **Alternative agents**
▪ Zonisamide
▪ Phenytoin
▪ Carbamazepine
▪ Oxcarbazepine
▪ Phenobarbital
▪ Primidone
▪ Felbamate

PART-III

5. Discuss the therapeutic uses and adverse effects of:

a. Enalapril

(Ref: https://www.medicines.org.uk/emc/product/562/smpc)

ANSWER

Enalapril

An angiotensin converting enzyme inhibitors

Therapeutic Uses

○ **Treatment of hypertension:** All grades of essential and renovascular hypertension

○ **Treatment of heart failure:** Along with non-potassium-sparing diuretics and, where appropriate digitalis

○ **Prevention of symptomatic heart failure:** In asymptomatic patients with left ventricular dysfunction, retarding development of symptomatic heart failure, and also reduces hospitalization for heart failure

Adverse Effects

○ **Gastrointestinal disorders:** Very common is nausea, commonly seen other adverse effects are diarrhoea, abdominal pain, alteration in taste

○ **Blood and the lymphatic system disorders:** Anemia (uncommon; including aplastic and hemolytic); rarely seen are neutropenia, decreased hemoglobin, decreased hematocrit, thrombocytopenia, agranulocytosis

○ **Nervous system and psychiatric disorders:** Headache and depression are common; uncommonly confusion, somnolence, insomnia, paresthaesia, vertigo

○ **Eye disorders:** Very commonly occurring is blurred vision

○ **Cardiac and vascular disorders:** Dizziness very commonly occurs; common: hypotension (including orthostatic hypotension), syncope, chest pain

○ **Respiratory disorders:** Cough and dyspnea, sore throat and hoarseness uncommonly seen

○ **Skin:** Rash, hypersensitivity/angioneurotic edema

○ **General:** Fatigue.

b. Physostigmine

(Ref: KD Tripathi, Essentials of Medical Pharmacology, 7th ed, pg. 105, 8th ed, pg. 122)

ANSWER

Physostigmine

○ This is an anticholinesterase agent which inhibit ChE and prevent hydrolysis of ACh

○ It can penetrate cornea easily

Therapeutic Uses

○ Used as miotic drops to decrease intraocular pressure in glaucoma

○ Breaking adhesions between cornea and iris, alternating with mydriatic drops

○ Belladonna poisoning and phenothiazine poisoning

○ Used to antagonize mydriatic effect of atropine

○ **Alzheimer's disease:** Presenile or senile dementia.

Adverse Effects

○ Gastric side effects are nausea, vomiting and hyperperistalsis

○ **Diaphoresis:** Excessive salivation occurs

○ Nervous effects include hallucinations and seizure

○ **Circulatory system:** Bradycardia and cardiovascular collapse

○ **Respiratory system:** Occurrence of wheezing, bronchospasm and dyspnea

○ **Eye:** Excessive watery eyes and decreased pupil size.

6. Write short notes on:

a. Dissociative anesthesia

(Ref: KD Tripathi, Essentials of Medical Pharmacology, 8th ed, pg. 411))

ANSWER

Dissociative Anesthesia

This is a type of anesthesia marked by catalepsy, catatonia, profound analgesia, and amnesia with light sleep

○ Loss of consciousness does not necessarily be present, and thus not always indicate state of general anesthesia

○ Examples of dissociative anesthetics include ketamine and phencyclidine

○ This state is produced by interfering with the transmission of incoming sensory signals to the cerebral cortex and also interfering with interaction between different parts of the central nervous system

Characteristics of Patients

○ Patient appears to be conscious, i.e., eyes opening, swallowing movements can be made, and stiff muscles

○ Sensory stimuli cannot be processed

○ Patient appears to be dissociated from his body and surroundings

○ Non-purposive movements of limbs occur

○ In up to 50% of cases, emergence delirium, hallucinations and involuntary movements at the time of recovery.

    b. Agonist and inverse agonist

(Ref: KD Tripathi, Essentials of Medical Pharmacology, 8th ed, pg. 49))

ANSWER

For answer, refer 2013 paper-I Q. 6 (b), Pg. 248

    c. Fixed dose drug combination

ANSWER

Fixed Dose Drug Combinations

○ Pharmaceutical preparations containing two or more drugs in a fixed dose ratio

○ **Merits:**

- **Convenience and better patient compliance:** All the components compiled in the FDC may actually needed by the patient. Cost-effective than both/all the components administered separately.

- **Synergistic combinations:** For example, amoxicillin + clavulanic acid, combination oral contraceptives, isoniazid + rifampin

- Additive therapeutic effects of two components while the side effects being different may not: The FDC components should act by different mechanisms, e.g., amlodipine + atenolol in hypertension

- Counteraction of side effect of one component by the other: For example, thiazide + potassium sparing diuretic

- Extreme significance in the treatment of tuberculosis, HIV-AIDS and falciparum malaria: As a single drug is not being administered.

○ **Demerits:**

- The patient is subjected to additional side effects and expense if all components are not required

- Dose of most drugs cannot be adjusted and individualized.

- Different time course of action of the components but administered at same intervals

- Adverse effects cannot be easily ascribed to the particular drug responsible for it

- Contraindication to any one component will lead to contraindication to the whole combination.

Name of the Paper	:	**Pharmacology Paper-II**
Name of the Course	:	**MBBS-2011**
Semester	:	**Annual**

Time: 3 Hours   M.M.: 40

INSTRUCTIONS

1. Write your Roll No. on the top immediately on receipt of this question paper
2. All questions are to be attempted
3. Answers to Parts I, II and III should be written in separate answer sheets provided
4. Attempt parts of a question in sequence

PART-I

1. **Explain why?**   [8]
   a. Multi drug therapy is advocated for the management of *H. Pylori* infection
   b. Low dose aspirin is administered in myocardial infarction
   c. Aminoglycoside antibiotics should be avoided in patients with myasthenia gravis
   d. Sulphonylureas are not useful in management of Type I diabetes mellitus

2. **Enumerate Beta lactam antibiotics. Discuss the mechanism of action, therapeutic uses, adverse effects and drug interactions of imipenem.**   [6]

PART-II

3. **Give the rationale for the use of**   [8]
   a. Ergotamine in postpartum hemorrhage
   b. Combination of antitubercular drugs in Tuberculosis
   c. Inhaled corticosteroids in bronchial asthma
   d. Fstro-progestin combination in contraceptives

4. **Discuss the drug treatment of:**   [6]
   a. Osteoporosis
   b. Chemotherapy induced anemia

PART-III

5. **Discuss the therapeutic status of:**   [6]
   a. Alteplase in myocardial infarction
   b. Artemisinin in malaria
   c. Aromatase inhibitor in breast cancer

6. **Write short notes on:**   [6]
   a. Cross resistance
   b. Tocolytic agents
   c. HAART in HIV

PART-I

1. Explain why?

a. Multi drug therapy is advocated for the management of *H. pylori* infection

ANSWER

H. pylori Infections

○ Most peptic ulcer disease occurs due to *H. Pylori*

○ Treatment aims at eradicating organisms to promote ulcer healing and recurrence risk as well as complications

Rationale to Multidrug Therapy in Management of *H. pylori* Infections:

○ Developing resistance to antimicrobials is the chief issue with *H. pylori* infections

○ Antimicrobial resistance along with incomplete treatment constitute to treatment failure

○ Thus, for eradicating organism and complete treatment, multidrug regimen and adequate duration of therapy become very significant

○ Continued multidrug therapy helps to overcome problem of antimicrobial resistance

○ Treatment continues for 2 weeks and is considered effective and reliable.

b. Low dose aspirin is administered in myocardial infarction

ANSWER

Aspirin

○ Cardio-protective effects are mediated through irreversible inhibition of platelet COX-1 and subsequent blockade of the production of TXA2, reducing thrombus formation

○ Prolongation of bleeding time is induced to last for 5–7 days

Low Doses of Aspirin is Used as an Antiplatelet Agent

○ Effects of aspirin at any given time are influenced by the aspirin doses as well as plasma exposure and rate of platelet renewal in body

○ Doses as low as 40 mg/day affects platelet aggregation

○ In the clinical settings, aspirin is used at doses from 75 to 1500 mg/day. Daily doses at or below 162 mg are usually referred as "low-dose" aspirin

○ Maximal inhibition of platelet function occurs at 75–150 mg aspirin given per day

○ Also at low doses, there is possibility of selective suppression of TXA2 formation, whereas higher doses (>900 mg/day) may cut both TXA2 and PGI2 production.

c. Aminoglycoside antibiotics should be avoided in patients with myasthenia gravis

ANSWER

Myasthenia Gravis

It an autoimmune disorder of neuromuscular transmission that involves synthesis of autoantibodies directed against the nicotinic AChR

Rationale to Avoid Aminoglycoside Antibiotics in Myasthenia Gravis

○ This class of antibiotics is associated with neuro-muscular transmission abnormalities, irrespective of administered by any route

○ Action via an extensive range of pre- and post-synaptic mechanisms

○ Aminoglycosides by impairing neuromuscular transmission, produce clinically significant weakness; thus exacerbating the symptoms of myasthenia gravis

○ Out of certain drugs like, amikacin, gentamicin, kanamycin, neomycin, netilmicin, streptomycin, and tobramycin, neomycin appears to be the most potent in interfering with neuromuscular transmission, whereas tobramycin to be the least noxious.

d. Sulphonylureas are not useful in management of Type I diabetes mellitus

(Ref: KD Tripathi, Essentials of Medical Pharmacology, 8th ed, pg. 295-97)

ANSWER

Sulfonylureas

These drugs cause blood glucose lowering in normal subjects and in type 2 DM, but not in type 1 DM

○ Primary drugs of this antidiabetic class include glibenclamide (glyburide), gliclazide, glipizide, and glimepiride

Rationale why Sulphonylureas cannot be Used to Treat Type 1 DM

○ This class is an insulin secretagogues, means they work by causing the body to secrete insulin

○ They exert their hypoglycemic effects by stimulating insulin secretion from the pancreatic β-cell

○ There is closure of ATP-sensitive K-channels in the β-cell plasma membrane

○ Thus initiate a chain of events resulting into insulin release

○ On the other hand, type 1 DM occurs due to autoimmune destruction of beta-cells

○ Thus, *the beta-cells which are the target cells for sulphonylureas are absent in type 1 diabetics*

○ This is the reason, direct administration of insulin forms drug of choice in these patients.

---

2. Enumerate Beta lactam antibiotics. Discuss the mechanism of action, therapeutic uses, adverse effects and drug interactions of Imipenem.

ANSWER

Beta-lactam Antibiotics

○ Antibiotic class of drugs with a beta-lactam ring in structure

(Ref: KD Tripathi, Essentials of Medical Pharmacology, 8th ed, pg. 731)

Classification

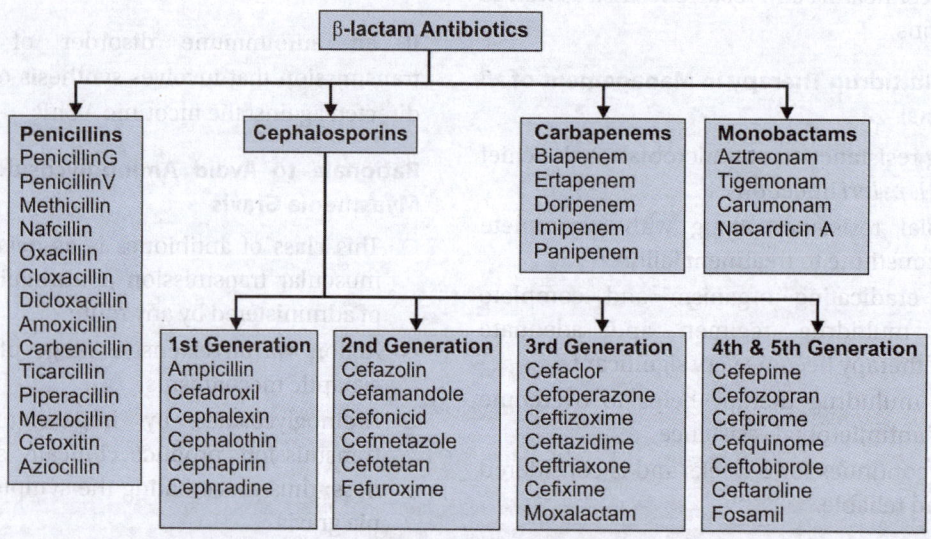

Fig. Classification of beta lactam antibiotics

Imipenem

A thienamycin derivative

○ An extremely potent and broad-spectrum β-lactam antibiotic

Mechanism of Action

○ It exerts bactericidal activity by inactivating the penicillin-binding proteins (PBP) and result in cell wall lysis, or interfering with formation of cell wall

○ Due to the capability of binding to a specific PBP (PBP-1), lead to more rapid lysis related to other beta-lactams

○ Hence, greater bactericidal activity and extensive postantibiotic effect

Therapeutic Uses

○ Severe hospital-acquired (nosocomial infections) respiratory, abdominal, urinary, pelvic, and skin and soft tissue infections

○ Patients in neutropenia, cancer and AIDS included

○ *Pseudomonas aeruginosa* infections

Drug Interactions

○ Imipenem undergoes rapid hydrolysis by the enzyme dehydropeptidase I, which is located on the brush border of renal tubular cells

○ Cilastatin (a reversible inhibitor of dehydropeptidase I)

○ Thus, it protects imipenem from hydrolysis

○ Combination of imipenem-cilastatin 0.5 g intravenously every 6 hour is effective in a wide range of conditions

○ For treating *Ps. aeruginosa* infections, should be combined with gentamicin.

Adverse Effects

○ Can induce seizures at larger doses and in predisposed patients

○ Diarrhea, very commonly seen

○ Vomiting

○ Skin rashes

○ Other hypersensitivity reactions.

PART-II

3. Give the rationale for the use of:

a. Ergotamine in postpartum hemorrhage

ANSWER

Ergotamine

Belongs to a group of drugs ergot alkaloids

Mechanism of Action

○ Works by partial agonist and antagonist action at α adrenergic and all subtypes of 5-HT$_1$ and 5-HT$_2$ receptors

Ergotamine in Postpartum Hemorrhage (PPH)

○ Uterotonics are used to prevent PPH during the third stage of labor

○ Oxytocin is recommended, but in settings if it is not available, ergotamine can be used

○ This drug produces continued and sustained vasoconstriction and contraction of visceral smooth muscle

○ It has specific action on uterus; contractions are tetanic and do not resemble normal physiological contractions, unlike oxytocin

○ It has moderate onset and long duration of action

■ Since the spasms are very powerful, therefore should not be used before delivery; should be used only to control late uterine bleeding.

b. Combination of antitubercular drugs in tuberculosis

ANSWER

For answer, refer 2016 paper-II Q. 1 (b), Pg. 209

c. Inhaled corticosteroids in bronchial asthma

(Ref: KD Tripathi, Essentials of Medical Pharmacology, 8th ed, pg. 230-31)

ANSWER

Inhaled corticosteroids

○ For example, beclomethasone, having high topical but low systemic actions

○ Low systemic activity is due to poor absorption as well as prominent first pass metabolism

Rationale to Use in Treatment of Bronchial Asthma

○ Inhaled steroids cause suppression of bronchial inflammation

○ Thus they increase peak expiratory flow rate, and chances of acute episodic asthma is reduced

○ Airways inflammation is seen even in early mild disease as well, and there is start of bronchial remodelling

○ This makes it significant to use inhaled beclomethasone to reduce this inflammation

○ Since it do not cause any bronchodilation, not used in an acute attack or status asthmaticus

○ Patients who are on oral steroid and need to be switched, inhaled steroid are given before additionally for 1 to 2 weeks before tapering doses of oral steroid to prevent withdrawal symptoms

○ Currently inhaled steroids are not considered cases with mild and episodic asthma.

d. Estro-progestin combination in contraceptives

(Ref: KD Tripathi, Essentials of Medical Pharmacology, 8th ed, pg. 345)

ANSWER

Rationale to Employ Estro-progestin Combination in Contraceptives

○ Progestin has potent antiovulatory action

○ When used alone, inhibitory dose for ovulation (per day) is estimated to be: levonorgestrel 60 µg, desogestrel 60 µg, norgestimate 200 µg

○ To attain complete 100% assurance, amount in the pill is 2 to 3 times higher

○ Both estrogens and progestins synergistic effect for inhibiting ovulation

○ Also, progestin confirms prompt bleeding at the end of a cycle and decrease risk of endometrial carcinoma which may develop due to the estrogen use

○ Normal cycle of 28 days has been maintained by customizing doses

○ **Dosing Regimen of Combined Oral Pill:**

■ One tablet to be taken daily for 21 days, this starts on the day 5 of menstruation

■ Next course begins after a gap of 7 days when bleeding occurs

■ Newer generations pills have improved action profile with reduced side effects but no compromise with efficacy.

4. Discuss the drug treatment of:

a. Osteoporosis

ANSWER

For answer, refer 2016 paper-II Q. 4 (b), Pg. 212

b. Chemotherapy induced anemia

(Ref: KD Tripathi, Essentials of Medical Pharmacology, 8th ed, pg. 933)

ANSWER

Patients with Cancer Receiving Chemotherapy Often Develop Anemia

○ Particularly, platinum-based chemotherapy caused reduction in production of the bone marrow-stimulating hormone erythropoietin

○ Frequent in lung cancers and gynecological malignancy, in part due to the fact that they require platinum-based regimens

Drug Treatment

○ Transfusion of packed red blood cells:
  ▪ Ideal for patients requiring rapid correction of anemia
  ▪ Affords a rapid surge in hemoglobin and hematocrit levels
  ▪ Transfusion of 1 unit of packed red blood cells estimated to lead to an increase in the hemoglobin level of 1 g/dl in a normal-sized adult

○ Administration of erythropoiesis-stimulating agents (ESAs), with or without iron supplementation:
  ▪ In patients receiving chemotherapy/radiotherapy, ESA therapy to be started at Hb levels of 9 to 11 g/dL based on the symptoms severity of symptoms
  ▪ Hb concentration to achieve is 12 to 13 g/dL for improving quality of life and avoid the need for RBC transfusions
  ▪ Therapy is associated to long-term gains
  ▪ **Note:** To be instituted only until target Hb is achieved, as risks of thromboembolic events are increased, when Hb levels exceed 14 g/dL.

PART-III

5. Discuss the therapeutic status of:

a. Alteplase in myocardial infarction

(Ref: KD Tripathi, Essentials of Medical Pharmacology, 8th ed, pg. 674-75)

ANSWER

Alteplase in Myocardial Infarction

○ Used to lyse thrombi/clot to recanalize blocked blood vessels (mainly coronary artery), thus significantly employed in subjects with myocardial infarction

○ It work by activating the natural fibrinolytic system

○ Therapeutic action profile than prophylactic

○ Produced from human tissue culture by using recombinant DNA technology, it shows moderate specificity to fibrin-bound plasminogen, thus lowering circulating fibrinogen only by around 50%

○ An accelerated regimen is used in cases of myocardial infarction; 15 mg bolus intravenous injection followed by 50 mg over 30 minutes, then 35 mg administered over the next 1 hour

○ Heparin coadministration is often required

○ Can also be used for ischemic stroke and pulmonary embolism.

b. Artemisinin in malaria

(Ref: KD Tripathi, Essentials of Medical Pharmacology, 8th ed, pg. 886)

ANSWER

For answer, refer 2015 paper-II Q. 1 (a), Pg. 223

c. Aromatase inhibitor in breast cancer

ANSWER

For answer, refer 2014 paper-II Q. 3 (a), Pg. 238

6. Write short notes on:

a. Cross resistance

(Ref: KD Tripathi, Essentials of Medical Pharmacology, 8th ed, pg. 744)

ANSWER

Cross Resistance

○ This is defined as attainment of resistance to one antimicrobial agent conferring resistance to another antimicrobial, to which the organism has not even been exposed

○ More commonly observed between drugs that are chemically or mechanistically related

Complete Cross Resistance

○ Resistance to any one sulfonamide means resistance to others, or resistance to one tetracycline means insensitivity to all drugs of this class.

Partial Cross Resistance

○ Unrelated drugs show this type of cross resistance, for example, tetracyclines and chloramphenicol

- At times, resistance to one aminoglycoside may not extend to other, e.g. strains resistant to gentamicin may respond to amikacin
- Cross resistance may be two-way, for example, between erythromycin and clindamycin and *vice versa*
- At times, it is one-way, for example, development of neomycin resistance by enterobacteriaceae makes them unresponsive to streptomycin but various streptomycin- resistant organisms persist vulnerable to neomycin.

b. **Tocolytic agents**

(Ref: KD Tripathi, Essentials of Medical Pharmacology, 8th ed, pg. 358-59)

ANSWER

For answer, refer 2012 paper-II Q. 5 (b), Pg. 268

c. **HAART in HIV**

(Ref: KD Tripathi, Essentials of Medical Pharmacology, 8th ed, pg. 868)

ANSWER

For answer, refer 2013 paper-II Q. 5 (b), Pg. 254

Your Roll No. ....

Name of the Paper : **Pharmacology Paper-I**

Name of the Course : **MBBS-2010**

Semester : **Annual**

Time: 3 Hours   M.M.: 40

INSTRUCTIONS

1. Write your Roll No. on the top immediately on receipt of this question paper
2. All questions are to be attempted
3. Answers to Parts I, II and III should be written in separate answer sheets provided
4. Attempt parts of a question in sequence

PART-I

1. **Explain why?**   [8]
   a. Spironolactone in use in the treatment of heart failure
   b. Ropinirole in used in the treatment of Parkinsonism
   c. Morphine should not be administered to patients with undiagnosed abdominal pain
   d. The subcutaneous route of drug administration is unsuitable in a patient of shock

2. **Classify sedative-hypnotic drugs. Explain the mechanism of action, adverse effects and therapeutic uses of diazepam.**   [6]

PART-II

3. **Discuss the therapeutic status of:**   [8]
   a. Erythropoietin in anemia
   b. Sumatriptain in migraine
   c. Aspirin in dengue fever
   d. Oximes in insecticide poisoning

4. **Describe the drug treatment of:**   [6]
   a. Glaucoma
   b. Manic depressive illness

PART-III

5. **Describe the drug treatment of:**   [6]
   a. Acute left ventricular failure
   b. Warfarin overdosage

6. **Explain the rationale use of the following:**   [6]
   a. Aspirin in myocardial infarction
   b. Bromhexine in cough
   c. Sulfasalazine in rheumatoid arthritis

PART-I

1. Explain why?

a. Spironolactone in use in the treatment of heart failure

(Ref: KD Tripathi, Essentials of Medical Pharmacology, 7th ed, pg. 520, 8th ed, pg. 567-68)

ANSWER

Spironolactone

- A potassium sparing diuretic
- Diuretics form important modality of treatment in symptomatic CHF
- Disease process is not influenced by diuretic therapy
- Diuretics (high-ceiling) are used in CHF for following purposes:
  - Reduce circulating volume and ventricular efficiency is improved
  - Mobilize edema fluid and pulmonary congestion is relieved

Rationale to Use Spironolactone in CHF

- Despite providing symptom relief in CHF by regulating volume overload, resistance may develop in cases where furosemide is used; this can be overcome by use of spironolactone
- Serum potassium concentration is improved, and thus counter the risk of hypokalemia and associated arrhythmic risk caused by non-potassium-sparing diuretics
- The addition of spironolactone to standard therapy can reduce the risk of both morbidity and mortality in patients with severe heart failure.

b. Ropinirole is used in the treatment of Parkinsonism

(Ref: KD Tripathi, Essentials of Medical Pharmacology, 7th ed, pg. 430, 8th ed, pg. 457-58)

ANSWER

Parkinsonism

Term used to describe the symptoms of tremors, slowness of movement, and muscle rigidity

Ropinirole in Treatment of Parkinsonism

- It is a dopamine agonist which can act on striatal dopamine receptors
- It contribute to selective activation of dopamine receptors; effective even in advanced cases in which capability to produce, collect, and release of dopamine is largely lost
- Chances of neuronal damage are reduced
- Can be used in Parkinson's disease as monotherapy also
  - Longer-acting; symptomatic relief provided can be compared to levodopa
  - Cases treated with ropinirole less commonly require levodopa supplemental therapy
  - Fewer cases develop dyskinesias and motor fluctuations, as compared to levodopa-carbidopa therapy.
- **Dose:** 0.25 mg thrice daily starting dose, titrated to a maximum of 4–8 mg thrice a day.

c. Morphine should not be administered to patients with undiagnosed abdominal pain

(Ref: KD Tripathi, Essentials of Medical Pharmacology, 8th ed, pg. 473-74)

ANSWER

Morphine in Pain Relief

- Better relief in nociceptive pain (due to stimulation of peripheral pain receptors) than neurotic pain (as in trigeminal neuralgia) which may occur due to inflammation or any damage to neural tissues or structures.
- Apprehension, fear, autonomic effects related to pain are also reduced
- Suppression of pain perception
- Analgesic effect constitutes both spinal and supraspinal components

Morphine should not be used in Undiagnosed Abdominal Pain

- It provides relief of moderate to severe pain in both acute and chronic conditions
- It should not be used in abdominal pain cases when diagnosis has not been established
- If the abdominal pain is due to biliary colic or inflamed appendix, it may worsen the condition
- The lesions may even rupture due to use of morphine.

d. **The subcutaneous route of drug administration is unsuitable in a patient of shock**

(Ref: KD Tripathi, Essentials of Medical Pharmacology, 8th ed, pg. 13, 22)

ANSWER

Subcutaneous Route of Drug Administration

○ Deposition of drug in loose subcutaneous tissue
○ The loose subcutaneous tissue has rich nerve supply and less vascular
○ Thus, irritant drugs cannot be injected; also, drug absorption is slower than intramuscular injections
○ It is easy to be self-administered as deep penetration is not required
○ **Unsuitable in a patient of shock since:**
  ▪ During shock, there is vasoconstriction
  ▪ Due to vasoconstriction, blood flow to subcutaneous tissue is reduced
  ▪ This will lead to delayed absorption of drug administered
  ▪ Drugs usually given by this route are: insulin, adrenaline, and local anesthetics.

2. **Classify sedative-hypnotic drugs. Explain the mechanism of action, adverse effects and therapeutic uses of diazepam.**

(Ref: KD Tripathi, Essentials of Medical Pharmacology, 7th ed, pg. 398, 402, 8th ed, pg. 424, 427-430)

ANSWER

Classification of Sedative-Hypnotic Drugs

Barbiturates

○ *Long acting*
  ▪ Phenobarbitone
○ Short acting
  ▪ Butobarbitone
  ▪ Pentobarbitone
○ Ultra-short-acting
  ▪ Thiopentone
  ▪ Methohexitone

Benzodiazepines

○ *Hypnotic*
  ▪ Diazepam
  ▪ Flurazepam
  ▪ Nitrazepam
  ▪ Alprazolam
  ▪ Temazepam
  ▪ Triazolam
○ *Antianxiety*
  ▪ Diazepam
  ▪ Chlordiazepoxide
  ▪ Oxazepam
  ▪ Lorazepam
  ▪ Alprazolam
○ *Anticonvulsant*
  ▪ Diazepam
  ▪ Lorazepam
  ▪ Clonazepam
  ▪ Clobazam

Newer Nonbenzodiazepine Hypnotics

○ Zopiclone
○ Zolpidem
○ Zaleplon

Diazepam

○ **Mechanism of action:**
  ▪ Preferential action on midbrain ascending reticular formation and limbic system
  ▪ Action on cerebellum results into ataxia and muscle relaxation via a primary medullary site of action
  ▪ Gamma amino butyric acid (GABA) is an inhibiting neurotransmitter; GABA promotes opening of a postsynaptic receptor, the GABA-A receptor
  ▪ This causes an increased conductance to chloride ions, and membrane hyperpolarization, and finally neuronal inhibition is induced
  ▪ Diazepam binds to the GABA-A receptor increases the affinity of GABA and its receptor, thereby elevating the opening frequency of GABA-A receptor
  ▪ Consequently, **it potentiate GABAergic neurotransmission**
  ▪ **Note:** No GABA mimetic action, only have GABA facilitatory action
○ **Therapeutic uses:**
  ▪ To control convulsions in status epilepticus (first choice drug)
  ▪ To treat anxiety disorder
  ▪ To treat sleeplessness (insomnia)
  ▪ In spastic disorders as skeletal muscle relaxant
  ▪ As pre-anesthetic medication
  ▪ To treat withdrawal effects of alcohol.
○ **Adverse effects:** Relatively safe drugs, however side effect profile include following:
  ▪ Dizziness

- Vertigo
- Disorientation
- Ataxia
- Amnesia
- Reaction time prolonged, thus psychomotor skills are impaired, hence driving not allowed
- Patients sometimes complain of weakness, blurring of vision, dry mouth, and urinary incontinence
- Flaccidity and respiratory depression in the neonate if given during labor, etc.

PART-II

3. **Discuss the therapeutic status of:**

a. **Erythropoietin in anemia**

(Ref: KD Tripathi, Essentials of Medical Pharmacology, 8th ed, pg. 611)

ANSWER

For answer, refer 2016 paper-II Q. 3 (b), Pg. 210

b. **Sumatriptan in migraine**

ANSWER

For answer, refer 2013 paper-II Q. 3 (c), Pg. 252

c. **Aspirin in dengue fever**

(Ref: KD Tripathi, Essentials of Medical Pharmacology, 8th ed, pg. 199)

ANSWER

Dengue

- Caused by a flavivirus; arthropod borne infections which is estimated to cause 390 million infections in a year
- The manifestations may vary from an asymptomatic infection, to undifferentiated acute febrile illness, to dengue hemorrhagic fever and severe dengue, may also include dengue shock syndrome

Aspirin in Dengue Fever

- It is recommended to use paracetamol/acetaminophen to treat fever and relieve other symptoms
- Aspirin, nonsteroidal anti-inflammatory drugs (NSAIDs), and corticosteroids should be avoided
- NSAIDs pose a danger of exacerbation of bleeding in view of depressed platelet levels during acute dengue

- Temporary withholding of aspirin should be considered in acute dengue cases where aspirin has been employed for antiplatelet therapy, until the thrombocytopenia improves, reason being there is increased risk of hemorrhage and reduced chances of thromboembolism during this period.

d. **Oximes in insecticide poisoning**

ANSWER

Organophosphorus (Organophosphate) Poisoning

Accidental, suicidal, or homicidal exposure to anti-ChE (carbamates and organophosphates) result into local muscarinic signs at the site of exposure (gastrointestinal (GI) tract, skin, and/or eye). The local manifestations are followed by complex systemic effects due to the central, nicotinic, and muscarinic actions.

- **These include:**
  - **Eye:**
    - Eye irritation, lacrimation, salivation, sweating, profuse tracheobronchial secretions
    - Miosis and blurring of vision
  - **Respiratory:** Bronchospasm and breathlessness
  - **GI:** Colic, involuntary defecation and urination.
  - **Cardiovascular:** Fall in blood pressure, tachycardia/bradycardia, cardiac arrhythmias, even vascular collapse.
  - **Others:**
    - Muscular fasciculations, weakness, respiratory paralysis
    - Disorientation, irritation, and unsteadiness
    - Tremor, ataxia (term for a group of disorders that affect coordination, balance and speech), convulsions, coma, and death (due to respiratory failure).

Oximes in Organophosphate Poisoning

- These are cholinesterase reactivators which are used to restore neuromuscular transmission (only in case of anti-ChE organophosphate poisoning)
- **Examples:** Pralidoxime (2-PAM), obidoxime (more potent than pralidoxime), and diacetyl-monoxime (DAM)
- Used secondary to that of atropine
- Rationale for use:
  - Positively charged quaternary nitrogen → attaches to anionic site of the enzyme (remains unoccupied in the presence of organophosphate inhibitors) → oxime end reacts with the phosphorus atom attached to esteratic site → oximephosphonate thus formed diffuses away → leaves reactivated ChE.

○ **Note:**

- 2-PAM is not effective as an antidote to carbamate anti-ChEs (physostigmine, neostigmine, carbaryl, propoxur) since the anionic site of the enzyme is not free.
- Contraindicated in carbamate poisoning as it not only does not reactivate carbamylated enzyme but also has weak anti-ChE activity of its own.

○ **Dose:** 2-PAM injected as IV slowly in a dose of 1–2 g (20–40 mg/kg in children). Other regimen is loading dose of 30 mg/kg IV, followed by continuous infusion 8–10 mg/kg/h till recovery.

○ Lower doses as symptoms improves.

---

4. **Describe the drug treatment of:**

a. **Glaucoma**

ANSWER

For answer, refer 2013 paper-I Q. 4 (a), Pg. 246

b. **Manic depressive illness**

(Ref: KD Tripathi, Essentials of Medical Pharmacology, 7th ed, pg. 447, 8th ed, pg. 442-44)

ANSWER

Manic Depressive Illness

Also known as bipolar disorder, and characterized by abnormal change in moods from highly elevated to depressive moods

Drug Treatment

○ **Lithium carbonate:**

- **Mechanism of action:** There are many methods proposed; when given in therapeutic levels, it causes inhibition of inositol-1-phosphate hydrolysis by inositol monophosphatase. Inositol supply for restoration of membrane phosphatidylinositides is reduced; thus affecting hyperactive neurones involved in the manic state as there is insufficient supply from outside cell
- Acts via mood stabilizing action in bipolar disorder
- Continued use inhibits cyclic changes in mood
- **Dose:** 0.5–0.8 mEq/L in maintenance therapy, 0.8–1.1 mEq/L in acute mania episodes
- Toxicity manifests frequently if levels exceed 1.5 mEq/L; thus monitoring of serum lithium concentration is very crucial

○ **Sodium valproate:**

- Forms first line of treatment
- Useful in cases showing no response or intolerance to lithium; doses being same as lithium
- When combined with an atypical antipsychotic, presents high efficacy in acute mania

○ **Carbamazepine:**

- Remission period in bipolar disorder is extended
- Less efficacy than lithium or valproate in acute mania

○ **Lamotrigine:**

- Not used in prevention or treatment; extensive used in the maintenance therapy of type II bipolar disorder

○ **Atypical antipsychotics:**

- Drugs like, olanzapine, risperidone, aripiprazole, quetiapine, used with or without a benzodiazepine help to control acute mania
- Aripiprazole employed in treatment of mania in bipolar I disorder, as monotherapy and also as adjuvant to lithium or valproate
- Olanzapine approved for maintenance therapy.

PART-III

5. **Describe the drug treatment of:**

a. **Acute left ventricular failure**

ANSWER

Acute Left Ventricular Failure

○ This presents as pulmonary edema due to elevated pressure in the pulmonary capillaries

○ **Drug treatment in acute management:**

- Oxygen should be given to all patients who are hypoxemic to maintain SaO_2 95–98%
- Diuretics use
  - ◆ Most patients with dyspnea in AHF caused by pulmonary edema; mobilize edema fluid and pulmonary congestion is relieved
  - ◆ They are indicated to provide symptomatic relief secondary to fluid retention
  - ◆ Start with individualized dose depending on clinical condition
- Opiates (Morphine)
  - ◆ Morphine as well as mild arterial dilatation; heart rate is also reduced
  - ◆ Morphine sulfate 2–5 mg intravenous over 2–3 minutes and can be repeated every 10–25

minutes until effect is seen

- ♦ Opiates induce nausea and depress respiratory drive potentially increasing the need for invasive ventilation

- ▪ **Vasodilators:**
  - ♦ First line therapy with an sufficient BP and signs of congestion with low diuresis
  - ♦ Nitrates lead to reduction in left ventricular preload and afterload, balanced vasodilation of vein and arteries without impairment of tissue perfusion

- ▪ **Inotropes:**
  - ♦ Reserved for cases cardiac output is severely reduced and there is compromised vital organ perfusion
  - ♦ Inotropes cause sinus tachycardia and may induce myocardial ischemia and arrhythmias
    - ▫ Effects of beta-blocker may be counteracted by levosimendan and milrinone

- ♦ **Vasopressors:**
  - ▫ They are employed if the combination of inotropic agent and fluid challenge get failed to restore adequate arterial pressure and organ perfusion
  - ▫ It may raise the after-load of a failing heart and further decrease end-organ blood flow

- ♦ **Cardiac glycosides:**
  - ▫ Employed in AF induced heart failure if there is inadequate ventricular rate-control by beta-blockers.

b. Warfarin Overdosage

ANSWER

Warfarin Overdose

This is the outcome of the administration of inappropriately high doses, altered protein binding, decreased intake of vitamin K, decreased production or increased clearance of vitamin K-dependent clotting factors and the concurrent usage of other drugs (e.g. Erythromycin, fluconazole, amiodarone, etc.) that compete with warfarin for protein binding

Drug Treatment

- ○ The goal of urgent warfarin reversal is to raise or replace vitamin K-dependent clotting factors
- ○ Vitamin K1 can be orally administered unless very rapid reversal of anticoagulation is not required, when slow intravenous infusion of vitamin K1 has to be administered
- ○ If INR is above the therapeutic range, but the

significant bleeding is not seen in patient, then just reduction of warfarin doses or omission and then remission (later at low doses) is considered

- ○ If INR is between 5 and 9, and any risk factor that may predispose to bleeding, is not present, then warfarin can be omitted, and vitamin K1 (in a dose of 1 to 2.5 mg) to be given orally
- ○ If in the above case, rapid reversal is required to allow some surgery or dental extraction, then dose of vitamin K1 can be increased and 2 to 5 mg is recommended
- ○ If INR is more than 9 but bleeding that is clinically significant has not occurred, then 3 to 5 mg dose of vitamin K1 orally is preferred
- ○ If INR is more than 20, and there is serious bleeding or major warfarin overdose, slow intravenous infusion of vitamin K1 in a dose of 10 mg, with fresh plasma or prothrombin complex concentrate transfused
- ○ In case of serious warfarin overdose or life-threatening bleeding, prothrombin complex concentrate replacement therapy is instituted.

6. Explain the rationale use of the following:

a. Aspirin in myocardial infarction

(Ref: KD Tripathi, Essentials of Medical Pharmacology, 8th ed, pg. 199)

ANSWER

Aspirin

General use is to treat mild to moderate pain and reduce fever or inflammation

Rationale to Use in Myocardial Infarction

- ○ Aspirin causes inhibition of platelet aggregation, thus lowering incidence of reinfarction
- ○ It also cause inhibition of thromboxane A2 synthesis in platelets at low doses
- ○ At a dose of 60–100 mg/day, incidence of myocardial infarction is reduced; thus now usually prescribed to postinfarct patients
- ○ At a dose of 100–150 mg/day for 12 weeks, reduces chances of "new onset" or "sudden worsening" angina to develop infarction
- ○ Not only reduces risk of transient ischemic attacks but also stroke incidence is reduced.

b. Bromhexine in cough

(Ref: KD Tripathi, Essentials of Medical Pharmacology, 7th ed, pg. 219, 8th ed, pg. 238)

PHARMACOLOGY

ANSWER

Bromohexine

A potent mucolytic and mucokinetic drug

Rationale to Use in Cough

○ Causes depolymerization of mucopolysaccharides directly and also by releasing lysosomal enzymes, this leads to breaking off of fibers network in tenacious sputum
○ It thus induces thin copious bronchial secretion
○ Especially used if mucus plugs are present

Side Effect Profile

○ Rhinorrhea
○ Lacrimation
○ Gastric irritation and nausea
○ Hypersensitivity.

c. **Sulfasalazine in rheumatoid arthritis**

(Ref: KD Tripathi, Essentials of Medical Pharmacology, 8th ed, pg. 228, 734)

ANSWER

Sulfasalazine

○ A compound of sulfapyridine and 5-aminosalicylic acid (5-ASA)
○ Also known as a disease modifying antirheumatic drug (DMARD)

Rationale to Use in Rheumatoid Arthritis (RA)

○ **Mechanism of action:** There is splitting of sulfapyridine in the colon by bacterial action. Followed by systemic absorption and is the active component in RA, unlike 5-ASA being active moiety in ulcerative colitis
○ Pain and swelling of inflammatory arthritis are reduced by use of sulfasalazine, along with preventing damage to joints
○ Disease is suppressed in many RA patients
○ Can also be used in juvenile arthritis and ankylosing spondylitis
○ **Note:** Second line drug for milder cases or given in combination with methotrexate.

Your Roll No. ....

Name of the Paper	:	**Pharmacology Paper-II**
Name of the Course	:	**MBBS-2010**
Semester	:	**Annual**

Time: 3 Hours   M.M.: 40

INSTRUCTIONS

1. Write your Roll No. on the top immediately on receipt of this question paper
2. All questions are to be attempted
3. Answers to Parts I, II and III should be written in separate answer sheets provided
4. Attempt parts of a question in sequence

PART-I

1. **Explain why?**   [8]
   a. Oral contraceptive failure can occur in patients treated with antitubercular chemotherapy
   b. Propranolol is prescribed to patients of thyrotoxicosis
   c. Cyclosporine is used in patients receiving organ transplants
   d. Penicillin is used in rheumatic fever

2. **Classify drugs used in the treatment of peptic ulcers. Describe the mechanism of action, adverse effects and therapeutic uses of omeprazole.**   [6]

PART-II

3. **Discuss the therapeutic status of:**   [8]
   a. Artesunate in malaria
   b. Albendazole in helminthiasis
   c. Acarbose in diabetes mellitus

4. **Describe the drug treatment of:**   [6]
   a. Gonococcal urethritis
   b. Acne vulgaris

PART-III

5. **Write short notes on:**   [6]
   a. Mast cell stabilizers
   b. Ritonavir
   c. 5-α reductase inhibitors

6. **Explain the rationale for the use of:**   [6]
   a. Clomiphene in infertility
   b. Acetyleysteine in paracetamol overdose
   c. Lugols iodine administered to patients prior to thyroidectomy

PART-I

1. Explain why?

a. Oral contraceptive failure can occur in patients treated with antitubercular chemotherapy

(Ref: KD Tripathi, Essentials of Medical Pharmacology, 8th ed, pg.768 PILs for rifampin on emc)

ANSWER

Antitubercular Chemotherapy

First line antitubercular drugs include: Isoniazid; Rifampicin; Pyrazinamide; Ethambutol; and Streptomycin

Antitubercular drugs lead to oral contraceptive (OCP) failure, especially with rifampicin.

Rationale of Failure in Antitubercular Chemotherapy

- Anti-TB drugs (particularly Rifampicin) are potent inducers of certain cytochrome P-450 enzymes
- When coadministering anti-TB drugs with other drugs that are also metabolized through the cytochrome P-450 enzymes; this may result in accelerating the metabolism of these drugs as well as reducing their drug activity
- Thus, when prescribing anti-TB drugs with drugs metabolized by cytochrome P-450, caution should be given
- These other drugs may need dose adjustment to maintain optimal therapeutic levels in blood, when starting or stopping parallel administered anti-TB drugs
- Examples of such drugs include: Oral contraceptives, corticosteroids, sulfonylureas, steroids, HIV protease inhibitors, nonnucleoside reverse transcriptase inhibitors (NNRTIs), theophylline, metoprolol, fluconazole, ketoconazole, clarithromycin, phenytoin, etc.
- This is the reason contraceptive failures have occurred
- It is advised to switch to an OCP having higher dose (50 µg) of estrogen or any alternative method should be practiced for contraception.

b. Propranolol is prescribed to patients of thyrotoxicosis

ANSWER

Thyrotoxicosis

- A common disorder characterized by excessive thyroid hormones, especially seen in women
- Most frequent cause is Graves' disease
- Other significant causes: toxic nodular hyperthyroidism, due to the presence of one or more autonomously functioning thyroid nodules, and thyroiditis caused by inflammation

Rationale to Use Propranolol (Not Atenolol) in Treating Thyrotoxicosis

- Propranolol nonselectively blocks β1 and β2 receptors; while atenolol is cardioselective (preferentially blocks β1 receptors)
- Without intrinsic sympathomimetic activity
- Rapidly controls symptoms due to sympathetic overactivity (palpitation, anxiety, tremor, nervousness, fixed gaze, severe myopathy, excessive perspiration) without significantly affecting thyroid status
  - Inhibition of peripheral conversion of T4 to T3
  - Dramatic symptomatic relief
  - Employed preoperatively and while awaiting response to antithyroid drugs/radioactive iodine
  - Extremely valuable to combat thyroid storm
  - **Dose:** 1–2 mg slow intravenously; may be followed by 40–80 mg oral every 6 hourly.

c. Cyclosporine is used in patients receiving organ transplants

ANSWER

For answer, refer 2016 paper-II Q. 3 (c), Pg. 211

d. Penicillin is used in rheumatic fever

(Ref: KD Tripathi, Essentials of Medical Pharmacology, 8th ed, pg. 766-67)

ANSWER

Penicillin G

Drug of choice, extensively used for infections caused by organisms that are susceptible, but anaphylactic reactions with this drug has limited the use

Rationale to use Penicillin in Rheumatic Fever

- Penicillin in low concentrations is capable to prevent colonization by streptococci that are indirectly accountable for rheumatic fever

○ Also, rheumatic fever is a streptococcal infection (like pharyngitis, otitis media, etc.). It responds to conventional doses of penicillin because *S. pyogenes* has not established significant resistance to the drug

○ **Dose:** Benzathine penicillin 1.2 MU every 4 weeks till patient attains 18 years of age or 5 years after an attack.

---

2. Classify drugs used in the treatment of peptic ulcers. Describe the mechanism of action, adverse effects and therapeutic uses of omeprazole.

(Ref: KD Tripathi, Essentials of Medical Pharmacology, 8th ed, pg. 700-01, 706)

ANSWER

Approaches for the Treatment of Peptic Ulcer

Reduction of Gastric Acid Secretion

○ **H2 antihistamines:** Cimetidine, ranitidine, famotidine, roxatidine

○ **Proton pump inhibitors:** Omeprazole, esomeprazole, lansoprazole, pantoprazole, rabeprazole, dexrabeprazole

○ **Anticholinergic drugs:** Pirenzepine, propantheline, oxyphenonium

○ **Prostaglandin analogue:** Misoprostol

Neutralization of Gastric Acid (Antacids)

○ **Systemic:** Sodium bicarbonate, sodium citrate

○ **Nonsystemic:** Magnesium hydroxide, magnesium trisilicate, aluminum hydroxide gel, magaldrate, calcium carbonate

Ulcer Protectives

○ Sucralfate, colloidal bismuth subcitrate (CBS)

Anti-*H. pylori* Drugs

○ Amoxicillin, clarithromycin, metronidazole, tinidazole, tetracycline

Omeprazole

Mechanism of Action

○ The most evident pharmacological action of omeprazole suppression of gastric acid secretion in a dose dependent manner; without any anticholinergic or H2 blocking activity

○ Resting as well as stimulated HCl secretion, can be both completely abolished, without much effect on pepsin, intrinsic factor, and gastric motility

○ **How PPIs work?**

PPIs

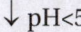

↓ pH<5

Rearrangement to two charged cationic forms
(a sulfenic acid and a sulfenamide configurations)

Covalent reaction with SH groups of the $H^+ K^+$ ATPase enzyme and irreversible inactivation

Acid secretion resumes only when new $H^+ K^+$ ATPase molecules synthesized

○ Inhibition of gastric mucosal carbonic anhydrase also occur

Therapeutic Uses

○ **Peptic ulcers:** Dose of 20 mg once daily. Healing is faster with 40 mg/day. Time taken by gastric ulcer usually is 4 to 8 weeks. Also prevents relapse

○ **Bleeding peptic ulcer:** Helps prevent bleeding from peptic ulcer as it causes suppression of acid production. Clot dissolution which promotes ulcer bleed is done due to acid

○ **Gastroesophageal reflux disease (GERD):** Higher than normally used doses administered twice daily. Continuous inhibition of gastric acid, thus causing rapid relief in pain and discomfort, etc. symptoms

○ **Zollinger-Ellison syndrome:** Dose of 60–120 mg/day given twice daily. Other gastric hypersecretory states, for example, systemic mastocytosis, etc. react well

○ **Aspiration pneumonia:** Employed for prophylaxis of aspiration pneumonia that has occurred due to persistent anesthesia.

Adverse Effects (High Safety Profile)

○ **Nausea:** Very commonly seen

○ **Diarrhea:** Commonly experienced with use of PPIs

○ Headache, pain abdomen, pain in muscles and joint
  ▪ Dizziness (in 3–5% of cases)
  ▪ Rashes
  ▪ Infrequently seen are leukopenia and hepatic dysfunction
  ▪ Atrophic gastritis infrequently on prolonged usage.

PART-II

---

3. Discuss the therapeutic status of:

a. Artesunate in malaria

Answer

Artesunate

An artemisinin derivative; water soluble while

Mechanism of Action

- It possess potent schizonticidal action
- Lethal damage to malarial gametes at early stage; but not mature ones
- Release of highly reactive free radical species, which binds to membrane proteins, leading to lipid peroxidation, damage to endoplasmic reticulum, and eventually parasite lysis

Artesunate in Malaria

- Reduction but no complete interruption in disease transmission
- No cross resistance with any other antimalarial class
- Short-acting or drug
- Can be administered orally, or as an intramuscular as well as intravenous injection.

    b. Albendazole in helminthiasis

Answer

Albendazole

- Antihelminthic drug with the broad-spectrum activity and excellent tolerability
- Single dose administration is effective in various infestations

Mechanism of Action

- Inhibits microtubule synthesis in intestinal roundworms
- This reversibly impairs glucose uptake
- Intestinal parasites are immobilized and slowly die

Therapeutic Uses

- *Ascaris,* hookworm, *Enterobius,* etc.: For adults and children more than 2 years of age, a dose of 400 mg is administered; 200 mg is suited for age group of 1–2 years)
- **Trichinosis:** Treatment causes expulsion of adult worms from intestine, but inadequate effect on larvae already migrated to muscles
- **Neurocysticercosis:** Generally a dose of 400 mg BD is given for 8–15 days
- **Cutaneous larva migrans:** A daily dose of 400 mg for 3 days is instituted to provide symptomatic relief
- **Hydatid disease and filariasis:** Preferred therapy employed before and after surgery as well as to inoperable cases. It also cause suppression of microfilaremia and disease transmission, etc.

Side Effect Profile

- Dizziness
- Prolonged use produces headache, fever, alopecia
- Jaundice and neutropenia
- **Note:** Contraindicated in pregnancy.

    c. Acarbose in diabetes mellitus

Answer

Acarbose

Alpha-glucosidase inhibitors, used in treatment of type 2 diabetes mellitus

Mechanism of Action

- Reversibly inhibit α-glucosidases, which is the final enzyme for the digestion of carbohydrates in small intestine
- It slows down and decreases digestion and absorption of polysaccharides
- Postmeal glycemia declines without significant rise in insulin levels

Pharmacological Effects

- They may be used as an adjuvant to diet (with or without metformin/SU) in obese diabetics
- Doses are taken at the start of each major meal

Side Effect Profile

- Flatulence
- Abdominal discomfort
- Loose stools.

4. **Describe the drug treatment of:**

    a. **Gonococcal urethritis**

Answer

Gonococcal Urethritis

Infection-induced inflammation of the urethra caused due to gonorrhea

Drug Treatment

- **Ciprofloxacin:** Gonor*rhea:* Initially 500 mg single dose was almost 100% curative in both non-PPNG and PPNG infections, resistance has developed, so it is not used as first line. But, still can be considered if strain is sensitive to it
- According to CDC, recommended for treatment for uncomplicated gonococcal infections, recommended regimen is:

Ceftriaxone 250 mg IM in a single dose
PLUS
Azithromycin 1 g orally

○ Both should be administered on the same day, if possible both together and under direct observation

○ A single injection (250 mg) of ceftriaxone offers persistent, high bactericidal levels in the blood

○ In case of need of any other single-dose injectable cephalosporin, ceftizoxime (500 mg IM), cefoxitin (2 g IM with probenecid 1 g orally), and cefotaxime (500 mg IM) can be considered

○ Efficacy of these alternatives in no way is superior to ceftriaxone in urethral gonococcal infections

○ Azithromycin is second preferred as prevalence of tetracycline resistance among isolates is high,

○ In case of allergy to azithromycin, doxycycline (100 mg oral twice daily for 7 days) can be used in combination with ceftriaxone or cefixime.

b. Acne vulgaris

(Ref: KD Tripathi, Essentials of Medical Pharmacology, 8th ed, pg. 952-56)

ANSWER

Acne Vulgaris

○ Most common skin disorder in adolescents

Drug Treatment

○ Topical Therapy

■ **Benzoyl peroxide:**

♦ Extensively used and most effective drugs in acne

♦ Works by gradual liberation of oxygen (in the presence of water) which kills bacteria, particularly anaerobic/microaerophilic ones

♦ Mild irritation like burning and stinging sensation is often felt initially

♦ Used as 5–10% cream, gel or lotion

■ **Retinoic acid**

♦ Comedones are horny impaction within follicles

♦ Retinoic acid acts as comedolytic

♦ Highly efficacious in acne, but response may take 6 to 10 weeks

♦ Used as 0.025–0.05% gel/cream

♦ Should not be applied together with benzoyl peroxide, application can be swapped; one at day and other at night

■ **Adapalene:**

♦ Very useful as it is equally effective but less irritating than tretinoin

♦ Can be used in presence of benzoyl peroxide; even in combination

♦ **Tazarotene** another topical retinoid which can be applied

■ Topical antibiotics

♦ Antibiotics like clindamycin, erythromycin, and tetracyclines are less efficacious

♦ **Nadifloxacin** (newer topical quinolone) exerts beneficial effects in inflamed acne and folliculitis

■ Azelaic acid

♦ Used as 10% or 20% cream

♦ Efficacy in acne is equivalent to benzoyl peroxide, but with a delayed response

○ **Systemic Therapy**

○ Employed only in severe cases with pustules and cysts

■ Antibiotics

♦ Tetracycline, minocycline or erythromycin

♦ Used for initial control, can be given in small maintenance doses

♦ Long-term treatment should not be used

■ Isotretinoin

♦ Orally administered retinoid which leads to reduction in sebum production

♦ Dose of 0.5–1 mg/kg daily for 20 weeks

♦ Due to numerous adverse effects, should be held in reserve for unresponsive cases of severe acne

PART-III

5. Write short notes on

a. Mast cell stabilizers

(Ref: KD Tripathi, Essentials of Medical Pharmacology, 8th ed, pg. 249)

ANSWER

Mast Cell Stabilizers

A synthetic chromone derivative; examples include sodium cromoglycate (ketotifen with H1 antihistaminic activity along with some cromoglycate actions)

Mechanism of Action

○ Inhibition of mast cells degranulation (including other inflammatory cells) by trigger stimuli

○ Inhibition of mediators release of asthma including histamine, leukotrienes, PAF, interleukins, etc.

○ Restriction of chemotaxis of inflammatory cells

Therapeutic Uses

○ **Allergic rhinitis:** Regular 4 times daily use; symptomatic improvement in some patients

○ **Bronchial asthma:** Sodium cromoglycate in long-term prophylaxis of mild-to-moderate asthma. Less effective than inhaled steroids

○ **Allergic conjunctivitis:** Helpful in some chronic uses when regularly used

Side Effect Profile

○ Fine powder inhalation may induce bronchospasm, irritation in throat, and cough

○ Nasal congestion and headache in rare cases

○ Dizziness, arthralgia and rashes

○ Sedation and dry mouth are commonly seen with ketotifen.

b. Ritonavir

(Ref: KD Tripathi, Essentials of Medical Pharmacology, 8th ed, pg. 865-66)

ANSWER

Ritonavir

○ An HIV protease inhibitor that works by interfering with the reproductive cycle of HIV

○ It also inhibits CYTOCHROME P-450 CYP3A

Mechanism of Action

○ Binding to the active site of protease molecule, inhibit its cleaving function

○ Efficacious in new as well as chronically infected cells as their action observed at late step of viral cycle

○ Lead to production of immature noninfectious viral progeny of HIV

Therapeutic Profile

○ Monotherapy reduced HIV viral levels and increased CD4 cell count

○ Improvement in clinical condition

○ Combination is more effective as resistance may develop to either drugs

○ Nucleoside reverse transcriptase inhibitor with protease inhibitors more effective than either drug given alone, and triple therapy is even better

○ **Current recommendations:** One PI in combination with either two nucleoside reverse transcriptase inhibitors or one Nucleoside reverse transcriptase inhibitor + one non-nucleoside reverse transcriptase inhibitor

○ Not used in first line treatment; instead reserved for failure cases

Side Effect Profile

○ Gastrointestinal intolerance

○ Asthenia (lack of muscle strength)

○ Headache and dizziness

○ Limb and facial tingling, numbness and rashes

○ Abdominal obesity and buffalo hump with wasting of limbs and face

○ Dyslipidemic action.

c. 5-α reductase inhibitors

ANSWER

5-α Reductase Inhibitors

○ Competitive inhibitor of 5α-reductase enzyme

○ Examples include finasteride and dutasteride

Mechanism of Action

○ 5α-reductase is the enzyme employed in conversion of testosterone into more active DHT responsible for androgen action in many tissues including the prostate gland and hair follicles

○ Comparatively selective for 5α-reductase type 2 isoenzyme which prevails in male urogenital tract

○ Reduces the static component of obstruction, while the dynamic component is overcome by a₁ blockers

○ Lowers the DHT concentration, but plasma LH and testosterone levels remain unchanged

Therapeutic Uses (Different Strength Imparts Specific Use)

○ Treatment of benign prostatic hyperplasia (enlarged prostate gland):
  ▪ In a strength of 5 mg
  ▪ Ensued a decrease in prostate size and increase in peak urinary flow rate

○ Male-pattern hair loss (androgenic alopecia)
  ▪ In a strength of 1 mg

Side Effect Profile

○ Decreased volume of ejaculate

○ Decreased libido

○ Impotence

○ Breast tenderness and testicular pain

○ Rash, pruritus, and urticaria.

6. Explain the rationale for the use of:

a. Clomiphene in infertility

(Ref: KD Tripathi, Essentials of Medical Pharmacology, 8th ed, pg. 337)

ANSWER

Clomiphene Citrate

○ Primarily used for infertility occurring due to failure of ovulation

○ Dose is 50 mg OD for 5 days; initiated from 5th day of cycle

○ Daily dose may be doubled for 2 to 3 cycles when treatment of 1–2 months fails to cause conception

Rationale to Use in Infertility

○ Acts as a pure estrogen antagonist

○ Induction of gonadotropin secretion in females by hindering estrogenic feedback inhibition of pituitary

○ Thus, increase in LH/FSH amount released at each secretory pulse, this causes ovaries to enlarge and if the ovaries are reactive to gonadotropin then, reovulation follows

○ It can also modify endometrium and cervical mucus

○ Menotropins or chorionic gonadotropin added to the therapy on the last 2 days of the course increases the success rate

○ **Note:** > 6 treatment cycles should not be tried.

b. Acetylcysteine in paracetamol overdose

ANSWER

For answer, refer 2014 paper-II Q. 1 (c), Pg. 237

c. Lugol's iodine administered to patients prior to thyroidectomy

(Ref: KD Tripathi, Essentials of Medical Pharmacology, 8th ed, pg. 277)

ANSWER

Lugol's Iodine

One of the most effective iodine preparations; preparations containing iodide have been used as an adjuvant treatment in patients with Graves' disease, etc.

Mechanism of Action

○ Thyroid hormone release inhibition

○ Attenuation of TSH and cAMP induced thyroid stimulation; interference with iodination residues of thyroglobulin, thus results in a decline in T_3/T_4 synthesis (Wolff-Chaikoff effect)

Rationale to Use Lugol's Iodine Prior to Thyroidectomy

○ Usually administered for 10 days just foregoing surgery

○ Goal of use is to make the gland firm and less vascular, thus making it easier to operate on

○ Thyroid status is lowered by iodide itself, attaining euthyroidism cannot be depended upon it

○ State of euthyroidism is achieved by carbimazole before starting iodide

○ To attain rapid control on symptoms, propranolol may also be added

○ Other uses include use in thyroid storm, prophylaxis of endemic goiter as iodized salt; also used as antiseptic (in form of tincture iodine).

Your Roll No. ....

Name of the Paper	:	**Pharmacology Paper-I**
Name of the Course	:	**MBBS-2009**
Semester	:	**Annual**

Time: 3 Hours   **M.M.: 40**

INSTRUCTIONS

1. Write your Roll No. on the top immediately on receipt of this question paper
2. All questions are to be attempted
3. Answers to Parts I, II and III should be written in separate answer sheets provided
4. Attempt parts of a question in sequence

PART-I

1. **Explain why?**   **[8]**
   a. Increasing doses of phenytoin may lead to sudden manifestations of toxic effects
   b. Low doses of aspirin is used as an antiplatelet agent in patients of ML
   c. Enalapril should be avoided in combination with triamterene for the management of CHF
   d. Allopurinol is used in chronic gout

2. **Classify antipsychotic drugs. Discuss the pharmacological actions, therapeutic uses and adverse effects of olanzapine.**   **[6]**

PART-II

3. **Discuss therapeutic status of following drugs:**   **[8]**
   a. Gold salts in the treatment of rheumatoid arthritis
   b. Aliskiren in hypertension
   c. Succinylcholine during electroconvulsive therapy
   d. Lignocaine in the management of ventricular arrhythmias

4. **Discuss the drug treatment of:**   **[6]**
   a. Hypertensive urgency
   b. Methyl alcohol poisoning

PART-III

5. **Discuss drug treatment of:**   **[6]**
   a. Thyroid storm
   b. Open angle glaucoma

6. **Discuss the rationale of the use of following drugs:**   **[6]**
   a. Atorvastatin in coronary artery disease
   b. Sumatriptan in migraine
   c. Corticosteroids in the treatment of bronchial asthma

PART-I

1. Explain why?

a. Increasing doses of phenytoin may lead to sudden manifestations of toxic effects

(Ref: KD Tripathi, Essentials of Medical Pharmacology, 8th ed, pg. 426)

ANSWER

Phenytoin

○ A hydantoin antiepileptic drug

○ Extensively distributed in body and is 80–90% bound to plasma proteins

Increasing Doses May Lead to Sudden Manifestations of Toxic Effects

○ Kinetics of phenytoin changes from first to zero order over the therapeutic range. Thus, even small increases in dose yields extremely high plasma concentrations

○ Phenytoin metabolism is dose dependent. So very small increments in dosage may result in adverse effects

○ Thus for tailoring dosage, plasma concentration monitoring is required

Dose Related Toxic Manifestations at High Plasma Levels

○ Ataxia, vertigo, nystagmus, diplopia

○ Drowsiness, alterations in behavior, mental confusion, rigidity, hallucinations, disorientation

○ Nausea, vomiting, pain in epigastric area

○ Edema and discoloration of the limb where intravenous injection has been given due to local vascular injury and thrombosis. Necrosis of the tissues in case of extravasation of the solution

○ Intravenous injection leads to fall in BP and cardiac arrhythmias.

b. Low doses of aspirin is used as an antiplatelet agent in patients of MI

(Ref: KD Tripathi, Essentials of Medical Pharmacology, 8th ed, pg. 677)

ANSWER

For answer, refer 2011 paper-II Q. 1 (b), Pg. 279

c. Enalapril should be avoided in combination with triamterene for the management of CHF

ANSWER

Enalapril

An angiotensin converting enzyme inhibitors

Indications

○ **Treatment of hypertension:** All grades of essential and renovascular hypertension

○ **Treatment of heart failure:** Along with non-potassium-sparing diuretics and, where appropriate digitalis

○ **Prevention of symptomatic heart failure:** In asymptomatic patients with left ventricular dysfunction, retarding development of symptomatic heart failure, and also reduces hospitalization for heart failure

Avoided in Combination with Triamterene for the Management of CHF

○ ACE inhibitors attenuate diuretic induced potassium loss. Triamterene is a potassium sparing diuretic, thus may (including potassium supplements, or potassium-containing salt substitutes) lead to significant increases in serum potassium

○ If concomitant use is indicated because of demonstrated hypokalemia, they should be used with caution and with frequent monitoring of serum potassium

○ It is recommended to temporarily discontinue the diuretics a few days before to avoid a hypotensive reaction after the first enalapril dose (lesser risk of hypovolemia).

d. Allopurinol is used in chronic gout

(Ref: KD Tripathi, Essentials of Medical Pharmacology, 8th ed, pg. 233-35)

ANSWER

For answer, refer 2013 paper-II Q. 3 (d), Pg. 253

2. Classify antipsychotic drugs. Discuss the pharmacological actions, therapeutic uses and adverse effects of olanzapine.

(Ref: KD Tripathi, Essentials of Medical Pharmacology, 8th ed, pg. 463-70)

ANSWER

Antipsychotic Drugs

Drugs that are employed to treat symptoms of many types of psychoses, such as delusions, hallucinations, paranoia, or confused thoughts, schizophrenia, and severe and severe anxiety

Classified as:

○ Phenothiazines
  ■ **Aliphatic side chain:** Chlorpromazine, triflupromazine
  ■ **Piperidine side chain:** Thioridazine
  ■ **Piperazine side chain:** Trifluoperazine, fluphenazine
○ **Butyrophenones:** Haloperidol, trifluperidol, penfluridol
○ **Thioxanthenes:** Flupenthixol
○ **Other heterocyclics:** Pimozide, loxapine
○ **Atypical antipsychotics:** Clozapine, risperidone, olanzapine, quetipine, aripiprazole, ziprasidone, amisulpiride, quetiapine, zotepine

For answer, refer 2017 paper-I Q. 5 (b), Pg. 191

PART-II

3. **Discuss therapeutic status of following drugs:**

   a. **Gold salts in the treatment of rheumatoid arthritis**

ANSWER

Rheumatoid Arthritis

An autoimmune disorder causing chronic inflammation of the joints throughout the body

Gold Salts in Treatment of Rheumatoid Arthritis

○ Mainstay in the management of patients with progressive rheumatoid disease for many years
○ Two forms of gold therapy are available: Injectable and oral routes
○ Indicated for the treatment of rheumatoid arthritis patients that are unresponsive to conventional chemotherapy
○ The most common hypothesis around anti-arthritic mechanism suggests that the accumulation of gold by macrophages inhibits both phagocytosis and of the activities of lysosomal enzymes
○ Help suppress the active stage of rheumatoid disease

○ May prevent damage progression in chronic advanced rheumatoid arthritis
○ Examples, auranofin, aurothioglucose, and sodium aurothiomalate
○ Now have been extensively replaced by methotrexate and other DMARDs.

   b. **Aliskiren in hypertension**

(Ref: KD Tripathi, Essentials of Medical Pharmacology, 8th ed, pg. 538)

ANSWER

Aliskiren

Direct renin inhibitors; selectively binds to catalytic site of renin and competitively blocks the access of angiotensinogen, thus Ang I is not produced and the RAS chain disturbed

Aliskiren in Hypertension

○ Recommended as an alternative antihypertensive drug (for unresponsive patients or those who do not tolerate first-line drugs
○ Used in combination with others for better control and lowering of BP
○ Aldosterone levels in plasma lowered attended by mild natriuresis
○ Antihypertensive effectiveness is comparable to that of ACE inhibitors or ARBs
○ Leads to reduction in hypertensive left ventricular hypertrophy and help patients of CHF
○ Holds renoprotective benefit in hypertensives and type 2 diabetics.

   c. **Succinylcholine during electroconvulsive therapy**

(Ref: KD Tripathi, Essentials of Medical Pharmacology, 8th ed, pg. 374, 376)

ANSWER

Succinylcholine

○ Most commonly used muscle relaxant for passing tracheal tube
○ Induces paralysis that is rapid, complete, and predictable; spontaneous recovery achieved around 5 minutes

Electroconvulsive Therapy

○ A procedure in which a brief application of electric stimulus is used to produce a generalized seizure, to improve upon some mental disorders
○ It may lead to convulsions and trauma
○ These unwanted effects can be avoided by the use of Succinylcholine (muscle relaxants)

○ Therapeutic benefit is not affected

○ An alternative can be mivacurium

○ Also used for other brief procedures, e.g. endotracheal intubation, laryngoscopy, bronchoscopy, esophagoscopy, etc.

d. Lignocaine in the management of ventricular arrhythmias

(Ref: KD Tripathi, Essentials of Medical Pharmacology, 8th ed, pg. 392)

ANSWER

Lignocaine

○ Most commonly used local anesthetic

○ No significant autonomic actions; has cardiac effects are all direct

○ A common antiarrhythmic in intensive care units

Management of Ventricular Arrhythmias

○ Most prominent cardiac action is automaticity suppression in ectopic foci

○ Employed to suppress VT and prevent VF

○ The action develops quite rapidly and is titratable, thus can be used in emergency settings, for example, arrhythmias following acute MI or during cardiac surgery

○ Futile in atrial arrhythmias

○ Poor efficiency in chronic ventricular arrhythmia, but effective in suppressing VT due to digitalis toxicity, as it does not worsen A-V block

○ Least cardiotoxic antiarrhythmic; no proarrhythmic potential

○ Cardiac depression and hypotension may result due to excessive doses.

4. Discuss the drug treatment of:

a. Hypertensive urgency

(Ref: KD Tripathi, Essentials of Medical Pharmacology, 8th ed, pg. 618-20)

ANSWER

Hypertensive Urgency

Elevation in BP with systolic BP more than 220 mmHg or diastolic BP more than 120 mm Hg without overt signs of end organ damage is termed "hypertensive urgency"

Drug Treatment

○ **Sodium nitroprusside:**
- Drug of choice in doses of 20–300 µg/min) for most such cases

- Superior option in case of associated MI or LVF
- Concurrent esmolol infusion in aortic dissection required
- Toxic when given in high doses and used for longer period

○ **Glyceryl trinitrate:**
- Less potent hypotensive given intravenously in doses of 5–20 µg/min
- Particularly appropriate to lower BP after cardiac surgery and in acute LVF, MI, unstable angina

○ **Hydralazine:**
- Less predictable and do not form first-line
- Intramuscular or slow intravenous in a dose of 10–20 mg
- Particularly used in eclampsia

○ **Esmolol:**
- Intravenous slow administration (50–100 µg/kg/min) follows 0.5 mg/kg bolus
- Especially used when cardiac contractility and work to be reduced, such as in aortic dissection
- Since BP lowering action is weak; nitroprusside given concurrently

○ **Phentolamine:**
- Drug of choice for hypertensive episodes in pheochromocytoma, cheese reaction or clonidine withdrawal
- Intravenously injected in a dose of 5–10 mg

○ **Labetalol:**
- Used for lowering BP in MI, unstable angina, eclampsia
- Since sedation or any increase in intracranial pressure is not seen, can be given to patients with altered consciousness

○ **Furosemide:**
- In case of volume overload, 20–80 mg orally or intravenously
- To be avoided when hypovolemia is caused due to pressure induced natriuresis.

b. Methyl alcohol poisoning

(Ref: KD Tripathi, Essentials of Medical Pharmacology, 8th ed, pg. 422-23)

ANSWER

Methyl Alcohol Poisoning

Uncommon and massively lethal intoxication; presenting with headache, epigastric pain, vomiting, tachypnea, bradycardia, acidosis, retinal damage, and disorientation, etc.

Drug Treatment

○ Patient to be kept in a quiet, dark room to provide protection from light to the eyes

○ Within 2 hours of methanol ingestion, gastric lavage with sodium bicarbonate; maintenance of BP and ventilation by supportive measures

○ Acidosis to be countered by intravenous sodium bicarbonate infusion. Large amounts may be needed. Serves as a significant measure as combats retinal damage and other symptoms

○ If alkali therapy results in hypokalemia, potassium chloride infusion is required

○ Ethanol (10% in water) administered through a nasogastric tube. Loading dose 0.7 mL/kg, followed by 0.15 mL/kg/h

  ▪ **How ethanol works?**
    ♦ Preferential metabolism of ethanol over methanol by the enzyme alcohol dehydrogenase.

  ▪ **Continuation of treatment for long**

○ Hemodialysis can clear off methanol and recovery is hastened

○ *Fomepizole* (4-methylpyrazole); drug of choice

  ▪ Specifically inhibits alcohol dehydrogenase

  ▪ Loading dose of intravenous 15 mg/kg, followed by 10 mg/kg every 12 hours till methanol levels in serum fall below 20 mg/dL

  ▪ Not available commercially in India

○ **Folate therapy:** Injection calcium leucovorin in a dose of 50 mg given 6 hourly is an adjuvant approach; enhances oxidation of blood formate.

Methanol Poisoning

○ Uncommon form of poisoning, however, a massively lethal intoxication.

○ Methanol is a multipurpose fuel. It has increasing use in an energy-driven society, thus high index of suspicion and immediate laboratory confirmation is required to manage the symptoms.

○ Methanol poisoning manifests as

  ▪ Headache
  ▪ Epigastric pain
  ▪ Vomiting
  ▪ Uneasiness
  ▪ Tachypnea
  ▪ Dyspnea
  ▪ **Bradycardia:** Hypotension also occurs in most cases.
  ▪ **Disorientation:** Delirium and seizures may occur. The patient may also suddenly pass into coma.

  ▪ **Acidosis:** There is production of formic acid. This is very significant.

  ▪ **Retinal damage:** This results as a specific toxicity of formic acid.

  ▪ Blurring of vision and congestion of optic disc, and finally followed by blindness before demise.

  ▪ Death due to respiratory failure.

Rationale for Ethanol to be used in Methanol Poisoning

○ Preferential metabolism of ethanol over methanol by the enzyme alcohol dehydrogenase.

○ This enzyme gets saturated by concentration 100 mg/dl of ethanol in blood. This slows down methanol metabolism and the rate of generation of formaldehyde and formic acid (conversion of methanol to these compounds is responsible for toxic manifestations) is reduced.

Dose

○ Ethanol (10% in water) administered through a nasogastric tube.

○ Loading dose 0.7 mL/kg, followed by 0.15 mL/kg/h.

○ **Note**: The enzyme saturating concentration of ethanol yields to intoxication and thus can lead to hypoglycemia.

PART-III

5. **Discuss drug treatment of:**

    a. **Thyroid storm**

        (Ref: KD Tripathi, Essentials of Medical Pharmacology, 8th ed, pg. 277)

ANSWER

For answer, refer 2014 paper-II Q. 4 (a), Pg. 239

    b. **Open angle glaucoma**

        (Ref: KD Tripathi, Essentials of Medical Pharmacology, 8th ed, pg. 165-70)

ANSWER

For answer, refer 2013 paper-I Q. 4 (a), Pg. 246

6. **Discuss the rationale of the use of following drugs:**

    a. **Atorvastatin in coronary artery disease**

        (Ref: KD Tripathi, Essentials of Medical Pharmacology, 8th ed, pg. 685-86)

ANSWER

Atorvastatin

- A HMG-CoA reductase inhibitor
- Other drugs of same class: Lovastatin, Simvastatin, Pravastatin, Atorvastatin, Rosuvastatin, Pitavastatin
- Considered as the first choice drugs for primary hyperlipidaemias with raised LDL and total cholesterol levels, with or without raised TG levels (Type IIa, IIb, V)
- Drugs of choice for secondary hypercholesterolemia (diabetes, nephrotic syndrome)
- Preferential drugs in dyslipidemia in diabetics

Rationale to Use in CAD

- Endothelial dysfunction and inflammation play significant roles in developing atherosclerosis
- **Atorvastatin exerts pleiotropic effects:** Improved endothelial function, reduced inflammation, and reduced thrombus formation, thus improves vascular health in CAD
- Intensive lipid-lowering therapy with statins not only improves survival rates and clinical outcomes but also reduces the progression of atherosclerosis.

b. Sumatriptan in migraine

ANSWER

For answer, refer 2013 paper-II Q. 3 (c), Pg. 252

c. Corticosteroids in the treatment of bronchial asthma

(Ref: KD Tripathi, Essentials of Medical Pharmacology, 8th ed, pg. 251, 253)

ANSWER

Corticosteroids

- Not bronchodilators
- Reduce hyper-reactivity of bronchi, mucosal edema and suppress inflammatory response to antigen-antibody reaction or other trigger stimuli
- Provide sustained symptomatic relief than bronchodilators or cromoglycate and reduce asthmatic exacerbations

Systemic Steroid Therapy Used in Following two Situations of Bronchial Asthma

- **Severe chronic asthma:**
  - Prednisolone 20–60 mg (or equivalent) daily, if not controlled by bronchodilators and inhaled steroids, frequently increased severity
  - Doses reduced after achieving optimum control and inhaled steroids are resorted to
- **Acute asthmatic exacerbation:**
  - High dose of rapidly acting glucocorticoid intravenous in patients not responding to intensive bronchodilator therapy
  - Shifted to oral therapy for 5–7 days; then abrupt discontinuation or rapid tapering.

Your Roll No. ....

Name of the Paper	:	**Pharmacology Paper-II**
Name of the Course	:	**MBBS-2009**
Semester	:	**Annual**

Time: 3 Hours   M.M.: 40

INSTRUCTIONS

1. Write your Roll No. on the top immediately on receipt of this question paper
2. All questions are to be attempted
3. Answers to Parts I, II and III should be written in separate answer sheets provided
4. Attempt parts of a question in sequence

PART-I

1. **Explain why?**   [8]
    a. Ferrous salts are preferred as a better salts than ferric salts in the treatment of mild anemia
    b. Intermittent pulse therapy is employed in cancer chemotherapy
    c. Low molecular weight heparin preparation are preferred over unfractionated heparin preparation
    d. Ergometrine should not be used for induction of labor

2. **Classify corticosteroids. Discuss the pharmacological actions, side effects and therapeutic uses of glucocorticoids.**
                                                                                                                [6]

PART-II

3. **Discuss therapeutic status of:**   [8]
    a. Aromatase inhibitors in breast cancer
    b. Domperidone as antiemetic agent
    c. Metronidazole in amoebic hepatitis

4. **Discuss the drug treatment of**   [6]
    a. Osteoporosis
    b. Peptic ulcer with *H. pylori* infection

PART-III

5. **Write short notes on:**   [6]
    a. Post antibiotic effects
    b. Lepra reaction
    c. Linezolid

6. **Give the rationale for the use of:**   [6]
    a. Management trisilicate as antacid
    b. Leuprolide in carcinoma prostrate
    c. Pyridoxine along with INH therapy of T-B

PART-I

1. Explain why?

a. Ferrous salts are preferred as a better salts than ferric salts in the treatment of mild anemia

(Ref: KD Tripathi, Essentials of Medical Pharmacology, 8th ed, pg. 648-50)

ANSWER

Iron Therapy

○ Can be given to anemic patients orally or parenterally

○ **Preferred route:** Oral

○ **Oral preparations can be:** Ferrous or ferric salts

○ Most significant side effects include gastric irritation and constipation, which are related to the amount of elemental iron administered

○ **Rationale to Prefer Ferrous Over Ferric Salts**

  ▪ Higher iron content in ferrous salts

  ▪ Better absorption than ferric salts, particularly at higher doses

  ▪ Dissociable ferrous salts are inexpensive, have

○ **Examples of oral preparations:**

  ▪ **Ferrous sulfate:** Hydrated salt 20% iron, dried salt 32% iron

  ▪ **Ferrous gluconate:** 12% iron

  ▪ **Ferrous fumarate:** 33% iron.

b. Intermittent pulse therapy is employed in cancer chemotherapy

ANSWER

For answer, refer 2014 paper-II Q. 1 (a), Pg. 237

c. Low molecular weight heparin preparation are preferred over unfractionated heparin preparation

(Ref: KD Tripathi, Essentials of Medical Pharmacology, 8th ed, pg. 663-67)

ANSWER

For answer, refer 2017 paper-II Q. 1 (d), Pg. 195

d. Ergometrine should not be used for induction of labor

(Ref: KD Tripathi, Essentials of Medical Pharmacology, 8th ed, pg. 176, 331)

ANSWER

Ergometrine

○ An amine ergot alkaloid

○ **Mechanism of action:** Agonistic action on 5-HT receptors partially in uterus, placental, and umbilical blood vessels, including certain brain areas

○ Causes contraction of myometrium which is used exclusively in obstetrics

○ Basal tone is increased with moderate increase in dose

○ **Rationale not to use ergometrine (oxytocin preferred) in induction of labor:**

  ▪ Control in intensity of action is better afforded by oxytocin due to its short half-life and slow intravenous infusion

  ▪ Since low concentrations do not allow normal relaxation in between contractions—foetal oxygenation suffer, which is not the case with oxytocin

  ▪ Stimulant action involves lower segment also; thus compromising fetal descent

  ▪ Consistent augmentation of uterine contractions cannot be achieved; oxytocin provides this consistency.

2. Classify corticosteroids. Discuss the pharmacological actions, side effects and therapeutic uses of glucocorticoids.

(Ref: KD Tripathi, Essentials of Medical Pharmacology, 8th ed, pg. 283, 308-17)

ANSWER

For answer, refer 2012 paper-II Q. 2, Pg. 265

PART-II

3. Discuss therapeutic status of:

a. Aromatose Inhibitors in breast cancer

(Ref: KD Tripathi, Essentials of Medical Pharmacology, 8th ed, pg. 339)

ANSWER

For answer, refer 2014 paper-II Q. 3 (a), Pg. 238

b. Domperidone as antiemetic agent

(Ref: KD Tripathi, Essentials of Medical Pharmacology, 8th ed, pg. 663, 666)

ANSWER

Domperidone

○ A dopamine D2-receptor antagonist developed as an antiemetic *and prokinetic* agent

○ **Mechanism of action:** Antiemesis caused due to chemoreceptor trigger zone in medulla oblongata, not protected by blood-brain barrier

○ **Antiemetic Profile:**

- Used in postoperative emesis and radiation sickness
- Disease-associated (for example, migraine) and drug-induced vomiting
- Less effect in motion sickness
- During emergency conditions when general anesthesia has to be given and the patient had taken meals less than 4 hours before as gastrokinetic for gastric emptying
- Might benefit mild cases of GERD, not as effectively as PPIs/H2 blockers

○ **Side effects:**

- Loose stools and dry mouth
- Rashes and headache
- Galactorrhea
- Rapid intravenous injection may cause cardiac arrhythmias.

c. Metronidazole in amoebic hepatitis

ANSWER

For answer, refer 2013 paper-II Q. 3 (a), Pg. 252

4. Discuss the drug treatment of:

a. Osteoporosis

(Ref: KD Tripathi, Essentials of Medical Pharmacology, 8th ed, pg. 325, 340-45, 352, 366, 370)

ANSWER

For answer, refer 2016 paper-II Q. 4 (b), Pg. 212

b. Peptic ulcer with *H. pyloric* infection

(Ref: KD Tripathi, Essentials of Medical Pharmacology, 8th ed, pg. 695, 706)

ANSWER

PART-III

5. Write short notes on:

a. Post antibiotic effects

(Ref: KD Tripathi, Essentials of Medical Pharmacology, 8th ed, pg. 748)

ANSWER

For answer, refer 2013 paper-II Q. 5 (a), Pg. 253

b. Lepra reaction

(Ref: KD Tripathi, Essentials of Medical Pharmacology, 8th ed, pg. 833)

ANSWER

Lepra Reaction

○ According to WHO, immunologically mediated episodes of acute or subacute inflammation known as reactions may occur during the course of leprosy, in up to 25% of patients with paucibacillary leprosy and as much as 40% with multibacillary leprosy

○ It is a Arthus (Jarisch Herxheimer) type of reaction which occurs when killing of bacilli results into release of antigens

○ **Manifests as:**

- Enlargement of existing lesions, redness, swelling and pain
- New lesions may appear
- Malaise and fever, etc.

○ May be mild, severe or life-threatening, i.e. erythema nodosum leprosum (ENL)

Note: Dapsone is temporarily discontinued only in severe cases.

Treatment

○ Prednisolone in a dose of 40–60 mg/day is started immediately and continued till the reaction subsides in severe cases

○ Thalidomide can be used as an alternative to prednisolone as cytokines play an important role in generating symptoms in lepra reaction.

c. Linezolid

(Ref: KD Tripathi, Essentials of Medical Pharmacology, 8th ed, pg. 808)

ANSWER

For answer, refer 2013 paper-II Q. 5 (c), Pg. 254

6. **Give the rationale for the use of:**

   a. **Magnesium trisilicate as antacid**

   (Ref: KD Tripathi, Essentials of Medical Pharmacology, 7th ed, pg. 654, 8th ed, pg. 703)

ANSWER

Magnesium Trisilicate

An antacid; which is slower acting than others, but exhibit more sustained effect

Rationale to Use Magnesium Trisilicate as Antacid

- There is a generation of $MgCl_2$ and also release of cholecystokinin is induced by Mg^{2+}
- The dissociation in stomach provides basic substances
- Gastric acid is neutralized and pH is increased
- Notably, acid production is not inhibited by antacids, only the antral pH is raised above 4
- Indirect reduction in Peptic activity at pH more than 4
- Used typically in unification with another antacid called aluminum hydroxide so as to neutralize acid in the stomach
- Magnesium trisilicate possess mild laxative action too, thus sometimes can lead to diarrhea if used all alone.

   b. **Leuprolide in carcinoma prostrate**

ANSWER

Leuprolide

- Synthetic analog of GnRh
- More potent and longer acting because of high affinity for GnRH receptor and resistance to enzymatic hydrolysis

Rationale to Use in Carcinoma Prostrate

- Effective in palliative treatment of advanced cases of prostatic cancer
- Leads to a decreased androgen production in testes
- Do not decrease adrenal androgens; flutamide may need to be added
- Cause desensitization and down regulation of GnRH receptors → inhibition of FSH and LH secretion
- Thus, leads to suppression of gonadal function after 1–2 weeks
- Within 2 months of stopping drug; gonads functioning is recovered

   c. **Pyridoxine along with INH therapy of T-B**

   (Ref: KD Tripathi, Essentials of Medical Pharmacology, 7th ed, pg. 776, 8th ed, pg. 818)

ANSWER

Rationale to Use Pyridoxine (Vitamin B6) with INH Therapy

- Isoniazid may probably lead to vitamin B6 deficiency by competing with pyridoxal phosphate for the enzyme apotryptophanase
- This deficiency is possibly noticed in elderly
- Due to disturbances in metabolism of vitamin B6, peripheral neuropathy may develop in few patients
- Classic clinical triad of acute isoniazid neurotoxicity includes seizures, metabolic acidosis, and coma
- Pyridoxine is given during whole therapy to counter neurotoxicity attributed to this drug regimen.

Your Roll No. ....

Name of the Paper : **Pharmacology Paper-I**

Name of the Course : **MBBS-2008**

Semester : **Annual**

Time: 3 Hours   M.M.: 40

INSTRUCTIONS

1. Write your Roll No. on the top immediately on receipt of this question paper
2. All questions are to be attempted
3. Answers to Parts I, II and III should be written in separate answer sheets provided
4. Attempt parts of a question in sequence

PART-I

1. **Explain why?**   [8]
   a. Diazepam though a drug of choice for status epilepticus is not recommended for maintenance therapy of epilepsy
   b. Halothane is frequently combined with nitrous oxide for general anesthesia
   c. Digoxin but not adrenaline is used in congestive heart failure
   d. Acetazolamide is not preferred as a diuretic agent

2. **Enumerate commonly used opioids. Write the mode of action, indications and contraindications for the use of morphine.**   [6]

PART-II

3. **Give the rationale for the therapeutic use of the following:**   [8]
   a. Sildenafil in erectile dysfunction
   b. Mannitol in cerebral edema
   c. Combining levodopa with carbidopa in parkinsonism
   d. Dopamine in cardiogenic shock

4. **Discuss the drug treatment of:**   [6]
   a. Generalized tonic-clonic seizures
   b. Acute gout

PART-III

5. **Discuss the therapeutic status of:**   [6]
   a. Sodium cromoglycate in bronchial asthma
   b. Clozapine in schizophrenia
   c. Terlipressin in bleeding esophageal varices

6. **Write short notes on:**   [6]
   a. Therapeutic window
   b. Midazolam
   c. Bioavailability

PART-I

1. **Explain why?**

    a. **Diazepam though a drug of choice for status epilepticus is not recommended for maintenance therapy of epilepsy**

    (Ref: KD Tripathi, Essentials of Medical Pharmacology, 8th ed, pg. 404-05, 427-30)

ANSWER

Diazepam

A benzodiazepine which exerts hypnotic, antianxiety, and anticonvulsant properties.

Mechanism of Action

- Preferential action on ascending reticular formation in midbrain (this center maintains wakefulness)
- Action on limbic system (control of thought and mental functions)
- Action on primary medullary site produces muscle relaxation
- Action on cerebellum leads to ataxia

Diazepam in Status Epilepticus

- Employed in status epilepticus in view of anti-convulsant actions
- Centrally mediated skeletal muscle relaxant property is exerted without impairment of voluntary activity
- Possess prominent muscle relaxant property though in very high doses can lead to depression of the neuromuscular transmission
- Forms the first-line therapy for emergency control in convulsions occurring in status epilepticus, convulsant drug poisoning, tetanus, eclampsia, etc.
- **Dose:** 0.2–0.5 mg/kg slow intravenously, followed by small doses repeated as needed; maximum 100 mg/day can be given

Rationale for not Using in Maintenance Therapy

- Sedative action of this drug is very prominent
- Tolerance to the antiepileptic effect develops very promptly

    b. **Halothane is frequently combined with nitrous oxide for general anesthesia**

    (Ref: KD Tripathi, Essentials of Medical Pharmacology, 7th ed, pg. 378, 8th ed, pg. 405-06)

ANSWER

Halothane

- A potent inhalational anesthetic agent
- Recommended concentration of 2–4% for induction and 0.5–1% for maintenance of anesthesia
- Possesses higher lipid solubility; continue to enter adipose tissue for hours and leaves it gradually
- Supplemental neuromuscular blocking agents may be needed as halothane may not harvest adequate muscle relaxation

Mechanism of Action

- Antagonizes NMDA receptors
- Reduces intracellular Ca^{2+} concentration and causes direct depression of myocardial contractility
- Sensitization of heart to the arrhythmogenic action of adrenaline

Rationale of Combining with Nitrous Oxide

- Good analgesic with quick and smooth onset of action
- Generally used as a carrier and adjuvant to other anaesthetics
- **Cardiostimulatory actions:**
    - Tends to increase sympathetic tone which counters weak the direct depressant action of halothane on heart and circulatory system
- **Anaesthetic sparing effect:**
    - The co-administration of N_2O with halothane allows lower concentration of the volatile agent, halothane, to be administered
    - Concentration of the other anesthetic to be used decreased to one-third to generate same effect
    - Mixture to be prepared: 70% N_2O + 25–30% O_2 + 0.2–2% Halothane.

    c. **Dignoxin but not adrenaline is used in congestive heart failure**

    (Ref: KD Tripathi, Essentials of Medical Pharmacology, 8th ed, pg. 136, 138, 556)

ANSWER

Digoxin

- A cardiac glycoside with positive inotropic charac-teristics
- Suppresses the neurohormonal activation, thus very useful in chronic heart failure (systolic) patients
- Employed for long-term therapy

PHARMACOLOGY

Mechanism of Action

Inhibits the Na-K adenosine triphosphatase (ATPase) pump at the cellular level

↓

Prevents Na-transport intracellularly to the extracellular space

↓

Effect on activity of Na-Ca

↓

Increased intracellular level of Ca, resulting in the inotropic effect of the drug.

Rationale for Using Digoxin but not Adrenaline in CHF

- ○ Systolic (ventricles are dilated, so adequate wall tension is not developed to eject sufficient quantity of blood) or diastolic dysfunction (ventricular filling is impaired, resulting in low cardiac output)
- ○ Digoxin has properties to directly improve myocardial contractility as well as electrophysiological properties
- ○ Moreover, it has vagomimetic action and alters sympathetic activity
- ○ The filling pressure is increased and tissue perfusion demands are also fulfilled
- ○ Thus, provides symptomatic relief in heart failure precipitated due to systolic dysfunction by reversing low ionotropic state of heart tissue
- ○ Instead, adrenaline acts directly as agonists on α and/or β adrenoceptors
- ○ It also improves upon cardiac output, but the vasoconstrictive effect pushes already damaged heart to work more, thus worsening symptoms.

  d. **Acetazolamide is not preferred as a diuretic agent**

(Ref: KD Tripathi, Essentials of Medical Pharmacology, 7th ed, pg. 586-87, 8th ed, pg. 634, 637)

ANSWER

Acetazolamide
- ○ Weak or adjunct diuretic
- ○ A sulfonamide derivative

Mechanism of Action

Noncompetitive but reversible inhibition of carbonic anhydrases (CAs) in renal proximal tubule cells

↓

CAs catalyze formation of HCO_3^- and H+ from H_2O and CO_2, which is inhibited

↓

Suppression of CO_2 reabsorption from glomerular filtrate

↓

Na^+ and HCO_3^- excretion is increased

- ○ Part of the Na· (not HCO3-) rejected in the proximal tubules are reabsorbed at the high capacity ascending limb of Henle's loop
- ○ Thus, resulting alkaline diuresis is only mild

Rationale for not Preferring as Diuretic

- ○ Acetazolamide continually depletes HCO_3^- and leads to acidosis
- ○ **Poses frequent side effects:** Acidosis, hypokalemia, drowsiness, paresthesias, fatigue, abdominal discomfort
- ○ In addition, diuretic action is self-limiting (less HCO_3^- is filtered at the glomerulus, thus less diuresis occurs, hence not preferred as diuretic
- ○ However, it has been used for several extrarenal conditions, which include following:
  - As an adjuvant to other ocular hypotensives in glaucoma
  - Symptomatic relief and prophylaxis in acute mountain sickness
  - As an adjuvant in absence seizures
  - In UTIs for alkalinizing urine

2. **Enumerate commonly used opioids. Write the mode of action, indications and contraindications for the use of morphine.**

(Ref: KD Tripathi, Essentials of Medical Pharmacology, 8th ed, pg. 497-506)

ANSWER

For answer, refer 2012 paper-I Q. 2, Pg. 258

PART-II

3. **Give the rationale for the therapeutic use of the following:**

   a. **Sildenafil in erectile dysfunction**

ANSWER

For answer, refer 2007 paper-II Q. 3 (c), Pg. 331

   b. **Mannitol in cerebral edema**

PHARMACOLOGY

ANSWER

Mannitol

An osmotic diuretic

Osmotic Diuretic

Pharmacological inert substances that are filtered in the glomerulus but not reabsorbed by the nephron

Mechanism of Action

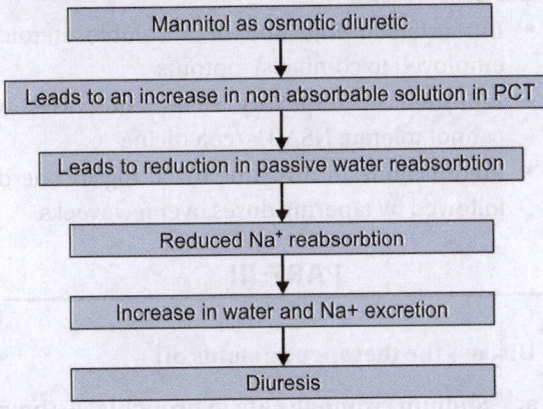

Mannitol as osmotic diuretic

↓

Leads to an increase in non absorbable solution in PCT

↓

Leads to reduction in passive water reabsorbtion

↓

Reduced Na⁺ reabsorbtion

↓

Increase in water and Na+ excretion

↓

Diuresis

Rationale for Employing Mannitol in Cerebral Edema

○ Never employed as natriuretic or for treating chronic edema

○ Employed in increased intracranial or intraocular tension (head injuries, stroke, acute congestive glaucoma, etc.)

○ It promotes water movement by osmotic action from CSF, brain parenchyma, and aqueous humour

○ Since it draws water out of the intracellular compartment, there is expansion of ECF volume, leading to reduction in edematous component

○ Although to increase urinary volume is the key action of mannitol, it also enhances excretion of all cations (Na_+, K_+, Ca_{2+}, Mg_{2+}) and anions (Cl^-, HCO_3^-, PO_{43}^-)

○ **Dose:** 1–1.5 g/kg is infused over 1 hour as 20% solution to momentarily raise osmolarity of plasma

○ Employed before and after ocular/brain surgery so as to avoid acute upsurge in intraocular/ intracranial pressure

○ **Note:** Mannitol is administered intravenously, as absorption is impeded via oral route.

c. **Combining levodopa with carbidopa in parkinsonism**

(Ref: KD Tripathi, Essentials of Medical Pharmacology, 8th ed, pg. 425, 460, 461)

ANSWER

Levodopa

○ Immediate precursor of the transmitter dopamine (DA), but inactive in itself

○ Approximately 1–2% of levodopa after administration reach the brain and is taken up by existing dopaminergic neurones, which then converted to DA

○ It acts on the CNS, CVS, and the CTZ to impart its effective therapeutic profile

Levodopa Combined with Carbidopa in Treating Parkinsonism

○ Chiefly employed in parkinsonian patients

○ Resolution of hypokinesia and rigidity, then tremor

○ Symptoms related to posture and gait, handwriting, speech, moods, self-care, and facial expression eventually normalize

○ Levodopa effects exerted on behavior entitled as "general alerting response"

○ **Carbidopa**: Extracerebral dopa decarboxylase inhibitors

○ Combination of levodopa with carbidopa known as "Co-careldopa"

○ **Merits of the combination:**

▪ Causes prolongation of plasma half-life of levodopa and dose reduction to approximately 1/4th.

▪ Nausea and vomiting are not much problematic since DA systemic concentration of DA declines

▪ Therapeutic doses of levodopa attained rapidly

▪ Inhibition of occurrence of pyridoxine reversal of levodopa

▪ Cardiac complications are curtailed

▪ Cerebral DA levels are better sustained

▪ Improvement in some patients not responding sufficiently to levodopa therapy

○ **Unresolved or accentuated issues:**

▪ Involuntary movements

▪ Abnormalities in behavior

▪ Too much daytime sleepiness in few patients

▪ Postural hypotension

▪ **Note:** Levodopa is essentially been used with carbidopa unless in cases which exhibit prominent involuntary movements due to the combination.

d. **Dopamine in cardiogenic shock**

(Ref: KD Tripathi, Essentials of Medical Pharmacology, 8th ed, pg. 146, 452)

ANSWER

For answer, refer 2017 paper-I Q. 1 (c), Pg. 186

PHARMACOLOGY

4. **Discuss the drug treatment of:**

   a. **Generalized tonic-clonic seizures**

ANSWER

For answer, refer 2011 paper-I Q. 4 (b), Pg. 275

   b. **Acute gout**

ANSWER

Gout

- A metabolic disorder when plasma urate levels exceeds the normal (2–6 mg/dL) value
- High levels of uric acid in blood results in its precipitation and deposition in joints, kidney, and subcutaneous tissues of body

Acute Gout

- Sudden flare-up of severe inflammation in a small joint due to accumulation of urate crystals in the joint space
- Redness, edema, and extreme pain results
- Most common joint affected is metatarsophalangeal joint of great toe

Drug Treatment

- **NSAIDs:**
  - Strong anti-inflammatory action is responsible for providing relief
  - Moderately effect in termination of the acute episode, but may take 12–24 hours
  - Response is slow, but are generally better tolerated
  - For examples, naproxen, piroxicam, diclofenac, indomethacin or etoricoxib can be used in relatively high and rapidly repeated doses
  - Inhibition of chemotactic migration of leucocytes into the inflamed joint is facilitated by naproxen and piroxicam
  - In view of high risk of toxicity, not recommended for long-term therapy
- **Colchicine:**
  - Fastest acting drug for controlling an acute gout attack of gout
  - **Dose:** 0.5 mg 1–3 hourly with a total of three doses in a day
  - Control achieved generally in 4–12 hours
  - For prophylaxis, NSAIDs are preferred
  - **Mechanism of action:**
    - No effect on phagocytosis of urate crystals
    - Inhibition of release of chemotactic factors and glycoprotein, hence subduing the following events
    - Inhibition of granulocyte migration into the affected joints by binding to fibrillar protein tubulin
      - Not recommended for chronic therapy as it grounds aplastic anemia, agranulocytosis, myopathy, and even hair loss.
- **Corticosteroids:**
  - Intraarticular injection of a soluble steroid is employed to combat symptoms
  - Indicated in refractory cases and cases who cannot tolerate NSAIDs/colchicine
  - Prednisolone in doses of 40–60 mg in one day, followed by tapering doses over few weeks.

PART-III

5. **Discuss the therapeutic status of:**

   a. **Sodium cromoglycate in bronchial asthma**

      (Ref: KD Tripathi, Essentials of Medical Pharmacology, 7th ed, pg. 229, 8th ed, pg. 249)

ANSWER

Sodium Chromoglycate

- Synthetic chromone derivative that causes inhibition of mast cells degranulation of mast cells by trigger stimuli
- Well tolerated, hence preferred in childhood asthma
- No absorption through oral route; hence administered by inhalation through metered dose inhaler

Mechanism of Action

Reduce accumulation of intracellular calcium ions induced by antigen

↓

Inhibit degranulation of mast cells

↓

Restriction on the release of asthma mediators, like histamine, PAF, interleukins, etc.

↓

Prevents bronchoconstriction (prophylactically)

Rationale to Use in Bronchial Asthma

- Since it does not antagonize constrictor activity of histamine and leukotriene, etc., so there is no bronchodilation
- Hence, futile when given during an asthma attack

○ Since it *prevents bronchoconstriction*, employed in long-term prophylaxis in mild-to-moderate asthma

○ Fall in the frequency and severity of attacks is probably more in patients of extrinsic (atopic) and exercise-induced asthma, notably in young age patients

○ Less effective than inhaled steroids.

b. Clozapine in schizophrenia

(Ref: KD Tripathi, Essentials of Medical Pharmacology, 8th ed, pg. 467, 468)

ANSWER

Clozapine in Schizophrenia

○ First atypical antipsychotic agent; weak D2 blocking action

○ Few/no extrapyramidal effects

○ Imparts improvement in both positive and negative symptoms of schizophrenia

○ Used as a reserve drug in resistant cases of schizophrenia (patients who do not respond to typical neuroleptics)

○ Tardive dyskinesia is rare and there is no rise in prolactin level

○ Moderately potent anticholinergic, quite sedating but paradoxically prompts hypersalivation

○ Substantial H_1 blocking property exists

○ **Side effect profile:**

  ▪ Higher incidence of agranulocytosis (0.8%) and other blood dyscrasias:

  ▪ Weight gain and hyperlipidemia

  ▪ Precipitation of diabetes

  ▪ Induction of seizures in nonepileptics when given in high doses

  ▪ Unstable BP and tachycardia

  ▪ Urinary incontinence

  ▪ Sedating effect.

c. Terlipressin in bleeding esophageal varices

(Ref: KD Tripathi, Essentials of Medical Pharmacology, 8th ed, pg. 643, 644 https://www.ncbi.nlm.nih.gov/pubmed/14562199)

ANSWER

Bleeding Esophageal Varices

One of the most common complications in gastroenterology and has a high mortality rate

Terlipressin

○ Synthetic prodrug of vasopressin

▪ Vasoactive drugs like terlipressin (somatostatin or octreotide) are indicated as drug of choice in emergency treatment

▪ Success rate of endoscopic treatments is also increased

How Terlipressin Works?

○ In view of vasoconstrictive effects on the dilated splanchnic blood vessels, terlipressin diminishes blood flow into the portal vein

○ Thus, leads to reduction in portal venous pressure and blood flow through portosystemic shunts

○ Consequently, arrest in variceal bleeding

○ Correction in central and arterial hypovolemia, and reduction in the stimulation of the renin-angiotensin-aldosterone system as well as the sympathetic nervous system, resulting in lower intrahepatic and intrarenal resistance

○ Improves organ perfusion, including perfusion of the kidneys and the liver.

6. Write short notes on:

a. Therapeutic window

(Ref: KD Tripathi, Essentials of Medical Pharmacology, 8th ed, pg. 65 HL Sharma, pg. 71)

ANSWER

Therapeutic Window

○ A dose regimen at times produces a high plasma concentration and toxicity in some patients, while the same dose regimen yields a low plasma concentration and inadequate response in the patient

○ There exists an optimal range of plasma concentration in which all patients will exhibit desired effects

○ This optimal dose bounded by dose producing minimal therapeutic effect and dose producing maximal acceptable adverse effects is known as "therapeutic window"

  ▪ Also known as therapeutic range

  ▪ Plasma concentrations of few drugs that falling within the therapeutic window:

    ♦ **Carbamazepine:** 4—10 mg/mL

    ♦ **Cyclosporine:** 100—400 ng/mL

    ♦ **Digoxin:** 0.8-2 ng/mL.

b. Midazolam

(Ref: KD Tripathi, Essentials of Medical Pharmacology, 7th ed, pg. 383, 8th ed, pg. 411)

ANSWER

Midazolam

- A water soluble benzodiazepine; faster and shorter acting
- Three times more potent than diazepam

Uses

- Sedation of intubated and mechanically ventilated patients
- Critical care anesthesia
- Preferred over diazepam for anesthetic use

Contraindications

- Use with caution in COPD, CHF, and elderly
- Known hypersensitive patients

Side effect Profile

- Headache
- Euphoria
- Confusion
- Coughing and laryngospasm
- Excessive sedation
- Retrograde amnesia, etc.

   c.   **Bioavailability**

   (Ref: KD Tripathi, Essentials of Medical Pharmacology, 8th ed, pg.22, HL Sharma 26)

ANSWER

Bioavailability

- Defined as the rate at which and extent to which the active concentration of the drug is available at the site of action.
- A measure of the fraction (F) of administered drug dose that will reaches the systemic circulation in the unchanged form
- Bioavailability is 100% for intravenously given drugs; frequently lower after oral administration due to:
  - Incompletely absorption of the drug
  - First pass metabolism
- Local binding of the drug may cause incomplete bioavailability in IM or SC routes.

Clinical Implications

Differences in bioavailability showing greater concern for drugs having steep dose response (rapidly and extensively absorbed and slowly eliminated)—switching different brands for same drugs may lead to:

- Therapeutic failure (decreased bioavailability)
- Drug intoxication (increased bioavailability)
- **Examples:** Phenytoin, warfarin, etc.

Your Roll No. ....

Name of the Paper	:	**Pharmacology Paper-II**
Name of the Course	:	**MBBS-2008**
Semester	:	**Annual**

Time: 3 Hours   **M.M.: 40**

INSTRUCTIONS

1. Write your Roll No. on the top immediately on receipt of this question paper
2. All questions are to be attempted
3. Answers to Parts I, II and III should be written in separate answer sheets provided
4. Attempt parts of a question in sequence

PART-I

1. **Explain why?**   [8]
   a. Ketoconazole is used in the treatment of cushing syndrome
   b. Propranolol and not atenolol is used in the treatment of thyrotoxicosis
   c. Chloramphenicol should not be used in premature neonates
   d. Clavulanic acid is used with amoxicillin

2. **Enumerate the drugs used in pulmonary tuberculosis. Discuss the pharmacology of Rifampicin. State WHO recommendations for short-and long-term antitubercular therapy.**   [6]

PART-II

3. **Discuss therapeutic status of:**   [8]
   a. Ondansetron as an antiemetic agent
   b. Metronidazole in amoebic hepatitis
   c. Corticosteroids in ulcerative colitis
   d. Fluoroquinolones in tuberculosis

4. **Write short notes on**   [6]
   a. Postcoital contraception
   b. Proton pump inhibitors
   c. Drugs for erectile dysfunction

PART-III

5. **Give the rationale for the use of:**   [6]
   a. Leuprolide in carcinoma prostate
   b. Cilastatin along with Imipenem
   c. Trimethoprim with sulfamethoxazole

6. **Discuss drug treatment of:**   [6]
   a. H1N1 influenza
   b. Chloroquine resistant malaria
   c. Acute gout

2008 PAPER-II

PART-I

1. Explain why?

a. Ketoconazole is used in the treatment of Cushing syndrome

(Ref: KD Tripathi, Essentials of Medical Pharmacology, 7th ed, pg. 792, 8th ed, pg. 844)

ANSWER

Cushing Syndrome

A collection of symptoms that develop as the result of very high levels of a hormone called cortisol in the body.

Ketoconazole

○ Broad-spectrum antifungal drug
○ Used to treat dermatophytosis and deep mycosis; ineffective in fungal meningitis
○ Useful in seborrhea of scalp and dandruff
○ Used in recurrent cases of monilial vaginitis or those who have not responded to topical agents
○ **Note:** Contraindicated in pregnant and lactating women

Rationale to Use in Cushing Syndrome

○ High doses are employed in Cushing's syndrome to reduce synthesis of corticosteroid
○ Effect is reported to be mediated by inhibiting adrenal 11 beta-hydroxylase and 17,20-lyase
○ Prevents the expected upsurge in ACTH secretion in patients with Cushing's disease
○ In effect for long term control of hypercortisolism of either pituitary or adrenal origin.

b. Propranolol and not atenolol is used in the treatment of thyrotoxicosis

(Ref: KD Tripathi, Essentials of Medical Pharmacology, 8th ed, pg. 162, 164, 195)

ANSWER

For answer, refer 2010 paper-II Q. 1 (b), Pg. 292

c. Chloramphenicol should not be used in premature neonates

(Ref: KD Tripathi, Essentials of Medical Pharmacology, 8th ed, pg. 762, 781)

ANSWER

Chloramphenicol

○ A broad-spectrum antibiotic
○ Predominantly bacteriostatic; in high concentrations exert bactericidal effect on some bacteria

Rationale for not Using in Premature Neonates

○ Newborns are unable to effectively metabolize and evacuate chloramphenicol
○ Results in blockage of electron transport in the liver, myocardium, and skeletal muscle at greater concentration
○ When high doses of chloramphenicol (~100 mg/kg) were administered prophylactically to premature neonates, following symptoms were developed in the baby:
  ▪ Feeding stopped
  ▪ Vomiting
  ▪ Hypothermia and hypotonia
  ▪ Abdominal distension
  ▪ Irregular respiration
  ▪ An ashen gray cyanosis, followed by cardiovascular collapse and even demise
     ◆ This condition is referred as ***Gray baby syndrome*** due to this characteristic cyanosis.

d. Clavulanic acid is used with amoxicillin

(Ref: KD Tripathi, Essentials of Medical Pharmacology, 8th ed, pg. 774, 811)

ANSWER

Amoxicillin

An extended spectrum penicillin

Clavulanic Acid

○ A β-lactamase inhibitor
○ The combination is known as coamoxiclav
○ **Indications:**
  ▪ Infections of skin and soft tissues
  ▪ Urinary, biliary and respiratory tract infections
  ▪ Intra abdominal and gynecological sepsis
  ▪ Gonorrhea (including PPNG)
○ **Rationale to use clavulanic acid with amoxicillin:**
  ▪ Re-establishment of amoxicillin action against β-lactamase producing resistant *S. aureus* (but not MRSA that have transformed cell wall

penicillin-binding proteins), *H. influenzae, N. gonorrhoeae, Klebsiella, E. coli,* etc.

- Combination inhibits species like, *B. Fragilis* and *Branhamella catarrhalis,* that do not respond to amoxicillin given alone
- Improved tolerance, when compared to both drugs used alone.

2. **Enumerate the drugs used in pulmonary tuberculosis. Discuss the pharmacology of rifampicin. State WHO recommendations for short- and long-term antitubercular therapy.**

(Ref: KD Tripathi, Essentials of Medical Pharmacology, 8th ed, pg. 818, 824, 826)

ANSWER

Drugs Used in Pulmonary Tuberculosis

- **First line:** High antitubercular efficacy and low toxicity; routinely used
  - Isoniazid (H)
  - Rifampin (R)
  - Pyrazinamide (Z)
  - Ethambutol (E)
  - Streptomycin (S)
- **Second line:** Either low efficacy or higher toxicity, or can exhibit both; reserve drugs
  - Ethionamide (Eto)
  - Prothionamide (Pto)
  - Cycloserine (Cs)
  - Terizidone (Trd)
  - Para-aminosalicylic acid (PAS)
  - Rifabutin
  - Thiacetazone (Thz)
  - **Injectable drugs:** Amikacin, capreomycin, kanamycin
  - **Fluoroquinolones:** Ofloxacin, levofloxacin, moxifloxacin, ciprofloxacin.

Pharmacology of Rifampicin

- Obtained from *Streptomyces mediterranei*
- Bactericidal action covering all subpopulations of TB bacilli, acts best on slowly or intermittently dividing bacilli
- Intra- and extracellular bacilli both are affected

Mechanism of Action

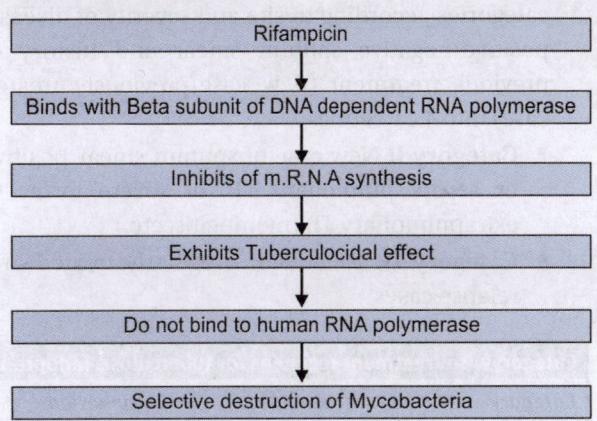

Indications Other than Tuberculosis

- **Leprosy:** Clinical benefits are attained very quickly; regression of skin lesions by 2 months and nasal symptoms (in case of lepromatous leprosy) between 2 and 3 weeks
- Prophylactically used in meningococcal and *H. influenzae* meningitis and carrier state
- First line treatment of brucellosis when combined with doxycycline
- Also employed in MRSA, Legionella, and diphtheroids infections

Adverse Effects Profile

- Failures of contraceptive measures (higher dose, 50 μg of estrogen are advised or switch to some other alternative method
- Hepatitis in patients with preexisting liver disease in a dose-related manner
- Jaundice develops, reversible after discontinuing the drug
- Flu syndrome, characterized by chills, fever, headache, malaise, etc.
- Cutaneous syndrome; rashes with pruritus mostly on face and scalp, flushing, red and watery eyes
- Abdominal syndrome; includes nausea, vomiting, abdominal cramps with or without diarrhea, etc.
- **Note:** Urine and secretions may appear orange-red in color; which is harmless

Short- and Long-term Therapy of Antitubercular Therapy

- A 6–8 months multidrug "short course" treatment regimen introduced by WHO in 1995 (DOTS program)

○ TB patients were assigned into four different categories according to site and severity of disease, positive/negative sputum smear and history of previous treatment (new case/previously treated case) into 4 categories:

- **Category I:** New case of sputum smear positive or severe pulmonary TB, or severe forms of extrapulmonary TB (meningitis, etc.)
- **Category II:** Defaulted, irregularly treated and relapse cases

- **Category III:** New sputum smear negative pulmonary TB and less severe forms of extrapulmonary TB (glandular/skin TB, etc.)
- **Category IV:** Chronic cases who remained or again became sputum smear positive after receiving fully supervised category II treatment

○ Later, clubbed into two main categories; new and previously treated patients

○ Standardization of dose of all first line drugs based on weight, valid to adults and children both

Categorywise treatment regimens for tuberculosis (adopted from WHO guidelines 2010)*

Category	Intensive phase	Continuation phase	Duration (months)	Comment
I New patient	2$ HRZE daily	4$ HR daily	6$	Optimal
	2 HRZE daily	4 HR thrice weekly	6	Acceptable if DOT ensured
	2 HRZE thrice weekly	4 HR thrice weekly	6	Acceptable it DOT ensured and no HIV coinfection or its risk
II Previously treated patients pending DST result	2 HRZES daily + 1 HRZE daily	5 HRE daily	8	For patient with low/medium risk of MDR-TB (failure, default, etc.)
	Empirical£ (standardized) MDR-regimen	Empirical (standardized) MDR regimen	18-24 or till DST result	For patient with high risk of MDR-TB (failure, 2nd default contact of MDR TB etc).

Abbreviations: DST, Drug sensitivity testing; DOT, Directly observed therapy
H, R, Z, E, S–Standard codes for isoniazid, rifampin, pyrazinamide, ethambutol and streptomycin, respectively.
$–The numerals indicate duration of a phase/total duration in months
£–Empirical (Standardized) MDR regimen is country specific depending upon local data and situation (Indian regimen on p.776)

* Treatment of tuberculosis: Guidelines, 4th edition (2010), WHO Geneva

○ **Multidrug resistance cases (MDR-TB):** Resistance to both isoniazid and rifampin, and even may include any number of other first line drugs

- Treatment is longer and complex, more expensive
- Multiple second line drug regimens to be employed
- **General principles:**
  ◆ At least 4 drugs to be included in the course certainly to be effective. As efficacy is undefined, often 5–6 drugs involved
  ◆ Avoidance to combine cross resistance drugs, e.g. two fluoroquinolones, kanamycin with amikacin, etc.
  ◆ Trust around efficacy may be formed on survey of similar patients earlier treated, DST results, and antitubercular drugs used previously in same patient
  ◆ Drugs from group I to group IV (alternative classification) to be included following hierarchy.

○ **DOTS-Plus guidelines:** Recommended by RNTCP in 2010 to be in sync with the current WHO guidelines:

- **Category IV regimen:** Intensive phase (6 drugs) lasting 6–9 months and continuation phase (4 drugs) of 18 months, employed in all confirmed or suspect MDR-TB cases
- Followed until an individualized regimen is mandated by DST results or other specifics (intolerance, etc.) in a patient
- Positive sputum culture at the end of 4th, 5th and 6th month, respectively: Intensive phase (6 months) extended by 1 month each time till a maximum of 9 months

Note: Pyridoxine 100 mg/day given during the entire course to all patients in order to prevent neurotoxicity of the antitubercular drugs.

PART-II

3. **Discuss therapeutic status of:**

a. **Ondansetron as an antiemetic agent**

(Ref: KD Tripathi, Essentials of Medical Pharmacology, 8th ed, pg. 186, 414)

Answer

Ondansetron

Developed to cater vomiting associated to chemotherapy/radiotherapy

Mechanism of Action

○ Peripheral 5-HT3 receptor blockade on vagal afferents in GIT, including nucleus tractus solitarius (NTS) and chemoreceptor trigger zone (CTZ)

Therapeutic Profile in Antiemesis

○ Vomiting induced by cisplatin and other highly emetogenic drugs employed in cancer chemotherapy

○ Also useful in postoperative nausea and vomiting; administered 4 h before surgery

○ Used in cases of acute vomiting than delayed vomiting

○ Effective in controlling vomiting which occurs as side effect of drugs or due to drug overdosage, uremia, neurological disorders and disorders of GI

○ Poor efficacy in motion sickness

○ Hyperemesis gravidarum (only given in pregnancy in unavoidable cases)

Advantages over Other Antiemetics

Does not produce dystonias or sedation.

b. Metronidazole in amoebic hepatitis

(Ref: KD Tripathi, Essentials of Medical Pharmacology, 8th ed, pg. 657, 705, 753, 772)

Answer

For answer, refer 2013 paper-II Q. 3 (a), Pg. 252

c. Corticosteroids in ulcerative colitis

(Ref: KD Tripathi, Essentials of Medical Pharmacology, 8th ed, pg. 734-37)

Answer

Ulcerative Colitis

A type of inflammatory bowel disease, involving only the colon beginning from the anal canal; mucosal lesions, which may be diffuse or even confluent

Corticosteroids in Ulcerative Colitis

○ Drugs of choice for moderately severe exacerbations

○ Relief in symptoms usually initiates within 3–7 days; induction of remission in 2–3 weeks

○ Intravenous methyl prednisolone to be initiated in case of in more severe disease with extraintestinal manifestations and to provide rapid relief

○ Mostly used for short term, and withdrawn after remission is induced

○ For topical treatment of proctitis and distal ulcerative colitis, hydrocortisone enema, or foam can be used

○ Many patients of severe IBD either do not respond to it (known as steroid-resistant) or show relapse on stoppage of the steroid (referred as steroid-dependent).

d. Fluoroquinolones in tuberculosis

(Ref: KD Tripathi, Essentials of Medical Pharmacology, 8th ed, pg. 759, 761)

Answer

Fluoroquinolones

○ New potent oral bactericidal drugs for TB

○ Second line therapy; well tolerated alternatives to first line antitubercular drugs

○ Show activity against MAC, *M. fortuitum,* and some other atypical mycobacteria

○ **Moxifloxacin:** Most active fluoroquinolone against *M. tuberculosis*

○ Primarily used for treatment of drug resistant TB

○ Usually employed in Group 3 patients (WHO recommendations for short term therapy); now have also been tried in first line regimens for new cases

○ Addition of moxifloxacin to RHZ regimen may possibly reduce the treatment duration from 6 months with RHZE used currently; however, not routinely used

○ Significantly introduced in all regimens for MDR-TB (except resistant cases)

Advantages

○ Penetration within cells and killing of mycobacteria lodged inside macrophages as well.

4. Write short notes on:

a. Postcoital contraception

(Ref: KD Tripathi, Essentials of Medical Pharmacology, 8th ed, pg. 344, 346)

Answer

For answer, refer 2017 paper-II Q. 6 (c), Pg. 200

b. Proton pump inhibitors

(Ref: KD Tripathi, Essentials of Medical Pharmacology, 8th ed, pg. 699-702)

ANSWER

Proton Pump Inhibitors

Examples include omeprazole, pantoprazole, etc.

Mechanism of Action

○ Dose dependent suppression of gastric acid secretion; without anticholinergic

○ or H_2 blocking action

○ HCl secretion, both resting as well as that stimulated by food or any of the secretagogues, can be abolished without considerable effect on pepsin, intrinsic factor, and gastric motility

Indications

○ Eradication of *H. pylori* (combined with anti-microbial drugs)

○ Resistant severe peptic ulcer (4 to 8 weeks) and prevent bleeding from ulcers

○ Reflux esophagitis

○ Hypersecretory conditions, such as Zollinger Ellison syndrome and gastrinoma

○ Prophylactically in stress ulcers, etc.

Side Effect Profile: (Minimal)

○ Nausea

○ Loose stools

○ Headache and pain abdomen

○ Muscle and joint pain

○ Rashes, leukopenia, and hepatic dysfunction infrequently

○ Atrophic gastritis on prolonged treatment.

c. Drugs for erectile dysfunction

(Ref: KD Tripathi, Essentials of Medical Pharmacology, 8th ed, pg. 327-29)

ANSWER

Erectile Dysfunction (ED)

Inability in attaining and maintaining an erect penis with sufficient rigidity to allow intercourse

Drugs Employed in Treatment

○ **Androgens:**

▪ This is useful only when loss of libido and ED have occurred due to androgen deficiency

▪ Parenteral testosterone esters or transdermal testosterone therapy

○ **Phosphodiesterase-5 (PDE-5) inhibitors:**

▪ Forms first-line therapy for ED

▪ Examples include sildenafil, Tadalafil and vardenafil (selective PDE-5 inhibitors) **Sildenafil:**

Belongs to group of phosphodiesterase-5 (PDE-5) inhibitors

▪ Selectively inhibits PDE-5 and enhances NO action in corpus cavernosum

▪ Thus erection of penis during sexual activity is improved, however, no such effect occur in the sexual arousal is absent

○ **Papaverine/Phentolamine induced penile erection (PIPE) therapy:**

▪ Papaverine (3–20 mg) injection with or without phentolamine (0.5–1 mg) in the corpus cavernosum

▪ Very risky uncertain results; priapism, which if not quickly treated results in permanent damage, etc.

PART-III

5. Give the rationale for the use of:

a. Leuprolide in carcinoma prostate

(Ref: KD Tripathi, Essentials of Medical Pharmacology, 8th ed, pg. 265)

ANSWER

For answer, refer 2009 paper-II Q. 6 (b), Pg. 307

b. Cilastatin along with Imipenem

(Ref: KD Tripathi, Essentials of Medical Pharmacology, 8th ed, pg. 782)

ANSWER

Imipenem

○ A thienamycin derivative

○ An extremely potent and broad-spectrum β-lactam antibiotic

○ Inhibition of some MRSA, not reliable for treatment of such infections

Rationale to Use with Cilastatin

○ Imipenem undergoes rapid hydrolysis by the enzyme dehydropeptidase I, which is located on the brush border of renal tubular cells

○ Cilastatin (a reversible inhibitor of dehydropeptidase I)

○ Thus, it protects imipenem from hydrolysis

○ Combination of imipenem-cilastatin 0.5 g intravenously every 6 hours is effective in a wide range of severe hospital-acquired respiratory, abdominal, urinary, pelvic, and skin and soft tissue infections

○ Patients in neutropenia, cancer and AIDS included

○ Though may induce diarrhea, vomiting, rashes on skin, etc., as side effects.

c. **Trimethoprim with sulfamethoxazole**

(Ref: KD Tripathi, Essentials of Medical Pharmacology, 8th ed, pg. 757-59)

ANSWER

For answer, refer 2012 paper-II Q. 6 (c), Pg. 270

6. **Discuss drug treatment of:**

a. **H1 N1influenza**

(Ref: KD Tripathi, Essentials of Medical Pharmacology, 8th ed, pg. 857-58)

ANSWER

H1N1 Influenza

○ Known as "Swine flu"
○ Transmitted from person to person mostly through contact with infected respiratory secretions during coughing and sneezing
○ Illness presents a range of symptoms: mild upper respiratory infection to an acute, life-threatening illness
○ If indicated, treatment with an antiviral agent, to be started as soon as possible after the start of typical influenza-like symptoms
○ Prompt empiric treatment recommended for progressive, severe cases, and illness needing hospitalizations (started before diagnostic confirmation)
○ An algorithm to treat H1N1 influenza is presented in figure 2
○ **Antiviral drugs**: Neuraminidase inhibitor: Oseltamivir (orally); zanamivir (inhaled)
○ **Dose:**
  ▪ Oseltamivir 75 mg twice daily for 5 days in adults during treatment and 75 mg once daily for 10 days in chemoprophylaxis
  ▪ Zanamivir 10 mg (two 5 mg inhalations) twice daily for 5 days during treatment in adults and 10 mg (two 5-mg inhalations) once daily given for 10 days during chemoprophylaxis

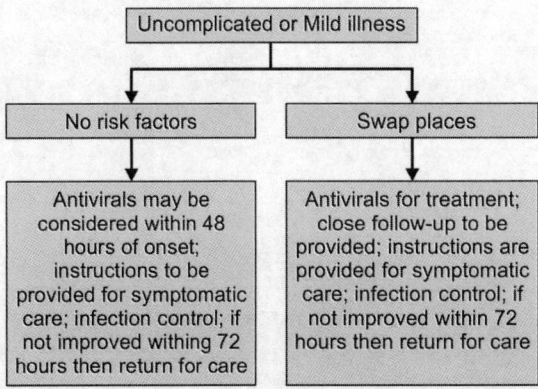

b. **Chloroquine resistant malaria**

(Ref: KD Tripathi, Essentials of Medical Pharmacology, 8th ed, pg. 874-76)

ANSWER

Chloroquine

Rapidly acting erythrocytic schizonticide against all species of plasmodia; most clinical attacks are controlled in 1–2 days

Treatment of Chloroquine Resistance among *P. vivax*

○ Quinine 600 mg (10 mg/kg) 8 hourly for 7 days + Doxycycline 100 mg daily for 7 days or + Clindamycin 600 mg 12 hourly for 7 days + Primaquine (15 mg daily for 14 days)

or

○ Artemisinin-based combination therapy + Primaquine

Treatment of Chloroquine Resistance among *P. falciparum:*

○ Artesunate 100 mg BD for 3 days + sulfadoxine 1500 mg + pyrimethamine 75 mg in single dose

or

○ Artesunate 100 mg BD for 3 days + mefloquine 750 mg on second day and 500 mg on third day

or

○ Artemether 80 mg + lumefantrine 480 mg BD for 3 days

or

○ Arterolane (as maleate) 150 mg + piperaquine 750 mg OD for 3 days

or

○ Quinine 600 mg 8 hourly for 7 days + doxycycline 100 mg daily for 7 days or + clindamycin 600 mg 12 hourly for 7 days.

c. **Acute gout**

ANSWER

For answer, refer 2008 paper-I Q. 4 (b), Pg. 312

Name of the Paper	:	**Pharmacology Paper-I**
Name of the Course	:	**MBBS-2007**
Semester	:	**Annual**

Time: 3 Hours   **M.M.: 40**

INSTRUCTIONS

1. Write your Roll No. on the top immediately on receipt of this question paper
2. All questions are to be attempted
3. Answers to Parts I, II and III should be written in separate answer sheets provided
4. Attempt parts of a question in sequence

PART-I

1. **Explain why?**   [8]
   a. Thiazide diuretics cause calcium retention while loop diuretics cause increase in calcium excretion
   b. Ethanol is used in methanol poisoning
   c. Plasma concentration of phenytoin rises disproportionately at higher doses
   d. First dose of prazosin should preferably be administered at bed time

2. **Classify antidepressant drugs. Write the mechanism of action, adverse effects and therapeutic uses of fluoxetine.**
                                                                                       [6]

PART-II

3. **Give rationale for the therapeutic use of the following:**   [8]
   a. Oximes in organophosphorus poisoning
   b. Sumatriptan in migraine
   c. Adenosine in the treatment of paroxysmal atrial tachycardia
   d. Tizanidine in spastic disorders

4. **Discuss the drug treatment of:**   [6]
   a. Status asthmaticus
   b. Paracetamol poisoning

PART-III

5. **Discuss the therapeutic status of:**   [6]
   a. ACE inhibitors in heart failure
   b. Statins in dyslipidemia
   c. Leukotriene antagonists in bronchial asthma

6. **Write short notes on:**   [6]
   a. Fixed dose drug combinations
   b. Drugs modulating cytochrome P450 enzymes
   c. Drug dependence

PART-I

1. Explain why?

a. Thiazide diuretics cause calcium retention while loop diuretics cause increase in calcium excretion

(Ref: KD Tripathi, Essentials of Medical Pharmacology, 8th ed, pg. 563)

ANSWER

Diuretics

Drugs that increase urine flow and induce urinary sodium loss.

- Diuretics are typically classified as:
  - Thiazide diuretics (chlorothiazide, chlorthalidone, hydrochlorothiazide, indapamide, metolazone and polythiazide)
  - Loop diuretics (bumetanide, ethacrynic acid, furosemide, and torsemide)
  - Potassium-sparing agents (amiloride, eplerenone, spironolactone, and triamterene).

- The thiazide diuretics are responsible for calcium retention and increased serum calcium levels during their use while loop diuretics lead to increased calcium excretion.

- This due to the different sites of action as well as mechanism of action of the two drugs.

Mechanism of Action for Thiazides

Site of action is the *early part of distal tubule* via inhibition of Na^+/Cl^- transport. They exert a direct distal tubular action and cause decreased renal Ca^{2+} excretion and increased Mg^{2+} excretion.

Mechanism of Action for Loop Diuretics

Site of action is *thick ascending limb of loop of Henle*. There is a transepithelial potential difference at this site of nephron. This leads to reabsorption of the divalent cations: Ca^{2+} and Mg^{2+}. The loop diuretics eliminate this potential difference and thus increase excretion of Ca^{2+} (as well as Mg^{2+}).

- This is why thiazides are used in treatment of *Hypercalciuria with recurrent calcium stones in the kidney* while loop diuretics are employed in the treatment of *Hypercalcemia of malignancy.*

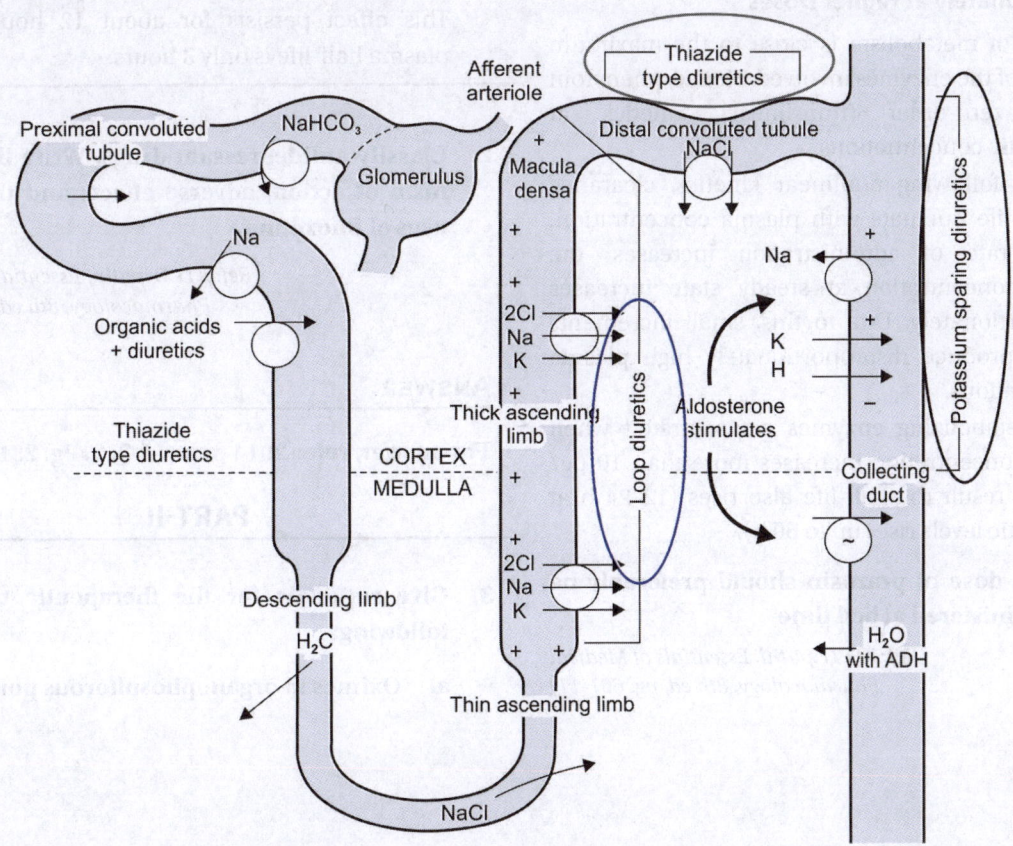

b. **Ethanol is used in methanol poisoning**

Answer

For answer, refer 2009 paper-I Q. 4 (b), Pg. 301

c. **Plasma concentration of phenytoin rises disproportionately at higher doses**

Answer

Phenytoin

- Synthesized in 1908 as a barbiturate analogue.
- It is a major **antiepileptic drug**.
- **Significant actions**:
  - Abolition of tonic phase of the maximal electroshock seizures, with no effect on or prolongation of clonic phase.
  - Restricting the spread of seizure activity.
  - Suppression of tonic-clonic epilepsy is suppressed, however, persistence of paroxysmal focal EEG discharge and "aura".
- Phenytoin elimination occurs mostly by its biotransformation to various inactive hydroxylated metabolites. Some of these metabolites are further metabolized by conjugation with glucuronic acid. These are then largely excreted in the urine.

Plasma Concentration of Phenytoin Rises Disproportionately at Higher Doses

- The rate of metabolism is close to the maximum capacity of the enzymes involved. Hence, phenytoin follows zero-order (non-linear) kinetics at therapeutic concentrations.
- In drugs following nonlinear kinetics, clearance and half-life fluctuate with plasma concentration. As the rate of administration increases, the plasma concentration at steady state increases disproportionately. Due to this, small increments in dose produce disproportionately high plasma concentrations.
- Since metabolizing enzymes get saturated when plasma concentration increases more than 10 μg/mL, as a result the half-life also rises (12–24 h at therapeutic levels rises up to 60 h).

d. **First dose of prazosin should preferably be administered at bed time**

(Ref: KD Tripathi, Essentials of Medical Pharmacology, 8th ed, pg. 601-11)

Answer

Prazosin

Selective α1 antagonist.

Mechanism of Action

- Prazosin causes dilatation of arterioles and veins (more pronounced on large resistance vessels i.e., arterioles), reduces total peripheral resistance as well as preload and afterload. Thus, it lowers blood pressure and used as an antihypertensive agent.
- The release inhibitory a2 (presynaptic) receptors are not blocked.
- Autoregulation of release of noradrenaline is preserved intact. However, central sympathetic tone is probably decreased.

First Dose Effect of Prazosin

- Postural hypotension and fainting may occur in the beginning and even with the dose increases.
- This usually get disappear as the therapy continues, but may persist in the elderly.
- Due to this first dose effect, prazosin is preferably given at bedtime. In addition, it is started at a low dose (0.5 mg) and gradually increased with twice daily administration (maximum dose 10 mg twice daily) to produce an adequate response.
- An oral dose causes peak fall in BP after 4–5 hours. This effect persists for about 12 hours, though plasma half-life is only 3 hours.

2. **Classify antidepressant drugs. Write the mechanism of action, adverse effects and therapeutic uses of fluoxetine.**

(Ref: KD Tripathi, Essentials of Medical Pharmacology, 8th ed, pg. 481-92)

Answer

For answer, refer 2014 paper-I Q. 2, Pg. 231

PART-II

3. **Give rationale for the therapeutic use of the following:**

a. **Oximes in organophosphorous poisoning**

ANSWER

For answer, refer 2010 paper-I Q. 3 (d), Pg. 287

b. Sumatriptan in migraine

(Ref: KD Tripathi, Essentials of Medical Pharmacology, 8th ed, pg. 193-94)

ANSWER

For answer, refer 2013 paper-II Q. 3 (c), Pg 252

c. Adenosine in the treatment of paroxysmal atrial tachycardia

ANSWER

Paroxysmal Atrial Tachycardia (PAT)

○ Also known as paroxysmal supraventricular tachycardia (PSVT) (this term better indicated the specific underlying abnormality)

○ Defined as sudden onset episodes of atrial tachycardia (@rate 150–200/min) with 1:1 atrioventricular (AV) conduction, largely due to circus movement type of re-entry that occurs within or around the AV node or can even use an accessory path between atria and ventricle

Adenosine in Treatment of PAT

○ Drug of choice in PAT

○ **Dose:** Administered by rapid IV injection over 1–3 seconds either as the free base (6–12 mg) or as ATP in a dose of 10–20 mg

○ **Mechanism of action**

○ Activation of ACh sensitive K· channel

○ Membrane hyperpolarization through interaction with A1 type of adenosine GPCRs on SA node (pacemaker depression leads to bradycardia), AV node (ERP prolongation resulting in slowing of conduction) and atrium (reduction in excitability)

○ Indirect decreases Ca_{2+} current in AV node

○ Depression of the reentrant circuit through AV node is accountable for terminating majority of PSVTs.

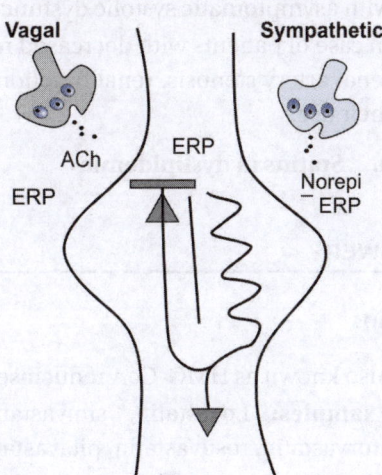

Increased AV node ERP breaks the reentrant cycle & restores sinus Rhythm

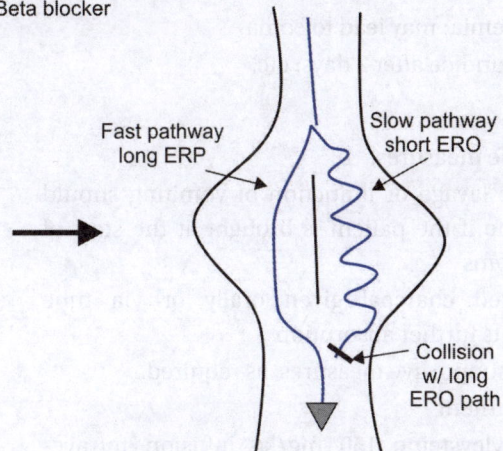

AVN ERP:
- Carotid massage
- Adenosine
- Verapamil or dilitazem
- Beta blocker

○ **Advantages:**
  - Better or equivalent efficacy when compared to verapamil.
  - Action lasting less than 1 min
  - Transient adverse effects
  - No hemodynamic deterioration observed
  - Can be given to patients with hypotension, CHF, wherein verapamil is contraindicated
  - Safe to use in wide QRS tachycardia (unlike verapamil)
  - Effective in patients not responding to verapamil.

○ **Side effect profile:**
  - Difficulty in breathing for short time
  - Chest pain
  - Fall in BP and flushing in 30–60% patients
  - Bronchospasm may be precipitated in asthmatics

○ **Note:** Not suitable for prophylaxis in recurrent cases.

d. Tizanidine in spastic disorders

ANSWER

For answer, refer 2014 paper-I Q. 1 (a), Pg. 231

PHARMACOLOGY

4. Discuss the drug treatment of:

a. Status asthmaticus

ANSWER

For answer, refer 2015 paper-I Q. 4 (b), Pg. 219

b. Paracetamol poisoning

(Ref: KD Tripathi, Essentials of Medical Pharmacology, 8th ed, pg. 223)

ANSWER

Paracetamol Poisoning

- Serious toxicity can occur with use of paracetamol if administered in large dose (>150 mg/kg or >10 g in adults).
- Occurs particularly in small children as their hepatic glucuronide conjugating ability is low.

Early Manifestations

- Nausea, vomiting
- Pain in abdomen and liver tenderness

Late Manifestations

- Centrilobular hepatic necrosis after 12–18 hours; renal tubular necrosis may also occur
- Hypoglycemia; may lead to coma
- Start of jaundice after 2 days, etc.

Treatment

- Supportive measures:
  - Gastric lavage or induction of vomiting should be done if the patient is brought at the start of symptoms
  - Activated charcoal given orally or via tube prevents further absorption
  - Other supportive measures, as required.
- Drug treatment
  - N-acetylcysteine 150 mg/kg infusion intravenously over 15 minutes
  - Same dose is followed IV over the next 20 hours
  - May be orally administered as an alternative in a dose 75 mg/kg every 4–6 hours for 2–3 days
  - **Aim of treatment:** Replenishing glutathione stores in liver and prevention of binding of the noxious metabolite to other cellular constituents.

Note: In 2009, the US-FDA recommended that amount of paracetamol in any single dosage form (tablet/capsule) to be reduced to 650 mg (earlier 1000 mg). The total daily dose should not exceed 2600 mg (earlier 4000 mg).

PART-III

5. Discuss the therapeutic status of:

a. ACE inhibitors in heart failure

ANSWER

ACE Inhibitors

- Produce vasodilation by impeding angiotensin II formation, a vasoconstrictor
- The proteolytic action of renin (released by the kidneys) acts on circulating angiotensinogen to form angiotensin I. Angiotensin I is then converted to angiotensin II by angiotensin converting enzyme (inhibited by ACE inhibitors)
- Plays role in providing symptomatic and disease modifying effects in congestive heart failure (CHF) by causing vasodilatation, preventing ventricular hypertrophy, apoptosis of myocardial cell, fibrosis intercellular matrix changes and remodeling.
- In addition, increase the level of kinins which stimulate generation of cardioprotective NO and PGs
- Symptomatically and prognostically effective in mild to severe (NYHA class I to IV) CHF and in subjects with asymptomatic systolic dysfunction
- In case of patients with decreased renal blood flow/renal artery stenosis, renal function deteriorates by their use.

b. Statins in dyslipidemia

ANSWER

Statins

- Also known as HMG-CoA reductase inhibitors
- **Examples:** Lovastatin, simvastatin, pravastatin, atorvastatin, rosuvastatin, pitavastatin
- Considered as the first choice drugs for primary hyperlipidemias with raised LDL and total cholesterol levels, with or without raised TG levels (Type IIa, IIb, V)
- Drugs of choice for secondary hypercholesterolemia (diabetes, nephrotic syndrome)
- Preferential drugs in dyslipidemia in diabetics
- All statins are administered at bed time to attain maximum efficacy since HMG-CoA reductase activity is maximum at midnight; same may not be very significant for atorvastatin and rosuvastatin, which have long plasma half-life.

c.   **Leukotriene antagonists in bronchial asthma**

(Ref: KD Tripathi, Essentials of Medical Pharmacology, 8th ed, pg. 248-49)

ANSWER

For answer, refer 2017 paper-I Q. 3 (d), Pg. 189

6.   **Write short notes on:**

a.   **Fixed dose drug combinations**

(Ref: KD Tripathi, Essentials of Medical Pharmacology, 8th ed, pg. 72)

ANSWER

For answer, refer 2011 paper-I Q. 6 (c), Pg. 277

b.   **Drugs modulating cytochrome P$_{450}$ enzymes**

(Ref: KD Tripathi, Essentials of Medical Pharmacology, 8th ed, pg. 30, 33)

ANSWER

Cytochrome P$_{450}$ enzyme

○   Cytochrome P$_{450}$ is Microsomal Enzyme Protein
○   Drugs modulating different cytochrome P$_{450}$ enzyme families:
  ▪   **CYP3A isoenzymes:** Anticonvulsants (phenobarbitone, phenytoin, carbamazepine), rifampin, glucocorticoids
  ▪   CYP2D6 by rifampin and CYP2B1 by phenobarbitone

  ▪   **CYP2E1:** Isoniazid and chronic alcohol consumption
  ▪   **CYP1A isoenzymes:** Polycyclic hydrocarbons like 3-methylcholanthrene and benzopyrene found in cigarette smoke, charcoal broiled meat, omeprazole and industrial pollutants induce.
  ▪   **Other important enzyme inducers:** Phenylbutazone, griseofulvin, DDT.
○   Induction includes microsomal enzymes in liver as well as other organs and this increases the rate of metabolism by 2–4 folds.
○   **Possible uses:**
  ▪   Congenital nonhemolytic jaundice: Due to deficient glucuronidation of bilirubin; clearance of jaundice hastened by phenobarbitone
  ▪   Chronic poisonings: More rapid metabolism of the collected poisonous substance.
  ▪   Liver disease
  ▪   Cushing's syndrome: Phenytoin may cause reduction in the manifestations by augmenting degradation of adrenal steroids which are formed in abundance.

c.   **Drug dependence**

(Ref: KD Tripathi, Essentials of Medical Pharmacology, 8th ed, pg. 98, 99)

ANSWER

For answer, refer 2016 paper-I Q. 6 (a), Pg. 206

Your Roll No. ....

Name of the Paper	:	**Pharmacology Paper-II**
Name of the Course	:	**MBBS-2007**
Semester	:	**Annual**

Time: 3 Hours   **M.M.: 40**

INSTRUCTIONS

1. Write your Roll No. on the top immediately on receipt of this question paper
2. All questions are to be attempted
3. Answers to Parts I, II and III should be written in separate answer sheets provided
4. Attempt parts of a question in sequence

PART-I

1. **Explain why?**   [8]
   a. Anaerobic microorganisms are resistant to aminoglycoside antibiotics
   b. Heparin and warfarin are started together in acute thromboemolic states
   c. Thalidomide is used for lepra reaction
   d. Dose of skeletal muscle relaxant should be lowered in patients receiving high doses of gentamicin

2. **Classify drugs used in diabetes mellitus. Describe the pharmacology of oral hypoglycemic drugs.**   [6]

PART-II

3. **Give rationale of the use of the following:**   [8]
   a. Hydroxychloroquine in systemic lupus erythematosis
   b. BAL in arsenic poisoning
   c. Sildenalfil in erectile dysfunction
   d. Finasteride in prostatic disease

4. **Discuss the drug treatment of:**   [6]
   a. HIV infection
   b. MDR tuberculosis

PART-III

5. **Discuss therapeutic status of:**   [6]
   a. Bisphosphonates in osteoporosis
   b. Cyclosporine in renal transplants
   c. Tamoxifen in breast cancer

6. **Write short notes on:**   [6]
   a. Albendazole
   b. Paclitaxel
   c. Emergency contraceptives

PART-I

1. Explain why?

a. Anaerobic microorganisms are resistant to aminoglycoside antibiotics

ANSWER

Aminoglycosides

Bactericidal antibiotics

- ○ **Mechanism of Action**

Aminoglycoside transported through the bacterial cell wall and cytoplasmic membrane

↓

Binds to ribosomes

↓

Inhibition of protein synthesis

- ■ Entrance from the periplasmic space through the cytoplasmic membrane is carrier mediated which is linked to the electron transport chain.
- ■ The penetration is dependent on the oxygen dependent active processes
- ■ *Under anaerobic conditions, there is lack of oxidative metabolism which drives uptake of aminoglycosides*
- ■ That is why, anaerobes are resistant to aminoglycosides.
- ○ Cidal (killing) action seems to be based on secondary variations in the integrity of bacterial cell membrane, since other antibiotics which hinder protein synthesis (tetracyclines, chloramphenicol, and erythromycin) are only static.

b. Heparin and warfarin are started together in acute thromboembolic states

ANSWER

Anticoagulants

Drugs used to reduce blood coagulability

Heparin

- ○ A parenteral anticoagulant, effective both *in vivo* and *in vitro*
- ○ **Mechanism of action**

Activates plasma antithrombin (AT III)

↓

Binding of heparin-AT III complex to clotting factors (Xa, IIa, IXa, XIa, XIIa, and XIIIa)

↓ Inactivation of clotting factors

Inhibition of factor Xa and thrombin (IIa) mediated conversion of fibrinogen to fibrin

- ■ Not absorbed orally as it is a large and highly ionized molecule.

Warfarin

- ○ Oral anticoagulants acting only *in vivo*, not *in vitro*
- ○ **Mechanism of action**

Act as competitive antagonists of vitamin K

↓

Interfere with the synthesis of vitamin K dependent clotting factors in liver

Rationale of Starting Heparin and Warfarin Together in Acute Thromboembolic States

- ○ Heparin is administered parenterally and used for *swift and short-lived action*
- ○ Warfarin is administered orally and suited for *maintenance therapy*
- ○ The objective of using these two anticoagulants is to impart immediate and fast action as well as prevent further thrombus extension and embolic complications by decreasing the rate of fibrin formation
- ○ **Note:** Clots which are already formed are not dissolved but recurrences are prevented
- ○ However started together, heparin is withdrawn after 4–7 days when warfarin has taken effect.

c. Thalidomide is used for lepra reaction

(Ref: KD Tripathi, Essentials of Medical Pharmacology, 8th ed, pg. 837)

ANSWER

Lepra Reaction

- ○ According to WHO, immunologically mediated episodes of acute or subacute inflammation known as reactions may occur during the course of leprosy, in up to 25% of patients with paucibacillary leprosy and as much as 40% with multibacillary leprosy
- ○ It is a Arthus (Jarisch Herxheimer) type of reaction which occurs when killing of bacilli results into release of antigens

- **Manifests as:**
  - Enlargement of existing lesions, redness, swelling and pain
  - New lesions may appear
  - Malaise and fever, etc.
- May be mild, severe or life-threatening, i.e. erythema nodosum leprosum (ENL)
- **Note:** Dapsone is temporarily discontinued only in severe cases.

Thalidomide in Lepra Reactions

- Prednisolone in a dose of 40–60 mg/day is started immediately and continued till the reaction subsides in severe cases
- Thalidomide imparts anxiolytic, antiemetic with anti-inflammatory actions. It also has cytokine (TNFα, ILs, interferon) modulatory property. Thus, can be used as an alternative to prednisolone as cytokines play an important role in generating symptoms in lepra reaction
- Also indicated in multiple myeloma
- **Dose for ENL**: 100–300 mg once daily at bed time.

  d. Dose of skeletal muscle relaxant should be lowered in patients receiving high doses of gentamicin

ANSWER

Gentamicin

- Antimicrobial drug obtained from *Micromonospora purpurea*
- Higher potency and broader spectrum of activity than streptomycin
- Most frequently used aminoglycoside for acute infections

Antibiotic Coverage of Gentamicin

- Active mainly against aerobic gram negative bacilli
- Few gram-positive bacteria including, especially *S. aureus*, *S. faecalis,* and some *Listeria*, however, *S. pyogenes*, *S. pneumoniae,* and enterococci usually show insensitivity
- No effect against *M. tuberculosis* and other mycobacteria

Dose of Skeletal Muscle Relaxant Decreased in View of Patients Receiving Gentamicin

- Aminoglycoside antibiotics possess neuromuscular blocking activity
- There is reduction in ACh release from the motor nerve endings as well as decrease in the sensitivity of the muscle endplates to Ach

- Myasthenic weakness is also accentuated
- The neuromuscular blockade may not be significant in the usual clinical use
- Nevertheless it becomes very important, when aminoglycosides are put into peritoneal or pleural cavity after a surgery, and particularly if a nondepolarizing muscle relaxant (curare-like effects; e.g., d-tubocurarine) was used during the same
- Nondepolarizing block is also known as a competitive block. These muscle relaxant drugs attach to cholinergic receptors, preventing acetylcholine from attaching to the receptor. Thus, the resultant neuromuscular blockade due to gentamicin and these muscle relaxants results in apnea and fatality in patients
- **Note:** Potency of those antibiotics tested appears to be as follows: gentamicin > streptomycin > amikacin > sisomicin > kanamycin = tobramycin > kendomycin = dibekacin.

2. Classify drugs used in diabetes mellitus. Describe the pharmacology of oral hypoglycemic drugs

(Ref: KD Tripathi, Essentials of Medical Pharmacology, 8th ed, pg. 294-302)

ANSWER

For answer, refer for classification of antidiabetic drugs, 2017 paper-II Q. 2, Pg. 196. For answer, refer 2015 paper-II. 2 of oral hypoglycemic drugs Mechanism of action and adverse effects, Pg. 224

PART-II

3. Give rationale of the use of the following:

  a. Hydroxychloroquine in systemic lupus erythematosis

ANSWER

Hydroxychloroquine

An antimalarial drug.

Mechanism of Action

- Reduce monocyte IL–I, consequently inhibition of B lymphocytes
- Interfering with antigen processing
- Lysosomal stabilization and scavenging free radicals

Rationale for Use in SLE

- Hydroxychloroquine leads to an increased pH within intracellular vacuoles and changes processes, such as protein degradation by acidic hydrolases in the lysosome, assembly of macromolecules in the endosomes, and post-translation modification of proteins in the Golgi apparatus

○ It is proposed that the antirheumatic properties results from the interference with "antigen processing" in macrophages and other antigen-presenting cells

○ This compound diminishes the formation of peptide-MHC protein complexes, which are required to stimulate CD4+ T cells and thus result in down regulation of the immune response against autoantigenic peptides

○ There is improvement of clinical and laboratory parameters, but have slow onset of action.

b. BAL in arsenic poisoning

(Ref: KD Tripathi, Essentials of Medical Pharmacology, 8th ed, pg. 928)

ANSWER

BAL (Dimercaprol)

An oily, pungent smelling, viscous liquid.

Mechanism of Action

○ Constitutes two SH groups which bind those metals that produce toxicity by interacting with sulfhydryl containing enzymes in the body

○ **For example:** As, Hg, Au, Bi, Ni, Sb, Cu

○ It is desirable to maintain BAL excess in plasma so as to allow formation of 2 : 1 complex in view of complex of two BAL molecules with one metal ion being more stable than 1:1 complex

Rationale for Use in Arsenic Poisoning

○ The two SH groups binds to the As molecule

○ BAL-metal complex impulsively dissociates releasing the metal at a slow rate; this emphasizes the BAL excess to treat metal toxicity

○ **Dose:** Given intramuscularly 5 mg/kg *stat*, followed by 2–3 mg/kg every 4–8 hours for 2 days, then once or twice a day for 10 days

○ **Note:** Contraindicated in Fe and Cd poisoning, as the BAL-Fe and BAL-Cd complexes are themselves toxic.

c. Sildenafil in erectile dysfunction

(Ref: KD Tripathi, Essentials of Medical Pharmacology, 8th ed, pg. 327-28)

ANSWER

Sildenafil

Belongs to group of phosphodiesterase-5 (PDE-5) inhibitors

Erectile Dysfunction (ED)

○ Inability in attaining and maintaining an erect penis with sufficient rigidity to allow intercourse

○ Variety of neurogenic, vascular, hormonal, pharmacologic or psychogenic causes may be responsible

Rationale for Use in ED

○ Penile erection occurs due to relaxation of smooth muscle in corpus cavernosum and the blood vessels supplying it

○ This is caused by nitric oxide (NO) released from parasympathetic nonadrenergic noncholinergic (NANC) nerves and vascular endothelium

○ Sildenafil selectively inhibits PDE-5 and enhances NO action in corpus cavernosum

○ Thus erection of penis during sexual activity is improved, however, no such effect occur in the sexual arousal is absent

○ **Dose:** Recommended in a dose of 50 mg (for men > 65 years 25 mg), if no effect, then 100 mg 1 hour before intercourse.

d. Finasteride in prostatic disease

ANSWER

Finasteride

Competitive inhibitor of 5α-reductase enzyme

Mechanism of Action

○ 5α-reductase is the enzyme employed in conversion of testosterone into more active DHT responsible for androgen action in many tissues including the prostate gland and hair follicles

○ Finasteride comparatively selective for 5α-reductase type 2 isoenzyme which prevails in male urogenital tract. Circulating and prostatic

Rationale for Use in Prostatic Disease

○ Reduces the static component of obstruction, while the dynamic component is overcome by a₁ blockers

○ Lowers the DHT concentration, but plasma LH and testosterone levels remain unchanged

○ Treatment with finasteride in benign hypertrophy of prostate (BHP) patients ensued a decrease in prostate size and increase in peak urinary flow rate

○ Provides symptomatic relief

○ Relief in symptoms is less pronounced as compared to surgery and adrenergic a₁ blockers though.

4. Discuss the drug treatment of:

a. HIV infection

(Ref: KD Tripathi, Essentials of Medical Pharmacology, 8th ed, pg. 860-67)

ANSWER

HIV Infection

Cure does not exists for HIV/AIDS, but strict adherence to antiretroviral regimens (ARVs) can dramatically slow the disease progression as well as prevent secondary infections and complications

Targets for Anti-HIV Attack

○ **Transcription of HIV-RNA into proviral DNA:** *HIV reverse transcriptase*

○ **Cleaving of the large virus directed polyprotein into functional viral proteins:** *HIV protease*

○ Fusion of plasma membrane of CD4 cells and viral envelope which allows entry of HIV-RNA into the cell

○ **Anchorage for the surface proteins of the virus:** Chemokine coreceptor (CCR5) on host cells

○ **Integration of the proviral DNA into host DNA:** Viral HIV-integrase.

Drugs Employed in Antiretroviral Therapy (Majorly)

○ *Nucleoside reverse transcriptase inhibitors* (NRTIs)

  ▪ For example, Zidovudine, lamivudine

  ▪ Prevents formation of double-stranded proviral DNA from single-stranded viral RNA by selectively inhibiting viral reverse transcriptase in preference to cellular DNA

  ▪ Used only in combination with at least two other ARV agents

  ▪ Decrease in occurrence of opportunistic infections

  ▪ Provides sense of well-being and weight gain

  ▪ Reduction in mortality among AIDS patients

○ *Non-nucleoside reverse transcriptase inhibitors* (NNRTIs)

  ▪ For example: Nevirapine and efavirenz

  ▪ Noncompetitive inhibitors which directly inhibit HIV reverse transcriptase

  ▪ No need for intracellular phosphorylation

  ▪ Not indicated in infections caused by HIV-2

  ▪ **Note:** If a patient fails to show response to any NNRTI regimen, another NNRTI should not be instituted

○ *HIV-protease inhibitors* (PIs)

  ▪ Acts at a late stage, i.e. while maturation of the new virus particles after the RNA genome acquires the core proteins and enzymes

  ▪ **For example:** Atazanavir, indinavir, nelfinavir, saquinavir, ritonavir (RTV) and lopinavir

  ▪ Effective in both lately as well as chronically infected cells

  ▪ Prevent further rounds of infection.

○ **Note:** ARV drugs are at all times used in combination of at least three drugs and over time regimens need to be altered due to development of resistance.

b. MDR tuberculosis

ANSWER

MDR-TB

○ Resistance to both isoniazid and rifampin, and may be any number of other (first line) drug(s)

○ Treatment involves use of complex multiple second line drugs

○ India, according to WHO, has the maximum number of MDR-TB cases in South-East Asia

○ **Principles of treatment of MDR-TB are:**

  ▪ The regimen should have at least 4 drugs certain to be effective. 5–6 drugs are often

  ▪ Combining cross resistance drugs to be avoided, for example, two FQs, Km with Am or Cs with terizidone

  ▪ Include drugs from group I to group IV following a hierarchical order

  ▪ Group I drugs (except isoniazid and rifampin) can be involved, adding one injectable drug (group II), one FQ (group III) and one or two group IV drugs.

○ The DOTS-plus program was initiated by RNTCP in 2000 to cover diagnosis as well as treatment of MDR-TB (updated in 2010)

○ **Standardized treatment regimen (also known as category IV regimen):** 6 drugs intensive phase lasts for 6–9 months and 4 drugs continuation phase of 18 months, which is used in all MDR-TB cases either confirmed or suspect, unless DST results or other specifics (intolerance, etc.) of an individual case demand practice of an customized regimen

○ If the sputum culture at the end of 4th, 5th and 6th months, respectively, are all positive, then extension of minimal 6 month intensive phase by 1 month each time till a maximum of 9 months

○ **Note:** Pyridoxine is given to all patients for prevention of neurotoxicity due to antitubercular drugs during the whole course of therapy.

PART-III

5. Discuss therapeutic status of:

a. Bisphosphonates in Osteoporosis

ANSWER

Bisphosphonates (BPNs)

Analogs of pyrophosphate

○ First choice therapy employed in osteoporosis

How They Work?

- Inhibition of bone resorption:
  - Accelerating apoptosis of osteoclasts reducing their number
  - Disrupting the cytoskeleton and ruffled border of osteoclasts
  - Affecting precursors of osteoclast and inhibiting their differentiation
  - Inactivating osteoclasts
- Second (Alendronate, etc.) and third generation (Zoledronate, etc.) drugs exhibit higher efficacy and potency than first generation drugs (Etidronate, etc.)
- BPNs employed in osteoporosis helps conserving bone mineral density
- Marked reduction in the risk of vertebral and hip fractures by 47–56%.
- Higher efficacy than calcitonin
- Provide protection for at least 5 years of continuous use.

b. Cyclosporine in renal transplants

(Ref: KD Tripathi, Essentials of Medical Pharmacology, 8th ed, pg. 940, 944)

ANSWER

Cyclosporine

- A highly selective immunosuppressant
- Specific T-cell inhibitor which has strikingly increased success in organ transplantations
- **How it works?**
  - Target T cell signal transduction
  - Inhibit expression of IL-2
  - Inhibit IL-2 mediated T cell activation, proliferation, and differentiation
  - Arrest at G_0 or G_1 phase of lymphocytes
- This compound preferentially suppresses cell-mediated immunity and prevents graft rejection
- Most effective drug for use in renal, hepatic, cardiac, bone marrow and other transplantations
- The recipient is yet left with sufficient immune activity to fight bacterial infection
- **Dose:**
  - Administered orally 12 hours before the transplant
  - Given intravenously if graft rejection has started as have low oral bioavailability
  - 10–15 mg/kg/day with milk or fruit juice till 1–2 weeks
  - Gradual reduction to maintenance dose of 2–6 mg/kg/day after transplant
- Effective therapy employs blood level monitoring is required for effective therapy as it is concentrated

in WBCs and RBCs, metabolized in liver by CYP3A4 and excreted in bile

- **Added advantages:**
  - No toxic effects on bone marrow and reticuloendothelial system
  - Humoral immunity remains intact.

c. Tamoxifen in breast cancer

(Ref: KD Tripathi, Essentials of Medical Pharmacology, 8th ed, pg. 337-38)

ANSWER

For answer, refer 2015 paper-II Q. 3 (d), Pg. 226

6. Write short notes on:

a. Albendazole

(Ref: KD Tripathi, Essentials of Medical Pharmacology, 8th ed, pg. 907-09)

ANSWER

For answer, refer 2010 paper-II Q. 3 (b), Pg. 294

b. Paclitaxel

(Ref: KD Tripathi, Essentials of Medical Pharmacology, 8th ed, pg. 924-25)

ANSWER

Paclitaxel

- Classified as a "plant alkaloid," a "taxane" and an "antimicrotubule agent."
- Employed in chemotherapy

Mechanism of Action

- Binding to β-tubulin and enhancement of its polymerization
- Stabilization of microtubules
- Inhibition of normal reorganization of the microtubules
- Production of abnormal arrays or bundles of microtubules all through the cell cycle

Therapeutic Uses

- Metastatic ovarian and breast carcinoma when first line chemotherapy fails and cases of relapse
- Small cell lung cancer, esophageal adenocarcinoma
- Advanced cases of head-neck cancer
- Urinary and hormone refractory prostate cancer
- Kaposi's sarcoma

Side Effect Profile

- Reversible myelosuppression
- "Stocking and glove" neuropathy
- Nausea
- Chest pain
- Edema
- Arthralgia
- Myalgia and mucositis.

c. Emergency contraceptives

(Ref: KD Tripathi, Essentials of Medical Pharmacology, 8th ed, pg. 345)

ANSWER

Emergency Contraception

These immediate measures are instituted to prevent unwanted pregnancy in cases of unprotected sexual intercourse

Standard Regimen

- *Levonorgestrel* in a dose of 0.75 mg (twice with a gap of 12 hours), or single dose of 1.5 mg

- It should be taken as soon as possible, but before 72 hours of unprotected sexual activity
- Milder side effects, for example, headache, nausea, vomiting, and less pronounced than estrogen + progestin therapy
- May result in delayed or disturbed menstrual cycles

- *Ulipristal* (recently approved)
  - This is also a well-tolerated method
  - It provides an extended window of protective action
  - Single dose of 30 mg single dose as soon as possible, within 120 hours of unprotected intercourse

- *Mifepristone*
  - Fewer side effects noted
  - Single dose of 600 mg within 72 hours of unprotected sexual activity

- **Note:** Emergency contraception should be held in reserve for cases of unexpected or accidental exposure (rape, condom rupture) only, as higher failure rate and more side effects than regular contraception are reported.

Microbiology

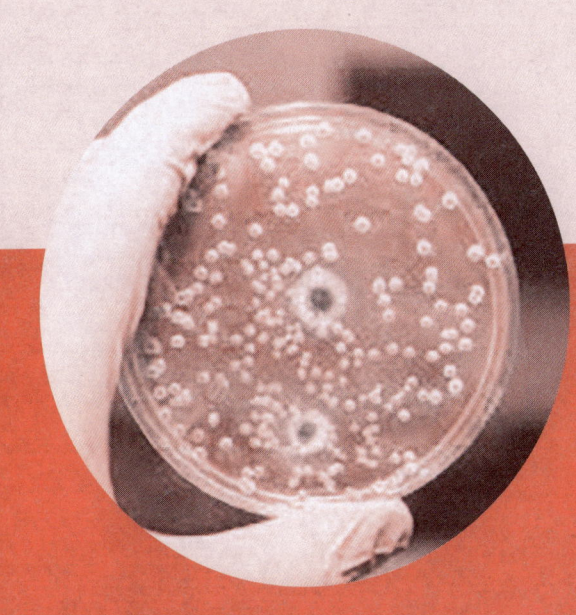

References Taken From:

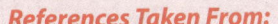

- *Textbook of Microbiology, Ananthanarayan & Paniker, 10th edition*
- *Medical Parasitology, D.R. Arora & Brij Bala Arora, 5th edition*

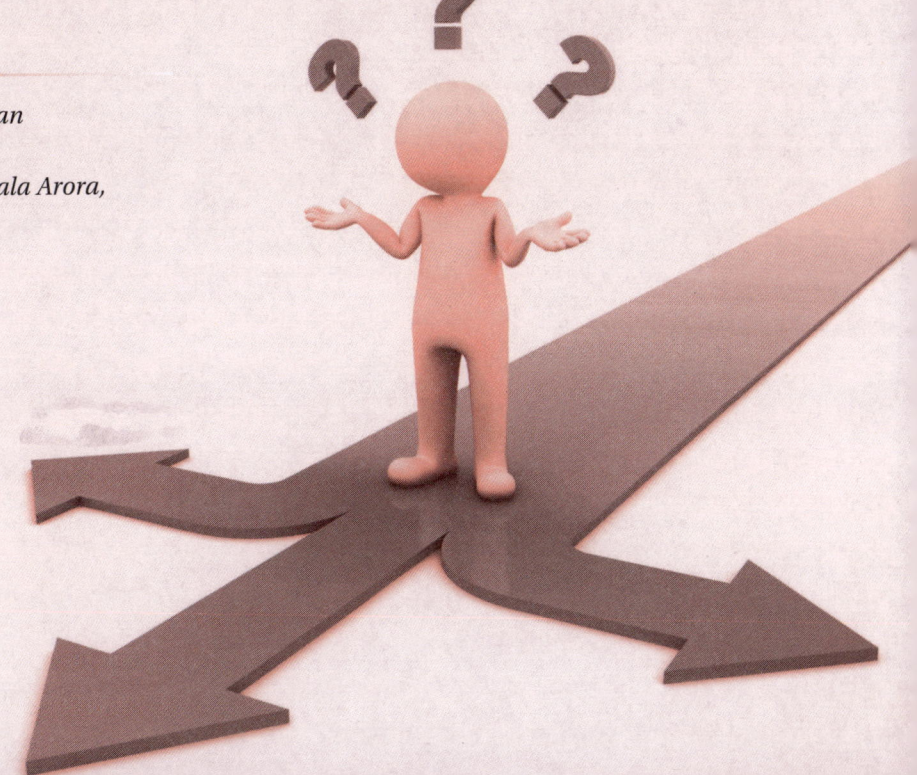

Name of the Paper	:	**Microbiology Paper-I**
Name of the Course	:	**MBBS-2017**
Semester	:	**Annual**

Time: 3 Hours   **M.M.: 40**

INSTRUCTIONS

1. Write your Roll No. on the top immediately on receipt of this question paper
2. All questions are to be attempted
3. Answers to Parts I, II and III should be written in separate answer sheets provided
4. Attempt parts of a question in sequence

PART-I

1. Classify hypersensitivity reactions. Describe in detail about type I hypersensitivity reactions.   [5]

2. Write short notes on: [10]
   a. Monoclonal antibodies
   b. Sterilization by moist heat

PART-II

3. Enumerate the agents causing enteric fever. Describe the laboratory diagnosis of enteric fever.   [5]

4. Write briefly on: [10]
   a. Elek's gel precipitation test
   b. Non–tuberculous mycobacteria

PART-III

5. Name the various water-borne pathogens. Describe briefly the bacteriological examination of water.   [5]

6. Describe briefly about the drug resistance in bacteria.   [5]

PART-I

1. **Classify hypersensitivity reactions. Describe in detail about type I hypersensitivity reactions.**

(Ref: Ananthanaryan & Paniker, Textbook of Microbiology, 10th ed, pg.163)

ANSWER

Classification of Hypersensitivity Reactions

	Type	Type II	Type III	Type IV
Immune reactant	IgE	IgE	IgE	T-cell
Antigen	Soluble molecule	Cell associated molecule	Soluble molecule	Soluble or cell associated molecule
Graphic				
Mechanism	IgE induced mast cell activation	Complement mediated phagocytosis	Tissue damage induced by immune complexes	T-cell mediated inflammation or cytotoxicity
Examples	Allergic rhinitis allergic asthma	Chronic urticaria (auto antibodies)	Serum sickness, arthus reaction	Multiple sclerosis, contact dermatitis, Crohn's disease, Rheumatoid arthritis

Type-I Hypersensitivity

○ It is an immediate immune reaction, i.e. it happens immediately after exposure to the particular substance.

○ Type I hypersensitivity is characterized by IgE mediated reaction. This reaction may occur in two types.

○ **Immediate reaction**
  ▪ Degranulation and release of vasoactive amines (i.e. histamine) and proteases

○ **Late-phase reaction**
  ▪ Synthesis and secretion of prostaglandins and leukotrienes
  ▪ Cytokine-induced inflammation and leukocyte recruitment

Mechanism	Effects	Examples
Ab- IgE (cytotropic) Cells- IgE B cell, mast cells, basophils, eosinophil Pivoted role- by TH2 cell Most important	Systemic acute anaphylaxis	• Bee sting • Insect bites • Anaphylactic shock • Answers with Explanation • Semisolved Question Bank
Vasoactive amine: Histamine Slow reacting substance of anaphylaxis (SRS-A) = leukotrienes (LT B$_4$, C$_4$, D$_4$, E$_4$)	Local anaphylaxis (Atopy)	• Urticaria • Angioedema • Hay fever • Some forms of asthma; eczema

Development of the Immediate Hypersensitivity Reaction

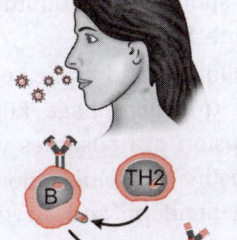

1. First exposure to allergen

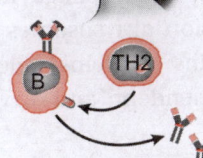

2. TH2 release of IL-4 and IL-13 stimulates B cell to produce IgE: class switching occurs

IgE antibody

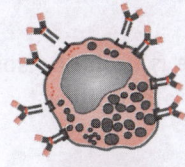

3. B cell produces IgE immunoglobulin: it attaches to Fc receptor on mast cell

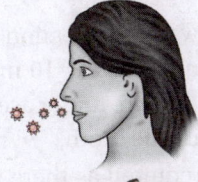

4. Second exposure to allergen

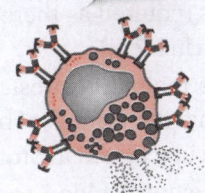

5. Allergen cross-links several IgE molecules on mst cell and cell degranulates, releasing

Fig. Development of the immediate hypersensitivity reaction

2. **Write short notes on:**

   a. **Monoclonal antibodies**

(Ref: Ananthanaryan & Paniker, Textbook of Microbiology,10th ed, pg.187, 190)

ANSWER

- Monoclonal antibodies are cells derived by cell division from a single ancestral cell.
- Kohler and Milstein (1975) found a method for production of monoclonal antibodies-They are awarded Nobel Prize for medicine in 1984.
- **Medium used for Monoclonal Antibody** production is HAT medium-hypoxanthine, Aminopterin and thymidine medium.
- Monoclonal antibodies target various proteins that influence cell activity such as receptors or other proteins present on the surface of normal and cancer cells.
- The specificity of Monoclonal Antibodies allows its binding to cancerous cells by coupling a cytotoxic agent such as a strong radioactive which then seek outs to destroy the cancer cells while not harming the healthy ones.

- Tumor cells that are able to replicate endlessly are fused with mammalian cells that produce a specific antibody which result in fusion called hybridoma that continuously produce antibodies. Those antibodies are named monoclonal because they come from only 1 type of cell, which is the hybridoma cell. Antibodies that are produced by conventional methods and derived from preparations containing many kinds of cells are called polyclonal Antibodies.
- Monoclonal antibodies are artificially produced against a specific antigen in order to bind to their target antigens. Laboratory production of monoclonal antibodies is produced from clones of only 1 cell which means that every monoclonal antibody produced by the cell is the same.

Types of Monoclonal Antibodies

- **Mouse mAb:** 100% mouse derived proteins
- **Chimeric mAb:** Recombination of mouse proteins (Variable region) and human proteins (Constant region).
- **Humanized mAb:** Only the antigen binding site is mouse derived; remaining part human derived.
- **Human mAb:** 100% human derived

   b. **Sterilization by moist heat**

(Ref: Ananthanaryan & Paniker, Textbook of Microbiology, 10th ed, pg.30)

ANSWER

- Moist heat kills microbes by coagulation of proteins i.e. denaturation. Boiling is most commonly used.
- Physical agents used in moist heat: Pasteurization, Inspissation, Boiling, Tyndallization and Autoclaves.
- Pasteurization is a process of making milk and milk products and other food stuffs safe for consumption by destroying all harmful microorganisms like Mycobacteria, *Brucella*, Diphtheria, *Staphylococcus* and *Salmonella* species. Spores and *Coxiella* burnetii are not destroyed because they are heat resistant. The temperature employed is either 63°C for 30 minutes known as Holder method, or 72°C for 10–15 seconds known as Flash method.

Holder method, or 72°C for 10–15 seconds known as Flash method.

Holder method	63°C for 30 minutes Coxiella burnetii are not destroyed because they are heat resistant
Flash method	72°C for 10–15 seconds followed by quickly cooling to 13°C.

- **Inspissation** Is a way to sterilize media like Lowenstein-Jensen or Loeffler's serum slopes by subjecting them to heat at 80–85°C for half an hour on three successive days in an inspissator First day heating destroys the vegetative forms of bacteria but allows the spores to germinate, which are killed on second time heating. Third heating ensures complete sterilization without destroying the constituents of the medium.

- **Boiling:** For 10–30 minutes at a temperature of 90–100°C kills vegetative bacterial cells, whereas spores need prolonged periods of boiling. To sterilize surgical instruments or needles boiling is not sufficient and autoclaving must be done to kill bacterial spores.

- Media containing sugars or gelatin needs to be exposed for 20 minutes at 100°C for three consecutive days and this method is known as **Tyndallization** or intermittent sterilization.

- **Autoclaves use pressurized** steam to destroy microorganisms, and are the most dependable systems available for the decontamination of laboratory waste and the sterilization of laboratory glassware, media and reagents. A variety of materials, such as dressings, instruments, laboratory ware, media and pharmaceutical products which can withstand high temperature, discarded media with growth can be sterilized or disposed of by this method. Transfusion equipment, glassware and metalware, intravenous equipment, applicators, syringes and items that can withstand high temperature and pressure can also be sterilized by this method

PART-II

3. **Enumerate the agents causing enteric fever. Describe the laboratory diagnosis of enteric fever.**

(Ref: Ananthanaryan & Paniker, Textbook of Microbiology,10th ed, pg. 300)

ANSWER

Agents Causing Enteric Fever

- *Salmonella typhi*
- *Salmonella paratyphi type A, B, or C*

Distinguishing Features from other organisms

- **Gram-negative rods, highly motile with the Vi capsule**
- **Facultative anaerobe, nonlactose fermenting**
- **Produces H2S**
- **Species identification with biochemical reactions**
- **Sensitive to acid**

- The sample can be collected from patient's blood, duodenal fluid, feces, suspected food, CSF, pus or sputum.

Direct microscopic examination shows Gram-negative bacteria.

- **In 1st week:** Patients have 80% positive blood cultures; 25% have rose spots (trunk/abdomen), signs of septicemia (mainly fever)

- S. typhi survives intracellularly and replicates in macrophages; resistant to macrophage killing because of decreased fusion of lysosomes with phagosomes and defensins (proteins) allow it to withstand oxygen-dependent and oxygen-independent killing

- **In 2nd week:** Serological tests like Widal test is helpful

- **In 3rd week:** Stool culture is useful to isolate S. typhi. 85% of stool cultures are positive

- **In 4th week:** Urine culture

- **Blood culture:**

- The test is positive in first week of infection and before starting course of antibiotics. 5–10 mL of blood is collected by vein puncture under aseptic conditions and inoculated in bile broth.

- Large quantity of blood is required as there may be less number of bacteria in blood.

- Moreover, blood contains inhibitory substances therefore it is necessary that the volume of blood is four times diluted when inoculated in broth.

- To nullify the bactericidal action of blood, sodium polyanethol sulfonate is added to broth.

- It is incubated at 37°C for overnight and then subcultured on MacConkey agar and incubated again.

- Pale, nonlactose fermenting colonies that appear on it are picked and identified by biochemical tests and slide agglutination test with specific antisera.

- **Treatment:** Fluoroquinolones or third-generation cephalosporins

- **Prevention:** Sanitation; 3 vaccines (attenuated oral vaccine of S. typhi strain 21 (Ty21a), parenteral heat-killed S. typhi (no longer used in U.S.), and parenteral ViCPS polysaccharide capsular vaccine)

4. **Write briefly on:**

a. **Elek's gel precipitation test**

(Ref: Ananthanaryan & Paniker, Textbook of Microbiology, 10th ed, pg. 108, 243)

ANSWER

- Elek test is an in vitro immunoprecipitation (immunodiffusion) test to determine whether or not a strain of

○ *Corynebacterium diphtheriae* is toxigenic.

○ A test strip of filter paper containing diphtheria antitoxin is placed in the center of the agar plate. Strains to be tested (patient's isolate), known positive and negative toxigenic strains are also streaked on the agar's surface in a line across the plate and at a right angle to the antitoxin paper strip.

○ Antitoxin diffuses away from the strip of filter paper whereas toxin produced by toxin-producing strains diffuse away from growth. At the zone of equivalence a precipitin line is formed.

Procedure

○ Mix a tube of melted nutrient agar with 2 mL of sterile horse serum.

○ Rotate the tube to mix the serum and agar. Do not shake the tube.

○ Pour the mixture into a sterile petri dish.

○ Using lightly flamed forceps, lay the strip of anti-toxin impregnated filter paper across the center of the petri dish allowing it to sink beneath the agar surface.

○ Allow the agar to set, then lift one corner of the lid and let the plate dry for 30-45 minutes in the incubator.

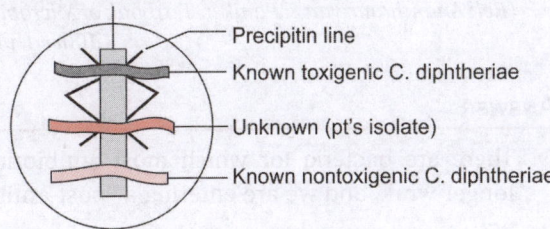

Filter paper strip with C. diphtheriae antitoxin

— Precipitin line
— Known toxigenic C. diphtheriae
— Unknown (pt's isolate)
— Known nontoxigenic C. diphtheriae

Fig. Elek's Test

○ When dry inoculate with a toxingenic strain of *C. diphtheriae* by streaking a single line of inoculum across the plate and paper strip at right angles to the strip.

○ Repeat this about 1 inch away from the *C. diphtheriae* inoculum with a test strain.

○ Incubate the plate for 24 hrs and observe the results.

b.   Nontuberculous mycobacteria

(Ref: Ananthanaryan & Paniker, Textbook of Microbiology,10th ed, pg. 352)

ANSWER

○ Nontuberculous mycobacteria (NTM) are naturally-occurring organisms found in water and soil. NTM lung infection occurs when a person inhales the organism from their environment

○ In some people, the organism infects the airways and lung tissue leading to disease. This causes inflammation in the respiratory system. Without treatment, many people, but not all, will develop a progressive lung infection characterized by cough, shortness of breath, fatigue, and weight loss.

○ It is also called atypical mycobacteria other than tuberculous (MOTT) or anonymous mycobacteria.

○ Classification of Nontuberculous mycobacteria

Runyon Classification

▪ **Photochromogens:** M. kansasii, M. marinum

▪ **Scotochromogens:** M. scrofulaceum, M. gordonae

▪ **Nonphotochromogens:** M. avium, M. intra-cellulare, M. ulcerans, M. xenopi

▪ **Rapid growers:** M. fortuitum, M. chelonae, M. phlei

○ Disease caused by non–tuberculous mycobacteria

▪ **M. marinum:** Fish tank granuloma or swimming pool granuloma

▪ **M. gordonae:** Tap water Scotochromogens

▪ **M. kansasii:** Cause chronic pulmonary disease. (DD:TB)

▪ **M. scrofulaceum:** Cervical adenitis in children

▪ **M. fortuitum:** Chronic abscess

▪ **M. chelonae:** Injection site abscess

▪ **M. ulcerans:** Buruli ulcer

▪ **M. avium:** It is called as Battey bacillus. Most common NTM isolated from lung disease. Causes pulmonary disease and disseminated lesions in AIDS patients.

Note: M. avium complex (MAC) typically occurs in AIDS patients with CD4 counts <50 cells/mm³ and presents as disseminated disease.

PART-III

5.   Name the various water-borne pathogens. Describe briefly the bacteriological examination of water.

ANSWER

Water Borne Pathogens

○ *Crytosporidium*

○ *Naegleria fowleri*

○ *Giardia*

○ *Salmonella typhimurium*

○ *Vibrio cholerae*

○ *Legionella*

- *Escherichia coli*
- *Campylobacter jejuni*

Bacteriological Examination of Water

- **Multiple tube method**
  - One of the oldest methods is called the multiple tube method. In this method a measured sub-sample (perhaps 10 mL) is diluted with 100 mL of sterile growth medium and an aliquot of 10 mL is then decanted into each of ten tubes. The remaining 10 mL is then diluted again and the process repeated. At the end of 5 dilutions this produces 50 tubes covering the dilution range of 1:10 through to 1:10000.
  - The tubes are then incubated at a pre-set temperature for a specified time and at the end of the process the number of tubes with growth in is counted for each dilution. This method can be enhanced by using indicator medium which changes color when acid forming species are present and by including a tiny inverted tube called a Durham tube in each sample tube. The Durham inverted tube catches any gas produced. The production of gas at 37°C is a strong indication of the presence of Escherichia coli.

- **ATP Testing**
  - An ATP test is the process of rapidly measuring active microorganisms in water through detection adenosine triphosphate (ATP). ATP is a molecule found only in and around living cells, and as such it gives a direct measure of biological concentration and health. ATP is quantified by measuring the light produced through its reaction with the naturally occurring enzyme firefly luciferase using a luminometer. The amount of light produced is directly proportional to the amount of biological energy present in the sample.

- **Plate count**
  - The plate count method relies on bacteria growing a colony on a nutrient medium so that the colony becomes visible to the naked eye and the number of colonies on a plate can be counted. To be effective, the dilution of the original sample must be arranged so that on average between 30 and 300 colonies of the target bacterium are grown. Fewer than 30 colonies makes the interpretation statistically unsound whilst greater than 300 colonies often results in overlapping colonies and imprecision in the count.

- **Membrane filtration**
  - Most modern laboratories use a refinement of total plate count in which serial dilutions of the sample are vacuum filtered through purpose made membrane filters and these filters are themselves laid on nutrient medium within sealed plates. The methodology is otherwise similar to conventional total plate counts. Membranes have a printed millimeter grid printed on and can be reliably used to count the number of colonies under a binocular microscope.

- **Pour plate method**
  - When the analysis is looking for bacterial species that grow poorly in air, the initial analysis is done by mixing serial dilutions of the sample in liquid nutrient agar which is then poured into bottles which are then sealed and laid on their sides to produce a sloping agar surface. Colonies that develop in the body of the medium can be counted by eye after incubation.
  - The total number of colonies is referred to as the Total Viable Count (TVC). The unit of measurement is cfu/mL (or colony forming units per milliliter) and relates to the original sample. Calculation of this is a multiple of the counted number of colonies multiplied by the dilution used.

---

6. **Describe briefly about the drug resistance in bacteria.**

(Ref: Ananthanaryan & Paniker, Textbook of Microbiology, 10th ed, pg.306)

ANSWER

- There are bacteria for which most antibiotics no longer work, and we are entering a "post-antibiotic era."
- There are 3 types of antibiotic resistance: intrinsic, chromosome-mediated, and plasmid-mediated. Drug resistance can be transferred from one genus of bacteria to another, e.g., from normal flora to a pathogen.

Intrinsic Drug Resistance

- Bacteria are intrinsically resistant to an antibiotic if they lack the target molecule for the drug or if their normal anatomy and physiology make them refractory to the drug's action.
- Bacteria that lack mycolic acids are intrinsically resistant to isoniazid.
- Bacteria such as Mycoplasma that lack peptidoglycan are intrinsically resistant to penicillin.

Chromosome-Mediated Resistance

- In chromosome-mediated resistance, resistance is conveyed by genes located on the bacterial chromosome.

- Most commonly, these genes modify the receptor for a drug so the drug can no longer bind (e.g., a mutation in a gene for a penicillin-binding protein).
- In general, drug resistance is low level.
- In methicillin-resistant Staphylococcus aureus, a major penicillin-binding protein was mutated.
- Even low-level resistance may be clinically significant, e.g., in Streptococcus pneumoniae meningitis.

Plasmid-Mediated Resistance

- The genes that determine this resistance are located on plasmids.
- Plasmid-mediated resistance is created by a variety of mechanisms, but often genes code for enzymes that modify the drug.
- R factors are conjugative plasmids carrying genes for drug resistance.
  - One section of the DNA (containing oriT and the tra gene region) mediates conjugation.
  - The other section (R determinant) carries genes for drug resistance.
- Multiple genes seem to have been inserted through trans positional insertion into a "hot spot."
- Multiple drug-resistance (MDR) plasmids arise from mobile DNA segments known as transposons (integrons) or gene cassettes. Transposons have the following features:
  - Are mobile genetic elements (DNA) that can move themselves or a copy from one molecule of DNA to another ("jumping genes")
  - Are found in eukaryotic and bacterial cells and viruses
  - Have at least 1 gene for a transposase (enzyme involved in the movement).
  - Create additional mutations with their insertion into another totally unrelated gene.

Name of the Paper	**:**	**Microbiology Paper-II**
Name of the Course	**:**	**MBBS-2017**
Semester	**:**	**Annual**

Time: 3 Hours   M.M.: 40

INSTRUCTIONS

1. Write your Roll No. on the top immediately on receipt of this question paper
2. All questions are to be attempted
3. Answers to Parts I, II and III should be written in separate answer sheets provided
4. Attempt parts of a question in sequence

PART-I

1. Name the various tissue nematodes and describe the pathogenesis and life cycle of *Wuchereria bancrofti*.   [5]

2. Write short notes on: [10]
   a.   Laboratory diagnosis of toxoplasmosis
   b.   Echinococcus granulosus

PART-II

3. Describe the laboratory diagnosis of fungal infections.   [5]

4. Write briefly on: [10]
   a.   Sporothrix schenckii
   b.   Prophylaxis against Hepatitis 'B' infections

PART-III

5. Describe the morphology of human immunodeficiency virus (HIV) and laboratory diagnosis of HIV infections.
                                                                                                                        [5]

6. Write briefly about the prophylaxis against rabies.   [5]

PART-I

1. **Name the various tissue nematodes and describe the pathogenesis and life cycle of *Wuchereria bancrofti*.**

ANSWER

(Ref: Arora parasitology 5th ed. P. 199, 200, 204)

Tissue Nematodes

- *Wuchereria bancrofti*
- *Brugia malayi*
- *Brugia timori*
- *Onchocerca volvulus*
- *Loa loa*

Life Cycle of Wuchereria bancrofti

- During a blood meal, an infected mosquito introduces third-stage filarial larvae onto the skin of the human host, where they penetrate into the bite wound.
- They develop in adults that commonly reside in the lymphatics.

- The female worms measure 80 to 100 mm in length and 0.24 to 0.30 mm in diameter, while the males measure about 40 mm by 0.1 mm.
- Adults produce microfilariae measuring 244 to 296 μm by 7.5 to 10 μm, which are sheathed and have nocturnal periodicity, except the South Pacific microfilariae which have the absence of marked periodicity.
- The microfilariae migrate into lymph and blood channels moving actively through lymph and blood.
- A mosquito ingests the microfilariae during a blood meal.
- After ingestion, the microfilariae lose their sheaths and some of them work their way through the wall of the proventriculus and cardiac portion of the mosquitoes midgut and reach the thoracic muscles.
- There the microfilariae develop into first-stage larvae and subsequently into third-stage infective larvae.
- The third-stage infective larvae migrate through the hemocoel to the mosquitoes prosboscis and can infect another human when the mosquito takes a blood meal.

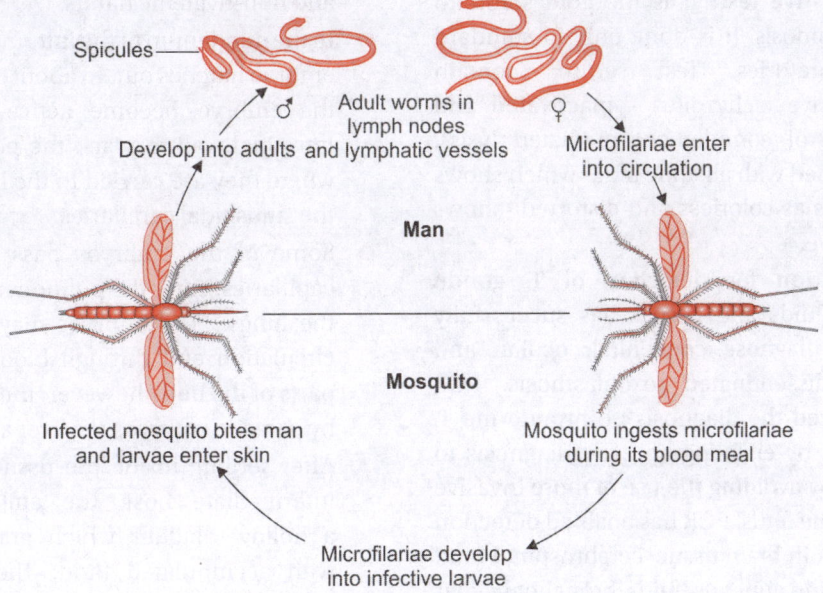

Fig. Life cycle of Wuchereria bancrofti

2. Write short notes on:

a. Laboratory diagnosis of toxoplasmosis

ANSWER

- *Toxoplasma gondii* is an obligate intracellular protozoan responsible for infections throughout the world in a wide range of hosts including humans. Primary infection is usually subclinical but in some patients cervical lymphadenopathy or ocular disease can be present.

- *T. gondii* infection can be diagnosed indirectly with serological methods and directly by polymerase chain reaction (PCR), hybridization, isolation, and histology. Whereas indirect serological methods are widely used in immunocompetent patients, definitive diagnosis in immunocompromised people is mostly undertaken by direct detection of the parasite.

- **Stain used is PAS or Giemsa:** Common shaped tachyzoites seen.

- **Animal inoculation:** Intraperitoneally into mice.

- **Serological test:** ELISA, IFA, IHA and Latex Agglutination Tests.

- **The use of serologic tests** for demonstration of specific antibody to T. gondii is the initial and primary method of diagnosis. Different serologic tests often measure different antibodies that possess unique patterns of rise and fall with time after infection.

- **Sabin-Feldman dye test:** It is the gold standard test for toxoplasmosis. It is done only in standard reference laboratories. Test serum (contain antibodies) + Live tachyzoites – inactivated and killed (because of complement mediated lysis). This is then stained with alkaline blue- which shows dead tachyzoites as colorless and distorted -shows the test is positive.

- **PCR amplification** for detection of T. gondii DNA in body fluids and tissues has successfully been used to diagnose congenital, ocular, and cerebral and disseminated toxoplasmosis. PCR has revolutionized the diagnosis of intrauterine T. gondii infection by enabling an early diagnosis to be made, thereby avoiding the use of more invasive procedures on the fetus. PCR has enabled detection of T. gondii DNA in brain tissue, cerebrospinal fluid (CSF), vitreous and aqueous fluids, bronchoalveolar lavage (BAL) fluid, and blood in patients with AIDS.

b. Echinococcus granulosus

ANSWER

Hydatid cyst disease is caused by Echinococcus granulosus. The worm completes its life cycle in two hosts. Primary or definitive hosts are dog, wolf, fox and jackal while the secondary or intermediate hosts are sheep, pig, cattle, horse, goat and man. The most common definite host is dog and the intermediate host is sheep.

- The adult worm which lies inside the small intestine of the definitive host is small in size and is supposed to be smallest among the tapeworms. It ranges from 2.5 to 9.0 mm in length.

- The eggs of Echinococcus contain within it a six hooked hexacanth larva. Egg covering along with the hexacanth larva is called "Onchosphere".

- The eggs are discharged into the lumen of the gut of the definitive host from the ruptured gravid proglottids from where they along with the feces of the host are carried outside the body.

- The eggs survive outside the body of the host for weeks, provided they are present in moist and shady places.

- They are unable to resist the high temperature and direct sun light.

- When the hexacanth containing eggs are swallowed by the intermediate host like sheep and other domestic animals while grazing in field, the oncosphere reaches the intestine of the secondary host. Infection may reach to man, particularly children, due to intimate handling of infected dogs and non-hygienic habits.

- In the duodenum of the intermediate host hexacanth embryo hatches out. In about 8 hours post infection, the embryo become active and bores through intestinal wall to reach the portal circulation from where they are carried to the liver to be lodged into the sinusoidal capillaries.

- Some of the embryos pass through the hepatic capillaries, enter the pulmonary circulation to reach the lungs. Few embryos may escape into general circulation and through blood reaches almost all parts of the body however; the chief organs infected by parasite embryos are liver and lungs.

- After settling inside the tissues and organs of the intermediate host, the embryo transform into a hollow bladder which gradually forms a cyst with accumulated fluid. The structure is called "hydatid cyst". The wall of the cyst is differentiated into an outer ectocyst and an inner endocyst. The diagrammatic representation is shown below:

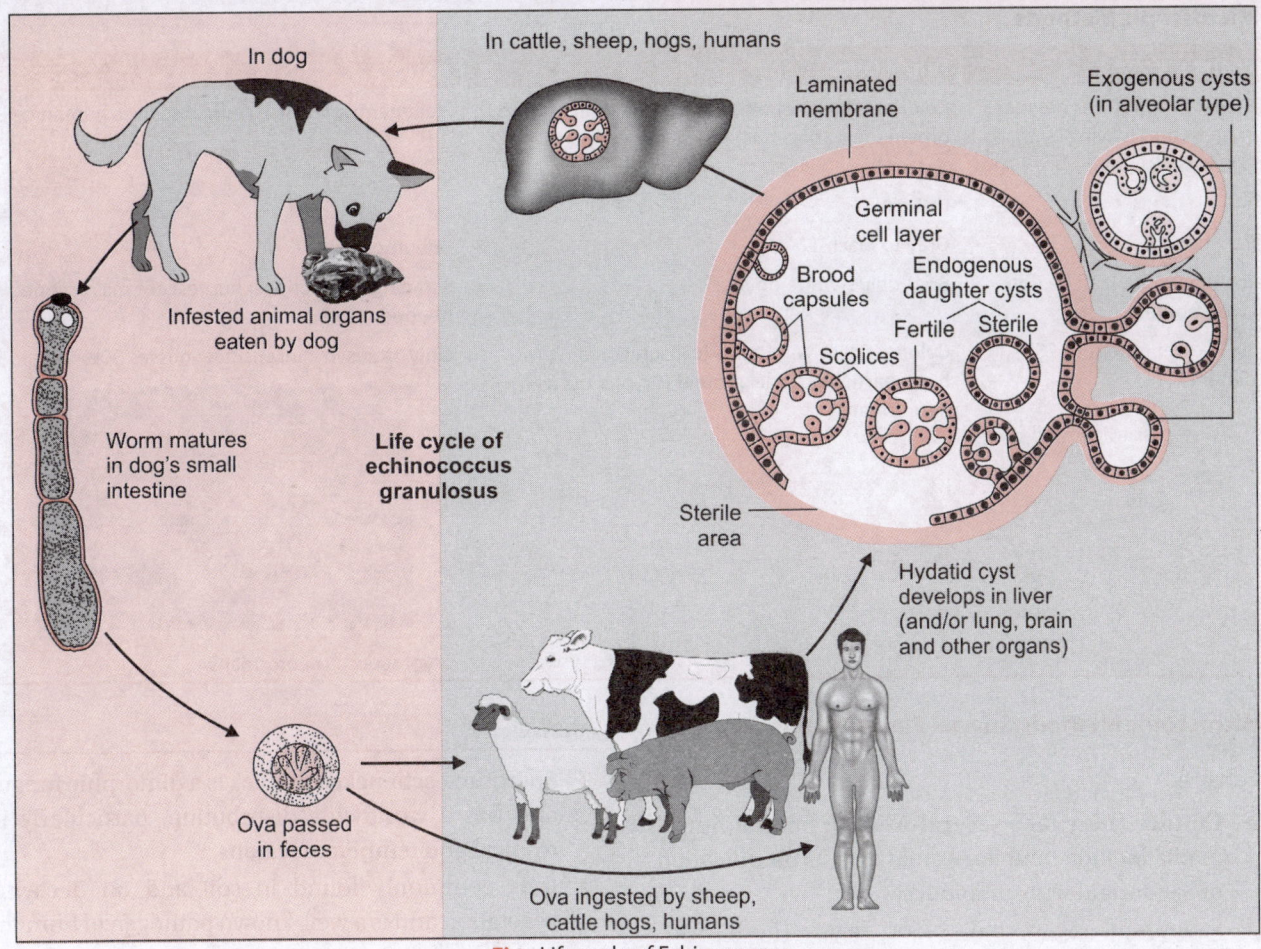

Fig. Life cycle of Echinococcus

Diagnosis of Echinococcus Diagnosis

- Laboratory diagnosis-post -surgical
- Microscopic demonstration of scolices in hydatid fluid
- Immunodiagnosis
- Casonis test, involves skin/intradermal injection of irradiated cystic fluid, which on presence of antibodies a burning swelling will be formed
- Serodiagnosis
- Detection of antibodies and antigens due to the parasite by ELISA, etc.
- Imaging methods
- X-ray helps in diagnosis of lung hydatid cyst, USG helps in diagnosis of liver and other organs.

PART-II

3. Describe the laboratory diagnosis of fungal infections

(Ref: Ananthanaryan & Paniker, Textbook of Microbiology, 10th ed, pg. 556)

ANSWER

Laboratory Diagnosis of Fungal Infections

I. Specimens

- Skin scrapings, nail clippings and hairs can be transported in an envelope, Petri dish, or other convenient conveyance.

II. Examination

Laboratory diagnosis of fungi

Clinical specimen E.g. Skin scrapings nail clippings and hairs

↓

First do microscopic examination with the small amount of clinical material in KOH-look for yeast cells or hyphae

↓

Inoculate the specimen in SDA or other specific media if needed and incubate at two different temperature 37°C and 25°C.

↓

After growth is visualized, take few colonies from the agar plate and put teased mount in LCBP and also do slide culture.

Microscopic Methods

Preparation	Fungal Color	Notes
KOH wet mount (KOH degrades human tissues leaving hyphae and yeasts visible)	Colorless (hyaline) refractive green or light olive to brown (dematiaceous) fungal elements	Heat gently; let sit 10 min; dissolves human cells
PAS	Hot pink	
Silver stain	Gray to black	Pneumocystis
Calcofluor white (can be done on wet mounts)	Bright blue-white on black	Scrapings or sections; fluorescent microscope needed
India ink wet mount of CSF sediment	Colorless cells with halos (capsule) on a black particulate background (Cryptococcus neoformans)	Only "rules in"; insensitive; misses 50%

Cryptococcus neoformans

Microscopic Methods/Special Fungal Stains

Culture

○ **Culture (may take several weeks):** Special fungal media include inhibitory mold agar as modification of Sabouraud with antibiotics:

○ Sabouraud agar and blood agar (both with antibiotics)

○ Culture identifies fungal morphology and PCR with nucleic acid probes.

○ Special addition in culture media-Chloramphenicol-to-suppress bacterial contamination; Cycloheximide (Actidione)-to suppress saprophytic fungi.

Serologic Tests

○ Serologic tests like ELISA for histoplasmosis, latex agglutination test and CFT have been devised.

Fungal antigen detection (CSF, serum): cryptococcal capsular polysaccharide detection by latex particle agglutination (LPA) or counter immunoelectrophoresis.

Skin test is most useful for epidemiology or demonstration of energy to an agent you know patient is infected with (grave prognosis); otherwise, like tuberculosis, skin test only indicates exposure to agent

---

4. **Write briefly on:**

   a. **Sporothrix schenckii**

   (Ref: Ananthanaryan & Paniker, Textbook of Microbiology, 10th ed, pg. 606)

ANSWER

○ Sporothrix schenckii complex is a dimorphic fungus and has a worldwide distribution, particularly in tropical and temperate regions.

○ It is commonly found in soil and on decaying vegetation and is a well-known pathogen of humans and animals.

○ Sporotrichosis is primarily a chronic mycotic infection of the cutaneous or subcutaneous tissues and adjacent lymphatics characterized by nodular lesions which may suppurate and ulcerate.

○ Most commonly affects gardeners, forest workers→ After a minor Traumatic implantation (rose or plum tree thorns, wire/sphagnum moss) → Nodule formed → Ulceration→ Necrosis→Fixed cutaneous Sporotrichosis→Spread to lymphatics→lymphocutaneous Sporotrichosis → Systemic spread to the bones, joints and meninges.

○ **Lab diagnosis:** KOH/HPE-shows asteroid Body.

○ **Culture:** Yeast phase in 37°C and mycelia in 25°C.

○ **Tissue form:** Cigar-shaped yeast in tissue

○ **Serology:** Slide agglutination test- Antigen in peptide-L-rhamno-D-mannan: ≥ 1:4 titer is positive (mainly helpful in pulmonary Sporotrichosis.

○ **Diseases include:**

  ▪ Sporotrichosis (rose gardener disease): subcutaneous or lymphocutaneous lesions; treatment: itraconazole or potassium iodide in milk

  ▪ Pulmonary (acute or chronic) sporotrichosis; urban alcoholics, particularly homeless (alcoholic rose-garden-sleeper disease)

Treatment is itraconazole for bone/joint infection and amphotericin B for severe/systemic infection.

b. Prophylaxis against Hepatitis 'B' infections

(Ref: Ananthanaryan & Paniker, Textbook of Microbiology, 10th ed, pg. 547)

ANSWER

Prophylaxis against Hepatitis B infections

- Currently used vaccine is prepared by cloning the S gene in baker's yeast.
- IM injection given in deltoid or anterolateral aspect of thigh in children-0, 1, 6 months.
- Due to low absorption rate which leading to poor immune response; So IM injection contraindicated in gluteal muscle.
- Seroconversion rate is around 90%.
- Immunoglobulin given for babies born too carrier mothers and for those who had exposure with unknown positive HBV persons.
- Disease can be prevented by immunization with two recombinant subunit vaccines (Recombivax HB and Energix-B) containing HBsAg: one HAV/HBV combination vaccine (Twinrix for those 18 years of age or older), and two pediatric vaccines (Comvax and Pediarix).
- Chronic infections can be treated with six drugs: standard and pegylated interferon-α and four reverse transcriptase inhibitors (lamivudine, cidofovir, dipivoxil, and entecavir) to improve survival and reduce progression to PHC.

Prophylaxis after exposure to Hepatitis B virus (HBV)

Type of exposure	Type of immunoprophylaxis
Perinatal	Vaccination + HBIG
Sexual– acute case	Vaccination + HBIG
Sexual–chronic HBV infection	Vaccination

Type of exposure	Type of immunoprophylaxis
Household (e.g., cell or dormitory) contact–to person with chronic HGV infection	Vaccination, If not previously vaccinated, also administer HBIG if known exposure§
Household (e.g., cell or dormitory) contact–acute case	Vaccination. If not previously vaccinated, also administer HBIG if known exposure§
Known percutaneous or permucosal (e.g., occupational)	Vaccination +/- HBIG,

Source: CDC, Hepatitis B vinus: a comprehensive strategy for eliminating transmission in the united states through universal childhood vaccination recommendation of the Advisory committee on Immunization Practices (ACIP). MMWR 1991; 40(No. RR-13):1-25.
† HBIG = hepatitis B immune globulin. Dosages; perinatal = 0.5 mL. intramuscular, all other = 0.06 mL/kg, intramuscular
§ Identifiable blood exposure to infected contract (e.g., by sharing toothbrushes or razors)

PART-III

5. Describe the morphology of Human immunodeficiency Virus (HIV) and laboratory diagnosis of HIV infections.

(Ref: Ananthanaryan & Paniker, Textbook of Microbiology,10th ed, pg.574)

ANSWER

Human Immunodeficiency Virus (HIV)

Morphology

The 3 structural genes (protein coded for):

- Env (gp120 and gp41):
- Formed from cleavage of gp160 to form envelope glycoproteins.
- Ep120—attachment to host CD4+ T cell.
- Ep41—fusion and entry.

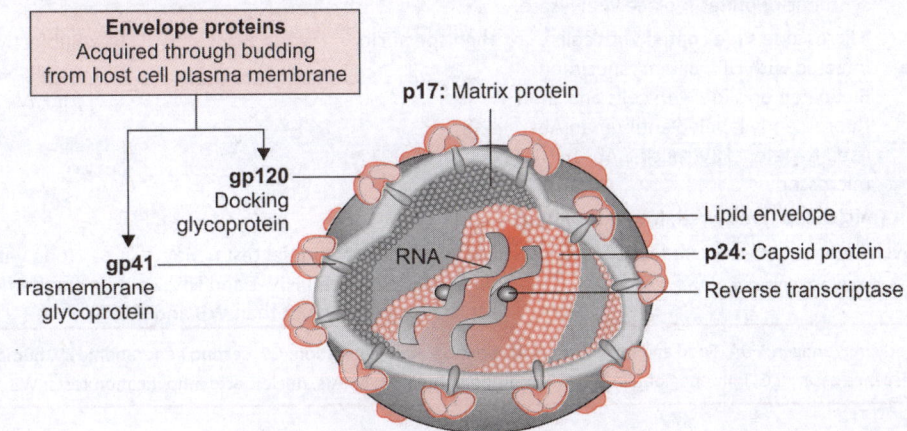

Fig. Structure of HIV virus

- ○ Gag (p24 and p17)—capsid and matrix proteins, respectively.
- ○ Pol—reverse transcriptase, aspartate protease, integrase.
- ○ Reverse transcriptase synthesizes dsDNA from genomic RNA; dsDNA integrates into host genome.
- ○ Virus binds CD4 as well as a co-receptor, either CCR5 on macrophages (early infection) or CXCR4 on T cells (late infection).

- ○ Homozygous CCR5 mutation = immunity.
- ○ Heterozygous CCR5 mutation = slower course

Laboratory Diagnosis

- ○ **Serological tests:**
  - ■ ELISAs
  - ■ Rapid test
  - ■ Western blots
- ○ **NAATs:** Sensitive tests for detection of HIV Infection- Viral Load can be detected.

Summary of Diagnostic Tests for HIV Infection

Technology	Principle	Strengths	Limitations
Initial HIV tests			
First- and second-generation immunoassays	Viral lysate (G1) or recombinant antigens (G2) capture anti-HIV Abs; specific IgGs detected using antihuman IgG	Detect HIV-specific IgG	Do not detect HIV- specific IgM and HIV antigens
Third-generation immunoassays	Recombinant antigens capture anti-HIV antibodies; IgG and IgM detected using antihuman IgG	Detect anti-HIV IgMs that may occur earlier in infection, in addition to IgG; improved seroconversion sensitivity; some have greater sensitivity in detecting HIV-2 and/or HIV-1 group O compared to earlier-generation assays	Do not detect HIV antigens
Fourth-generation immunoassays	Recombinant antigens capture anti-HIV antibodies; IgG and IgM detected using antihuman antibodies plus direct detection of p24 Ag	Detect antibodies and antigame simultaneously, allowing recognition of HIV infection prior to seroconversion	May miss early HIV infection (prior to antigenemia)
Rapid tests	Immunoassays that employ lateral flow, immunoconcentration, or particle agglutination technologies	Completed in <30 min often at point of care; performance characteristics similar to lab-based immunoassays (generation dependent)	Similar to lab-based immunoassays (generation dependent)
NAATs	Nucleic acids (DNA or RNA) amplified using specific primers and detected using labeled probes	Detect acute HIV infection prior to seroconversion	Most detect HIV-1 only; HIV-1 RNA may be undetectable in some Ab-positive
HIV-infected persons; technically complex and expensive			
Western blot	Viral lysate separated by electrophoresis, transferred to membrane and patient specimen is incubated with membrane to identify specific Ag/Ab complexes	High specificity due to Ag separation and concentration	Less sensitive than third- and fourth-generation immunoassays,
Technically complex, opportunities for technical error			
Line immunoassays	Similar to WB, recombinant Ags or synthetic peptides replace viral lysate.	High specificity	Similar to WB
Indirect immunofluorescence assays	Microscope slide coated with cells infected with HIV, patient specimen incubated on slide with cells and then fluorescently labeled antihuman Abs used to detect HIV specific Abs by microscopy	High specificity	Subjective interpretation of results; assays only approved for HIV- 1 detection in US;
Expensive instrument (microscope) required; low throughput			
Enzyme immunoassays	Same as above for initial HIV tests	Same as above for initial tests. May distinguish between HIV-1 and HIV-2. More simple and rapid than WB and IFAs	None yet FDA approved for supplemental testing

Abbreviations: Ab, antibody; Ag, antigen; FDA, Food and Drug Administration; G1, first generation; G2, second generation; HIV, human immunodeficiency virus; IFA, immunofluorescence assay; IgG, immunoglobulin G; IgM, immunoglobulin M; NAATs, nucleic acid amplification tests; WB, Western blot.

6. Write briefly about the prophylaxis against rabies

ANSWER

Prophylaxis of Rabies

- It is prevented by vaccination with a killed vaccine (HDCV, commercially called Imovax-Rabies) or treated with rabies immunoglobulin (RIG, commercially called Imogam-Rabies).
- **Types of vaccine**

Neural Vaccines	Non-neural Vaccines
• Sample vaccine	• Drug e.g. vaccine
• Beta propiolactone vaccine	• Live attenuate chick embryo vaccine
• Suckling mouse brain vaccine	• Tissue culture vaccine
	• Sub-unit vaccine (in experimental stage)

- **In India, tissue culture vaccine are used:**
  - Human Diploid cell vaccine (HDC)
  - Purified chick embryo cell vaccine (PCEC)
  - Purified Vero Cell Vaccine
- Vaccination Schedule

Pre-exposure prophylaxis	0, 7, 21 or 0, 28, 56; Booster after 1 year and then after 5 years
Post-exposure prophylaxis	0., 3, 7, 14, 30 and optionally 90.

Prophylaxis of Rabies

Post Exposure Prophylaxis

Wound Treatment

- Should be immediate
- Is essential even if the person presents long after exposure
- Consists of:
  - Immediate washing and flushing wound for 15 minutes with soap and water, or water alone
  - Disinfection with detergent, ethanol (700 ml/l), iodine (tincture or aqueous solution), or other substances with virucidal activity
  - Bleeding at any wound site indicates potentially severe exposure and must be infiltrated with either human or equine rabies immunoglobulin

- Other treatments include: Administration of antibiotics and tetanus prophylaxis
- Administration of rabies immunoglobulin (RIG) to wounds classified as category III exposure, is of upmost importance in wound management.
- Bites to the head, neck, face hand and genitals are category III exposures
- Infiltrate RIG into the depth of the wound and around the wound
- RIG should be infiltrated around the wound as much as anatomically feasible
- Remaining RIG should be injected at an intramuscular site distant from that of vaccine inoculation (e.g. into the anterior thigh)

Preexposure Prophylaxis

It is recommended for anyone who is at continual, frequent or increased risk for exposure to the rabies virus, as a result of their occupation or residence such as:

- Groups of persons at high risk of exposure to live rabies virus (laboratory staff, veterinarians, animal handlers and wildlife officers)
- Children living in or visiting rabies affected areas may be immunized preventively on a voluntary individual basis or in mass campaigns when there are no economic, programmatic or logistical obstacles
- Travellers to rabies-affected areas according to the level of risk in that area.

Pre-exposure rabies prophylaxis regimens with vaccines fulfilling WHO requirements Intramuscular:

- One intramuscular dose is given on each of days 0, 7 and 21 or 28
- Site of injection: deltoid area of the arm for adults; anterolateral area of the thigh is recommended for children aged less than 2 years

Intradermal

- One intradermal injection of 0.1 ml is given on each of days 0, 7, and 21 or 28
- If antimalarial chemoprophylaxis is applied concurrently, intramuscular injections must be used The vaccination series listed above must be completed at the stipulated times. However, there is no need to restart the series if the doses are not given on the exact schedule

Name of the Paper : **Microbiology Paper-I**

Name of the Course : **MBBS-2016**

Semester : **Annual**

Time: 3 Hours   M.M.: 40

INSTRUCTIONS

1. Write your Roll No. on the top immediately on receipt of this question paper
2. All questions are to be attempted
3. Answers to Parts I, II and III should be written in separate answer sheets provided
4. Attempt parts of a question in sequence

PART-I

1. **Enumerate various antigen antibody reactions. Describe the principle and application of any two of them.**   [5]

2. **Write short notes on:**   [10]
   a. Classical complement pathway
   b. Difference between exotoxin and endotoxin

PART-II

3. **Enumerate the agents causing gas gangrene. Outline its laboratory diagnosis.**   [5]

4. **Write briefly on:**   [10]
   a. Laboratory diagnosis of cholera
   b. Drug resistance in tuberculosis

PART-III

5. **Enumerate the probable etiological agents of a case of fever of unknown origin and describe the laboratory diagnosis of brucellosis.**   [5]

6. **Write the different color codes for the various biomedical wastes generated in a hospital and their respective methods of disposal:**   [5]

PART-I

1. Enumerate various antigen antibody reactions. Describe the principle and application of any two of them.

(Ref: Ananthanaryan & Paniker, Textbook of Microbiology,10th ed, pg. 105, 106)

ANSWER

○ Antigens, antibodies, antigen-antibody reactivity, cytokines, drugs, and cells can be detected in vitro or in vivo, and some even in the nanogram and picogram range.

■ The union of antigen with antibody is very sensitive, specific, and firm, but reversible; multiple short-range forces are involved.

■ Binding occurs in seconds but is not visible until a lattice forms, which occurs more slowly. Since antibodies are bivalent, they form the lattice through cross-linkages. The composition of the lattice depends on the ratio of antigen to antibody.

■ Affinity measures the binding energy between an antibody and a univalent epitope; avidity is the total binding energy between an antibody and a multivalent antigen.

■ Changing the position of atoms, double bonds, structural conformation, or the composition of amino acids or sugars of the epitope changes specificity.

Types of Antigen–Antibody Reactions

○ **Conventional techniques:** Precipitation, Agglutination reaction, Complement fixation test and Neutralization test.

○ **Newer techniques:** ELISA, IFA, RIA, CLIA, Immunohistochemistry, Rapid test (Lateral flow assay or ICT and Flow through assay) Western blot and Immunoassay using electron microscope.

Precipitation Reaction

When a soluble antigen reacts with its antibody in the presence of optimal temperature, pH and electrolytes (NaCl), it leads to formation of the antigen-antibody complex in the form of :-

○ Insoluble precipitate band when gel containing medium used or

○ Insoluble floccules when liquid medium is used.

Agglutination Tests

It is used to detect antibody union with large, particulate antigens.

○ Rapid, slide identification of bacteria can occur by mixing a loopful of bacteria from the patient's culture with a battery of specific antibacterial antisera and noting which antiserum causes agglutination.

○ Semi quantitative diagnostic test for bacterial diseases involves addition of the suspect bacterium (killed) to dilutions of the patient's serum. The highest dilution that results in visible agglutination is called the titer. A fourfold increase in titer is necessary for diagnosis due to low levels of "natural" antibodies occurring in the serum of most normal human beings.

Diagnostic Application of Agglutinations Tests

○ **Slide agglutination**

■ It is used in blood grouping to determine qualitatively whether the donor's cells or serum possess antigens or antibodies that are reactive with the recipient's serum or cells.

○ **Tube Agglutination**

It is routinely used for

■ Typhoid fever (Widal test) Detects Ab against both H (Flagellar) and O (Somatic) Ag

■ Acute Brucellosis (Standard agglutination test)

■ **Coombs test or Antiglobulin test:**
  ♦ Detects incomplete Rh antibodies.
  ♦ Two variations of the Coombs test exist.
    ▫ **Direct Coombs Test:** is designed to identify maternal anti-Rh antibodies that are already bound to infant RBCs or antibodies bound to RBCs in patients with autoimmune hemolytic anemia.

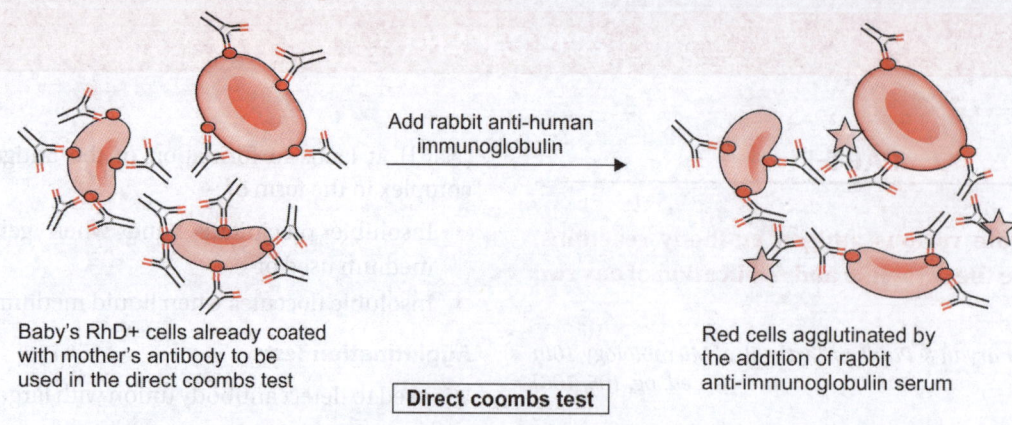

Baby's RhD+ cells already coated with mother's antibody to be used in the direct coombs test

Add rabbit anti-human immunoglobulin

Red cells agglutinated by the addition of rabbit anti-immunoglobulin serum

Direct coombs test

Fig. Direct Coombs test

- **Indirect Coombs test:** It is designed to identify Rh-negative mothers who are producing anti-Rh antibodies of the IgG isotype, which may be transferred across the placenta harming Rh-positive fetuses. The indirect Coombs is also used in the diagnosis of transfusion reactions.

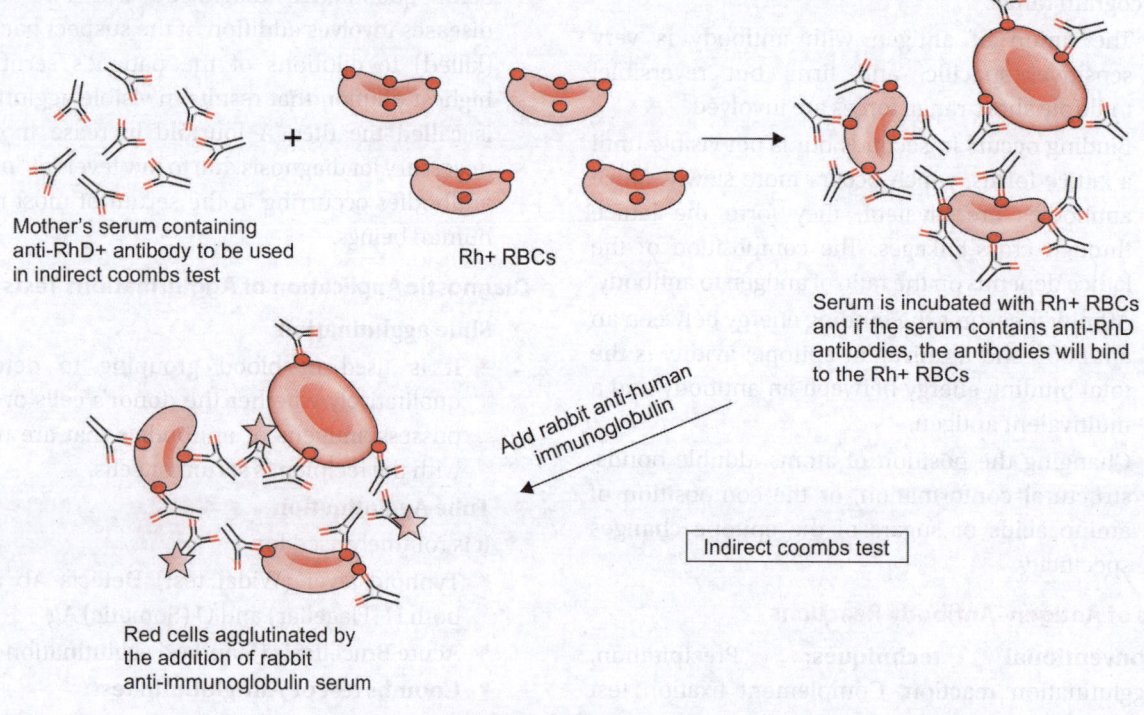

Mother's serum containing anti-RhD+ antibody to be used in indirect coombs test

Rh+ RBCs

Serum is incubated with Rh+ RBCs and if the serum contains anti-RhD antibodies, the antibodies will bind to the Rh+ RBCs

Add rabbit anti-human immunoglobulin

Red cells agglutinated by the addition of rabbit anti-immunoglobulin serum

Indirect coombs test

Fig. Indirect coombs test

- **Indirect or passive agglutination test:**
  Antigen is coated on carriers such as Latex or RBCs to detect Antibody in serum. Examples:
  - Indirect hemagglutination test (IHA)
  - Latex agglutination Test (LAT) for antibody detection e.g. ASO
- **Reverse passive agglutination test:**
  Antibody is coated on carriers such as Latex or RBCs to detect Antigen in serum. Examples:
  - RPHA (Reverse Passive Hemagglutination Assay), e.g. HBsAg detection

- Latex agglutination test (LAT) for antibody detection, e.g. CRP, RA actor, Capsular antigen in CSF and streptococcal grouping.
- **Coagglutination Test**
- It another type of Passive agglutination test, where Staphylococcus aureus act as carrier molecule.
- Some strains of S. aureus (Cowan 1strain) possess protein A on the surface, which has a property of binding to Fc portion of any IgG molecule (except IgG3) making the Fab portion free, which can agglutination with the corresponding antigen present in the clinical sample.

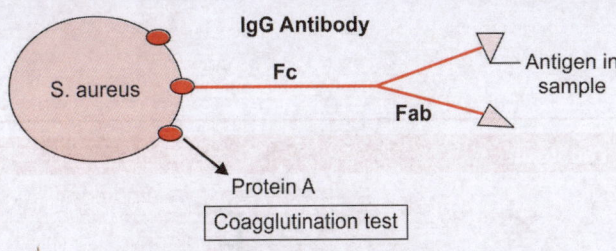

Fig. Coagglutination test

Complement Fixation Test

CFT detects complement fixing antibodies in patient's serum. It is now almost obsolete.

○ Wasserman test was the most popular CFT, used for the diagnosis off syphilis.

○ CFT was also widely used for detection of antibodies in Rickettsia, Chlamydia, Brucella, Mycoplasma infections and some viral infections such as arboviruses, rabies, etc.

○ **Indirect complement fixation test:** Detects certain avian (e.g. duck, Parrot) and mammalian (e.g. horse, cat) serum antibodies cannot fix guinea pig complement.

○ **Conglutination test:** To perform CFT using non hemolytic complements, e.g. horse complements.

Complements are also used for various serological tests, Other than CFT such as:

○ Treponema pallidum immobilization test

○ (For detecting antibodies to T. pallidum)

○ Sabin-Feldman dye test for detecting toxoplasma antibodies.

○ Vibriocidal antibody test foe V. cholerae

Neutralization Test

Neutralization test are also less commonly used in Morden days. Examples include:

○ **Viral neutralization test:** Detects viral neutralizing antibodies

○ **Plaque inhibition text:** Done for bacteriophages

○ **Toxin-Antitoxin neutralization test:**

■ Schick test for Corynebacterium diphtheriae.

■ **Nagler's reaction:** Due to toxin of clostridium perfringens

■ ASLO detection in past (Now it is done by latex agglutination)

■ Hemagglutination Inhibition (HAI) test

---

2. **Write short notes on:**

(Ref: Ananthanaryan & Paniker, Textbook of Microbiology,10th ed, pg.123

a. **Classical complement pathway**

ANSWER

Classical complement pathway: It is an important component of both innate and adaptive immunity.

○ It is comprised of nine major factors (C1 to C9), most of which are pro-enzymes present in normal serum and not increased by antigenic stimulation. It is effective via three pathways:

■ The classical pathway results in lysis of microbial or mammalian cells to which IgM or a doublet of IgG1, IgG2, or IgG3 antibody has been bound to the membrane, followed by sequential "fixation" of C to the antigen–antibody complex.

◆ C1qrs is bound initially via C1q, resulting in enzymatic cleavage and fragmentation of C4 and C2.

◆ C4b and C2a bind to the cell surface as C4b2a, becoming a C3 convertase that cleaves C3 into fragments C3a and C3b.

◆ C3b complexes with C4b2a to become a C5 convertase, which cleaves C5 into C5a and C5b.

◆ C5b combines with C6 and C7 and inserts into the cell membrane.

◆ C8 and C9 combine with the C5 b, 6, 7 complex to form the MAC, resulting in increased permeability, changes in osmotic pressure, and cell lysis.

▫ The alternate pathway is activated by cell walls of certain Gram-negative and Gram-positive bacteria, viruses, yeasts, and aggregated IgA.

◆ It acts independent of antibody or C1, C4, or C2.

◆ It is initiated by cell wall absorption of small amounts of C3b existing in normal serum.

◆ Binding of a serum protein, factor B, follows, which serves as a substrate for an enzyme, factor D. The resulting complex, C3bBb, is stabilized by properdin and has C3 convertase activity, which generates additional C3b.

◆ A complex, C3bBbC3b, forms, which becomes a C5 convertase, leading to the further reactions resulting in the MAC.

▫ The mannan-binding lectin pathway follows the binding by an acute phase protein, mannose-binding lectin (MBL), onto mannose residues on the cell walls of certain bacteria, fungi, and viruses.

◆ This complex acts similar to CI and thus follows the classical pathway, forming C3 and C5 convertases that result in cell lysis via MAC.

◆ It is an adjunct to innate immunity, independent of antibody.

b. **Difference between exotoxin and endotoxin**

ANSWER

Property	Exotoxin	Endotoxin
Bacterial source	Mostly from gram-positive bacteria	Gram-negative bacteria
Relation to microorganism	Metabolic product of growing cell	Present i LPS of outer membrane of cell wall and released with destruction of cell or during cell division
Chemistry	Proteins, usually with two parts (A-B)	Lipid portion (lipid A) of LPS of outer membrane (lipopolysaccharide)
Pharmacology (effect on body)	Specific for a particular cell structure or function in the host (mainly affects cell functions, nerves, nerves, and gastrointestinal tract)	General, such as fever, weaknesses, aches, and shock; all produce the same effects
Heat stability	Unstable: can usually be destroyed at 60-80°C	Stable; can withstand autoclaving (121°C for 1 hour)
Toxicity (ability to cause disease)	High	Low
Fever-producing	No	Yes
Immunology (relation to antibodies)	Can be converted to toxoids to immunize against toxin; neutralized by antitoxin	Not easily neutralized by antitoxin; therefore, effective toxoids cannot be made to immunize against toxin
Lethal dose	Small	Considerably larger
Representative diseases	Gas gangrene, tetanus, botulism, diphtheria, scarlet fever	Typhoid fever, urinary tract infections, and meningococcal meningitis

PART-II

3. **Enumerate the agents causing gas gangrene. Outline its laboratory diagnosis.**

(Ref: Ananthanaryan & Paniker, Textbook of Microbiology, 10th ed, pg. 258)

ANSWER

Gas Gangrene

Gas gangrene is a bacterial infection that produces gas in tissues in gangrene. This deadly form of gangrene usually is caused by Clostridium perfringens bacteria. It is a medical emergency

Agents Causing Gas Gangrene

○ Clostridium perfringens
○ Group A streptococcus,
○ Staphylococcus aureus
○ Vibrio vulnificus.

Laboratory Diagnosis

○ **Specimens:** Wound swab, discharge and affected tissue
○ **Direct smear:** Shows rectangular gram positive bacilli; spores are usually not seen
○ **Culture:** Specimen are incoulated into cooked meat media as well as in a blood agar media and the latter is incubated anaerobically for 48–72 hours. In blood agar medium there is hemolysis around the colony. The bacterial culture is used for Nagler reaction and biochemical tests.
○ **Animal pathogenicity:** For demonstration of toxigenicity of the strain, 0.1 mL of 24 hours culture of the bacteria in cooked meat broth is injected intramuscularly on the right thigh of a healthy guinea pig. Animal dies within 24 hours. A control animal prior to test is to be included. On autopsy, the injected limb shows swelling with crepitation and the muscles appear pink. Bacteria can be recovered from heart and spleen of the animal.

4. Write briefly on:

(Ref: Ananthanaryan & Paniker, Textbook of Microbiology, 10th ed, pg. 313)

a. Laboratory diagnosis of cholera

ANSWER

- **Macroscopic examination:** Rice watery stool with mucus flecks
- The laboratory diagnosis of cholera is based on colony morphology, culture characteristics, biochemical reactions and serological identification by slide agglutination using specific antisera. However, a presumptive diagnosis of cholera can be made by an immobilization test.
- **Immobilization test:** A rapid presumptive diagnosis of cholera can be made by observing the wet smear for the distinctive rapid to and fro movement (darting movement) of V. cholerae O1 and O139 due to their single polar flagellum. The movement can be stopped by adding one drop of V. cholerae O1 and O139 antiserum respectively.
- Hanging drop method for Vibrio cholerae is one of the easy but most popular test used for the presumptive diagnosis. Read details about this test here
- **Oxidase test:** On performing oxidase test from a pure culture on Macconkey agar or nutrient agar, positive reaction is observed. (Note: However, Aeromonas spp also gives a positive oxidase test result so further confirmation is necessary by culture and serotyping)
- **Cultural characteristics:**
  - Fresh stool can be directly plated on a non-selective medium like MacConkey agar and a selective medium such as Thiosulphate Citrate Bile Salt Sucrose (TCBS) agar.
  - However, in case of rectal swab, the swab stick should be dipped in 10 mL of alkaline peptone water (APW) and incubate for 6-8 hours. After incubation, inoculation on solid media should be done only from the pellicle formed at the upper layer of the broth. (Note: The broth should not be shake before plating)
  - After 18–24 hours of incubation at 37°C observe the colony morphology.
    - **MacConkey agar:** Appearance of pale, non lactose fermenting, 1-2 mm in diameter, flat with a serrated margin.
    - **TCBS:** Button shaped yellow colonies of 1-2 mm diameter.
- Biochemical Reactions:
  - **Gram stain:** Gram negative, curved rods

- **Catalase/Oxidase:** Both positive
- **Citrate:** Positive or negative
- **Indole:** Positive
- **Urea hydrolysis:** Negative
- **Motility:** Motile
- **Methyl Red:** Positive
- **Voges Proskauer:** Negative
- **String Test:** Positive
- **TSI:** Alkali/Acid (R/Y) or Acid/Acid (Y/Y) without gas and H2S.

- **Serological Reactions:**
  - Pick up the colonies resembling *V. cholerae* and perform a slide agglutination test using polyvalent and serotype specific antisera for V. cholerae O1, if negative perform agglutination test with O139 antiserum.
  - Place two drops of normal saline on a slide side by side and emulsify colonies resembling V. cholerae from a non selective medium on both.
  - Add a drop of polyvalent O1 antisera to one of the suspension and tilt the slide to and fro. Observe for agglutination within a minute.
  - If positive continue the same procedure with mono specific Ogawa and Inaba antisera. If any one is positive report as Ogawa or Inaba. If both positive report as Hikojima.
  - If none of the above shows positive reaction, perform agglutination test with O139 antiserum.

b. Drug resistance in tuberculosis

(Ref: Ananthanaryan & Paniker, Textbook of Microbiology, 10th ed, pg. 357)

ANSWER

- Multi drug-resistant TB (MDR-TB) and extensively drug-resistant TB (XDR-TB) are major global health threats.
- Drug-resistant forms of TB can develop if treatment is incorrect or incomplete. This can happen for several reasons.
- Because treatment for TB takes six months and can have difficult side effects, people may be tempted to stop taking their medication before they have completed treatment, particularly if they are starting to feel better.
- They may be given the incorrect treatment or may fear the stigma of having TB. People with infectious drug- resistant TB can then also pass this drug-resistant strain on to others.
- There are two main types of drug resistant TB, MDR-TB and XDR-TB.

- MDR TB is the type of drug resistant TB, when the bacteria are resistant to the TB drugs rifampicin and isoniazid

- MDR (multi drug resistant) TB is the name given to TB when the bacteria that are causing it are resistant to at least isoniazid and rifampicin, two of the most effective TB drugs.

- In May 2016 WHO issued guidance that people with TB resistant to rifampicin, with or without resistance to other drugs, should be treated with an MDR-TB treatment regimen.

- This group of patients (effectively an expanded MDR-TB group), is sometimes referred to as MDR/RR-TB).

- When a person is described as having MDR-TB, it is not clear whether they may also be resistant to other drugs as well.

- So the World Health Organization has now started to refer to "uncomplicated MRD-TB". This is TB which is resistant to isoniazid and rifampicin (making it MDR TB) but it is known that the bacteria are not resistant to any of the second line TB drugs.

- XDR-TB (extensively drug resistant TB) is defined as strains resistant to at least rifampicin and isoniazid. This is in addition to strains being resistant to one of the fluoroquinolones, as well as resistant to at least one of the second line injectable TB drugs amikacin, kanamycin or capreomycin.

- MDR-TB and XDR-TB do not respond to the standard six months of TB treatment with "first line" anti TB drugs.

Treatment of Drug Resistant TB

Definition	Treatment
MDR TB: resistant to the TB drugs rifampicin and isoniazid	
XDR-TB: resistant to rifampicin, isoniazid any Fluoroquinolones and at least one injectable second line drugs	Kanamycin + Ofloxacin + Ethionamide + Pyrazinamide + Ethambutol + Cycloserine (6-9 months) followed by
	Ofloxacin + Ethionamide + Ethambutol + Cycloserine for 18 months

PART-III

5. **Enumerate the probable etiological agents of a case of fever of unknown origin and describe the laboratory diagnosis of brucellosis.**

ANSWER

Bacterial Causes of PUO

- **Abscesses:**
  - They are most commonly in the subphrenic space, liver, right lower quadrant, retroperitoneal space or the pelvis in women.

- **Tuberculosis:** When dissemination has occurred (e.g. in patients who are immunocompromised) the initial presentation is more likely to consist of constitutional symptoms than localizing signs. CXR may be normal.

- **Urinary tract infections (UTIs):** These are rare causes perinephric abscesses occasionally fail to communicate with the urinary system, resulting in a normal urinalysis.

- Endocarditis (this is a rare cause of PUO):
  - **Culture:** Negative endocarditis is reported in 5-10% of endocarditis cases.

- **Hepatobiliary infections (e.g. cholangitis):** These can occur without local signs and with only mildly elevated or normal LFTs, especially in the elderly.

- **Osteomyelitis:** This usually causes localized pain or discomfort at least sporadically.

- **Brucellosis:** This should be considered in patients with persistent fever and a history of contact with cattle, swine, goats or sheep, or in patients who consume raw milk products.

- **Borrelia recurrentis:** This is transmitted by ticks. It is responsible for causing relapsing fever.

- **Other spirochetal diseases that can cause PUO:** These include Spirillum minor (rat-bite fever), Borrelia burgdorferi (Lyme disease) and Treponema pallidum (syphilis).

Viral Causes

- **Herpes viruses (such as cytomegalovirus (CMV) and Epstein-Barr virus (EBV):** These can cause prolonged febrile illnesses with constitutional symptoms and no prominent organ manifestations, particularly in the elderly.

Parasites

- **Toxoplasmosis:** This should be considered in patients who are febrile with lymph node enlargement.

Fungi

Immunosuppression, the use of broad-spectrum antibiotics, the presence of intravascular devices and total parenteral nutrition all predispose people to disseminated fungal infections.

Diagnosis of Brucellosis

- Complete blood count
  - A complete blood count (CBC) typically is ordered routinely as part of an evaluation for a patient with potential infectious disease.
  - Leukocytosis is rare in brucellosis, and a significant number of patients are neutropenic.
  - Anemia is reported in 75% of patients (particularly with chronic infection), thrombocytopenia is reported in 40% (secondary to hepatosplenomegaly or from immune thrombocytopenia), and pancytopenia is reported in 6% of patients.
- Liver enzymes
  - A slight elevation in liver enzyme levels is a very common finding. These elevated levels may reflect the severity of hepatic involvement and correlate clinically with hepatomegaly.
- Culture
  - Diagnosis of brucellosis is definitive when *Brucella* organisms are recovered from blood, bone marrow, or other tissue. Some *Brucella* species require 5-10% carbon dioxide for primary isolation. Because of the ease of aerosol transmission, any potential *Brucella* specimens should be handled under a biohazard hood.
  - The sensitivity of blood cultures with improved techniques such as the Castaneda bottles is further improved by the lysis-centrifugation technique. With these methods, the sensitivity is approximately 60%.
  - Subcultures are still advised for at least 4 weeks; thus, if brucellosis is suspected, the laboratory should be alerted to keep the cultures for 3-4 weeks, which is not done routinely for most bacterial cultures.
  - Because the reticuloendothelial system holds a high concentration of brucellae, bone marrow culture is thought to be the criterion standard. Sensitivity is usually 80-90%.
  - Any fluid (e.g. synovial fluid, pleural fluid, or cerebrospinal fluid [CSF]) can be cultured, but the yield is usually low.
- Castaneda's bottle with both solid and liquid medium increases the chance of isolation.
- Serologic test includes standard agglutination test (SAT)- in this test the blocking antibodies in the sera should be removed by prior treatment with saline or y heating. A titer of 160 is considered as positive test; these blocking antibodies are IgA type.
- ELISA test to detect IgM and IgG available.
- Polymerase chain reaction
  - Polymerase chain reaction (PCR) tests have been developed for the detection and rapid diagnosis of *Brucella* species in human blood specimens

---

6. **Write the different color codes for the various biomedical wastes generated in a hospital and their respective methods of disposal.**

ANSWER

New Biomedical Waste Management Guidelines 2015-16

Category	Type of wastes	Bag/container	Treatment/disposal
Yellow	Human anatomical waste Animal anatomical waste	Yellow non-chlorinated plastic bags	Incineration/Plasma pyrolysis/Deep burial
	Solid waste		Incineration/Plasma pyrolysis/Deep burial OR autoclaving/microwaving/Hydroclaving THEN Shredding/Mutilation
	Discarded medicine Chemical waste	Yellow non-chlorinated plastic bags	Incineration/Encapsulation/Plasma pyrolysis
	Chemical liquid waste	Separate collection system leading to effluent treatment system.	Pretreatment THEN Drain
	Discarded linen, mattresses, bedding contaminated with blood or body fluid	Yellow non-chlorinated plastic bags or suitable packing material	Non-chlorinated chemical disinfection THEN Incineration/Plasma pyrolysis/Energy recovery or Shredding/Mutilation

Category	Type of wastes	Bag/container	Treatment/disposal
	Microbiology Biotechnology clinical laboratory waste	Autoclave safe plastic bags or containers	Pre-treat with Non-chlorinated chemicals THEN, Incineration
		Red non-chlorinated	Autoclaving/microwaving/Hydroclaving THEN
Red	**Contaminated waste (Recyclable)**	Plastic bags or containers	Shredding/Mutilation THEN Energy recovery/Plastic to diesel or fuel oil/ Road making
White (Translucent)	Waste sharp including metal's	Puncture proof, leak proof, Tamper proof container	Autoclaving/Dry heat THEN Shredding/Mutilation/Encapsulation THEN Iron foundries/Sanitary landfill/Waste sharp pit
Blue	Glassware Metallic Body Implants	Cardboard boxes with blue colored marking	Sodium hypochlorite/Autoclaving/Microwaving/ Hydroclaving THEN Recycling

Your Roll No. ....

Name of the Paper	:	**Microbiology Paper-II**
Name of the Course	:	**MBBS-2016**
Semester	:	**Annual**

Time: 3 Hours   M.M.: 40

INSTRUCTIONS

1. Write your Roll No. on the top immediately on receipt of this question paper
2. All questions are to be attempted
3. Answers to Parts I, II and III should be written in separate answer sheets provided
4. Attempt parts of a question in sequence

PART-I

1. **Enumerate the free living amoebae. Describe their pathogenesis and laboratory diagnosis.**   [5]

2. **Write short notes on:**   [10]
    a. Laboratory diagnosis of kala-azar
    b. Stool concentration methods

PART-II

3. **List various species of candida causing human infections. Mention its pathogenicity and outline the laboratory diagnosis.**   [5]

4. **Write briefly on:**   [10]
    a. Prophylaxis against rabies
    b. Aspergillosis

PART-III

5. **Enumerate four vector borne viral diseases in India. Describe the laboratory diagnosis of any one of these.**   [5]

6. **Outline the various approaches to laboratory diagnosis of viral infections.**   [5]

PART-I

1. Enumerate the free living amoebae. Describe their pathogenesis and laboratory diagnosis.

ANSWER

Free Living Amoebae

- Free-living amoebae (FLA) are found in soil and water habitats throughout the world.
- It does not have human carrier state: no vector
- These are neuropathogenic.
- These are four species
  - *Acanthamoeba spp*
  - *Balamuthia mandrillaris*
  - *Naegleria fowleri*
  - *Sappinia diploidea*

Characteristics of Free- Living Amoeba

Free-living amoebae	Characteristics
Acanthamoeba spp	**Transmission:** Free living ameba in contaminated contact lens solution (airborne cysts). Not certain for **GAE:** inhalation or contact with contaminated soil or water **Disease:** Keratitis; granulomatous amebic encephalitis (GAE) in immunocompromised patients; insidious onset but progressive to death. **Diagnosis:** Star-shaped cysts on biopsy; rarely seen in CSF culture as above **Treatment:** Keratitis: topical miconazole and propamidine isethionate; GAE: ketoconazole, sulfamethazine (rarely successful)
Naegleria fowleri	Infection is acquired while swimming in contaminated water. Amoeboid trophozoite enters through nasal mucosa goes to brain. It causes Primary amebic meningoencephalitis (PAM): severe **Diagnosis:** Motile trophozoites in CSF, Culture on plates seeded with gram-negative bacteria; ameba will leave trails **Treatment:** Amphotericin B (rarely successful)
Sappinia	Only one case of Sappinia causing amoebic encephalitis has been reported.
Balamuthia mandrillaris	Infection is transmitted through respiratory tract or skin lesions It causes GAE. Presence of multiple nucleoli in trophozoites helps in diagnosis. Not reported in India yet.

2. Write short notes on:

a. Laboratory diagnosis of kala-azar

Arora parasitology 5th ed p 53

ANSWER

- Smear prepared from spleen, BM, lymph nodes or peripheral smear shows amastigotes seen inside macrophages (LD bodies).
- Most sensitive method to detect LD bodies in splenic smear.
- But the most common method of diagnosis is bone marrow aspiration and microscopy.
- Culture can be done by NNN medium.

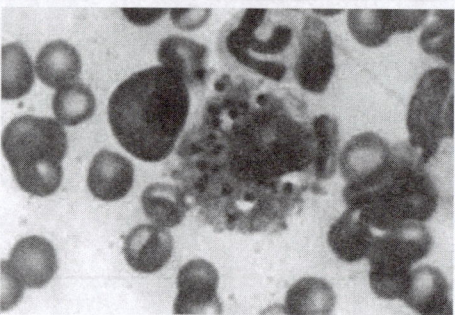

Fig. Amastigotes of L. donovani in microscopy

- Animal inoculation done in Chinese and golden hamster (Intraperitoneal inoculation).
- **Serodiagnosis:**
  - Complement fixation test
  - Direct agglutination test
  - Rapid immunochromatographic test (RTD)- for detection of antibodies againstrK39 antigen-rK39 dipstick test is widely used now and it is very sensitive.
  - **Napier's aldehyde teat:** 1–2 mL of the serum from patient is added with 40% formalin; a milky white jellification is seen means that indicates positive test. But this test is nonspecific.
- **Leishmanin skin test:** Montenegro test (Used for epidemiological studies). This test is usually positives 4-6 weeks after onset in case of cutaneous and Mucocutaneous leishmaniasis.

b. Stool concentration methods

ANSWER

Concentration procedure separate parasites from fecal debris and increase the chances of detecting parasitic organisms when these are in small numbers. They are divided into flotation techniques and sedimentation techniques.

- ○ **Flotation techniques (most frequently used:** Zinc sulfate or Sheather's sugar) use solutions which have higher specific gravity than the organisms to be floated so that the organisms rise to the top and the debris sinks to the bottom. The main advantage of this technique is to produce a cleaner material than the sedimentation technique. The disadvantages of most flotation techniques are that the walls of eggs and cysts will often collapse, thus hindering identification. Also, some parasite eggs do not float.

- ○ Sedimentation techniques use solutions of lower specific gravity than the parasitic organisms, thus concentrating the latter in the sediment. Sedimentation techniques are recommended for general diagnostic laboratories because they are easier to perform and less prone to technical errors. The sedimentation technique used at CDC is the formalin-ethyl acetate technique, a diphasic sedimentation technique that avoids the problems of flammability of ether, and which can be used with specimens preserved in formalin, MIF or SAF.

PART-II

3. List various species of candida causing human infections. Mention its pathogenicity and outline the laboratory diagnosis.

(Ref: Ananthanaryan & Paniker, Textbook of Microbiology, 10th ed, pg. 615)

ANSWER

Candida Causing Human Infections

- ○ Candida albicans
- ○ Candida tropicalis
- ○ Candida glabrata
- ○ Candida parapsilosis
- ○ Candida krusei
- ○ Candida lusitaniae

Pathogenicity

- ○ **Fibronectin receptor** on *Candida albicans* facilitates its adherence to the (fibronectin, a component of the host extracellular matrix) epithelium of the gastrointestinal or urinary tract.
- ○ **Hydrophobic molecules** on the surface of Candida also helps in adhesion.

- ○ **Aspartyl proteases** found in C. albicans has shown increased ability to cause disease in animal models.
- ○ **Phenotypic switching** and presence of **phospholipase** also play a role in pathogenesis.

Laboratory Diagnosis

- ○ **Microscopy and Staining**
  - ▪ Candida yeast cells can be detected in unstained wet preparations or Gram stained preparations of sample. In Gram stained smears, Candida appears as gram positive budding yeast cells (blastoconidia) and/or pseudohyphae showing regular points of constriction.

- ○ **Culture:**
  - ▪ *Candida albicans* grows well on Sabouraud dextrose agar and most routinely used bacteriological media. Cream colored pasty colonies usually appear after 24-48 hours incubation at 25-37°C. The colonies have a distinctive yeast smell and the budding cells can be easily seen by direct microscopy in stained or unstained preparations.
  - ▪ In blood agar, *candida albicans* gives white, creamy colored colonies which can be mistaken for Staphylococcus spp. Whenever you are analyzing the culture report of 'high vaginal swab', take extra care as the colony you are observing can be of Candida albicans instead of Staphylococcus aureus or vice versa (quick solution for this is to perform wet mount or gram staining and observing under microscope).

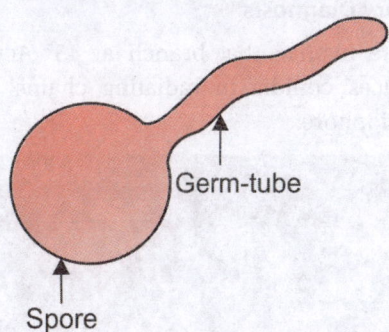

Fig. Germ tube test of Candida albicans

- ○ Further tests from culture isolate:
  - ▪ *Candida albicans* can be identified presumptively by a simple germ tube test.

---

4. Write briefly on:

a. Prophylaxis against rabies

(Ref: Ananthanaryan & Paniker, Textbook of Microbiology, 10th ed, pg. 536)

ANSWER

Prophylaxis of Rabies

For answer, refer 2017 paper-I Q. 6, Pg. 351

b.   Aspergillosis

ANSWER

○ Aspergillosis is a disease caused by a fungus (or mold) called Aspergillus.

○ The species that grows at 37°C can cause invasive infections and other can cause only allergic manifestations.

○ Mopst common species are Aspergillus fumigatus, Aspergillus flavus, Aspergillus niger and Aspergillus terreus.

○ Incubation Period of invasive aspergillosis after inhalation is 2 to 90 days.

Clinical Features

○ **Allergic bronchopulmonary aspergillosis (ABPA):** hypersensitivity response associated with asthma and cystic fibrosis; may cause bronchiectasis and eosinophilia.

○ Causes invasive aspergillosis in immunocompromised, patients with chronic granulomatous disease.

○ Can cause aspergillomas in pre-existing lung cavities, especially after TB infection.

○ Some species of Aspergillus produce Aflatoxins (associated with hepatocellular carcinoma).

Laboratory Diagnosis

○ Septate hyphae that branch at 45° Acute Angle. Produces conidia in radiating chains at end of conidiophore.

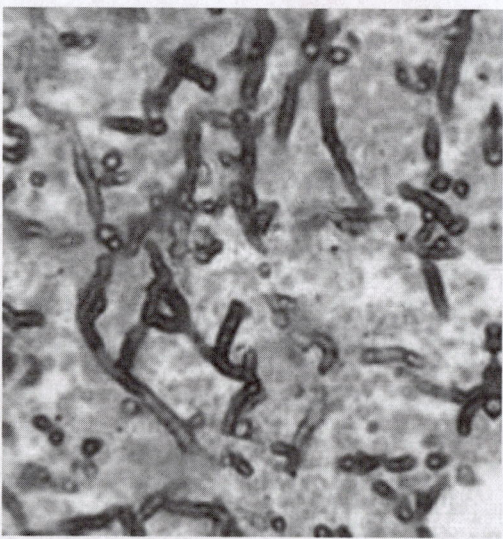

Fig. 45° acute angle

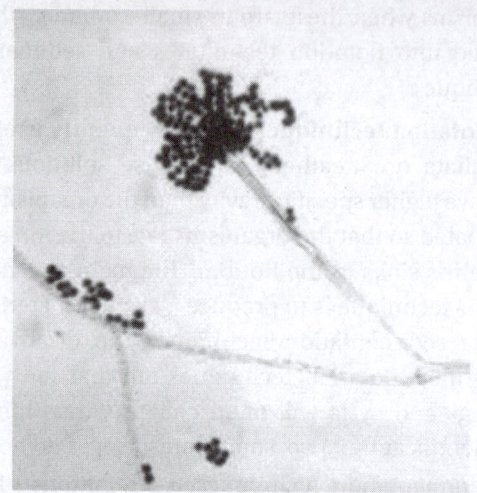

Fig. Conidiophore

PART-III

5.   **Enumerate four vector borne viral diseases in India. Describe the laboratory diagnosis of any one of these.**

ANSWER

Three viruses that spread through mosquito are:

○ Yellow fever

○ Dengue fever

○ Zika fever

○ Chikungunya

Important Features about Zika Virus

○ It is a flavivirus most commonly transmitted by Aedes mosquito bites.

○ Vertebrates Sexual and vertical transmission possible

○ Outbreaks more common in tropical and subtropical climates.

○ It causes conjunctivitis, low-grade pyrexia, and itchy rash in 20% cases.

○ It can lead to congenital microcephaly or miscarriages if transmitted in utero.

○ Supportive care, no definitive treatment.

Laboratory Diagnosis of Zika Virus

○ Zika virus has been detected in whole blood, urine,, CSF, amniotic fluid, semen and saliva.

○ Zika virus that is present in urine and semen can be seen for longer periods than whole blood or saliva.

○ Whole blood, serum collected in a dry tube and/or urine collected from patients presenting with onset of symptoms ≤ 7 days should be subjected from nucleic acid tests.

- Whole blood collected in a dry tube and serum collected from patients presenting with onset of symptoms ≥ days need to be done with serological test.
- RT-PCR is the gold standard test.

---

6. Outline the various approaches to laboratory diagnosis of viral infections

(Ref: Ananthanaryan & Paniker, Textbook of Microbiology, 10th ed, pg. 445)

ANSWER

- **In general, diagnostic tests can be grouped into 3 categories:**
  - Direct detection
  - Indirect examination (virus isolation)
  - Serology.
- In direct examination, the clinical specimen is examined directly for the presence of virus particles, virus antigen or viral nucleic acids.
- In indirect examination, the specimen into cell culture, eggs or animals in an attempt to grow the virus: this is called virus isolation.
- Serology actually constitute by far the bulk of the work of any virology laboratory.
- A serological diagnosis can be made by the detection of rising titers of antibody between acute and convalescent stages of infection, or the detection of IgM.
- In general, the majority of common viral infections can be diagnosed by serology. The specimen used for direction detection and virus isolation is very important.
- A positive result from the site of disease would be of much greater diagnostic significance than those from other sites.

- For example, in the case of herpes simplex encephalitis, a positive result from the CSF or the brain would be much greater significance than a positive result from an oral ulcer, since reactivation of oral herpes is common during times of stress.

Direct Examination of Specimen

- Electron Microscopy morphology/immune electron microscopy
- Light microscopy histological appearance e.g. inclusion bodies
- Antigen detection immunofluorescence, ELISA etc.
- Molecular techniques for the direct detection of viral genomes

Indirect Examination

- **Cell culture:** Cytopathic effect, hemadsorption, confirmation by neutralization, interference, immunofluorescence etc.
- **Eggs pocks on CAM:** Hemagglutination, inclusion bodies
- Animals disease or death confirmation by neutralization

Serology

Detection of rising titers of antibody between acute and convalescent stages of infection, or the detection of IgM in primary infection.

Classical Techniques	Newer Techniques
Complement fixation tests (CFT)	Radioimmunoassay (RIA)
Hemagglutination inhibition tests	Enzyme linked immunosorbent assay (EIA)
Immunofluorescence techniques (IF)	Particle agglutination
Neutralization tests	Western Blot (WB)
Single Radial Hemolysis	Recombinant immunoblot assay (RIBA), line immunoassay (Liatek) etc.

Name of the Paper	:	**Microbiology Paper-I**
Name of the Course	:	**MBBS-2015**
Semester	:	**Annual**

Time: 3 Hours   **M.M.: 40**

INSTRUCTIONS

1. Write your Roll No. on the top immediately on receipt of this question paper
2. All questions are to be attempted
3. Answers to Parts I, II and III should be written in separate answer sheets provided
4. Attempt parts of a question in sequence

PART-I

1. Define and classify hypersensitivity. Describe the mechanism of anaphylaxis.   [5]

2. Write short notes on   [10]
   a. Gram-negative cell wall
   b. IgM

PART-II

3. Describe the laboratory diagnosis of pulmonary tuberculosis.   [5]

4. Write briefly on: [10]
   a. Treponema palladum hemagglutination assay (TPHA)
   b. Toxins and enzymes produced by Streptococcus pyogenes

PART-III

5. Define hospital acquired infections. Elaborate the factors contributing in development of these infections.   [5]

6. Define biomedical waste. Mention the categories of biomedical waste and their disposal.   [5]

PART-I

1. **Define and classify hypersensitivity. Describe the mechanism of anaphylaxis.**

(Ref: Ananthanaryan & Paniker, Textbook of Microbiology, 10th ed, pg. 163)

ANSWER

Hypersensitivity Reaction

○ A state of **altered reactivity** in which the body reacts with an exaggerated immune response to a foreign agent

○ These reactions may be damaging, uncomfortable, or occasionally fatal

○ Coombs and Gell classified hypersensitivity into 4 types

	Type	Type II	Type III	Type IV
Immune reactant	IgE	IgE	IgE	T-cell
Antigen	Soluble molecule	Cell associated molecule	Solube molecule	Soluble or cell associated molecule
Graphic	Allergen — Allergen-specific IgE — Fc receptor for IgE — Degranulation	NK cell — Fc receptor for IgG — Surface antigen — Abnormal cell — Antibody-dependent cellular cytotoxicity	Neutrophils — Enzymes from neutrophils damage endothelial cell	Antigen presenting cell — Antigen — Sensitized Th1 cell — Cytokines — Activated macrophage — Delayed-type hypersensitivity
Mechanism	IgE induced mast cell activation	Complement mediated phagocytosis	Tissue damage induced by immune complexes	T-cell mediated inflammation or cytotoxicity
Examples	Allergic rhinitis allergic asthma	Chronic urticaria (auto antibodies)	Serum sickness, arthus reaction	Multiple sclerosis, contract dermatitis, Crohn's disease, Rheumatoid arthritis

Mechanism of Anaphylaxis

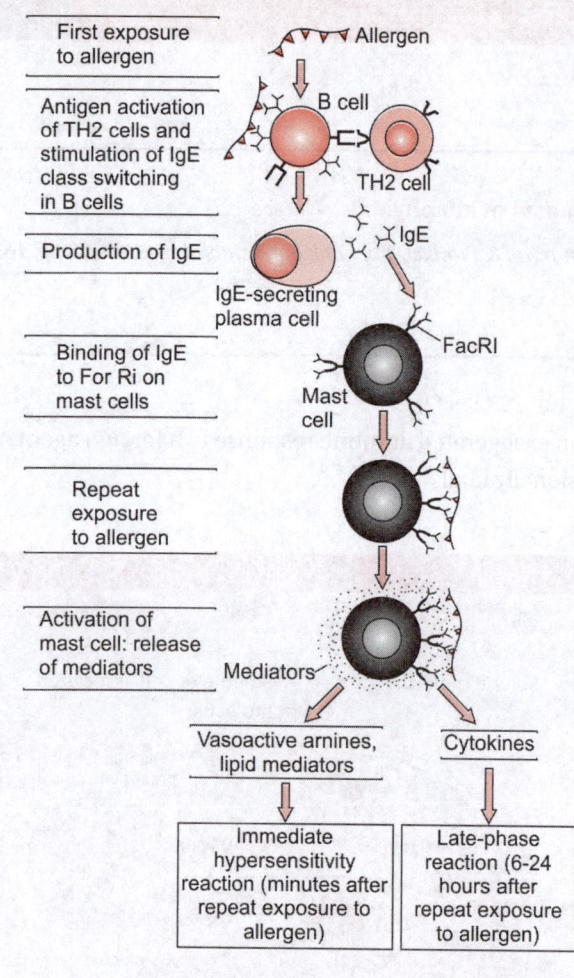

Fig. Mechanism of anaphylaxis

Phospholipids are located mainly in the inner layer of the outer membrane, as are the lipoproteins that connect the outer membrane to the peptidoglycan.

○ The lipopolysaccharides, located in the outer layer of the outer membrane, consist of a lipid portion called lipid A embedded in the membrane and a polysaccharide portion extending outward from the bacterial surface.

○ The LPS portion of the outer membrane is also known as endotoxin.

○ In addition, pore-forming proteins called porins span the outer membrane.

○ The porins function as channels for the entry and exit of solutes through the outer membrane of the Gram-negative cell wall.

○ The outer membrane of the Gram-negative cell wall is studded with surface proteins that differ with the strain and species of the bacterium.

Gram (+) cell-wall   Gram (−) cell-wall

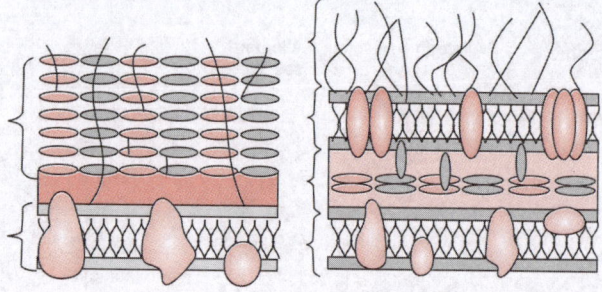

Fig. Cell wall of gram-positive and gram-negative cell wall

2. Write short notes on:

a. Gram-negative cell wall

(Ref: Ananthanaryan & Paniker, Textbook of Microbiology, 10th ed, pg. 274)

ANSWER

○ In electron micrographs, the Gram-negative cell wall appears multilayered. It consists of a thin, inner wall composed of peptidoglycan and an outer membrane.

○ The peptidoglycan portion of the Gram-negative cell wall is generally 2–3 nanometers (nm) thick and contains just 2–3 layers of peptidoglycan.

○ Chemically, only 10–20% of the Gram-negative cell wall is peptidoglycan.

○ The outer membrane of the Gram-negative cell wall appears as a lipid bilayer about 7 nm thick.

○ It is composed of phospholipids, lipoproteins, lipopolysaccharides (LPS), and proteins.

b. IgM

(Ref: Ananthanaryan & Paniker, Textbook of Microbiology, 10th ed, pg. 98)

ANSWER

○ Serum IgM exists as a pentamer in mammals and comprises approximately 10% of normal human serum Ig content.

○ It predominates in primary immune responses to most antigens and is the most efficient complement-fixing immunoglobulin.

○ IgM is also expressed on the plasma membrane of B lymphocytes as a monomer. In this form, it is a B cell antigen receptor, with the H chains each containing an additional hydrophobic domain for anchoring in the membrane.

○ Monomers of serum IgM are bound together by disulfide bonds and a joining (J) chain.

○ Immunoglobulin M is the third most common serum Ig and takes one of two forms:

- A pentamer where all heavy chains are identical and all light chains are identical
- A monomer (e.g., found on B lymphocytes as B cell receptors)

○ The large pentameric structure allows for building of bridges between encountered epitopes on molecules that are too distant as to be connected by smaller IgG antibodies.

○ IgM is the first antibody built during an immune response.

○ It is responsible for agglutination and cytolytic reactions since in theory, its pentameric structure gives it 10 free antigen-binding sites as well as it possesses a high avidity.

○ Due to conformational constraints among the 10 Fab portions, IgM only has a valence of 5. Additionally, IgM is not as versatile as IgG.

○ However, it is of vital importance in complement activation and agglutination.

○ IgM is predominantly found in the lymph fluid and blood and is a very effective neutralizing agent in the early stages of disease.

○ Elevated levels can be a sign of recent infection or exposure to antigen.

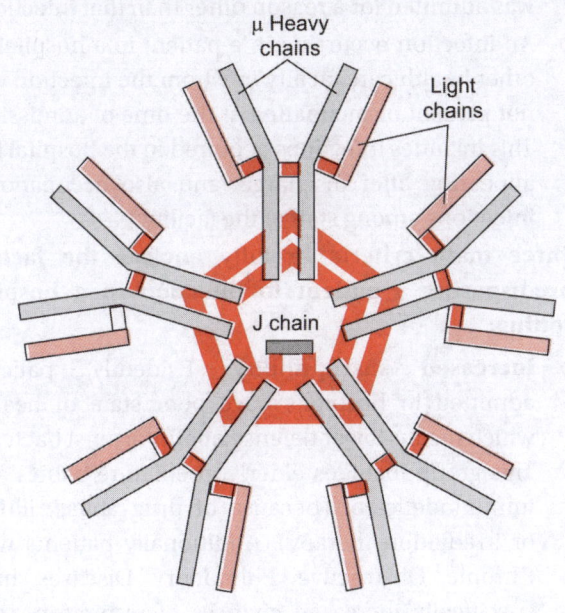

Fig. Structure of IgM

PART-II

3. Describe the laboratory diagnosis of Pulmonary Tuberculosis:

(Ref: Ananthanaryan & Paniker, Textbook of Microbiology, 10th ed, pg.357)

ANSWER

Distinguishing Features

○ Auramine-rhodamine staining bacilli (fluorescent apple green); no antibody involved (sensitive but not specific)

○ Acid fast

○ Aerobic, slow growing on Lowenstein-Jensen medium; new culture systems (broths with palmitic acid) faster

○ Produces niacin

○ Produces a heat-sensitive catalase: catalase-negative at 68.0°C (154.4 F) (standard catalase test); catalase active at body temperature.

Diagnosis

○ Microscopy of sputum: screen with auramine-rhodamine stain (fluorescent apple-green); no antibody involved; very sensitive; if positive, confirm with acid fast stain

○ PPD skin test (Mantoux): measure zone of induration at 48–72 hours; positive if:

- ≥5 mm in HIV+ or anyone with recent TB exposure; AIDS patients have reduced ability to mount skin test.
- ≥10 mm in high-risk population: IV drug abusers, people living in poverty, or immigrants from high TB area
- ≥15 mm in low-risk population

○ Positive skin test indicates only exposure but not necessarily active disease.

○ Quantiferon-TB Gold Test: measures interferon-gamma production when leukocytes exposed to TB antigens

○ Slow-growing (3–6 weeks) colonies on Lowenstein-Jensen medium (faster new systems)

○ Organisms produce niacin and are catalase-negative (68°C).

○ No Serodiagnosis

4. Write briefly on:

a. Treponema palladim hemagglutination assay (TPHA)

(Ref: Ananthanaryan & Paniker, Textbook of Microbiology, 10th ed, pg. 378)

ANSWER

○ Treponema pallidum Hemagglutination Assay (TPHA) is a treponemal test for the serologic diagnosis of syphilis, a sexually transmitted infection caused by a Spirochetes, Treponema pallidum.

○ Based on the principle of **passive hemagglutination**, this test detects anti-treponemal **antibodies** (IgG and IgM antibodies) in serum or CSF.

○ TPHA has been used as a confirmatory test for the diagnosis of Treponema pallidum infection since the mid 1960's.

○ TPHA is a good primary screening test for syphilis at all stages beyond the early primary stage.

○ TPHA test is a passive hemagglutination assay based on hemagglutination of erythrocytes sensitized with T. pallidum **antigen by antibodies found in the patient's serum or plasma**.

○ It is used for both qualitative and semi-quantative detection of Anti-treponemal antibodies.

○ TPHA Test Principle

  ▪ The test sample is diluted in absorbing diluent to remove possible cross-reacting heterophile antibody and to remove, block, or absorb potentially cross-reacting, nonpathogenic treponemal antibodies.

  ▪ Sera containing antibodies to T. pallidum **react with erythrocytes (chicken or avian) sensitized with sonicated** T. pallidum, Nichols strain (the antigen), **to form a smooth mat of agglutinated cells in the microtiter tray well.**

  ▪ If antibodies are not present the cells settle to the bottom of the tray well, forming a compact button **of unagglutinated cells.**

  b. **Toxins and enzymes produced by Streptococcus pyogenes.**

(Ref: Ananthanaryan & Paniker, Textbook of Microbiology, 10th ed, pg. 210)

ANSWER

○ **Erythrogenic, Dick or scarlational toxin:**

  ▪ Intradermal injection into susceptible individuals.

  ▪ Produce an erythematous reaction (Dick test).

  ▪ Effects of toxin are seen by induce fever.

  ▪ Three types are there-A, B and C

  ▪ A and C are phase coded; B is chromosomal

○ **Hemolysins**- Streptolysin O and S

  ▪ **Streptolysin O:** Antibody to this appears post infections; ASO titer helps to diagnose; Oxygen labile.

  ▪ **Streptolysin S:** Responsible for hemolysis seen around streptococcal colonies on the surface of blood agar plates; Oxygen stable.

○ **Streptokinase:** Fibrinolysin-It is responsible for breaking down of fibrin barrier and spread of infections.

○ **Deoxyribonuclease (Streptodornase, DNAse)**- depolymerization of DNA; helps to liquefy the thick pus; four types A, B, C and D; type B is the most antigenic, demonstration of anti DNAse B antibody- retrospective diagnosis of S. pyogenes infection- especially in skin infections

○ **Hyaluronidase** helps in the spread of infection along the intercellular spaces.

PART-III

5. **Define Hospital acquired infections. Elaborate the factors contributing in development of these infections.**

(Ref: Ananthanaryan & Paniker, Textbook of Microbiology, 10th ed, pg. 648)

ANSWER

A nosocomial infection–also called "hospital acquired infection" can be defined as:

○ An infection acquired in hospital by a patient who was admitted for a reason other than that infection .

○ An infection occurring in a patient in a hospital or other health care facility in whom the infection was not present or incubating at the time of admission. This includes infections acquired in the hospital but appearing after discharge, and also occupational infections among staff of the facility.

Three main criteria broadly enclose the factors predisposing a patient to infection in a hospital setting:

○ **Increased susceptibility:** Evidently, patients admitted in hospitals have poor state of health, which means lower defense quality against bacteria. This group includes elderly, premature babies and immunodeficient (because of drug abuse, illness or irradiation therapy). Additionally patients with Chronic Obstructive Pulmonary Diseases have specifically increased chances of respiratory tract infection.

○ **Invasive devices:** For instance intubation tubes, catheters, surgical drains, and tracheotomy tubes as they have already overcome bodies primary defense line. Patients already colonized on admission are instantly put at greater risk when they undergo an invasive procedure.

○ Medications or treatment (e.g. repeated blood transfusions) themselves make the patient vulnerable to infections, e.g. antacid treatment or antimicrobial therapy (which eliminates competitive flora and allows flourishing of resistant organisms)

6. **Define Biomedical waste. Mention the categories of Biomedical waste and their disposal.**

ANSWER

Bio-medical Waste

○ Bio-medical waste means "any solid and/or liquid waste including its container and any intermediate

product, which is generated during the diagnosis, treatment or immunization of human beings or animals or research activities pertaining thereto or in the production or testing of biological or in health camps.

○ Biomedical waste poses hazard due to two principal reasons – the first is infectivity and other toxicity.

○ **Biomedical waste consists of:**

Categories of Biomedical Waste and their Disposal

For answer, refer 2016, paper-I Q. 6 , Pg. 359

Your Roll No. ....

Name of the Paper : **Microbiology Paper-II**

Name of the Course : **MBBS-2015**

Semester : **Annual**

Time: 3 Hours   M.M.: 40

INSTRUCTIONS

1. Write your Roll No. on the top immediately on receipt of this question paper
2. All questions are to be attempted
3. Answers to Parts I, II and III should be written in separate answer sheets provided
4. Attempt parts of a question in sequence

PART-I

1. Enumerate the intestinal nematodes infecting humans. Describe the life cycle of any one of them.   [5]

2. Write short notes on: [10]
   a. Laboratory diagnosis of malaria
   b. Evolution and pathogenesis of hydatid cyst

PART-II

3. Enumerate the fungi causing dermatophytosis. Briefly describe the laboratory diagnosis of this condition.   [5]

4. Write briefly on: [10]
   a. Ebola virus
   b. Cell culture techniques

PART-III

5. Draw a labeled diagram depicting the morphology of human immunodeficiency virus and briefly describe the strategies used for diagnosis of infections caused by this virus.   [5]

6. Tabulate the viral vaccines mentioning the type, preparation and schedule as used in the National Immunization Schedule of India.   [5]

PART-I

1. **Enumerate the intestinal nematodes infecting humans. Describe the life cycle of any one of them**

ANSWER

(Ref: Arora Parasitology 5th ed 194, 195)

Intestinal Nematodes

- *Ascaris lumbricoides*
- *Trichuris trichiura*
- *Ancylostoma duodenale*
- *Necator americanus*
- *Enterobius vermicularis*
- *Strongyloides stercoralis.*

Life Cycle of Ascaris Lumbricoides

The life cycle of Ascaris completes in single host. Human.

- **Stage I:** Eggs in feces
  - Sexually mature female produces as many as 200,000 eggs per day, which are shed along with feces in unembryonated form. They are non-infective.
- **Stage II:** Development in soil
  - Embryonation occurs in soil as optimum temperature of 20–25°C with sufficient moisture and oxygen
  - Infective larva develops within egg in about 3-6 weeks.

- **Stage III:** Human infection and liberation of larvae
  - Human get infection with ingestion of embryonated egg contaminated food and water
  - Within embryonated state inside egg, first stage larvae develops into second stage larvae. This second stage larvae is known as rhabditiform larvae
  - Second stage larvae is stimulated to hatch out by the presence of alkaline pH in small intestine and solubilization of its outer layer by bile.
- **Stage IV:** Migration of larvae through lungs
  - Hatched out larvae penetrates the intestinal wall and carried to liver through portal circulation
  - It then travels via blood to heart and to lungs by pulmonary circulation within 4–7 days of infection.
  - The larvae in lungs molds twice, enlarge and breaks into alveoli.
- **Stage V:** Re-entry to stomach and small intestine
  - From alveoli, the Larvae then pass up through bronchi and into trachea and then swallowed.
  - The larvae passes down the esophagus to the stomach and reached into small intestine once again.
  - Small intestine is the normal habitat of Ascaris and it colonizes here.
  - Within intestine parasite molds twice and mature into adult worm.
  - Sexual maturation occurs with 6–10 weeks and the mature female discharges its eggs in intestinal lumen and excreted along with feces, continuing the life cycle.
  - The life span of parasite is 12–18 months

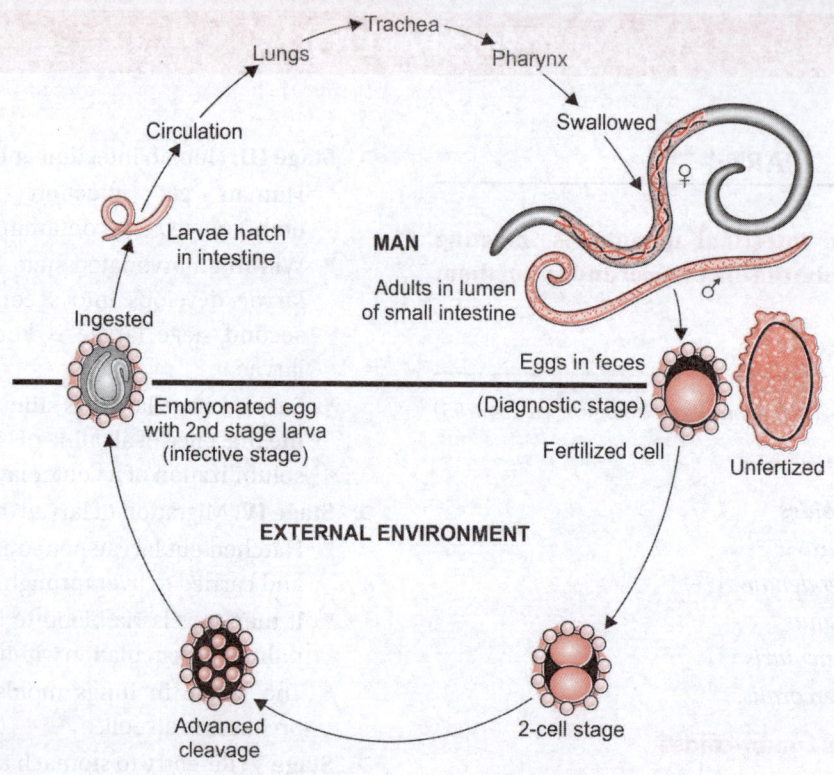

Fig. Life cycle of ascaris lumbricoides

2. Write short notes on:

a. Laboratory diagnosis of malaria

ANSWER

- Microscopy of peripheral smear-thick and thin smear method.
- Conventional light microscopy is the gold standard for confirmation of malaria.
- Thick smear is helpful for species identification.
- Fluorescence method using acridine orange staining is also helpful
- QBC-Quantitative Buffy Coat:
  - Principle is based on acridine orange which stain the nucleic acid in the parasites
  - More sensitive method than thick blood smear-can detect as low as 3-4 parasites/μL of blood.
- Serodiagnosis:
  - Immunochromatographic test-rapid diagnostic test-detects HRP-2 and pLDH and aldolase.
- PCR-helpful to diagnosis P. knowlesi.

Note:

- **P. vivax:** Schüffner's dots
- **P. falciparum:** Maurer's dots
- **P. malariae:** Ziemann's dots
- **P. ovale:** James's dots

Summaries Table for Diagnosis of Malaria

Standard methods for diagnosis of malaria	Features
Thick blood film	Sensitive method that will detect even 0.0001% of parasitemia; but it needs experience to look the parasites.
Thin blood film	Rapid and specific method bur it can detect only 0.05% parasitemia.
PfHRP2 dipstick test	Rapid and inexpensive tests. Help in field survey. Detects inly plasmodium falciparum.
Plasmodium LDH dipstick test	Rapid test; can detect all species
Microtube concentration methods (with acridine orange staining)	Sensitive tests and superior to thick films; helps to identify and process large number of sample; but it needs fluorescence microscopy.

b. Evolution and pathogenesis of hydatid cyst

ANSWER

(Ref: Arora parasitology 5th ed p 143, 144)

Hydatid Cyst: (Larval Stage of the Tapeworm)

- It represents the scolex of adult worm
- Outer layer–Ectocyst–Cuticular layer
- Inner layer–Endocyst–Germinal layer

○ *Brood capsules are formed from germinal layer*

○ When brood capsules are not formed–called as *acephalocysts*

○ This causes unilocular hydatid disease

○ *Hydatid fluid:*

▪ Antigenic in nature and highly toxic; if when secreted into the human body by rupture of cysts–it leads to anaphylaxis

▪ *Hydatid sand* indicates brood capsules and protoscolices which are floating in the hydatid fluid gives an appearance of sand grains;

○ Hydatid cyst can occur anywhere in the body; *M/c is liver followed by lung*

○ *Lab diagnosis:*

▪ *Wet mount of the hydatid fluid:* Demonstration of protoscolices

▪ Casoni's test–immediate hypersensitivity test

▪ Antigen detection by ELISA

▪ Antibody detection has low sensitivity

▪ X-ray–helps in diagnosis of lung hydatid cyst, USG–helps in diagnosis of liver and other organs

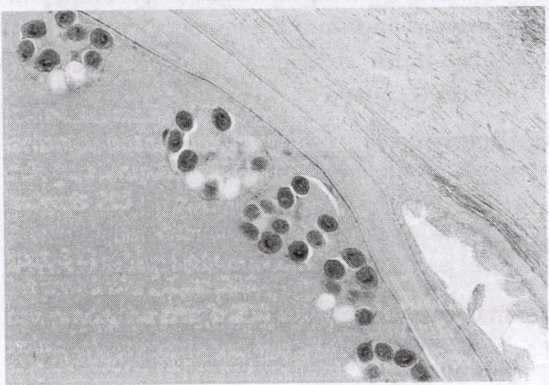

Fig: Hydatid cyst
(*Courtesy:* CDC/Dr Mae Melvin)

○ Main modality of treatment is *surgical removal of the cyst followed by albendazole or mebendazole* for a minimum of three months

PART-II

3. Enumerate the fungi causing Dermatophytosis. Briefly describe the laboratory diagnosis of this condition:

(*Ref: Ananthanaryan & Paniker, Textbook of Microbiology, 10th ed, pg. 599, 600*)

ANSWER

○ Dermatophytes are aerobic fungi that can invade and infect the keratinized layers of skin, hair, and nails

○ There are three genera of dermatophytes, recognized by the nature of their macroconidae (asexual spores):

▪ Trichophyton (abbreviated as "T")

▪ Microsporum ("M")

▪ Epidermophyton ("E")

Diagnosis of Dermatophyte Infections

It is done primarily by 2 methods

○ Direct microscopic examination

○ Culture

Clinical Material

Skin scrapings, nail scrapings, scalp and hairs. For a laboratory diagnosis, clinicians should be aware of the need to generate an adequate amount of suitable clinical material. The laboratory needs enough specimen to perform both microscopy and culture

Slide Preparation with KOH

○ Place a drop of potassium hydroxide solution on a slide

○ Transfer the specimen (small pieces) to the drop of KOH, and cover with cover glass

○ **Note:** To assist clearing, hairs should note be more than 5 mm long, and skin scales, crusts and nail snips should not be more than 2 mm across.

○ Hairs clear within 5-10 minutes. Skin scales and crusts usually take 20-30 minutes. Pieces of nail, however, may take several hours to clear

Culture

○ Useful to confirm the diagnosis of dermatophyte when long term oral therapy is being considered, and to identify dermatophyte species

○ Specimen are cultured as follows:

○ Skin scales, crusts, pieces of nail:

▪ Using a sterile blade or scissors, cut the specimens into pieces as small as possible

▪ Using sterile, inoculate the small pieces (a few millimeters apart), on the surface of a plate of sabouraud dextrose agar (SDA)

▪ Incubate at incubator (25-30°C). for up to 3 weeks, examining every few days for growth

4. Write briefly on:

a. Ebola virus

(*Ref: Ananthanaryan & Paniker, Textbook of Microbiology, 10th ed, pg. 562*)

ANSWER

- Ebola virus named after Ebola river, where the first cases were noticed.
- **Mode of Infection:** Person to person transmission through blood and body fluids.
- Causes fever with hemorrhagic illness- Highly fatal
- Three distinct strains:
    - **Zaire:** CFR 90%
    - **Sudan:** CFR 90%
    - Reston
- Recent outbreak- West Africa-2013 to 2016
- **Vaccine:** rVSV-ZEBOV
- Symptoms may appear anywhere from 2 to 21 days after contact with the virus, with an average of 8 to 10 days.

b.   Cell culture techniques

ANSWER

- Cell culture is one of the major tools used in cellular and molecular biology, providing excellent model systems for studying the normal physiology and biochemistry of cells (e.g., metabolic studies, aging), the effects of drugs and toxic compounds on the cells, and mutagenesis and carcinogenesis.
- It is also used in drug screening and development, and large scale manufacturing of biological compounds (e.g., vaccines, therapeutic proteins).
- Cell culture refers to the removal of cells from an animal or plant and their subsequent growth in a favorable artificial environment.
- The cells may be removed from the tissue directly and disaggregated by enzymatic or mechanical means before cultivation, or they may be derived from a cell line or cell strain that has already been established.
- Primary culture refers to the stage of the culture after the cells are isolated from the tissue and proliferated under the appropriate conditions until they occupy all of the available substrate (i.e., reach confluence).

- At this stage, the cells have to be subcultured (i.e., passaged) by transferring them to a new vessel with fresh growth medium to provide more room for continued growth.
- After the first subculture, the primary culture becomes known as a cell line or subclone.
- Cell lines derived from primary cultures have a limited life span (i.e., they are finite; see below), and as they are passaged, cells with the highest growth capacity predominate, resulting in a degree of genotypic and phenotypic uniformity in the population.
- If a subpopulation of a cell line is positively selected from the culture by cloning or some other method, this cell line becomes a cell strain.
- A cell strain often acquires additional genetic changes subsequent to the initiation of the parent line.

PART-III

---

5. **Draw a labeled diagram depicting the morphology of human immunodeficiency Virus and briefly describe the strategies used for diagnosis of infections caused by this virus:**

(Ref: Ananthanaryan & Paniker, Textbook of Microbiology, 10th ed, pg.574)

ANSWER

Human Immunodeficiency Virus (HIV)

Morphology

The 3 structural genes (protein coded for):

- Env (gp 120 and gp41):
    - Formed from cleavage of gp160 to form envelope glycoproteins.
    - gp120—attachment to host CD4+ T cell.
    - gp41—fusion and entry.

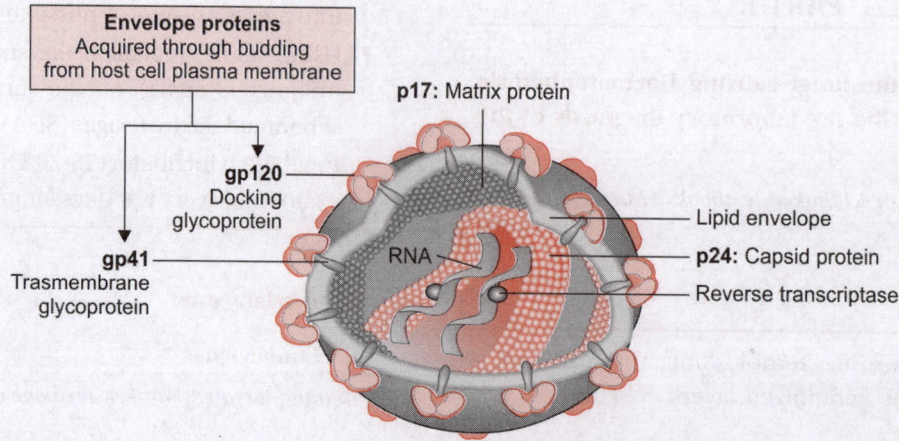

- gag (p24 and p17)—capsid and matrix proteins, respectively.
- pol—reverse transcriptase, aspartate protease, integrase.
- Reverse transcriptase synthesizes dsDNA from genomic RNA; dsDNA integrates into host genome.
- Virus binds CD4 as well as a co-receptor, either CCR5 on macrophages (early infection) or CXCR4 on T cells (late infection).
- Homozygous CCR5 mutation = immunity.
- Heterozygous CCR5 mutation = slower course

Laboratory Diagnosis

- Serological tests:
  - ELISAs
  - Rapid test
  - Western blots
- **NAATs:** Sensitive tests for detection of HIV Infection-Viral Load can be detected.

Summary of Diagnostic Tests for HIV Infection

Technology	Principle	Strengths	Limitations
Initial HIV tests			
First- and second-generation immunoassays	Viral lysate (G1) or recombinant antigens (G2) capture anti-HIV Abs; specific IgGs detected using antihuman IgG	Detect HIV-specific IgG	Do not detect HIV-specific IgM and HIV antigens
Third-generation immunoassays	Recombinant antigens capture anti-HIV antibodies; IgG and IgM detected using antihuman antibodies	Detect anti-HIV IgMs that may occur earlier in infection, in addition to IgG; improved seroconversion sensitivity; some have greater sensitivity in detecting HIV-2 and/or HIV-1 group O compared to earlier-generation assays	Do not detect HIV antigens
Fourth-generation immunoassays	Recombinant antigens capture anti-HIV Abs; IgG and IgM detected using antihuman antibodies plus direct detection of p24 Ag	Detect Antibodies and antigua simultaneously, allowing recognition of HIV infection prior to seroconversion	May miss early HIV infection (prior to antigenemia)
Rapid tests	Immunoassays that employ lateral flow, immunoconcentration, or particle agglutination technologies	Completed in <30 min often at point of care; performance characteristics similar to lab-based immunoassays (generation dependent)	Similar to lab-based immunoassays (generation dependent)
NAATs	Nucleic acids (DNA or RNA) amplified using specific primers and detected using labeled probes	Detect acute HIV infection prior to seroconversion	Most detect HIV-1 only; HIV-1 RNA may be undetectable in some Ab-positive HIV-infected persons; technically complex and expensive
Supplemental HIV tests			
Western blot	Viral lysate separated by electrophoresis, transferred to membrane and patient specimen is incubated with membrane to identify specific Ag/Ab complexes	High specificity due to Ag separation and concentration	Less sensitive than third- and fourth-generation immunoassays, technically complex, opportunities for technical error
Line immunoassays	Similar to WB, recombinant antigua or synthetic peptides replace viral lysate.	High specificity	Similar to WB
Indirect immunofluorescence assays	Microscope slide coated with cells infected with HIV, patient specimen incubated on slide with cells and then fluorescently labeled antihuman antibodies used to detect HIV specific Antibodies by microscopy	High specificity	Subjective interpretation of results; assays only approved for HIV-1 detection in US; expensive instrument (microscope) required; low throughput

MICROBIOLOGY

Technology	Principle	Strengths	Limitations
NAATs	Nucleic acids (DNA or RNA) amplified using specific primers and detected using labeled probes	High specificity; detect HIV infection prior to seroconversion; may be used when WB is indeterminate	Most detect HIV-1 only; HIV-1 RNA may be undetectable in some Ab positive HIV-infected persons; technically complex and expensive
Enzyme immunoassays	Same as above for initial HIV tests	Same as above for initial tests. May distinguish between HIV-1 and HIV-2. More simple and rapid than WB and IFAs	None yet FDA approved for supplemental testing

Abbreviations: Ab, antibody; Ag, antigen; FDA, Food and Drug Administration; G1, first generation; G2, second generation; HIV, human immunodeficiency virus; IFA, immunofluorescence assay; IgG, immunoglobulin G; IgM, immunoglobulin M; NAATs, nucleic acid amplification tests; WB, Western blot.

6. **Tabulate the viral vaccines mentioning the type, preparation and schedule as used in the National Immunization Schedule of India**

ANSWER

(Ref: Ananthanaryan & Paniker, Textbook of Microbiology, 10th ed, pg.643, 644 and 645)

Types of Vaccines

Live attenuated	Measles, mumps, rubella, varicella zoster, BCG, rotavirus, oral polio (Sabin)
Killed vaccine	Rabies, pertussis, cholera, hepatitis A, killed polio (Salk)
Recombinant subunit	Hepatitis B
Toxoid	Tetanus, diphtheria
Protein conjugated	H. influenzae type-b (Hib), meningococcal, pneumococcal (13PCV)
Polysaccharide	Meningococcal and pneumococcal vaccines

National Immunization Schedule of India

Ideal age	Vaccine	Special comments
At birth (for institutional deliveries)	BCG and OPV -0 dose, Hep B	• OPV -0 dose can be given till 15 days after birth • Hep B (Within 24 hours)
At 6 weeks	BCG (if not given at birth), OPV-1, Pentavalent Vaccine and Rotavirus Vaccine* IPV@, Pneumococcal vaccine ***	• BCG can be given up to 1 year of age. • **Rotavirus vaccine**- Dose is 5 drops, Storage conditions similar to OPV (Up to district level -20°C and below district 2–8°C), No Open Vial policy (open vial to be discarded in 4 hours), it can be initiated maximum by 1 year age
At 10 weeks	OPV-2, Pentavalent Vaccine and Rotavirus Vaccine*, Pneumococcal vaccine ***	• Interval between 2 doses should not be less than one month • Pentavalent Vaccine protects against – Diphtheria, Pertussis, Tetanus, Hepatitis B, *H. Influenza* type B associated Pneumonia and Meningitis
At 14 weeks	OPV-3, Pentavalent Vaccine* and Rotavirus Vaccine*, IPV@ Pneumococcal vaccine ***	• If 2nd or 3rd dose in an immunization is delayed, immunization schedule need not be started all over again
At 9 months (complete)	Measles and JE Vaccine**	• Along with Vitamin A- 1st dose 9th month, 2nd 18 month, 3rd to 9th dose at 6 monthly intervals till 5 years of age
At 16–24 months	DPT Booster, OPV Booster, 2nd dose Measles, 2nd dose of JE vaccine**	
At 5 years	DPT booster	• 2nd dose of DPT should be given at 1-month interval if there is no clear history or documented evidence of previous immunization with DPT

Ideal age	Vaccine	Special comments
At 10 and at 16 years	Tetanus Toxoid	• 2nd dose of TT vaccine should be given at 1-month interval if there is no clear history or documented evidence of previous immunization with DPT, DT or TT vaccines
National Immunization Schedule (Pregnant Women)		
As early as possible in pregnancy (16 weeks)	TT -1 or Booster	• 1 dose if previously vaccinated with 2 doses of TT one month apart in the last 3 previous year
One month after TT -1 and ideally before the last month of gestation	TT-2	Interval between 2 doses should not be less than 1 month

* Rotavirus vaccine- At present in Andhra Pradesh, Himachal Pradesh, Odisha and Haryana from 2016.
** JE vaccination in 110 endemic districts.
***Pneumococcal Vaccine – in 5 states Himachal Pradesh, Bihar, Uttar Pradesh, Rajasthan and Madhya Pradesh.
 @IPV given as fractional dose (0.1 mL) intradermal route (Right upper arm deltoid) Measles, Vitamin A and OPV is to be given maximum by 5 years, BCG, Pentavalent and Rotavirus (initiation) by 1 year, DPT given maximum by 7 years, Measles-Rubella (MR) vaccination campaign initiated in five states/UTs Karnataka, Tamil Nadu, Puducherry, Goa and Lakshadweep. Following the campaign, measles-rubella vaccine will be introduced in routine immunization, replacing the currently given two doses of measles vaccine, at 9–12 months and 16–24 months of age.

Name of the Paper : **Microbiology Paper-I**

Name of the Course : **MBBS-2014**

Semester : **Annual**

Time: 3 Hours   M.M.: 40

INSTRUCTIONS

1. Write your Roll No. on the top immediately on receipt of this question paper
2. All questions are to be attempted
3. Answers to Parts I, II and III should be written in separate answer sheets provided
4. Attempt parts of a question in sequence

PART-I

1. Enumerate the various methods of antigen antibody reactions. Describe briefly the principle and applications of agglutination reactions.   [5]

2. Write short notes on: [10]
   a. IgA
   b. Contribution of Robert Koch

PART-II

3. Enumerate the bacterial causes of urinary tract infection. Describe briefly the laboratory diagnosis of this condition.   [5]

4. Write briefly on: [10]
   a. Chlamydia trachomatis
   b. Nontuberculous mycobacteria

PART-III

5. Name the bacterial pathogens that may cause acute pyogenic meningitis. Describe the laboratory diagnosis of this condition.   [5]

6. Write briefly about drug resistance in bacteria.   [5]

PART-I

1. Enumerate the various methods of antigen antibody reactions. Describe briefly the principle and applications of agglutination reactions.

(Ref: Ananthanaryan & Paniker, Textbook of Microbiology, 10th ed, pg. 105, 106)

ANSWER

For answer, refer 2016 paper-I Q. 1, Pg. 353

2. Write short notes on:

(Ref: Ananthanaryan & Paniker, Textbook of Microbiology, 10th ed, pg.98)

a. IgA

ANSWER

○ It is present in breast milk, mucus, saliva, sweat and serum. IgA constitutes about 10-15% of serum immunoglobulins and occurs in two subclasses - IgA1 and IgA2.

○ IgA1 is mainly a monomer, synthesized in the bone marrow and constitutes major portion of IgA.

○ IgA2 is synthesized by B cells present in MALT.

○ IgA in breast milk interferes with colonization of harmful bacteria in the gut for first few months of life.

○ IgA may activate the alternate complement pathway and promote phagocytosis. These are the characteristics of IgA:

○ It is the second most abundant immunoglobulin in serum

○ It is the major class of immunoglobulin that is found in secretions like, tears, saliva, colostrum and mucus

○ It binds to cells like polymorphonuclear cells and lymphocytes

○ Normally it does not fix complement although may activate the alternate complement pathway.

b. Contribution of Robert Koch

(Ref: Ananthanaryan & Paniker, Textbook of Microbiology, 10th ed, pg.4)

ANSWER

Robert Koch is regarded as 'Father of medical Microbiology and Bacteriology'.

Robert Koch – Notable Contributions	
1876	Koch demonstrated that anthrax is caused by *Bacillus anthracis*
1877	Methods for staining bacteria, photographing and preparing permanent visual records on slides
1881	Koch developed solid culture media and the methods for studying bacteria in pure cultures
1882	Isolated the bacterium—*Mycobacterium tuberculosis*—that causes tuberculosis
1882	Use of agar as a support medium for solid culture in Koch's lab by Hesse
1883	Isolation of *Vibrio cholerae*, the cause of cholera
1883	Verification of the germ theory of disease by relating a specific organism to the specific disease
1884	Koch put forth his postulates—known as Koch's postulates

PART-II

3. Enumerate the bacterial causes of urinary tract infection. Describe briefly the laboratory diagnosis of this condition.

(Ref: Ananthanaryan & Paniker, Textbook of Microbiology, 10th ed, pg. 260)

ANSWER

Bacterial Causes of Urinary Tract Infection

○ *E. coli*

○ *Klebsiella*

○ *Proteus*

○ *Pseudomonas aeruginosa*

○ *Staphylococcus saprophyticus*

○ *Enterococcus faecalis*

○ *Streptococcus agalactiae*

Type infection	Case vignette/key clues	Most common causal agents
Urethritis	Gram-negative diplococci in PMNs in urethral exudate	Neisseria gonorrhoeae
	Culture negative, inclusion bodies	Chlamydia trachomatis
	Urease positive, no cell wall	Ureaplasma urealyticum
	Flagellated protozoan with corkscrew motility	Trichomonas vaginalis
Cystitis	Frequent and painful urination, hematuria, and fever	E. coli, other gram-negative enterics, Pseudomonas, Proteus

Type infection	Case vignette/key clues	Most common causal agents
	Young, newly sexually active individual; gram-positive cocci	Staphylococcus saprophyticus
Pyelone-phritis	As above, with flank pain and prominent fever	E. coli, Staphylococcus
Pyelone-phritis	As above, with flank pain and prominent fever	E. coli, Staphylococcus
Genital lesions	Genital warts	Human papilloma virus (most common U.S. STD), Treponema pallidum, molluscum contagiosum
	Multiple painful vesicular, coalescing, recurring	Herpes simplex virus
	Non-tender, indurated ulcer healing spontaneously 2–10 weeks	Treponema pallidum
	Non-indurated, painful papule, Suppurative with adenopathy, slow to heal	Haemophilus ducreyi
	Soft, painless ulcer, patient from Caribbean or New Guinea, gram-negative intracellular bacilli	Klebsiella granulomatis (granuloma inguinale)

Laboratory Diagnosis of Urinary Tract Infection

○ Detection of bacteriuria by urine microscopy. Bacteriuria can be detected microscopically using Gram staining of uncentrifuged urine specimens, Gram staining of centrifuged specimens, or direct observation of bacteria in urine specimens.

○ Detection of bacteriuria by nitrite test. Bacteriuria can be detected chemically when bacteria produce nitrite from nitrate. The biochemical reaction that is detected by the nitrite test is associated with members of the family Enterobacteriaceae

○ Routine bacterial urine cultures. Urine culture may not be necessary as part of the evaluation of outpatients with uncomplicated UTIs. However, urine cultures are necessary for outpatients who have recurrent UTIs, experience treatment failures, or have complicated UTIs.

○ A specimen for culture is generally collected as a midstream urine (MSU) sample.

4. Write briefly on:

(Ref: Ananthanaryan & Paniker, Textbook of Microbiology, 10th ed, pg. 424)

a. Chlamydia trachomatis

ANSWER

○ *Chlamydia trachomatis* is the organism responsible for diseases such as trachoma and the STD

○ *Chlamydia* are obligate intracellular parasites, and are among the smallest living organisms.

○ There are two stages in the life of *Chlamydia*: elementary bodies and reticulate bodies. Another feature of *Chlamydia* is that they are unable to synthesize their own energy (ATP) and are completely dependent on their host for energy.

○ The organism is in the elementary stage of its life when it encounters its host and is taken up by phagocytosis.

○ It prevents the fusion of the phagosome and lysosome; this is what normally kills pathogens.

○ Once the phagolysosome formation is stopped, the bacteria secrete glycogen and transform into the reticulate body.

○ Reticulate bodies obtain their energy by sending forth "straw-like" structures into the host cell cytoplasm, and they divide by binary fission.

○ Each phagolysosome produces about 100-1000 reticulate bodies.

○ The cell wall of *Chlamydia* has been characterized as gram-negative with a notable difference: it lacks muramic acid that is found in the cell walls of most other bacteria.

○ This makes *Chlamydia* resistant to β-lactam antibiotics such as penicillin, because such antibiotics disrupt the

○ "typical" cell wall, which includes muramic acid.

○ Being gram-negative, it also contains LPS, which helps cause damage to the host's body(mainly due to the host's immune response).

b. See the explanation of 2017 paper-I Ques No-4 (b), Pg. 341

PART-III

5. Name the bacterial pathogens that may cause acute pyogenic meningitis. Describe the laboratory diagnosis of this condition.

(Ref: Ananthanaryan & Paniker, Textbook of Microbiology, 10th ed, pg. 250)

ANSWER

Bacterial Causes of Meningitis

○ *Streptococcus pneumoniae*

○ *Group B Streptococcus*

○ *Neisseria meningitidis*

○ *Haemophilus influenzae*

○ *Listeria monocytogenes*

Laboratory Diagnosis of Acute Pyogenic Meningitis

Microscopy and Staining: CSF Gram stains should be prepared after cytocentrifugation and positive results reported immediately to clinicians. If Cryptococcal meningitis is suspected, India ink preparation should be done.

○ N. meningitidis may occur intracellularly or extracellularly in PMN leukocytes and will appear as gram-negative, coffee-bean shaped diplococci.

○ S. pneumoniae may occur intracellularly or extracellularly and will appear as gram-positive, lanceolate diplococci, sometimes occurring in short chains.

○ H. influenzae are small, pleomorphic gram-negative rods or coccobacilli with random arrangements

Culture and Sensitivity: Identification and susceptibility testing of bacteria recovered from cultures is routinely performed by growing the organisms in their specific culture media unless contamination during collection or processing is suspected. Following media are routinely used in the diagnostic microbiology laboratory for the isolation of common bacterial agents;

○ **Chocolate Agar**
  ▪ On chocolate agar plate, H. influenzae appear as large colorless to gray, opaque colonies with no discoloration of the surrounding medium.

○ **Blood Agar N. meningitidis on blood agar plate**
  ▪ Overnight growth of N. meningitidis on blood agar plate appears as round, moist, glistening and convex colonies.
  ▪ S. pneumoniae appear as small grayish mucoid (watery) colonies with a greenish zone of alpha-hemolysis surrounding them on the blood agar plate.

○ **MacConkey Agar**
  ▪ Antigen-antibody reactions
  ▪ **Antigen Testing:** Cryptococcal Antigen latex agglutination test is preferred method in the suspected cases of Cryptococcal meningitis. Bacterial antigen testing on CSF is not recommended
  ▪ **Serology:** Serologic diagnosis is based on CSF to serum antibody index, 4- fold rise in acute to convalescent immunoglobulin G (IgG) titer, or a single positive immunoglobulin M (IgM). Submission of acute (3–10 days after onset of symptoms) and convalescent (2–3 weeks after acute) serum samples is recommended

6. **Write briefly about drug resistance in bacteria.**

ANSWER

For answer, refer 2017 paper-I Q. 6, Pg. 342

Your Roll No. ....

Name of the Paper	:	**Microbiology Paper-II**
Name of the Course	:	**MBBS-2014**
Semester	:	**Annual**

Time: 3 Hours   M.M.: 40

INSTRUCTIONS

1. Write your Roll No. on the top immediately on receipt of this question paper
2. All questions are to be attempted
3. Answers to Parts I, II and III should be written in separate answer sheets provided
4. Attempt parts of a question in sequence

PART-I

1. Describe the life cycle of *Wuchereria bancrofti* and the laboratory diagnosis of filariasis.   [5]

2. Write short notes on: [10]
   a. Laboratory diagnosis of Kala-azar
   b. Visceral larva migrans (VLM)

PART-II

3. Enumerate the dimorphic fungi. Describe the laboratory diagnosis of histoplasmosis.   [5]

4. Write briefly on: [10]
   a. Epstein–Barr virus (EBV)
   b. Non–neural rabies vaccines

PART-III

5. Enumerate the viruses causing diarrhea and write briefly about Rotavirus.   [5]

6. Enumerate the arboviruses prevalent in India. Describe briefly the laboratory diagnosis of dengue fever.   [5]

PART-I

1. Describe the life cycle of Wuchereria bancrofti and the laboratory diagnosis of filariasis:

(Ref: Arora parasitology 5ᵗʰ ed. P. 199, 200, 204)

ANSWER

For answer, refer 2017 paper–II Q. 1, Pg. 345

2. Write short notes on:

(Ref: Arora parasitology 5ᵗʰ ed p 53)

a. Laboratory diagnosis of Kala-azar

ANSWER

For answer, refer 2016 paper-II Q. 2 (a), Pg. 362

b. Visceral larva migrans (VLM)

(Ref: Arora parasitology 5ᵗʰ edition p 215, 219)

ANSWER

○ It is a condition in humans caused by the migratory larvae of certain nematodes, humans being a *dead-end host.*

○ Nematodes causing such zoonotic infections Toxocara canis, *Toxocara cati,* and *Ascaris suum.*

○ These nematodes can infect but not mature in humans and after migrating through the intestinal wall, travel with the blood stream to various organs where they cause inflammation and damage.

○ Affected organs can include the *liver, heart* (causing myocarditis) and the CNS (causing dysfunction, seizures, and coma).

○ A special variant is *ocular larva* migrans where usually T. canis larvae travel to the eye.

PART-II

3. Enumerate the dimorphic fungi. Describe the laboratory diagnosis of Histoplasmosis:

(Ref: Ananthanaryan & Paniker, Textbook of Microbiology,10th ed, pg. 609)

ANSWER

Dimorphic Fungi

○ *Histoplasma capsulatum*
○ *Blastomyces dermatitidis*
○ *Paracoccidioides brasiliensis*
○ *Coccidioides immitis*

Laboratory Diagnosis of Histoplasmosis

○ **Obtain appropriate specimens**

Sputum	Bone marrow
Blood	Lesion scrapings
Urine	Biopsy specimens

○ **Direct examination**
  ▪ Tissue specimens
    ♦ Stains for fungi-PAS, GMS, GIEMSA
    ♦ Routine histology- H & E
    ♦ Small yeast (2-4 m) intracellular in macrophages
    ♦ Granulomas-non
    ♦ Caseating
      ▫ Caseating
  ▪ Speutum-KOH or calcofluor

○ **Culture**
  ▪ Sabouraud's agar
    ♦ White-brown mould
    ♦ Typical microscopic morphology
  ▪ Slow growth 2-8 weeks
  ▪ Rapid ID confirmation
    ♦ Exo-antigen
    ♦ Molecular probe
  ▪ Traditional ID confirmation
    ♦ Conversion mould to yeast
    ♦ Animal inoculation

4. Write briefly on:

(Ref: Ananthanaryan & Paniker, Textbook of Microbiology,10th ed, pg.570)

a. Epstein-Barr virus (EBV)

ANSWER

○ **Reservoir:** Humans
○ **Transmission:** Saliva, 90% of adult population is seropositive

○ **Pathogenesis**
  ▪ Virus infects nasopharyngeal epithelial cells, salivary and lymphoid tissues → latent infection of B cells (EBV binds to CD21 and acts as a B-cell mitogen) → results in production of atypical reactive T cells (Downey cells), which may constitute up to 70% of WBC count
  ▪ Heterophile antibodies are produced (due to B cell mitogenesis)

○ **Diseases**
  ▪ **Heterophile-positive mononucleosis, "kissing disease":** Fatigue, fever, sore throat, lymphadenopathy, splenomegaly; latency in B cells
  ▪ **Lymphoproliferative disease:** Occurs in immunocompromised patients; T cells can't control B-cell growth
  ▪ **Hairy oral leukoplakia:** Hyperproliferation of lingual epithelial cells; occurs in AIDS patients

○ **Malignancies**
  ▪ **Burkitt lymphoma:** Cancer of the maxilla, mandible, abdomen; Africa; malaria cofactor; AIDS patients; translocation juxtaposes c-myc oncogene to a very active promoter such as immunoglobulin gene promoter
  ▪ **Nasopharyngeal carcinoma:** Asia (most common cancer in southern China); tumor cells of epithelial origin
  ▪ Hodgkin and non-Hodgkin lymphoma

○ **Diagnosis:** Heterophile-antibody positive (IgM antibodies that recognize Paul-Bunnell antigen on sheep and bovine RBCs)

○ **Treatment:** Symptomatic, for uncomplicated mononucleosis

  b. **Non–Neural rabies vaccines**

(Ref: Ananthanaryan & Paniker, Textbook of Microbiology, 10th ed, pg.539)

ANSWER

○ **Types of vaccine**

Neural vaccines	Non- neural vaccines
• Sample vaccine	• Drug e.g. vaccine
• Beta propiolactone vaccine	• Live attenuate chick embryo vaccine
• Suckling mouse brain vaccine.	• Tissue culture vaccine
	• Sub-unit vaccine (in experimental stage)

○ **Vaccination schedule**

Pre-exposure prophylaxis	0, 7, 21 or 0, 28, 56; Booster after 1 year and then after 5 years
Post- exposure prophylaxis	0., 3, 7, 14, 30 and optionally 90.

○ Cell Culture Vaccines (CCV)
  ▪ Human diploid cell vaccine (HDCV) contains the Pitman-Moore L503 or Flury strain of rabies virus grown on MRC-5 human diploid cell culture, concentrated by ultrafiltration and inactivated with ß-propiolactone. This vaccine is licensed for intra-muscular use. It contains no preservative or stabilizer.
  ▪ Purified chick embryo cell vaccine (PCECV) is a sterile lyophilized vaccine obtained by growing the fixed rabies virus strain Flury LEP-25 in primary cultures of chick fibroblasts. The virus is inactivated with ß-propiolactone, purified and concentrated by zonal centrifugation .
  ▪ Purified Vero cell rabies vaccine (PVRV) contains inactivated and lyophilized Wistar strain of rabies virus grown on Vero cell cultures in fermenters allowing mass cultivation. These are inactivated by ß-propriolactone and purified by ultracentrifugation.
  ▪ Primary Hamster Kidney Cell vaccine (PHKCV) uses the Beijing strain and is inactivated with formalin and adsorbed to aluminum hydroxide. It also contains 0.01% thiomersal and 10 mg human albumin.

○ Embryonated egg-based vaccines (EEV)
  ▪ Purified duck embryo vaccine (PDEV) uses duck embryo cells as substrate. These are inactivated by ß-propiolactone and purified by ultracentrifugation. PDEV contains thiomersal.

PART-III

5. Enumerate the viruses causing diarrhea and write briefly about rotavirus:

(Ref: Ananthanaryan & Paniker, Textbook of Microbiology, 10th ed, pg.564)

ANSWER

Viruses Causing Diarrhea

○ Rotavirus
○ Adenovirus
○ Astrovirus
○ Norovirus
○ Calicivirus

Rotavirus

○ **Genome:** Have 11 segments of double-stranded RNA; virion has wheel-and-spoke morphology.

○ **Classification:** Exist in at least seven serotypes, with type A being involved in most human infections.

- **Clinical disease:** Cause infantile diarrhea and are the most common cause of gastroenteritis in children; are frequent causes of nosocomial infections
- **Diagnosis:** Diagnosed by demonstrating virus in the stool or by serologic tests, particularly ELISA.
- **Prevention:** Have been modified and genetically manipulated for preparation of live attenuated vaccines (RotaTeq and Rotarix).

---

6. **Enumerate the arboviruses prevalent in India. Describe briefly the laboratory diagnosis of dengue fever:**

(Ref: Ananthanaryan & Paniker, Textbook of Microbiology, 10th ed, pg.529)

ANSWER

Arboviruses Prevalent in India

- Chikungunya
- Dengue
- Japanese encephalitis
- Kyasanur forest disease

Laboratory Diagnosis of Dengue Fever

- **Microscopy and staining:** In this case, direct visualization of the virus in the sample (using electron microscopy or via fluorescent staining technique) is not done in diagnostic laboratories.
- **Culture:** Virus isolation in cell culture is difficult and is not the commonly used method in diagnostic laboratories because it is demanding procedure (both in terms of infrastructure and technical expertise). Virus may be recovered from serum, plasma and peripheral blood mononuclear cells. Inoculation of a mosquito cell line with patient serum, coupled with nucleic acid assays to identify the recovered virus is commonly used approach.
- **Serological test:** Serological tests are the mainstay in the diagnosis of viral infections.
  - **Detection of viral antigen:** Dengue NS1 Antigen detection useful for the diagnosis of acute dengue infections. Has been detected in the serum of DENV infected patients as early as 1 day post onset of symptoms (DPO), and up to 18 DPO. NS1 ELISA based antigen assay is commercially available NS1 assay may also be useful for differential diagnostics between flaviviruses because of the specificity of the assay
  - Detection of Anti-dengue antibodies in serum or other body fluids by ELISA or other rapid tests. Various methods (IgM/IgG ELISA, Hemagglutination Inhibition Test, or Rapid diagnostic kits) are available to detect Anti-Dengue Antibodies; IgM detection: Useful for the diagnosis of primary Dengue infection and in distinguishing dengue from other flavivirus infections. IgM antibodies are detectable in 99% of patients by day 10 after onset of illness. IgM levels peak about two weeks after the onset of symptoms and then decline to undetectable levels over 2–3 months. Sensitivity: 65-75% sensitive in single acute serum sample.
  - **IgG detection:** Tests that detect IgG are useful in diagnosing secondary disease (IgG is the dominant immunoglobulin type in secondary infection). The test is complicated by cross-reactivity of IgG antibodies to heterologous flavivirus antigens (West Nile virus, tick-borne encephalitis virus, yellow fever virus, Zika virus).
  - **Molecular diagnosis:** Detection of viral RNA in plasma or serum or tissues using Nucleic Acid Amplification Tests (NAAT). RT-PCR based methods for rapid identification and serotyping of dengue virus in acute phase serum are available.

Name of the Paper   :   **Microbiology Paper-I**

Name of the Course   :   **MBBS-2013**

Semester   :   **Annual**

Time: 3 Hours   M.M.: 40

INSTRUCTIONS

1. Write your Roll No. on the top immediately on receipt of this question paper
2. All questions are to be attempted
3. Answers to Parts I, II and III should be written in separate answer sheets provided
4. Attempt parts of a question in sequence

PART-I

1. Describe the principle of anaerobiosis. Enumerate various methods used to culture anaerobic bacteria. Describe their advantages and disadvantages.   [5]

2. Write short notes on: [10]

   a. Transposons
   b. Determinants of virulence in microorganisms

PART-II

3. Enumerate the agents causing enteric fever. Describe its laboratory diagnosis.   [5]

4. Write briefly on: [10]

   a. Scrub typhus
   b. Drug resistant tuberculosis

PART-III

5. Write briefly short the biomedical Waste, its classification, categories and methods of disposal.   [5]

6. Write in brief method of detection of MRSA.   [5]

PART-I

1. Describe the principle of anaerobiosis. Enumerate various methods used to culture anaerobic bacteria. Describe their advantages and disadvantages.

(Ref: Ananthanaryan & Paniker, Textbook of Microbiology,10th ed, pg. 273)

ANSWER

Principle of Anaerobiosis

The anaerobic jar employs a chemical reaction to generate hydrogen gas. In the presence of a palladium catalyst, the hydrogen gas will react with free oxygen in the air to form water. This reaction removes the oxygen from the sealed atmosphere. The jar is then incubated at the desired temperature. There will be slight negative pressure inside.

Various Methods to Culture Anaerobic Bacteria

- Producing a vacuum
- Oxygen displacement
- Oxygen absorption
- Reducing agents
- Anaerobic chambers–(have catalyst, desiccant, H_2, CO_2, N_2 + indicator; airtight gloves)

2. Write short notes on:

a. Transposons

(Ref: Ananthanaryan & Paniker, Textbook of Microbiology,10th ed, pg. 63)

ANSWER

Transposons are segments of DNA that can move around to different positions in the genome of a single cell. In the process, they may

- Cause mutations
- Increase (or decrease) the amount of DNA in the genome of the cell, and if the cell is the precursor of a gamete, in the genomes of any descendants.

These mobile segments of DNA are sometimes called **"jumping genes"**.

There are two distinct types:

- **Class II transposons**. These consist of DNA that moves directly from place to place.

- **Class I transposons**. These are **retrotransposons** that
  - First transcribe the DNA into RNA and then
  - Use reverse transcriptase to make a DNA copy of the RNA to insert in a new location.

PART-II

3. Enumerate the agents causing enteric fever. Describe its laboratory diagnosis.

(Ref: Ananthanaryan & Paniker, Textbook of Microbiology,10th ed, pg. 300)

ANSWER

For answer, refer 2017 paper-I Q. 3, Pg. 340

4. Write briefly on:

(Ref: Ananthanaryan & Paniker, Textbook of Microbiology,10th ed, pg. 415)

a. Scrub typhus

ANSWER

- Scrub typhus is an acute febrile illness caused by *orientia tsutsugamushi*, transmitted to humans by the bite of the larva of trombiculid mites.
- It causes a disseminated vasculitis and perivascular inflammatory lesions resulting in significant vascular leakage and end-organ injury.
- It affects people of all ages and even though scrub typhus in pregnancy is uncommon, it is associated with increased fetal loss, preterm delivery, and small for gestational age infants.
- After an incubation period of 6-21 days, onset is characterized by fever, headache, myalgia, cough, and gastrointestinal symptoms.
- A primary popular lesion which later crusts to form a flat black eschar, may be present. If untreated, serious complications may occur involving various organs.
- Laboratory studies usually reveal leukopenia, thrombocytopenia, deranged hepatic and renal function, proteinuria and reticulonodular infiltrate.
- Owing to the potential for severe complications, diagnosis, and decision to initiate treatment should be based on clinical suspicion and confirmed by serologic tests

MICROBIOLOGY

Infections Caused by Rickettsiae and Close Relatives

Group disease	Bacterium	Arthropod vector	Reservoir host
Rocky mountain spotted fever	R. rickettsii	Ticks	Ticks, dogs, rodents
Epidemic typhus	R. prowazekii	Human louse	Humans
Endemic typhus	R. typhi	Fleas	Rodents
Scrub typhus	Orientia tsutsugamushi	Mites	Rodents
Ehrlichiosis	E. chaffeensis A. phagocytophilum	Tick	Small mammals

b.　Drug resistant tuberculosis

(Ref: Ananthanaryan & Paniker, Textbook of Microbiology,10th ed, pg.356)

ANSWER

For answer, refer 2016 paper-I Q. 4 (b), Pg. 357

PART-III

5.　Write briefly about biomedical Waste, its classification, categories and methods of disposal.

ANSWER

Biomedical Waste

Biomedical waste means "any solid and/or liquid waste including its container and any intermediate product, which is generated during the diagnosis, treatment or immunization of human beings or animals". Biomedical waste poses hazard due to two principal reasons–the first is infectivity and the other, toxicity.

Biomedical Waste Categories and Methods of Disposal

According to the new rules of biomedical waste management—there are only four waste categories

Color of the bag	Type of waste	Waste treatment
Yellow	Human anatomical waste	Incineration or plasma pyrolysis or deep burial
	Animal anatomical waste	Incineration or plasma pyrolysis or deep burial
	Soiled waste	Incineration or plasma pyrolysis or deep burial
	Expired or discarded medicines	Return back to the manufacturer or supplier for incineration at temperature >1200°C
	Chemical waste	Incineration or plasma pyrolysis or deep burial or encapsulation
	Chemical liquid waste	Pretreatment and then disposal

Biomedical waste consists of:

○ Human anatomical waste like tissues, organs and body parts

○ Animal wastes generated during research from veterinary hospitals

○ Microbiology and biotechnology wastes

○ Waste sharp instruments like hypodermic needles, syringes, scalpels and broken glass

○ Discarded medicines and cytotoxic drugs

○ Soiled waste such as dressing, bandages, plaster casts, material contaminated with blood, tubes and catheters

○ Liquid waste from any of the infected areas

○ Incineration ash and other chemical wastes

Classification

The World Health Organization (WHO) has classified medical wastes according to their weight, density and constituents into different categories. These are:

○ **Infectious**: Material-containing pathogens in sufficient concentrations or quantities that, if exposed, can cause diseases. This includes waste from surgery and autopsies on patients with infectious diseases, sharps, disposable needles, syringes, saws, blades, broken glasses, nails or any other item that could cause a cut

○ **Pathological**: Tissues, organs, body parts, human flesh, fetuses, blood and body fluids, drugs and chemicals that are returned from wards, spilled, outdated, contaminated, or are no longer required

○ **Radioactive**: Solids, liquids and gaseous waste contaminated with radioactive substances used in diagnosis and treatment of diseases like toxic goiter

○ **Others**: Waste from the offices, kitchens, rooms, including bed linen, utensils, paper, etc.

Color of the bag	Type of waste	Waste treatment
	Discarded linen, mattresses, beddings, contaminated with blood or body fluids	Nonchlorinated chemical disinfection followed by Incineration or plasma pyrolysis
	Microbiology, biotechnology and other clinical laboratory waste	Pretreat to sterilize with nonchlorinated chemicals on site
Red	Contaminated waste like plastic bag, bottles, pipes or containers	Autoclaving or microwaving/hydroclaving followed by shredding or mutilation
White translucent	Waste sharps included needles, syringes with fixed needles, needles from needle tip cutter or burner, scalpels and blades	Autoclaving or dry heat sterilization followed by shredding or mutilation or encapsulation in metal container or cement concrete
Blue cardboard box with blue label	Glassware: Broken or discarded and contaminated glass including medicine vials and ampoules except those contaminated with cytotoxic wastes; metallic body implants	Disinfection with sodium hypochlorite treatment or autoclaving or microwaving or hydroclaving then sent for recycling

6. Write in brief methods of detection of MRSA.

(Ref: Ananthanaryan & Paniker, Textbook of Microbiology, 10th ed, pg. 202)

ANSWER

Phenotypic Detection Systems
- Disc diffusion test
  - Colony suspension prepared from colonies and plated on muller hinton agar containing 2-4% NaCl at neutral pH
  - Oxacillin disc (1 ug) Placed and incubated t 35°C for 24 hours
  - <10 mm is considered resistant, >13mm is considered sensitive
  - For isolates with intermediate results
    - Test for mec A, PBP2a
    - Cefoxitin disc test
    - Oxacillin MIC test or
    - Oxacillin salt agar screen test may be performed
  - Any growth within the zone of inhibition indicates oxacillin resistance

Molecular Methods
- Detection of mecA gene by PCR is considered gold standard

- DNA extraction
- mecA gene amplified using specific primers
  - 30 cycles of denaturation at 94°C for 45 seconds
  - Annealing at 50°C for 45 seconds
  - Extension at 72°C for 1 minute
  - Final extension step at 72°C for 3 minutes
- PCR products visualized on 2% agarose gel with ethidium bromide dye under U-V transilluminator

Other Detection Methods
- Agar dilution test
  - 0.5 McFarland preparation of isolate is spot inoculated on MHA with 2% NaCl containing 256-0.125 ug oxacillin/mL in serial doubling dilutions
  - MIC of >4 ug/mL is considered resistant, MIC <2 ug/mL is considered susceptible
- Broth microdilution
  - Muller hinton broth inoculated with inoculum density of 5×10^5 cfu/mL
- Breakpoint methods
  - Includes both agar and broth methods but test only the breakpoint concentration (2 mg/L oxacillin, 4 mg/L methicillin)
- E-test oxacillin MIC test
  - Easy to set up as a disc diffusion test

Name of the Paper	:	**Microbiology Paper-II**
Name of the Course	:	**MBBS-2013**
Semester	:	**Annual**

Time: 3 Hours   **M.M.: 40**

INSTRUCTIONS

1. Write your Roll No. on the top immediately on receipt of this question paper
2. All questions are to be attempted
3. Answers to Parts I, II and III should be written in separate answer sheets provided
4. Attempt parts of a question in sequence

PART-I

1. **Enumerate vector borne parasitic diseases. Discuss the life cycle and pathogenesis of any one of them.**   [5]

2. **Write short notes on the life cycles of:**   [10]
   a. Taenia solium
   b. Ancylostoma duodenale

PART-II

3. **Enumerate the yeasts causing human infections. Describe the pathogenicity of *Candida albicans*.**   [5]

4. **Write briefly on:**   [10]
   a. Swine influenza
   b. Human Herpes virus Type 4

PART-III

5. **Discuss the laboratory diagnosis and prophylaxis of rabies.**   [5]

6. **Describe the strategies of HIV testing as per NACO guidelines.**   [5]

PART-I

1. **Enumerate vector borne parasitic diseases. Discuss the life cycle and pathogenesis of any one of them.**

(Ref: Arora parasitology 5th ed p 73, 74)

ANSWER

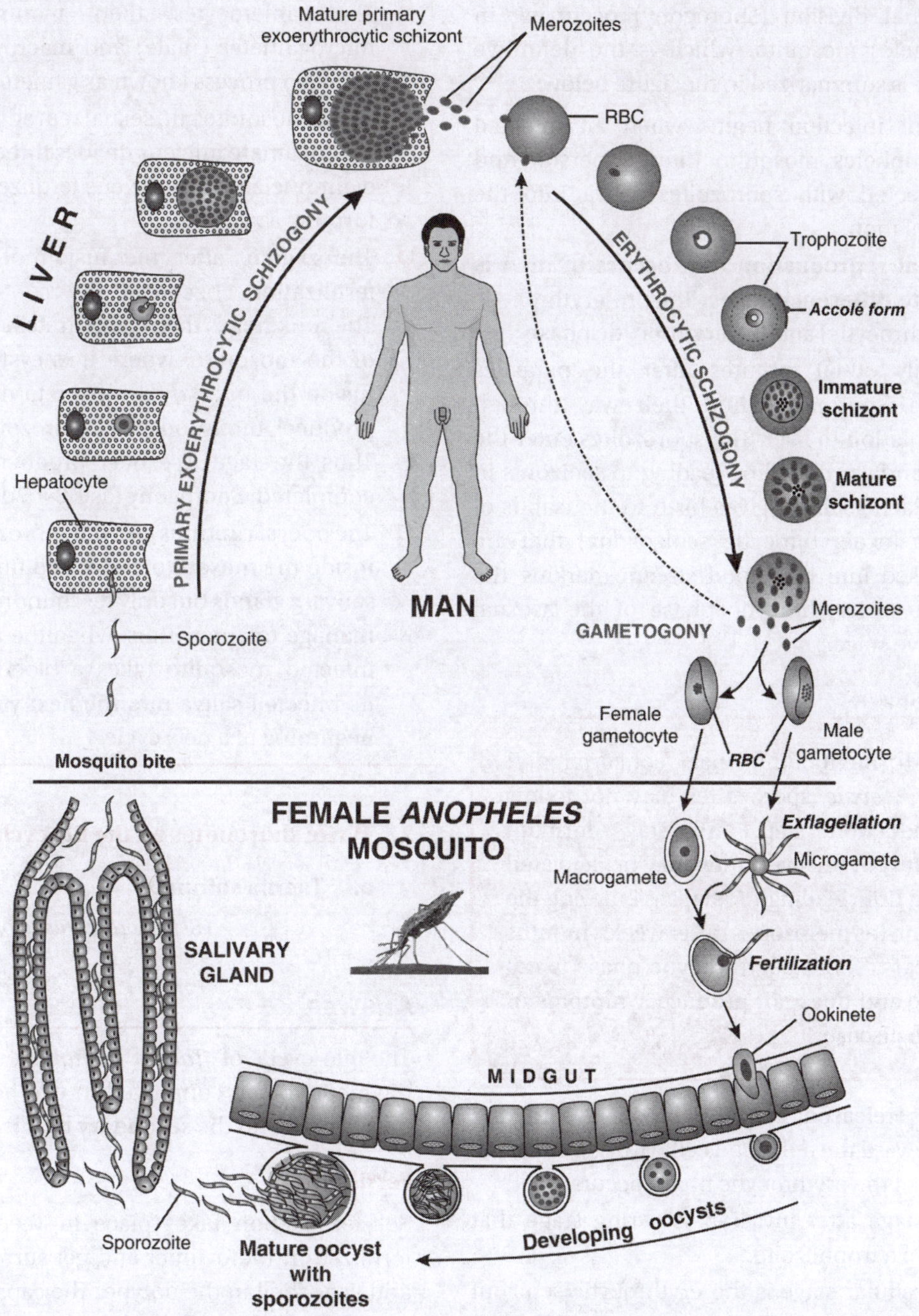

Mature primary
exoerythrocytic schizont

Merozoites

RBC

LIVER

Hepatocyte

PRIMARY EXOERYTHROCYTIC SCHIZOGONY

Sporozoite

Mosquito bite

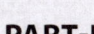

MAN

Trophozoite

Accolé form

Immature schizont

Mature schizont

ERYTHROCYTIC SCHIZOGONY

Merozoites

GAMETOGONY

Female gametocyte

RBC

Male gametocyte

FEMALE *ANOPHELES* MOSQUITO

SALIVARY GLAND

Macrogamete

Exflagellation

Microgamete

Fertilization

Ookinete

MIDGUT

Developing oocysts

Sporozoite

Mature oocyst with sporozoites

Fig. Life cycle of malaria parasite

Vector Borne Parasitic Diseases

○ Leishmaniansis
○ Filariasis
○ Malaria
○ Chagas disease
○ Onchocerciasis

Life Cycle of Malarial Parasite

Malarial parasite or *Plasmodium* has a complex life cycle. It involves alternating cycles of asexual division (schizogony) occurring in man, who is the intermediate host and sexual division (sporogony) occurring in female Anopheles mosquito, which is the definitive host. The cycle is summarized in the figure below:

○ The human infection begins when an infected female anopheles mosquito bites a person and injects infected with sporozoites saliva into the blood circulation.

○ **The asexual reproduction that occurs in man is divided into different phases:** The pre-erythrocytic (or exoerythrocytic) and the erythrocytic phase.

○ Within only 30-60 minutes after the parasites inoculation, sporozoites find their way through blood circulation to liver. The sporozoites enter the liver cells and start dividing leading to schizonts in 6-7 days. Each schizont gives birth to thousands of merozoites (exoerythrocytic schizogony) that are then released into the blood stream marking the end of the exoerythrocytic phase of the asexual reproductive stage.

🔖 Also Know

It is worth mentioning that, concerning *P. vivax* and *P. ovale*, sporozoites may not follow the reproduction step and stay dormant (hypnozoites) in the liver; they may be activated after a long time leading to relapses entering the blood stream (as merozoites) after weeks, months or even years. The exoerythrocytic phase is not pathogenic and does not produce symptoms or signs of the disease.

○ Merozoites released into the blood stream, are directed toward the red blood cells (RBCs). Thus, the beginning of the erythrocytic phase occurs.

○ The first stage after invasion is a ring stage that evolves into a trophozoite.

○ The next cellular stage is the erythrocytic schizont (initially immature and then mature schizont). Each mature schizont gives birth to new generation merozoites (erythrocytic schizogony) that, after RBCs rupture, are released in the blood stream

in order to invade other RBCs. This is when parasitaemia occurs and clinical manifestations appear.

○ The parasite differentiates into male and female gametocytes that is a nonpathogenic form of parasite.

○ When a female anopheles mosquito bites an infected person, it takes up these gametocytes with the blood meal (mosquitoes can be infected only if they have a meal during the period that gametocytes circulate in the human's blood).

○ The gametocytes, then, mature and become microgametes (male) and macrogametes (female) during a process known as gametogenesis.

○ In the mosquito gut, sexual reproduction occurs. The microgamete nucleus divides three times producing eight nuclei; each nucleus fertilizes a macrogamete forming a zygote.

○ The zygote, after the fusion of nuclei and the fertilization, becomes the so- called ookinete. The ookinete, then, penetrates the midgut wall of the mosquito, where it encysts into an oocyst. Inside the oocyst, the ookinete nucleus divides to produce thousands of sporozoites (sporogony). Thus, the stage of sexual reproduction/ sporogony is completed. Sporogony lasts 8-15 days.

○ The oocyst ruptures and the sporozoites are released inside the mosquito cavity and find their way to its salivary glands but only few hundreds of sporozoites manage to enter. Thus, when the above mentioned infected mosquito takes a blood meal, it injects its infected saliva into the next victim marking the beginning of a new cycle.

---

2. **Write short notes on the life cycles of:**

    a. **Taenia solium**

        (Ref: Arora Parasitology 5th ed ition p 131)

ANSWER

The life-cycle of *Taenia solium* is complicated and digenetic, being completed in two hosts. The primary host is man and the secondary host is pig.

Fertilization

Self-fertilization takes place in Taenia. The eggs are fertilized in the oviduct and get surrounded with yolk and egg- shell in the ootype. The capsulated egg enters the uterus and is collected there. The uterus enlarges in size, gets branched and occupies the whole space. The eggs are very small in size measuring about 40 microns in diameter.

Cleavage

The division in the eggs start, while these are- still inside the uterus. The first cleavage is unequal so that a large vitelline cell and a small embryonic cell is formed. The embryonic cell undergone repeated divisions and a solid ball of cells, the morula is formed. The divisions are unequal so the morula consists of a few larger cells, the macromeres forming an outer or peripheral layer and inner mass of small cells or micromeres.

Hexacanth Larva

The micromeres develop into a hexacanth or oncosphere larva.

Infection to Secondary Host

The development of egg up to the formation of oncosphere takes place inside the uterus of gravid proglottid. The further development is not possible inside the host body. The gravid proglottids detach from the body of the parasite and come out along with the host feces. These infect the secondary host when pig feeds upon the contaminated feces.

Cysticercus or Hydatid Larva or Bladder Worm Stage

The numerous hexacanths are set free in the stomach, where the embryonic membranes of onchospheres is dissolved. These bore through the intestinal wall the help of hooks and enter the blood stream or lymph vessels. Travelling through the heart, these enter the muscles of various parts in the body. The usual site where the hexacanths gey encysted is the voluntary muscles of tongue, heart, liver and shoulder.

Infection of Final Host

Further development of the bladder worm takes place only inside the definitive host. Infection of man occurs when inadequately cooked pork infected with bladder worms is eaten. The cysticerci become active in the intestine. The scolex takes a firm hold of intestinal wall of the host. The bladder is thrown off and the neck starts budding off segments an adult tapeworm is formed.

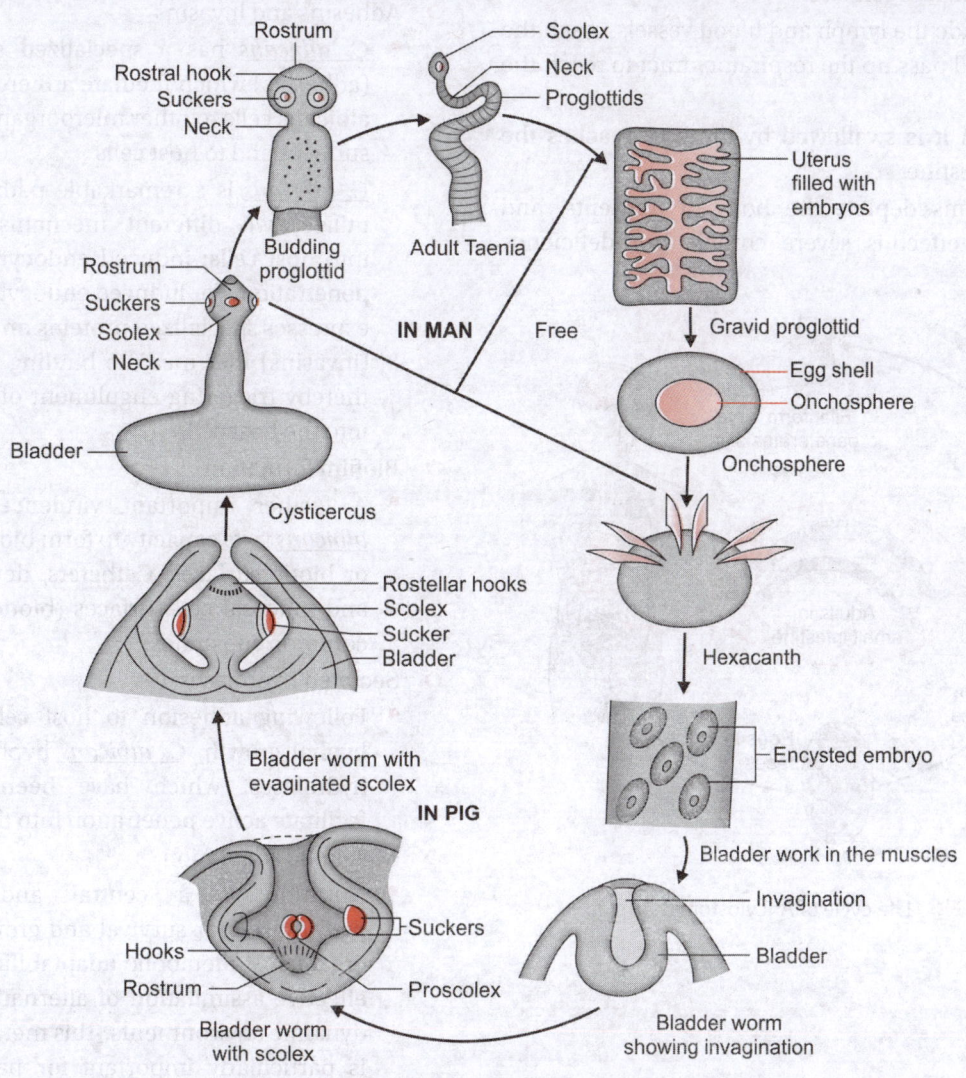

Fig. Life cycle of Taenia solium

b. Ancylostoma duodenale

(Ref: Arora parasitology 5th ed p 185)

ANSWER

- Hookworm infection begins when the worm is in the larval stage. The infective stage of hookworm is known as filariform larva. It penetrates the skin and migrates during its life cycle through the liver and the lungs, and it attaches to the mucosa of the small intestine.

- The larva matures into adult in the small intestine, where the female worms may produce several thousand eggs a day.

- The eggs are released into the feces and live on soil.

- Embryonated egg on soil hatch into juvenile 1 stage (rhabditiform or noninfective stage) and mature into filariform larvae. It starts a new reproductive cycle.

- The filariform larvae penetrate exposed skin of human host, usually that of the foot by the sweat glands and hair follicles.

- They invade the lymph and blood vessels, reach the lungs, and pass up the respiratory tract to reach the mouth.

- In mouth it is swallowed by the host reaches the small intestine.

- Hookworms deplete the body of nutrients, and a major effect is severe chronic iron-deficiency anemia.

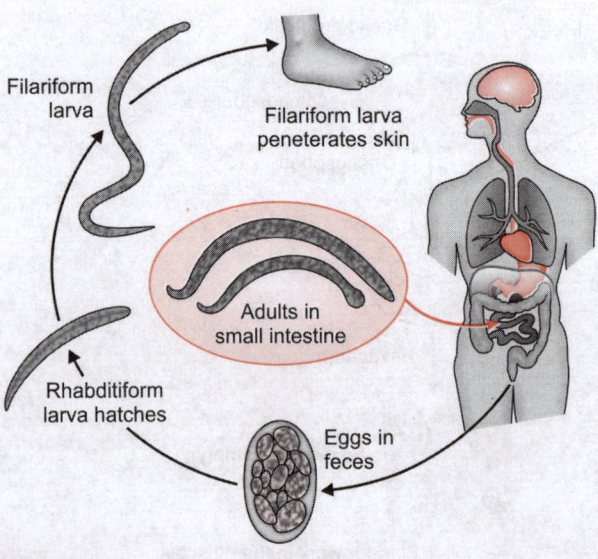

Fig. Life cycle of Ancylostoma

PART-II

3. Enumerate the yeasts causing human infections. Describe the pathogenicity of *Candida albicans*.

(Ref: Ananthanaryan & Paniker, Textbook of Microbiology,10th ed, pg. 615)

ANSWER

Yeasts Causing Human Infections

- Candida albicans
- Malassezia furfur

Pathogenicity of Candida Albicans

- Polymorphism
  - *C. albicans* is a polymorphic fungus that can grow either as ovoid-shaped budding yeast, as elongated ellipsoid cells with constrictions at the septa (pseudohyphae) or as parallel-walled true hyphae.

- Adhesins and invasins
  - *C. albicans* has a specialized set of proteins (adhesins) which mediate adherence to other C. albicans cells to other microorganisms, to abiotic surfaces and to host cells
  - *C. albicans* is a remarkable pathogen as it can utilize two different mechanisms to invade into host cells: induced endocytosis and active penetration. For induced endocytosis, the fungus expresses specialized proteins on the cell surface (invasins) that mediate binding to host ligands thereby triggering engulfment of the fungal cell into the host cell.

- Biofilm formation
  - A further important virulence factor of <u>C. albicans</u> is its capacity to form biofilms on abiotic or biotic surfaces. Catheters, dentures (abiotic) and mucosal cell surfaces (biotic) are the most common substrates.

- Secreted hydrolases
  - Following adhesion to host cell surfaces and hyphal growth, *C. albicans* hyphae can secrete hydrolases, which have been proposed to facilitate active penetration into these cells.

- Metabolic adaptation
  - Nutrition is a central and fundamental prerequisite for survival and growth of all living organisms. Metabolic adaptability mediates the effective assimilation of alternative nutrients in dynamic environments. This metabolic flexibility is particularly important for pathogenic fungi during infection of different host niches

○ Environmental stress response
  ▪ A robust stress response contributes to the survival and virulence of *C. albicans* by facilitating the adaptation of the fungus to changing conditions and protecting it against host-derived stresses.

4. Write briefly on:

a. Swine influenza

(Ref: Ananthanaryan & Paniker, Textbook of Microbiology, 10th ed, pg. 509)

ANSWER

○ Swine influenza is a highly contagious acute respiratory disease of pigs caused by one of the several strains of swine influenza A.

○ The virus is spread among pigs by aerosols, through direct and indirect contact, and also by asymptomatic carrier pigs.

○ In humans, the symptoms of swine flu are similar to those of influenza namely chills, fever, sore throat, muscle pains, severe headache, coughing, weakness, and general discomfort.

○ The influenza virus changes over time because of the imperfect replication by RNA polymerase and the propensity of antigenic shift and reassortment of viral RNA segments.

○ These genetic and antigenic changes are some of the most important factors affecting the epidemiology of swine influenza throughout the world

b. Human Herpes virus Type 4

ANSWER

(Ref: Ananthanaryan & Paniker, Textbook of Microbiology, 10th ed, pg. 570)

○ Epstein-Barr virus (EBV), also known as human herpes virus 4.

For answer, refer 2014 paper-II Q. 4 (a), Pg. 385

PART-III

5. Discuss the laboratory diagnosis and prophylaxis of rabies.

(Ref: Ananthanaryan & Paniker, Textbook of Microbiology, 10th ed, pg.536)

ANSWER

Laboratory Diagnosis of Rabies

Laboratory Diagnosis

○ **Histopathology:** Negri bodies are pathogenomonic of rabies. However, Negri bodies are only present in 71% of cases

○ **Rapid virus antigen detection:** In recent years, virus antigen detection by If had become widely used. Corneal impressions or neck skin biopsy are taken. The direct fluorescent antibody test (DFA) is commonly used.

○ **Virus cultivation:** The most definitive means of diagnosis is by virus cultivation from saliva sand infected tissue. Cell cultures may be used or more commonly, the specimen is inoculated intracerebrally into infant mice. Because of the difficulties involved, this is rarely offered by diagnostic laboratories

○ **Serology:** Circulating antibodies appear slowly in the course of infection but they are usually present by the time of onset of clinical symptoms

Prophylaxis of Rabies

For answer, refer 2017 paper-II Q. 6, Pg. 351

6. Describe the strategies of HIV testing as per NACO guidelines

(Ref: Ananthanaryan & Paniker, Textbook of Microbiology, 10th ed, pg. 583)

ANSWER

Strategy I

○ Used to screen blood/blood products
○ Sample is reported subjected once to E/R for HIV
○ NACO recommends use of ELISA kits with a sensitivity of >99.5% and specificity of >98%

Strategy IIA

○ Used for surveillance (2A) and diagnosis (2B) if AIDS indicator disease is present.
○ If a serum sample is positive in first ELISA, another ELISA is performed. If the result in second ELISA is positive, then it is considered positive, otherwise test results are considered negative.

Strategy IIB

- Used to determine the HIV status of clinically symptomatic suspected AIDS cases in which blood/serum/plasma is tested with highly sensitive screening and confirmatory tests based on different principles or antigens as compared to first test.

Strategy 3

- Used in asymptomatic individuals
- Similar to strategy 2, with an additional third positive ELISA test being required for a sample to be reported HIV reactive

Summaries Table

Strategies	Samples
Strategy-I	To screen blood, blood products, organ, tissue and sperms
Strategy-IIA	For surveillance
Strategy-IIB	For diagnosis to determine the HIV status of clinically symptomatic suspected AIDS patients
Strategy-III	For diagnosis in asymptomatic individuals

Name of the Paper	:	**Microbiology Paper-I**
Name of the Course	:	**MBBS-2012**
Semester	:	**Annual**

Time: 3 Hours   **M.M.: 40**

INSTRUCTIONS

1. Write your Roll No. on the top immediately on receipt of this question paper
2. All questions are to be attempted
3. Answers to Parts I, II and III should be written in separate answer sheets provided
4. Attempt parts of a question in sequence

PART-I

1. Enumerate the various methods of gene transfer in bacteria and discuss any one method in detail.   [5]

2. Write short notes on   [10]
   a. Biological effects of complement activation
   b. Principle and uses of ELISA

PART-II

3. Enumerate agents causing gas gangrene. Describe the laboratory diagnosis of gas gangrene.   [5]

4. Write briefly on: [10]
   a. Mycoplasma pneumonia
   b. Typhoid vaccine

PART-III

5. Enumerate the bacterial causes of community acquired pneumonia and describe its laboratory diagnosis.   [5]

6. What are hospital associated infections? What is the role of a microbiologist in their control?   [5]

PART-I

1. Enumerate the various methods of gene transfer in bacteria and discuss any one method in detail.

ANSWER

○ Bacterial reproduction is by the asexual process of binary fission. With the exception of a de novo mutation, the resultant daughter cells are genetically identical to the parent cell. This lends itself to the question, "How then have bacteria undergone genetic variation resulting in the different virulence factors and antibiotic resistances?"

○ Three mechanisms have been observed to transfer novel genetic material into bacteria: Transformation, conjugation, and transduction.

▪ **Conjugation:** Transfer of genes between cells that are in physical contact with one another

▪ **Transduction:** Transfer of genes from one cell to another by a bacteriophage

▪ **Transformation:** Transfer of cell-free or "naked" DNA from one cell to another

○ Upon reception of the new genes, the genetic material must be stabilized either by reformation of a plasmid or by recombination. Linear DNA is always stabilized by homologous recombination.

○ Occasionally, a plasmid will be an episome and integrate into the bacterial chromosome by the process of site-specific recombination

Transformation

○ Transformation is the uptake of naked (free) DNA from the environment by competent cells.

○ Cells become competent (able to bind short pieces of DNA to the envelope and import them into the cell) under certain environmental conditions (which you do not need to know).

○ Some bacteria are capable of natural transformation (they are naturally competent): Haemophilus influenzae, Streptococcus pneumoniae, Bacillus species, and Neisseria species.

○ DNA (released from dead cells) is taken up

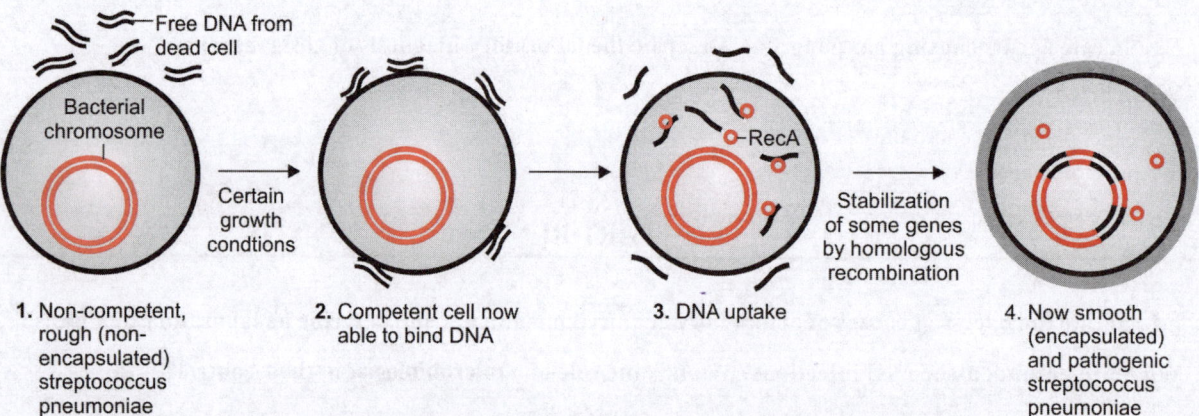

Fig. Transformation of a Non-encapsulated Streptococcus pneumoniae

○ Newly introduced DNA is generally linear, homologous DNA; a similar type of cell but perhaps one that is genetically diverse.

○ The linear DNA is then stabilized by homologous recombination.

Conjugation

○ Conjugation was the first extensively studied method of gene transfer

○ Conjugation requires donor cell-to-recipient cell contact and is mediated by sex pilus

○ Process occurs between two living cells

○ Requires mobilization of donor bacterium's chromosome/plasmid

○ Plasmid are genetic elements most frequently transferred by conjugation

Transformation

○ Phage mediated genetic recombination in bacteria i.e. phage is used to transfer DNA from one bacterium to another

- Transducing particle: Bacterial nucleic acid in phage coat
- There are two broad categories of Transduction
  - Generalized transduction: Where virtually any genetic marker can be transferred
  - Specialized transduction: Bacterial DNA who are adjacent to viral DNA in the prophage get transferred
- For artificial Genetic recombination purpose Temperate phage are preferred vehicle for gene transfer
- Transduction has been found to occur in a variety of bacterial populations including:
  - *Escherichia coli*
  - Pseudomonas spp
  - Salmonella spp
  - Staphylococcus spp

2. Write short notes on:

a. Biological effects of complement activation

(Ref: Ananthanaryan & Paniker, Textbook of Microbiology,10th ed, pg. 123)

ANSWER

Biological Effects of Complement Activation

Activity	Components and fragments
Increase of vascular permeability Smooth muscle contraction Degranulation of mast cells and basophils	C5a, C3a, C5 C4a
Neutrophil activation and chemotaxis Stimulation of prostaglandin and leukotriene production	C5a, C5
Opsonization of bacteria and immune complexes leading to phagocytosis	C3b, C4b
Stimulation of the respiratory burst of professional phagocytes	C3b, C5a, C5, C1q
Lysis of bacteria and foreign cells	C5b678 (9)n
Solubilization of circulating immune complexes	C3b, CR1

- **Cell lysis:** The most important purpose of complement activation is to lyse the microbes that have entered into the host. Complement activation leads to the lysis of bacterial, viral, fungal, protozoal, and many other cells through the membrane attack complexes. However, cells such as cancer cells are more resistant to complement mediated lysis.
- **Inflammation:** During complement activation, some of the complement components are split into complement fragments. In general, the larger fragments

continue the complement cascade, while the smaller fragments play important roles in inflammation.

- The binding of antibodies to antigens results in the formation of antigen-antibody complexes or immune complexes. In certain autoimmune diseases and certain microbial infections large amounts of immune complexes are formed.
- Complement fragments play an important role in the development of secondary B cell immune responses against antigens.

b. Principle and uses of ELISA

(Ref: Ananthanaryan & Paniker, Textbook of Microbiology,10th ed, pg.349)

ANSWER

- ELISA is a plate based assay technique which is used for detecting and quantifying substances such as peptides, proteins, antibodies and hormones.
- An enzyme conjugated with an antibody reacts with colorless substrate to generate a colored product. Such substrate is called chromogenic substrate.
- A number of enzymes have been used for ELISA such as alkaline phosphatase, horse radish peroxidase and beta galactosidase.
- Specific substrate such as ortho-phenylenediamine dihydrochloride (for peroxidase), paranitrophenyl phosphate (for alkaline phosphatase) are used which are hydrolyzed by above enzymes to give colored end product.

Principle

- ELISAs are typically performed in 96-well polystyrene plates.
- The serum is incubated in a well, and each well contains a different serum.
- A positive control serum and a negative control serum would be included among the 96 samples being tested.
- Antibodies or antigens present in serum are captured by corresponding antigen or antibody coated on to the solid surface.
- After some time, the plate is washed to remove serum and unbound antibodies or antigens with a series of wash buffer.
- To detect the bound antibodies or antigens, a secondary antibodies that are attached to an enzyme such as peroxidase or alkaline phosphatase are added to each well.
- After an incubation period, the unbound secondary antibodies are washed off.

○ When a suitable substrate is added, the enzyme reacts with it to produce a color.

○ This color produced is measurable as a function or quantity of antigens or antibodies present in the given sample.

○ The intensity of color/optical density is measured at 450 nm. The intensity of the color gives an indication of the amount of antigen or antibody.

Applications of ELISA

○ Serum antibody concentration

○ Detecting potential food allergens
  ▪ (Milk, peanuts, walnuts, almonds and eggs)

○ Disease outbreaks-tracking the spread of disease
  ▪ e.g. HIV, bird flu, common, colds, cholera, sexually transmitted diseases etc.

○ Detections of antigens
  ▪ e.g. pregnancy hormones, drug allergen, GMO, mad cow disease

○ Detection of antibodies in blood sample for past exposure to disease
  ▪ e.g. Lyme disease, trichinosis, HIV, bird flu

PART-II

3. Enumerate agents causing gas gangrene. Describe the laboratory diagnosis of gas gangrene.

(Ref: Ananthanaryan & Paniker, Textbook of Microbiology, 10th ed, pg. 258)

ANSWER

Gas gangrene is a bacterial infection that produces *gas* in tissues in *gangrene*. This deadly form of *gangrene* usually is caused by Clostridium perfringens bacteria. It is a medical emergency

Agents Causing Gas Gangrene

○ *Clostridium perfringens*
○ *Group A streptococcus*
○ *Staphylococcus aureus*
○ *Vibrio vulnificus.*

Laboratory Diagnosis

○ **Specimens:** Wound swab, discharge and affected tissue

○ **Direct smear:** Shows rectangular gram positive bacilli; spores are usually not seen

○ **Culture:** Specimen are inoculated into cooked meat media as well as in a blood agar media and the latter is incubated anaerobically for 48–72 hours. In blood agar medium there is hemolysis around the colony. The bacterial culture is used for Nagler reaction and biochemical tests.

○ **Animal pathogenicity:** For demonstration of toxigenicity of the strain, 0.1 mL of 24 hours culture of the bacteria in cooked meat broth is injected intramuscularly on the right thigh of a healthy guinea pig. Animal dies within 24 hours. A control animal prior to test is to be included. On autopsy, the injected limb shows swelling with crepitation and the muscles appear pink. Bacteria can be recovered from heart and spleen of the animal.

4. Write briefly on:

a. Mycoplasma pneumonia

(Ref: Ananthanaryan & Paniker, Textbook of Microbiology, 10th ed, pg. 393)

ANSWER

○ Mycoplasma pneumonia is a common respiratory pathogen that produces diseases of varied severity ranging from mild upper respiratory tract infection to severe atypical pneumonia.

○ Although rarely fatal, *M. pneumoniae* is an important cause of acute respiratory tract infection, especially as a potential etiology of the clinical entity termed "atypical pneumonia".

○ Of the many species of Mycoplasma known to infect man, *M. pneumoniae* is an important cause of respiratory tract infections.

○ Apart from respiratory tract infections, this organism is also responsible for producing a wide spectrum of non- pulmonary manifestations including neurological, hepatic, cardiac diseases, hemolytic anemia, polyarthritis and erythema multiform.

○ Of the non-pulmonary manifestation, neurological manifestations are thought to be the most common.

○ The absence of cell wall structure makes these organisms insensitive to beta-lactam antimicrobial agents, prevents them from staining by gram's stain, and is largely responsible for their polymorphism.

○ Mycoplasmas are more closely related to gram positive bacteria.

b. Typhoid vaccine

(Ref: Ananthanaryan & Paniker, Textbook of Microbiology, 10th ed, pg. 646)

ANSWER

Several typhoid vaccines are currently available and these can be administered orally or parenterally and are safe and efficacious for preventing typhoid fever

○ **Live attenuated vaccine:** (Ty21a) This vaccine was developed in the early 1970s, requires at least three doses for optimal protection, and is supplied as gelatin capsules coated with phthalate or sachets containing lyophilised Ty21a, a mutant strain of Salmonella enterica serovar Typhi (S. typhi).

○ **Parenteral vaccines**

- **Monovalent typhoid vaccines:** Vi polysaccharide is a well-standardized antigen that is effective in a single parenteral dose, is safer than whole-cell vaccine, and may be used in children 2 years of age or older. The following vaccines contain the Vi antigen.

  ◆ **Capsular polysaccharide vaccines:** Is a one-dose injectable solution consisting 25 μg Vi antigen prepared from the surface polysaccharide of S. typhi strain Ty2.

  ◆ **Conjugate vaccine:** (Vi-TT), where the Vi antigen is coupled to a carrier protein. there is only one licensed conjugate vaccine (Peda-typhTM, BioMed). It consists of Vi coupled to tetanus toxoid (TT). This vaccine has been licensed only in India and only limited clinical data are available to document its safety and immunogenicity. Multiple other conjugates are in development consisting of Vi linked to tetanus toxoid or to other carrier proteins.

  Multivalent combination vaccines: Combined ViCPS and hepatitis A vaccines contain 25 μg Vi polysaccharide antigen of S. typhi combined with either 1440 EL.U. or 160 AU of inactivated hepatitis A virus grown in human diploid cells and adsorbed onto aluminium hydroxide.

PART-III

---

5. **Enumerate the bacterial causes of community acquired pneumonia and describe its laboratory diagnosis**

(Ref: Ananthanaryan & Paniker, Textbook of Microbiology, 10th ed, pg. 321)

ANSWER

Bacterial Causes of CAP

○ *Streptococcus pneumoniae,*
○ *Haemophilus influenzae,*
○ *Moraxella catarrhalis*

Laboratory Diagnosis of CAP

○ Diagnostic testing other than CBC and metabolic profiles rarely affects therapy for CAP, except in cases of severe CAP requiring hospitalization

- Most patients are treated empirically without having etiology identified

- **CBC:** Leukocytosis with left shift suggests bacterial etiology

- **Complete metabolic and electrolyte profile:** Use only in patients >55 years or with suspected toxicity

- **Urine antigen tests for Legionella and pneumococcus:** Available and recommended in select situations

- Nasal screening

  ◆ High specificity and negative predictive value for methicillin-resistant *Staphylococcus aureus* (MRSA)

  ◆ Consider in antimicrobial decision-making for CAP and healthcare-associated pneumonia

Imaging Studies

○ **Chest X-ray:** Gold standard for confirmation of pneumonia

- **Single or several lobe patterns:** Bacterial

- **Diffuse or interstitial pattern:** Viral or atypical organism

- **Cavitary:** More common in gram negative, fungi, acid-fast bacilli

- **Miliary:** Acid-fast bacilli, fungi, atypical pneumonia agents

○ **Computed tomography (CT):** Better imaging approach for small pneumonias; however, cost, radiation exposure, and time contraindicate its use for most patients

---

6. **What are hospital associated infections? What is the role of a microbiologist in their control.**

(Ref: Ananthanaryan & Paniker, Textbook of Microbiology, 10th ed, pg. 648)

ANSWER

Those infections which were not present in a person at the time of admission to a hospital but are acquired during a stay in a hospital are considered as hospital-acquired infections (HAIs).

Role of Microbiologist

○ Specimen Collection

- Educate on proper specimen collection and transport

- Sputum versus spit (oropharyngeal flora)

- Monitor specimen quality

  ◆ Sputum gram stains

- Reject improper specimens

- Sputums with > 25 squamous epithelial cells, low PMNs, oropharyngeal flora

- Accurate Identification of Healthcare-Associated Pathogens
- Identify causative organisms rapidly and accurately to species level.
- Accurate Identification of Pathogens
  - Educated and well trained personnel
  - Automated systems
    - Know the limitations of each system
    - Good for Identification of aerobic gram positive and gram-negative bacteria, not good for many nonfermentative gram-negatives
- Molecular testing
  - Live versus dead
  - Cross-reactivity
- Identify causative organisms rapidly and accurately to species level.

- Susceptibility Testing of Healthcare-Associated Pathogens
- Perform accurate susceptibility testing
  - Survey for MDR organisms
  - Detect unexpected antimicrobial resistance
- Participates as a member of the infection control committee
  - Provides expertise in the interpretation of culture results
  - Advice about the appropriateness and feasibility of microbiological approaches
  - Input regarding the laboratory resources necessary to accomplish the goals of the committee
  - Inform the committee of the strengths and limitations of methods employed to detect and characterize HAI pathogens

Your Roll No. ....

Name of the Paper	:	**Microbiology Paper-II**
Name of the Course	:	**MBBS-2012**
Semester	:	**Annual**

Time: 3 Hours   M.M.: 40

INSTRUCTIONS

1. Write your Roll No. on the top immediately on receipt of this question paper
2. All questions are to be attempted
3. Answers to Parts I, II and III should be written in separate answer sheets provided
4. Attempt parts of a question in sequence

PART-I

1. **Describe life cycle of Balantidium coli.**   [5]

2. **Write short notes on**   [10]
   a. Fungi causing oculomycosis
   b. Enterobius vermicularis

PART-II

3. **Write briefly on nongonococcal urethritis.**   [5]

4. **Write briefly on:**   [10]
   a. Coxsackie viruses
   b. Differences between Salk and Sabin vaccines

PART-III

5. **Describe pathogenesis and complications of Measles.**   [5]

6. **Write a note on larval forms of Diphyllobothrium latum.**   [5]

PART-I

1. Describe life cycle of Balantidium coli.

ANSWER

- *Balantidium coli* is an intestinal protozoan parasite. It is the protozoan parasite of humans. It is a species of ciliate protozoan.

- Ciliates have 2 nuclei, a macronuclei and a micronuclei. The macronucleus is a long, kidney-shaped structure while the micronucleus is spherical. The micronucleus is usually next to the macronucleus.

- *Balantidium* coli is the only known ciliated parasite that is infectious to humans. **Balantidium** coli has two contractile vacuoles.

- Balantidium coli has two developmental stages called the trophozoite stage (reproductive stage) and the cyst stage (infectious stage).

- In the trophozoite stage, Balantidium coli can measure between 50-130 µm long by 20-70 µm wide. When observing Balantidium coli unstained, it has a short ciliary covering and has spiraling motility.

- The two nuclei of *Balantidium coli* are clearly visible in this stage when the specimens are stained. The peristome, which is an opening at the anterior end of cell, is also visible. The peristome leads to the cytostome (cell mouth).

- *Balantidium* coli reproduces either by asexual transverse binary fission or sexual conjugation. In asexual transverse binary fission the bacteria grows in volume until it divides in half to make two identical daughter cells. This is how most bacteria typically grow. In sexual conjugation, a transfer of genetic material between bacteria through direct cell-to-cell contact happens. During sexual conjugation in bacteria is not an equal exchange of genetic material.

- There is usually a donor and a recipient. The motile trophozoite lives in the lumen of the large intestine. It feeds on intestinal bacterial flora and nutrients. The trophozoite can invade into the mucosa of the large intestine by penetrating through it. The trophozoites are released in the host's feces and this is when the cyst stage (infectious stage) begins

- The cyst stage begins right when the trophozoite is released in feces. Encystation begins. Encystation is the process of becoming enclosed in a cyst. This process takes place in the rectum.

- This is done by Balantidium coli as a survival technique. After the release of trophozoites in the feces the feces starts to dehydrates right away.

- Cysts can be spherical of ellipsoid and range from 50-70 µm long, 40-60 µm across, which makes it smaller than trophozoites.

- When a stool sample if first observed, the cysts may still have cilia, but after encystation the cilia disappear. The macronucleus and the micronucleus can still be seen in stained specimens.

- Because cysts exists in fecal matter, this is when contamination comes into play. Feces can contaminate water or food. Once the contaminated food or water has entered the host's digestive system, cysts can start infecting.

- Cysts can have cyst walls made of one or two layers, which make them tough and heavy. This allows them to pass through the digestive system without being destroyed.

- Once in the large intestine excystation occurs. This is when trophozoites are produced from cysts. Cysts multiply by transverse binary fission.

2. Write short notes on:

a. Fungi causing oculomycosis

ANSWER

Oculomycosis is a type of fungal eye infection. Eye infections can be caused by many different irritants, including bacteria, viruses, amoeba, and fungi. Eye infections caused by fungi are extremely rare, but they can be very serious. Fungal infections can affect different parts of the eye.

There are two primary types of oculomycosis:

- **Keratitis:** This is an infection of the clear, front layer of the eye (the cornea).

- **Endophthalmitis:** This is an infection of the inside of the eye (the vitreous and/or aqueous humor). There are two types of endophthalmitis: exogenous and endogenous. Exogenous fungal endophthalmitis occurs after fungal spores enter the eye from an external source. Endogenous endophthalmitis occurs when a bloodstream infection (for example, candidemia) spreads to one or both eyes.

It is believed that many of different types of fungi can cause eye infections. Common types include:

- **Fusarium:** A fungus that lives in the environment, especially in soil and on plants.
- **Aspergillus:** A common fungus that lives in indoor and outdoor environments
- **Candida:** A type of yeast that normally lives on human skin and on the protective lining inside the body called the mucous membrane.

b. Enterobius vermicularis

ANSWER

- The worms are small, white, and threads like, with the larger females ranging between 8 and 13 mm x 0.3 and 0.5 mm and the smaller males ranging between 2 and 5 mm x 0.1 and 0.2 mm. Females also possess a long, pin-shaped posterior end from which the parasite's name is derived. They dwell primarily in the cecum of the large intestine, from where the gravid females migrate at night to lay up to 15,000 eggs on the perineum.
- Pinworm eggs are flattened asymmetrically on one side, ovoid, approximately 55 x 25 mm in size, and embryonate in six hours. These eggs can remain viable for about twenty days in a moist environment, and viable eggs and larvae were even found in the sludge of sewage treatment plants in Czechoslovakia in 1992.

Life Cycle

- Eggs are deposited at night by the gravid females.
- Eggs are ingested via person-to-person transmission through the handling of contaminated surfaces (such as clothing, linen, curtains, and carpeting), or airborne eggs may be inhaled and swallowed. Self-infection may also occur if eggs are transferred from to the mouth by fingers that have scratched the perianal area.
- After ingestion, larvae hatch from the eggs in the small intestine. The adults then migrate to the colon. The life span of the adults is about two months. Adults mate in the colon, and the males die after mating.
- Gravid females migrate nocturnally to the anus and ovideposit eggs in the perianal area. The females die after laying their eggs. The time period from ingestion of infective eggs to the oviposition of eggs by females is approximately one month.
- The larvae develop and the eggs become infection within 4–6 hours. Newly hatched larvae may also migrate back into the anus, and this is known as retroinfection.

PART-II

3. Write briefly on non gonococcal urethritis.

(Ref: Ananthanaryan & Paniker, Textbook of Microbiology, 10th ed, pg. 260)

ANSWER

NGU (nongonococcal urethritis) is an infection of the urethra caused by pathogens (germs) other than gonorrhea. Several kinds of pathogens can cause NGU, including:

- *Chlamydia trachomatis*
- *Ureaplasma urealyticum*
- *Trichomonas vaginalis (rare)*
- *Herpes simplex virus (rare)*
- *Adenovirus*
- *Haemophilus vaginalis*
- *Mycoplasm genitalium*

NGU is most often caused by chlamydia, a common infection in men and women. The diagnosis of NGU is more commonly made in men than women, primarily due to anatomical differences.

Symptoms

Men (Urethral Infection)

- Discharge from the penis
- Burning or pain when urinating (peeing)
- Itching, irritation, or tenderness
- Underwear stain

Women (Vaginal/Urethral Infection)

The germs that cause NGU in men might cause other infections in women. These might include vaginitis or mucopurulent cervicitis (MPC). Women may also be asymptomatic (have no symptoms).

Symptoms of NGU in women can include:

- Discharge from the vagina
- Burning or pain when urinating (peeing)
- Abdominal pain or abnormal vaginal bleeding may be an indication that the infection has progressed to pelvic inflammatory disease (PID)

4. Write briefly on:

(Ref: Ananthanaryan & Paniker, Textbook of Microbiology, 10th ed, pg. 497)

a. Coxsackie Viruses

ANSWER

- Coxsackie virus is a member of the Picornaviridae family of viruses in the genus termed Enterovirus.

- Coxsackie viruses are subtype members of Enterovirus that have a single strand of ribonucleic acid (RNA) for its genetic material.
- The enteroviruses are also referred to as picorna viruses (pico means "small," so "small RNA viruses")
- Coxsackie viruses are separable into two groups, A (CVA) and B (CVB), which are based on their effects on newborn mice (coxsackie virus A results in muscle injury, paralysis, and death; coxsackie virus B results in organ damage but less severe outcomes.)
- There are over 24 different serotypes of the virus (having distinct proteins on the viral surface). Coxsackie viruses infect host cells and cause host cells to break open (lyse).

b. Differences between Salk and Sabin vaccines

ANSWER

Salk versus Sabin vaccine

IPV (Salk)	OPV (Sabin)
Killed formolised virus	Live attenuated virus
Given SC or IM	Given orally
Induces circulating antibodies, but not local (Intestinal immunity)	Immunity is both humoral and intestinal. Induces antibody quickly
Prevents paralysis but does not prevent re-infection	Prevents paralysis and prevents reinfection
Not useful in controlling epidemics	Can be effectively used in controlling epidemics
More difficult to manufacture & is relatively costly	Easy to manufacture and is cheaper
Does not require stringent conditions during storage transportation. Has a longer shelf life	Requires to be stored & transported at subzero temperatures, & is damaged easily

PART-III

5. Describe pathogenesis and complications of Measles.

(Ref: Ananthanaryan & Paniker, Textbook of Microbiology, 10th ed, pg.518)

ANSWER

Pathogenesis

- In temperate areas, the peak incidence of infection occurs during late winter and spring. Infection is transmitted via respiratory droplets, which can remain active and contagious, either airborne or on surfaces, for up to 2 hours. Initial infection and viral replication occur locally in tracheal and bronchial epithelial cells.

- After 2–4 days, measles virus infects local lymphatic tissues, perhaps carried by pulmonary macrophages. Following the amplification of measles virus in regional lymph nodes, a predominantly cell-associated viremia disseminates the virus to various organs prior to the appearance of rash.

- Measles virus infection causes a generalized immunosuppression marked by decreases in delayed-type hypersensitivity, interleukin (IL)-12 production, and antigen-specific lymphoproliferative responses that persist for weeks to months after the acute infection. Immunosuppression may predispose individuals to secondary opportunistic infections particularly bronchopneumonia, a major cause of measles-related mortality among younger children.

- In individuals with deficiencies in cellular immunity, measles virus causes a progressive and often fatal giant cell pneumonia.

- In immunocompetent individuals, wild-type measles virus infection induces an effective immune response, which clears the virus and results in lifelong immunity.

Complications

Common infectious complications include otitis media, interstitial pneumonitis, bronchopneumonia, laryngotracheobronchitis (ie, croup), exacerbation of tuberculosis, transient loss of hypersensitivity reaction to tuberculin skin test, encephalomyelitis, diarrhea, sinusitis, stomatitis, subclinical hepatitis, lymphadenitis, and keratitis, which can lead to blindness. In fact, measles remains a common cause of blindness in many developing countries.

Summary Table

- **Description:** Exists in one serotype.
- **Components:** Has hemagglutinin, but no neuraminidase activity (H protein rather than HN protein).
- **Pathobiology:** Uses the CD46 molecules as its cellular receptor.
- **Replication:** Frequently forms giant multinucleated cells (syncytia) as part of its replication process (called Warthin-Finkeldey cells in nasal secretions).
- **Clinical disease:** Causes an acute generalized disease characterized by a maculopapular rash, fever, respiratory distress, and Koplik's spots on the buccal mucosa.
- **Prevention:** Infections can be prevented by a live attenuated measles vaccine (Moraten strain) that is part of the trivalent (measles, mumps, and rubella) vaccine given to children.

6. Write a note on larval forms of Diphyllobothrium latum.

ANSWER

The eggs mature in water within three weeks and form oncospheres. Larvae called coracidia hatch and get eaten by freshwater crustaceans such as copepod. After ingestion coracidia develop into procercoid larvae. If the copepod is eaten by a small fish (second intermediate host), the procercoid larvae penetrate the gut and migrate to muscle tissue where they develop into plerocercoid larvae (sparganum), the infective stage for humans. Usually a third intermediate host is needed because humans do not usually eat raw fish this small. If a trout, walleyed pike or perch eats the smaller fish, the plerocercoid larvae once again penetrate the gut and migrate to fish flesh. If a human eats the infected fish raw or undercooked the plerocercoid larvae develop into adults in the small intestine.

Your Roll No. ....

Name of the Paper : **Microbiology Paper-I**

Name of the Course : **MBBS-2011**

Semester : **Annual**

Time: 3 Hours   M.M.: 40

INSTRUCTIONS

1. Write your Roll No. on the top immediately on receipt of this question paper
2. All questions are to be attempted
3. Answers to Parts I, II and III should be written in separate answer sheets provided
4. Attempt parts of a question in sequence

PART-I

1. Describe the virulence factors of bacteria and differentiate between exotoxins and endotoxins.   [5]

2. Write short notes on: [10]
   a. Coagglutination
   b. Type III hypersensitivity reaction

PART-II

3. Tabulate various rickettsial diseases of man along with their causative agent and vector responsible of transmission of the disease.   [5]

4. Write briefly on: [10]
   a. Enterococcus
   b. Helicobacter pylori

PART-III

5. Enumerate the bacterial causes of meningitis and outline the laboratory diagnosis of acute pyogenic meningitis.   [5]

6. Name various bacterial agents causing water-borne diseases. Describe briefly about bacterial examination of water.   [5]

PART-I

1. **Describe the virulence factors of bacteria and differentiate between exotoxins and endotoxins.**

(Ref: Ananthanaryan & Paniker, Textbook of Microbiology, 10th ed, pg.258)

ANSWER

Virulence Factors of Bacteria

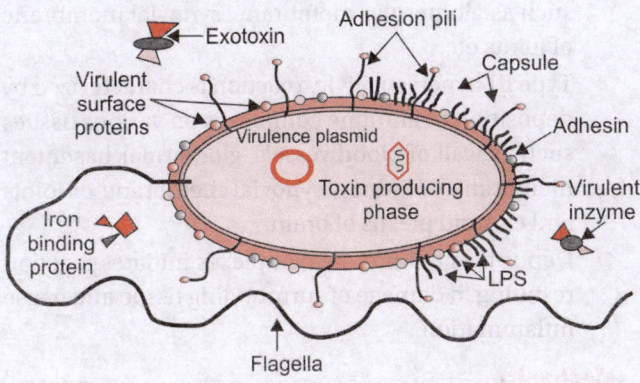

Fig. Virulence factors of bacteria LPS, lipopolysaccharides

Virulence Factors

○ **Virulence factors help bacteria to:**
- Invade the host
- Cause disease
- Evade host defenses.

The following are types of virulence factors:

- **Adherence factors:** Many pathogenic bacteria colonize mucosal sites by using pili (fimbriae) to adhere to cells.
- **Invasion factors:** Surface components that allow the bacterium to invade host cells can be encoded on plasmids, but more often are on the chromosome.
- **Capsules:** Many bacteria are surrounded by capsules that protect them from opsonization and phagocytosis.
- **Endotoxins:** The lipopolysaccharide endotoxins on Gram-negative bacteria cause fever, changes in blood pressure, inflammation, lethal shock, and many other toxic events.
- **Exotoxins:** Exotoxins include several types of protein toxins and enzymes produced and/ or secreted from pathogenic bacteria. Major categories include cytotoxins, neurotoxins, and enterotoxins.
- **Siderophores:** Siderophores are iron-binding factors that allow some bacteria to compete with the host for iron, which is bound to hemoglobin, transferrin, and lactoferrin.

Differences Between Exotoxins and Endotoxins

Property	Exotoxin	Endotoxin
Bacterial Source	Mostly from gram-positive bacteria	Gram-negative bacteria
Relation to Microorganism	Metabolic product of growing cell	Present i LPS of outer membrane of cell wall and released with destruction of cell or during cell division
Chemistry	Proteins, usually with two parts (A-B)	Lipid portion (lipid A) of LPS of outer membrane (lipopolysaccharide)
Pharmacology (Effect on Body)	Specific for a particular cell structure or function in the host (mainly affects cell functions, nerves, nerves, and gastrointestinal tract)	General, such as fever, weakness, aches, and shock; all produce the same effects
Heat stability	**Unstable:** Can usually be destroyed at 60–80°C	**Stable:** Can withstand autoclaving (121°C for 1 hour)
Toxicity (Ability to Cause Disease)	High	Low

Property	Exotoxin	Endotoxin
Fever-Producing	No	Yes
Immunology (Relation to Antibodies)	Can be converted to toxoids to immunize against toxin; neutralized by antitoxin	Not easily neutralized by antitoxin; therefore, effective toxoids cannot be made to immunize against toxin
Lethal Dose	Small	Considerably larger
Representative Diseases	Gas gangrene, tetanus, botulism, diphtheria, scarlet fever	Typhoid fever, urinary tract infections, and meningococcal meningitis

2. Write short notes on:

a. Coagglutination

ANSWER

○ It another type of Passive agglutination test, where staphylococcus aureus act as carrier molecule.

○ Some strains of S. aureus (Cowan 1strain) possess protein A on the surface, which has a property of binding to Fc portion of any IgG molecule (except IgG3) making the Fab portion free, which can agglutination with the corresponding antigen present in the clinical sample

○

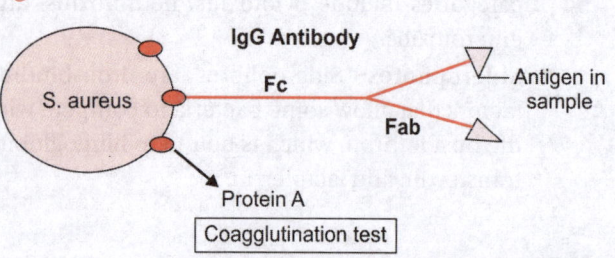

Fig. Coagglutination test

b. Type III hypersensitivity reaction

(Ref: Ananthanaryan & Paniker, Textbook of Microbiology,10th ed, pg.163)

ANSWER

○ The reaction of antibody with antigen generates immune complex. In most of the cases, these immune complexes are removed from blood circulation. Some immune complexes are removed by phagocytic action of phagocytic cells in blood. Most other immune complexes are first carried by blood to spleen where they are destroyed by macrophages. Complement system is also needed for removal of immune complexes from blood to spleen.

○ In some cases large amount of immune complexes are formed and deposited on various body parts and leads to tissue damage resulting in Type III hypersensitivity reaction.

○ If immune complexes are not removed from blood, they accumulate on wall of blood vessels and on tissue where filtration of blood and plasma occurs such as glomerular membrane, synovial membrane of joints etc.

○ Type III hypersensitivity reaction is characterized by deposition of immune complexes on various tissues such as wall of blood vessels, glomerular basement membrane of kidney, synovial membrane of joints and choroid plexus of brain.

○ Deposition of immune complexes initiates reaction resulting in damage of surrounding tissue and cause inflammation.

Mechanism

○ Type III hypersensitivity reaction develops when immune complex activates C3a and C5a components of complement system.

○ C3a and C5a are lymphotoxin (anaphylotoxin) that causes localized mast cell degranulation.

○ Degranulation of mast cell releases histamine which increases vascular permeability of blood capillaries. This facilitates deposition of immune complexes on wall of blood vessel.

○ C5a, C3a and C5b67 also act as chemotactic factors for neutrophils, So it attracts neutrophils at the site of immune complex deposition.

○ C3b acts as opsonin by binding with immune complex. Neutrophil binds to C3b coated immune complex by means of type I complement receptor which is specific for C3b.

○ The neutrophils attempt to phagocytose the immune complex but phagocytosis is not possible because immune complexes are deposited on basement membrane, so the neutrophil releases lytic enzymes to destroy immune complex.

○ The lytic enzymes cause tissue damage surrounding of immune complex deposits, resulting hypersensitivity reaction. Furthermore complement proteins can also contribute to tissue destruction.

PART-II

3. **Tabulate various rickettsial diseases of man along with their causative agent and vector responsible of transmission of the disease.**

(Ref: Ananthanaryan & Paniker, Textbook of Microbiology, 10th ed, pg.412)

ANSWER

Organism	Disease	Arthropod vector	Vertebrate reservoir
Spotted fevers[c]			
R. rickettsii	Rocky Mountain spotted fever	Tick[a]	Dogs, rodents
R. akari	Rickettsial/pox	Mite[a]	Mice
R. conorii	Mediterranean spotted fever	Tick	Dogs
Typhus			
R. prowazekii	Epidemic typhus	Louse	Human[b]
R. typhi	Endemic typhus	Flea	Rodents
Orientia tsutsugamushi	Scrub typhus	Mite[a]	Rodents
Other			
Coxiella burnetii	Q fever	None	Sheep, goats, Cattle
Bartonella quintana	Trench fever	Louse	Human
Ehrlichia chaffeensis[c]	Fever (ehrlichiosis)	Tick	?

[a]Vertically transmitted in arthropod
[b]Non-human vertebrates are possibly also involved
[c]Other rickettsiae cause similar tick-borne fevers in Africa, India, Australia

4. **Write briefly on:**

a. Enterococcus

(Ref: Ananthanaryan & Paniker, Textbook of Microbiology, 10th ed, pg.219)

ANSWER

- Enterococci are ubiquitous Gram-positive cocci, catalase-negative, non-spore-forming, facultative anaerobic organisms, that belong to the Lancefield group D streptococci.
- Enterococci are normally present, as colonizers, in the intestinal tract of human beings and animals, and can be recovered from feces in large quantities.
- Enterococci may occasionally reside in the vagina and oral cavity. They also may be found in food and water.
- The two predominant enterococcal species in humans are *E. faecalis* and *E. faecium*, while other species are occasionally found.

- Enterococci may survive in adverse environmental conditions, such as high temperature, drying, and in some antiseptic agents.
- This property helps enterococci contaminate surfaces and medical equipment, enabling it to be transmitted to patients via healthcare workers, causing outbreaks.

b. Helicobacter pylori

(Ref: Ananthanaryan & Paniker, Textbook of Microbiology, 10th ed, pg. 407)

ANSWER

- Helicobacter pylori (H. pylori) is a Gram negative, curved or spiral shaped bacteria.
- It is the major cause of peptic ulcer disease and gastritis.
- Approximately two-thirds of the world's population is infected with H. pylori.
- H.pylori is found in the gastric mucous layer or adherent to the epithelial lining of the stomach and

causes more than 90% of duodenal ulcers and up to 80% of gastric ulcers.

○ Persons with active gastric or duodenal ulcers or documented history of ulcers should be tested for H. pylori.

○ Various tests are available to diagnose H. pylori infection. These tests can be categorized into those that are based on direct assessment of gastric biopsies (endoscopic testing) and indirect tests (nonendoscopic testing) that detect an immunological response (i.e. antibodies against H. pylori) or metabolic products (i.e. urease activity) of H. pylori

PART-III

5. Enumerate the bacterial causes of meningitis and outline the laboratory diagnosis of acute pyogenic meningitis.

(Ref: Ananthanaryan & Paniker, Textbook of Microbiology, 10th ed, pg. 250)

ANSWER

For answer, refer 2014 paper-I Q. 5, Pg. 382

6. Name various bacterial agents causing water-borne diseases. Describe be briefly about bacterial examination of water.

ANSWER

Bacterial agents causing water-borne diseases

○ *Clostridium botulinum*
○ *Campylobacter jejuni*
○ *Vibrio cholerae*
○ *Escherichia coli*
○ *Shigella*
○ *Salmonella*
○ *Legionella*

For answer, refer 2017 paper-I Q. 5, Pg. 341

Your Roll No. ....

Name of the Paper   :   **Microbiology Paper-II**

Name of the Course   :   **MBBS-2011**

Semester   :   **Annual**

Time: 3 Hours   M.M.: 40

INSTRUCTIONS

1. Write your Roll No. on the top immediately on receipt of this question paper
2. All questions are to be attempted
3. Answers to Parts I, II and III should be written in separate answer sheets provided
4. Attempt parts of a question in sequence

PART-I

1. **Enumerate the different species of Leishmania. Outline the laboratory diagnosis of a case of kala-azar.**   [5]

2. **Write short notes on**   [10]
   a. Visceral larva migrans
   b. Free living amoebae

PART-II

3. **Enumerate fungi implicated in systemic mycoses. Discuss the methods used in the laboratory diagnosis of fungal infections.**   [5]

4. **Write briefly on:**   [10]
   a. Rhinosporidiosis
   b. Post-exposure prophylaxis of HIV

PART-III

5. **Name the mosquito-borne viruses and infections caused by them. Briefly describe the laboratory diagnosis of any one of them.**   [5]

6. **Discuss prophylaxis against polio and write briefly about Pulse Polio program.**   [5]

PART-I

1. Enumerate the different species of leishmania. Outline the laboratory diagnosis of a case of kala-azar.

ANSWER

Leishmania is widely distributed in nature. All it species are morphologically identical nearly

Leishmania species
• *L. aethiopica*
• *L. tropica minor*
• *L. tropica major*
• *L. peruviana*
• *L. mexicana*
• *L. mexicana amazonensis*
• *L. mexicana pifanoi*
• *L. braziliensis*
• *L. donovani*
• *L. donovani infantum*
• *L. donovani chagasi*

Laboratory Diagnosis of Kala-azar

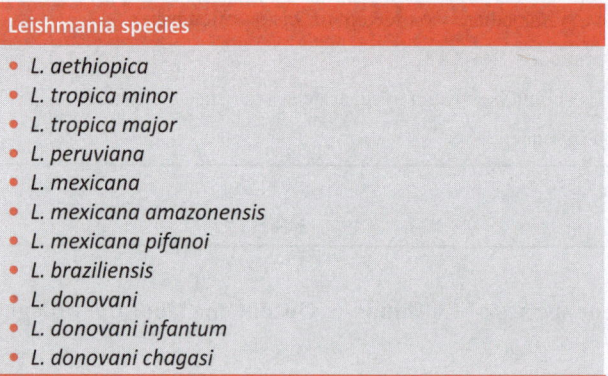

- Serologic testing is useful with the indirect fluorescent antibody (IFA) test, which is 80-100% sensitive in patients with visceral leishmaniasis who are not infected with human immunodeficiency virus (HIV). However, IFA may cross-react in patients who have leprosy, tuberculosis, malaria, schistosomiasis, Chagas disease, and African trypanosomiasis.

- An enzyme-linked immunosorbent assay (ELISA) can be combined with IFA and/or Western blot to increase sensitivity and specificity. Polymerase chain reaction (PCR) is being used more frequently; it is more accurate in determining new-onset leishmaniasis than serum tests (92-99% sensitivity; 100% specificity).

- **Complete blood cell (CBC) count:** In patients with visceral leishmaniasis, the presence of (1) normocytic normochromic anemia, (2) leukopenia with decreased neutrophils and a relative monocytosis and lymphocytosis, and (3) thrombocytopenia may occur due to parasitic bone-marrow infiltration. The severity of pancytopenia may vary with only 1 or 2 cell lines decreased.

- **Coagulation studies:** Prothrombin and partial thromboplastin times are generally normal in visceral leishmaniasis.

- Amastigotes are revealed inside the circulating monocytes and neutrophils. However, these are often difficult to locate because of their small numbers.

○ The aldehyde test and the antimony test were the initial tests used to detect hypogammaglobulinemia and diagnose visceral leishmaniasis. Findings include elevated gamma globulin levels and a reversal of the albumin-globulin ratio.

○ Patients with visceral leishmaniasis may exhibit mild elevations in alkaline phosphatase, aspartate aminotransferase (AST), and alanine aminotransferase (ALT) levels.

○ The safest and most common way to obtain tissue is through bone-marrow aspiration obtained from the sternum or the iliac crest, although splenic aspiration may be used in cases that are difficult to diagnose. Amastigote forms are revealed in plain film, and the promastigote forms are revealed in culture.

○ The Leishmanin skin test (LST), also known as the Montenegro skin test (for its introduction in Montenegro, South America) is similar to the purified protein derivative (PPD) used for Mycobacterium tuberculosis. This test has been used in the developing world to determine delayed-type hypersensitivity reactions.

○ Killed promastigotes are injected intradermally; a 5-mm area of induration over 48-72 hours suggests past infection (i.e, results are negative during active visceral leishmaniasis; positive results occur 2-3 months after infection, usually after successful therapy. The test results are also positive in patients with post–kala-azar dermal leishmaniasis).

2. Write short notes on:

a. Visceral Larva migrans

ANSWER

For answer, refer 2014 paper–II Q. 2 (b), Pg. 385

b. Free living amoebae

ANSWER

For answer, refer 2016 paper–II Q. 1, Pg. 362

PART-II

3. Enumerate fungi implicated in systemic mycoses. Discuss the methods used in the laboratory diagnosis of fungal infections.

(Ref: Ananthanaryan & Paniker, Textbook of Microbiology, 10th ed, pg.609)

ANSWER

Fungi Implicated in Systemic Mycoses

○ *Blastomyces dermatitidis*
○ *Paracoccidioides*
○ *Histoplasma*
○ *Pneumocystis jirovecii*
○ *Candida*
○ *Cryptococcus neoformans*

Laboratory Diagnosis of Fungal Infections

○ Direct Examination of Clinical Specimen
  ▪ Direct microscopic examination of fungal cells within the clinical specimen is a valuable diagnostic procedure for the following reasons:
  ▪ In many instances, a tentative or even a definitive diagnosis can be made before the growth of fungal cells would be apparent in culture.
  ▪ Observing fungal cells in a clinical specimen may be more valuable as a criterion for diagnosis than isolating in a culture.
  ▪ Preparations for direct examination of clinical specimen include KOH, India ink, and calcofluor white; in addition, a few staining techniques such as Giemsa and periodic acid-Schiff are effective.

○ **Preparations with KOH (Unstained):** Patches from the mucous membrane of the mouth, vagina, skin, or nails scrapping, sputum etc. are collected in a sterile container. These are examined in a KOH wet mount or gram stain. Yeast cells of 4-8 μm with budding mixed pseudohyphae are seen. The presence of pseudohyphae shows colonization and tissue invasion and so their demonstration is significant. For detection of Candida, wet smear microscopy has been positive in the majority, but not in all cases with positive culture.

○ **Preparations with Potassium Hydroxide (KOH):** The specimen should first be examined microscopically for necrotic, purulent, bloody, or caseous areas. Because these are the areas most likely to yield evidence of fungal growth, they are selected for direct examination. Preparation with KOH clears the tissue and cellular debris from all types of clinical specimens without damaging the fungal cells. This clearing process requires only 5 to 10 min, after which one can observe the fungal morphology as well as the pigment of the fungal cell wall.

○ **Preparations with calcofluor white and KOH:** Calcofluor white is used as a whitening agent in the textile and paper industry. The dye is useful for demonstrating the presence of fungal cells in clinical specimens because it binds to β 1-3, β 1-4 polysaccharides. The dye then fluoresces as it is exposed to the shorter wavelengths of ultraviolet light. A Fluorescence microscope is needed for detecting fungal cells prepared with Calcofluor white.

○ **Preparation With India Ink:** India ink is useful for indicating the presence or absence of extra cellular polysaccharide capsules of fungal cells. The technique is particularly helpful for detecting Cryptococcus neoformans in CSF. Because India ink serves as a negative stain, the encapsulated yeast cells can readily be detected against the dark back ground. The ink should be free from artifacts or granular carbon particles to ensure a good preparation.

○ **Preparations With Periodic Acid-schif (PAS) Stain:** The PAS stain one of the most widely used stains for fungal histopathology. In a direct examination of clinical specimen, PAS stain is sometimes used when a KOH preparation do not reveal fungi that are suspected to be present.

○ **Culture Medias:** All fungi require several specific elements for growth and reproduction. The requirements for growth are generally less stringent than for sporulation, so it is often necessary to try several types of media when attempting to identify a fungus in culture.[12]

○ Common media for primary fungal isolation include Sabouraud dextrose agar and brain-heart infusion agar, either in petri dishes or screwtop tubes. The media may be enriched with 5% to 10% sheep blood to support the growth of certain fungi.

---

4. Write short notes on

a. Rhinosporidiosis

(Ref: Ananthanaryan & Paniker, Textbook of Microbiology,10th ed, pg.607)

ANSWER

○ Rhinosporidiosis is a disease caused by the organism Rhinosporidium seeberi, which was once thought to be a fungus but is now believed to be a rare aquatic protistan parasite of fish.

○ First described in 1900 by Guillermo Seeber, it generally presents as swollen, pink or red polyps in the nasal cavity or the ocular conjunctivae. Other sites of infection are rare.

○ Infection generally occurs after swimming in stagnant freshwater ponds, lakes, or rivers, but is also suspected to occur from dust or air.

○ The disease is most often seen in individuals ages 15–40, with preferential occurrence in boys.

○ *R. seeberi* progresses through several stages of development and can be easily diagnosed via traditional fungal stains.

○ Although there is no effective antibiotic therapy, surgical excision of the polyps is often successful in treating the disease.

○ *R. seeberi* has a worldwide distribution with a proclivity for warm, tropical environments

b. Post-exposure prophylaxis of HIV

(Ref: Ananthanaryan & Paniker, Textbook of Microbiology,10th ed, pg.574)

ANSWER

Strategy of Post-Exposure Prophylaxis
Assessment

○ Clinical assessment of exposure

○ Eligibility assessment for HIV post-exposure prophylaxis

○ HIV testing of exposed people and source if possible

○ Provision of first aid in case of broken skin or other wound

Counseling and Support

○ Risk of HIV

○ Risks and benefits of HIV post-exposure prophylaxis

○ Side effects of treatment to be told

○ Enhanced adherence counselling if post-exposure prophylaxis to be prescribed

○ Specific support in case of sexual assault

Prescription

○ Post-exposure prophylaxis should be initiated as early as possible following exposure

○ 28-day prescription of recommended age-appropriate ARV drugs

○ Drug information should be shared

Follow-up

○ Assessment of underlying comorbidities and possible drug-drug interactions

○ HIV test at 3 months after exposure

○ Link to HIV treatment if possible

○ Provision of prevention intervention as appropriate

PART-III

5. Name the mosquito-borne viruses and infections caused by them. Briefly describe the laboratory diagnosis of any one of them.

(Ref: Ananthanaryan & Paniker, Textbook of Microbiology,10th ed, pg.530)

ANSWER

For answer, refer 2016 paper-II Q. 5, Pg. 364

6. **Discuss prophylaxis against polio and write briefly about Pulse Polio program.**

(Ref: Ananthanaryan & Paniker, Textbook of Microbiology, 10th ed, pg.496)

ANSWER

Pulse Polio Program

O India committed to the resolution passed by World Health Assembly for global polio eradication in 1988.

O Country introduced polio vaccine under Expanded Programme on Immunization (EPI, 1978), and subsequently in Universal Immunization Program (UIP, 1985), but started carrying out special polio campaigns from 1995.

O At present in routine immunization, bivalent oral polio vaccine (bOPV) drops are being provided to all children less than five years of age and Inactivated Polio Vaccine (IPV) to children less than one year of age.

O National Immunization Days (NIDs) commonly known as Pulse Polio Immunization program was launched in India in 1995, and is conducted twice in early part of each year.

O Additionally, multiple rounds (at least two) of sub - National Immunization Days (SNIDs) have been conducted over the years in high risk states/areas. o In these campaigns, children in the age group of 0-5 years are administered polio drops. Over 170 million children are immunized during each NID and 77 million in SNID.

O WHO, on 24th February 2012, removed India from the list of "endemic countries with active polio virus transmission".

O On 27th March 2014, the Regional Certification Commission of World Health Organization certified South-East Asia Region of WHO, which includes India, as polio free.

O This is a remarkable achievement considering the fact that in 2009 India accounted for half of the total number of polio cases globally and there were an estimated 2 lakh cases of polio every year in the country in the year 1978.

Name of the Paper	:	**Microbiology Paper-I**
Name of the Course	:	**MBBS-2010**
Semester	:	**Annual**

Time: 3 Hours   **M.M.: 40**

INSTRUCTIONS

1. Write your Roll No. on the top immediately on receipt of this question paper
2. All questions are to be attempted
3. Answers to Parts I, II and III should be written in separate answer sheets provided
4. Attempt parts of a question in sequence

PART-I

1. Enumerate the different methods of sterilization by heat. Add a short note on the principle of working and application of the autoclave.   [5]

2. Write short notes on: [10]
   a. Complement fixation Test
   b. Monoclonal antibodies

PART-II

3. Discuss morphology and cultural characteristics of V. cholerae. Outline the laboratory diagnosis of cholera.   [5]

4. Write briefly on: [10]
   a. Listerosis
   b. Mycoplasma

PART-III

5. Discuss the laboratory diagnosis of a case of Enteric fever in the first week of illness.   [5]

6. Discuss genetic mechanisms of transfer of drug resistance in bacteria.   [5]

PART-I

1. Enumerate the different methods of sterilization by heat. Add a short note on the principle of working and application of the autoclave.

(Ref: Ananthanaryan & Paniker, Textbook of Microbiology,10th ed, pg.31)

ANSWER

Thermal (Heat) Methods

○ **Dry heat sterilization**
  ▪ Incineration
  ▪ Red heat
  ▪ Flaming
  ▪ Hot air Oven

○ **Moist heat sterilization**
  ▪ Dry saturated steam–Autoclaving
  ▪ Boiling water/steam at atmospheric pressure
  ▪ Hot water below boiling point

Autoclave

A device used to sterilize equipment and supplies by subjecting them to high pressure saturated steam at 121 degrees Celsius for around 15-20 minutes depending on the size of the load and the contents.

Principle of Working

○ Water boils when its vapor pressure equals that of the surrounding atmosphere.

○ When pressure inside the closed vessel increases, the temperature at which water boils also increases.

○ Steam is condensed to water and gives up latent heat to that surface when it comes in contact with the cooler surface.

○ The energy available from this latent heat is considerable. For example 1600 mL steam at 100°C and releases 518 calories of heat.

○ The large reduction in the volume sucks in more steam in the area and the process continuous till the temperature of the surface is raised to that of the steam.

○ The water formed due to condensation ensures moisture conditions for killing microorganisms.

○ It is a better sterilizing agent than dry heat because the saturated steam has penetrative power.

○ Bacteria are more susceptible to moist heat as bacterial proteins coagulate rapidly and condensed water ensures moist conditions for killing the present microbes.

Application of Autoclave

○ A variety of materials, such as dressings, instruments, laboratory ware, media and pharmaceutical products which can withstand high temperature, discarded media with growth can be sterilized or disposed of by this method.

○ Transfusion equipment, glassware and metalware, intravenous equipment, applicators, syringes and items that can withstand high temperature and pressure can also be sterilized by this method.

2. Write short notes on:

a. Complement fixation test

(Ref: Ananthanaryan & Paniker, Textbook of Microbiology,10th ed, pg.112)

ANSWER

Complement Fixation Test

○ CFT detects complement fixing antibodies in patient's serum. It is now almost obsolete.
  ▪ Wasserman test was the most popular CFT, used for the diagnosis off syphilis.
  ▪ CFT was also widely used for detection of antibodies in Rickettsia, Chlamydia, Brucella, Mycoplasma infections and some viral infections such as arboviruses, rabies, etc.
  ▪ **Indirect complement fixation test:** Detects certain avian (e.g. duck, Parrot) and mammalian (e.g. horse, cat) serum antibodies cannot fix guinea pig complement.
  ▪ **Conglutination test:** To perform CFT using non hemolytic complements, e.g. horse complements.

Complements are also used for various serological tests, Other than CFT such as:

○ **Treponema pallidum immobilization test**
  For detecting antibodies to T. pallidum)

○ **Sabin-Feldman dye test** for detecting Toxoplasma antibodies.

○ **Vibriocidal antibody** test foe V.cholerae

b. Monoclonal antibodies

(Ref: Ananthanaryan & Paniker, Textbook of Microbiology,10th ed, pg.187)

ANSWER

For answer, refer 2017 paper–I Q. 2 (a), Pg. 339

PART-II

3. Discuss morphology and culture characteristies of V. cholerae. Outline the laboratory diagnosis of cholera.

(Ref: Ananthanaryan & Paniker, Textbook of Microbiology, 10th ed, pg.309)

ANSWER

- Cholerae is caused by *Vibrio cholerae*, a gram-negative, rod-shaped bacteria with a small bend in the middle and a long tail-like flagella.
- *V. cholerae* looks basically like a bratwurst with a tail.
- Gram-negative refers to its thin cell wall, which is surrounded by a protective outer membrane.
- The bacteria swim quickly about in infested water using their flagella in a whip-like manner to propel forward.

Culture Characteristics

- On alkaline nutrient agar, the colonies are moist, translucent, round disks (1-2 mm in diameter) with a bluish tinge in transmitted light and a distinctive odour
- On MacConkey's agar, their colonies become reddish on prolonged incubation as V. cholerae are late lactose fermenters.
- On blood agar, the greenish zone initially appears around the colonies and later becomes clear due to haemodigestion.
- In alkaline peptone water, a fine surface pellicle appears within 6 hours and breaks on shaking.
- On alkaline bile salt agar (BSA), Colonies are similar to those on nutrient agar.
- On Monsur's gelatin taurocholate trypticase tellurite agar (GTTA) medium the colonies are small translucent with a greyish black centre (due to tellurite reduction) and a turbid halo due to gelatin liquefaction.

Laboratory Diagnosis

- Macroscopic examination: Rice watery stool with mucus flakes
- The laboratory diagnosis of cholera is based on colony morphology, culture characteristics, biochemical reactions and serological identification by slide agglutination using specific antisera. However, a presumptive diagnosis of cholera can be made by an immobilization test.

4. Write briefly on:

(Ref: Ananthanaryan & Paniker, Textbook of Microbiology, 10th ed, pg.402)

a. Listeriosis

ANSWER

- Listeriosis is an infection caused by Listeria bacteria, named after Joseph Lister, the surgeon and pioneer of antiseptic surgery.
- There are 10 distinct species of Listeria; the variant that most commonly impacts humans is Listeria monocytogenes.
- The initial symptoms of listeriosis might not become apparent for some time;
- The incubation period is variable and can be anything from 11-70 days after consuming food with Listeria.
- The following symptoms of Listeria infection are likely to last 1–3 days:
  - Muscle aches
  - Fever
  - Flu-like symptoms
  - Nausea
  - Diarrhea
- For many people, a Listeria infection will pass unnoticed. However, in some individuals, the infection will spread to the nervous system where symptoms might include:
  - Headache
  - Confusion
  - Stiff neck
  - Tremors and convulsions
  - Loss of balance
  - In susceptible individuals, listeriosis can lead to a serious blood infection (septicemia) or inflammation of the membranes around the brain (meningitis).

b. Mycoplasma

(Ref: Ananthanaryan & Paniker, Textbook of Microbiology, 10th ed, pg. 393)

ANSWER

- Mycoplasmas are spherical to filamentous cells with no cell walls.
- There is an attachment organelle at the tip of filamentous M. pneumoniae, M. genitalium, and several other pathogenic mycoplasmas.
- Fried-egg-shaped colonies are seen on agar.
- The mycoplasmas presumably evolved by degenerative evolution from Gram-positive bacteria

and are phylogenetically most closely related to some clostridia.

○ Mycoplasmas are the smallest self-replicating organisms with the smallest genomes (a total of about 500 to 1000 genes); they are low in guanine and cytosine.

○ Mycoplasmas are nutritionally very exacting. Many require cholesterol, a unique property among prokaryotes.

○ Mycoplasmas have surface antigens such as membrane proteins, lipoproteins, glycolipids, and lipoglycans.

○ Some of the membrane proteins undergo spontaneous antigenic variation. Antibodies to surface antigens inhibit growth; various serological tests have been developed and are useful in classification.

○ Mycoplasmas are surface parasites of the human respiratory and urogenital tracts.

PART-III

---

5. **Discuss the laboratory diagnosis of a case of Enteric fever in the first week of illness.**

(Ref: Ananthanaryan & Paniker, Textbook of Microbiology,10th ed, pg. 300)

ANSWER

For answer, refer 2017 paper–I Q. 3, Pg. 340

---

6. **Discuss genetic mechanisms of transfer of drug resistance in bacteria.**

ANSWER

For answer, refer 2017 paper–I Q. 6, Pg. 342

Name of the Paper : **Microbiology Paper-II**

Name of the Course : **MBBS-2010**

Semester : **Annual**

Time: 3 Hours   M.M.: 40

INSTRUCTIONS

1. Write your Roll No. on the top immediately on receipt of this question paper
2. All questions are to be attempted
3. Answers to Parts I, II and III should be written in separate answer sheets provided
4. Attempt parts of a question in sequence

PART-I

1. Enumerate the parasites seen in peripheral blood smear. Outline the laboratory diagnosis of malaria.   [5]

2. Write short notes on: [10]
   a. Various laboratory procedures for the diagnosis of HIV infection
   b. Life cycle of Ascaris lumbricoides

PART-II

3. Classify dermatophytes. Discuss laboratory diagnosis in brief.   [5]

4. Write short notes on: [10]
   a. Histoplasmosis
   b. Dengue fever

PART-III

5. Name five agents (both DNA and RNA) causing diarrhea. Briefly describe the laboratory diagnosis of viral diarrhea.   [5]

6. Discuss various stool concentration techniques.   [5]

PART-I

1. **Enumerate the parasites seen in peripheral blood smear. Outline the laboratory diagnosis of malaria.**

ANSWER

Parasites seen in Peripheral Blood Smear

- Malaria
- Babesia
- Leishmania
- Filaria
- Trypanosoma cruzi

Laboratory Diagnosis of Malaria

Laboratory diagnosis of malaria requires the identification of the parasite or its antigens/ products in the patient's blood.

Microscopy

- Thick and thin blood smear study is the gold standard method for malaria diagnosis. The procedure follows these steps: collection of peripheral blood, staining of smear with Giemsa stain and examination of red blood cells for malaria parasites under the microscope.
- Thick smear. It is not fixed in methanol; this allows the red blood cells to be hemolyzed, and leukocytes and any malaria parasites present will be the only detectable elements. However, the hemolysis may lead to distorted plasmodial morphology making plasmodium species differentiation difficult. Therefore, thick smears are mainly used to detect infection and to estimate parasitemia.
- Thin smear. It is fixed in methanol. Thin smears allow the examiner to identify malaria species, quantify parasitemia, and recognize parasite forms like schizonts and gametocytes.

Quantitative Buffy Coat (QBC) Test

- This method involves centrifuged and compressed red blood cell layer stained with acridine orange and then examined under an ultraviolet light source. The whole procedure takes place in a glass hematocrit tube which is precoated internally with acridine orange stain and potassium oxalate; it is filled with 55–65 µl of blood. The tube is centrifuged and so the components separate according to their densities forming bands
- Fluorescing parasites are then observed, with a UV microscope, at the red blood cell/white blood cell interface
- QBC test is easier and faster than classic peripheral blood smear microscopy but the equipment required is expensive and species identification and accurate enumeration are impossible.

Rapid Diagnostic Test (RDT)

- RDT is a device that can detect malaria antigen in a small amount of blood (5µl) by immunochromatographic assay (colour change in an absorbing nitrocellulose strip) with monoclonal antibodies directed against the parasite antigen. Depending on the target antigen, rapid tests that now exist may involve combinations of the following:
  - HRP-2 (Histidine Rich Protein-2) is a protein produced by the asexual stages and gametocytes of P. falciparum, expressed on the membrane of red blood cells (sensitivity: detects parasitemia of >40 parasites/ µl). It often persists in patient's blood for weeks after successful treatment.
  - Plasmodium aldolase is an enzyme of the parasite glycolytic pathway expressed by all malaria species (pan malarial antigen- PMA).
  - Lactate dehydrogenase (LDH) is a glycolytic enzyme produced by asexual and sexual stages of parasites and released by infected red blood cells. (sensitivity: detects parasitemia of >100 parasites/ µl)

2. **a. Write briefly on the various laboratory procedures for the diagnosis of HIV infection**

(Ref: Ananthanaryan & Paniker, Textbook of Microbiology, 10th ed, pg.574)

ANSWER

Summary of Diagnostic Tests for HIV Infection

Technology	Principle	Strengths	Limitations
Initial HIV tests			
First- and second-generation immunoassays	Viral lysate (G1) or recombinant antigens (G2) capture anti-HIV antibodies; specific IgGs detected using antihuman IgG	Detect HIV-specific IgG	Do not detect HIV-specific IgM and HIV antigens
Third-generation immunoassays	Recombinant antigens capture anti-HIV antibodies; IgG and IgM detected using antihuman antibodies	Detect anti-HIV IgMs that may occur earlier in infection, in addition to IgG; improved seroconversion sensitivity; some have greater sensitivity in detecting HIV-2 and/or HIV-1 group O compared to earlier-generation assays	Do not detect HIV antigens
Fourth-generation immunoassays	Recombinant antigens capture anti-HIV antibodies; IgG and IgM detected using antihuman antibodies plus direct detection of p24 Ag	Detect antibodies and Ags simultaneously, allowing recognition of HIV infection prior to seroconversion	May miss early HIV infection (prior to antigenemia)
Rapid tests	Immunoassays that employ lateral flow, immunoconcentration, or particle agglutination technologies	Completed in <30 min often at point of care; performance characteristics similar to lab-based immunoassays (generation dependent)	Similar to lab-based immunoassays (generation dependent)
NAATs	Nucleic acids (DNA or RNA) amplified using specific primers and detected using labeled probes	Detect acute HIV infection prior to seroconversion	Most detect HIV-1 only; HIV-1 RNA may be undetectable in some Ab-positive HIV-infected persons; technically complex and expensive
Supplemental HIV tests			
Western blot	Viral lysate separated by electrophoresis, transferred to membrane and patient specimen is incubated with membrane to identify specific Ag/Ab complexes	High specificity due to Ag separation and concentration	Less sensitive than third- and fourth-generation immunoassays, technically complex, opportunities for technical error
Line immunoassays	Similar to WB, recombinant antigen or synthetic peptides replace viral lysate.	High specificity	Similar to WB
Indirect immunofluorescence assays	Microscope slide coated with cells infected with HIV, patient specimen incubated on slide with cells and then fluorescently labeled antihuman antibodies used to detect HIV specific antibodies by microscopy	High specificity	Subjective interpretation of results; assays only approved for HIV-1 detection in US; expensive instrument (microscope) required; low throughput
Enzyme immunoassays	Same as above for initial HIV tests	Same as above for initial tests. May distinguish between HIV-1 and HIV-2. More simple and rapid than WB and IFAs	None yet FDA approved for supplemental testing

Abbreviations: Ab, antibody; Ag, antigen; FDA, Food and Drug Administration; G1, first generation; G2, second generation; HIV, human immunodeficiency virus; IFA, immunofluorescence assay; IgG, immunoglobulin G; IgM, immunoglobulin M; NAATs, nucleic acid amplification tests; WB, Western blot.

b. Describe in brief the Life cycle of Ascaris lumbricoides.

ANSWER

Ascaris lumbricoides is an intestinal round worm. It is the largest intestinal nematode to infect Human. The adult worm lives in small intestine and grow to a length of more than 30 cm. Human is only the natural host and reservoir of infection.

Life Cycle

The life cycle of Ascaris completes in single host. Human.

○ **Stage I:** Eggs in feces
  ▪ Sexually mature female produces as many as 200,000 eggs per day, which are shed along with feces in unembryonated form. They are non infective.

○ **Stage II:** Development in soil
  ▪ Embryonation occurs in soil as optimum temperature of 20–25C with sufficient moisture and O_2
  ▪ Infective larva develops within egg in about 3–6 weeks.

○ **Stage III:** Human infection and liberation of larvae
  ▪ Human get infection with ingestion of embryonated egg contaminated food and water
  ▪ Within embryonated state inside egg, first stage larvae develops into second stage larvae. This second stage larvae is known as rhabditiform larvae
  ▪ Second stage larve is stimulated to hatch out by the presence of alkaline pH in small intestine and solubilization of its outer layer by bile.

○ **Stage IV:** Migration of larvae through lungs
  ▪ Hatched out larvae penetrates the intestinal wall and carried to liver through portal circulation
  ▪ It then travels via blood to heart and to lungs by pulmonary circulation within 4–7 days of infection.
  ▪ The larvae in lungs molds twice, enlarge and breaks into alveoli.

○ **Stage V:** Re-entry to stomach and small intestine
  ▪ From alveoli, the Larvae then pass up through bronchi and into trachea and then swallowed.
  ▪ The larvae passes down the esophagus to the stomach and reached into small intestine once again.
  ▪ Small intestine is the normal habitat of Ascaris and it colonises here.
  ▪ Within intestine parasite molds twice and mature into adult worm.
  ▪ Sexual maturation occurs with 6–10 weeks and the mature female discharges its eggs in intestinal lumen and excreted along with feces, continuing the life cycle.
  ▪ The life span of parasite is 12–18 months

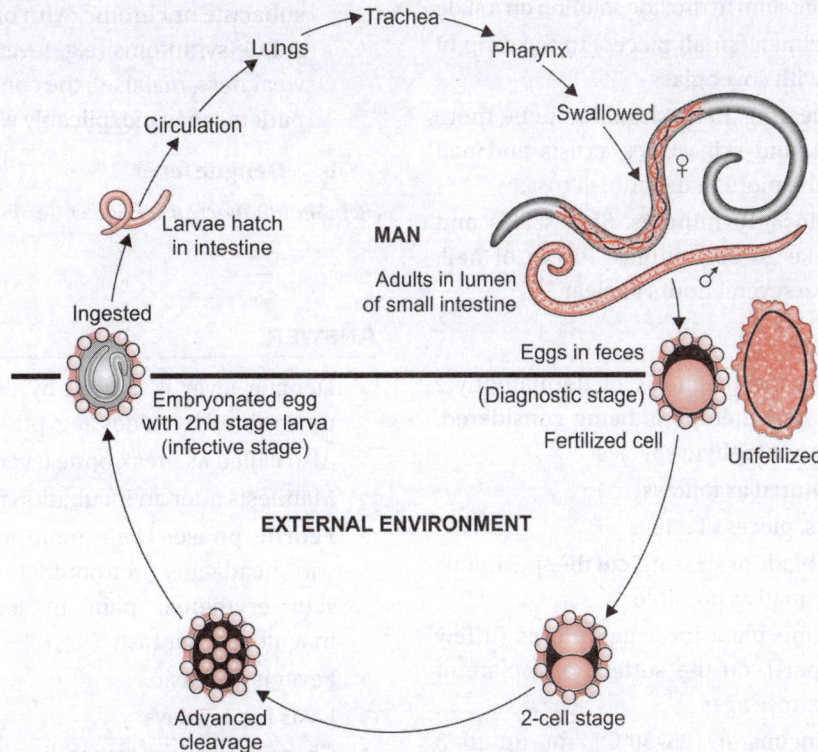

Fig. Life cycle of ascaris lumbricoides

PART-II

3. Classify Dermatophytes. Discuss Laboratory diagnosis in brief.

(Ref: Ananthanaryan & Paniker, Textbook of Microbiology,10th ed, pg.600)

ANSWER

Dermatophytes are aerobic fungi that can invade and infect the keratinized layers of skin, hair, and nails

There are three genera of dermatophytes, recognized by the nature of their macroconidae (asexual spores):

○ Trichophyton (abbreviated as "T")
○ Microsporum ("M")
○ Epidermophyton ("E")

Diagnosis of dematophyte infections:

○ It is done primarily by 2 methods
  ▪ Direct microscopic examination
  ▪ Culture

Clinical Material

Skin scrapings, nail scrapings, scalp and hairs. For a laboratory diagnosis, clinicians should be aware of the need to generate an adequate amount of suitable clinical material. The laboratory needs enough specimen to perform both microscopy and culture

Slide Preparation with KOH

○ Place a drop of potassium hydroxide solution on a slide
○ Transfer the specimen (small pieces) to the drop of KOH, and cover with cover glass
○ **Note:** To assist clearing, hairs should note be more than 5 mm long, and skin scales, crusts and nail snips should not be more than 2 mm across.
○ Hairs clear within 5–10 minutes. Skin scales and crusts usually take 20–30 minutes. Picces of nail, however, may take several hours to clear

Culture

○ Useful to confirm the diagnosis of dermatophyte when long-term oral therapy is being considered, and to identify dermatophyte species
○ Specimen are cultured as follows:
○ Skin scales, crusts, pieces of nail:
  ▪ Using a sterile blade or scissors, cut the specimens into pieces as small as possible
  ▪ Using sterile, inoculate the small pieces (a few millimeters apart), on the surface of a plate of sabouraud dextrose agar
  ▪ Incubate at incubator (25–30°C). for up to 3 weeks, examining every few days for growth

4. Write short notes on:

a. Histoplasmosis

(Ref: Ananthanaryan & Paniker, Textbook of Microbiology,10th ed, pg.609)

ANSWER

○ Histoplasmosis is a pulmonary and hematogenous disease caused by Histoplasma capsulatum; it is often chronic and usually follows an asymptomatic primary infection.

○ Histoplasmosis has 3 main forms.

  ▪ Acute primary histoplasmosis is a syndrome with fever, cough, myalgias, chest pain, and malaise of varying severity. Acute pneumonia (evident on physical examination and chest X-ray) sometimes develops.

  ▪ Chronic cavitary histoplasmosis is characterized by pulmonary lesions that are often apical and resemble cavitary TB. Manifestations are worsening cough and dyspnea, progressing eventually to disabling respiratory dysfunction. Dissemination does not occur.

  ▪ Progressive disseminated histoplasmosis characteristically includes generalized involvement of the reticuloendothelial system, with hepatosplenomegaly, lymphadenopathy, bone marrow involvement, and sometimes oral or GI ulcerations. The course is usually subacute or chronic, with only nonspecific, often subtle symptoms (e.g, fever, fatigue, weight loss, weakness, malaise); the condition of HIV-positive patients may inexplicably worsen

b. Dengue fever

(Ref: Ananthanaryan & Paniker, Textbook of Microbiology,10th ed, pg. 529)

ANSWER

○ Dengue fever is caused by dengue virus which is transmitted by Aedes aegypti.
○ Also called as break bone fever
○ Manifests after an incubation period of 3–14 days
○ **Febrile phase:** High grade fever of sudden onset wit headache, retrobulbar pain, photophobia, skin erythema, pain in back and limbs and maculopapular rash
○ Fever is biphasic
○ Lasts for 2–7 days
○ Characterized by generalized body ache, myalgia, arthralgia

PART-III

5. Name five agents (both DNA & RNA) causing diarrhea. Briefly describe the laboratory diagnosis of viral diarrhea.

(Ref: Ananthanaryan & Paniker, Textbook of Microbiology, 10th ed, pg.632)

ANSWER

Viruses Causing Diarrhea

- Rotavirus
- Adenovirus
- Astrovirus
- Norovirus
- Calcivirus

Laboratory Diagnosis of Viral Diarrhea

Diagnosis

- **Electron microscopy:** This is the only catch-all method currently available. Faecal extracts, preferably after undergoing concentration, are stained and placed onto grids. For the virus to be recognizable, it should be present in quantities exceeding 106 /ml. All diarrhoeal viruses were first discovered by electron microscopy. The drawback for electron microscopy is its cost and the requirement for trained staff. The sensitivity and specificity of EM may be enhanced by the use of immune electron microscopy techniques.
- **PAGE:** Stool extracts may contain levels of viral nucleic acid high enough to be demonstrated by PAGE. Many types of viruses can be recognized e.g. rotaviruses have 11 segments which could be recognized readily, as can a single line corresponding to the double stranded DNA for adenoviruses. It may be possible to apply restriction endonucleases to further characterize the DNA or RNA. There is no reason why other viruses cannot be demonstrated by this method. This method may eventually be considered as a cheaper alternative to EM as a catch-all method for the detection of diarrhoeal viruses.
- **Culture:** None of the fastidious viruses will grow readily in cell culture. However, it may be possible in the foreseeable to find culture systems for many of these viruses.
- **Virus antigen detection:** These tests are specific tests using polyclonal and monoclonal antibodies. Most of these tests are homemade tests by individual laboratories although commercial tests are becoming available. ELISA and Latex Agglutination are the most commonly used tests.

- **PCR:** PCR has become the method of choice for diagnosing norovirus infections, particularly in outbreak situations.

6. Discuss various stool concentration techniques.

ANSWER

Stool Concentration Techniques

- **Sedimentation method:** Use solutions of lower specific gravity than the parasitic organisms, thus concentrating the latter in the sediment. Sedimentation techniques are recommended for general diagnostic laboratories because they are easier to perform and less prone to technical errors. The formalin-ethyl acetate technique is a diphasic sedimentation technique that avoids the problems of flammability of ether, and which can be used with specimens preserved in formalin, MIF or SAF.
  - Modified Formal- Ether sedimentation technique
  - Acid- Ether sedimentation technique
- **Flotation method:** Flotation use solutions which have higher specific gravity than the organisms to be floated so that the organisms rise to the top and the debris sinks to the bottom. The main advantage of this technique is to produce a cleaner material than the sedimentation technique. The disadvantages of most flotation techniques are that the walls of eggs and cysts will often collapse, thus hindering identification. Also, some parasite eggs do not float.
  - Saturated Salt Solution technique
  - Sheather's Sugar Centrifugal Flotation technique
  - Zinc Sulfate Centrifugal Flotation Technique

Modified Formal- Ether Sedimentation Technique

- **Formalin:** Ether or Formalin- Ethyl acetate method is the recommended concentration procedures.
- Most types of worm eggs (round worms, tapeworms, schistosomes, and other fluke eggs), larvae, and protozoan cysts may be recovered by this method.
- **Advantages:**
  - **Speed:** One sample can be processed in 5 minutes.
  - **Broad spectrum:** It will recover most ova, cyst and larvae.
  - The morphology of most parasites is retained for easy identification.
- **Disadvantages:**
  - Requires several pieces of apparatus which does not make it an easy.
  - The preparation contains some debris.
  - Ether is flammable. Formalin is an irritant.
  - Hymenolepis nana and Fasciola spp. do not concentrate well

Name of the Paper	:	**Microbiology Paper-I**
Name of the Course	:	**MBBS-2009**
Semester	:	**Annual**

Time: 3 Hours   **M.M.: 40**

INSTRUCTIONS

1. Write your Roll No. on the top immediately on receipt of this question paper
2. All questions are to be attempted
3. Answers to Parts I, II and III should be written in separate answer sheets provided
4. Attempt parts of a question in sequence

PART-I

1. Enumerate various methods of gene transfer in bacteria and discuss any one method in detail.   [5]
2. Write short notes on: [10]
   a. Type I hypersensitivity
   b. Biological effects of complement activation

PART-II

3. Discuss the laboratory diagnosis of primary syphilis.   [5]
4. Write briefly on: [10]
   a. Virulence factors of streptococcus pyogenes
   b. Clostidium perfringens

PART-III

5. Enumerate the bacterial causes of PUO and discuss its laboratory diagnosis.   [5]
6. Discuss about significant bacteriuria.   [5]

PART-I

1. **Enumerate various methods of gene transfer in bacteria and discuss any one method in detail.**

ANSWER

For answer, refer 2012 paper–I Q. 1, Pg. 400

2. **Write short notes on:**

   a. **Type I hypersensitivity**

   (Ref: Ananthanaryan & Paniker, Textbook of Microbiology,10th ed, pg.163)

ANSWER

For answer, refer 2017 paper–I Q. 1, Pg. 338

   b. **Biological effects of complement activation**

   For answer, refer 2012 paper–I Q. 2 (a), Pg. 401

PART-II

3. **Discuss the laboratory diagnosis of primary syphilis:**

   (Ref: Ananthanaryan & Paniker, Textbook of Microbiology,10th ed, pg.380)

ANSWER

Syphilis is a sexually transmitted infection caused by the spirochete Treponema pallidum.

Primary Syphilis

This stage is characterized by a painless genital, anal, or less commonly oral ulcer or chancre. This lesion occurs at the site of inoculation. The ulcer is typically indurated and is usually without exudate. There may be regional lymphadenopathy.

Direct Diagnosis

- Direct laboratory methods used for the laboratory diagnosis of syphilis includes the detection of Treponema pallidum by microscopic examination of fluid or smears from lesions, histological examination of tissues or nucleic acid amplification methods such as polymerase chain reaction (PCR).

- **Tests used for the direct detection of Treponema pallidum are:**
  - Dark-field microscopy
  - Direct fluorescent antibody test for Treponema pallidum
  - Nucleic acid amplification (PCR based) methods

Indirect Diagnosis/Serological Methods

- It is based on serological tests for the detection of antibodies.
- Serological testing is the mainstay in the laboratory diagnosis and follow-up of syphilis.
- **Serological tests fall into two categories:** Nontreponemal tests for screening, and treponemal tests for confirmation.
  - **Nontreponemal tests:** They measure both immunoglobulin (IgG and IgM) antiphospholipid antibodies formed by the host in response to lipoidal material released by damaged host cells early in infection and lipid from the cell surfaces of the treponeme itself. Commonly used nontreponemal tests are
    - Rapid plasma reagin (RPR) test
    - Toluidine red unheated serum test (TRUST)
    - Venereal Disease Research Laboratory (VDRL) test
  - Treponemal tests are used as confirmatory tests to verify reactivity in non-treponemal tests. Once positive, treponemal tests remain positive throughout life with or without treatment, so these tests cannot be used to know response to treatment. Commonly used treponemal tests are:
    - Fluorescent treponemal antibody absorption test (FTA-ABS) test
    - Treponema pallidum particle agglutination (TP-PA) test
    - Treponema pallidum Hemagglutination Assay (TPHA)

4. **Write briefly on:**

   a. **Virulence factors of streptococcus pyogenes**

   (Ref: Ananthanaryan & Paniker, Textbook of Microbiology,10th ed, pg.212)

ANSWER

Virulence Factors of Streptococcus Pyogenes

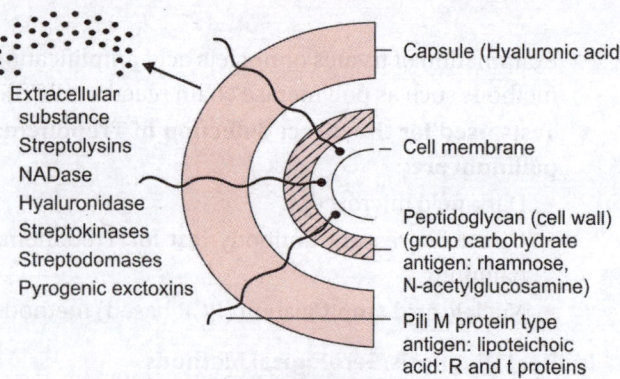

Fig. Virulence factors of streptococcus pyogenes

○ **Hyaluronic acid capsule:** The hyaluronic acid capsule of S. pyogenes is non antigenic because of its chemical similarity to host connective tissue. Capsule of S. pyogenes thus assists the bacterium to hide its own antigens and to go unrecognized as antigenic by its host. The hyaluronic acid capsule also prevents opsonized phagocytosis.

○ **Adhesins:** Adhesion of S. pyogenes in the epithelial cells of oral, nasal cavities and skin is the first step for infection. S. pyogenes produces various adhesins; Fibronectin (Fn) binding protein, lipoteichoic acids (LTA), M protein, Protein F etc.

○ **Hemolysins:** Two hemolytic and cytolytic toxins-streptolysin O (SLO) and Streptolysin S (SLS) are produced by most strains of group A streptococci. Blood agar showing β-hemolysis

  ▪ **Streptolysin O:** The oxygen labile cytolysin is responsible for beta hemolysis seen around Group A streptococcus (GAS) colonies in blood agar. It is believed to be toxic to leukocytes. Streptolysin O is strongly immunogenic. The concentration of antistreptolysin O antibodies is used diagnostically as an indicator of prior or recent streptococcal infection.

  ▪ **Streptolysin S:** It is oxygen stable and non-immunogenic cytolysin. However, like streptolysin O, streptolysin S is hemolytic and cytotoxic.

○ Pyrogenic exotoxins of streptococcus pyogenes (SPEs) types A, B and C These toxins acts as superantigens (not requiring processing by antigen presenting cells). SPEs A and C are produced when S. pyogenes is lysogenized strains (bacteria carrying an integrated phage i.e. prophage). Non lysogenized strains are atoxic. SPE B is encoded by a bacterial chromosome. These toxins act directly on the hypothalamus to exert their pyrogenic (fever producing) properties, and they cause the rash characteristics of scarlet fever.

○ **Streptokinase:** (Fibrinolysin) Streptokinase acts on plasminogen, which is converted to plasmin, an active proteolytic enzymes that lyse fibrin. Thus streptokinase appears to play a biological role in streptococcal infections by breaking down the fibrin barrier around the lesions and facilitates the spread of infection. Antistreptokinase antibodies provide retrospective evidence of streptococcal infection.

○ **Hyaluronidase:** Hyaluronidase splits hyaluronic acid, an important component of connective tissue. Thus hyaluronidase aids in spreading of the microorganisms along the intercellular spaces.

b. Clostidium perfringens

(Ref: Ananthanaryan & Paniker, Textbook of Microbiology, 10th ed, pg. 256)

ANSWER

○ Clostridium perfringens is a rod-shaped Gram-positive bacterium, which is a mesophile that has an optimal growing temperature of 37 °C.

○ It is a non-motile pathogen that produces endospores.

○ Although C. perfringens is an inhabitant of human normal intestinal flora, it is a pathogen responsible for many gastrointestinal illnesses with severity ranging from mild enterotoxaemia to fatal gas gangrene

○ It possesses the typical characteristics of Gram-positive bacteria, such as a protective thick cell wall, which is made up of peptidoglycan, surrounding an inner membrane.

○ C. perfringens is an anaerobic bacterium, who acquires energy by performing anaerobic respiration using Nitrate as its electron acceptor.

○ There is an increase in growth when this bacterium is grown in the presence of Nitrate, because this inorganic acceptor allows more metabolites molecules to undergo substrate-level phosphorylation reactions, leading to an increase yield in energy production

PART-III

5. Enumerate the bacterial causes of PUO and discuss its laboratory diagnosis.

ANSWER

Bacterial Causes of PUO

○ Abscesses

○ They are most commonly in the subphrenic space, liver, right lower quadrant, retroperitoneal space or the pelvis in women.

○ **Tuberculosis:** When dissemination has occurred (eg, in patients who are immunocompromised) the initial presentation is more likely to consist of constitutional symptoms than localising signs. CXR may be normal.

○ **Urinary tract infections (UTIs):** These are rare causes. Perinephric abscesses occasionally fail to communicate with the urinary system, resulting in a normal urinalysis.

○ **Endocarditis (this is a rare cause of PUO):**
  ▪ **Culture:** Negative endocarditis is reported in 5-10% of endocarditis cases.

○ **Hepatobiliary infections (eg, cholangitis):** These can occur without local signs and with only mildly elevated or normal LFTs, especially in the elderly.

○ **Osteomyelitis:** This usually causes localised pain or discomfort at least sporadically.

○ **Brucellosis:** This should be considered in patients with persistent fever and a history of contact with cattle, swine, goats or sheep, or in patients who consume raw milk products.

○ **Borrelia recurrentis:** This is transmitted by ticks. It is responsible for causing relapsing fever.

○ **Other spirochetal diseases that can cause PUO:** These include Spirillum minor (rat-bite fever), Borrelia burgdorferi (Lyme disease) and Treponema pallidum (syphilis).

Laboratory Diagnosis

○ FBC, erythrocyte sedimentation rate (ESR), U and Es, C-reactive protein (CRP), LFTs, antinuclear antibody (ANA), Rh factor and TFTs should be taken.

○ Labelled white cell scan; in this investigation white cells are labelled extracorporeally and then re-injected into the patient. It is used to identify areas of sepsis. If the patient is neutropenic then donor white cells may be used. False positive scans may occur with haematomas and inflammatory disease. False negatives may occur in chronic sepsis.

○ Blood cultures (preferably having been off antibiotics for several days) should be taken at differing times and from different sites. Culture for two weeks to detect slow-growing organisms and on special media if necessary.

○ Culture urine, sputum, stool, CSF and morning gastric aspirates (if tuberculosis is suspected).

○ CXR, abdominal CT scan and echocardiography (if endocarditis or atrial myxoma is suspected) should be considered.

○ CT, intravenous pyelogram (IVP), MRI and positron emission tomography (PET) scanning all have a place in diagnosis.

○ Invasive procedures for abnormal findings:
  ▪ Lumbar puncture for headache.
  ▪ Skin biopsy for rash.
  ▪ Lymph aspiration or biopsy for lymphadenopathy.
  ▪ **In an HIV-positive patient:** Bone marrow aspiration or biopsy.
  ▪ Abnormal LFTs should prompt a liver biopsy (even if normal size).

○ Laparoscopy or laparotomy is rarely necessary in the light of modern diagnostic techniques but may be required in patients who are deteriorating

---

6. Significant bacteriuria

ANSWER

○ Significant bacteriuria traditionally refers to the laboratory finding of >105 colony-forming units (CFU) of bacteria per mL of urine.

○ Urine cultures from patients with symptomatic UTI usually show >105 CFU/mL of urine, whereas asymptomatic patients whose cultures have been contaminated usually show < 103 CFU/mL of urine.

○ Limitations of the ">105 per mL rule" have become increasingly apparent.

○ In fewer than 105 CFU/mL often assume significance when the pre-test probability of UTI is high because of the clinical setting.

○ These cases are sometimes called low colony-count UTI.

○ Stated differently, 104 or even fewer bacteria per mL of urine represent "significant bacteriuria" when there is strong clinical evidence of UTI.

Your Roll No. ....

Name of the Paper	:	**Microbiology Paper-II**
Name of the Course	:	**MBBS-2009**
Semester	:	**Annual**

Time: 3 Hours   **M.M.: 40**

INSTRUCTIONS

1. Write your Roll No. on the top immediately on receipt of this question paper
2. All questions are to be attempted
3. Answers to Parts I, II and III should be written in separate answer sheets provided
4. Attempt parts of a question in sequence

PART-I

1. Classify human herpes viruses. Write briefly on Epstein-Barr virus (EBV). [5]

2. Write briefly on: [10]
   a. Laboratory diagnosis of toxoplasmosis
   b. Cryptosporidium

PART-II

3. Discuss pathogenesis and laboratory diagnosis of Cryptococcus neoformans. [5]

4. Write short notes on: [10]
   a. Rhinosporidiosis
   b. Slow virus diseases

PART-III

5. Write briefly on amoebic liver abscess. [5]

6. Write briefly on prophylaxis against rabies. [5]

PART-I

1. Classify human herpes viruses. Write briefly on Epstein-Barr virus (EBV).

(Ref: Ananthanaryan & Paniker, Textbook of Microbiology,10th ed, pg. 568)

ANSWER

Classification of Human Herpes Virus

Classification of human herpes viruses					
Sub family	Growth cycle	Cytopathology	Latent infections	Official name	Common name
Alpha herpes virus	Short	Cytolytic	Neurons	Human herpes virus 1 Human herpes virus 2 Human herpes virus 3	Herpes simplex virus type 1 Herpes simplex virus type 2 Varicella zoster virus
Beta herpes virus	Long	Cytomegalic	Glands Kidneys	Human herpes virus 5	Cytomegalovirus
		Lymphotropic	Lymph node	Human herpes virus 6	Human B cell Lymphotropic virus
				Human herpes virus 7	RK virus
Gamma herpes virus	Variable	Lymphoproliferative	Lymphoid tissue	Human herpes virus 4	Epstein Barr (EB) virus
				Human herpes virus 8	**Kaposi's sarcoma associated herpes virus**

Epstein-Barr Virus

For answer, refer 2014 paper-II Q. 4 (a), Pg. 385

2. Write briefly on:

a. Laboratory diagnosis of toxoplasmosis

ANSWER

For answer, refer 2017 paper-II Q. 2 (a), Pg. 346

b. Cryptosporidium

ANSWER

○ Cryptosporidium is a protozoan that is responsible for causing cryptosporidiosis, one of the most important opportunistic infections in AIDS patients.
○ Out of 16 species, only C. parvum and C. hominis are infectious to man.
○ Developmental stages of C. parvum do not occur within host cells but are confined to an intracellular, extracytoplasmic location. Each stage is within a parasitophorous vacuole in the microvilli of small intestines.

○ The parasite released in the feces is called oocyst, which is colorless, spherical or oval. The anterior end is pointed and posterior end is rounded and contains nucleus.
○ Humans get infected either by direct contact with infected animals or ingestion of fecally contaminated food or water.
○ Oocysts of C. parvum are not eliminated by chlorination of water and can persist for a longer time in post-treatment water supplies.
○ The most common symptom of cryptosporidiosis is **watery diarrhea.**

PART-II

3. Discuss pathogenesis and laboratory diagnosis of Cryptococcus neoformans.

(Ref: Ananthanaryan & Paniker, Textbook of Microbiology,10th ed, pg.617)

ANSWER

Cryptococcus neoformans is a yeast with prominent polysaccharide capsule. It is an opportunistic fungal pathogen notoriously known as the most common cause of fungal meningitis (infection and inflammation of the meninges) in immunocompromised patients (such as people with AIDS).

Pathogenesis

Infection is initiated by inhalation of the yeast cells. The primary pulmonary infection may be asymptomatic or may mimic influenza like respiratory infection often resolving spontaneously. In immune-compromised patients with impaired T cell immunity, the yeasts may multiply and disseminate to other parts of the body but preferentially to the central nervous system (neurotropic), causing cryptococcal meningitis. Other common sites of dissemination include the skin, adrenals, bone, eye and prostate gland. The inflammatory reaction is usually minimal or granulomatous.

Laboratory Diagnosis

Specimens

Specimens depends on clinical presentation and suspected disease conditions. Common specimens include spinal fluid (CSF), tissue, exudates, sputum, blood and urine.

○ **Microscopy and staining:** Cryptococcus neoformans appear as a spherical, single or multiple budding, thick walled yeast that is 2-15 μm (wide variation in size) in diameter. It is usually surrounded by a wide refractile capsule.

○ India ink preparation is used as a rapid and inexpensive diagnostic tools of detecting cryptococcal infection in many institutions and resource poor settings. Demonstration of heavily capsulated yeast cells (see the image) in CSF, exudates and urine establishes the diagnosis. India ink preparation when positive in CSF is diagnostic of cryptococcal meningitis but its sensitivity is low. Many diagnostic laboratories have replaced this test with more sensitive cryptococcal latex agglutination test.

○ **Culture:** Colonies develop within a few days on most media (e.g., Sabouraud's dextrose agar) at room temperature or 37 °C. Cryptococcus neoformans is sensitive to cycloheximide so media containing cycloheximide should be avoided. Other culture media are Blood Agar, BHI Agar, Bird seed agar etc. Colonies in SDA are creamy, white and mucoid (because of capsule).

  ▪ **Identification:** Cryptococcus neoformans is identified by urease production and carbohydrate assimilation test, and confirmed by direct immunofluorescence using a fluorescein-labelled anti-neoformans antibody.

○ Detection of Antigen and/or Antibody

  ▪ **Detection of antigen:** Tests for capsular antigen can be performed on CSF and serum. Latex agglutination test is most useful in detection of cryptococcal polysaccharide antigen. Slide latex agglutination test has sensitivity of 90% in the cases of cryptococcal meningitis.

  ▪ **Detection of antibody:** Serum antibodies can be detected by agglutination and immunofluorescence.

---

4. **Write short notes on:**

   a. **Rhinosporidiosis**

(Ref: Ananthanaryan & Paniker, Textbook of Microbiology,10th ed, pg.607)

Answer

For answer, refer 2011 paper-II Q. 4 (a), Pg. 418

   b. **Slow Virus diseases**

Answer

It is applied to a group of infections in animals and human beings, characterized by a very long incubation period and a slow course, terminating fatally.

Characteristics

○ Incubation period–months to years
○ Course of illness lasting for months or years, with remissions and exacerbations.
○ Predilection for involvement of the central nervous system
○ Absence of immune response or an immune response that does not arrest the disease, but may actually contribute to pathogenesis
○ Genetic predisposition
○ Invariable fatal termination

Classification

Group A

○ Slowly progressive infections of sheep, caused by lentivirus

Group B

○ Prion diseases of CNS (Transmissible spongiform viral encephalopathies)

Group C

○ Subacute sclerosing panencephalitis
○ Progressive multifocal leukoencephalopathy

PART-III

5. Write briefly on Amoebic liver abscess.

ANSWER

- Amoebic liver abscess is an uncommon but potentially life-threatening complication of infection with the protozoan parasite *Entamoeba histolytica*.
- Trophozoites of E. histolytica are carried as emboli by the radicles of portal vein.
- Capillary system of liver acts as an excellent filter to hold these parasites
- Their multiplication occurs in liver and leads to cytolutic action
- Amoebae obstruct the portal venules and result in anemic necrosis of hepatic cells.
- Necrosis is followed by cytolysis
- Small military abscesses coalesce to form big liver abscesses

- They predominate in the age group of 20-60 years
- It has marked preference for right lobe of the liver.
- A section through the margins of liver abscess can be differentiated into 3 zones:
  - Necrotic center with thick pus and no amoebae
  - Intermediate zone of degenerated liver cells, a few red cells and occasionally trophozoites of E. histolytica
  - Outer zone of nearly normal hepatic tissues just being invaded by amoebae

6. Write briefly on prophylaxis against rabies.

(Ref: Ananthanaryan & Paniker, Textbook of Microbiology, 10th ed, pg.536)

ANSWER

For answer, refer 2017 paper-II Q. 6, Pg. 351

Name of the Paper   :   **Microbiology Paper-I**

Name of the Course   :   **MBBS-2008**

Semester   :   **Annual**

Time: 3 Hours   M.M.: 40

INSTRUCTIONS

1. Write your Roll No. on the top immediately on receipt of this question paper
2. All questions are to be attempted
3. Answers to Parts I, II and III should be written in separate answer sheets provided
4. Attempt parts of a question in sequence

PART-I

1. Describe the methods and applications of sterilization using moist heat.   [5]
2. Write short notes on: [10]
   a. Cell mediated immunity
   b. Immunofluorescence

PART-II

3. Discuss the various methods of detecting antimicrobial resistance in the laboratory.   [5]
4. Write short notes on: [10]
   a. Leptospirosis
   b. Diphtheria toxin

PART-III

5. Enumerate the bacterial causes of community acquired pneumonia and discuss its laboratory diagnosis.   [5]
6. Describe the pathogenesis and laboratory diagnosis of bacillary dysentery.   [5]

PART-I

1. Describe the methods and applications of sterilization using moist heat.

(Ref: Ananthanaryan & Paniker, Textbook of Microbiology,10th ed, pg.30)

ANSWER

For answer, refer 2017 paper-I Q. 2 (a), Pg. 339

2. Write short notes on:

a. Cell-mediated immunity

(Ref: Ananthanaryan & Paniker, Textbook of Microbiology,10th ed, pg.147)

ANSWER

- This system is important when antigens do not come in body fluids and remain confined to some cells.
- After maturation in thymus, if T lymphocyte encounter an antigen, they get differentiated into cytotoxic, helper, suppressor and Memory T cells – together known as lymphoblasts.
- They release lymphokines that attract immune cells like macrophages and other lymphocytes to the site of infection and prepare them for immune response.
- The lymphokines help B cells to prepare antibodies too.
- Cytotoxic T cells are meant to kill the infected cells with the help of perforin, which is a protein secreted by them.
- The perforin makes a hole in the membrane of affected cell and the cell bursts due to hydration.
- Helper T cells help the killer cells and also help the B cells to produce antibodies.
- Suppressor cells control the immune response after the infection is countered.
- Memory T cells remember the previous contact with the same antigen and helps to boost up the action in future.
- Functions of Cellular Immunity
  - It helps in activating antigen-specific cytotoxic T-lymphocytes that are able to induce apoptosis in body
  - Cells having receptors on their surface, such as virus-infected cells, cells with intracellular bacteria, and cancer cells displaying tumor antigens.

- It also activates macrophages and natural killer cells and enables them to destroy intracellular pathogens.
- It stimulates cells to secrete a variety of cytokines that influence the function of other cells involved in adaptive immune responses and innate immune responses

b. Immunofluorescence

(Ref: Ananthanaryan & Paniker, Textbook of Microbiology,10th ed, pg.483)

ANSWER

- The antigens and antibodies possess a property of specificity for each other and when they are attached or tagged with a suitable fluorescence molecule like fluorescein and rhodamine dyes, they absorb light of shorter wave length (UV light) and emit light of longer wave length (visible light).
- As a result, the antigen-antibody complexes fluoresce and can be detected by fluorimeter or a UV/ fluorescence microscope.
- The fluorescence molecules like propidium iodide that binds to DNA in dead cells or Evans blue which binds to nonfluorescence cells are used in the tests.
- The other fluorescence molecules include fluorescein, rhodamine and Texas red.

PART-II

3. Discuss the various methods of detecting antimicrobial resistance in the laboratory.

ANSWER

- Dilution methods
  - The Broth dilution method involves subjecting the isolate to a series of concentrations of antimicrobial agents in a broth environment.
  - Microdilution testing uses about 0.05 to 0.1 mL total broth volume and can be conveniently performed in a microtiter format.
  - Macrodilution testing uses broth volumes at about 1.0 mL in standard test tubes.
  - For both of these broth dilution methods, the lowest concentration at which the isolate is completely inhibited (as evidenced by the absence of visible bacterial growth) is recorded as the minimal inhibitory concentration or MIC.

- **Disk Diffusion test**
  - Because of convenience, efficiency and cost, the disk diffusion method is probably the most widely used method for determining antimicrobial resistance in private veterinary clinics.
- **E-test**
  - E-test is a commercially available test that utilizes a plastic test strip impregnated with a gradually decreasing concentration of a particular antibiotic.
  - The strip also displays a numerical scale that corresponds to the antibiotic concentration contained therein.
  - This method provides for a convenient quantitative test of antibiotic resistance of a clinical isolate.
  - However, a separate strip is needed for each antibiotic, and therefore the cost of this method can be high.
- **Automated antimicrobial susceptibility testing systems**
  - Most automated antimicrobial susceptibility testing systems provide automated inoculation, reading and interpretation.
- **Mechanism specific tests**
  - Resistance may also be established through tests that directly detect the presence of a particular resistance mechanism.
  - For example, beta lactamase detection can be accomplished using an assay such as the chromogenic cephalosporinase test
- **Genotypic methods**
  - Since resistance traits are genetically encoded, we can sometimes test for the specific genes that confer antibiotic resistance.
  - However, although nucleic acid-based detections systems are generally rapid and sensitive, it is important to remember that the presence of a resistance gene does not necessarily equate to treatment failure, because resistance is also dependent on the mode and level of expression of these genes.
  - Commonly used methods are: PCR and DNA hybridization.

4. **Write short notes on:**

a. **Leptospirosis**

(Ref: Ananthanaryan & Paniker, Textbook of Microbiology,10th ed, pg.390)

ANSWER

- Leptospirosis is an infectious zoonotic disease of vertebrates, except humans.

- The wild rats act as reservoir of infection and is one of the commonest zoonotic diseases in areas with poor sanitation, moisture and soil exposure.
- The organisms localize in the convoluted tubules of kidneys of animal and are excreted with urine.
- Infection in humans is transmitted with contaminated food, water or cuts and abrasions on the skin.
- After an incubation period of 1–8 weeks, the organism disseminates in the body with blood stream causing severe jaundice or Weil's disease.
- The patient complains headache, fever, retro-orbital pain with photophobia, rigors, conjunctivitis, nausea, vomiting, diarrhea, myalgia especially in calf muscles or in lumbar region and dry cough.
- In severe form of Weil's disease, the patient suffers from icterus jaundice, hemorrhage, renal failure with oliguria and systemic inflammatory syndrome.

b. **Diphtheria toxin**

(Ref: Ananthanaryan & Paniker, Textbook of Microbiology,10th ed, pg.239)

ANSWER

- Diphtheria toxin is an exotoxin secreted by Corynebacterium diphtheriae, the pathogenic bacterium that causes diphtheria.
- Unusually, the toxin gene is encoded by a bacteriophage (a virus that infects bacteria).
- The toxin causes the disease in humans by gaining entry into the cell cytoplasm and inhibiting protein synthesis.
- It is an acidic, globular protein (PH 4.1) with a molecular weight most recently estimated at 62,000 to 63,000.
- As far as is known, it contains no unusual amino acids, no nonprotein moieties, and no other gross features to distinguish it from a wide variety of other nontoxic proteins.
- It is not as potent on a weight or molar basis as certain other bacterial toxins, such as those of the botulinum and tetanus bacilli, but its toxicity is remarkable nonetheless.

PART-III

5. **Enumerate the bacterial causes of community acquired pneumonia and discuss its laboratory diagnosis.**

(Ref: Ananthanaryan & Paniker, Textbook of Microbiology,10th ed, pg.321)

ANSWER

For answer, refer 2012 paper–I Q. 5, Pg. 403

6. **Describe the pathogenesis and laboratory diagnosis of bacillary dysentery.**

(Ref: Ananthanaryan & Paniker, Textbook of Microbiology,10th ed, pg.293)

ANSWER

Bacillary Dysentery

Bacillary Dysentery is caused by infection with Shigella Spp.

Pathogenesis

○ Infection is initiated by ingestion of shigellae (usually via fecal-oral contamination).

○ An early symptom, diarrhea (possibly elicited by enterotoxins and/or cytotoxin), may occur as the organisms pass through the small intestine.

○ The hallmarks of shigellosis are bacterial invasion of the colonic epithelium and inflammatory colitis.

○ These are interdependent processes amplified by local release of cytokines and by the infiltration of inflammatory elements.

○ **Colitis in the rectosigmoid mucosa, with concomitant malabsorption, results in the characteristic sign of bacillary dysentery:** Scanty, unformed stools tinged with blood and mucus.

Laboratory Diagnosis

○ **Hematology**

  ▪ The total WBC count reveals no consistent findings. A shift to the left (increased number of band cells) in the differential WBC count in a patient with diarrhea suggests bacillary dysentery. Leukopenia or leukemoid reactions are occasionally detected.

  ▪ In HUS, anemia and thrombocytopenia occur.

  ▪ Bacteremia is rare, even in severe disease, possibly due to the superficial nature of Shigella infection; the organism rarely penetrates beyond the mucosa.

  ▪ Blood culture should be obtained in children who appear toxic, very young, severely ill, malnourished, or immunocompromised because of their increased risk of bacteremia.

○ **Stool examination**

  ▪ Isolation of Shigella from feces or rectal swab specimen is diagnostic but lacks specificity. Routine microscopy may reveal sheets of leukocytes on methylene-blue stained stool smear, which is a sensitive test for colitis but not specific for Shigella species.

  ▪ In approximately 70% of patients with shigellosis, fecal blood or leukocytes (confirming colitis) are detectable in the stool.

○ **Stool culture**

  ▪ A sample for stool culture should be obtained in all suspected cases of shigellosis.

  ▪ The yield from stool cultures is greatest early in the course of disease. Guidelines for obtaining specimens to improve the yield are as follows:

    ◆ Process specimens immediately after collection.

    ◆ If processing is delayed, use a transport medium (e.g, buffered glycerol saline).

    ◆ Collect more than one stool or rectal (not anal) swab and inoculate them promptly on at least 2 different culture media.

    ◆ Specimens should be plated lightly onto MacConkey, xylose-lysine-deoxycholate, Hektoen enteric, or Salmonella-Shigella, or eosin-methylene blue agars.

  ▪ If processing is delayed, a rectal-swab sample can be placed in Cary-Blair transport medium or buffered glycerol saline.

  ▪ After overnight incubation, colorless, nonlactose-fermenting colonies may be tested by means of latex agglutination to establish a preliminary identification of Shigella infection.

  ▪ Antimicrobial susceptibility tests of all confirmed isolates should be performed by using the agar diffusion technique. The agar and broth-dilution methods are also widely used. The new Epsilometer strip method (E test) is used to accurately determine the minimum inhibitory concentration (MIC).

  ▪ Despite meticulous care in obtaining and processing specimens from patients infected with Shigella species, approximately 20% may fail to yield Shigella organisms.

○ **Enzyme immunoassay:** An enzyme immunoassay for Stx is used to detect S *dysenteriae* type 1 in the stool.

Your Roll No. ....

Name of the Paper	:	**Microbiology Paper-II**
Name of the Course	:	**MBBS-2008**
Semester	:	**Annual**

Time: 3 Hours   M.M.: 40

INSTRUCTIONS

1. Write your Roll No. on the top immediately on receipt of this question paper
2. All questions are to be attempted
3. Answers to Parts I, II and III should be written in separate answer sheets provided
4. Attempt parts of a question in sequence

PART-i

1. Describe the life cycle and diagnosis of the agent causing hydatid disease.   [5]

2. Write short notes on: [10]
   a. The differences between Plasmodium vivax and Plasmodium falciparum on peripheral blood smear examination
   b. Larva migrans

PART-II

3. Discuss the opportunistic fungal infection in HIV/AIDS.   [5]

4. Write short notes on: [10]
   a. Cryptococcus neoformans
   b. Direct demonstration of fungi in clinical samples

PART-III

5. Enumerate 3 viruses transmitted by mosquito. Discuss the laboratory diagnosis of any one of these.   [5]

6. Describe the principles and strategies for prevention and eradication of poliomyelitis.   [5]

PART-I

1. Describe the life cycle and diagnosis of the agent causing hydatid disease.

ANSWER

For answer, refer 2017 paper–II Q. 2 (b), Pg. 446

2. Write short notes on:

a. **The differences between Plasmodium vivax and Plasmodium falciparum on peripheral blood smear examination**

ANSWER

	P. Vivax	P. falciparum
Forms in peripheral blood	Trophozoites, schizonts and gametocytes	Rings and crescents (gametocytes)
Early trophozoite or ring stage	Large, 2.5 µm in diameter, usually one prominent chromatin dot, sometimes two, cytoplasm opposite the chromatin dot thicker, usually one and occasionally two rings in one red blood cell.	Small, delicate, 1.25–1.5 µm in diameter, often with two chromatin dots, two rings in one red blood cell common. Some parasites lie along the red cell membrane. These are known as accole forms
Late trophozoite	Large, markedly amoeboid, prominent vacuole	Medium-sized, compact and rounded
Schizont	Large, 9–10 µm in diameter, almost fills an enlarged red cell	Small, 4.5–5.0 µm in diameter, fills two-thirds of normal-sized red blood cell which is not enlarged
Number of merozoites	12–24	14-32
Microgametocytes	Spherical, 9–10 µm in diameter, compact, no vacuole, diffuse chromatin, cytoplasm stains light blue or reddish	Crescent-shaped (banana-shaped), 8–10 µm × 2–3 µm, chromatin diffuse
Macrogametocytes	Spherical, 10–12 µm in diameter, compact, larger than microgametocyte, compact chromatin, cytoplasm stains dark blue	Crescent-shaped, longer and more slender, 10–12 µm chromatin compact, cytoplasm stains dark blue
Malaria pigment	Yellowish-brown; fine granules	Dark brown; one or two solid blocks
Age of red blood cells invaded	Young	All ages (young and old)
Alterations in infected red cell	Enlarged, pale and the portion of the cytoplasm not occupied by the parasite shows a dotted or stippled appearance, called Schuffner's dots. With Leishman stain they appear as fine pink granules	Normal size and possesses 6–12 Maurer's dots which stain brick-red with Leishman stain
Duration of erythrocytic schizogony	48 hours	36–48 hours
Presence of secondary exoerythrocytic cycle	Yes	No

MICROBIOLOGY

b. Larva migrans

Answer

Larva Migrans is of 2 Types:

○ **Visceral larva migrans:** It is a condition in humans caused by the migratory larvae of certain nematodes, humans being a dead-end host. Nematodes causing such zoonotic infections Toxocara canis, Toxocara cati, and Ascaris suum. These nematodes can infect but not mature in humans and after migrating through the intestinal wall, travel with the blood stream to various organs where they cause inflammation and damage. Affected organs can include the liver, heart (causing myocarditis) and the CNS (causing dysfunction, seizures, and coma). A special variant is ocular larva migrans where usually T. canis larvae travel to the eye.

○ **Cutaneous larva migrans:** Cutaneous larva migrans is a parasitic skin infection caused by hookworm larvae that usually infest cats, dogs and other animals. Humans can be infected with the larvae by walking barefoot on sandy beaches or contacting moist soft soil that have been contaminated with animal faeces. It is also known as creeping eruption as once infected, the larvae migrate under the skin›s surface and cause itchy red lines or tracks..

PART-II

3. Discuss the opportunistic fungal infection in HIV/AIDS.

(Ref: Ananthanaryan & Paniker, Textbook of Microbiology,10th ed, pg.574)

Answer

Fungi contribute greatly to opportunistic infections in patients with late-stage HIV infection. Pneumocystis jirovecii is the most common cause of respiratory infection and Cryptococcus neoformans the most common cause of CNS infection in patients with AIDS across large parts of the world. Histoplasma capsulatum (especially common in parts of the Americas) and Talaromyces (formerly Penicillium) marneffei (endemic in south and southeast Asia) are thermally dimorphic fungi that cause disseminated infections.

○ Pneumocystis pneumonia has emerged as a major cause of infection in those with HIV/AIDS. during periods of immune suppression such as in patients with HIV who have CD4 counts lower than 200 cells per μL, the organism proliferates, leading to life-threatening pneumonia. In the absence of effective CD4-based immunity, innate inflammatory responses promote the accumulation of inflammatory cells, including neutrophils and CD8 lymphocytes, which strongly contribute to lung injury.

○ Patients with cryptococcal meningitis present with headache and fever, with a median duration of 2 weeks between symptom onset and first presentation. Many patients develop nausea, vomiting, diplopia due to cranial nerve VI palsies, and reduced visual acuity related to raised cerebrospinal fluid pressure. If untreated, symptoms progress to abnormal mental status, reduced conscious level, seizures, and finally coma.

○ HIV-associated histoplasmosis is more widespread than was previously thought and is probably neglected, undiagnosed, or misdiagnosed as tuberculosis. fragments, which are inhaled and, at body temperature, convert into yeasts in the lungs. Infection might also develop when, years after the primary infection, quiescent organisms are reactivated during immunosuppression. Once in the lungs, H. capsulatum survives phagocytosis in macrophages, facilitating its dissemination throughout the mononuclear phagocyte system. people with HIV are at higher risk of disseminated histoplasmosis, an AIDS-defining disease, which is lethal if left untreated.

○ Most infections with talaromycosis occur in patients with CD4 counts lower than 100 cells per μL. Patients typically develop disseminated disease with fever, weight loss, hepatosplenomegaly, lymphadenopathy, and respiratory and gastrointestinal abnormalities. Papulonecrotic skin lesions are present in 60–70% of patients.

4. Write short notes on:

a. **Cryptococcus neoformans**

(Ref: Ananthanaryan & Paniker, Textbook of Microbiology,10th ed, pg.617)

Answer

○ Cryptococcus neoformans is a round or oval yeast (4–6 μm in diameter), surrounded by a capsule that can be up to 30 μm thick.

○ The organism grows readily on fungal or bacterial culture media and is usually detectable within 1 week after inoculation, although in some circumstances up to 4 weeks are required for growth.

○ Cryptococcus neoformans var. neoformans is the major cause of cryptococcal disease worldwide.

○ C. neoformans is the most common cause of meningitis in HIV patients, occurring when CD4 + counts decline below 100 cells/mm³.

○ Because signs and symptoms of meningitis can be subtle in HIV-infected persons, isolation of Cryptococcus from any site must be followed by a lumbar puncture to rule out meningitis.

b. Direct demonstration of fungi in clinical samples

ANSWER

Almost all the specimens are processed for direct microscopic examination. This provides the presumptive diagnosis for the physician and also aid in the selection of appropriate culture media. Various methods for direct examinations are

○ **India Ink:** Used for negative staining of capsulated yeast e.g. cryptococcus

○ **KOH:** Skin crapings and other tissue specimens are examined as wet mounts after treatment with 10% KOH. It digests the tissue materials and fungal elements can be hence visualized easily

○ **Calcofluorl mounts:** it is a sensitive technique that provides good visualization of fungal morphology

○ Lactophenol cotton blue (LPCB) mounts: It is used for microscopic study of fungal colonies teased on to a slide and mounted.

○ **Gram stain:** It is used to visualize yeast and yeast-like fungi

○ **Methenamine silver and periodic acid Schiff:** Valuable methods for visualizing fungi in tissues.

PART-III

5. Enumerate 3 viruses transmitted by mosquito. Discuss the laboratory diagnosis of any one of these.

(Ref: Ananthanaryan & Paniker, Textbook of Microbiology,10th ed, pg.530)

ANSWER

3 Viruses that spread through mosquito are:

○ Yellow fever,
○ Dengue fever,
○ Zika fever
○ Chikungunya

Laboratory Diagnosis of Zika Virus

○ Molecular Test for Zika Virus
▪ For symptomatic persons with Zika virus infection, Zika virus RNA can sometimes be detected early in the course of illness. RNA NAT (nucleic acid testing) should be performed on paired serum and urine specimens.

▪ NAT testing of symptomatic non-pregnant individuals should be performed on specimens collected <14 days post-symptom onset. NAT testing is not recommended for asymptomatic non-pregnant individuals. A negative NAT result does not exclude Zika virus infection.

○ The Trioplex rRT-PCR is a laboratory test designed to detect Zika virus, dengue virus, and chikungunya virus RNA.

○ Serologic Test for Zika Virus

▪ Zika virus-specific IgM and neutralizing antibodies typically develop toward the end of the first week of illness. IgM levels are variable, but generally are positive starting near day 4 after onset of symptoms and continuing for up to 12 weeks post symptom onset or exposure, but may persist longer.

○ **Zika MAC-Elisa:** The Zika IgM Antibody Capture Enzyme-Linked Immunosorbent Assay (Zika MAC-ELISA) is used for the qualitative detection of Zika virus IgM antibodies in serum or cerebrospinal fluid; however, due to cross-reaction with other flaviviruses and possible nonspecific reactivity, results may be difficult to interpret. Consequently, presumed positive, equivocal, or inconclusive tests must be forwarded for confirmation by plaque-reduction neutralization testing (PRNT).

6. Describe the principles and strategies for prevention and eradication of poliomyelitis.

(Ref: Ananthanaryan & Paniker, Textbook of Microbiology,10th ed, pg.492)

○ It was considered possible to eradicate the disease by global immunization with OPV.

○ Successful poliomyelitis prevention depends upon the epidemiological characteristics of the infection and the immune status of the population in the area.

○ Presently available polio vaccines may prove very useful for progress with polio control, provided the prevention program has been adequately chosen and the limitations of the vaccine used have been taken into consideration.

○ In the present and near future, polio prevention should aim at the containment and local elimination of the paralytic disease, which can be obtained with either OPV or E-IPV.

○ Since its launch at the World Health Assembly (WHA) in 1988, the Global Polio Eradication Initiative (GPEI) has reduced the global incidence of polio by more than 99% and the number of countries with endemic polio from 125 to 3. More than 10 million people are walking today who otherwise would have been paralyzed

o The year 2012 saw tremendous advances for the programme, setting up the possibility to end polio for good.

o Among the most significant advances is India which, in February 2012, celebrated a full year without a child paralyzed by indigenous wild poliovirus (WPV).

o India was arguably the most technically challenging place to eliminate polio. The country's success was due to the ability of the program to repeatedly reach all children; the use of a new bivalent oral polio vaccine (bOPV); sustained political commitment and accountability; societal support; and the availability of resources needed to complete the job. The country remains polio-free today.

Name of the Paper	:	**Microbiology Paper-I**
Name of the Course	:	**MBBS-2007**
Semester	:	**Annual**

Time: 3 Hours   M.M.: 40

INSTRUCTIONS

1. Write your Roll No. on the top immediately on receipt of this question paper
2. All questions are to be attempted
3. Answers to Parts I, II and III should be written in separate answer sheets provided
4. Attempt parts of a question in sequence

PART-I

1. Describe briefly principle and functions of hot air oven.   [5]

2. Write short notes on: [10]
   a. IgM Antibody
   b. Adjuvants

PART-II

3. Classify mycobacteria. Write briefly about the laboratory diagnosis of Pulmonary tuberculosis.   [5]

4. Write short notes on: [10]
   a. TRIC agents
   b. Helicobacter pylori

PART-III

5. Define biomedical waste. Discuss briefly methods of disposal.   [5]

6. Describe briefly principle and use of Polymerase chain reaction (PCR).   [5]

PART-I

1. Describe briefly principles and functions of hot air oven.

(Ref: Ananthanaryan & Paniker, Textbook of Microbiology,10th ed, pg. 29-30)

ANSWER

Hot Air Oven

○ Hot air oven is the most widely used method of sterilization

○ Uses dry heat for sterilization and it is achieved by conduction

Principle

○ Inside the chamber, the air flows in a forced circulation manner that allows appropriate heat distribution in the chamber.

○ As the air becomes hot inside the chamber, it becomes lighter and moves in upward direction. As it reaches the top, the fan inside pushes it back to the bottom.

○ The creates a circular motion inside the cabinet and a consistent flow of the air is maintained. Eventually, with this process, optimum temperature is reached.

○ The heat is absorbed by the outside surface of the item, then passes towards the centre of the item, layer by layer. The entire item will eventually reach the temperature required for sterilization to take place.

○ The commonly-used temperatures and time that hot air ovens need to sterilize materials is 180°C for 30 minutes, 170°C for 60 minutes, and 160°C for 120 minutes.

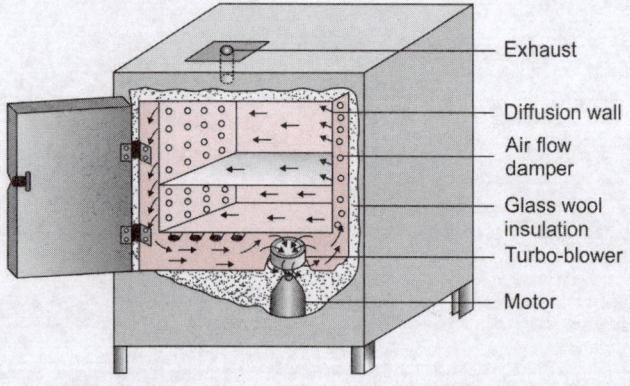

Exhaust
Diffusion wall
Air flow damper
Glass wool insulation
Turbo-blower
Motor

Fig. Hot air oven

2. Write short notes on:

a. IgM Antibody

(Ref: Ananthanaryan & Paniker, Textbook of Microbiology,10th ed, pg. 100)

ANSWER

For answer, refer 2015 paper–I Q. 2 (b), Pg. 34

b. Adjuvants

ANSWER

○ Any substance that increases the immunogenicity of an antigen is an adjuvant.

○ They may confer

  ▪ Immunogenicity on non antigenic substances,

  ▪ Increases the concentration and persistence of circulating antibody,

  ▪ Induce or enhance the degree of cellular immunity

  ▪ Lead to production of adjuvant diseases such as allergic disseminated encephalomyelitis.

○ The most potent adjuvant is Freund's complete adjuvant, which is the incomplete adjuvant along with a suspension of killed tubercle bacilli

PART-II

3. Classify mycobacteria. Write briefly about the laboratory diagnosis of Pulmonary tuberculosis.

(Ref: Ananthanaryan & Paniker, Textbook of Microbiology,10th ed, pg. 351)

ANSWER

Classification of Mycobacteria

○ Tubercle bacilli

  ▪ Human– MTB

  ▪ Bovine– M. bovis

  ▪ Murine– M. microti

  ▪ Avian– M. avium

  ▪ Cold blooded–M. marinum

○ Lepra bacilli

  ▪ Human–M. leprae

  ▪ Rat–M. Lepraemurium

○ Mycobacteria causing skin ulcers

- M. ulcerans
- M. belinelli
○ Atypical Mycobacteria (Runyon Groups)
  - Photochromogens
  - Scotochromigens
  - Nonphotochromogens
  - Rapid growers
○ Johne's bacillus
  - M. paratuberculosis
○ Saprophytic mycobacteria
  - M. butyricum
  - M. phlei
  - M. stercoralis
  - M. smegmatis
  - Others

Laboratory Diagnosis of Pulmonary Tuberculosis

○ Chest X-ray: Anyone with a cough that lasts for two weeks or more or with unexplained chronic fever and/ or weight loss should be evaluated for TB11. Chest X-ray is the primary radiologic evaluation of suspected or proven pulmonary TB. Radiological presentation of TB may be variable but in many cases is quite characteristic. Radiology also provides essential information for management and follow-up of these patients and is extremely valuable for monitoring complications.

○ For pulmonary TB, sputum is the most critical sample for laboratory testing. Direct sputum smear microscopy is the most widely used method for diagnosing pulmonary TB and is available in most primary health-care laboratories

○ Conventional light microscopy of Ziehl-Neelsen-stained smears prepared directly from sputum specimens is the most widely available test for diagnosing TB in resource-limited settings. Ziehl-Neelsen microscopy is highly specific, but its sensitivity is variable

○ The Xpert MTB/RIF assay (Cepheid, Sunnyvale, CA, USA; hereafter referred to as Xpert MTB/RIF) is a novel, rapid, automated, and cartridge-based NAA test that can detect TB along with rifampicin resistance directly from sputum within 2 hours of collection

---

4. **Write short notes on:**

   a. **TRIC agents**

   (Ref: Ananthanaryan & Paniker, Textbook of Microbiology,10th ed, pg.424)

ANSWER

○ TRIC is derived from words Trachoma and Inclusion Conjunctivitis.

○ Both of these ophthalmic diseases are produced by a bacterium Chlamydia trachomatis. Serotypes of C. trachomatis A to K are together called TRIC agents.

○ Chlamydiae are obligate intracellular parasitic organisms that exclusively infect humans. They were once considered as viruses.

○ Though they can't be stained well with Gram's stain, they are considered gram negative on the basis of cell wall structure.

○ The cell wall is proposed to be gram-negative in that it contains an outer lipopolysaccharide membrane, but it lacks peptidoglycan in its cell wall.

○ They exist in two forms, namely elementary body and reticulate body.

○ Elementary body is considered to be the extracellular infective form while reticulate body is the reproductive form that is seen in infected host cells.

○ Once inside, elementary body reorganizes into reticulate body. Over a 24-hour period, these reticulate bodies divide and begin to reorganize back into elementary bodies.

○ About 48–72 hours after infection, the cell is lysed and numerous infectious elementary bodies are released.

b. **Helicobacter pylori**

(Ref: Ananthanaryan & Paniker, Textbook of Microbiology,10th ed, pg. 407)

ANSWER

○ Helicobacter pylori (H. pylori) is a gram negative, curved or spiral shaped bacteria.

○ It is the major cause of peptic ulcer disease and gastritis.

○ Approximately two-thirds of the world's population are infected with H.pylori.

○ H.pylori is found in the gastric mucous layer or adherent to the epithelial lining of the stomach and causes more than 90% of duodenal ulcers and up to 80% of gastric ulcers.

○ Persons with active gastric or duodenal ulcers or documented history of ulcers should be tested for H. pylori.

○ Various tests are available to diagnose H. pylori infection. These tests can be categorized into those that are based on direct assessment of gastric biopsies (endoscopic testing) and indirect tests (nonendoscopic testing) that detect an immunological response (i.e. antibodies against H. pylori) or metabolic products (i.e. urease activity) of H. pylori

PART-III

5. Define biomedical waste. Discuss briefly methods of disposal.

(Ref: Ananthanaryan & Paniker, Textbook of Microbiology,10th ed, pg. 657)

ANSWER

Biomedical Waste

○ Any waste which is generated during the diagnosis, treatment or immunization of human beings or animals or in research activities pertaining thereto or in the production or testing of biological.

Methods of Disposal

○ **Incineration Technology**

▪ This is a high temperature thermal process employing combustion of the waste under controlled condition for converting them into inert material and gases.

▪ Incinerators can be oil fired or electrically powered or a combination thereof.

▪ Broadly, three types of incinerators are used for hospital waste: multiple hearth type, rotary kiln and controlled air types.

▪ All the types can have primary and secondary combustion chambers to ensure optimal combustion.

▪ These are refractory lined.

○ **Non-Incineration Technology**

▪ Non-incineration treatment includes four basic processes: Thermal, chemical, irradiative, and biological.

▪ The majority of non-incineration technologies employ the thermal and chemical processes.

▪ The main purpose of the treatment technology is to decontaminate waste by destroying pathogens.

○ **Autoclaving**

▪ The autoclave operates on the principle of the standard pressure cooker.

▪ The process involves using steam at high temperatures.

▪ The steam generated at high temperature penetrates waste material and kills all the microorganisms

▪ Autoclave treatment has been recommended for microbiology and biotechnology waste, waste sharps, soiled and solid wastes.

○ **Microwave Irradiation**

▪ The microwave is based on the principle of generation of high frequency waves

▪ These waves cause the particles within the waste material to vibrate, generating heat.

▪ This heat generated from within kills all pathogens.

○ **Chemical methods:** 1% hypochlorite solution can be used for chemical disinfection

○ Plasma Pyrolysis

▪ Plasma pyrolysis is a state-of-the-art technology for safe disposal of medical waste. It is an environment-friendly technology, which converts organic waste into commercially useful byproducts.

▪ The intense heat generated by the plasma enables it to dispose all types of waste including municipal solid waste, biomedical waste and hazardous waste in a safe and reliable manner.

▪ Medical waste is pyrolysed into CO, H_2, and hydrocarbons when it comes in contact with the plasma-arc.

▪ These gases are burned and produce a high temperature (around 1200°C).

6. Describe briefly principle and use of Polymerase chain reaction (PCR).

ANSWER

Principle

○ Polymerase chain reaction is method for amplifying particular segments of DNA. It is an enzymatic method and carried out in vitro. PCR technique was developed by Kary mullis in 1983. PCR is very simple, inexpensive technique for characterization, analysis and synthesis of specific fragments of DNA or RNA from virtually any living organisms.

Denaturation

○ Two strand of DNA separates (melt down) to form single stranded DNA

○ This step is generally carried out at 92°C–96°C for 2 minutes.

Annealing

○ Annealing of primer to each strand is carried out at 45°C–55°C

Extension

○ DNA polymerase adds dNTPs complementary to templates strands at 3'end of primer.

○ It is carried out at temperature of 72°C.

○ These three steps are repeated 20–30 times in an automated thermalcycler that can heat and cool the reaction mixture in tube within very short time. This results in exponential accumulation of specific DNA fragments.

○ The doubling of number of DNA strands corresponding to target sequences can be estimated by amplification number associated with each cycle using the formula.

Uses of PCR

○ PCR can amplify a desired DNA sequences of any origin hundred or millions time in a matter of hour, which is very short in comparison to recombinant DNA technology.

○ PCR is especially valuable because the reaction is highly specific, easily automated and very sensitive.

○ It is widely used in the fields like- clinical medicine for medical diagnosis, diagnosis of genetic diseases, forensic science; DNA finger printing, evolutional biology

Your Roll No. ....

Name of the Paper : **Microbiology Paper-II**

Name of the Course : **MBBS-2007**

Semester : **Annual**

Time: 3 Hours   M.M.: 40

INSTRUCTIONS

1. Write your Roll No. on the top immediately on receipt of this question paper
2. All questions are to be attempted
3. Answers to Parts I, II and III should be written in separate answer sheets provided
4. Attempt parts of a question in sequence

PART-I

1. Describe the life cycle of malarial parasite in details.   [5]

2. Write short notes on: [10]
    a. Amoebic liver abscess
    b. Casoni's test

PART-II

3. Name various genera of Dermatophytes. Discuss the laboratory diagnosis of infections caused by Dermatophytes.   [5]

4. Write short notes on: [10]
    a. Rhinosporidiosis
    b. Inclusion bodies

PART-III

5. Describe briefly various methods of viral cultivation.   [5]

6. Discuss the laboratory markers associated with progression of HIV infection.   [5]

PART-I

1. Describe the life cycle of malarial parasite in details.

(Ref: Arora parasitology 5th ed p 73,74)

ANSWER

For answer refer 2013 paper–II Q. 1, Pg. 393

2. Write short notes on:

a. Amoebic liver abscess

(Ref: Arora parasitology 5th ed p 25, 26)

ANSWER

For answer, refer 2009 paper–II Q. 5, Pg. 437

b. Casoni's test

(Ref: Arora parasitology 5th ed p 143, 144)

ANSWER

○ Intradermal test, used for diagnosis of hydatid cyst disease caused by Echinococcus granulosus (Dog tapeworm). Introduced by Casoni in 1911.

○ **Antigen used:** Hydatid fluid collected from animal/ human cyst and sterilized by Seitz filtration.

○ **Control:** Sterile saline.

○ **Principle of the test:** Immediate type of hypersensitivity primarily. Type IV Delayed hypersensitivity also plays a part.

○ **Test:** 0.2 ml of antigen injected intradermally on forearm and equal volume of saline injected on the other forearm. Observations made for next 30 mins and after 1 to 2 days.

○ **Positive test:** Appearance of wheal within 30 minutes on test forearm about 5 cm in diameter, with multiple pseudopodia like projections, fading in about an hour. There must not be any such a reaction on the control side.

○ Secondary reaction consisting of oedema and induration (Type IV–Tuberculin type Delayed type of hypersensitivity) after 8 hrs.

○ The test is very sensitive, but not specific. False positive reactions known to occur in other related parasitic infections.

○ **Precaution:** Being a type I hypersensitivity reaction, anaphylactic reaction tray must be kept ready before carrying out the test.

PART-II

3. Name various genera of Dermatophytes. Discuss the laboratory diagnosis of infections caused by Dermatophytes

(Ref: Ananthanaryan & Paniker, Textbook of Microbiology,10th ed, pg. 599, 600)

ANSWER

For answer, refer 2010 paper–II Q. 3, Pg. 428

4. Write short notes on:

a. Rhinosporidiosis

(Ref: Ananthanaryan & Paniker, Textbook of Microbiology,10th ed, pg. 607)

ANSWER

For answer refer 2009 paper–II Q. 4 (a), Pg. 436

b. Inclusion bodies

ANSWER

○ Inclusion bodies are distinctive abnormal structures in cells that are the result of viral infection. They require staining to make them visible and can then be observed through an optical microscope.

○ Inclusion bodies are distinctive for different viruses and so were useful in disease identification before molecular and genetic diagnostics were available

○ Examples of viral inclusion bodies in animals include
  - Negri bodies in Rabies
  - Henderson-Peterson bodies in Molluscum contagiosum
  - Cowdry type A in Herpes simplex virus and Varicella zoster virus
  - "Owl eyes" in cytomegalovirus

○ Inclusion bodies for different viruses can represent different structures resulting from the infection, they may appear within the cell cytoplasm, cell nucleus, or both.

○ Some inclusion bodies are known to be infective, these likely represent aggregates of virus particles in combination with cellular material; others are apparently not infective and are probably abnormal structures formed in the cell in response to infection.

PART-III

5. Describe briefly various methods of viral cultivation.

(Ref: Ananthanaryan & Paniker, Textbook of Microbiology,10th ed, pg. 440)

ANSWER

Viruses are obligate intracellular parasites so they depend on host for their survival. They cannot be grown in non- living culture media or on agar plates alone, they must require living cells to support their replication.

The primary purpose of virus cultivation is:

○ To isolate and identify viruses in clinical samples.
○ To do research on viral structure, replication, genetics and effects on host cell.
○ To prepare viruses for vaccine production.

Cultivation of viruses can be discussed under following headings:

○ Animal inoculation
○ Inoculation into embryonated egg
○ Cell culture

Animal Inoculation

○ Viruses which are not cultivated in embryonated egg and tissue culture are cultivated in laboratory animals such as mice, guinea pig, hamster, rabbits and primates are used.
○ The selected animals should be healthy and free from any communicable diseases.
○ Suckling mice (less than 48 hours old) are most commonly used.
○ Suckling mice are susceptible to togavirus and coxsackie viruses, which are inoculated by intracerebral and intranasal route.
○ Viruses can also be inoculated by intraperitoneal and subcutaneous route.
○ After inoculation, virus multiply in host and develops disease. The animals are observed for symptoms of disease and death.
○ Then the virus is isolated and purified from the tissue of these animals.
○ Live inoculation was first used on human volunteers for the study of yellow fever virus.

Inoculation Into Embryonated Egg

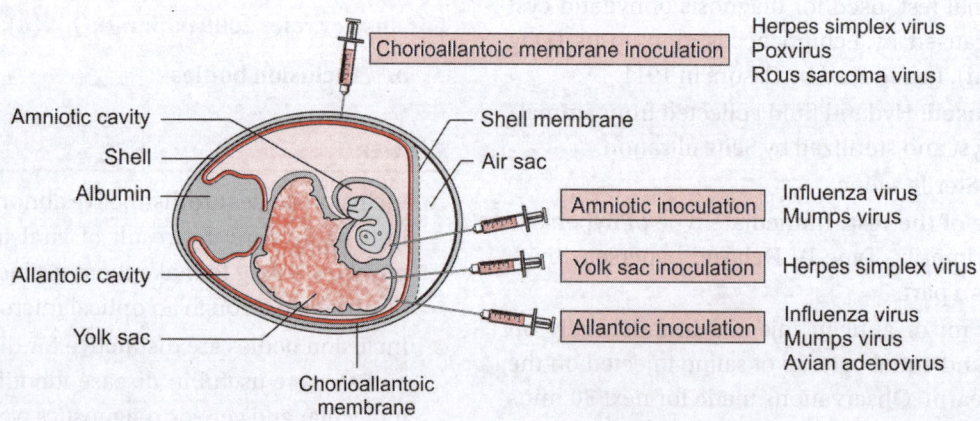

Fig. Inoculation into embryonated Egg

○ Good pasture in 1931 first used the embryonated hen's egg for the cultivation of virus.
○ The process of cultivation of viruses in embryonated eggs depends on the type of egg which is used.
○ Viruses are inoculated into chick embryo of 7–12 days old.
○ For inoculation, eggs are first prepared for cultivation, the shell surface is first disinfected with iodine and penetrated with a small sterile drill.

○ After inoculation, the opening is sealed with gelatin or paraffin and incubated at 36°C for 2–3 days.
○ After incubation, the egg is broken and virus is isolated from tissue of egg.
○ Viral growth and multiplication in the egg embryo is indicated by the death of the embryo, by embryo cell damage, or by the formation of typical pocks or lesions on the egg membranes

- Viruses can be cultivated in various parts of egg like chorioallantoic membrane, allantoic cavity, amniotic sac and yolk sac.

Cell Culture (Tissue Culture)

There are three types of tissue culture; organ culture, explant culture and cell culture. Cell culture is mostly used for identification and cultivation of viruses.

- Cell culture is the process by which cells are grown under controlled conditions.
- Cells are grown in vitro on glass or a treated plastic surface in a suitable growth medium.
- At first growth medium, usually balanced salt solution containing 13 amino acids, sugar, proteins, salts, calf serum, buffer, antibiotics and phenol red are taken and the host tissue or cell is inoculated.
- On incubation the cell divide and spread out on the glass surface to form a confluent monolayer.

---

6. **Discuss the laboratory markers associated with progression of HIV infection.**

(Ref: Ananthanaryan & Paniker, Textbook of Microbiology, 10th ed, pg.580, 581)

ANSWER

- Infection with HIV may develop to AIDS at different rates in different individuals, with a spectrum varying from rapid progression to long term non-progression.
- Markers of AIDS development include HIV related symptoms, depletion of CD4+ T cells, cutaneous energy, elevated serum b2-microglobulin (b2-m) and neopterin levels, HIV-1 p24 (core) antigenaemia, and syncytium inducing HIV-1 phenotype.

- None of these markers are ideal; all have limitations in sensitivity, specificity, or predictive power. The single best predictor of AIDS onset identified thus far, is the percentage or absolute number of circulating CD4+ T cells.
- Plasma viral load (HIV RNA) quantification is presently considered the most representative and sensitive laboratory test for monitoring progression of HIV infection and response to antiretroviral therapy.
- Active replication of virus occurs in all clinical stages of infection. It is possible to detect and quantify virus throughout the course of HIV infection. The viral load usually ranges between 102 and 107 HIV RNA copies/ mL in untreated individuals though it may be lower in those on treatment.
- A number of non HIV specific cellular markers, have been used for staging, monitoring progression of HIV infection and assessing response to therapy but the most commonly used cellular marker is the CD4 lymphocyte count.
- CD4 count can be measured by flow cytometry, microsphere assay, and Enzyme immunoassay (EIA). Antibodies to these antigens allow a rapid and accurate measurement by flow cytometry of the number of cells expressing each antigen.
- CD4 also serves as a receptor for HIV, and cells expressing this protein usually decline in number with progressive HIV infection. The number of cells that express the CD4 antigen is therefore a useful guide to the pathological effects of HIV on the immune system.
- Its decline is the hallmark of HIV infection and the rate of loss in each person is unique.

Forensic
Medicine & Toxicology

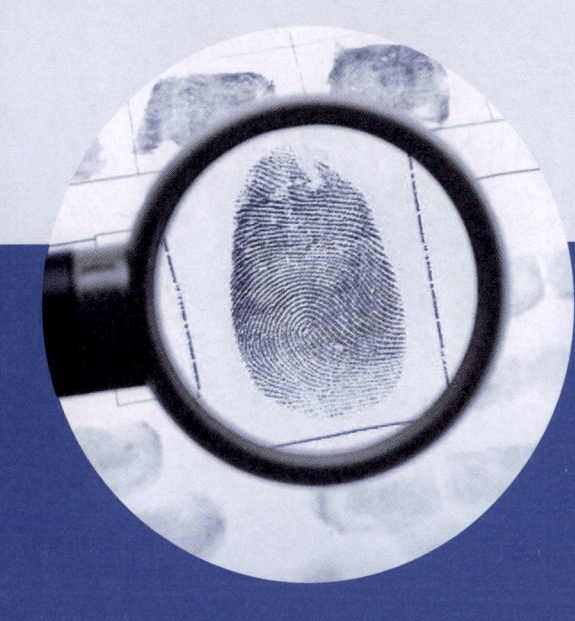

References Taken From:

- *The Essentials of Forensic Medicine & Toxicology, KS Narayan Reddy, & O.P. Murty, 34th edition*
- *Parikh's Textbook of Medical Jurisprudence, Forensic Medicine and Toxicology 7th edition*

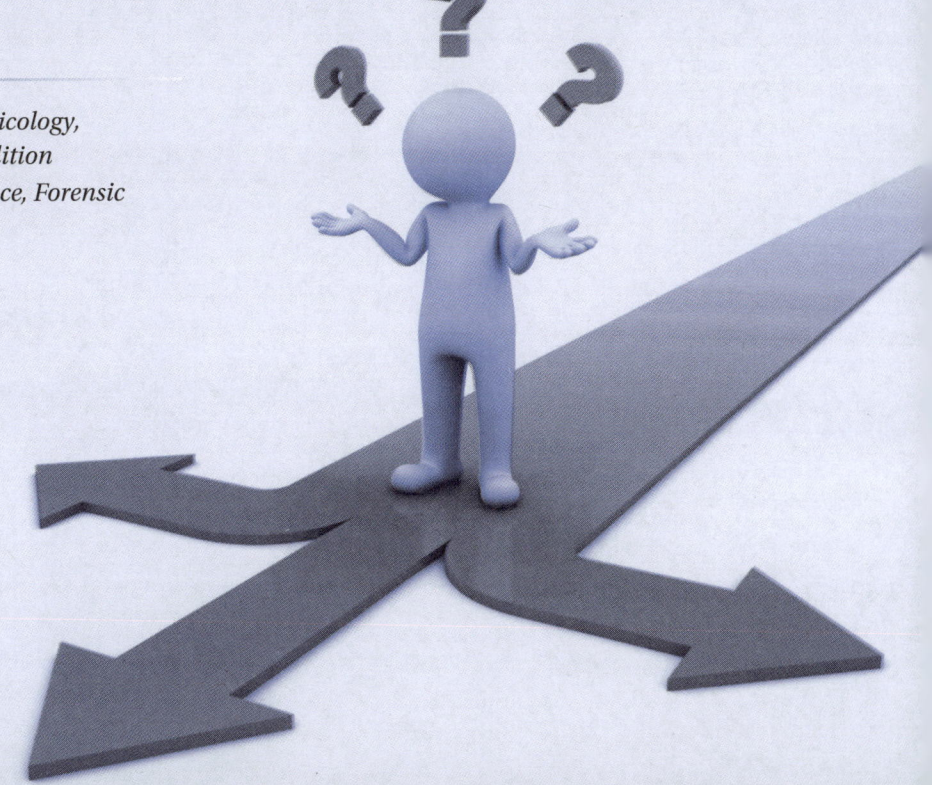

Your Roll No. ....

Name of the Paper	:	**Forensic Medicine & Toxicology**
Name of the Course	:	**MBBS-2017**
Semester	:	**Annual**

Time: 3 Hours   M.M.: 40

INSTRUCTIONS

1. Write your Roll No. on the top immediately on receipt of this question paper
2. All questions are to be attempted
3. Answers to Parts I, II and III should be written in separate answer sheets provided
4. Attempt parts of a question in sequence

PART-I

1. What are the findings and medicolegal importance when it is stated that: [8]
   a. The girl is 18 years of age
   b. The body is showing adipocere
   c. The death is due to Battered baby syndrome
   d. The boy is a habitual passive agent

2. Write short notes on: [6]
   a. Modern concept of moment of death
   b. Complications of criminal abortion
   c. Extradural hematoma

PART-II

3. Define stupefying agents. Describe clinical features and management of acute datura poisoning.   [7]

4. Differentiate between: [6]
   a. Male and female pelvis
   b. Homicidal and suicidal cut throat injury
   c. Civil negligence and criminal negligence

PART-III

5. Classify firearms. Discuss the findings of entry wounds caused by rifled firearms from various ranges.   [7]

6. Write short notes on: [6]
   a. Delirium
   b. Clinical features of chronic mercurial poisoning
   c. Cross examination

PART I

1. What are the findings and medicolegal importance when it is stated that?

a. The girl is 18 years of age

(Ref: Parikh's Textbook of Medical Jurisprudence, Forensic Medicine and Toxicology, 7/e, Pg. 59; The Essentials of Forensic Medicine & Toxicology, K.S. Narayan Reddy-34/e, pg. 78)

ANSWER

A Girl is of 18 Years Age

Findings

○ **Teeth:**
  ▪ Presence of 2 wisdom teeth
  ▪ On X-ray of wisdom teeth, roots are not calcified
○ **Ossification of bones:**
  ▪ All the epiphyses at the elbow, head of femur and lower end of tibia join the respective shafts
  ▪ All epiphyses at the wrist, knee, crest of ilium and lateral end of clavicle are united
  ▪ Acromion appeared but yet to unite
  ▪ Upper end of humerus is fused
  ▪ Inner end of clavicle appeared
○ **Sex:**
  ▪ Possession of developed breasts
  ▪ Female distribution of hair
  ▪ Distribution of subcutaneous fat
  ▪ Vagina is present

Interpretation

○ Union of epiphysis in cartilaginous bones takes place earlier by 2 years in females than in males except in case of skull sutures where obliteration sets in little later and proceeds more slowly in female than in males
○ Epiphyses at elbow join their respective shafts by 13–14 years in females

Medicolegal Importance

○ **Criminal responsibility**
  ▪ Child under 12 years of age cannot give valid consent to suffer harm which can occur from an act done in good faith and for its benefit e.g. consent for operation
  ▪ Person under 18 years of age cannot give valid consent whether express or implied to suffer any harm which may result from an act not intended to cause any grievous hurt e.g. consent for wrestling

○ **Judicial punishment**
  ▪ Children (boys below 16 years and girls below 18 years of age), who have committed a crime, are tried by Juvenile court and if convicted, are entrusted to parents for special care or sent to correctional school with facilities for education, vocational training and rehabilitation
○ **Employment**
  ▪ Child below 14 years of age cannot be employed for any type of work
○ **Kidnapping**
  ▪ Kidnapping or abducting a minor, if boy is under 16 and girl is under 18 years is an offence
○ **Marriage**
  ▪ The Child Marriage Restraint Act lays down that a girl under 18 years of age and a boy under 21 years of age cannot contract a valid marriage
○ **Attainment of majority**
  ▪ Under Indian Majority Act, persons domiciled in India attain majority on completion of 18 years, except when under a guardian appointed by a court or under a court of wards, when the individual attains majority on completion of 21 years
  ▪ Persons under this age are minors and they cannot make a valid will, sell his property or serve a jury
○ **Rape**
  ▪ Under section 375 IPC, sexual intercourse by a man with a girl under 18 years of age constitutes the offence of rape

b. The body is showing adipocere

(Ref: Parikh's Textbook of Medical Jurisprudence, Forensic Medicine and Toxicology, 7/e, Pg. 160; The Essentials of Forensic Medicine & Toxicology, K.S. Narayan Reddy-34/e, pg. 162)

ANSWER

The Body is Showing Adipocere

Findings

○ Yellowish white, greasy, wax-like substance with a rancid smell
○ Floats as specific gravity is less than water
○ Cuts easily and burns with faint yellow flame and produces offensive smell due to ammonia and traces of sulfur compounds
○ Fresh adipocere is soft and moist, old one is dry and brittle
○ **Forms in fatty tissues:** Cheeks, breasts, buttocks and abdomen

Interpretation

○ A body which has been immersed in water or in damp soil undergoes adipocere formation

Medicolegal Importance

○ Identification of person when external features are well preserved
○ Indication of the cause of death when injuries are recognizable
○ Indication of the time passed since death
○ **Indication of the place:** Water or moist ground– from which body has been recovered

c. The death is due to "Battered baby syndrome"

(Ref: Parikh's Textbook of Medical Jurisprudence, Forensic Medicine and Toxicology, 7/e, Pg. 360; The Essentials of Forensic Medicine & Toxicology, K.S. Narayan Reddy-34/e, pg. 417)

ANSWER

The Death is due to "Battered Baby Syndrome"

Findings

○ Bruises on face, trunk, extremities with grip marks
○ Tearing of frenum of upper lip and of alveolar margin of gums
○ Head injury
○ Fractured skull, subdural hematoma
○ Liver rupture, mesenteric hemorrhages
○ Fresh burns with cigarettes
○ Subconjunctival hemorrhages, detached retina, displaced lenses
○ Injuries to hyoid bone, thyroid cartilages
○ **Fractured ribs, vertebral bodies:** Nobbing fractures
○ Rupture of viscera
○ Incisions on soles of feet, avulsion and chipping of epiphyses at knee and elbow
○ Asymmetry of arms and legs

Medicolegal Importance

○ Victim may be unwanted child, an illegitimate child or a child whose father's paternity is in doubt
○ Result of sudden loss of temper
○ Accused may have low IQ, history of family discord, long standing emotional problems, financial stress or criminal background
○ Sometimes, it is seen that such parents had received similar treatment from their parents in their own childhood

d. The boy is a habitual passive agent

(Ref: Parikh's Textbook of Medical Jurisprudence, Forensic Medicine and Toxicology, 7/e, Pg. 408; The Essentials of Forensic Medicine & Toxicology, K.S. Narayan Reddy-34/e, pg. 399)

ANSWER

The Boy is a Habitual Passive Agent

Pediatric passive agent' is called catamite

Findings

○ **Anal skin:** Smooth and thick
○ **Anal opening:** Deeper than usual due to absorption of fat – appearance of funnel shaped depression
○ **Anal sphincter:** Lax, patulous opening, dilated canal, loss of rugosity of the anal mucosa
○ Presence of fissure or fissure scar, external and internal hemorrhoids
○ Incriminating stains on clothes
○ Anal hair may be shaved
○ Signs of implanted venereal disease

Medicolegal Importance

○ Evidence of sodomy is the presence of semen in anus
○ Medical examination of both active and passive agents is required for investigation of crime
○ False charges can be made for purpose of blackmail

2. Write short notes:

a. Modern concept of moment of death

(Ref: Parikh's Textbook of Medical Jurisprudence, Forensic Medicine and Toxicology, 7/e, Pg. 137; The Essentials of Forensic Medicine & Toxicology, K.S. Narayan Reddy-34/e, pg. 91)

ANSWER

Modern Concept of Moment of Death

Definition

○ Traditionally, death means irreversible and permanent cessation of life as evidenced by stoppage of brain function, respiratory activity and cardiac function

Modern Concept of Moment of Death

○ Since organ retrieval and scavenging for transplantation has started, brainstem death is considered death legally

Characteristics of Brainstem Death

○ Pupils are fixed in diameter
○ All reflexes are absent or lost i.e. light reflex, corneal reflex, oculocephalic reflex, heat and cold response, vestibulo-ocular reflex
○ Gag reflex is absent
○ Respiratory movements are absent on withdrawal of mechanical respirator
○ According to Organ Transplantation Act in India, brainstem death is legal death

Stages of Death

○ Somatic, systemic or clinical
  ▪ Due to complete and irreversible cessation of vital functions of the brain, followed by cessation of the functions of heart and lungs

○ Cellular or molecular

  ▪ After somatic death, tissues and cells survive for a varying period depending upon their oxygen requirements

  ▪ When these individual tissues and cells die, it is termed as cellular death

  ▪ Occurs piecemeal i.e. nervous tissue dies rapidly within 5 minutes whereas muscles survive up to about 3 to 4 hours

  ▪ Accompanied by cooling of the body, changes in the eye, skin and muscles

  ▪ It takes around 3–4 hours after somatic death

b. Complications of criminal abortion

(Ref: Parikh's Textbook of Medical Jurisprudence, Forensic Medicine and Toxicology, 7/e, Pg. 420)

ANSWER

Complications of Criminal Abortion

Complications of criminal abortions are as follows:

○ **Shock**

  ▪ Occur immediately from reflex vagal inhibition due to stimulation of the trigger area, namely, the cervix of the uterus by attempts at dilatation without an anesthetic

○ **Hemorrhage**

  ▪ Due to internal injuries or perforation of the vagina or the uterus

  ▪ May follow incomplete separation of membranes of the placenta from the uterine wall

  ▪ Uterus and pelvic organs are pale and anemic, if death occurred due to hemorrhage from criminal abortion, but are congested if death occurred during menstruation

○ **Air and fat emboli**

  ▪ Occur when a liquid or soapy solution is ingested under pressure by means of a syringe into the uterus

  ▪ Causes separation of the membranes and consequent exposure of the uterine raw surface through which air and fat may enter the maternal circulation leading to death in few minutes or hours

○ **Sepsis**

  ▪ Death may occur due to sepsis (clostridium welchii, hemolytic streptococci, anaerobic streptococci), tetanus or renal failure

IPC Relate to Criminal Abortion

○ **312 IPC:** Criminal abortion with consent (3yrs imprisonment and if woman is quick 7yrs imprisonment)

○ **313 IPC:** Criminal abortion without consent (10yrs imprisonment)

○ **314 IPC:** Criminal abortion leading to death (10yrs imprisonment and if act is done with her consent then he is punished with life imprisonment)

c Extradural hematoma

(Ref: Parikh's Textbook of Medical Jurisprudence, Forensic Medicine and Toxicology, 7/e, Pg. 295; The Essentials of Forensic Medicine & Toxicology, K.S. Narayan Reddy-34/e, pg. 242)

ANSWER

Extradural Hematoma

○ Least Common intracranial hemorrhage (10%).

Causes

○ Mostly traumatic in origin, and unilateral.

Salient Feature

○ It occurs usually on the side of the impact (coup injury).

○ Never a contrecoup injury.

Age Group

○ Common in adults between 20 and 40 years.

○ Rare in elderly and children due to greater adherence of dura to the skull.

○ Fracture (fissure type) is present in most of the cases.

○ Site and vessels

○ Blow impact over lateral convexity of head → fissure fracture of squamous temporal bone → rupture of underlying middle meningeal artery.

Common Vessels Involved

○ Anterior branch of middle Meningeal artery, Posterior branch of middle meningeal artery, Middle meningeal veins

Clinical Features

○ Loss of consciousness due to concussion.

○ Dilation of pupil on the side of hemorrhage with conjugate deviation of eyes to opposite side.

○ **Lucid interval:** It is a state of consciousness between two episodes of unconsciousness.

○ **CT scan:** Biconvex lenticular-shaped hemorrhage.

Medicolegal Aspects

○ Patient may be discharged from hospital during lucid interval and may die at home; doctor may be charged with negligence.

○ Extradural hemorrhage my resemble drunkenness and patient may die in police custody.

PART II

3. **Define stupefying agents. Describe clinical features and management of acute datura poisoning**

  a. Stupefying agents

  (Ref: Parikh's Textbook of Medical Jurisprudence, Forensic Medicine and Toxicology, 7/e, Pg. 633)

ANSWER

Definition

○ Substances which cause (someone) to be unable to think clearly or be sensitive to the surroundings

○ **Examples:** Datura, alcohol, cannabis, atropa belladonna, hyoscyamus

b. Acute datura poisoning

(Ref: Parikh's Textbook of Medical Jurisprudence, Forensic Medicine and Toxicology, 7/e, Pg. 634; The Essentials of Forensic Medicine & Toxicology, K.S. Narayan Reddy-34/e, pg. 91)

ANSWER

Clinical Picture

○ Symptoms appear within half an hour

○ Initial symptom is bitter taste in mouth

○ Dryness of the mouth and throat (dry as a bone)

○ Difficulty in talking, dysphagia and unquenchable thirst

○ Flushed face due to dilatation of cutaneous blood vessels (red as a beet)

○ Dilated pupils, insensitive to light, power for accommodation for near vision is paralyzed (blind as a bat)

○ Body temperature increased

○ **Skin:** Dry and hot (hot as a hare)

○ Vomiting followed by unsteady gait, giddiness, staggering like drunkard

○ Patient becomes restless and confused and later becomes delirious, mutters indistinct words (mad as a wet hen)

○ **Hallucinations:** Visual and auditory–appears to grasp imaginary things, picks at his clothes, tries to pull imaginary threads from tips of his fingers

○ When delirium passes off, patient becomes drowsy

○ Scarlatiniform rash appears

○ Drowsiness leads to stupor or coma and rarely death from respiratory paralysis

○ When patient recovers, secondary delirium occurs

Fatal Dose

○ 100–125 seeds

○ **Lethal dose for alkaloids:** 60 mg for adults and 4 mg for children

Fatal Period

○ Death occurs within 24 hours

Management

○ Stomach wash with either a weak solutions of potassium permanganate or 4–5% tannic acid

○ **Physostigmine:** 1–4 mg (repeated, if necessary, at intervals of 1–2 hours), or

○ **Neostigmine:** 2.5 mg IV every 3 hours

○ Purgatives are helpful

○ Rest is symptomatic treatment

○ Moistening of the tongue and change in size of pupils towards normal are significant points in treatment

Postmortem Appearances

○ Datura seeds are seen in stomach

○ Congestion of gastrointestinal tract

○ Datura seeds resist putrefaction and are observed even when body is decomposed

○ Signs of asphyxia are seen

Medicolegal Importance

○ In India, mainly used as stupefying poison prior to robbery, kidnapping and rape

○ **Also known as road poison:** Powdered seeds are mixed with food, tea, drink or paan (betel leaf) and given to innocent traveler by apparently considerate person and on ingestion of such things, person becomes drowsy, and his pockets are picked, belongings are stolen and police consider such person as drunkard owing to drunken gait and difficulty in talking

○ Children can be easily kidnapped by giving candy mixed with datura as they comply with the instructions of poisoner to follow him

○ Women can be abducted, robbed and raped

○ Accidental cases can occur by eating raw fruit or seeds mistaking them for edible fruits or capsicum seeds

4. Differentiate between

a. Male and female pelvis

(Ref: Parikh's Textbook of Medical Jurisprudence, Forensic Medicine and Toxicology, 7/e, Pg. 78; The Essentials of Forensic Medicine & Toxicology, K.S. Narayan Reddy-34/e, pg. 60)

ANSWER

Male and Female Pelvis

Male pelvis	Female pelvis
• Massive bony framework	• Less massive bony framework
• Deep and narrow inlet	• Shallow and wide inlet
• Less expanded ilium therefore walls are not separated	• More expanded ilium therefore walls are separated
• Anterior superior iliac spines not widely separated	• Anterior superior iliac spines widely separated
• V-shaped and narrow suprapubic arch, angle not more than 70°; distance between ischia is less	• U-shaped and wide suprapubic arch, angle more than right angle; distance between ischia is more
• Inverted ischial tuberosities	• Everted ischial tuberosities

Male pelvis	Female pelvis
• Ovoid obturator foramina	• Triangular obturator foramina
• Greater sciatic notch narrow, deep and less than a right angle	• Greater sciatic notch wide, shallow and almost a right angle
• Preauricular sulcus narrow, shallow and without marked edges	• Preauricular sulcus broad and deep in parous women
• Wider and deeper acetabula	• Narrower and shallower acetabula
• Sacrum long and narrow, with five or more segments and well-marked promontory	• Sacrum wide and short, with five segments, and promontory less marked

b. Homicidal and suicidal cut throat injury

(Ref: Parikh's Textbook of Medical Jurisprudence, Forensic Medicine and Toxicology, 7/e, Pg. 305)

ANSWER

Suicidal and Homicidal Cut Throat Injuries

Suicidal cut throat	Homicidal cut throat
• Left side of the neck in a right handed person, rarely both sides, usually above the thyroid cartilage	• Usually on the sides, usually below the thyroid cartilage
• Hesitation cuts are present either at the beginning, above, or below the main wound	• No hesitation cuts but one or more deep cuts
• Gradual deepening and shallowing with tailing on the right in right handed persons	• Boldly cut in at commencement without tailing
• Main wound may contain many cuts	• Main wound usually deep and solitary but sometimes repeated almost parallel wounds
• Sloped down, when seen	• Sloped up, when seen
• Often accompanied by wounds across wrists or vital parts elsewhere and healed scars	• Unaccompanied by wounds to wrists but often associated with other severe injuries
• No cuts on hands unless from open razor blades between the fingers	• Frequent 'protective' cuts, that is, defense wounds in wrinkled skin of grasping surfaces of hands, or on back of forearms
• As head is thrown back, carotid artery usually escapes injury	• Carotid artery and jugular veins are likely to be cut
• Weapon is usually present, occasionally firmly grasped by cadaveric spasm	• Weapon is usually removed by the culprit
	• No grasping by cadaveric spasm

c. Civil negligence and Criminal negligence

(Ref: Parikh's Textbook of Medical Jurisprudence, Forensic Medicine and Toxicology, 7/e, Pg. 35; The Essentials of Forensic Medicine & Toxicology, K.S. Narayan Reddy-34/e, pg. 41)

ANSWER

Civil Negligence and Criminal Negligence

Civil negligence	Criminal negligence
• Simply absence of required care and skill	• Gross negligence, lack of attention and mismanagement
• Arises when a patient or his relative sue the doctor for compensation of injury or when doctor brings a civil suit for realization of his professional fees	• Arises when patient gets seriously injured or dies due to criminal negligence or undue interference by doctor in treatment
• Trial is done in civil court	• Trial is done in criminal court
• Strong evidence is needed	• Guilt has to be proved apart from reasonable doubt
• Litigation is between 2 parties	• Litigation is between State and Doctor
• Punishment is liability to pay compensation for damage done	• Punishment is imprisonment with or without fine

PART III

5. Classify firearms. Discuss the findings of entry wounds caused by rifles firearms from various ranges.

a. Firearms

(Ref: Parikh's Textbook of Medical Jurisprudence, Forensic Medicine and Toxicology, 7/e, Pg. 233; The Essentials of Forensic Medicine & Toxicology, K.S. Narayan Reddy-34/e, pg. 204)

ANSWER

Definition
○ Specialized device designed to propel a projectile by the expansive force of gases generated as a result of combustion of the propellant at its base in a closed space
○ Combustion results in building up of optimum pressure which forces the missile out of the muzzle with sufficient velocity resulting in firearm injury
○ Consists of
  ■ Barrel, Action and Grip or butt stock

Classification
○ Smooth-bored firearms (shotgun)
  ■ Cylinder bore, Choke bore, Paradox, Breech loader, Muzzle loader and Country made

- Rifled firearms
  - Rifles
    - Air and gas operated, 0.22 rifle and Military sporting rifles
  - Single-shot target practice pistols
    - Revolvers, Automatic pistols and True automatic weapons (machine guns)

Findings of Entry Wounds Caused by Rifled Firearms from Various Ranges

- **Contact range shot:**
  - No burning, no tattooing, so soot around the wound
  - Physical imprint of the muzzle may occasionally be found on the skin
  - Muscles around the track of the bullet may be bright pink due to carboxyhemoglobin
  - Entry wound may be small and regular or large and irregular, depending upon the underlying structures
  - For example skin wound is large and irregular in head wounds where gases may expand between the scalp and skull causing undermined, ragged, cruciform opening with everted margins
  - Semi explosive tearing type of soft tissue injury associated with bursting fractures of the skull
  - Soot deposits n the bone underlying a contact gunshot
- Close range shot:
  - Entry wound is circular, singed by flame, surrounded by soot, shows tattooing
  - Hair burnt and shriveled, singeing is absent if body is covered with clothes
  - Usual abraded collar or contact ring is present in which the superficial skin layers are abraded – contusion collar
  - Skin if this ring dries quickly and becomes dark
  - Smudge ring or dirt collar is seen on the entry wound
- **Near range shot:**
  - Tattooing is present
  - No singeing of hair
  - No charring of skin
  - Entry wound has appearance of distant shot with abrasion collar and grease collar
- **Distant range shot:**
  - No burning, no soot, no tattooing
  - Circular wound with inverted margins
  - Smaller in size due to initial stretching of skin
  - Slightly contused edges
  - Adjacent skin may be abraded and soiled and presents 2 zones
    - **Outer abraded zone:** Dark red or red in color when fresh–abrasion collar

- **Inner zone:** Soiled by grease–grease collar
  - Fibers of clothes may be turned in at entry

6. Write short notes:

a. Delirium

(Ref: Parikh's Textbook of Medical Jurisprudence, Forensic Medicine and Toxicology, 7/e, Pg. 609)

ANSWER

Person is Showing Delirium Tremens
Findings

- Waxing and waning" level of consciousness with acute onset; rapid decreases in attention span and level of arousal.
- Characterized by disorganized thinking, hallucinations (often visual), illusions, misperceptions, disturbance in sleep wake cycle, cognitive dysfunction.
- Usually 2° to other illness (e.g, CNS disease, infection, trauma, substance abuse/withdrawal, metabolic/ Electrolyte disturbances, hemorrhage, urinary/fecal retention).
- Most common presentation of altered mental status in inpatient setting, especially in the intensive care unit and with prolonged hospital stays.
- Commonly, diffuse slowing EEG.

Interpretation

- Treatment is aimed at identifying an addressing underlying condition. Antipsychotics may be used acutely as needed.
- Delirium = changes in sensorium.
- May be caused by medications (eg, anticholinergics), especially in the elderly.
- Reversible.

Medicolegal Importance

- Under section 84 IPC, person is not held responsible for his acts, if he lost consciousness to such an extent as would prevent him from knowing the nature of the act or distinguishing between right and wrong

b. Clinical features of chronic mercury poisoning

(Ref: Parikh's Textbook of Medical Jurisprudence, Forensic Medicine and Toxicology, 7/e, Pg. 556; The Essentials of Forensic Medicine & Toxicology, K.S. Narayan Reddy-34/e, pg. 504)

ANSWER

Causes

- Consequences of an acute attack
- Careless medical administration

- Continuous accidental absorption in those working with metal or its salts as in manufacture of thermometers, barometers, fur felt, mirrors, and ultraviolet apparatus or in police officers engaged in finger print detection as finger print powder contains mercury

Clinical Features

- Excessive salivation with metallic taste in mouth
- Loosening of teeth with painful inflamed gums
- Occasional blue-black line on the gums as occurs in lead poisoning
- Irritation of skin
- In serious cases, Nephritis may occur
- Abortion
- Discoloration of capsule of lens of eye due to deposition of mercury (Mercuria Lentis), as observed through a slit lamp
- No observed effect on Visual acuity
- **Nervous symptoms:** Tremors, known as hatter's shake–common in workers of that industry–coarse, intentional and affects hands, arms, tongue and legs
- **Mental symptoms:** Erethism–peculiar disturbance of personality characterized by shyness, irritability, tremors, loss of memory and insomnia – common in workers of mirror industry

Management

- Removal of the patient from exposure to mercury
- Promoting elimination of the mercury by bowels and kidneys
- Symptomatic treatment

Postmortem Findings

- Changes in large intestine due to re-excretion with necrosis involving whole lower bowel
- **Kidney damage:** Tubular nephritis
- Fatty degeneration of liver and cardiac muscle
- Chemical analysis of viscera, bones, teeth, hair and nails in case of death due to mercury poisoning

Medicolegal Importance

- Accidental poisoning occurs from
  - Accidental intake of antiseptic solutions containing perchloride or cyanide or of antiseptic tablets of perchloride or iodide
  - Soluble salts employed as vaginal douches

  - Absorption of mercurial preparations applied to the skin
  - Intravenous administration of organic mercurial as diuretics
- In children, accidental poisoning occurs from
  - Use of ammoniated mercury in some bleaching creams
  - Swallowing the sulphocyanide of mercury stick or tablet, the chief constituent of Pharaoh's serpents, which when ignited, produces pungent smell and ash in the form of a long tortuous figure resembling a snake
- Suicidal and homicidal poisoning is rare
- Occurs in industrial workers due to continued inhalation of volatalized mercury

c. Cross examination

(Ref: Parikh's Textbook of Medical Jurisprudence, Forensic Medicine and Toxicology, 7/e, Pg. 10; The Essentials of Forensic Medicine & Toxicology, K.S. Narayan Reddy-34/e, pg. 14)

ANSWER

Cross Examination

- Counsel of the opposite side, that is counsel of the accused, enquires from the witness any facts which appear beneficial to his client and which he believes to be within the knowledge of the witness
- Leading questions are allowed
- Aim is to weaken the evidence of the witness by showing that his details are inaccurate, conflicting, contradictory or that his opinions are ill founded and opposed to that of well recognized authorities
- Witness must be prepared to face questions regarding his qualifications, experience and professional knowledge
- Cross examination need not be confined to the statements made by the witness in the examination-in-chief
- Questions can be asked which may challenge the character of the witness, if appropriate material is available
- Court can forbid any questions which may be insulting, annoying or needlessly offensive
- No limit is decided for cross examinations, however, presiding officer can overrule irrelevant questions

Your Roll No. ....

Name of the Paper	:	**Forensic Medicine & Toxicology**
Name of the Course	:	**MBBS-2016**
Semester	:	**Annual**

Time: 3 Hours   **M.M.: 40**

INSTRUCTIONS

1. Write your Roll No. on the top immediately on receipt of this question paper
2. All questions are to be attempted
3. Answers to Parts I, II and III should be written in separate answer sheets provided
4. Attempt parts of a question in sequence

PART-I

1. What are the findings and medicolegal importance when it is stated that: **[8]**
   a. Defense wounds are present on the body
   b. Death is due to stampede
   c. Newborn child shows umbilical cord strangulation
   d. Tattooing is present in firearm injury

2. Write short notes on: **[6]**
   a. Infamous conduct
   b. Aims and objectives of medicolegal autopsy
   c. Dying declaration

PART-II

3. Classify poisons. Describe clinical features, management and medicolegal importance in a case of organo-Phosphorus poisoning.   **[7]**

4. Differentiate between: **[6]**
   a. Antemortem and postmortem drowning
   b. Heat hematoma and extradural hematoma
   c. Antemortem and postmortem burns

PART-III

5. Define medical negligence. Discuss the precautions that a physician should take to prevent medical negligence suits.   **[7]**

6. Write short notes on: **[6]**
   a. Recording of evidence in a court of law
   b. M'Naghten rules
   c. Contraindications of gastric lavage

PART I

1. What are the findings, interpretation and medicolegal importance when it is stated that?

a. Defense wounds are present on the body

(Ref: Parikh's Textbook of Medical Jurisprudence, Forensic Medicine and Toxicology, 7/e, Pg. 229)

ANSWER

Defense Wound are Present Over the Body

Findings

- Nature of injury depending upon the type of weapon used
- Sharp defense cuts or stabs against sharp weapon
- Defense wounds on grasping surfaces of hands, ulnar borders of forearms, or raised upper limb, dorsum of palm while trying to cover face or head
- May use legs to defend himself hence injuries on lower limbs are present

Interpretation

- Sustained by a person while warding off an attack i.e. while trying to save himself/herself
- Injuries on lower limb indicates, person could have fallen down and used his legs to protect himself
- Any part of the body may get injured depending upon the method of defense
- In case of female, injuries on lower limb suggest sexual assault

Medicolegal Importance

- Indicate a homicidal attack
- Helps to assess victim's presence of mind, awareness, consciousness, ability to resist, nature of attack and type of weapon used
- Cannot be found if hands and feet were tied or he was unaware, or unconscious or unable to protect himself
- Injuries to arms and hands or wrists caused by restraint should be revealed during postmortem
- If hands and arms were placed by the side of the body and become fixed due to rigor mortis with fingers in flexion, defense wounds could not be found at autopsy

b. Death is due to stampede

(Ref: Parikh's Textbook of Medical Jurisprudence, Forensic Medicine and Toxicology, 7/e, Pg. 187; The Essentials of Forensic Medicine & Toxicology, K.S. Narayan Reddy-34/e, pg. 370)

ANSWER

Death is Due to Stampede

Findings

- Deep cyanosis of face and neck
- Eyes are blood shot
- Numerous petechiae on scalp, face, neck and shoulders
- Demarcation line between discolored upper body and lower normal colored body

Interpretation

- Occurs due to pressure on the chest from unconcerted movements of persons in a crowd
- Trauma to chest, abdomen and back preventing normal respiratory movements resulting in death

Medicolegal Importance

- Death due to stampede is usually accidental

c. Newborn child shows umbilical cord strangulation

(Ref: Parikh's Textbook of Medical Jurisprudence, Forensic Medicine and Toxicology, 7/e, Pg. 435)

ANSWER

Newborn Child Shows Umbilical Cord Strangulation

Findings

- Vernix caseosa present
- Examination of umbilical cord shows evidence of displacement of Wharton's jelly
- Evidence of rough handling of umbilical cord
- Umbilical cord tightly twisted around the neck
- No excoriation in and around ligature mark
- Lungs: Found in fetal condition

Interpretation

- Death was due to strangulation by umbilical cord

Medicolegal Importance

- Accidental death
- Occasionally umbilical cord can be used in homicidal death as a ligature to simulate accident

d. Tattooing is present in firearm injury

(Ref: Parikh's Textbook of Medical Jurisprudence, Forensic Medicine and Toxicology, 7/e, Pg. 246; The Essentials of Forensic Medicine & Toxicology, K.S. Narayan Reddy-34/e, pg. 204)

ANSWER

Tattooing is Present in Firearm Injury

Tattooing is due to the deposition of gun powder. (Antemortem phenomenon).

Findings

- Ragged tear
- Burning, blackening and tattooing of skin
- Scorching of skin, singeing of hair
- Clothes trap most of the soot and powder grains
- Wound track and adjacent tissues appear pink due to absorption of carbon monoxide
- Wound is circular or elliptical depending upon the angle of firing
- **Edge:** Smooth or crenated depending upon the size of pellets

Interpretation

- Close discharge shot, entry wound

Medicolegal Importance

- **Suicide:** Wound is rarely of close discharge or distant shot, usually contact shot
- **Homicide:** Close discharge or distant shot is seen
- **Accident:** Rare

2. **Write short notes on:**

    a. **Infamous conduct**

    (Ref: Parikh's Textbook of Medical Jurisprudence, Forensic Medicine and Toxicology, 7/e, Pg. 24; The Essentials of Forensic Medicine & Toxicology, K.S. Narayan Reddy-34/e, pg. 26)

ANSWER

Infamous Conduct

    (Ref: Parikh's Textbook of Medical Jurisprudence, Forensic Medicine and Toxicology, 7/e, Pg. 24; The Essentials of Forensic Medicine & Toxicology, K.S. Narayan Reddy-34/e, pg. 26)

Definition

- Conduct or behavior on part of medical practitioner during his practice which would be reasonably considered as disgraceful or dishonorable by his professional colleagues of good repute and competence
- State medical councils take cognizance of any offence of misconduct committed by a registered medical practitioner only
  - When they receive a written complaint in this respect
  - When a medical practitioner is convicted by a court of law
- Council decides whether any Disciplinary action is required or not after hearing the complainant as well as the medical practitioner

- Depending upon the seriousness of the offence, the action may be
  - A warning or
  - Erasure of the name from the Register either for a temporary period or permanently, known as penal erasure and when it permanent, it is called as professional death sentence depriving the practitioner of all privileges

Unethical Practices Constituting Professional Misconduct

- Association with unqualified persons
  - Employment of unqualified assistants
  - Assisting unqualified person in some procedure
  - Having relations with uncertified persons enabling them to practice midwifery or issuing of certificates enabling such practices to occur
- **Advertising:** Direct or indirect
  - Unusually big-name plate
  - Inserting name in telephone directory in a special place or in bold type
  - Prescription paper containing anything other than his name, qualifications, speciality, address, telephone number and service timings
  - Appearances on broadcasting or television which may have the effect of advertising
  - Allowing the use of his name on the price list of publicity materials
- **Adultery:** Doctor should not abuse his position to seduce a female patient or some other member of the family
- **Abortion:** Procuring, assisting or attempting to procure an illegal abortion
- Disregard of personal responsibilities to patients by
  - Using unsterile instruments
  - Not providing adequate information to patients about drug or diet
  - Giving wrong information e.g. a benign tumor is cancer and performing unnecessary surgeries
  - Ordering unnecessary laboratory tests
  - Not attending a patient who is already under his treatment
  - Attending a patient while under the influence of drink or drugs
  - Suddenly terminating services to a patient
  - Arranging for a substitute without prior intimation to the patient
  - Experimenting on a patient without his valid consent
- Avoiding consultations in certain conditions such as poisoning, when diagnosis is in doubt, a case has taken a serious turn etc.

- Attending a patient who is under treatment of another doctor
- Refusing to provide professional service on religious grounds
- Contravening the provisions of the Drugs Act and Regulations made thereunder e.g. by selling schedule poisons to the public under cover of his own qualifications except to his patients
- Writing prescriptions in a secret formula known to some particular pharmacy only
- Commercialization of a secret remedy
- Running an open shop for sale of medicines, for dispensing prescriptions of other doctors or for sale of medical or surgical appliances
- Improper association with drug manufacturing firms
- Receiving or giving commission or other benefits from or to a professional colleague, a manufacturer, trader, chemist etc.
- Issuing a false certificate in respect of births, cause of death, illness, vaccination, injury
- Talking disparagingly about other colleagues or doing anything that means unfair competition
- **Conviction:** By court of law for offenses involving moral turpitude

b. Aims and objectives of medicolegal autopsy

(Ref: Parikh's Textbook of Medical Jurisprudence, Forensic Medicine and Toxicology, 7/e, Pg. 87)

ANSWER

Aims and Objectives of Medicolegal Autopsy

Definition

- **Medicolegal autopsy:** Special type of scientific examination of a dead body carried out under the laws of the State mainly for the protection of its citizens and to assist the identification and prosecution of the guilty in cases of unnatural death
- Requires State permission and must meet with certain essential requirements

Objectives

- To identify the person
- To determine
  - **Cause of death:** Whether natural or unnatural
  - **If unnatural:** Whether suicide, homicide or accident
  - To collect and document trace evidence, if any, left by the accused on the victim, in all cases, especially in homicidal cases
  - To identify weapon used, person or poison responsible for death

- In case of fatal wounds, to determine the volitional activity possible after such trauma
- To estimate the approximate time since death
- To determine the question of live birth and viability of the child in case of new born infants
- In case of mutilated, fragmented or skeletal remains, to determine if they are human and if human, the probable cause of death and approximate time since death
- To restore the body to the best possible cosmetic appearance before it is released to the relatives

Essential Requirements

- Only a registered medical practitioner (licensed) having special training or experience in forensic medicine (forensic pathology) should perform it
- Examination should be meticulous and complete; all important positive and negative findings should be routinely recorded i.e. absence of skull fracture in a case of head injury, absence of defense wounds in a case of struggle, condition of coronaries arteries in sudden death
- All information should be preserved by written records with relevant photographs, sketches on body diagrams, measurements and weights
- Proper documentation and preservation of the trace evidence material should be done, when recovered
- Medical officer should provide a factual and objective medical report from the data obtained, for the law enforcement agencies as he may have to explain his findings and opinions at the time of cross examination in a court of law

c. Dying declaration

(Ref: Parikh's Textbook of Medical Jurisprudence, Forensic Medicine and Toxicology, 7/e, Pg. 15; The Essentials of Forensic Medicine & Toxicology, K.S. Narayan Reddy-34/e, pg. 10)

ANSWER

Dying Declaration

- **Definition:** Written or verbal statement made by a dying person narrating the cause of his condition or the circumstances resulting in his impending death
- If time allows, Executive Magistrate should be arranged to record the dying declaration of the person who is likely to die as a result of criminal violence
- If the condition of patient is grave that death or unconsciousness may ensue before the arrival of magistrate, the doctor should record the statement keeping in mind the following points

- **Doctor issues 2 certificates**
  - Firstly, certifying that person is conscious and his mental condition is sound to make the declaration
  - When concluding the declaration, certifying that it was made while declarant was compos mentis (sound mental condition), it was read over to him and that he accepted it as having been correctly recorded
- Declaration can be made verbally but person receiving it should commit it to writing at that time
- Should be recorded in presence of 2 witnesses and the questions asked to him and his answers should be written down in his own words without any alteration of terms or phrases
- Leading questions should not be asked from the victim and nothing should be suggested to him
- In cases where victim is unable to speak such as in extreme weakness or cut-throat injuries, but is able to make signs in answer to questions, these should be recorded in form of questions and answers
- After conclusion, declaration should be read over to victim who should affix his signature or left thumb impression to it and should also be signed by the doctor recording it as well as by the witnesses
- If the declarant dies or becomes unconscious during the recording, the doctor himself should record as much information as he has received and sign it himself
- Declaration should be forwarded to the magistrate in a sealed cover
- Investigating officer should not be allowed to enter while recording the declaration
- **Medicolegal importance:**
  - Forms an important evidence in criminal trial in case of victim's death
  - Has no legal value if the victim survives
    - Declarant has to come to the court to give oral evidence and be cross examined for it
    - Declaration has corroborative value

Dying Declaration Vs Dying Deposition

Features	Dying declaration	Dying deposition
Statement	Recorded buy anyone- Magistrate/ Doctor/ Village head man/ Police/ Any member of public	Always recorded buy magistrate
Oath	Not required	Must needed

Features	Dying declaration	Dying deposition
Accused or his counsel	Not present	Always present
Cross-examination	Not done	Done
Legal value	Comparatively less	Much more
Admissibility, if declarant survives	Not admitted, but has corroborative value	Fully admitted
Nature	Merely recording of statement	Complete court procedure
Type of evidence	Documentary	Oral
Role of doctor	• Assess compos mentis	• Assess compos mentis
	• Record the statement in absence of magistrate but in presence of witness	• Statement always recorded by the magistrate
Status in India	Followed	Not Followed

PART II

3. **Classify poisons. Describe clinical features, management and medicolegal importance in a case of organophosphorus poisoning.**

   a. Poisons

   (Ref: Parikh's Textbook of Medical Jurisprudence, Forensic Medicine and Toxicology, 7/e, Pg. 507)

ANSWER

Poisons

Definition

- A substance which, when administered, inhaled or ingested is capable of acting deleteriously on the human body, therefore almost everything is a poison

Classification

- **Corrosives**
  - **Mineral acids**: Sulfuric acid, nitric acid, hydrochloric acid
  - **Organic acids**: Oxalic acid, carbolic acid, acetic acid, salicylic acid
  - **Vegetable acid**: Hydrocyanic acid
  - **Concentrated alkalis:** Caustic soda, caustic potash and carbonates of ammonium, sodium and potassium
- **Irritants**
  - **Inorganic**
    - **Non-metallic**
      - Phosphorus, Chlorine, Bromine, Iodine.

- ♦ **Metallic**
  - ▫ Arsenic, Antimony, Mercury, Lead, Copper, Thallium, Zinc, Manganese, Barium and Radioactive substances
- ▪ **Organic**
  - ♦ **Vegetable poisons**
    - ▫ Castor seeds, Croton seeds, Abrus precatorius, Colocynth, Ergot, Capsicum, Semecarpus anacardium, Calotropis, Plumbago rosea and Plumbago zeylanica
  - ♦ **Animal poisons**
    - ▫ Cantharides, Snakes, Scorpions, Spiders and Poisonous insects
  - ♦ **Mechanical**
    - ▫ Coarsely powdered glass, Chopped hair, Dried sponge and Diamond dust
- ○ **Neurotics**
  - ▪ **Cerebral–act on cerebrum**
    - ♦ **Somniferous**
      - ▫ Opioids
    - ♦ **Inebriant**
      - ▫ Alcohol, Anesthetics, Sedatives, Hypnotics, Fuels and Agrochemical compounds
    - ♦ **Deliriant**
      - ▫ Datura, Belladonna, Hyoscyamus and Cannabis indica
  - ▪ **Spinal:** Act on spinal cord
    - ♦ Nux vomica and its alkaloids
    - ♦ Gelsemium
  - ▪ **Peripheral:** Act on peripheral nerves
    - ▫ Curare and Conium
- ○ **Cardiac:** Act on heart
  - ▪ Digitalis Oleander Aconite Nicotine
- ○ **Asphyxiants:** Act on lungs
  - ▪ Irrespirable gases
    - ♦ Carbon monoxide and Carbon dioxide
  - ▪ War gases
  - ▪ Sewer gas
- ○ **Miscellaneous**
  - ▪ Analgesics, Antipyretics, Antihistaminics, Tranquillizers, Antidepressants, Stimulants, Hallucinogens, Street drugs and Designer drugs

b. Organophosphorus poisoning

(Ref: Parikh's Textbook of Medical Jurisprudence, Forensic Medicine and Toxicology, 7/e, Pg. 625 ; The Essentials of Forensic Medicine & Toxicology, K.S. Narayan Reddy-34/e, pg. 484)

ANSWER

Clinical Picture
Toxic Effects are of 3 Types

- ○ Muscarine-like effects–signs and symptoms are:
  - ▪ Bronchial tree
    - ♦ Tightness in chest with prolonged wheezing expiration – suggestive of bronchospasm and increased secretion
    - ♦ Discomfort or pain in chest
    - ♦ Dyspnea
    - ♦ Cough
    - ♦ Pulmonary edema
    - ♦ Froth at mouth and nose
    - ♦ Cyanosis
  - ▪ Gastrointestinal
    - ♦ Anorexia
    - ♦ Nausea
    - ♦ Vomiting
    - ♦ Abdominal cramps
    - ♦ Epigastric and substernal tightness
    - ♦ Heartburn and eructation
    - ♦ Diarrhea
    - ♦ Tenesmus
    - ♦ Involuntary defecation
  - ▪ Sweat glands
    - ♦ Increased sweating
  - ▪ Salivary glands
    - ♦ Increased salivation
  - ▪ Lacrimal glands
    - ♦ Increased lacrimation
    - ♦ Tears can be red owing to porphyrin in lacrimal glands
  - ▪ Heart
    - ♦ Slight bradycardia
  - ▪ Pupils
    - ♦ Slight miosis
  - ▪ Ciliary body
    - ♦ Blurring or dimness of vision
  - ▪ Urinary bladder
    - ♦ Frequency of micturition
    - ♦ Involuntary micturition
- ○ Nicotine-like effects
  - ▪ Striated muscle
    - ♦ Easy fatigue
    - ♦ Mild weakness
    - ♦ Muscular fasciculations
    - ♦ Cramps
    - ♦ Generalized weakness of muscles of respiration with dyspnea and cyanosis
  - ▪ Sympathetic ganglia
    - ♦ Pallor
    - ♦ Occasional elevation of blood pressure
- ○ **CNS effects**
  - ▪ Irritability, apprehension and restlessness
  - ▪ Fine fibrillary tremors of hands, eye lids, face or tongue

- Mental confusion progressing to stupor and muscular weakness with tremors and convulsions
- Coma with absence of reflexes and depression of respiratory and circulatory centers

Management

○ **Decontamination:**
  - Physician and nurses should wear rubber gloves
  - Patient must be separated from the source of exposure and all clothes should be removed
  - Exposed areas should be washed with tap water and soap or some alkaline solution
  - In case of ingestion of poison, stomach should be washed with tap water

○ **Care of airway**
  - Foot end of the bed is raised to ensure drainage of respiratory muscles
  - Secretions should be aspirated and tracheostomy is required
  - Artificial respiration given, if required
  - Positive pressure oxygen should be given in case of pulmonary edema

○ **Antidote**
  - Atropine blocks the peripheral actions of the excessive acetylcholine levels built up by the cholinesterase inhibitors
  - Dose–2 mg every 15-30 minutes IM or IV till signs of atropinization appear i.e. flushed face, dry mouth, dilated pupils, fast pulse and warm skin

○ **Cholinesterase reactivators**
  - ♦ Act by dephosphorylating the inactivated cholinesterase
  - ♦ Act as specific antidotes, used to supplement atropine therapy
  - ♦ **Dose:** 1–2 g IV for adults and 25–50 mg/kg for children, as 5% solution in isotonic saline; repeated every 12 hours or if as required

○ **Other measures**
  - Diuretic and brisk saline purgative can be beneficial
  - Restlessness can be prevented by quick acting barbiturates or diazepam

Postmortem Findings

○ **External**
  - Cyanosed face
  - Blood stained froth at nose and mouth
  - Kerosene-like smell can be perceived

○ **Internal**
  - Stomach contains greenish oily substances used as diluents
  - **Kerosene:** Like or garlic smell is perceived
  - Blood stained contents of stomach

- Congested mucosa
- Submucous petechial hemorrhages are found
- Pulmonary edema
- Capillary dilatation
- Petechial hemorrhages
- Hyperemia of lungs, brain and other organs
- In delayed paralysis of extremities induced by parathion, malathion and other compounds – demyelination of ascending and descending spinal tracts with degeneration of motor horn cells

Medicolegal Importance

○ **Suicide:** Due to easy availability of pesticides, rodenticides and vermicides
○ **Homicide:** Mixed with alcohol to mask the smell and can be used for homicidal purpose
○ **Accidental:** Through contamination of edible things with these compounds

---

4. **Differentiate between:**

    a. **Antemortem and postmortem drowning**

    (Ref: Parikh's Textbook of Medical Jurisprudence, Forensic Medicine and Toxicology, 7/e, Pg. 188)

ANSWER

Antemortem and Postmortem Drowning

Antemortem drowning	Postmortem drowning
• Death was due to immersion during life	• Body was immersed Postmortem i.e. after death
• Presence of diatoms in tissues such as bone marrow, brain, liver, blood or kidneys	• Absence of diatoms in tissues such as bone marrow, liver, blood etc.
• Froth at the nose and mouth	• No froth is observed if death occurred before immersion in water
• Presence of weeds, mud etc. in clenched hand due to cadaveric spasm	• Absence of cadaveric spasm
• Water in stomach and intestine swallowed during struggle for life	• In dead bodies thrown in water, it cannot get beyond the cardiac sphincter
• Ballooning of lungs i.e. emphysema aquosum, covering heart and bulging out of the chest	• No such changes are observed in postmortem drowning

b. **Heat hematoma and extradural hematoma**

(Ref: Parikh's Textbook of Medical Jurisprudence, Forensic Medicine and Toxicology, 7/e, Pg. 295; The Essentials of Forensic Medicine & Toxicology, K.S. Narayan Reddy-34/e, pg. 302)

ANSWER

Heat Hematoma and Extradural Hematoma

Heat hematoma	Extradural hematoma
• It is due to rupture of vessels with subsequent escape and coagulation of blood in the extradural space	• Due to bleeding between dura and skull
• Caused by exposure to heat; heating of the skull	• Caused by trauma as in falls and accidents; fracture of skull
• Soft, friable clot, light chocolate colored or can be pink if blood contains carbon monoxide, spongy	• Jelly like clot
• Not closely related to heat fracture site	• Occurs at the site of traumatic fracture
• It is a purely postmortem finding	• Not a postmortem finding as caused by trauma
• No medicolegal significance	• Medicolegally significant

c. Antemortem and postmortem burns

(Ref: Parikh's Textbook of Medical Jurisprudence, Forensic Medicine and Toxicology, 7/e, Pg. 340)

ANSWER

Antemortem and Postmortem Burns

Antemortem burns	Postmortem burns
• Line of redness is present	• Line of redness is absent
• Vesicles contain albuminous fluid and chlorides	• Vesicles contain air
• Pus and sloughing is present	• Pus and sloughing is absent
• Granulation due to healing	• No granulation is seen
• Soot in upper respiratory tract is present	• No soot in upper respiratory tract is seen
• Carboxyhemoglobin in blood is absent	• Carboxyhemoglobin in blood is present
• Increase in enzymes	• **No such increase**

PART III

5. **Define medical negligence. Discuss the precautions that a physician should take to prevent medical negligence.**

a. Medical Negligence

(Ref: Parikh's Textbook of Medical Jurisprudence, Forensic Medicine and Toxicology, 7/e, Pg. 35; The Essentials of Forensic Medicine & Toxicology, K.S. Narayan Reddy-34/e, pg. 41)

ANSWER

Medical Negligence

Definition

○ Lack of reasonable care and skill or wiliful negligence on the part of a medical practitioner in the treatment

of a patient whereby the health or life of a patient is at risk

○ Neglect or carelessness where there is a legal duty to take care and failure in that duty causes damage/injury

○ Legally, any want to proper care or skill that causes the patient's death, reduces his chances of recovery, prolongs his illness or increases his sufferings constitutes injury

○ If no damage has occurred, even if the doctor has been negligent, the patient is not entitled to any compensation

○ Damage to the patient may be physical, mental or financial and includes pain and suffering and are assessed by the court as
  ▪ Loss of present and future earning capacity of the damaged person
  ▪ Actual medical and surgical care costs
  ▪ Reduction in quality of life which may be caused by lameness, deafness, blindness and so on

Types of Medical Negligence

○ **Civil negligence**
  ▪ When a patient or his relative, in the event of his death, sue the doctor in civil court for compensation for the damages or death of the patient as the case may be due to negligence of the doctor
  ▪ When the doctor brings a civil suit for realization of his professional fees from the patient or his relative who refuse to pay on the grounds of malpractice

○ **Criminal negligence**
  ▪ In case of death or serious injury to patient attributable to criminal negligence or undue interference by the doctor in treatment of a patient
  ▪ Doctor may be prosecuted by the police and charged in a criminal court with having caused the death of his patient by a rash and negligent act amounting to culpable homicide, if death by due to gross ignorance, gross carelessness, gross negligence or undue interference by him

Various Medicolegal Issues in Case of Negligence by a Doctor

○ Failure in regard to the contractual obligations by a doctor if he agreed to treat a person – burden of proving negligence and resulting damage lies with the patient

○ **Diagnosis:** It is difficult to justify failure to X-ray in which there is doubt about diagnosis, such a failure is generally basis of a successful plea in an action for negligence

- Failure to use an ophthalmoscope or refer to a specialist can be considered as negligence
- **Treatment:** Use of dangerous drugs and unnecessary exposure of the patient to radiation should be avoided
- **Failure to warn:** If the practitioner fails to warn the patient regarding side effects of a drug or procedure renders him liable for harm suffered by patient
- **Certificates:** Doctor should be fully satisfied about the accuracy of the statement contained and should be true to the best of his knowledge e.g. in mental disorders
- **Workmen's Compensation Act:** Under this act, provision is made for disabilities suffered as a result of industrial accidents or occupational diseases, given the fact, the worker himself was not responsible for the injury or was negligent; therefore, doctors who may be called to look after such workmen should have a clear understanding of the provisions of this act
- Carelessness during treatment, anesthesia, operation or postoperative period
- Mismanagement of delivery under the influence of alcohol or drugs
- When indicated, not doing sensitivity testing
- Injection of basal anesthetics in a fatal dose or in wrong tissues
- Amputation of wrong finger or limb, or removal of wrong organ
- Surgery on wrong patient
- Leaving instruments or sponges in the abdomen or any other part of the body
- Giving wrong or infected blood

Precautions Physician Should Take to Prevent Medical Negligence

- Health care professional/physician should keep up-to-date with the latest technologies and advances
- Wherever possible and necessary, diagnosis should be confirmed by laboratory tests including biopsy
- In cases of suspected cancer, precaution should be taken to determine early diagnosis
- When diagnosis is doubtful or in case of injury to bones or joints, X-ray should be routinely advised
- In doubtful cases, consultation with specialist should be advised
- When there is danger of infection, immunization/prophylactic cover should be considered essential
- Sensitivity tests should be done before injecting preparations expected to cause anaphylactic shock
- Verification of drugs to be administered by injection or otherwise should be done

- No procedure should be undertaken beyond one's skill
- Experimental methods should not be implemented without prior consent
- Instruments to be used for any procedure should be properly sterilized, safe and in proper working condition

---

6. **Write short notes on:**

a. **Recording of evidence in court of law**

(Ref: Parikh's Textbook of Medical Jurisprudence, Forensic Medicine and Toxicology, 7/e, Pg. 10; The Essentials of Forensic Medicine & Toxicology, K.S. Narayan Reddy-34/e, pg. 13)

ANSWER

Recording of Evidence in Court of Law

Procedure of Recording of Evidence in Court of Law

- **Examination-in-chief or direct examination**
  - **In private cases:** Questions put to the witness by the counsel for the side who has called him or summoned him
  - **In government prosecutions:** Public prosecutor begins this examination
  - Aim is to place all the facts before the court that relate to the case and if witness be an expert, his interpretation of these facts
  - No leading questions are allowed except in those cases where judge is satisfied that a witness is hostile
  - Witness is expected to tell the truth but if he is influenced, intimidated or bribed, he may purposely conceal a part of the truth or give outright false evidence and is then liable to be found guilty of perjury
  - Court in its discretion declare such witness as hostile
  - Leading questions may be asked in the examination-in-chief when hostile witness is being examined to produce the facts

Cross Examination

For answer, refer 2017 paper Q. 6 (c), Pg. 466
- **Re-examination**
  - Witness may be re-examined by the counsel who has called him, after cross examination
  - **Aim is to**
    - Clear up any doubts that may have arisen during cross examination
    - Explain some subject that may seem damaging his direct testimony in proper perspective so that unnecessary importance or possible misinterpretation can be evaded

- Leading questions are not allowed
- New issue cannot be introduced without permission of the judge and consent of the opposing counsel
- Opposing side has right of cross examination on the new points

- **Court questions**
  - Judge may ask any question to the witness at any stage of trial to clear any doubtful points
  - Evidence recorded by the presiding judge or magistrate should be read by the witness and signed by him after getting any corrections, if needed, done by the court under its initials
  - Subsequent to discharge, witness may be recalled if his evidence needs any clarification or explanation

b. M'Naghten Rules

(Ref: Parikh's Textbook of Medical Jurisprudence, Forensic Medicine and Toxicology, 7/e, Pg. 461; The Essentials of Forensic Medicine & Toxicology, K.S. Narayan Reddy-34/e, pg. 459)

ANSWER

M'Naghten Rules

According to M'Naghten Rules

- In order to establish defense on the ground on insanity, it must be clearly shown that at the time of committing act, the accused was laboring under such defect of reason from disease of the mind as not to know the nature and quality of the act he was doing, or if he knew this, that he did not know that what he was doing was wrong or contrary to law
- It must be kept in mind that the defense can be founded only on a known and identifiable disease of mind
- Lesser conditions prevailing temporarily at the time of act do not suffice which includes rage, jealousy, transient loss of control and others including unresisted impulse
- Legal test of insanity has been accepted in India and included in Section 84 IPC – nothing is an offence which is done by a person who at the time of doing it is by reason of unsoundness of mind, is incapable of knowing the nature of act, or that he is doing what is either wrong or contrary to law

Examples

- If a person in delusion thinks that somebody wants to kill him and in defense, he kills somebody, then he has no criminal responsibility
- Or if he thinks that another person is a dangerous animal and kills him in defense, he has no criminal responsibility

Criticism of M'Naghten Rules

- This criterion of deciding that a person is insane is purely intellectual and there is no place for emotional factors of ability of mind to control his impulses
- It has been understood that there is no mental disorder, however partial, which does not have its repercussions throughout the rest of affected mind
- It has been accepted that intellectual defect is actually deficient emotional control

c. Contraindications of gastric lavage

(Ref: Parikh's Textbook of Medical Jurisprudence, Forensic Medicine and Toxicology, 7/e, Pg. 515; The Essentials of Forensic Medicine & Toxicology, K.S. Narayan Reddy-34/e, pg. 489)

ANSWER

Contraindications of Gastric Lavage

Definition

- Gastric lavage (stomach washing) is the technique of cleaning out contents of the stomach
- Life-saving process if performed within 4-6 hours of ingestion of poison

Indications

- To remove unabsorbed poison from the body
- Only if poison is life threatening and can be removed within 6 hours of ingestion
- Treatment for duodenal atresia in new born

Indications with Precautions

- Strychnine poisoning, control of convulsions should be taken care of
- Kerosene or volatile poisons or comatose conditions, airway should be sealed by cuffed intubation to avoid high risk of aspiration into air passages
- In hypothermia, body temperature should be checked regularly

Contraindications

- In compromised, unprotected airway
- In risk of gastrointestinal hemorrhage or perforation
- When the poisoning is due to corrosive substance (strong acids or strong bases) (T54), hydrocarbons (T53)
- In case of aluminum phosphide poisoning

Your Roll No. ....

Name of the Paper : **Forensic Medicine & Toxicology**

Name of the Course : **MBBS-2015**

Semester : **Annual**

Time: 3 Hours   M.M.: 40

INSTRUCTIONS

1. Write your Roll No. on the top immediately on receipt of this question paper
2. All questions are to be attempted
3. Answers to Parts I, II and III should be written in separate answer sheets provided
4. Attempt parts of a question in sequence

PART-I

1. What are the findings and medicolegal importance when it is stated that: [8]
    a. Dribbling of saliva from angle of mouth
    b. Dead body is showing mummification
    c. Skull is showing signature fracture
    d. A girl is of 18 years age

2. Write short notes on: [6]
    a. Treatment of methyl alcohol poisoning
    b. Privileged communication
    c. Universal antidote

PART-II

3. Classify poisons. Discuss clinical features, management and autopsy findings in a case of phenol poisoning. What viscera will you preserve in such a case?   [7]

4. Differentiate between: [6]
    a. Artificial and true bruise
    b. Strychnine poisoning and tetanus
    c. Male and female skulls

PART-III

5. Define medical negligence. Discuss various medicolegal issues in the case of negligence by a doctor.   [7]

6. Write short notes on: [6]
    a. Whiplash injury
    b. Frost bite
    c. Sadism

PART I

1. **What are the findings, interpretation and medicolegal importance when it is stated that?**

   a. **Dribbling of saliva from angle of mouth**

   (Ref: Parikh's Textbook of Medical Jurisprudence, Forensic Medicine and Toxicology, 7/e, Pg. 171; The Essentials of Forensic Medicine & Toxicology, K.S. Narayan Reddy-34/e, pg. 315)

ANSWER

Dribbling of Saliva From Angle of Mouth

- **Findings:**
  - Dribbling of saliva from corner of mouth opposite to the side on the knot due to pressure on salivary glands by the ligature
  - Neck is stretched due to upward pull of ligature and head is inclined to opposite side on knot
  - Pale face or congested and swollen with profuse petechiae in head and neck
  - Cyanosed hands and nail beds
  - Eyeballs prominent due to congestion
  - Tongue turgid or protruded and becomes dark brown or almost black
  - Petechial hemorrhages on arms and legs
  - Postmortem lividity seen on arms and legs and face and neck
  - Ligature mark on the neck

Interpretation

- Death was due to hanging

Medicolegal Importance

- Whether death was due to hanging
- Whether it was suicidal, accidental or homicidal hanging

   b. **Dead body is showing mummification**

   (Ref: Parikh's Textbook of Medical Jurisprudence, Forensic Medicine and Toxicology, 7/e, Pg. 161)

ANSWER

Mummification

Definition

- Modified process of putrefaction
- Sometimes, process of Putrefaction may become arrested at some stage and body tissues may undergo mummification

- Characterized by dehydration or desiccation of the body tissues and viscera after death
- Body desiccates by losing its moisture from evaporation
- **Ideal conditions for mummification:** High atmospheric temperature devoid of moisture with a free circulation of air around the body
- Not common in adults but can be found in bodies that have been buried in dry soil e.g. in desert sand
- Tissues of infants are generally free from organizations at birth and they do not develop normal putrefactive changes, hence it is usually observed in infants who were exposed to warm and dry atmosphere shortly after death such as when kept perched up on trees, roof rafters or concealed in trunks
- Chronic arsenic or antimony poisoning is favorable for the process of mummification

Process of Mummification

- Exposed parts of the body such as lips, nose, fingers and toes mummify first, extends to the rest of the body
- Mummified body appears shriveled, odorless and often very dark (almost black) in color and has lost weight
- Skin is hard, dry leathery and adheres to the shrunken body
- Viscera are shrunken, dark brown or black and blend together or can be invisible
- Unless attacked by animals or insects, result of process of mummification is the preservation of the anatomical features of the deceased for many years

Time Required for Mummification

- **3 months to 1 year or longer:** Depending upon the size of body and atmospheric temperature

Medicolegal Significance

- Helps in identification of person as features are well preserved
- Indicates the cause of death as injuries are recognizable
- Indicates the time since death
- **Indicates the place:** Hot or dry, from where the body has been recovered

Chemical Favoring Mummification

- Arsenic poisoning
- Antimony poisoning
- Concentrated Salt-NATRON

c. Skull is showing signature fracture

(Ref: Parikh's Textbook of Medical Jurisprudence, Forensic Medicine and Toxicology, 7/e, Pg. 290; The Essentials of Forensic Medicine & Toxicology, K.S. Narayan Reddy-34/e, pg. 230)

ANSWER

Skull is Showing Signature Fracture

Findings

○ Fractured bone is driven inward into skull cavity

○ Outer table is pushed into the diploe, inner table is fractured erratically and to a larger extent and may be comminuted

○ Resembles the shape of weapon used

Interpretation

○ Caused by heavy weapon with a small striking surface for example a hammer

○ Shape of fracture indicates type of weapon used

○ Differences in depth of various portions of depression suggests relative position of the assailant and victim when the blow was made

○ Deepest part of the depression usually marks the most advanced part of the striking surface

Medicolegal Importance

○ Given indication about the position of the victim and the assailant

○ Suggests homicidal attack

○ Indicates the kind of weapon used e.g. firearm, hammer, stone

d. A girl is of 18 years age

(Ref: Parikh's Textbook of Medical Jurisprudence, Forensic Medicine and Toxicology, 7/e, Pg. 59; The Essentials of Forensic Medicine & Toxicology, K.S. Narayan Reddy-34/e, pg. 78)

ANSWER

For answer, refer 2017 paper Q. 1 (a) Pg. 460

2. Write short notes on:

a. Treatment of methyl alcohol poisoning

(Ref: Parikh's Textbook of Medical Jurisprudence, Forensic Medicine and Toxicology, 7/e, Pg. 616; The Essentials of Forensic Medicine & Toxicology, K.S. Narayan Reddy-34/e, pg. 540)

ANSWER

Treatment of Methyl Alcohol Poisoning

Clinical Picture

○ Symptoms usually get delayed but may appear within an hour

○ Headache

○ Nausea and vomiting

○ Dizziness

○ Pain in abdomen

○ Profound muscular weakness

○ Depressed cardiac action

○ Breath has spirit like odor

○ Dyspnea

○ Cyanosis

○ Acidosis due to accumulation of acid metabolites

○ **Effects in eyes:** Temporary blindness; optic nerve atrophy causing permanent blindness

○ Convulsions may occur

○ **Intestinal contraction:** Small or large bowel or sometimes, both

○ Death due to respiratory failure

Fatal Dose

○ 60–240 mL in adults kills

○ 15 mL causes blindness

○ 1 mL/kg of denatured alcohol containing methyl alcohol in children causes serious symptoms

Fatal Period

○ Death may occur within 24 hours to 36 hours or 3–4 days

Management

○ Gastric lavage to prevent absorption with 5% solution of sodium bicarbonate in warm water

○ For acidosis, oral administration of sodium bicarbonate in a dose of 2 g in 250 mL of water every 2 hours is required to maintain neutral or slightly alkaline urine

○ In case, where oral therapy is not possible, 50 g of sodium bicarbonate dissolved in 1 L of 5% dextrose solution can be given intravenously along with 10-15 units of insulin

○ Plasma bicarbonate level should be maintained at around 20 mEq/L

○ Intravenous administration of molar sodium lactate is beneficial

○ 50% ethyl alcohol in a dose of 0.75–1 mL/kg body weight should be given orally for 3-4 days to prevent methanol oxidation to formaldehyde and formic acid and helps in its excretion in urine and breath

○ **Hemodialysis is indicated in:** Ocular findings, metabolic acidosis, renal failure and a blood methanol level above 50 mg%

○ Eyes should be covered to protect from strong light

○ Rest treatment is symptomatic

Postmortem Findings

○ Cyanosis is profound
○ **Dark:** Fluid blood
○ Cerebral and pulmonary edema can be observed
○ Inflamed gastrointestinal mucosa
○ Necrobiosis of liver
○ Kidneys show tubular degeneration
○ Viscera and postmortem blood should be preserved

Medicolegal Significance

○ Accidental poisoning may occur
○ Most commonly due to ingestion of liquor containing methyl alcohol by drinking cheap illicit liquor or accidently methanol getting into liquor

b. Privileged communication

(Ref: Parikh's Textbook of Medical Jurisprudence, Forensic Medicine and Toxicology, 7/e, Pg. 29; The Essentials of Forensic Medicine & Toxicology, K.S. Narayan Reddy-34/e, pg. 32)

ANSWER

Privileged Communication

○ **Definition**
  ■ When a doctor is justified in disclosing information about the patient and the communication made by the doctor to a proper authority having corresponding legal, social and moral duties to protect the public

○ **Circumstances in which disclosure of professional secrets are justified**
  ■ When the doctor is directed by the judge to do so as a witness in the court
    ◆ Doctor must disclose any secret information about his patients received in the course of his professional relationship
    ◆ Failure to do so can be treated as contempt of court
    ◆ Information can be written and handed over to judge
  ■ When the doctor has moral or social duty to perform under circumstances such as
    ◆ If a bar maid has developed chancre or tuberculosis and is unfit to serve drinks to public
    ◆ If a bus driver has noticeable hypertension or brittle diabetes and is unsafe to be charge of a public vehicle
    ◆ An engine driver being color blind or epileptic is unfit for his job
    ◆ To warn the partners of patients with AIDS
    ◆ To report cases of suspected child abuse
    ◆ To warn parents if patient has a tendency to any violent act such as suicide or homicide
  ■ In order to protect doctor's own interests
    ◆ In cases where he has a statutory duty to public health authorities or the state
    ◆ Has to notify births, deaths, communicable diseases, case with a danger to public such as food poisoning after eating from a restaurant or drinking water from a public source
    ◆ Has to notify to the police, cases of homicidal poisoning
  ■ When the doctor's duty as a citizen to assist in the apprehension of a person who has committed a serious crime compensates his obligation to his patients
    ◆ If doctor has been called for the treatment of a patient who he believes to be victim or accused of a serious crime such as murder, robbery, jail breaking
    ◆ Patient with a stab wound or firearm injury, which could have been inflicted during deadly scuffle
  ■ In certain other cases
    ◆ When a servant is sent by owner
    ◆ In relation to insurance reports

c. Universal antidote

(Ref: Parikh's Textbook of Medical Jurisprudence, Forensic Medicine and Toxicology, 7/e, Pg. 518; The Essentials of Forensic Medicine & Toxicology, K.S. Narayan Reddy-34/e, pg. 481)

ANSWER

Universal Antidote

Definition

○ Antidote which is beneficial in those cases where the nature of consumed poison is unknown or where intake of combination of 2 or more poisons is suspected
○ Consists of mixture of readily available substances
○ **Administration of mixture:** 1 tablespoon stirred up in 200 mL of water (tumblerful), can be repeated once or twice
○ Not very effective even when given immediately after ingestion of poison
○ Despite the name as universal antidote, it is not a Panacea in all cases of poisoning
○ Has been replaced by activated charcoal in many institutions

FORENSIC MEDICINE & TOXICOLOGY

Constituents	Purpose	Quantity
• Powdered charcoal (burnt toast)	• Adsorbs alkaloids	• 2 parts
• Magnesium oxide (milk of magnesia)	• Neutralizes acids	• 1 part
• Tannic acid (strong tea)	• Precipitates alkaloids, certain glucosides and many metals	• 1 part

PART II

3. **Classify poisons. Discuss clinical features, management and autopsy findings in a case of phenol poisoning. What viscera will you preserve in such a case?**

(Ref: Parikh's Textbook of Medical Jurisprudence, Forensic Medicine and Toxicology, 7/e, Pg. 507)

ANSWER

For answer, refer 2016 paper Q. 3 (a), Pg. 471

b.   Phenol poisoning or carbolic acid poisoning

(Ref: Parikh's Textbook of Medical Jurisprudence, Forensic Medicine and Toxicology, 7/e, Pg. 535; The Essentials of Forensic Medicine & Toxicology, K.S. Narayan Reddy-34/e, pg. 497)

ANSWER

Clinical Picture

Poisoning by carbolic acid is termed as Carbolism

○ **Local action**
  ▪ **Skin**
    ♦ Necrosis and sloughing of tissues
    ♦ Mild corrosive
    ♦ Anesthetic upon skin and mucous membranes
    ♦ Eschar formation occurs
  ▪ **Alimentary tract**
    ♦ Hot burning pain extending from mouth to stomach
    ♦ Tingling sensation and anesthesia
    ♦ Painful swallowing
    ♦ Difficult speech
    ♦ No vomiting due to anesthetic action on stomach
    ♦ Corrosion of lips, tongue, mouth
    ♦ Burnt cheeks and chin–appear white, bleached and hard
    ♦ Burns later become brown
    ♦ Rapid sloughing of dead tissue
○ **Remote action**
  ▪ Shock develops

▪ Rapid establishment of local and remote action of phenol
▪ Giddiness
▪ Cold and clammy skin
▪ Weak and thread pulse
▪ Contracted and pinpoint pupils
▪ **Temperature:** Subnormal
▪ **Breathing:** Stertorous and labored
▪ Breath smells of carbolic acid
▪ **Carboluria:** Nephrotoxic action–irritation of kidneys, oliguria
▪ Coma
▪ Death due to paralysis of respiratory or cardiac center

Fatal Dose
○ 20 drops of pure phenol results in death

Fatal Period
○ Death occurs in 3–4 hours

Management
○ Gastric lavage with 10% solution of Glycerin in water or plain water with magnesium sulfate – continued washing until phenolic odor disappears
○ About one ounce of magnesium sulfate or 2 ounces of medicinal liquid paraffin may be left in the stomach
○ Magnesium sulfate forms an insoluble sulphocarbolate
○ Alcohol tends to prevent cauterizing action of phenol and can be given in 10% solution
○ Demulcents such as egg white or milk can be beneficial
○ In order to render urine alkaline, intravenous saline with sodium bicarbonate should be given
○ Surface burns should be washed with water and castor oil should be applied

Postmortem Findings
○ Greyish white stains at the angles of mouth and on chin
○ Perceptible odor
○ Mucous membranes of mouth and esophagus are swollen, hardened and discolored
○ White and swollen tongue
○ Mucous membranes of stomach forms projecting folds and prominent rugae–thickened, brownish, lethargy appearance
○ Contents of stomach–dark brown mucoid with characteristic phenolic smell
○ Injection of vessels in peritoneal surface of stomach, duodenum, upper part of small intestine

- Liver and spleen present whitish hard patch
- Swelling and congestion of glottis
- Congestion of lungs and brain
- Parenchymal degenerative changes in kidneys

Medicolegal Importance

- Used in antiseptics, disinfectants and surface anesthetics
- Used in past to commit suicide
- Rarely used for homicide due to its smell and taste
- Sometimes used to cause abortion
- Accidental poisoning may occur due to indiscriminate medicinal use

4. Differentiate between

a. Artificial bruise and True bruise

(Ref: Parikh's Textbook of Medical Jurisprudence, Forensic Medicine and Toxicology, 7/e, Pg. 571; The Essentials of Forensic Medicine & Toxicology, K.S. Narayan Reddy-34/e, pg. 179)

ANSWER

Artificial Bruise and True Bruise

Artificial bruise	True bruise
• Caused by chemical	• Caused by trauma
• Located on accessible parts of the body	• Located anywhere
• Blisters are formed	• No blisters are formed
• No color change occurs	• Color change characteristic
• Ecchymosis is absent	• Ecchymosis is present
• Contents are acrid serum	• Contents are extravasated blood
• Itching present	• Itching absent
• May show marks due to scratching	• No marks present
• On analysis chemical found in the blister fluid	• No chemical found on analysis

b. Strychnine poisoning and Tetanus

(Ref: Parikh's Textbook of Medical Jurisprudence, Forensic Medicine and Toxicology, 7/e, Pg. 640)

ANSWER

Strychnine Poisoning and Tetanus

Strychnine poisoning	Tetanus
• History of poisoning	• History of injury
• Sudden onset	• Gradual onset
• Generalised convulsions	• Lock jaw
• Chest fixed during convulsions	• Not so

Strychnine poisoning	Tetanus
• Complete relaxation in between seizures	• Relaxation between the spasms is never complete
• Ends fatally in a few hours	• Death rare within a few few hours
• Chemical analysis reveals the poison	• Not so

c. Male and Female Skulls

(Ref: Parikh's Textbook of Medical Jurisprudence, Forensic Medicine and Toxicology, 7/e, Pg. 79; The Essentials of Forensic Medicine & Toxicology, K.S. Narayan Reddy-34/e, pg. 59)

ANSWER

Male and Female Skulls

Male skull	Female skull
• Bigger, heavier and more rugged	• Smaller, lighter and less rugged
• Cranial capacity almost 10% more	• Cranial capacity almost 10% less
• Frontal sinuses more developed	• Frontal sinuses less developed
• Frontonasal angulation distinct	• Frontonasal angulation not well marked
• Glabella, supraorbital ridges, zygomatic arch, mastoid processes, occipital protuberance, occipital condyles and muscle attachments are more pronounced	• Glabella, supraorbital ridges, zygomatic arch, mastoid processes, occipital protuberance, occipital condyles and muscle attachments are less pronounced
• Orbital opening comparatively big and rectangular	• Orbital opening comparatively small and rounded
• Facial bones more massive and not delicate in texture	• Facial bones less massive and delicate in texture

PART III

5. Define medical negligence. Discuss various medicolegal issues in the case of negligence by a doctor.

(Ref: Parikh's Textbook of Medical Jurisprudence, Forensic Medicine and Toxicology, 7/e, Pg. 35)

ANSWER

Medical Negligence

For answer, refer 2016 paper Q. 5 (a), Pg. 474

6. Write short notes on:

a. Whiplash injury

(Ref: Parikh's Textbook of Medical Jurisprudence, Forensic Medicine and Toxicology, 7/e, Pg. 263)

ANSWER

Whiplash Injury

- **Definition:** Injury occurred from a blow on brow or chin or when vehicle comes to a sudden stop, the forward thrust dashes the head against the windscreen of a car resulting in hyperextension of the head and consequent injury to the cervical column
- A momentary dislocation of the cervical spine in the region of C4 – C6 occurs resulting in contusion of the spinal cord, leading to self-reduction
- Occurs in occupants of front seat
- This injury is likely to be missed and paralysis resulting therefrom regarded as hysterical unless the cord in this region is carefully examined
- On autopsy:
  - Area of hemorrhagic discoloration on the surface or in substance of the cord, or subthecal effusions of blood is seen
  - Extent of hemorrhage must be demonstrated by serial sections of the cord, in case of hemorrhage

b. Frost bite

(Ref: Parikh's Textbook of Medical Jurisprudence, Forensic Medicine and Toxicology, 7/e, Pg. 201; The Essentials of Forensic Medicine & Toxicology, K.S. Narayan Reddy-34/e, pg. 295)

ANSWER

Frost Bite

Definition

- Tissue necrosis from vascular spasm or thrombosis resulting from local effect of cold on exposed parts of the body such as tip of nose, ears, fingers and toes
- Skin on exposed parts of body is patchy red with a general pallor elsewhere
- Occurs due to exposure to extremes of cold, develops rapidly and extends to extremities

Symptoms and Signs

- Edema
- Redness
- Necrosis of tissue beyond a line of demarcation of inflammation

- Necrosis with blister formation
- Gangrene may occur
- Skin becomes hard and black after 2 weeks

Mechanism

- As cold grips, metabolism is lowered
- Respiratory rate is slowed and heart rate is slowed
- Striking fall in peripheral circulation so as to maintain core body temperature by reducing heat loss
- Surface of body becomes pale (vasospasm)
- Dilatation of capillaries causes stasis of blood and thrombosis
- Therefore, blood vessels are blocked resulting in tissue necrosis
- Exposed parts such as tip of nose, ears, fingers and toes are rapidly affected

c. Sadism

(Ref: Parikh's Textbook of Medical Jurisprudence, Forensic Medicine and Toxicology, 7/e, Pg. 411)

ANSWER

Sadism

Definition

- Type of Sexual perversion in which, infliction of pain is necessary or sometimes the sole aspect for sexual gratification
- More common in males
- Sadist usually bites, injures, ill-treats his partner
- Injuries may be inflicted on any part of body but more common are on breasts and external genitalia

Examples

- Sadist sometimes use cigarettes to cause burns to their partners to get an erection
- May perform sexual intercourse on a dead body or dying person – necrophilia
- May tear out genitals or other organs and drink blood or eat flesh in order to satisfy sexual desire – necrophagia
- May get fit to commit violent acts – lust murder

Your Roll No. ....

Name of the Paper	:	**Forensic Medicine & Toxicology**
Name of the Course	:	**MBBS-2014**
Semester	:	**Annual**

Time: 3 Hours   M.M.: 40

INSTRUCTIONS

1. Write your Roll No. on the top immediately on receipt of this question paper
2. All questions are to be attempted
3. Answers to Parts I, II and III should be written in separate answer sheets provided
4. Attempt parts of a question in sequence

PART-I

1. **What are the findings and medicolegal importance when it is stated that:**   [8]

   a. The boy is 21 years of age
   b. Body is showings pugilistic attitude
   c. Burtonian line is present on the gums
   d. The female is a false virgin

2. **Write short notes on:**   [6]

   a. Defense wounds
   b. Legal duties of a doctor in a case of suspected poisoning
   c. Gustafson's method

PART-II

3. **Classify irritant poisons. Discuss clinical features, management and autopsy findings in a case of acute Malathion poisoning. What viscera will you preserve such a case?**   [7]

4. **Differentiate between:**   [6]

   a. Antemortem and postmortem drowning
   b. Heat hematoma and Traumatic extradural hematoma
   c. Professional negligence and professional misconduct

PART-III

5. **Define and classify injuries. Describe in details various causes of death due to injuries and factors that will help in determining age of injury**   [7]

6. **Write short notes on:**   [6]

   a. Subpoena
   b. Exhumation
   c. Modern concept of the moment of death

PART I

1. What are the findings and medicolegal importance when it is stated that

a. The boy is 21 years of age

(Ref: Parikh's Textbook of Medical Jurisprudence, Forensic Medicine and Toxicology, 7/e, Pg. 59; The Essentials of Forensic Medicine & Toxicology, K.S. Narayan Reddy-34/e, pg. 78)

ANSWER

The Boy is 21 Years of Age

Findings

- **Teeth**
  - Presence of 3 wisdom teeth
  - On X-ray of wisdom teeth, roots are not calcified
- **Ossification of bones**
  - All the epiphyses at wrist, knee, crest of ilium and lateral end of clavicle are united
  - Acromion process is united to scapula
  - Articular facets of ribs are united
  - Basiocciput is fused with basisphenoid

Interpretation

- Boy is around 21 years of age
- Union of epiphysis in cartilaginous bones takes place earlier by 2 years in females than in males except in case of skull sutures where obliteration sets in little later and proceeds more slowly in female than in males

Medicolegal Importance

- **Criminal responsibility**
  - Child under 12 years of age cannot give valid consent to suffer harm which can occur from an act done in good faith and for its benefit e.g. consent for operation
  - Person under 18 years of age cannot give valid consent whether express or implied to suffer any harm which may result from an act not intended to cause any grievous hurt e.g. consent for wrestling
- **Judicial punishment**
  - Children below 18 years of age, who have committed a crime, are tried by Juvenile court and if convicted, are entrusted to parents for special care or sent to correctional school with facilities for education, vocational training and rehabilitation

- **Employment**
  - Child below 14 years of age cannot be employed for any type of work
- **Kidnapping**
  - Kidnapping or abducting a minor, if boy is under 16 and girl is under 18 years is an offence
- **Marriage**
  - The Child Marriage Restraint Act lays down that a girl under 18 years of age and a boy under 21 years of age cannot contract a valid marriage
- **Attainment of majority**
  - Under Indian Majority Act, persons domiciled in India attain majority on completion of 18 years, except when under a guardian appointed by a court or under a court of wards, when the individual attains majority on completion of 21 years
  - Persons under this age are minors and they cannot make a valid will, sell his property or serve a jury

b. Body is showing pugilistic attitude

(Ref: Parikh's Textbook of Medical Jurisprudence, Forensic Medicine and Toxicology, 7/e, Pg. 337)

ANSWER

Body is Showing Pugilistic Attitude

- **Findings**
  - Legs are flexed at the hips and knees
  - Arms are flexed at the elbows and wrists and held out in front of body
  - Fingers are hooked like claws
  - Head is slightly extended
  - Contraction of paraspinal muscles often causes a marked opisthotonus
- **Interpretation**
  - Occurs due to heat stiffening due to coagulation of proteins of the muscles and dehydration causing contraction
  - Differs from rigor mortis as it is permanent and does not pass off
  - Skin is tense, leathery, hard and frequently shows splits due to tension
  - Condition is distinguished from violence by
    - Presence of nerves, blood vessels and connective tissue, running across split from side to side

- No clotted blood in fissures and no extravasation of blood in surrounding tissues as heat coagulates blood in vessels
    - No bruising or other signs of vital reaction in margins of heat rupture split
  - Fractures may occur due to sudden contraction of muscles as a result of heat
○ **Medicolegal importance**
  - Has no medicolegal importance as attitude is present whether a living or dead body is burnt

c. Burtonian line is present on the gums

(Ref: Parikh's Textbook of Medical Jurisprudence, Forensic Medicine and Toxicology, 7/e, Pg. 559)

ANSWER

Burtonian Line is Present on the Gums

Findings

○ Bluish-black line on the gums at the junction with teeth (but not on teeth)
○ Facial pallor
○ **Anemia with punctate basophilia:** Presence of dark blue colored pinhead like spots in cytoplasm of RBCs
○ Colic pain, relieved by pressure on abdomen
○ Constipation
○ **Onset of Paralysis in later stages may be seen:** Wrist drop or foot drop
○ **Encephalopathy:** Convulsions, mental deterioration, optic atrophy
○ Vascular constriction
○ **Menstrual disorders:** Dysmenorrhea, amenrrhea, menorrhagia

Interpretation

○ Lead poisoning is suspected
○ Occasionally case of mercury poisoning

Medicolegal Importance

○ Acute poisoning is rare as lead is rarely used for homicidal purpose
○ Accidental poisoning may occur in children from eating paint on cribs or beds or toys
○ Chronic lead poisoning may occur due to contamination of food or drink or use of lead monoxide for treatment of syphilis

d. The female is a false virgin

(Ref: Parikh's Textbook of Medical Jurisprudence, Forensic Medicine and Toxicology, 7/e, Pg. 376)

ANSWER

A Female is a False Virgin

Findings

○ Intact hymen but edges are undulated
○ Hymenal opening admits 2 fingers to pass through easily
○ Labia majora are fleshy and do not completely close the vaginal orifice
○ Labia minora are cutaneous and not covered by labia majora
○ Clitoris is enlarged
○ Vestibule is gaping
○ Fourchette is torn
○ Vagina is roomy

Interpretation

○ If hymen is thick and distensible, sexual intercourse may not rupture hymen
○ Hymen may be ruptured in a true virgin by digital and sanitary pad insertions, by trauma and by perineal injury

Medicolegal Importance

○ Defamation
○ Sexual offences
○ Divorce
○ Nullity of marriage

2. Write short notes on:

a. Defense wounds

(Ref: Parikh's Textbook of Medical Jurisprudence, Forensic Medicine and Toxicology, 7/e, Pg.229)

ANSWER

Defense Wounds

For answer, refer 2016 paper Q. 1 (a), Pg. 468

b Legal duties of a doctor in a case of suspected poisoning

(Ref: Parikh's Textbook of Medical Jurisprudence, Forensic Medicine and Toxicology, 7/e, Pg. 514; The Essentials of Forensic Medicine & Toxicology, K.S. Narayan Reddy-34/e, pg. 477)

ANSWER

Legal Duties of a Doctor in a Case of Suspected Poisoning

In all cases of poisoning, the doctor must:

○ Record preliminary details such as Name in full, age, sex, occupation, address, date and time, brought by whom, history, dying declaration necessary or not

○ Treat the patient is the first duty of the doctor
  ▪ If doctor in private practice is sure that it is the case of accidental or suicidal poisoning, he is not bound to provide information of his own accord to the police or magistrate
  ▪ If he is summoned by investigating officer for such information, then he should do so

○ Notify the public health authorities immediately if there is any indication of danger to general public in case of accidental poisoning such as food poisoning from eating at a public eating joint or drinking contaminated water meant for public use

○ Inform the nearest police officer or magistrate, in case of homicidal poisoning
  ▪ As a precautionary measure, he should try to prevent the likelihood of further administration of poison to the patient

In every case of suspected poisoning, the doctor must:

○ Keep the records of the case in meticulous detail

○ Collect and preserve the stomach washings and samples of vomit and urine passed in his presence only, and blood likely to contain poison, properly and in separate containers, for transmission to the forensic science laboratory

○ Any suspicious article for example.
  ▪ Utensils used for preparing the poison
  ▪ Bottles or containers of solid or liquid medicine found at the scene
  ▪ Food or drink lying near the patient
  ▪ Clothes or bed sheet soiled by vomit, urine or feces, should be preserved for possible future examination

○ Make arrangements for taking dying declaration, if the patient is serious

○ In the event of death, a death certificate should not be issued but the fact of death must be communicated to the nearest police officer for necessary investigation

○ Opinion about the nature of poison can only be given after report from forensic science laboratory

○ Doctor in charge of government or public hospital must report to police all cases of poisoning admitted to the institution, either suicidal, homicidal or accidental

c. Gustafson's method

(Ref: Parikh's Textbook of Medical Jurisprudence, Forensic Medicine and Toxicology, 7/e, Pg. 60; The Essentials of Forensic Medicine & Toxicology, K.S. Narayan Reddy-34/e, pg. 67)

ANSWER

Gustafson's Method

Definition

○ Method of age estimation

○ Comprises of microscopic examination of the longitudinal section of the central part of the tooth to determine the changes in teeth as a result of wear and tear with advancing age

○ Beneficial for estimation of age between 25 to 60 years

Type of Grading of Changes in Teeth

○ Attrition or gradual wearing out of teeth

○ Periodontosis or loosening of teeth

○ Secondary dentition formation or infilling of normal root cavity

○ Cement apposition or increase in the tissue holding the root in place

○ Root resorption

○ Root transparency

PART II

3. **Classify Irritant poisons. Discuss clinical features, management and autopsy findings in a case of acute malathion poisoning. Which viscera will you preserve in such a case?**

(Ref: Parikh's Textbook of Medical Jurisprudence, Forensic Medicine and Toxicology, 7/e, Pg. 510)

ANSWER

Definition

○ Poisons which produce symptoms of pain in abdomen, vomiting and purging

○ Postmortem appearances are generally apparent to the naked eye and produce redness or ulceration of the gastrointestinal tract

Classification

○ **Inorganic**
  ▪ **Nonmetallic**
    ◆ Phosphorus
    ◆ Chlorine
    ◆ Bromine
    ◆ Iodine
  ▪ **Metallic**
    ◆ Arsenic
    ◆ Antimony
    ◆ Mercury
    ◆ Lead
    ◆ Copper
    ◆ Thallium

- ◆ Zinc
- ◆ Manganese
- ◆ Barium
- ◆ Radioactive substances
- ○ **Organic**
  - ▪ **Vegetable poisons**
    - ◆ Castor seeds
    - ◆ Croton seeds
    - ◆ Abrus precatorius
    - ◆ Colocynth
    - ◆ Ergot
    - ◆ Capsicum
    - ◆ Semecarpus anacardium
    - ◆ Calotropis
    - ◆ Plumbago rosea
    - ◆ Plumbago zeylanica
  - ▪ **Animal poisons**
    - ◆ Cantharides
    - ◆ Snakes
    - ◆ Scorpions
    - ◆ Spiders
    - ◆ Poisonous insects
- ○ **Mechanical**
  - ▪ Coarsely powdered glass
  - ▪ Chopped hair
  - ▪ Dried sponge
  - ▪ Diamond dust

b.   Acute malathion poisoning

(Ref: Parikh's Textbook of Medical Jurisprudence, Forensic Medicine and Toxicology, 7/e, Pg. 625)

ANSWER

Malathion Poisoning or Organophosphorus Poisoning

For answer, refer 2016 paper Q. 3 (b), Pg. 472

Viscera to be Preserved

- ○ Stomach and its contents
- ○ Upper part of small intestine
- ○ Liver – 200 g
- ○ Kidney – half of each
- ○ Blood – 30 ml
- ○ Urine – 30 ml

4.   Differentiate between

a.   Antemortem and Postmortem drowning

(Ref: Parikh's Textbook of Medical Jurisprudence, Forensic Medicine and Toxicology, 7/e, Pg. 188; The Essentials of Forensic Medicine & Toxicology, K.S. Narayan Reddy-34/e, pg. 41)

ANSWER

For answer, refer 2016 paper Q. 4 (a), Pg. 473

b.   Heat hematoma and Traumatic extradural hematoma

(Ref: Parikh's Textbook of Medical Jurisprudence, Forensic Medicine and Toxicology, 7/e, Pg. 295)

ANSWER

Heat Hematoma and Traumatic Extradural Hematoma

For answer, refer 2016 paper Q. 4 (b), Pg. 474

c.   Professional negligence and professional misconduct

ANSWER

Professional Negligence and Professional Misconduct

(Ref: Parikh's Textbook of Medical Jurisprudence, Forensic Medicine and Toxicology, 7/e, Pg. 35; The Essentials of Forensic Medicine & Toxicology, K.S. Narayan Reddy-34/e, pg. 41)

Professional negligence	Professional misconduct
• Lack of reasonable care and willful negligence	• Violation of code of ethics
• Action against negligence is brought in civil or criminal court, depending upon the case	• State medical council take charge of any offence of misconduct committed
• Nature of action may be Fine or Imprisonment	• Nature of action may be a warning or erasure of name from Register
• Damages to the patient must be present	• Damages to patient may not be present
• Duty of care towards patient is always present which he neglected	• Duty of care towards patient may not be present
• Appeal is made to higher court	• Appeal is made to state or central government

PART III

5.   Define and classify injuries. Describe in detail various causes of death due to injuries and factors that will help in determining age of injury

(Ref: Parikh's Textbook of Medical Jurisprudence, Forensic Medicine and Toxicology, 7/e, Pg. 211)

ANSWER

Injuries

Definition

○ A solution or disruption of the anatomical continuity of any of the tissues of the body

○ Any harm whatever illegally caused to any person in body, mind, reputation, or property

Classification

○ Mechanical:
○ Based on cause
○ Abrasions
○ Bruises
○ Lacerations
○ Fractures
○ Incised wounds
○ Stab wounds
○ Firearm wounds

Based on Nature

○ Defense wounds
○ Self-inflicting wounds
○ Injury patterns
○ Thermal

Due to Cold

○ Frostbite
○ Trench foot
○ Immersion foot

Due to Heat

○ **Simple burns:** Caused by dry heat – by hot substances, by flames

○ **Scalds:** Caused by moist heat

○ **Corrosive burns:** By chemicals

○ **Electric burns:** By electric contact, electric spark, flashes of lightning

○ **Radiation burns:** Caused by X-rays, ultraviolet rays, radium, laser, microwave oven

b. **Causes of death due to injuries**

(Ref: Parikh's Textbook of Medical Jurisprudence, Forensic Medicine and Toxicology, 7/e, Pg. 266)

ANSWER

Immediate or Direct

○ Hemorrhage

Site of hemorrhage	Cause of death
• Extradural, subdural or subarachnoid	• Cerebral compression
• Medulla	• Failure of vital functions

Site of hemorrhage	Cause of death
• Pericardial sac	• Cardiac tamponade
• Pleural cavity	• Collapse of lung and displacement of mediastinum
• Respiratory passages, e.g. in cut throat injury or tonsillectomy	• Asphyxia

■ **Injury to vital organ:** Brain, heart and lungs is fatal

■ **Neurogenic shock:** Primary shock or vagal inhibition is characterized by sudden stoppage of heart and respiration as a result of reflex stimulation of the vagus nerve and consequent paralysis of cardiac and respiratory centers

■ Combination of any of these

Remote or indirect causes

○ **Infection**

■ Local sepsis or septicaemia and pyaemia

■ **Infective processes in internal organs:** Penetrating wounds in abdomen, risk of peritonitis, bladder infection, pyelonephritis, suppurative meningitis

■ **Necrosis or sloughing:** Due to loss of blood supply as seen in cut throat injury

■ **Tetanus:** In all wounds and especially in lacerated wounds, deep stab wounds

○ **Renal failure (Crush syndrome)**

■ Due to extensive muscle damage, burns, poisons

■ Due to damage to juxtaglomerular apparatus, renin-angiotensin system, effect on glomeruli of disseminated intravascular coagulation

○ **Thrombosis:** Delayed complication of trauma, person confined to bed develops phlebothrombosis in leg veins

○ **Embolism**

■ **Fat embolism:** Intrinsic and extrinsic
   ◆ Pulmonary fat embolism
   ◆ Systemic or arterial fat embolism

■ **Air embolism**
   ◆ Pulmonary or venous air embolism
   ◆ Systemic or arterial air embolism

○ **Secondary shock**

■ Due to reduction of total circulating blood volume

■ Due to loss of fluid at the site of injury, increased capillary permeability, hypotension etc.

■ Infection

■ Exposure to cold

○ **Consumptive coagulopathy:** Due to series of insults such as crush injuries, sepsis and other acute events

○ **Indirect effects:** Onset of delirium tremens after fracture of leg in an alcoholic person; transfusion hepatitis due to accidental introduction of virus from blood or serum used to treat shock

- **Acceleration of pre-existing disease:** If injury hastens or precipitates death, responsibility of the consequences rests on the assailant
- **Supervention of new disease:** If symptoms of disease appear within a reasonable time in a previously healthy person, there is presumption that the injury is a causal factor and the attacker is responsible for the consequences of his violent act
- **Operative treatment:** If death follows anesthesia or surgical operation, the assailant is responsible for the result, if the wound was such as would have proved dangerous without such interference
- **Neglect of treatment:** It is not obligatory for the assaulted person to submit himself for treatment, even if death occurs from this omission or through disobedience of the physician's instructions by the victim, the assailant is responsible for his act

Factors Help in Determining the Age of Injury

- Vitality of the injured person
- Extent of damage
- Vascularity of the part
- Infection
- Mobility of the part
- Nutrition
- Diabetes
- Other factors interfering with healing

---

6. **Write short notes on:**

    a. **Subpoena**

    (Ref: Parikh's Textbook of Medical Jurisprudence, Forensic Medicine and Toxicology, 7/e, Pg. 9; The Essentials of Forensic Medicine & Toxicology, K.S. Narayan Reddy-34/e, pg. 8)

ANSWER

Subpoena

Definition

- **Subpoena or summons:**
    - Document compelling the attendance of a witness, on a specified day and at a specified time, in a court of law under a penalty
    - Issued by the court in writing, in duplicate and signed by the presiding officer of the court
    - Served on the witness by a police officer or officer of the court or other public servant
    - Witness retains one copy and returns the other one duly signed by him in acknowledgement of its receipt

- When a summons or subpoena is served on a witness, he has to attend the court punctually, provide evidence, and produce such documents or other articles as required by the court
- Failure to obey summons without a just cause renders the witness liable to an action for damages in a civil case and fine, imprisonment or warrant of arrest and compulsory attendance in a criminal one

Conduct Money

- A fee is tendered in civil cases, to cover the expenses to attend the court when summons is served
- Paid by the party which has called him as a witness
- In case where medical witness considers that the tender of fees is inadequate, he may inform the court accordingly and get it enhanced
- However, no such tender is made in criminal cases, where summons is served but a medical witness must always obey the summons, otherwise he will be charged with contempt of court

    b. **Exhumation**

    (Ref: Parikh's Textbook of Medical Jurisprudence, Forensic Medicine and Toxicology, 7/e, Pg. 133; The Essentials of Forensic Medicine & Toxicology, K.S. Narayan Reddy-34/e, pg. 126)

ANSWER

Exhumation

Definition

- Lawful disinterment or digging out of a buried body from the grave
- Becomes necessary for
    - Identification purposes
    - Determination of cause of death, when foul play is suspected

Procedure

- **General precautions**
    - Carried out under supervision of the medical officer and in the presence of a police officer
    - Police officer provides witnesses to identify the grave, the coffin and the dead body
    - Should be carried out in early morning so that the whole process of digging and autopsy, if required can be completed during the day
- **Identification and opening the grave**
    - Formally identified by the warden of the cemetery from the records, and the exact site by friends and relatives who were present at the time of burial
    - Sexton and caretaker may confirm this identification procedure

- In a suspected case of poisoning, samples of earth in a quantity of about 500 g are collected from above, below and sides of coffin and control samples at some distance from it, in separate clean dry, glass bottles for chemical analysis

○ **Identification of the coffin**

- Coffin top should be cleaned up and the plate exposed
- Should be identified by the original caretaker who made it and a photograph of it is valuable
- Coffin can then be raised to the surface and before examining the contents, the lid is lifted to allow the escape of gases
- One should stand on the windward side in order to avoid inhaling offensive gases
- Samples of earth from above, below and sides should be taken
- If coffin contains water, it should be drained off, the total volume with sludge measured and a sample collected for analysis
- Samples should be collected from coffin wood and burial clothes to rule out any possibility of contamination from external sources

○ **Identification of the body**

- Attempt should be made to identify the body by any person who was present when the body was placed in the coffin
- Magistrate or coroner views the body and orders a reburial or an autopsy

○ **Autopsy**

- Strict attention to health and safety of the participants in the exhumation should be taken care of
- Gloves should be worn and should be perfect condition
- Doctor should have complete history of the case so that his attention is properly directed to important points
- Photograph of the body should be taken and if required X-ray examination should be done
- Injuries, if present should be explained in detail
- Since soft tissue injuries disappear due to decomposition, fracture of bones such as skull, hyoid and ribs should be checked
- Any organ which may offer any evidence should be kept for further examination and/or chemical analysis by forensic laboratory
- Whole procedure should be videographed
- Medical officer should make sure that he has taken all specimens before leaving the place that may be required for later examinations

c.   **Modern concept of the moment of death**

(Ref: Parikh's Textbook of Medical Jurisprudence, Forensic Medicine and Toxicology, 7/e, Pg. 137; The Essentials of Forensic Medicine & Toxicology, K.S. Narayan Reddy-34/e, pg. 128)

ANSWER

For answer, refer 2017 paper Q. 2 (a), Pg. 461

Your Roll No. ....

Name of the Paper : **Forensic Medicine & Toxicology**

Name of the Course : **MBBS-2013**

Semester : **Annual**

Time: 3 Hours   M.M.: 40

INSTRUCTIONS

1. Write your Roll No. on the top immediately on receipt of this question paper
2. All questions are to be attempted
3. Answers to Parts I, II and III should be written in separate answer sheets provided
4. Attempt parts of a question in sequence

PART-I

1. What are the findings, interpretations and medicolegal importance, when it is stated that: [8]
   a. Defense wound are present over the body
   b. Boy examined is of 14 years
   c. Blue line is present on the gums
   d. Body showing filigree burns

2. Write short notes on: [6]
   a. Informed consent
   b. Delusion
   c. Sadism

PART-II

3. Define poison. Discuss the clinical features, management, postmortem findings and medicolegal significance of "Methyl Alcohol" poisoning   [7]

4. Differentiate between: [6]
   a. Suicidal and homicidal cut throat injuries
   b. Acute arsenic poisoning and cholera
   c. Antemortem and postmortem burns

PART-III

5. Define infanticide. Describe in detail the postmortem findings on the body of a new born: [7]

6. Write short notes on: [6]
   a. Vicarious responsibility
   b. Burking
   c. Statutory rape

PART I

1. What are the findings, interpretation and medicolegal importance, when it is stated that?

a. Defense wound are present over the body

(Ref: Parikh's Textbook of Medical Jurisprudence, Forensic Medicine and Toxicology, 7/e, Pg. 229; The Essentials of Forensic Medicine & Toxicology, K.S. Narayan Reddy-34/e, pg. 194)

ANSWER

For answer, refer 2016 paper Q. 1 (a), Pg. 468

b. Boy examined is of 14 years

(Ref: Parikh's Textbook of Medical Jurisprudence, Forensic Medicine and Toxicology, 7/e, Pg. 59; The Essentials of Forensic Medicine & Toxicology, K.S. Narayan Reddy-34/e, pg. 78)

ANSWER

Boy Examined is of 14 Years

Findings

○ **Teeth**
  - Period of mixed dentition has passed and permanent teeth present in lower jaw and then upper jaw
  - Bicuspids are most irregular
  - Second molars have been erupted
  - Space for last molar can be seen

○ **Ossification of bones – as seen on X-ray studies**
  - Lateral epicondyle of the humerus has been united with trochlea and capitulum
  - Olecranon united with ulna
  - Pisiform already ossified
  - Heads of metacarpals and phalanges not yet fused

Interpretation

○ Union of epiphysis in cartilaginous bones takes place earlier by 2 years in females than in males except in case of skull sutures where obliteration sets in little later and proceeds more slowly in female than in males

Medicolegal Importance

○ **Criminal responsibility**
  - Child under 12 years of age cannot give valid consent to suffer harm which can occur from

an act done in good faith and for its benefit e.g. consent for operation
  - Person under 18 years of age cannot give valid consent whether express or implied to suffer any harm which may result from an act not intended to cause any grievous hurt e.g. consent for wrestling

○ **Employment**
  - Child below 14 years of age cannot be employed for any type of work

○ **Kidnapping**
  - Kidnapping or abducting a minor, if boy is under 16 and girl is under 18 years is an offence

c. Blue line is present on the gums

(Ref: Parikh's Textbook of Medical Jurisprudence, Forensic Medicine and Toxicology, 7/e, Pg. 559; The Essentials of Forensic Medicine & Toxicology, K.S. Narayan Reddy-34/e, pg. 507)

ANSWER

Blue Line is Present on the Gums

For answer, refer 2014 paper Q. 1 (c), Pg. 486

d. Body showing filigree burns

(Ref: Parikh's Textbook of Medical Jurisprudence, Forensic Medicine and Toxicology, 7/e, Pg. 357; The Essentials of Forensic Medicine & Toxicology, K.S. Narayan Reddy-34/e, pg. 312)

ANSWER

Body Showing Filigree Burns

Findings

○ Superficial, thin, trivial lesions, involving only epidermal layer of skin (filigree burns or arborescent markings)
○ Erythema with pattern like branches of tree
○ Appears within minutes to hours of accident

Interpretation

○ Indicate path taken by the discharge and disappears within a day or two if patient survives
○ Caused due to natural electrical discharge from cloud to earth

Medicolegal Importance

○ Depends on exclusion of any other cause of death
○ History of thunderstorm in the vicinity

FORENSIC MEDICINE & TOXICOLOGY

○ Evidence of lightning such as damaged trees, dead cattle, appearance of various lesions on body such as filigree burns (arborescent markings), fractures, wounds, torn clothes, burns on body

○ Death from lightning stoke are accidental

2. Write short notes on:

a. Informed consent

(Ref: Parikh's Textbook of Medical Jurisprudence, Forensic Medicine and Toxicology, 7/e, Pg. 30; The Essentials of Forensic Medicine & Toxicology, K.S. Narayan Reddy-34/e, pg. 49)

ANSWER

Informed Consent

Definition

○ The consent to be legally valid must be informed and intelligent which means, consent must be given after understanding what is given for and the risks involved with it.

○ Doctor must provide reasonable information to his patient about
  ▪ Diagnosis
  ▪ Nature of treatment procedure
  ▪ Risks involved with the procedure
  ▪ Prospects of success
  ▪ Prognosis and risks if the procedure is not performed
  ▪ Alternative methods of treatment

○ Law states that
  ▪ Patient must be fully informed of every risk and factual material for making of a proper consent
  ▪ Consent should be based upon such material disclosure

○ All disclosures of the consent must be in such language which patient can understand

○ Therapeutic exceptions to the informed consent
  ▪ Apprehensive or neurotic patients
  ▪ Emergency

b. Delusion

(Ref: Parikh's Textbook of Medical Jurisprudence, Forensic Medicine and Toxicology, 7/e, Pg. 442)

ANSWER

Delusion

Definition

○ False but firm belief in something which is not a fact despite proof to the contrary

○ Indicates a serious disorder such as schizophrenia or GPI

Types of Delusions

○ **Hypochondriacal delusion:** Most common in depressions in later life e.g. if a person says he has cancer and is not able to swallow food

○ **Delusions of poverty:** Common in depressions e.g. person believes he has left with no money and worries about his relatives that they are starving or sick

○ **Nihilistic delusions:** Common in involutional melancholia and patient believes that there is no world, He does not exist or that he is dead

○ **Delusions of infidelity:** Occur in chronic alcoholism and schizophrenia e.g. patient suspects the fidelity of his wife although she is chaste and assaults her

○ **Delusions of grandeur:** GPI, mania and schizophrenia e.g. patient believes that he has untold wealth, is related to ministers, has divine powers etc.

○ **Delusions of persecution (paranoid delusions):** As in schizophrenia, paranoid states, affective disorders (disorders of mood) e.g. mania and depression, organic syndromes and alcoholic and drug psychoses – patient believes that his relatives are attempting to poison him or kill him

○ **Delusion of reference:** Patient believes that people, things or events refer to him in a special way

○ **Delusion of influence:** Patient believes that his thoughts, feelings and actions are being influenced via radio, hypnotism, or other means in order to harm him

Medicolegal Importance

○ Affects the conduct and actions of the sufferer who may try to commit suicide, murder or some other crime therefore such person is not held responsible for his actions

c. Sadism

(Ref: Parikh's Textbook of Medical Jurisprudence, Forensic Medicine and Toxicology, 7/e, Pg. 411; The Essentials of Forensic Medicine & Toxicology, K.S. Narayan Reddy-34/e, pg. 402)

ANSWER

For answer, refer 2015 paper Q. 6 (c), Pg. 483

PART II

3. Define poisons. Discuss the clinical features, management, postmortem findings and medicolegal significance of Methyl Alcohol poisoning.

(Ref: Parikh's Textbook of Medical Jurisprudence, Forensic Medicine and Toxicology, 7/e, Pg. 507)

a. Poisons

ANSWER

Definition

○ Poison is any substance solid, liquid or gas, which when introduced, ingested, inhaled, injected or brought in contact with body causes ill health or death by its local or remote action.

○ Substances which when administered, inhaled or ingested, are capable of acting deleteriously on the human body

○ Almost everything or anything is a poison

○ Actual difference between a medicine and a poison is the intent with which it is given

○ If given with intention to save life, it is medicine but if given with intention to harm somebody, it is poison

b. Methyl alcohol poisoning

(Ref: Parikh's Textbook of Medical Jurisprudence, Forensic Medicine and Toxicology, 7/e, Pg. 616; The Essentials of Forensic Medicine & Toxicology, K.S. Narayan Reddy-34/e, pg. 540)

ANSWER

For answer, refer 2015 paper Q. 2 (a), Pg. 479

4. Differentiate between:

a. Suicidal and homicidal cut throat injuries

(Ref: Parikh's Textbook of Medical Jurisprudence, Forensic Medicine and Toxicology, 7/e, Pg. 305)

ANSWER

For answer, refer 2017 paper Q. 4 (b)

b. Acute Arsenic poisoning and Cholera

(Ref: Parikh's Textbook of Medical Jurisprudence, Forensic Medicine and Toxicology, 7/e, Pg. 550; The Essentials of Forensic Medicine & Toxicology, K.S. Narayan Reddy-34/e, pg. 502)

ANSWER

Acute Arsenic Poisoning and Cholera

Acute arsenic poisoning	Cholera
• Throat pain before vomiting	• Throat pain after vomiting
• After vomiting, there is purging	• Before vomiting, there is purging
• At first, stools are dark colored and bloody which later becomes rice-watery	• Stools are rice-watery with no blood, continuous involuntary passage of stools

Acute arsenic poisoning	Cholera
• Patient has tenesmus and irritation in anus	• No tenesmus or anal irritation is seen
• Vomitus contains mucus, blood and bile	• Vomitus is watery and without any mucus, bile or blood
• In Stool analysis, arsenic is found	• In stool analysis, cholera vibrio is found
• Inflammation of conjunctivae is present	• Inflammation of conjunctivae is absent

c. Antemortem and postmortem burns

(Ref: Parikh's Textbook of Medical Jurisprudence, Forensic Medicine and Toxicology, 7/e, Pg. 340)

ANSWER

Antemortem and postmortem Burns

For answer, refer 2016 paper Q. 4 (c), Pg. 474

PART III

5. Define Infanticide. Describe in detail the postmortem findings on the body of a new born.

a. Infanticide

(Ref: Parikh's Textbook of Medical Jurisprudence, Forensic Medicine and Toxicology, 7/e, Pg. 424; The Essentials of Forensic Medicine & Toxicology, K.S. Narayan Reddy-34/e, pg. 409)

ANSWER

Definition

○ Unlawful destruction of a new born child, and is regarded as a murder in law

○ Punishable under section 302IPC, by death or transportation for life and also fine

○ Differs from ordinary murder, as it is essential to prove that the child was born alive

○ New born child means infant who is in first year of life

○ Most commonly, infant is killed soon after birth

○ Committed by
  ▪ Unmarried women
  ▪ Widows
  ▪ Sometimes by married women also
  ▪ In communities where dowry is prevalent, female infanticide is common
  ▪ Male infanticide is resorted to by prostitutes

Postmortem Findings on the Body of a NewBorn

○ **External examination**
  ▪ **Clothes and wrappings:** Torn old clothes of mother, newspaper, blanket, plastic bag etc. which helps in identification

- **Appearance of body**
  - **Vernix caseosa:** Can't be removed easily hence its presence or absence suggests if body has been washed or not
  - Violence marks around mouth, nose, neck or head may be present in the form of nail marks or contusions
  - Foreign bodies may be seen in mouth or upper respiratory passages
  - Other natural orifices should be checked
  - **Caput succedaneum:** Presence/absence and position and character should be checked
  - Nape of neck should be observed carefully for any punctured wounds
  - Decomposition changes indicates time since death
  - Any maceration or mummification indicates intrauterine death
- **Maturity:** Helps to calculate intrauterine age; crown heel length of mature ne born infant is around 48-52 cm, crown rump length—28-32 cm, head circumference—30-35 cm and weight 2.5-3.3 kg
- Malformations and birth injuries
  - Any bulging fontanelles (hydrocephalus) or spina bifida should be examined
  - Hands and feet should be observed for abnormal number of digits
  - Mouth and palate for cleft palate
  - Rectum for patency
  - Irregularities in consistency of bone
  - Any evidence of birth injury should be looked for
- **Umbilical cord:** Normally, it is 50–55 cm long and 1 cm thick, fleshy with normal spiral twist and glistening surface
  - **Check to assess length:** Unduly short or long
  - Whether has been cut, tied (determines that someone attended the delivery), torn or still attached to placenta
  - Cut ends should be checked for vital signs, abnormal twists, knots or any evidence of displacement of Wharton's jelly
  - Signs of vital reaction suggest interval between birth and death
  - Displacement of Wharton's jelly suggests that cord has been used as ligature to strangulate the new born
  - To check for infections, umbilical region should be observed and histological examination of cord should be carried out

- **Placenta:** 22 cm in diameter, central thickness is 1.5 cm, weight—500 g
  - **Abnormalities include:** Placental infarcts, retroplacental hematomas, acute chorioamnionitis, hemorrhagic endovasculitis, hydrops
- **Internal examination**
- **Head**
  - **Injuries to fontanelles:** Punctured wounds through anterior fontanelle
  - Meningeal tears (in forceps delivery)
  - Hemorrhages or lacerations of brain
- **Mouth:** Interior of mouth should be observed as new born is usually smothered by stuffing wads of paper or cloth into mouth
- **Neck:** Observed for internal injuries and trachea should be looked for any foreign body, froth, mucus, amniotic fluid; nape of neck requires special attention
- **Thorax**
  - **Shape of chest is examined:** Dome shaped or flat
  - **Lungs:** Observe volume, color, consistency, weight and presence of petechial hemorrhages
  - **Heart:** 4 chambers should be observed–color of blood is checked; patency of foramen ovale and ductus arteriosus is noted
  - **Abdomen:** Stomach is ligated at both ends to check for floatation; contents of stomach are examined for presence of milk, poison, blood, amniotic fluid and squamous epithelium
  - **Intestines:** Examined for presence of air, presence of meconium and its position helps to calculate intrauterine age of fetus
- Other viscera should be observed for development, malformations, asphyxial signs and injuries
- **Genitals:** Any malformations; position of testes-descended or not
- **Limbs and sternum:** Observed for presence of ossific centers to calculate the age of fetus

302 IPC	Punishment for murder (death or imprisonment for life)	
312 IPC	Criminal abortion with consent (3 years imprisonment and if woman is quick 7 years imprisonment)	
Offence against children	317 IPC	Exposure and abandonment of child under twelve years, by parent or person having care of it (upto 7 years)
	317 IPC	Concealment of birth (2 years imprisonment)

6. Write short notes on:

a. Vicarious responsibility

(Ref: Parikh's Textbook of Medical Jurisprudence, Forensic Medicine and Toxicology, 7/e, Pg. 43; The Essentials of Forensic Medicine & Toxicology, K.S. Narayan Reddy-34/e, pg. 45)

ANSWER

Vicarious Responsibility

- **Definition:** Liability exists in spite of the absence of culpable conduct on the part of the master
- According to law, the master is held responsible for the negligent acts of his servants within the scope of his employment but in not so liable where he has employed an independent person to do something for him
- Hospital and nursing homes are liable for the negligent acts and omissions of their non-medical staff and full time junior medical staff but senior medical staff and honorary medical staff are in different position as there is not true relationship of a master and servant between them and managers of hospital
- Hospital management is held responsible for negligent acts of resident physicians and interns in training as they are considered employees while performing their normal duties
- Hospital management is not held responsible for negligent acts of senior medical staff, as they had employed well qualified and experienced staff
- Physician is held responsible for the acts of residents and interns carried out under his immediate direction and control
- Physicians and surgeons are not responsible for acts of qualified nurses unless such acts are carried out under their guidance
- Physician is held responsible under the doctrine of negligent choice, if he refers his patient to an incompetent or inappropriate doctor, otherwise he is not so responsible

b. Burking

(Ref: Parikh's Textbook of Medical Jurisprudence, Forensic Medicine and Toxicology, 7/e, Pg. 185; The Essentials of Forensic Medicine & Toxicology, K.S. Narayan Reddy-34/e, pg. 341)

ANSWER

Burking

Definition

- Type of asphyxia resulting from a procedure adopted by the murderers Burke and Hare, for murdering their victims and selling their bodies for dissection to the Edinburgh medical students for a living.

- Burke used to sit on the chest of the inebriated victim covering his mouth and nose with one hand and pushing up the jaw using the other hand whereas Hare used to pull him round the room by the feet
- It is a mixed example of homicidal smothering and traumatic asphyxia

b. Statutory rape

(Ref: Parikh's Textbook of Medical Jurisprudence, Forensic Medicine and Toxicology, 7/e, Pg. 389; The Essentials of Forensic Medicine & Toxicology, K.S. Narayan Reddy-34/e, pg. 387)

ANSWER

Statutory Rape

Definition

- Unlawful sexual intercourse by a man with a minor past the age of puberty, who is under the age of consent

Examination of Rape Victim

- **Preliminary data**
  - Name in full, address, age, occupation and social status, date, time of arrival, consent for examination, identification marks, by whom examination is requested, name of female nurse present at the time of examination
- **Statement of the victim and others separately**
  - Statement of victim in her own words must be written down as much as possible word for word
  - Amount of violence used, position of the assailant and mode of attack should be obtained
  - Inquiry should be made if vaginal, oral or rectal contact occurred
  - Statement should be recorded with reference to pain, hemorrhage, sensation as to penetration and emission and appearance of any discharge
  - Enquiry should be made if she cried for any help or was too terrified to do so or she fainted
  - Events after the alleged assault should be enquired i.e. if she changed her clothes, bathed or passed urine
  - Delay in making complaint to the authorities should be properly explained
  - Statement of others accompanying her should be recorded separately
- **Signs of struggle on clothes and body**
  - **Clothing should be checked**—if they are same as that worn during the crime should be examined for evidence of struggle such as tears in fabrics, marks of mud or grass, stains of blood or semen
  - If clothes are torn, corresponding injuries to the body should be looked for

- Mud and blood stains are usually found on the back clothes whereas seminal stains are found on front clothes
- Stains may be present on material used for cleaning after assault such as handkerchief
- Blood stains must be ascertained if they are due to menstruation
- Other physical evidence such as foreign hairs, pieces of clothing that could have been came from victim, any trouser button identical with those of assailant who has one missing
- Any injury to the nails of victim while scratching the assailant during struggle, debris under nails should be examined
- Whole body should be examined for marks of violence
  - Cheeks, lips and neck to stifle the victim's cries for help
  - Wrists and arms to restrain her
  - On the back from impact of gravel or hard ground while pinning her
  - Inner sides of thighs, knees while separating her legs
  - **Breasts from mishandling**—bitten nipples
- Examination of genitals, urethra, mouth or anus for:
  - **Local signs of violation**
    - Presence or absence of blood stains about the legs or vagina, urethra, mouth, anus should be noted and if present, it should be determined whether such stains could be due to menstruation or blood from victim or assailant
    - Pubic hair should be examined for matting from seminal fluid or blood and for foreign hairs
  - **Genital injuries**
    - Vulva, hymen, vagina and perineum should be examined for injuries
    - Signs of recent rupture of hymen are ragged tears with lack of epithelial healing but with edema and hemorrhage
    - Redness due to long standing inflammation or to irritation by a chronic discharge must be distinguished from the effect of recent injury
    - Gait is broad-based and painful

- Distensibility of vagina should be noted in relation to the number of fingers it can admit without causing discomfort, if it admits 2 fingers easily, sexual intercourse has probably occurred
- Extent of violence to private parts depends upon the age of victim
- **Rape on virgin**—findings in a 15-year-old girl alleged to have been raped 12 hours ago
  - Swelling and bruising of vulva
  - Laceration of labia
  - Hymen is torn posteriorly at one or other side or in middle
  - Semilunar hymen often ruptures on both sides
  - Annular hymen suffers several tears
  - Fourchette is torn and fossa navicularis disappears
  - Posterior commissure could be ruptured
  - Torn margins are sharp and red and bleed on touch, immediately after the act
  - Edges of laceration are congested and swollen even after 3-4 days of offence
  - Surrounding tissues are swollen and tender
  - Laceration of vaginal wall invariably occurs posteriorly or slightly posteriorly
- **Presence of spermatozoa and other microorganisms**
  - If motile sperms are found in vagina, it would mean that intercourse has taken place within about 12 hours
  - If sperms found inside the vagina are nonmotile, it may be over 12 hours and within 24-48 hours
  - Presence of smegma bacilli suggests intercourse has taken place
- **Any evidence of sexually transmitted disease**
  - Presence or absence of any urethral or vaginal discharge is examined
  - Presence of sores should be observed
  - Blood should be examined for T cells

Name of the Paper   :   **Forensic Medicine & Toxicology**

Name of the Course   :   **MBBS-2012**

Semester   :   **Annual**

Time: 3 Hours   M.M.: 40

INSTRUCTIONS

1. Write your Roll No. on the top immediately on receipt of this question paper
2. All questions are to be attempted
3. Answers to Parts I, II and III should be written in separate answer sheets provided
4. Attempt parts of a question in sequence

PART-I

1. **What are the findings, interpretations and medicolegal importance when it is stated that:**   [8]
    a. Person is more than 12 years of age
    b. Dead body is showing mummification
    c. Hesitational cuts are present
    d. Person is in lucid interval

2. **Write short notes on:**   [6]
    a. Hostile witness
    b. Sodomy
    c. Dying declaration

PART-II

3. **Classify irritant poisons. Describe clinical features, management and autopsy findings in case of organophosphorus poisoning**   [7]

4. **Differentiate between:**   [6]
    a. Temporary and permanent dentition
    b. Poisonous and nonpoisonous snakes
    c. Respired and nonrespired lungs

PART-III

5. **Define and classify strangulation. Describe the autopsy findings in case of ligature strangulation**   [7]

6. **Write short notes on:**   [6]
    a. Res ipsa loquitur
    b. Dactylography
    c. Joule burn

2012 PAPER

PART I

1. **What are the findings, interpretations and medicolegal importance when it is stated that?**

   a. Person is more than 12 years of age

   (Ref: Parikh's Textbook of Medical Jurisprudence, Forensic Medicine and Toxicology, 7/e, Pg. 59; The Essentials of Forensic Medicine & Toxicology, K.S. Narayan Reddy-34/e, pg. 78)

ANSWER

Person is More than 12 Years of Age

Findings

○ **Teeth**
  ▪ Period of mixed dentition has passed and permanent teeth present in lower jaw and then upper jaw
  ▪ Bicuspids are most irregular
  ▪ Second molars have been erupted
  ▪ Space for last molar can be seen

○ **Ossification of bones—as seen on X-ray studies**
  ▪ Lateral epicondyle of the humerus has been united with trochlea and capitulum
  ▪ Olecranon united with ulna
  ▪ Pisiform already ossified
  ▪ Heads of metacarpals and phalanges not yet fused

Interpretation

○ Union of epiphysis in cartilaginous bones takes place earlier by 2 years in females than in males except in case of skull sutures where obliteration sets in little later and proceeds more slowly in female than in males

Medicolegal Importance

○ **Criminal responsibility**
  ▪ Child under 12 years of age cannot give valid consent to suffer harm which can occur from an act done in good faith and for its benefit e.g. consent for operation
  ▪ Person under 18 years of age cannot give valid consent whether express or implied to suffer any harm which may result from an act not intended to cause any grievous hurt e.g. consent for wrestling

○ **Judicial punishment**
  ▪ Children (boys below 16 years and girls below 18 years of age), who have committed a crime,

are tried by Juvenile court and if convicted, are entrusted to parents for special care or sent to correctional school with facilities for education, vocational training and rehabilitation

○ **Employment**
  ▪ Child below 14 years of age cannot be employed for any type of work

○ **Kidnapping**
  ▪ Kidnapping or abducting a minor, if boy is under 16 and girl is under 18 years is an offence

   b. Dead body is showing mummification

   (Ref: Parikh's Textbook of Medical Jurisprudence, Forensic Medicine and Toxicology, 7/e, Pg. 161)

ANSWER

Dead Body is Showing Mummification

For answer, refer 2015 paper Q. 1 (b), Pg. 478

   c. Hesitation cuts are present

   (Ref: Parikh's Textbook of Medical Jurisprudence, Forensic Medicine and Toxicology, 7/e, Pg. 222; The Essentials of Forensic Medicine & Toxicology, K.S. Narayan Reddy-34/e, pg. 184)

ANSWER

Hesitation Cuts are Present

Findings

○ Tentative cuts are present which are small, multiple, superficial, somewhat parallel and usually skin deep
○ Found close to incised wound and may even merge with main incision

Interpretation

○ Person who tries to commit suicide generally makes preliminary cuts in order to gather enough courage to make a final incision
○ Right handed person will hold razor or knife in his right hand and will start incision from left to right, therefore tailing of the wound will be present on the right side

Medicolegal Importance

○ Hesitation cuts are present in suicidal deaths and not found in homicidal assaults
○ Generally seen at wrists, groin, elbows, throat
○ Always multiple, superimposed and with varying depth

○ Doctor treating a case of hesitation cuts should keep in mind that such a person might need psychiatric help to avert the possibility of future attempts

d. Person is in lucid interval

(Ref: Parikh's Textbook of Medical Jurisprudence, Forensic Medicine and Toxicology, 7/e, Pg. 443; The Essentials of Forensic Medicine & Toxicology, K.S. Narayan Reddy-34/e, pg. 243)

ANSWER

Person is in lucid Interval

Findings

○ Sequence of symptoms follows as
  ▪ Unconsciousness due to concussion
  ▪ Consciousness due to recovery
  ▪ Unconsciousness due to raised intracranial tension due to bleeding

Interpretation

○ Traumatic brain injury
○ Epidural hematoma
○ Cerebral edema
○ Heat stroke
○ Epileptic seizure

Medicolegal importance

○ Patient can make a valid will during this period and also can provide valid evidence
○ He can judge his actions well and is held responsible for his conducts
○ In criminal cases, however, it is difficult to state whether any mental abnormality was present at the time of committing crime, therefore it is advisable to treat the person as insane
○ Also observed in head injuries for e.g. in extradural hemorrhage, when it is necessary to arrange for a dying declaration

2. Write short notes on:

a. Hostile witness

(Ref: Parikh's Textbook of Medical Jurisprudence, Forensic Medicine and Toxicology, 7/e, Pg. 11; The Essentials of Forensic Medicine & Toxicology, K.S. Narayan Reddy-34/e, pg. 13)

ANSWER

Hostile Witness

○ **Definition:** When a witness purposely makes statements contrary to facts or to what he has already stated in lower court or in same court on previous occasion, the court declares such a witness as a hostile witness

○ Reasons of witness turning hostile
  ▪ He may be influenced, intimidated or bribed
  ▪ He may purposely conceal part of truth or give outright false evidence and is then liable to be found guilty of perjury

○ While examining a hostile witness, leading questions can be asked in the examination-in-chief to elicit the facts

○ Medical witnesses are not declared hostile as they are court witnesses.

b. Sodomy

(Ref: Parikh's Textbook of Medical Jurisprudence, Forensic Medicine and Toxicology, 7/e, Pg. 407; The Essentials of Forensic Medicine & Toxicology, K.S. Narayan Reddy-34/e, pg. 399)

ANSWER

Sodomy

Definition

○ Anal intercourse between 2 males (homosexual sodomy), or between a male and a female (heterosexual sodomy)
○ Also known as buggery
○ **Gerontophilia:** When passive agent is an adult
○ **Pederasty:** When passive agent is a young boy, boy being known as catamite
○ **Active agent:** Who performs the act
○ **Passive agent:** On whom the act is performed
○ Can be performed by 2 men acting alternately as active and passive agent
○ Question of consent does not arise and it is no defense that passive agent is accused's wife but if offence is done without consent of passive agent, then the active agent is held guilty
○ Most common in people who are sex-starved due to circumstances such as prisoners, members of armed forces and sailors

Medicolegal Importance

○ Act is difficult to perform against the will unless the person is drugged or drunk
○ Medical examination of both active and passive agents is required for investigation of crime
○ False charges can be made for purpose of blackmail
○ Men can be tricked into homosexual relationship by men masquerading as women whilst on shore, especially in eastern seas

c. Dying Declaration

(Ref: Parikh's Textbook of Medical Jurisprudence, Forensic Medicine and Toxicology, 7/e, Pg. 15)

ANSWER

Dying Declaration

For answer, refer 2016 paper Q. 2 (c), Pg. 470

PART II

3. **Classify Irritant Poisons. Describe clinical Features, management and autopsy findings in case of organophosphorus poisoning.**

a. Irritant Poisons

(Ref: Parikh's Textbook of Medical Jurisprudence, Forensic Medicine and Toxicology, 7/e, Pg. 510)

ANSWER

Classification

For answer, refer 2016 paper Q. 3, Pg. 471

b. Organophosphorus Poisoning

(Ref: Parikh's Textbook of Medical Jurisprudence, Forensic Medicine and Toxicology, 7/e, Pg. 625)

ANSWER

For answer, refer 2016 paper Q. 3 (b), Pg. 472

4. **Differentiate between**

a. Temporary and permanent dentition

(Ref: Parikh's Textbook of Medical Jurisprudence, Forensic Medicine and Toxicology, 7/e, Pg. 59; The Essentials of Forensic Medicine & Toxicology, K.S. Narayan Reddy-34/e, pg. 66)

ANSWER

Temporary and Permanent Dentition

Temporary teeth	Permanent teeth
• Small, narrow, light and delicate	• Big, broad, heavy and strong
• Crowns china-white in color	• Crowns ivory-white in color
• Junction of the crown with the fang	• Junction of the crown with the fang not often marked by a ridge
• Neck more constricted	• Neck less constricted

Temporary teeth	Permanent teeth
• Edges serrated	• Edges not serrated
• Anterior teeth vertical	• Anterior teeth usually inclined somewhat forward
• Molars are usually larger. Their crowns are flat, and their roots are smaller and more divergent	• Bicuspids which replace the temporary molars are usually smaller, their crowns have cusps which sharply differentiate them. Their roots are bigger and relatively Straight

b Poisonous and nonpoisonous snakes

(Ref: Parikh's Textbook of Medical Jurisprudence, Forensic Medicine and Toxicology, 7/e, Pg. 574)

ANSWER

Poisonous and Nonpoisonous Snakes

	Poisonous shakes	Nonpoisonous snakes
• Belly scales as seen by turning the snake with belly upwards	• Large, and cover the entire breadth of the belly. Some harmless snakes also have such belly scales	• Small like those on the back or moderately large but do not cover the entire breadth of the belly
• Head scales	• Small (vipers)	
	a. Large with conspicuous pit between the eye and nostril (pit vipers) b. Third labial touches the eye and nasal shields (cobra, king cobra, or coral) c. Central row of scales on back enlarged, and under surface of the mouth with only four infralabials, the fourth being the largest kraits, and perhaps bands or half rings across the back	• Large with the exceptions as outlined under the poisonous snakes, viz. pit vipers, cobra, king cobra, coral, and kraits
• Tail	• Compressed	• Not markedly compressed
• Fangs	• Long and canalized like hypodermic needle	• Short and solid
• Bite	• Two fang marks with or without small marks of other teeth	• A number of small teeth marks in a row
• Habits	• Generally nocturnal	• Not so

c. Respired and non-respired lungs

(Ref: Parikh's Textbook of Medical Jurisprudence, Forensic Medicine and Toxicology, 7/e, Pg. 429; The Essentials of Forensic Medicine & Toxicology, K.S. Narayan Reddy-34/e, pg. 441)

ANSWER

Respired and Nonrespired Lungs

Respired lung	Nonrespired lung
• Distended lungs fill the thoracic cavity overlapping the heart and thymus gland and covering pleura becomes taut	• Lungs are found lying at the back of the thoracic cavity behind the heart and thymus gland and covered with wrinkled loose pleura
• Voluminous with uneven surface due to expanded air vesicles and becomes light red alternating with dark bluish- red areas	• Small, smooth, of uniform dark blue-red color and appear liver-like
• Crepitate on squeezing	• Non-crepitant on squeezing
• Round edges	• Sharp edge
• On section, they exude frothy blood	• On section, exude blood but not froth
• When placed in water, they usually float	• When placed in water, they usually sink
• Specific gravity is 950	• Specific gravity is 1050

PART III

5. **Define and classify strangulation. Describe the autopsy findings in case of ligature strangulation**

(Ref: Parikh's Textbook of Medical Jurisprudence, Forensic Medicine and Toxicology, 7/e, Pg. 177; The Essentials of Forensic Medicine & Toxicology, K.S. Narayan Reddy-34/e, pg. 416)

ANSWER

Strangulation

Definition

○ Form of asphyxia caused by constricting neck by some means other than body weight
○ Means can be a ligature, hand, elbow, stick

Classification

○ Ligature strangulation
○ Mugging or choke hold strangulation (using elbow)
○ Bansdola (using stick)
○ Throttling (using hand) or manual strangulation
○ Garrotting

Signs and Symptoms

○ When windpipe is completely occluded
  ▪ Sudden and violent compression of windpipe often renders a person powerless and may cause immediate insensibility and death
○ If windpipe is not completely occluded
  ▪ Face becomes cyanosed
  ▪ Bleeding occurs from mouth and nose due to congestion and rupture of various venous plexuses

▪ Hands are clenched
▪ Convulsions precede death
▪ Rapid loss of consciousness

Cause of Death

○ Death usually occurs from asphyxia and compression of cervical vasculature in ligature strangulation

Autopsy Findings

○ External appearances

Cause of Death	Signs
• Vagal inhibition	• Instantaneous death • No asphyxial signs

• Slight vagal effect and some venous constriction	• Slight asphyxial signs
	  ▪ Cyanosed face
	  ▪ Occasional petechiae
	  ▪ Suffused eyes
	  ▪ Dilated pupils

• Moderate venous constriction and some respiratory obstruction	• Moderate asphyxia signs
	  ▪ Cyanosed face
	  ▪ Bulging eyes
	  ▪ Ecchymosed conjunctivae
	  ▪ Few petechiae

• Pronounced venous and respiratory obstruction	• Well-marked asphyxial signs
	  ▪ Deeply cyanosed face
	  ▪ Blood shot eyes
	  ▪ Bruised, bitten, swollen and protruded tongue
	  ▪ Many petechiae in eyelids, conjunctivae and face

○ **Injuries on the neck:** Vary with the means used for strangulation
  ▪ **Ligature**
    ◆ Ligature mark is seen round the neck as a depression
    ◆ Initially it looks pale but later becomes dry, hard, yellowish brown, hard and parchment like
    ◆ Abrasions and ecchymoses are often seen, along the edges of depression, indicating that the mark was made during life
    ◆ Ligature mark is situated at the level of thyroid cartilage or below, is almost horizontal and encircles the neck completely or nearly so
    ◆ Absent at the back due to interposition of hair or clothing
    ◆ Character of mark depends upon nature of ligature used but is also affected by number of turns round the neck and length of time it remains applied
    ◆ Pattern of ligature may be imprinted on neck as a pressure abrasion or bruise
  ▪ **Stick**
    ◆ Bruise in front of neck in the center and when two sticks are used, one in front and other behind the neck as in bansdola

- **Foot**
  - Irregular widespread bruising with local injuries to neck depending on the force applied
  - Foot with boot on, causes more abrasions than when a bare foot is used, which causes contusions
- **Internal appearances**
  - V-shaped incision is made and evisceration of cranial, thoracic and abdominal viscera is done
  - Severe congestion and hemorrhage into tissues in and around the area of compression
  - Injuries to deeper tissues of neck is more common due to considerable force used
  - Subcutaneous connective tissue under the ligature mark is ecchymosed
  - Neck muscles, laryngeal cartilages, tracheal rings and carotid arteries are injured
  - Superior horns of thyroid cartilage are fractured but hyoid is rarely injured due to level of constriction being below this bone unless considerable force is applied

6. Write short notes on:

a. Res ipsa loquitur

(Ref: Parikh's Textbook of Medical Jurisprudence, Forensic Medicine and Toxicology, 7/e, Pg. 35; The Essentials of Forensic Medicine & Toxicology, K.S. Narayan Reddy-34/e, pg. 37)

ANSWER

Res Ipsa Loquitur

Definition

- Rule of evidence which in reality belongs to the law of torts
- Professional negligence of a doctor must be proved in court by expert evidence of another doctor
- Patient need not prove negligence in case where the rule of res ipsa loquitur applies, which means, "the thing or fact speaks for itself"
- Patient just has to state what according to him was the act of negligence

Conditions to be Satisfied

- In the absence of negligence, the injury would not have occurred
- That the doctor had exclusive control over the injury producing instrument or treatment
- That the patient was not guilty of contributory negligence, enabling the patient's lawyer to prove his case without medical evidence

Application

- Applied to both to civil and criminal negligence
- Does not apply where common knowledge or experience is not sufficiently extensive to know that the patient's condition would not have existed but for the doctor's negligence
- Cannot be applied against several defendants only one of whom, who cannot be identified could have caused patient's injury
- Rarely used successfully by patients

Examples

- Prescribing an overdose of medicine producing ill effects
- Prescribing poisonous medicine carelessly
- Failure to give anti-tetanic serum in cases of injury causing tetanus
- Burns from application of hot water bottles or from X-ray therapy
- Breaking of needles
- Failure to remove swabs during operation which may lead to complications or cause death
- Blood transfusion misadventure
- Loss of use of hand due to prolonged splinting

b. Dactylography

(Ref: Parikh's Textbook of Medical Jurisprudence, Forensic Medicine and Toxicology, 7/e, Pg. 67; The Essentials of Forensic Medicine & Toxicology, K.S. Narayan Reddy-34/e, pg. 82)

ANSWER

Dactylography

Definition

- Study of fingerprints for the purpose of identification
- A fingerprint means impression made by ball of a finger
- Fingerprint system is based on the principle that skin of the balls of the fingers and thumbs are covered with ridges and grooves, the pattern of which varies between individuals and makes absolute identification possible
- Causes of impression of ridges: Moistening of skin by sweat and sebum from skin glands
  - At crime scene, impressions are found on door knobs, furniture, weapons and various other articles, unless gloves are worn by criminal
  - Fingers soiled with blood or grease
- If fingerprints are faded, the fingerprint expert can make them visible by special techniques, e.g. by the use of dusting powder

- In a dead body, if the fingerprints are dried up, the prints can be taken by soaking the fingers in an alkaline solution for some time
- In case of skin peeling due to burns, putrefaction or drowning, the prints can be recorded either from dermis or from the peeled off skin hardened by formalin

Features of Ridges

- Present from birth, both on epidermis and dermis
- Remain constant for the life of the individual and cannot be altered except by destruction of the true skin
- Form patterns that are absolutely individual, they are not entirely alike, even in identical twins

Classification

- **On the basis of arrangement of ridges:**
  - Loops
  - Whorls
  - Arches
  - Composites or compounds

Advantages

- Applicable to persons of all ages
- Can be obtained even from putrefied bodies
- Absolute identification is possible
- No special training or expensive instruments are required
- Easy classification
- Actual print is always available to check for any suspected error
- Print can be transmitted from one place to another as a coded or digitalized message
  - Development of computerized automated fingerprint identification system now permits rapid entry, comparison and identification in minutes to hours as opposed to weeks to months using conventional manual search methods

Practical Application

- Recognition of chance impressions left at a scene of crime
- Identification of weapon used for committing suicide or homicide e.g. firearm
- Identification of habitual criminals, suicides, deserters, persons suffering from loss of memory or those dead or unconscious after being involved in an accident
- Identification of decomposing or mummified bodies of unknown persons
- Prevention of impersonation
- As an extra precaution on cheques, bank notes and other legal documents which may bear a fingerprint in addition to manual signature

c. **Joule burn**

ANSWER

Joule Burn

(Ref: Parikh's Textbook of Medical Jurisprudence, Forensic Medicine and Toxicology, 7/e, Pg. 349; The Essentials of Forensic Medicine & Toxicology, K.S. Narayan Reddy-34/e, pg. 308)

Definition

- Endogenous burn occurred due to heat generated by electric current
- Found at the entry of the current
- Diagnostic point of contact with electricity

Clinical Picture

- Burnt area is dry, charred and insensitive
- Site of entry is devoid of common signs of inflammation and red line of demarcation
- Grayish white ulcer-like opening appears with everted and corrugated margins and necrosed tissue
- Resemble in shape the object causing electrocution
- Finger print pattern is lost with flattened skin ridges, if tip of fingers is the site of entry
- Compression of stratum corneum and flattening of the papillae of the corium with occurrence of spaces of varying size giving lace like or honey comb appearance
- At site of exit, tissues are usually split in the form of punctured or lacerated wounds
- Microscopically, the exit wound is similar to the entrance burn except for presence of metallization at the wound of entry
- Small lesions may sometimes be seen at the plexuses of a limb where the current has jumped across the bend instead of passing round it
- Due to intense and sustained spasm of arteries, gangrene of a part of limb followed by thrombosis, may sometimes occur
- In rare instances, victim may completely be charred with heat coagulation of muscles – Zenker's degeneration with spiraling and fragmentation of muscle fibers
- **In recovery phase, symptoms are:** Restlessness, irritability and excitement–from insurance point of view, these sequelae are significant
- Angina pectoris may immediately occur or after a few days and may disappear or can lead to myocardial necrosis leading to death
- Due to thrombosis of arteries, edema and gangrene of limbs ensues
- After few months of the incident, delayed effects may arise which comprises of necrosis and secondary hemorrhage, disturbance of central nervous system owing to cell degeneration

Name of the Paper	:	**Forensic Medicine & Toxicology**
Name of the Course	:	**MBBS-2011**
Semester	:	**Annual**

Time: 3 Hours   **M.M.: 40**

INSTRUCTIONS

1. Write your Roll No. on the top immediately on receipt of this question paper
2. All questions are to be attempted
3. Answers to Parts I, II and III should be written in separate answer sheets provided
4. Attempt parts of a question in sequence

PART-I

1. What are the findings, interpretation and medicolegal importance when it is stated that: [8]
   a. A girl is 16 years old
   b. Death is from café coronary
   c. A female is a false virgin
   d. Person showing delirium tremens

2. Write short notes on: [6]
   a. Infamous conduct
   b. Cadeveric rigidity
   c. Lochia

PART-II

3. Classify neurotic poisons. Describe the signs, Symptoms, management and Postmortem findings in Carbolic acid poisoning: [7]

4. Differentiate between: [6]
   a. Strychnine poisoning and tetanus
   b. Antemortem and postmortem burns
   c. True and feigned insanity

PART-III

5. Define medical negligence. Discuss various medicolegal issue in case of negligence by a Doctor [7]

6. Write short notes on: [6]
   a. Treatment of organophosphate poisoning
   b. Arborescent burns
   c. Perjury

PART I

1. What are the findings, interpretation and medicolegal importance when it is stated that

a. A girl is 16 years old

(Ref: Parikh's Textbook of Medical Jurisprudence, Forensic Medicine and Toxicology, 7/e, Pg. 59)

ANSWER

A Girl is 16 years Old

Findings

○ **Teeth:**
  - Complete root calcification of second molars
  - Wisdom tooth has not yet erupted
○ Ossification of bones
  - All epiphyses at elbow, head of femur and lower end of tibia have joined respective shafts
  - Pisiform ossified
  - Heads of metacarpals and phalanges have fused
  - Lower ends of radius and ulna fused
  - Coracoid process fused
  - Inner end of clavicle has appeared
  - Acromion appeared
  - Upper end of humerus partially fused
  - All the epiphyses at wrist, knee, crest of ilium and lateral end of clavicle have not yet united which unites at around 18 years

Interpretation

○ In females, union of epiphysis in cartilaginous bones takes place earlier by 2 years than in males except in case of skull sutures where obliteration sets in little later and proceeds more slowly in female than in males

Medicolegal Importance

○ **Criminal responsibility**
  - Child under 12 years of age cannot give valid consent to suffer harm which can occur from an act done in good faith and for its benefit e.g. consent for operation
  - Person under 18 years of age cannot give valid consent whether express or implied to suffer any harm which may result from an act not intended to cause any grievous hurt e.g. consent for wrestling

○ **Judicial punishment**
  - Children (boys below 16 years and girls below 18 years of age), who have committed a crime, are tried by Juvenile court and if convicted, are entrusted to parents for special care or sent to correctional school with facilities for education, vocational training and rehabilitation
○ **Employment**
  - Child below 14 years of age cannot be employed for any type of work
○ **Rape**
  - Sexual intercourse by a man with a girl under 15 years of age even if she is his own wife, or with any girl under 18 years of age even with her consent is rape
○ **Kidnapping**
  - Kidnapping or abducting a minor, if boy is under 16 and girl is under 18 years

b. Death is from café coronary

(Ref: Parikh's Textbook of Medical Jurisprudence, Forensic Medicine and Toxicology, 7/e, Pg. 186; The Essentials of Forensic Medicine & Toxicology, K.S. Narayan Reddy-34/e, pg. 340)

ANSWER

Death is from Café Coronary

Findings

○ Bolus of unchewed food impacted in larynx
○ Marked cyanosis

Interpretation

○ Occurs generally when a gag reflex is suppressed especially in intoxicated persons after large dose of tranquillizers
○ Death is due to asphyxia from inability to breathe or reflex cardiac arrest due to stimulation of laryngeal nerve endings

Medicolegal Importance

○ Additional insurance benefits to surviving relatives as accidental death occurs

c. A female is a false virgin

(Ref: Parikh's Textbook of Medical Jurisprudence, Forensic Medicine and Toxicology, 7/e, Pg. 376; The Essentials of Forensic Medicine & Toxicology, K.S. Narayan Reddy-34/e, pg. 367)

ANSWER

For answer, refer 2014 paper Q. 1 (d), Pg. 486

d. **Person is showing delirium tremens**

(Ref: Parikh's Textbook of Medical Jurisprudence, Forensic Medicine and Toxicology, 7/e, Pg. 609; The Essentials of Forensic Medicine & Toxicology, K.S. Narayan Reddy-34/e, pg. 509)

ANSWER

For answer, refer 2017 paper Q. 6 (a), Pg. 465

2. **Write short notes on:**

a. **Infamous conduct**

ANSWER

For answer, refer 2016 paper Q. 2 (a), Pg. 469

b. **Cadaveric rigidity**

(Ref: Parikh's Textbook of Medical Jurisprudence, Forensic Medicine and Toxicology, 7/e, Pg. 147; The Essentials of Forensic Medicine & Toxicology, K.S. Narayan Reddy-34/e, pg. 154)

ANSWER

Cadaveric Rigidity

Definition

- Condition characterized by stiffening and shortening of muscles following the period of primary relaxation due to chemical changes involving structural proteins of muscle fibers indicating molecular death of its cells
- Also known as Rigor mortis, reaction of muscle changes from slightly alkaline to distinctly acid due to local formation of lactic acid
- Persists until autolysis of myosin and actin filaments occurs as a part of putrefaction, when autolysis occurs, muscles become soft and secondary relaxation occurs
- It can be broken by mechanical force, therefore, when a limb is stiff due to rigidity, it is flexed forcibly at a joint, becomes flaccid and remains so after that-breaking of rigor mortis
- All voluntary and involuntary muscles are affected by rigor–appearing first in involuntary muscles and then in voluntary muscles
- Does not depend upon nerve supply and therefore, also develops in paralyzed limbs
- **Tested by:**
  - Attempt to lift eyelids
  - Depress the jaw
  - Gently bend the neck and various other joints of body

- Rigidity passes off in the same order of appearance
- When arrector pili muscles of skin are affected, it presents a granular puckered appearance-cutis anserine, affecting mainly extremities

Sequence of Appearance of Rigor Mortis

- In involuntary muscles, appears in heart within an hour after death
- In voluntary muscles
  - Muscles of eyelids in 3–4 hours
  - Muscles of face in 4–5 hours
  - Neck and trunk in 5–7 hours
  - **Muscles of upper extremities:** 7–9 hours
  - **Muscles of legs:** 9–11 hours
  - Small muscles of fingers and toes in 11–12 hours

Medicolegal Importance

- Sign of death
- Helps in estimation of time since death
- Provides information about position of body at the time of death

Factors Affecting Rigor Mortis (Cadaveric Rigidity)

- **Age and condition of body:**
  - in children and old people, onset is earlier than adults
  - in strong muscular person, onset is late with prolonged duration
- Mode of death
  - In chronic diseases and convulsive disorders, onset is early and duration is short
  - In sudden death, onset is late with prolonged duration
  - In drowning, onset is early with prolonged duration
- Surroundings
  - Delayed by cold and accelerated by heat

c. **Lochia**

(Ref: Parikh's Textbook of Medical Jurisprudence, Forensic Medicine and Toxicology, 7/e, Pg. 383; The Essentials of Forensic Medicine & Toxicology, K.S. Narayan Reddy-34/e, pg. 372)

ANSWER

Lochia

Definition

- Vaginal discharge with peculiar sour odor after delivery
- Contains red cells, leucocytes, decidual debris, vaginal epithelium, peptones and cholesterol crystals

○ Discharge in postpartum period which is part of healing process of uterus after child birth

○ Characteristic of full term delivery rather than premature birth

Three Stages of Lochia

○ **Lochia rubra:** Blood stained during first 3 days

○ **Lochia serosa:** Paler and serous for next 3 days

○ **Lochia alba:** Yellowish or greenish and then whitish for another 3 days, disappears after 15 days

Medicolegal Importance

○ Disappears within 10 days in strong, vigorous women or in multipara

○ Can indicate size of fetus and rapidity of the birth, from the extent of stretching and lacerations of parts

○ Sooner the woman is examined after delivery, more are the chances of getting useful information

PART II

3. **Classify neurotic poisons. Describe the signs, symptoms, management and postmortem findings in carbolic acid poisoning.**

   a. **Neurotic poisons**

   (Ref: Parikh's Textbook of Medical Jurisprudence, Forensic Medicine and Toxicology, 7/e, Pg. 510)

Answer

Definition

○ Poisons which act mainly on nervous system

Classification

○ **Cerebral:** Act on cerebrum

  ▪ Somniferous

    ◆ Opioids

  ▪ Inebriant

    ◆ Alcohol

    ◆ Anesthetics

    ◆ Sedatives

    ◆ Hypnotics

    ◆ Fuels

    ◆ Agrochemical compounds

  ▪ Deliriant

    ◆ Datura

    ◆ Belladonna

    ◆ Hyoscyamus

    ◆ Cannabis indica

○ **Spinal:** Act on spinal cord

  ▪ Nux vomica and its alkaloids

  ▪ Gelsemium

○ **Peripheral:** Act on peripheral nerves

  ▪ Curare

  ▪ Conium

   b. **Carbolic acid poisoning**

   (Ref: Parikh's Textbook of Medical Jurisprudence, Forensic Medicine and Toxicology, 7/e, Pg. 535)

Answer

For answer, refer 2015 paper Q. 3 (b), Pg. 481

4. **Differentiate between**

   a. **Strychnine poisoning and tetanus**

   (Ref: Parikh's Textbook of Medical Jurisprudence, Forensic Medicine and Toxicology, 7/e, Pg. 640; The Essentials of Forensic Medicine & Toxicology, K.S. Narayan Reddy-34/e, pg. 570)

Answer

For answer, refer 2015 paper Q. 4 (b), Pg. 482

   b. **Antemortem and postmortem burns**

   (Ref: Parikh's Textbook of Medical Jurisprudence, Forensic Medicine and Toxicology, 7/e, Pg. 340)

Answer

For answer, refer 2016 paper Q. 4 (c), Pg. 474

   c. **True and feigned insanity**

   (Ref: Parikh's Textbook of Medical Jurisprudence, Forensic Medicine and Toxicology, 7/e, Pg. 453; The Essentials of Forensic Medicine & Toxicology, K.S. Narayan Reddy-34/e, pg. 455)

Answer

True and Feigned Insanity

True unsoundness of mind	Feigned unsoundness of mind
• Gradual onset or rarely sudden but usually without any motive	• Sudden onset and not without some motive
• Predisposing or exciting cause may be present, e.g. family history of insanity, grief, sudden loss of money, etc.	• No predisposing or exciting cause is usually present

True unsoundness of mind	Feigned unsoundness of mind
• Well-developed cases of insanity have a peculiar facial expression	• Facial expression is generally normal even when the person pretends to be mad outright.
• The individual shows signs and symptoms of insanity irrespective of his conduct being observed or not	• The individual pretends to be insane only when he is observed and there is total absence of symptoms when he is alone and unobserved
• Signs and symptoms usually suggest a particular type of mental illness	• Signs and symptoms are not uniform and do not suggest any particular type of mental illness
• Can stand violent exertion for several hours or days without exhaustion, or sleep	• Violent exertion leads to exhaustion, and sleep
• Physical manifestations of true insanity, viz. dry, harsh skin, furred tongue, constipation, anorexia, and insomnia are present	• Physical manifestations of true insanity, viz. dry, harsh tongue, furred tongue, constipation, anorexia, and insomnia are not present
• Not worried about being repeatedly examined	• Dislike for repeated examination is obvious

PART III

5. Define Medical Negligence. Discuss various medicolegal issue in case of negligence by a doctor

(Ref: Parikh's Textbook of Medical Jurisprudence, Forensic Medicine and Toxicology, 7/e, Pg. 35)

ANSWER

For answer, refer 2016 paper Q. 5 (a), Pg. 474

6. Write short notes on:

   a. Treatment of organophosphorus poisoning

(Ref: Parikh's Textbook of Medical Jurisprudence, Forensic Medicine and Toxicology, 7/e, Pg. 625)

ANSWER

Treatment of Organophosphorus Poisoning

For answer, refer 2016 paper Q. 3 (b), Pg. 472

   b. Arborescent burns

(Ref: Parikh's Textbook of Medical Jurisprudence, Forensic Medicine and Toxicology, 7/e, Pg. 357)

ANSWER

Arborescent Burns

○ Also known as Filigree burns

For answer, refer 2013 paper Q. 1 (d), Pg. 493

   c. Perjury

(Ref: Parikh's Textbook of Medical Jurisprudence, Forensic Medicine and Toxicology, 7/e, Pg. 10)

ANSWER

Perjury

○ **Definition:** Giving wilful false or fabricated evidence or statement

○ If a witness, after taking oath or making a solemn affirmation, wilfully makes a statement that he knows or believes to be false is guilty of the crime of Perjury under section 1933 IPC

○ Witness is liable to be prosecuted for perjury and his imprisonment may extend to 7 years

○ If the person's earlier statement regarding the facts on oath and subsequent statement on oath are opposed to each other, they cannot be reconciled

Name of the Paper : **Forensic Medicine & Toxicology**

Name of the Course : **MBBS-2010**

Semester : **Annual**

Time: 3 Hours   M.M.: 40

INSTRUCTIONS

1. Write your Roll No. on the top immediately on receipt of this question paper
2. All questions are to be attempted
3. Answers to Parts I, II and III should be written in separate answer sheets provided
4. Attempt parts of a question in sequence

PART-I

1. What are the findings, interpretations and medicolegal importance when it is stated that: [8]

   a. Death is due to traumatic asphyxia
   b. Patterned injuries are present on the body
   c. Child is dead born
   d. Dead body is showing mummification

2. Write short notes on: [6]

   a. Lucid interval
   b. Scar marks
   c. Tattoo marks

PART-II

3. Define positions. Discuss the sign, symptoms, management, and postmortem findings in a case of morphine poisoning: [7]

4. Differentiate between: [6]

   a. Cobra and viper bite marks
   b. Human and animal hair
   c. Male and female femur

PART-III

5. What are the functions of Delhi Medical Council? How do they differ from the functions of Medical council of India? [7]

6. Write short notes on: [6]

   a. Carboluria
   b. Hallucination
   c. MTP Act, 1971

PART I

1. **What are the findings, interpretations and medicolegal importance when it is stated that**

   a. **Death is due to traumatic asphyxia**

   (Ref: Parikh's Textbook of Medical Jurisprudence, Forensic Medicine and Toxicology, 7/e, Pg. 187)

ANSWER

The Death is Due to Traumatic Asphyxia

Findings and Interpretation

○ Deep cyanosis of face
○ Numerous petechiae over scalp, face, neck and shoulders
○ Demarcation line between discolored upper body and normally colored lower part of body
○ Eyes are blood shot
○ In mild cases, injury to lungs may be in form of traumatic emphysema wherein the air in the lungs is forcible redistributed producing small bullae along the edges of the lung
○ In severe cases, injuries to chest include

Medicolegal Significance

○ In most of the cases it is accidental but rarely can be homicidal as in burking or bansdola
○ In very instance, an obese mother or father can roll over a child in sleep causing the death of the child from traumatic asphyxia, who is sharing the same bed
   ▪ **Fracture of ribs:** Bilateral, multiple and at their angles with damage to diaphragm occasionally
   ▪ Injuries to lungs and heart

   b. **Patterned injuries are present on the body**

   (Ref: Parikh's Textbook of Medical Jurisprudence, Forensic Medicine and Toxicology, 7/e, Pg. 319)

ANSWER

Patterned Injuries

○ **Definition:** Injuries with a distinct pattern that often reproduce the characteristics of the object causing the injury
○ Caused by impact of a weapon or other object on the body, or by contact of the body with a patterned surface

○ Assume a definite and distinguishing pattern in case of pedestrian and a driver or a passenger, depending on the type of impact

Injuries can be subdivided according to the type of force involved:

○ Blunt force injuries
   ▪ Most common type of patterned injuries
   ▪ Abrasions may preserve patterns well, especially if the force is applied at or near perpendicular to the skin surface
   ▪ Bruises may also reproduce patterns well, particularly if they are mainly intradermal
   ▪ Lacerations less frequently show a well-defined reproduction of the shape of the injuring object
○ Sharp force injuries
   ▪ Knife wounds produce characteristics of a specific type of blade (e.g., 'fish-tail' appearance of a stab wound)
   ▪ Stab wounds due to other types of patterned objects (e.g., Phillips head screwdrivers, scissors) may produce typical patterns
○ Gunshot wounds
   ▪ Contact entry wounds (which may have sight marks) and shotgun wounds (e.g., with wad marks) may produce distinct patterned injuries
○ Other miscellaneous wounds and marks e.g., fern-like pattern with lightning strikes, tool marks on internal structures (such as cartilage)

Medicolegal Importance

○ Linking a particular weapon or other object to an injury
○ Allows a perpetrator to be linked to the crime and/or enable better understanding of the events surrounding a death

   c. **Child is dead born**

   (Ref: Parikh's Textbook of Medical Jurisprudence, Forensic Medicine and Toxicology, 7/e, Pg. 427; The Essentials of Forensic Medicine & Toxicology, K.S. Narayan Reddy-34/e, pg. 409)

ANSWER

Child is Dead Born

Findings

○ **Rigor mortis:** May occur in dead fetus before birth
○ **Maceration:** Aseptic autolysis of a fetus in utero
   ▪ **Spalding's sign:** Overriding of skull bones enabling diagnosis of condition when fetus is inside the uterus

- **Putrefaction:** Nauseating and unpleasant odor, green color of skin and formation of gases
- **Mummification:** When death of fetus results from deficient supply of blood or scanty liquor amnii and no air entered the uterus

Interpretation

- Death may occur due to antenatal hemorrhage in mother
- Fetus was dead for 3-4 days in the uterus

Medicolegal Importance

- Charge of infanticide does not stand in such cases

c. Dead body is showing mummification

(Ref: Parikh's Textbook of Medical Jurisprudence, Forensic Medicine and Toxicology, 7/e, Pg. 161)

ANSWER

Dead Body is Showing Mummification

For answer, refer 2015 paper Q. 1 (b), Pg. 478

2. Write short notes:

a. Lucid interval

(Ref: Parikh's Textbook of Medical Jurisprudence, Forensic Medicine and Toxicology, 7/e, Pg. 443)

ANSWER

Lucid Interval

- **Definition:** Period in the passage of mental illness during which there is complete termination of symptoms of insanity
- Generally met with in depression and mania i.e. bipolar disorder
- Patient can make a valid will during this period and also can provide valid evidence
- He can judge his actions well and is held responsible for his conducts
- In criminal cases, however, it is difficult to state whether any mental abnormality was present at the time of mitting crime, therefore it is advisable to treat the person as insane
- Also observed in head injuries for e.g. in extradural hemorrhage, when it is necessary to arrange for a dying declaration

b. Scar marks

(Ref: Parikh's Textbook of Medical Jurisprudence, Forensic Medicine and Toxicology, 7/e, Pg. 71; The Essentials of Forensic Medicine & Toxicology, K.S. Narayan Reddy-34/e, pg. 88)

ANSWER

Scar Marks

Definition

- Permanent cicatricial mark resulting from healing of a wound
- Superficial injury involving only epidermis does not produce a scar such as an abrasion
- Devoid of hair follicles, sweat glands, pigment and elastic tissue and covered by few layers of epithelium

Time Required for Scar Formation Depends On

- Nature, size and method of wound healing
- Presence or absence of sepsis
- Vascularity of part affected
- Age and general well-being of person

Types of Scar and Cause

- **Linear scar:** Caused by incised wound e.g. surgical operations
- **Elliptical scar:** Caused by stab wound
- **Puckered scar:** Caused by punctured wound
- **Irregular scar:** Caused by lacerated wound e.g. burns, corrosives
- **Circular, oval or elongated depressed scar:** Caused by bullet wound e.g. smallpox vaccination

Medicolegal Significance

- Helps in identification
- Shape of scar generally corresponds to the type of wound sustained, e.g. linear scar of incised wound
- Age of scar corresponds to the time of occurrence of the event e.g. in pleas of self defense in cases of murder
- Old scars on wrist or throat indicate previous attempt of suicide
- Linea albicantes indicate certain diseased conditions such as ascites or previous pregnancy in a female
- Linear needle track scars indicate intravenous drug abuser
- Wounds may be kept infected or sometimes covered with irritants deliberately to promote slow healing and to obtain unsightly big scars in order to bring injury within the purview of grievous hurt

c. **Tattoo marks**

(Ref: Parikh's Textbook of Medical Jurisprudence, Forensic Medicine and Toxicology, 7/e, Pg. 70; The Essentials of Forensic Medicine & Toxicology, K.S. Narayan Reddy-34/e, pg. 70)

ANSWER

Tattoo Marks

○ **Definition:** Designs caused by multiple small puncture wounds produced through the skin using needles or similar penetrating tools dipped in dye

○ Permanency of tattoo marks depends on:
  ▪ Type of dye used
  ▪ Depth of penetration
  ▪ Part of body tattooed

○ Optimum depth of penetration is up to superficial layers of dermis

○ Commonly used dyes are black, blue and red as these are more durable and almost permanent

○ In order to reveal latent tattoo marks, high contrast photography, computer image enhancement, ultraviolet lamp or infrared photography is beneficial

○ Tattoo marks on unidentified putrefied bodies may be photographed with sharp definition, if the loose epidermis is first removed and design on the dermis recorded

○ In order to conceal identity, various artificial methods have been used for elimination of tattoo mark
  ▪ Dermabrasion
  ▪ Application of caustic substances or carbon dioxide snow
  ▪ Electrolysis
  ▪ Surgery
  ▪ Exposure to laser beam

○ Dermabrasion, application of caustic substances and electrolysis leave a visible scar, whereas surgical removal with skin grafting will leave a less obvious scar

○ Laser beam exposure will destroy the pigmented cells and evaporates the dye from tattooed areas without any pain, damage or alteration of skin structure

○ Chronic eczema and confluent smallpox can cause disappearance of tattoo designs

Complications

○ Sepsis
○ Transmission of diseases such as
  ▪ Syphilis
  ▪ Leprosy
  ▪ Tuberculosis
  ▪ Hepatitis

  ▪ AIDS

Medicolegal Importance

○ **Helps in indicating:**
  ▪ **Identity of person:** Special design, one's own name, name of spouse or close relation, date of birth or marriage etc.
  ▪ **Race:** Extensive tattooing of chest and limbs is common in Japanese
  ▪ **Religion:** Design of Hanuman, Lord Krishna, Cross or Christ
  ▪ **Profession/Occupation:** Some criminal gangs have certain specific emblems of tattoo marks; coalminer's leave visible tattoo marks on hands and face due to material handled
  ▪ **Behavioral characteristics:** Erotic tattoos of sexual fanatics
  ▪ **Social status:** In India, lower social class generally practices tattoos
  ▪ **Fashion statement:** Models, sports persons

PART II

3. **Define poisons. Discuss the signs, symptoms, management and postmortem findings in a case of morphine poisoning**

   a. **Poisons**

   (Ref: Parikh's Textbook of Medical Jurisprudence, Forensic Medicine and Toxicology, 7/e, Pg. 507; The Essentials of Forensic Medicine & Toxicology, K.S. Narayan Reddy-34/e, pg. 543)

ANSWER

For answer, refer 2013 paper Q. 3 (a), Pg. 495

   b. **Morphine poisoning**

   (Ref: Parikh's Textbook of Medical Jurisprudence, Forensic Medicine and Toxicology, 7/e, Pg. 595)

ANSWER

Acute Morphine Poisoning

Clinical Features

○ Appears within half an hour after ingestion and within 3-5 minutes after injection

○ Initially affects central nervous system, at first causing stimulation and later depression and then narcosis

○ **Stages:**
  ▪ **Stage of excitement**
    ♦ In case of large dose, the stage doesn't appear
    ♦ Adults go through a sense of wellbeing for short duration

- ◆ Laughter, hallucination, rapid heart rate
- ◆ Convulsions may occur in children
- ▪ **Stage of stupor**
  - ◆ Weariness, headache, giddiness
  - ◆ Sense of weight in the limbs
  - ◆ Reduced sensibility
  - ◆ Strong tendency to sleep from which patient can be roused by painful stimuli
  - ◆ Contracted pupils
  - ◆ Cyanosed face and lips
  - ◆ Itching sensation all over the skin
  - ◆ Normal pulse and respiration
- ▪ **Stage of narcosis**
  - ◆ Patient passes into deep coma from which he cannot be aroused
  - ◆ Relaxed muscles
  - ◆ Abolished reflexes
  - ◆ Pupils contracted to pin point and do not react to light
  - ◆ Low Blood pressure
  - ◆ Rapid and feeble pulse
  - ◆ Breathing slow and gradually diminishing in rate
  - ◆ Cold skin with profuse perspiration
  - ◆ **Temperature:** Subnormal
  - ◆ **In fatal cases:**
    - ▫ Marked cyanosis
    - ▫ Froth coming out of mouth
    - ▫ **Irregular breathing with sighing:** Cheyne-stokes breathing
    - ▫ **Rate of respiration:** 2-4 per minute
    - ▫ Imperceptible pulse
    - ▫ Dilated pupils when asphyxia ensues but do not react to light
    - ▫ Coma deepens
    - ▫ Death from asphyxia due to respiratory paralysis
    - ▫ Smell of opium from breath
- ○ **Fatal dose:** 200 mg of morphine and equivalent of opium is fatal
- ○ **Fatal period:** 9-12 hours

Management

- ○ Washing of stomach first with tepid water (if patient is brought in early stages), then with solution of potassium permanganate, 1:5000 strength till the water turns to original pink color
- ○ Some solution should be left in stomach to oxidize the alkaloid that might be excreted in the stomach after absorption
- ○ If potassium permanganate is not available, infusion of tea or tannic acid or mixture of finely powdered animal charcoal and water can be used

- ○ Alkaloid is re-excreted into stomach after absorption therefore gastric lavage should be carried out even after hypodermic injection of drug
- ○ Intestines should be cleared with enemata or by purgatives such as magnesium sulfate 15 g only
- ○ **Nalorphine:** Antidote to morphine should be administered intravenously 5-10 mg every 15 minutes till the pupils begin to dilate, respiration becomes normal and the patient is aroused; or maximum of 40 mg is given
- ○ Naloxone can be given intravenously or intramuscularly 0.4 -0.8 mg every 10-15 minutes or maximum 10 mg
- ○ In initial stages, the patient should be made to walk in open air to keep him awake, supporting him during procedure and care should be taken so that he is not exhausted
- ○ Artificial respiration and oxygen can be given depending upon his condition
- ○ Body warmth has to be maintained
- ○ Antibiotics should be given in cases of prolonged coma
- ○ Symptomatic treatment should be continued till patient is conscious and care should be taken so that relapse does not occur

Postmortem Findings

- ○ Comato-asphyxia
  - ▪ External
    - ◆ Smell of opium is present
    - ◆ Deeply cyanosed face – almost black
    - ◆ Blue colored finger nails
    - ◆ Engorged and distended neck veins
    - ◆ Postmortem lividity is almost black and is better visible in fair skinned body
    - ◆ Froth present at nose and mouth
    - ◆ Internal
    - ◆ Small, soft, brownish lumps of opium may be present in the stomach
    - ◆ Pronounced degree of venous congestion at trachea, bronchi, lungs and brain
    - ◆ Trachea and bronchi filled with froth and lungs become edematous

Medicolegal Importance

- ○ As death is painless from its use, opium is the choice for suicidal purposes
- ○ Rarely used for homicidal purposes owing to black color, characteristic odor and bitter taste
- ○ **Sometimes used for infanticide:** Breastfeeding after application of opium tincture on nipples causes death of the infant

○ Accidental poisoning in case of drugging infants and children to keep them quiet or after overdose of a medicinal preparation

4. Differentiate between

a. Cobra and viper bite marks

(Ref: Parikh's Textbook of Medical Jurisprudence, Forensic Medicine and Toxicology, 7/e, Pg. 580; The Essentials of Forensic Medicine & Toxicology, K.S. Narayan Reddy-34/e, pg. 524)

ANSWER

Cobra and Viper Bite Marks

Cobra bite marks	Viper bite marks
• Mild local symptoms—redness, slight burning pain, slight oozing of blood	• Severe local symptoms—intense local pain, ecchymosis, severe oozing of blood
• Swelling—minimal or absent	• Swelling involves limb and spreads up to trunk
• Appearance of blisters - absent	• Serous or serosanguinous blisters appear
• During recovery—skin and cellular tissues surrounding the bite mark undergo necrosis	• During recovery—local lesion suppurates and undergoes superficial necrosis

c. Human and animal hair

(Ref: Parikh's Textbook of Medical Jurisprudence, Forensic Medicine and Toxicology, 7/e, Pg. 499; The Essentials of Forensic Medicine & Toxicology, K.S. Narayan Reddy-34/e, pg. 93)

ANSWER

Human and Animal Hair

Differences between Human and Animal Hair

Human hair	Animal hair
• Fine and thin texture	• Coarse and thick texture
• Cuticle scales are small, flattened (type VII), serrated, and surround the shaft completely (coronal)	• Cuticle scales are large, polyhedral (types I to VI), wavy, and do not surround the shaft completely (imbricate)
• Medulla is narrow. May be absent, fragmented, or discontinuous	• Medulla is broad, always present, and continuous
• Cortex is thick. 4–10 times as broad as medulla	• Cortex is thin. Rarely more than twice the breadth of medulla
• Medullary index is less than 0.3	• Medullary index is more than 0.5
• Precipitin test with intact root is specific for human	• Precipitin test with intact root is specific for animal

d. Male and female femur

(Ref: Parikh's Textbook of Medical Jurisprudence, Forensic Medicine and Toxicology, 7/e, Pg. 61)

ANSWER

Male and Female Femur

Male femur	Female femur
• Head of the femur is larger and forms about 2/3 of a sphere	• Head is smaller and forms less than 2/3 of a sphere
• Vertical diameter is more than 47 mm	• Vertical diameter is less than 45 mm
• Neck forms obtuse angle with the shaft, about 125 degrees	• Neck forms less obtuse angle with the shaft
• Bicondylar width is 74–89 mm	• Bicondylar width 67–76 mm
• Angulation of shaft with condyles is around 80°	• Around 76°

PART III

5. What are the functions of Delhi Medical Council? How do they differ from the functions of Medical Council of India?

(Ref: Parikh's Textbook of Medical Jurisprudence, Forensic Medicine and Toxicology, 7/e, Pg. 21; The Essentials of Forensic Medicine & Toxicology, K.S. Narayan Reddy-34/e, pg. 24)

ANSWER

Functions of Delhi Medical Council

Main functions of state (Delhi) medical council are:

○ To maintain a medical register

- The Registrar or Secretary of the Council maintains a Register to provide for registration of medical practitioners within its jurisdiction
- Any doctor possessing required medical qualifications as prescribed by the Indian Medical Council is eligible for Registration on payment of prescribed fee
- Provisional registration is given to a doctor who has passed qualifying examination but has to complete certain training in an approved institution before such qualification is awarded to him
- Registrar informs the Indian Medical Council, about the additions and deletions from the Delhi Medical Register, from time to time
- To ensure doctors update their skills regularly, Delhi Medical Council has decided that doctors practising in Delhi have to apply for fresh registration every 5 years

- ○ **Medical etiquette and Medical ethics**
  - ■ **Medical etiquette**
    - ◆ Concerned with conventional laws and customs of courtesy which are generally followed between members of same profession
    - ◆ A doctor should behave with his colleagues as he wants them to behave with him
    - ◆ He should treat his colleague as his brother and therefore not charge him or his family members for professional service
  - ■ **Medical ethics**
    - ◆ Concerned with moral principles for the members of medical profession in their dealings with each other, their parents and the state
    - ◆ Aim is to honor and maintain the noble traditions of medical profession
    - ◆ **For example:** Medical practitioner should not take charge of a patient who is under the care of another practitioner
    - ◆ He should not refuse to give professional service on religious grounds
    - ◆ Must remember his responsibility to the State in relation to notifiable diseases and to the public to provide emergency care on humanitarian grounds
- ○ **Disciplinary control**
  - ■ Delhi medical council exercise disciplinary control over their members by reprimanding or erasing temporarily or permanently from the Register, the name of practitioner found guilty of infamous conduct in any professional respect (professional misconduct).
  - ■ They also have the power to direct the restoration of any removed name.
  - ■ Takes cognizance of any offence of misconduct committed by a registered medical practitioner only
    - ◆ When a written complaint in this respect is received by them
    - ◆ Or, when a medical practitioner is convicted by court of law
- ○ **Warning notice**
  - ■ Depending on the gravity of offence, the action may be in the nature of warning notice or erasure of name from register either temporarily or permanently
  - ■ Such erasure is called Penal erasure and when permanent, it is called as Professional death sentence
  - ■ It deprives the practitioner of all the privileges of a registered medical practitioner

Functions of Medical Council of India

- ○ **Medical education**
  - ■ Maintains standards of undergraduate medical education and lays down the requirements i.e. accommodation, equipment, teaching staff and their qualifications and other facilities
  - ■ Appoints inspectors for inspection of these requirements and standard of examination held by medical institutions in India for recommending recognition of medical qualifications awarded by them
  - ■ Prescribes standards for postgraduate medical education
- ○ **Medical qualifications**
  - ■ Recognizes Medical Act under three schedules of qualifications
    - ◆ First schedule includes recognized medical qualifications granted by medical institutions in India
    - ◆ Second schedule includes recognized medical qualifications granted by medical institutions outside India
    - ◆ Part I includes recognized medical qualifications granted by medical institutions in India not included in first schedule, Part II includes recognized medical qualifications granted by medical institutions outside India not included in second schedule
    - ◆ Can enter into negotiations for setting up of schemes for reciprocal recognition of medical qualifications with authority in any state or country outside India, entrusted by its constitution with maintenance of a register of medical practitioners
- ○ **Medical register**
  - ■ Maintains in a prescribed manner a register of medical practitioners known as Indian medical register containing the names of all persons enrolled in any state medical council and registered after recognized medical qualifications
- ○ **Advice on disciplinary action**
  - ■ Advises Central Health Ministry when an appeal is made by a registered medical practitioner against the decision of the state medial council on disciplinary matters
- ○ **Warning notices**
  - ■ Can issue warning notice in relation to certain unethical practices which are considered as falling within the meaning of term Infamous Conduct in a professional conduct
- ○ **Certificates**
  - ■ Empowered to issue certificates of good conduct and character to medical students or doctors going abroad for higher studies/service

- CME programs
  - Sponsors and organizes continuing medical education programs for medical practitioners to help in updating their knowledge
- Code of ethics
  - Follows Declaration of Geneva as modified by World Medical Association

6. Write short notes on:

a. Carboluria

(Ref: Parikh's Textbook of Medical Jurisprudence, Forensic Medicine and Toxicology, 7/e, Pg. 536; The Essentials of Forensic Medicine & Toxicology, K.S. Narayan Reddy-34/e, pg. 497)

ANSWER

Carboluria

Definition

- Presence of carbolic acid (phenol) in the urine
- Carbolic acid has nephrotoxic action, as observed in carbolic acid poisoning
- Presence of carbolic acid in urine is indicated by addition of little ferric chloride when the urine turns blue or little bromine water when urine forms a white precipitate of tribromo phenol
- Urine containing carbolic acid also reduces Benedict's and Fehling's solution

Symptoms Perceived are

- Irritation of kidneys in the form of suppression of urine or oliguria
- Urine contains albumin, blood casts and metabolic products of carbolic acid i.e. hydroquinone and pyrocatechol
- On standing or when exposed to air, these products are oxidized producing dark green and smoky appearance of urine–known as carboluria
- Served as a warning sign of the toxic action of carbolic acid when used as an antiseptic dressing
- It is followed by coma and death from paralysis of respiratory or cardiac center

b. Hallucination

(Ref: Parikh's Textbook of Medical Jurisprudence, Forensic Medicine and Toxicology, 7/e, Pg. 443; The Essentials of Forensic Medicine & Toxicology, K.S. Narayan Reddy-34/e, pg. 448)

ANSWER

Hallucination
Definition

- Seeing, smelling, hearing, tasting or touching something which is actually not present

- It is a false perception without a sensory stimuli, therefore any sensation can be involved
- Common hallucinations are Visual, Auditory, Olfactory, Gustatory, Tactile

Visual Hallucinations

- Occur in states of altered consciousness and epilepsy
- More common than auditory hallucinations
- Consist of–flashes of light, frightening faces, wild animals, terrifying scenes

Auditory Hallucinations

- Occur in schizophrenia and severe depressive disorders
- Patient often hears people abusing him or demanding his death

Olfactory or Hallucinations of Smell and Gustatory or Hallucinations of Taste

- Occur in schizophrenia and temporal lobe epilepsy
- Both are generally associated
- Patient states that his room has unpleasant smell or his food has peculiar taste
- Form basis for persecutory delusions e.g. patient feels that his room is filled with gas or his food has been poisoned

Tactile or Touch Hallucinations

- Occur in state of altered consciousness i.e. organic psychosis and schizophrenia
- Occur in cocaine psychosis
- Patient may try to commit suicide or some violent act

c. MTP Act, 1971

(Ref: Parikh's Textbook of Medical Jurisprudence, Forensic Medicine and Toxicology, 7/e, Pg. 413; The Essentials of Forensic Medicine & Toxicology, K.S. Narayan Reddy-34/e, pg. 374)

ANSWER

MTP Act, 1971

Medical Termination of Pregnancy Act, 1971 Legalizes abortion on following grounds:

- **Therapeutic grounds:** Relate to conditions where continuation of pregnancy would risk
  - The life of pregnant woman
  - Grave injury to her physical or mental health
    - Organic heart disease with failure, active tuberculosis, severe diabetes
    - Hypertension complicated with cardiac or renal failure
    - Nephrotic syndrome
    - Pulmonary hypertension
    - Hepatocellular failure, acute hepatitis, acute pancreatitis

- Toxemia of pregnancy
- Hydatidiform mole or acute hydramnios
- Uterine hemorrhage or infected uterus after attempts at criminal abortion
- Malignant neoplasms of breast or female genital tract
- Repeated caesareans or irreducible prolapse of gravid uterus
- Threatened insanity

○ **Eugenic grounds:** Conditions when there is substantial risk to the child, if born, will suffer from serious mental or physical abnormalities to be seriously handicapped

- German measles, smallpox, chickenpox, viral hepatitis or other serious viral infections, if contracted within the first trimester of pregnancy
- Exposure to X-rays and other radiation
- When pregnant woman has received cytotoxic drugs, thalidomide, LSD etc.
- When the parents have some inheritable mental condition or chromosomal abnormalities

○ **Humanitarian grounds**

- When pregnancy has been caused by rape, the anguish caused by such pregnancy is presumed to produce grave injury to her mental health

○ **Social grounds**

- Where pregnancy in a married woman is result of contraceptive failure
- When the environment of pregnant woman, during the continuance of pregnancy and at the time when the child would be born and thereafter

so far as is foreseeable would involve risk of injury to her health

Requirements for termination of pregnancy:

○ In an emergency, any registered medical practitioner, irrespective of his experience or training in obstetrics and gynecology can terminate pregnancy at any place, irrespective of its duration, if he is of opinion formed in good faith that the termination of such pregnancy is immediately necessary to save the life of the pregnant woman

○ Except in an emergency, where duration of pregnancy does not exceed 12 weeks, a pregnancy can be terminated on the opinion of one registered medical practitioner and where the duration exceeds 12 weeks but is less than 20 weeks, opinion from 2 registered medical practitioners is necessary. It is essential that

- Opinion must be formed in good faith
- Registered medical practitioner must have specified experience or training in gynecology and obstetrics
- Such practitioner must have been registered with a certifying board for this purpose
- Termination must be carried out in a hospital maintained by government or at a place approved by the government
- Written consent of the woman only is essential
- Consent of woman is not necessary
- Written consent from her guardians in case where she is a minor or mentally defective

Name of the Paper   :   **Forensic Medicine & Toxicology**

Name of the Course   :   **MBBS-2009**

Semester   :   **Annual**

Time: 3 Hours   **M.M.: 40**

INSTRUCTIONS

1. Write your Roll No. on the top immediately on receipt of this question paper
2. All questions are to be attempted
3. Answers to Parts I, II and III should be written in separate answer sheets provided
4. Attempt parts of a question in sequence

PART-I

1. What are findings, interpretations and medicolegal importance when it is stated that: [8]

   a. Body is showing pugilistic attitude
   b. The boy is 14 years of age
   c. The person has died of air embolism
   d. Person is intersex

2. Write short notes on: [6]

   a. Mummification
   b. Perjury
   c. Vicarious liability

PART-II

3. Classify insecticides. Discuss the signs, symptoms, management, and postmortem findings and medicolegal importance of acute organophosphorus poisoning: [7]

4. Differentiate between: [6]

   a. Examination-in-chief and cross examination
   b. Poisonous and nonpoisonous snakes
   c. Animal and human teeth bites

PART-III

5. Classify injuries. Discuss in detail the pattern of injuries in fall from height case. How will you differentiate between suicide, homicidal and accidental fall?   [7]

6. Write short notes: [6]

   a. DNA profiling
   b. Warning notice
   c. Eye change after death

PART I

1. **What are the findings, interpretations and medicolegal importance when it is stated that:**

   a.   Body is showing pugilistic attitude

   (Ref: Parikh's Textbook of Medical Jurisprudence, Forensic Medicine and Toxicology, 7/e, Pg. 337)

ANSWER

Body is Showing Pugilistic Attitude

For answer, refer 2014 paper Q. 1 (b), Pg. 485

   b.   The boy is 14 years of age

   (Ref: Parikh's Textbook of Medical Jurisprudence, Forensic Medicine and Toxicology, 7/e, Pg. 59)

ANSWER

For answer, refer 2013 paper Q. 1 (b), Pg. 493

   c.   The person has died of air embolism

   (Ref: Parikh's Textbook of Medical Jurisprudence, Forensic Medicine and Toxicology, 7/e, Pg. 271; The Essentials of Forensic Medicine & Toxicology, K.S. Narayan Reddy-34/e, pg. 104)

ANSWER

The Person has Died of Air Embolism

Findings

- In pulmonary or venous air embolism
  - Distension of right ventricle with air under pressure
  - Bright red frothy blood on the right side of heart, inferior vena cava, pulmonary arteries and coronary veins
  - Bubbles can be traced back to the site of entry
- Systemic or arterial air embolism
  - Cerebral and coronary arteries appear segmented due to presence of air

Interpretation and Medicolegal Importance

- About 10–20 mL of air has been introduced into circulation
- Pulmonary air embolism could have occurred due to
  - Faulty technique of giving intravenous injection such as saline drip

- Cut throat or incised wounds of neck
- Injury to superior sagittal sinus
- Crush injuries of chest resulting in penetration of lung
- Systemic air embolism could have occurred due to:
  - Penetrating wound of the chest
  - Crush injuries of the thorax
  - Surgical procedures on the chest

   d.   Intersex

   (Ref: Parikh's Textbook of Medical Jurisprudence, Forensic Medicine and Toxicology, 7/e, Pg. 58)

ANSWER

Intersex

Findings and Interpretation

- **In Gonadal agenesis**
  - Sexual organs i.e. testes or ovaries, have not developed
  - Chromatin negative
- **In Gonadal dysgenesis**
  - **In Klinefelter syndrome, a boy has:**
    - Small testicles, firm consistency
    - Gynecomastia
    - **Eunuchoidism:** Long arms and legs, scanty pubic hair, scanty axillary hair, poor or no beard growth
    - Chromatin positive like female and sex chromosome pattern is XXY
  - **In turner syndrome**
    - **Sexual infantilism:** Primary amenrrhea and consequent sterility
    - Short stature
    - **Congenital abnormalities:** Webbing of neck, cubitus valgus, coarctation of aorta, red green color blindness, renal abnormalities, osteoporosis
    - Lack of breast development with widely spaced nipples
    - Hypoplastic areolae
    - Scanty pubic hair
    - Infantile external genitalia, uterus and fallopian tubes
    - Streak ovaries with no ovarian follicles
    - Chromatin negative like a male and sex chromosome pattern is XO

○ **True hermaphroditism**
- External genitalia of both sexes
- Internal genitalia has both ovaries and testes or ovotestes
- Hypospadias
- Cryptorchidism
- Inguinal hernia

○ **Pseudohermaphroditism**
- External genitalia lacks clear cut differentiation
- Internal genitalia has only one sex

Medicolegal Importance

Complications pertain to:

○ Marriage
○ Inheritance
○ Civil rights

2. Write short notes on:

a. Mummification

(Ref: Parikh's Textbook of Medical Jurisprudence, Forensic Medicine and Toxicology, 7/e, Pg. 161; The Essentials of Forensic Medicine & Toxicology, K.S. Narayan Reddy-34/e, pg. 163)

ANSWER

For answer, refer 2015 paper Q. 1 (b), Pg. 478

b. Perjury

(Ref: Parikh's Textbook of Medical Jurisprudence, Forensic Medicine and Toxicology, 7/e, Pg. 10; The Essentials of Forensic Medicine & Toxicology, K.S. Narayan Reddy-34/e, pg. 13)

ANSWER

For answer, refer 2011 paper Q. 6 (c), Pg. 510

c. Vicarious liability

(Ref: Parikh's Textbook of Medical Jurisprudence, Forensic Medicine and Toxicology, 7/e, Pg. 43)

ANSWER

Vicarious Liability

For answer, refer 2013 paper Q. 6 (a), Pg. 497

PART II

3. Classify insecticides. Discuss signs, symptoms, management and postmortem findings and medicolegal importance of acute organophosphorus poisoning.

(Ref: Parikh's Textbook of Medical Jurisprudence, Forensic Medicine and Toxicology, 7/e, Pg. 625)

ANSWER

Classification of Insecticides

○ Vegetable origin
- Nicotine
- Pyrethrins
- Rotenone

○ Chemical
- **Inorganic:** Phosphorus and compounds of antimony, arsenic, barium, mercury, thallium, zinc and fluorides

○ Synthetic organic chemical
- Phosphorus esters
- Carbamates
- Chlorinated hydrocarbons
  - **Indane derivatives:** chlordane, heptachlor, aldrin, dieldrin, endrin, dieldrin
  - **Chlorobenzene derivatives:** DDT, chlorophenothane
  - **Benzene hexachloride:** Lindane, gammexane
  - **Chlorinated camphene:** Toxaphene, strobane

b. Acute Organophosphorus Poisoning

(Ref: Parikh's Textbook of Medical Jurisprudence, Forensic Medicine and Toxicology, 7/e, Pg. 625)

ANSWER

For answer, refer 2016 paper Q. 3 (b), Pg. 472

4. Differentiate between:

a. Examination-in-chief and cross examination

(Ref: Parikh's Textbook of Medical Jurisprudence, Forensic Medicine and Toxicology, 7/e, Pg. 11; The Essentials of Forensic Medicine & Toxicology, K.S. Narayan Reddy-34/e, pg. 13)

ANSWER

Examination-in-Chief and Cross Examination

Examination-in-chief	Cross examination
• Questions put by the counsel for the side who has summoned him	• Questions put by counsel for the opposite side that is counsel for the accused
• Object is to place before the court all the relevant facts that relate to the case	• Object is to weaken the evidence of the witness by showing that the details are inaccurate, conflicting, contradictory or that his opinions are ill-founded and opposed to that of well recognized authorities
• If witness tries to modify any of his findings or conclusions, lawyer should point out	• Lawyer tries to modify what witness has said
• Leading questions are not allowed	• Leading questions are allowed

b. Poisonous and nonpoisonous snakes

(Ref: Parikh's Textbook of Medical Jurisprudence, Forensic Medicine and Toxicology, 7/e, Pg. 574; The Essentials of Forensic Medicine & Toxicology, K.S. Narayan Reddy-34/e, pg. 519)

ANSWER

For answer, refer 2012 paper Q. 4 (b), Pg. 502

c. Animal and human teeth bites

(Ref: Parikh's Textbook of Medical Jurisprudence, Forensic Medicine and Toxicology, 7/e, Pg. 83; The Essentials of Forensic Medicine & Toxicology, K.S. Narayan Reddy-34/e, pg. 95)

ANSWER

Animal and Human Teeth Bites

Animal teeth bite	Human teeth bite
• Clear cut, Narrow in anterior aspect, V-shaped and elongated	• Semi-circular or crescentic, caused by front teeth, U-shaped
• Bite marks are deep resembling stab wounds and small in area	• Bite marks are abrasions, contusions or lacerations
• Intercanine distance is 32-43 mm	• Intercanine distance is 29-30 mm
• Tooth numbering system is Modified Triadan tooth numbering system	• Tooth numbering system is Fédération Dentaire Internationale

PART III

5. Classify injuries. Discuss in detail the pattern of injuries in fall from height case. How will you differentiate between suicide, homicide and accidental fall?

(Ref: Parikh's Textbook of Medical Jurisprudence, Forensic Medicine and Toxicology, 7/e, Pg. 211)

ANSWER

Injuries

Classification

- ○ **Mechanical:**
  - ▪ **Based on Cause:**
    - ◆ Abrasions
    - ◆ Bruises
    - ◆ Lacerations
    - ◆ Fractures
    - ◆ Incised wounds
    - ◆ Stab wounds
    - ◆ Firearm wounds
  - ▪ **Based on Nature:**
    - ◆ Defense wounds
    - ◆ Self-inflicting wounds
    - ◆ Injury patterns
- ○ **Thermal:**
  - ▪ **Due to cold:**
    - ◆ Frostbite
    - ◆ Trench foot
    - ◆ Immersion foot
  - ▪ **Due to heat:**
  - ▪ **Simple burns:** Caused by dry heat – by hot substances, by flames
  - ▪ **Scalds:** Caused by moist heat
  - ▪ **Corrosive burns:** By chemicals
  - ▪ **Electric burns:** By electric contact, electric spark, flashes of lightning
  - ▪ **Radiation burns:** Caused by X-rays, ultraviolet rays, radium, laser, microwave oven

b. Pattern of injuries in fall from height

(Ref: Parikh's Textbook of Medical Jurisprudence, Forensic Medicine and Toxicology, 7/e, Pg. 287)

ANSWER

- ○ When falling from a high building, the displaced air tends to act as a cushion which drives the body from the wall
- ○ A simple fall can result in a body impact some distance from the foot of building, which is not an evidence of a push or of a deliberate Jump
- ○ **Pattern of injuries after fall depends on:**
  - ▪ **Height:** From which the body falls
  - ▪ **Orientation of body at point of impact:** Generally, vertical landing with feet first is seen and next common is vertical landing with head first
  - ▪ **Impact of surface:** On which the body falls
  - ▪ **Deceleration:** Quicker the body is brought to rest, greater will be forces acting on it

○ **Most commonly seen injuries with body landing with feet first are:**
- Fractures of bones of feet (calcaneus and other tarsal and metatarsal bones)
- Tibias may be driven through soles of feet
- Fracture-dislocation of ankles
- Oblique or comminuted fractures of tibiae and fibulae
- Fractures of femur
- Fractures of pelvis
- Fractures of spine
- Lacerations of vertebral column
- Ring or comminuted fractures of base of skull
- Injuries to brainstem

- Lacerations of spleen and liver
- Rupture of aortic arch
- Ruptures and lacerations of pulmonary trunk, arteries and veins

○ **Injuries with head first are**
- Open comminuted or depressed fracture of skull
- Brain lacerations
- Partial or complete extrusion of brain

○ Abrasions and contusions are common when body hits hard patterned surfaces

○ Bruises of palms and fingers

○ Perineal bruises

○ Ribs fractures

Difference between Suicidal, Homicidal and Accidental Fall

Features	Suicidal fall	Homicidal fall	Accidental fall
• Grab marks	• Not present	• May be present on the inner surface of arms	• Not present
• Suicide note	• May be present	• Not present	• Not present
• Psychiatric history	• May be present	• Not present	• Not present
• Heights of fall	• Greater	• May be Greater	• May be less
• Site of fall	• Bridges or high rise apartments	• Homes of deceased	• Usually Buildings or construction sites
• Marks of assault	• Not present	• May be present	• Not present
• Hesitation marks	• May be present	• Not present	• Not present
• Position of fall	• Usually falls Forward	• If pushed from front, falls on back	• If unconscious while standing or walking, Usually falls forward

6. Write short notes:

a. DNA profiling

(Ref: Parikh's Textbook of Medical Jurisprudence, Forensic Medicine and Toxicology, 7/e, Pg. 478)

ANSWER

DNA Profiling

○ **Definition:** Technique involving chemically dividing the DNA into fragments which form a unique pattern and then matching that identity profile with the pattern obtained from similarly testing a suspect's blood specimen

○ Looks directly at person's genetic make-up

○ DNA molecule is made up of sugars, phosphates and nitrogenous bases which form the functional unit known as nucleotide

○ Essence of DNA profiling in forensic work is comparison between 2 samples

○ Samples for DNA profiling must contain nucleated cells e.g. leucocytes, seminal fluid, brain, bone marrow, muscle, skin, dental pulp, hair with root sheath cells, dried stains

○ Identity of a criminal is determined by comparing the accused man's DNA profile with a biological item e.g. blood or seminal stain, found at the scene of crime

○ If tests are performed properly, identification is absolute

Medicolegal Importance

○ Blood or few hair roots on crime weapon can be matched with victim's blood

○ Seminal fluid in vagina of a rape and murder victim can be matched against blood DNA pattern of a suspect

Applications

○ **Paternity testing:** Absolute identification can be made

○ Linking body parts

○ Baby mix-ups

○ Identification of person with loss of memory

○ Allied situations

○ Sex of the fetus can be determined by looking at DNA sequences from Y chromosome in fetal cells present in mother's blood as early as fifth week of pregnancy

○ Can be useful to identify physical attributes such as eye color, hair color and appearance of a skeleton

b **Warning notice**

(Ref: Parikh's Textbook of Medical Jurisprudence, Forensic Medicine and Toxicology, 7/e, Pg. 22; The Essentials of Forensic Medicine & Toxicology, K.S. Narayan Reddy-34/e, pg. 26)

ANSWER

Warning Notice

○ **Definition:** The Medical Council of India may prescribe standards of professional conduct and etiquette and a Code of Ethics for medical practitioners

○ It can issue Warning notice containing certain practices which are considered as falling within the meaning of the term, "serious professional misconduct" or infamous conduct in a professional respect.

○ Warning notice can also be issued by State Medical Council

c. **Eye change after death**

(Ref: Parikh's Textbook of Medical Jurisprudence, Forensic Medicine and Toxicology, 7/e, Pg. 143; The Essentials of Forensic Medicine & Toxicology, K.S. Narayan Reddy-34/e, pg. 145)

ANSWER

Eye Change After Death

Changes in the Eye after Death

○ Cornea
  ▪ Becomes dry, cloudy and opaque due to failure of production of tears

▪ Clear glistening appearance is vanished
▪ Corneal reflex is lost but not a reliable sign as it can also be lost in brainstem death
▪ Light reflex is lost

○ **Eyeballs**
  ▪ Become flaccid, flaccidity can be appreciated by palpation
  ▪ Tend to sink into orbits
  ▪ Intraocular tension falls

○ **Retina**
  ▪ Bloodstream in retinal vessels become dotted at first and then segmented (cattle truckling) and then optic disc becomes pale

○ **Pupils**
  ▪ Generally dilate at the time of death and then becomes constricted through the development of rigor mortis
  ▪ Their state after death doesn't indicate their antemortem appearance
  ▪ Early state of pupil is significant in suspected narcotic poisoning
  ▪ Unequal pupils

○ **Sclera**
  ▪ If eyes remain open, Taches Noires appear on sclera within 3 hours of death
  ▪ Taches Noires are brownish-black discolored areas on exposed sclera between eyelids due to formation of cellular debris and settling of dust
  ▪ Potassium content of vitreous humor rises gradually

Your Roll No. ....

Name of the Paper   :   **Forensic Medicine & Toxicology**

Name of the Course   :   **MBBS-2008**

Semester   :   **Annual**

Time: 3 Hours   M.M.: 40

INSTRUCTIONS

1. Write your Roll No. on the top immediately on receipt of this question paper
2. All questions are to be attempted
3. Answers to Parts I, II and III should be written in separate answer sheets provided
4. Attempt parts of a question in sequence

PART-I

1. What are the findings, interpretations and medicolegal importance when it is stated that: [8]
   a. Hydrostatic test is positive
   b. The death is due to traumatic asphyxia
   c. Cadaveric spasm is present
   d. The person is in lucid interval

2. Explain why: [6]
   a. Contributory negligence
   b. True and Feigned mental illness
   c. Testamentary capacity

PART-II

3. What are somniferous poisons? Describe the clinical features, management, postmortem findings and medicolegal significance in a case of acute morphine poisoning   [7]

4. Differentiate between: [6]
   a. Entry and exit wounds of rifled firearm
   b. Heat hematoma and extradural hematoma
   c. Ligature marks of hanging and strangulation

PART-III

5. Classify thermal injuries. Describe in detail the cause of death, postmortem finding in a case of carbon monoxide poisoning: [7]

6. Write short notes on: [6]
   a. Patterned injuries
   b. Delusion
   c. Hostile witness

PART I

1. What are the findings, interpretation and medicolegal importance when it is stated that:

a. Hydrostatic test is positive

(Ref: Parikh's Textbook of Medical Jurisprudence, Forensic Medicine and Toxicology, 7/e, Pg. 429; The Essentials of Forensic Medicine & Toxicology, K.S. Narayan Reddy-34/e, pg. 411)

ANSWER

Hydrostatic Test is Positive

Findings

○ **Piece of lung floats in water:** Respiration has taken place

○ If some pieces float while others sink that means feeble respiration

Interpretation

○ Hydrostatic test depends on changes in specific gravity of lungs due to respiration

○ Specific gravity of non-respired lung is about 1050 i.e. heavier than water and that of a respired lung is about 950 i.e. lighter than water

○ Non respired lung sink in water and respired lungs float

○ **If the test is positive:** i.e. piece of lung floats in water then it means respiration has taken place

Medicolegal Importance

○ **Not of much importance as:**
  ▪ No value in forensic medicine as lungs of liveborn who has lived for few days may sink and lungs of still born may float
  ▪ Slightest degree of decomposition invalidates any interpretation of the floatation test
  ▪ Resuscitation attempts make evaluation of test difficult or even impossible
  ▪ Some expansion of air sacs of lungs in fetus does occur towards the end of pregnancy as a result of amniotic fluid moving in and out of bronchial tree

b The death is due to traumatic asphyxia

(Ref: Parikh's Textbook of Medical Jurisprudence, Forensic Medicine and Toxicology, 7/e, Pg. 187)

ANSWER

For answer, refer 2010 paper Q. 1(a)

c. Cadaveric spasm is present

(Ref: Parikh's Textbook of Medical Jurisprudence, Forensic Medicine and Toxicology, 7/e, Pg. 150; The Essentials of Forensic Medicine & Toxicology, K.S. Narayan Reddy-34/e, pg. 154)

ANSWER

Cadaveric Spasm is Present

Findings

○ Stiffening of a particular group of muscles such as forearm, hands

○ Some object remains firmly grasped after death when it is held in the hand of person at the time of death foe e.g. knife or grass weeds or hair

Interpretation

○ Somatic death occurred with extreme rapidity

○ Person was in a state of excessive emotional pressure

○ Muscles were in physical activity at the time of death

○ **In case of object found in hand:** It is obvious that object was gripped at the time of death

Medicolegal Importance

○ Indicates sudden death associated with profound emotional stress

○ Indicates muscles in physical activity at the time of death

○ May indicate nature of death i.e. suicide, homicide or accident
  ▪ **Suicide:** In case of weapon of light weight is seen tightly clenched in hand such as blades or razors in cut throat or pistol in firearm injury
  ▪ **Homicide:** If some part of clothing or hair belonging to assailant is found in victim's hand; or in soldiers killed in action–helps in identification of murderer
  ▪ **Accident:** In mountain fatalities or some branches of trees are seized by deceased

d. Person is in lucid interval

ANSWER

For answer, refer 2012 paper Q. 1(d), Pg. 501

FORENSIC MEDICINE & TOXICOLOGY

2. **Explain why?**

a. **Contributory negligence**

(Ref: Parikh's Textbook of Medical Jurisprudence, Forensic Medicine and Toxicology, 7/e, Pg. 43; The Essentials of Forensic Medicine & Toxicology, K.S. Narayan Reddy-34/e, pg. 38)

ANSWER

Contributory Negligence

Definition

○ Simultaneous negligence by the patient and doctor resulting in delayed recovery or harm to the patient

○ Negligence of both parties has contributed to this harm

Types of Negligence

○ **Failure on the part of patient to give accurate medical history:** Incomplete information could result in misdiagnosis and wrong treatment thus causing harm

○ Failure to cooperate with the doctor in following all instructions properly such as laboratory tests, proper diet

○ Refusal to take adequate medication

○ Leaving the hospital premises against doctor's advice

Liability of Doctor

○ If negligence on the part of patient is proved, patient has no right to claim the damage against doctor for any harm occurred

○ Doctor has to foresee that the patient may harm himself and should warn him accordingly. Failing to do that, doctor cannot plead contributory negligence

○ Responsibility of proving the negligence depends entirely on the doctor

Example

○ While injecting a patient using a thin hypodermic needle, doctor had warned him to keep his arm steady otherwise the needle would break but the patient moved suddenly. The needle broke and had to be removed surgically. Patient could not succeed in getting any compensation from the doctor

b. **True and feigned mental illness**

(Ref: Parikh's Textbook of Medical Jurisprudence, Forensic Medicine and Toxicology, 7/e, Pg. 453)

ANSWER

True and Feigned Mental Illness

True unsoundness of mind	Feigned unsoundness of mind
• Gradual onset or rarely sudden but usually without any motive	• Sudden onset and not without some motive
• Predisposing or exciting cause may be present, e.g. family history of insanity, grief, sudden loss of money, etc.	• No predisposing or exciting cause is usually present
• Well-developed cases of insanity have a peculiar facial expression	• Facial expression is generally normal even when the person pretends to be mad outright.
• The individual shows signs and symptoms of insanity irrespective of his conduct being observed or not	• The individual pretends to be insane only when he is observed and there is total absence of symptoms when he is alone and unobserved
• Signs and symptoms usually suggest a particular type of mental illness	• Signs and symptoms are not uniform and do not suggest any particular type of mental illness
• Can stand violent exertion for several hours or days without exhaustion, or sleep	• Violent exertion leads to exhaustion, and sleep
• Physical manifestations of true insanity, viz. dry, harsh skin, furred tongue, constipation, anorexia, and insomnia are present	• Physical manifestations of true insanity, viz. dry, harsh tongue, constipation, anorexia, and insomnia are not present
• Not worried about being repeatedly examined	• Dislike for repeated examination is obvious

c. **Testamentary capacity**

(Ref: Parikh's Textbook of Medical Jurisprudence, Forensic Medicine and Toxicology, 7/e, Pg. 458; The Essentials of Forensic Medicine & Toxicology, K.S. Narayan Reddy-34/e, pg. 458)

ANSWER

Testamentary Capacity

Definition

○ Capacity of a person to prepare a valid will

○ Possession of a sound disposing mind (compos mentis), which must be certified by a doctor

Conditions Fulfilling the Validity of Will

○ Testator must be a major

○ Must possess sound disposing mind at the time of making will

○ Must understand nature and consequence of his act

○ Must know what property he has, to whom he is giving it and has good reason for his action

○ Executing it voluntarily and without any undue influence by any other person

○ Must sign it in presence of two witnesses of which one should be a medical man

  ▪ Both witnesses should also sign in the presence of each other and of testator

○ None of the witnesses should be beneficiaries from the will

○ Mentally ill patient can prepare a valid will only during lucid intervals

○ Person affected by delusions can also prepare valid will as long as the delusions are not related to property

○ Will can also be made during fits of drunkenness unless the person was so drunk as not to know what he was doing and unless it was repudiated in sober moments

○ Person can also make valid will despite of extreme age, feeble health and mental sluggishness unless his mind has become so weakened to understand the nature of the act

PART II

3. **What are somniferous poisons? Describe the clinical features, management, postmortem findings and medicolegal significance in a case of acute morphine poisoning.**

(Ref: Parikh's Textbook of Medical Jurisprudence, Forensic Medicine and Toxicology, 7/e, Pg. 595)

ANSWER

Somniferous Poisons

Definition

○ Poisons used to reduce pain and induce sleep knows as somniferous or narcotic effect

  ▪ Opium and Morphine

  ▪ Heroin

  ▪ Pethidine

○ Action is characterized by two sets of symptoms i.e. excitement and narcosis

For answer, refer 2010 paper Q. 3 (b), Pg. 514

4. **Differentiate between:**

a. **Entry and exit wounds of rifled firearm**

(Ref: Parikh's Textbook of Medical Jurisprudence, Forensic Medicine and Toxicology, 7/e, Pg. 252; The Essentials of Forensic Medicine & Toxicology, K.S. Narayan Reddy-34/e, pg. 215)

ANSWER

Entry and Exit Wounds of Rifled Firearm

Exit wound	Entry wound
• The wound is smaller in size (except at contact range when the skin may be torn by blast or rarely when the bullet ricochets, or loses its gyroscopic stability)	• The missile tears out the tissues and has sharply defined outwardly split edges
• In flat bone, like skull, the entry wound is clean cut on the outer surface and chipped inward	• In flat bone, like skull, the exit wound is beveled and everted
• Edges are inverted because the missile penetrates from outside. In fat persons, they may be everted due to protrusion of fat	• Edges are everted because the missile forces its way out
• Abrasion collar is present; grease collar may or may not be present	• Abrasion collar is absent except in shored exit wounds when irregular abrasion will be seen. Grease collar is never seen
• Burning, blackening, singeing, and tattooing may be seen at appropriate distances	• Burning, blackening, singeing, and tattooing cannot be seen
• Clothing may be turned in and carried into the wound	• Clothing may or may not be turned out
• Track near the entry wound may be bright pink due to carboxy-hemoglobin in the case of near discharge	• Not usually so but very exceptionally gas can be blown along a wound track
• Lead ring may be present on radiological or micro chemical examination	• Lead ring absent

b. **Heat hematoma and extradural hematoma**

(Ref: Parikh's Textbook of Medical Jurisprudence, Forensic Medicine and Toxicology, 7/e, Pg. 295; The Essentials of Forensic Medicine & Toxicology, K.S. Narayan Reddy-34/e, pg. 242)

ANSWER

Heat Hematoma and Extradural Hematoma

For answer, refer 2016 paper Q. 4 (b), Pg. 474

c. Ligature marks of hanging and strangulation

(Ref: Parikh's Textbook of Medical Jurisprudence, Forensic Medicine and Toxicology, 7/e, Pg. 171; The Essentials of Forensic Medicine & Toxicology, K.S. Narayan Reddy-34/e, pg. 328)

ANSWER

Ligature Marks of Hanging and Strangulation

Ligature marks of hanging	Ligature marks of strangulation
• Situated above the level of thyroid cartilage between larynx and chin	• Situated at the level of thyroid cartilage or below
• Directed obliquely upward along the line of the mandible and reaches the mastoid process behind the ears	• Almost horizontal and encircles the neck completely or nearly so
• Injuries to deeper tissues are not considerable	• Injuries to deeper tissues are common due to amount of force used

PART III

5. Classify thermal injuries. Describe in detail the cause of death, postmortem finding in a case of carbon monoxide poisoning.

a. Thermal injuries

(Ref: Parikh's Textbook of Medical Jurisprudence, Forensic Medicine and Toxicology, 7/e, Pg. 332)

ANSWER

Definition

○ Injury to tissue caused by application of heat in any form to external or internal body surfaces

Classification

○ **Simple burns:** Caused by dry heat–by hot substances, by flames
○ **Scalds:** Caused by moist heat
○ **Corrosive burns:** By chemicals
○ **Electric burns:** By electric contact, electric spark, flashes of lightning
○ **Radiation burns:** Caused by X-rays, ultraviolet rays, radium, laser, microwave oven

b. Carbon monoxide poisoning

(Ref: Parikh's Textbook of Medical Jurisprudence, Forensic Medicine and Toxicology, 7/e, Pg. 651; The Essentials of Forensic Medicine & Toxicology, K.S. Narayan Reddy-34/e, pg. 544)

ANSWER

Cause of Death

○ Reduces oxygen carrying capacity of blood
○ Results in tissue anoxia
○ Interferes with vital cellular enzymes

Signs and Symptoms

Symptoms of saturation of carbon monoxide in blood	
Saturation of hemoglobin with CO	Symptoms
• 0–10%	• No appreciable symptoms
• 10–20%	• Shortness of breath on exertion, mild headache, lassitude and flushed skin
• 20–30%	• Throbbing headache, buzzing in the ears. Breathlessness. muscular weakness and in coordination, dulling of senses
• 30–40%	• Severe headache, dizziness, nausea, vomiting, collapse on slight exertion. Breathlessness. Mental confusion, impaired judgment, muscular weakness and incoordination. Dim vision
• 40–50%	• All symptoms intensified. May be mistaken with drunkenness. Incoordination, staggering, mental confusion, loss of memory, palpitation and dyspnea
• 50–70%	• Intermittent asphyxial convulsions, coma, Cheyne-Stokes respiration, respiratory paralysis and death
• Above 70%	• Rapidly fatal due to respiratory arrest

Fatal Dose and Fatal Period

○ **At rest:** 0.1% CO in atmosphere results in stupor and coma in 2.5 to 3 hours
○ **With exercise:** 1 hour
○ **A 1% concentration will result in stupor and coma:** 15-20 minutes
○ Debilitated, diseased or drunk may surrender to lower saturations

Treatment

○ Patient must be removed to open air at once and body warmth should be maintained
○ If patient is conscious and breathing, no further treatment is necessary
○ CO is speedily eliminated by giving oxygen

○ If breathing is even slightly irregular, artificial respiration is required

○ Whole blood transfusion is required in severe cases

○ Prophylactic antibiotics are given for lung infection

○ Till all acute symptoms are disappeared, patient has to be kept at absolute rest, even after respiration becomes normal

Postmortem Findings

○ **External:**

  ▪ Fine froth seen at mouth and nose

  ▪ If saturation of CO in blood is higher than 30%, the color of the skin is bright cherry red

  ▪ No coloration is seen below 20%

  ▪ Skin blisters due to hypoxia are found on axillae, inner side of thighs etc. areas where skin is in contact with ground or where skin is in apposition

○ **Internal**

  ▪ In case of more than 5 g CO Hb/100 mL of blood, blood, tissues and viscera are of bright cherry red color

  ▪ Serous effusions

  ▪ Edematous brain and petechial hemorrhages on meninges are found

  ▪ Necrosis and cavitation of basal ganglia, especially putamen and globus pallidus in cases of prolonged hypoxia

  ▪ Edematous lungs or show bronchopneumonia

  ▪ Myocardial degeneration and necrotic patches in cardiac muscle

  ▪ Carboxyhemoglobin can be found in highly putrefied bodies

Medicolegal Significance

○ **Suicidal exposure:** By sitting in car and connecting tube from exhaust to nostril or remaining near exhaust pipe in his garage with doors closed

○ **Accidental exposure:** Due to leakage from sources of domestic supply, lime burning, burning buildings and explosions in confined spaces such as mines

○ Persons with history of epilepsy, convulsions may lose consciousness

6. **Write short notes on:**

  a. **Patterned Injuries**

  (Ref: Parikh's Textbook of Medical Jurisprudence, Forensic Medicine and Toxicology, 7/e, Pg. 319)

ANSWER

For answer, refer 2010 paper Q. 1 (b), Pg. 512

  b. **Delusion**

  (Ref: Parikh's Textbook of Medical Jurisprudence, Forensic Medicine and Toxicology, 7/e, Pg. 442; The Essentials of Forensic Medicine & Toxicology, K.S. Narayan Reddy-34/e, pg. 477)

ANSWER

For answer, refer 2013 paper Q. 2 (b), Pg. 494

  c **Hostile Witness**

  (Ref: Parikh's Textbook of Medical Jurisprudence, Forensic Medicine and Toxicology, 7/e, Pg. 11)

ANSWER

For answer, refer 2012 paper Q. 2 (a), Pg. 501

Your Roll No. ....

Name of the Paper	:	**Forensic Medicine & Toxicology**
Name of the Course	:	**MBBS-2007**
Semester	:	**Annual**

Time: 3 Hours   **M.M.: 40**

INSTRUCTIONS

1. Write your Roll No. on the top immediately on receipt of this question paper
2. All questions are to be attempted
3. Answers to Parts I, II and III should be written in separate answer sheets provided
4. Attempt parts of a question in sequence

PART-I

1. **What are the findings, interpretation and medicolegal importance when it is stated that:** [8]
   a. Skull is having a ring fracture
   b. Body is showing pugilistic attitude
   c. Person is 12 years of age
   d. Diatoms are present in bone marrow

2. **Write short notes on:** [6]
   a. Dying declaration
   b. Whiplash injury
   c. Privileged communication

PART-II

3. **Classify irritant poisons. Describe clinical features, management postmortem findings and medicolegal importance in case of chronic mercury poisoning.** [7]

4. **Differentiate between:** [6]
   a. Datura and capsicum seeds
   b. Burns and scalds
   c. Antemortem and postmortem contusions

PART-III

5. **Define rape. What will be findings in a 15-year-old alleged to have been raped 12 hours ago?** [7]

6. **Write short notes on:** [6]
   a. Concussion
   b. DNA fingerprinting
   c. Impulse

PART I

1. **What are the findings, interpretation and medicolegal importance when it is stated that:**

    a.   Skull is having a ring fracture

    (Ref: Parikh's Textbook of Medical Jurisprudence, Forensic Medicine and Toxicology, 7/e, Pg. 291; The Essentials of Forensic Medicine & Toxicology, K.S. Narayan Reddy-34/e, pg. 321)

ANSWER

Skull is Having a Ring Fracture

○ **Findings**
  - Any fracture encircling the skull separating the anterior third at its junction with the middle and posterior third
  - Fissured fracture about 3.5 cm outside the foramen magnum at the back, involving middle ear sideways and roof of nose anteriorly separating the skull from the spine
  - In severe cases, skull may be driven into skull cavity and the vault of the skull may burst open giving the impression of an original massive fracture

○ **Interpretation**
  - Rare and requires a lot of force to occur
  - Produces after
    - Falls from height on to feet or buttocks
    - Sudden violent turn of the head on the spine
    - Severe blow on vertex which drives the skull downwards on the vertebral column
    - Heavy blow directed below the occiput or chin as in traffic accident

○ **Medicolegal importance**
  - Autopsy findings in a victim of an accidental or suicidal fall from a height may be indistinguishable from a homicidal fall where victim was deliberately pushed or thrown off a roof or out of window

    b.   Body is showing pugilistic attitude

    (Ref: Parikh's Textbook of Medical Jurisprudence, Forensic Medicine and Toxicology, 7/e, Pg. 337; The Essentials of Forensic Medicine & Toxicology, K.S. Narayan Reddy-34/e, pg. 300)

ANSWER

For answer, refer 2014 paper Q. 1 (b), Pg. 485

    c.   Person is 12 years of age

    (Ref: Parikh's Textbook of Medical Jurisprudence, Forensic Medicine and Toxicology, 7/e, Pg. 59)

ANSWER

○ **Findings**
  - **Teeth**
    - **Mixed dentition:** Second molars have erupted
    - Lengthening of the ramus of the lower jaw behind the second molar
  - **Ossification of bones:** As seen on X-ray studies
    - Ossification of pisiform but lateral epicondyle of humerus has not yet united with trochlea and capitulum
    - Heads of metacarpals and phalanges are not fused which generally fuse at 15-16 years
    - Lower ends of radius and ulna are not fused
    - Olecranon not united with ulna

○ **Interpretation**
  - In females, union of epiphysis in cartilaginous bones takes place earlier by 2 years than in males except in case of skull sutures where obliteration sets in little later and proceeds more slowly in female than in males

○ **Medicolegal importance**
  - Criminal responsibility
    - Child under 12 years of age cannot give valid consent to suffer harm which can occur from an act done in good faith and for its benefit e.g. consent for operation
    - Person under 18 years of age cannot give valid consent whether express or implied to suffer any harm which may result from an act not intended to cause any grievous hurt e.g. consent for wrestling
  - Judicial punishment
    - Children (boys below 16 years and girls below 18 years of age), who have committed a crime, are tried by Juvenile court and if convicted, are entrusted to parents for special care or sent to correctional school with facilities for education, vocational training and rehabilitation
  - Employment
    - Child below 14 years of age cannot be employed for any type of work

- Rape
  - Sexual intercourse by a man with a girl under 15 years of age even if she is his own wife, or with any girl under 18 years of age even with her consent is rape
- Kidnapping
  - Kidnapping or abducting a minor, if boy is under 16 and girl is under 18 years

d. Diatoms are present in bone marrow

(Ref: Parikh's Textbook of Medical Jurisprudence, Forensic Medicine and Toxicology, 7/e, Pg. 193; The Essentials of Forensic Medicine & Toxicology, K.S. Narayan Reddy-34/e, pg. 347)

ANSWER

- ○ **Findings**
  - Microscopic unicellular or colonial algae varying in size from 2 microns to 1mm in length or diameter enter pulmonary circulation during drowning
  - Drowning fluid and particles pass from ruptured alveolar wall into lymph channels and pulmonary veins and therefore enter left heart
  - Only a live body with a circulation could transport diatoms from the lungs to the bone marrow
  - Bone marrow of long bones such as femur, tibia and humerus or sternum is examined for diatoms
  - Shape of diatoms can be circular, triangular, oval, rectangular, linear, crescentic or boat-shaped
- ○ **Interpretation**
  - Death was caused due to drowning
  - Diatom test is valid only if
    - Person did not drink this water immediately after submersion
    - Species obtained from specimen are all present in sample from site of drowning
    - Various species are present in same order of dominance for admissible size range and in approximately same proportions
- ○ **Medicolegal importance**
  - Diatom test can be valuable in examination of decomposed bodies since diatoms resist putrefaction
  - Test is negative in dead bodies thrown in water
  - Test is negative in dry drowning
  - Test is negative in undoubted cases of drowning in water full of diatoms
  - Diatoms enter circulatory system from alimentary canal and may reach various organs of body, therefore can be found in other cases apart from drowning

2. **Write short notes on:**

a. Dying declaration

(Ref: Parikh's Textbook of Medical Jurisprudence, Forensic Medicine and Toxicology, 7/e, Pg. 15)

ANSWER

For answer, refer 2016 paper Q. 2 (c), Pg. 470

b. Whiplash injury

(Ref: Parikh's Textbook of Medical Jurisprudence, Forensic Medicine and Toxicology, 7/e, Pg. 302; The Essentials of Forensic Medicine & Toxicology, K.S. Narayan Reddy-34/e, pg. 250)

ANSWER

For answer, refer 2015 paper Q. 6 (a), Pg. 482

c. Privileged communication

(Ref: Parikh's Textbook of Medical Jurisprudence, Forensic Medicine and Toxicology, 7/e, Pg. 29)

ANSWER

For answer, refer 2015 paper Q. 2 (b), Pg. 480

PART II

3. **Classify irritant poisons. Describe clinical features, management, postmortem findings and medicolegal importance in case of chronic mercury poisoning.**

a. Irritant poisons

(Ref: Parikh's Textbook of Medical Jurisprudence, Forensic Medicine and Toxicology, 7/e, Pg. 510)

ANSWER

For answer, refer 2014 paper Q. 3, Pg. 487

b. Chronic Mercury Poisoning

(Ref: The Essentials of Forensic Medicine & Toxicology, K.S. Narayan Reddy-34/e, pg. 504)

ANSWER

For answer, refer 2017 paper Q. 6 (b), Pg. 465

4. **Differentiate between:**

a. Datura and capsicum seeds

(Ref: Parikh's Textbook of Medical Jurisprudence, Forensic Medicine and Toxicology, 7/e, Pg. 570)

ANSWER

Datura and Capsicum Seeds

Dhatura seeds	Chilli seeds/Capsicum seeds
• Large and thick in size	• Small and thin
• Brown or black in color	• Pale yellow in color
• Seeds are Kidney-shaped, finely pitted and reticulated	• Smooth and round seeds
• Odourless in smell	• Smell is Pungent
• Taste Bitter	• Pungent taste
• Double edge convex border	• Single edge convex border
• Embryo curved outward on sectioning	• On sectioning, embryo is curved inward

b Burns and scalds

(Ref: Parikh's Textbook of Medical Jurisprudence, Forensic Medicine and Toxicology, 7/e, Pg. 344)

ANSWER

Burns and Scalds

Burns	Scalds
• Present at and above the site of flame	• Present at and below the site of contact
• Occur as a result of flame, heated solid substance or radiant heat	• Occurs as a steam or any liquid at or near boiling point
• Skin is dry, shrivelled and charred	• Skin is bleached and sodden
• Clothing burnt and may be adherent to the body	• Clothing urinary wet but not burnt
• Vesicles present at circular reference of burnt area	• Mostly over burnt area
• Trickle marks present	• Trickle marks present
• Scar is thick and results in disfigurement	• Scar is thin and causes less disfigurement

c. Antemortem and postmortem contusions

(Ref: Parikh's Textbook of Medical Jurisprudence, Forensic Medicine and Toxicology, 7/e, Pg. 217)

ANSWER

Antemortem and Postmortem Contusions

Antemortem contusion	Postmortem contusion
• Swelling of tissues present	• Swelling of tissues is absent
• Damage to epithelium	• No damage to epithelium

Antemortem contusion	Postmortem contusion
• Extravasation of blood	• No extravasation of blood is present
• Coagulation of blood	• Coagulation of blood is absent
• Infiltration of tissues with blood	• No infiltration of tissues with blood
• Change of color	• No change of color is observed
• Margins are less sharp or indistinct	• Margins are quite sharply defined

PART III

5. Define rape. What will be the findings in a 15-year-old girl alleged to have been raped 12 hours ago?

(Ref: Parikh's Textbook of Medical Jurisprudence, Forensic Medicine and Toxicology, 7/e, Pg. 389; The Essentials of Forensic Medicine & Toxicology, K.S. Narayan Reddy-34/e, pg. 391)

ANSWER

Definition

○ Unlawful sexual intercourse by a man with his wife under the age of 15 years, with any other woman under the age of 18 years, or above, against her will, without her consent, or with her consent when it has been obtained by unlawful means i.e. fraud, putting her in fear of death or hurt, drugging, or impersonation.

○ **Custodial rape:** Rape by persons, such as police officers, jail wardens, hospital staff etc., who abuse their position to commit the offence when the woman is in their custody or care.

○ **Gang rape:** When a woman is raped by one or more in a group of persons acting in furtherance of their common intention, each is deemed to have committed gang rape

For answer, refer 2013 paper, Q. 6 (c), Pg. 498

6. Write short notes on:

a. Concussion

(Ref: Parikh's Textbook of Medical Jurisprudence, Forensic Medicine and Toxicology, 7/e, Pg. 293; The Essentials of Forensic Medicine & Toxicology, K.S. Narayan Reddy-34/e, pg. 238)

ANSWER

Concussion

○ **Definition:** Cerebral concussion or stunning occurs after head injury, characterized by gross physiological disturbance of brain function due to diffuse neuronal injury but with little or no noticeable anatomical changes

- Occurs after traffic accidents and injuries to head sustained in industry
- Severe injury occurs in case of damage to moving head than from blows to skull
- Sudden loss of consciousness and tendency to spontaneous recovery
- Intensified by repeated blows
- Depending on the physical stress on the neurons, the neuronal injury may be wholly or partly reversible or may be fatal in case of complex concussion

Signs and Symptoms

- **On autopsy, in fatal cases**
  - No naked eye lesions can be seen in brain
  - On histological examination, microscopic hemorrhages are seen in tissues
  - Bruises, lacerations and intracranial hemorrhages are found in some cases
- **In less severe cases**
  - Patient regains consciousness after a varying period showing signs of cerebral irritation
  - Patient lies curled up in bed, with face buried beneath clothes
  - Resents all types of interference and exposure to light
  - Pays no regard to surrounding, although not unconscious
  - Becomes violent and abusive if disturbed
  - Symptoms are followed by postconcussional syndrome
    - Dizziness
    - Headache
    - Insomnia
    - Mental irritability
- **Retrograde amnesia occurs after recovery from concussion**
  - Inability to recollect the exact manner of injury
  - Loss of memory extends over a period of a fortnight to a month or more
- **Post-traumatic automatism**
  - Injured person may speak or act in an apparently purposeful manner but has n recollection about it afterwards
  - Associated with amnesia and duration is proportional to the severity of injury

Medicolegal Importance

- Postconcussional syndrome should be distinguished from malingering in cases where symptoms are prolonged especially where compensation is involved

- Retrograde amnesia is significant in the case of litigation, as the prosecution or defense may suggest that this selective loss of memory is just a pretence to escape answering inconvenient questions

b. DNA fingerprinting

(Ref: Parikh's Textbook of Medical Jurisprudence, Forensic Medicine and Toxicology, 7/e, Pg. 478; The Essentials of Forensic Medicine & Toxicology, K.S. Narayan Reddy-34/e, pg. 429)

ANSWER

For answer, refer 2009 paper Q. 6 (a), Pg. 524

c. Impulse

(Ref: Parikh's Textbook of Medical Jurisprudence, Forensic Medicine and Toxicology, 7/e, Pg. 460; The Essentials of Forensic Medicine & Toxicology, K.S. Narayan Reddy-34/e, pg. 449)

ANSWER

Impulse

Definition

- Sudden and irresistible force compelling the person to the conscious performance of acts without motive or forethought
- Sudden and temporary lapse of sanity during which period a person may commit some horrible act without realizing that it is wrong or contrary to law
- Irresistible impulse would be such as none would be able to resist for e.g. impulse to get out of the house when fire breaks
- Providing the patient is able to realize the difference between right and wrong and the nature and consequences of the act, defense plea of irresistible impulse for committing a crime is not acceptable
- Exemption from criminal responsibility is not extended to such persons except in mental disorder

Causes

- Impulses may be due to mental subnormality, dementia, schizophrenia, mania-depressive states, obsessive-compulsive neurosis, epileptic psychosis
- Most crimes are due to impulses such as rage, jealousy that are not resisted–Unresisted impulses

Types of Impulses

- **Kleptomania:** Stealing articles of little value
- **Pyromania:** Setting things on fire
- **Multimania:** Maiming animals
- **Sexual impulses:** Sexual perversions
- Suicidal or homicidal acts

Extra Edge

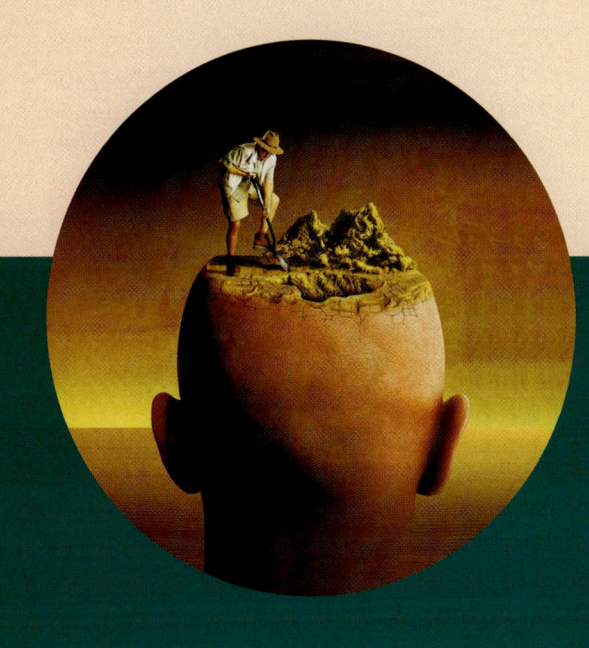

Subject-wise Spotters, Important Tables and Important MCQs with Answer Keys

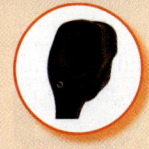 Spotters

 Important Tables

 Important MCQs

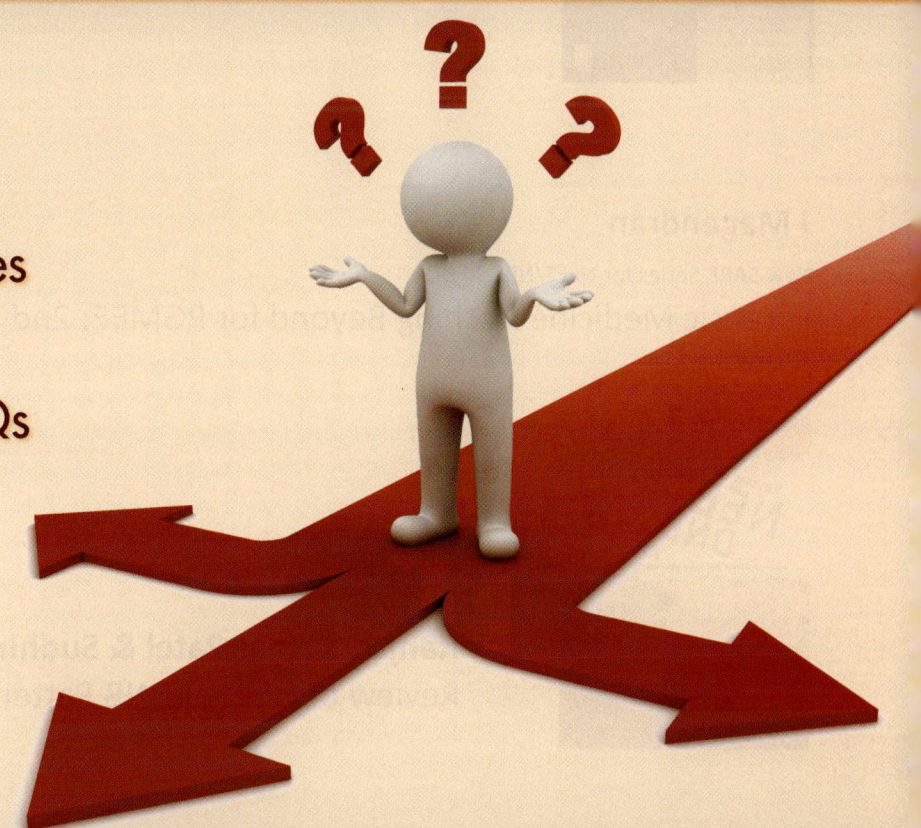

This whole section is the compilation of the important contents from CBS Exam books as follows:

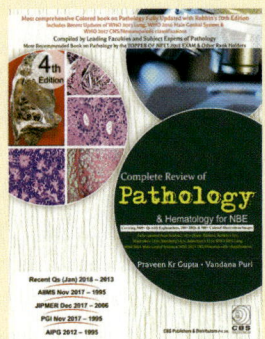

Praveen Kumar Gupta, Vandana Puri
Complete Review of Pathology & Hematology
for NBE; 4th Edition

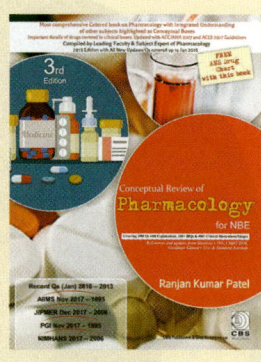

Ranjan Kumar Patel
Conceptual Review of Pharmacology for NBE; 3rd Edition

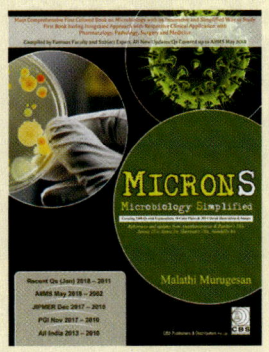

Malathi Murugesan
Microns Microbiology Simplified; 1st Edition

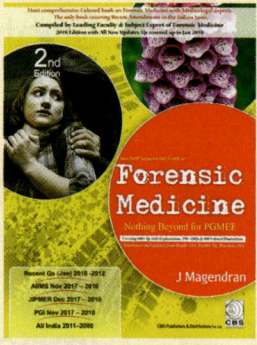

J Magendran
New SARP Series for NEET/NBE/AI
Forensic Medicine Nothing Beyond for PGMEE; 2nd Edition

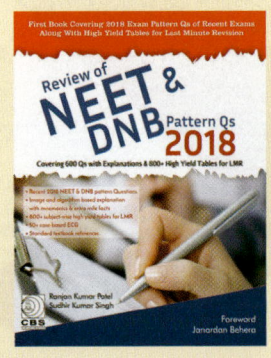

Ranjan Kumar Patel & Sudhir Kumar Singh
Review of NEET & DNB Pattern Qs 2018; 1st Edition

Pathology

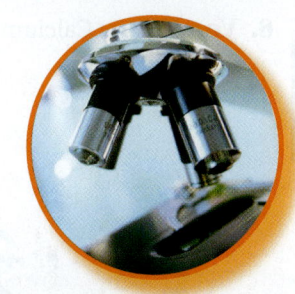

 Spotters

1. **Periodic acid Schiff:** Glycogen and Fungi
   - It is often used to show glomeruli, basement membranes, and glycogen in the liver.

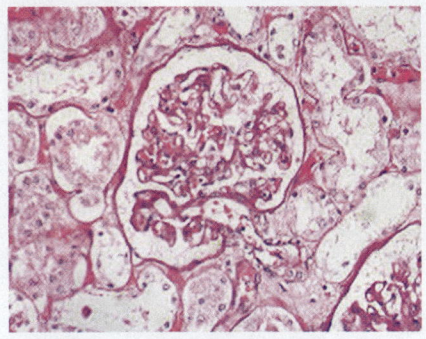

2. **Hematoxylin and Eosin:** Routine tissue sections

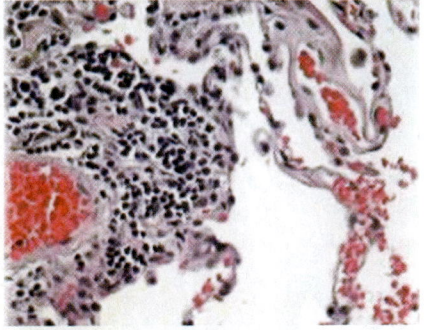

3. **Acid fast stain:** Mycobacterial organisms

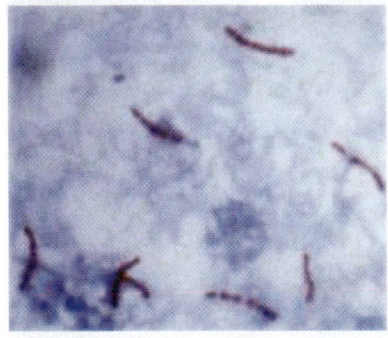

4. **Alcian blue:** Mucins andMuco substances

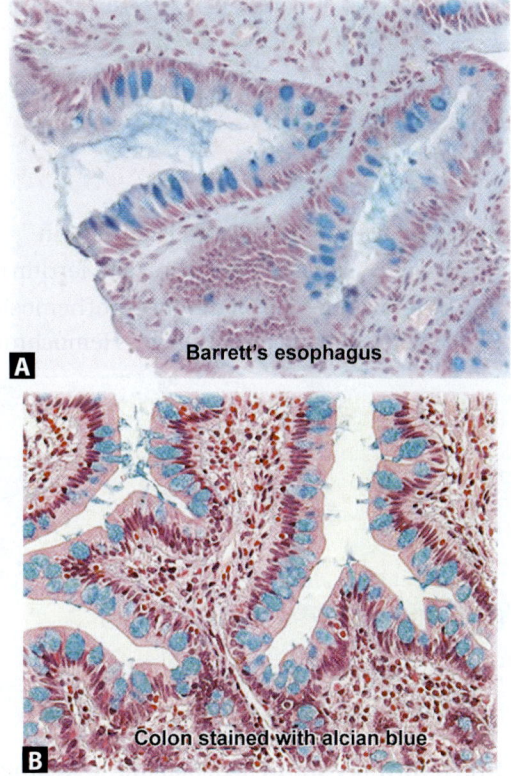

A

Barrett's esophagus

B

Colon stained with alcian blue

5. **Congo red:** Amyloid

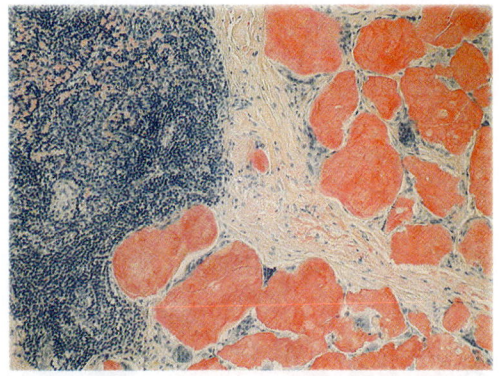

Praveen Kumar Gupta, Vandana Puri, Complete Review of Pathology & Hematology for NBE; 4th Edition

6. Von Kossa: Calcium salts

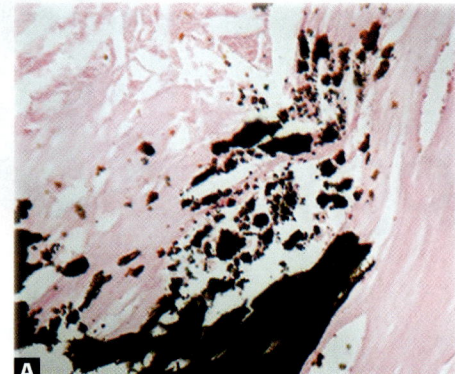

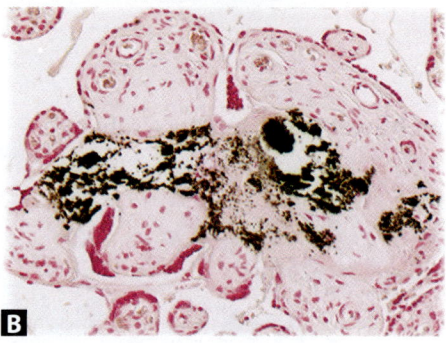

7. Perl's prussian blue stain: Hemisiderin

- Used to stain iron (ferric iron and ferritin).
- Demonstrates the blue granules of hemosiderin in hepatocytes and Kupffer cells.- Hemochromatosis

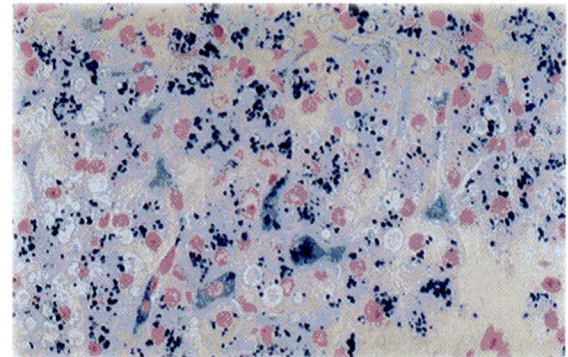

8. Bielschowsky stain: Reticular fibres, Neurofibrillary tangles and Senile plaques

Plaques

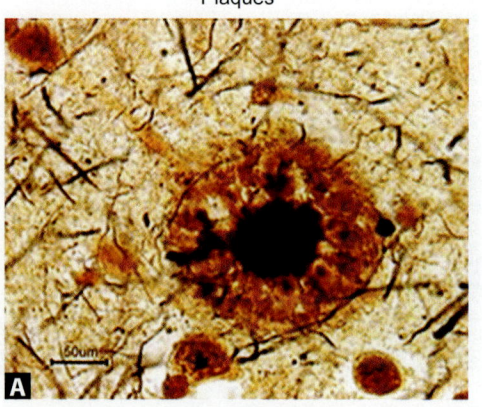

Neurofibrillary tangles

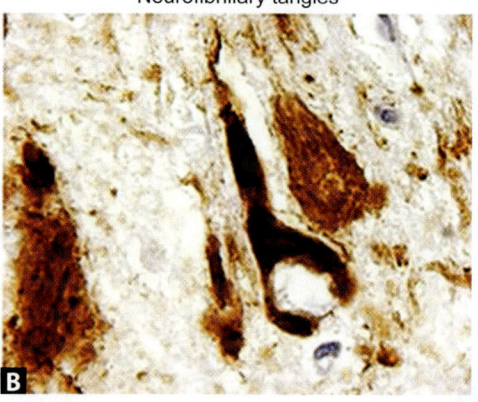

9. India ink stain: Cryptococcus neoformans; mucicarmine can also be used to stain thick polysaccharide capsule red.

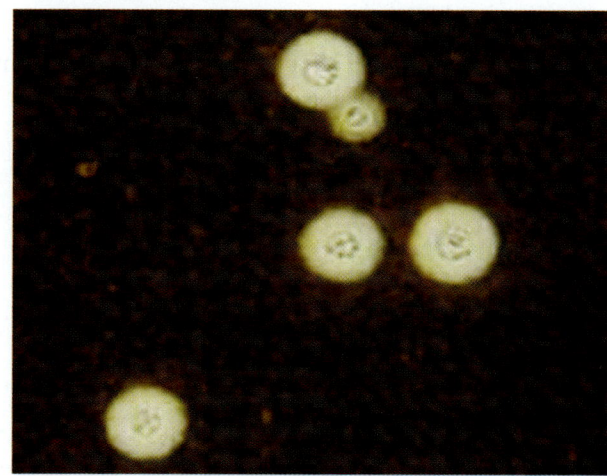

10. Verhoeff Van Gleeson: Elastic fibres

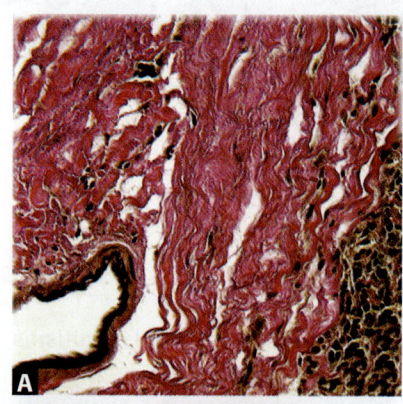

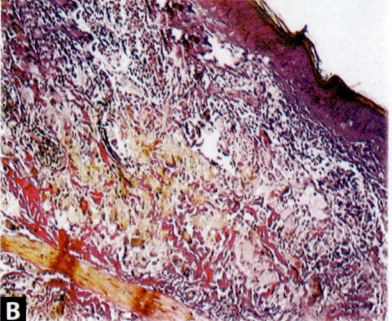

HEMATOLOGY

TYPE: Target Cell

Example:

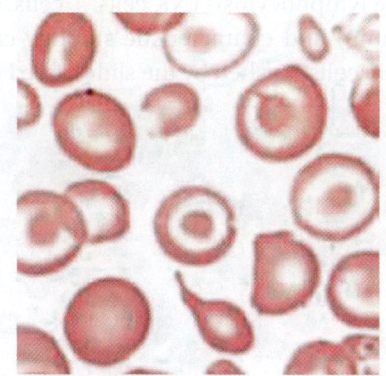

Associated pathology: HbC disease, **A**splenia, **L**iver disease, **T**halassemia.

Notes: "**HALT**," said the hunter to his **target**

Type: Heinz Bodies

Example:

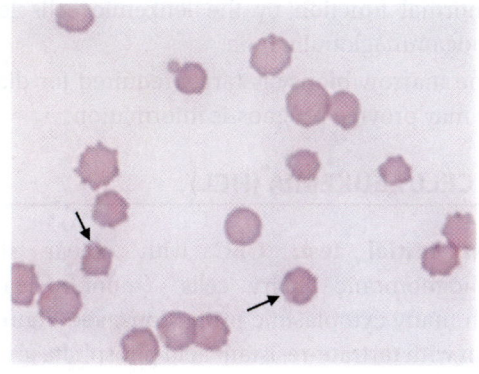

Associated pathology: Seen in G6PD deficiency

NOTES: Oxidation of Hb-SH group to -S—S- → Hb precipitation (Heinz bodies), with subsequent phagocytic damage to RBC membrane → bite cells.

Type: Howell-Jolly Bodies

Example:

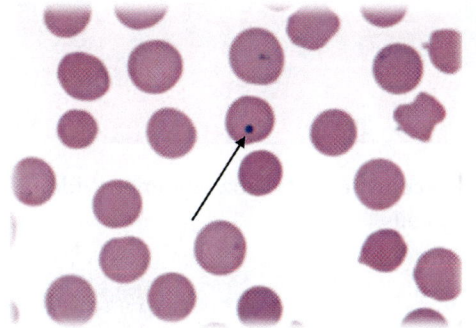

Associated Pathology: Seen in patients with functional hyposplenia or asplenia

Notes: Basophilic nuclear remnants found in RBCs. Howell-Jolly bodies are normally removed from RBCs by splenic macrophages.

SIDEROBLASTIC ANEMIA

○ **Causes:** genetic (e.g. X-linked defect in ALA synthase gene), acquired (myelodysplastic syndromes), and reversible (alcohol is most common; also lead, vitamin B6 deficiency, copper deficiency, isoniazid).

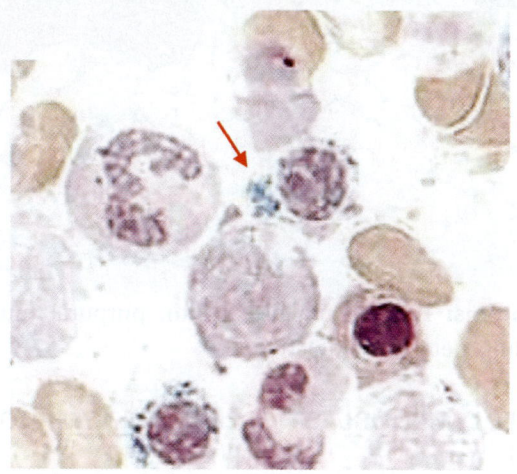

○ **Lab findings:** ↑iron, normal/ ↓TIBC, ↑ferritin. Ringed sideroblasts (with iron-laden, Prussian blue–stained mitochondria) seen in bone marrow. Peripheral blood smear: basophilic stippling of RBCs.

MEGALOBLASTIC ANEMIA

○ Impaired DNA synthesis → maturation of nucleus of precursor cells in bone marrow delayed relative to maturation of cytoplasm.

○ RBC macrocytosis, hypersegmented neutrophils, glossitis.

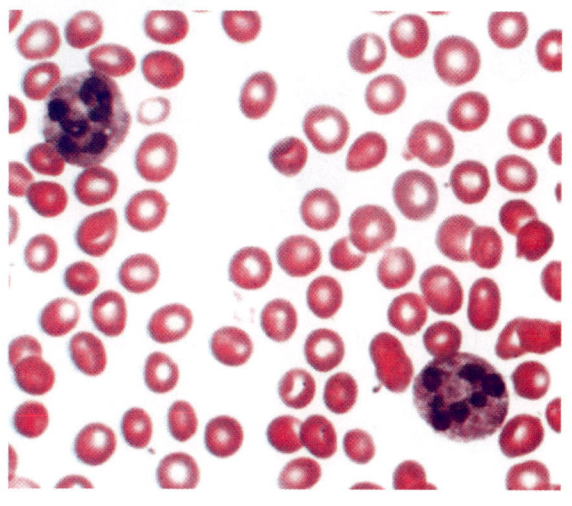

Praveen Kumar Gupta, Vandana Puri, Complete Review of Pathology & Hematology for NBE; 4th Edition

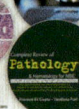

Praveen Kumar Gupta, Vandana Puri, Complete Review of Pathology & Hematology for NBE; 4th Edition

APLASTIC ANEMIA

Findings

○ ↓reticulocyte count, ↑EPO.

○ Pancytopenia characterized by severe anemia, leukopenia, and thrombocytopenia. Normal cell morphology, but hypocellular bone marrow with fatty infiltration (dry bone marrow tap).

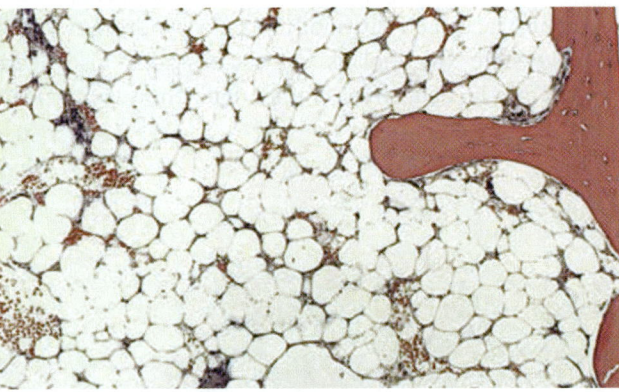

Symptoms: Fatigue, malaise, pallor, purpura, mucosal bleeding, petechiae, infection.

ACUTE LYMPHOBLASTIC LEUKEMIA/LYMPHOMA (ALL)

○ Most frequently occurs in children; less common in adults (worse prognosis). T-cell ALL can present as mediastinal mass (presenting as SVC-like syndrome). Associated with Down syndrome.

○ Peripheral blood and bone marrow have ↑↑↑ lymphoblasts (See figure).

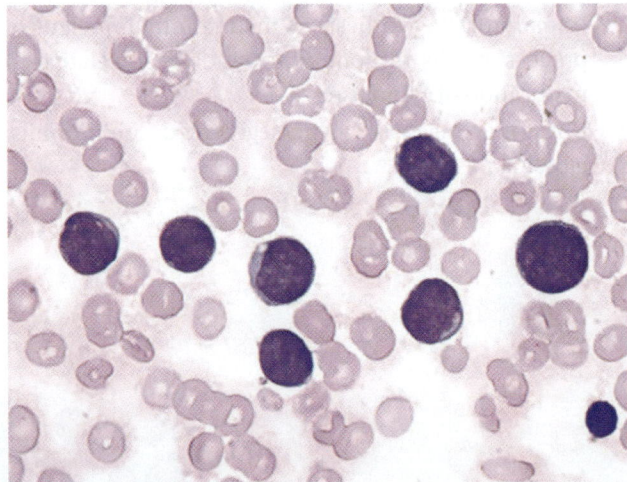

○ TdT+ (marker of pre-T and pre-B cells), CD10+ (marker of pre-B cells).

CHRONIC LYMPHOCYTIC LEUKEMIA/SMALL LYMPHOCYTIC LYMPHOMA (CLL)

○ **Best initial test:** CBC with differential and smear showing lymphocytosis (NK cells, T cells, or B cells > 5000/mm3) and characteristic smudge cells (fragile leukemia cells crushed by the slide). **See Figure.**

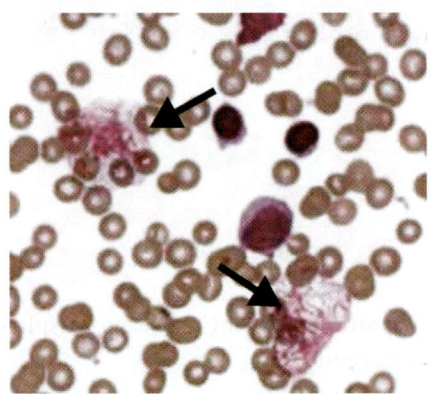

○ **Most accurate test:** Flow cytometry showing the CD5 marker on B cells (normally found on T cells).

○ Granulocytopenia, anemia, and thrombocytopenia are common as leukemic cells infiltrate bone marrow. Abnormal function by the leukemic cells leads to hypogammaglobulinemia.

○ Bone marrow biopsy is rarely required for diagnosis but may provide prognostic information.

HAIRY CELL LEUKEMIA (HCL)

○ **Best initial test:** CBC with smear showing pathognomonic "hairy cells" (mononuclear cells with many cytoplasmic projections, **see Figure**) that stain with tartrate-resistant acid phosphatase (TRAP). Leukopenia can sometimes be seen as well.

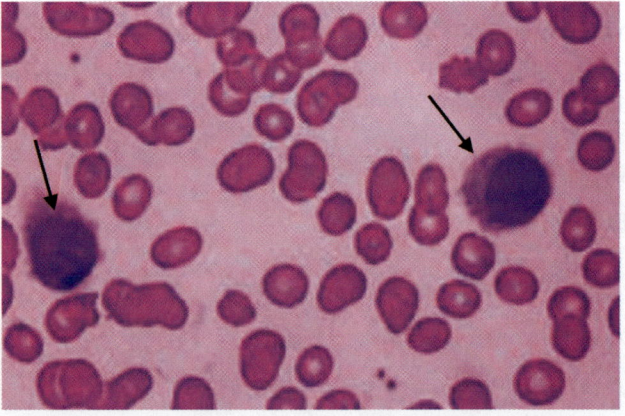

○ **Most accurate test:** Flow cytometry identifying the "hairy cells."

ACUTE MYELOGENOUS LEUKEMIA (AML)

○ Median onset 65 years.

○ Auer rods **(See figure)**; myeloperoxidase ⊕ cytoplasmic inclusions seen mostly in APL (formerly M3 AML); ↑↑↑ circulating myeloblasts on peripheral smear; adults.

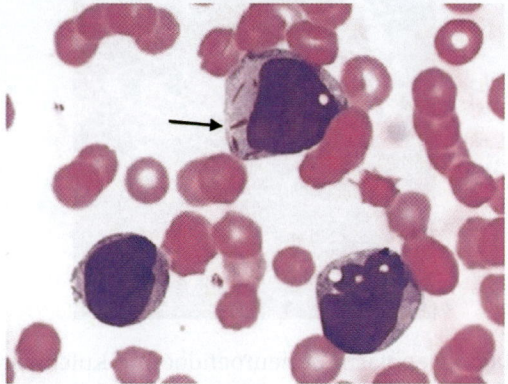

CHRONIC MYELOGENOUS LEUKEMIA (CML)

○ Most accurate test: Philadelphia chromosome via PCR or FISH analysis showing the t(9,22) translocation, although some cases lack the translocation.

○ CBC often shows a **very high WBC count**—often > 100,000/mm3 at diagnosis, sometimes reaching > 500,000/mm3. The differential shows granulocytes in all stages of maturation. Rarely, the WBC count will be so elevated as to cause a **hyperviscosity syndrome.**

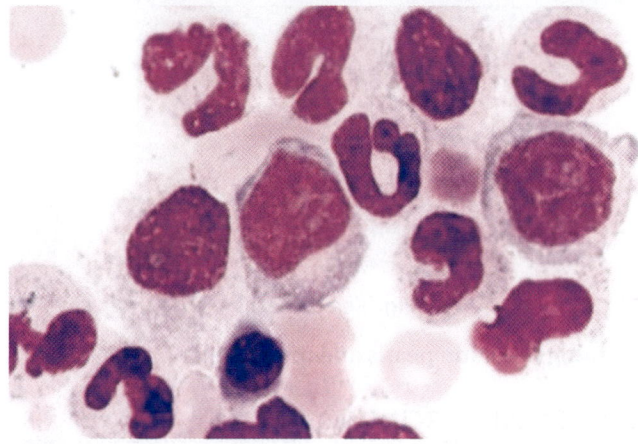

Fig. The figure shows blast cells, promyelocytes, myelocytes, and band forms.

○ CML can be confused clinically with a **leukemoid** reaction (acute in amatory response to infection with ↑ neutrophils and a left shift). In CML and other hematologic malignancies, **LAP is low** while in leukemoid reactions **LAP is high.**

○ LDH, uric acid, and B12 levels are also often elevated in CML

HODGKIN LYMPHOMA (HL)

○ Best initial step is an excisional lymph node biopsy showing the classic Reed-Sternberg cells (giant abnormal B cells with bilobar nuclei and huge, eosinophilic nucleoli, which create an "**owl's-eye**" appearance; see Figure).

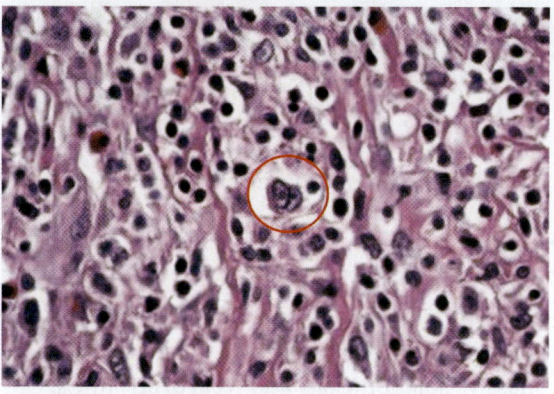

○ Staging is based on the number of nodes, the presence of B symptoms, and whether the disease involves sites on both sides of the diaphragm.

BURKITT LYMPHOMA

○ **Occurs:** In Adolescents or young adults

○ **Genetics:** t(8;14)—translocation of c-myc (8) and heavy-chain Ig (14)

○ High grade, "starry sky" appearance on lesion biopsy; sheets of lymphocytes with interspersed "tingible body" macrophages.

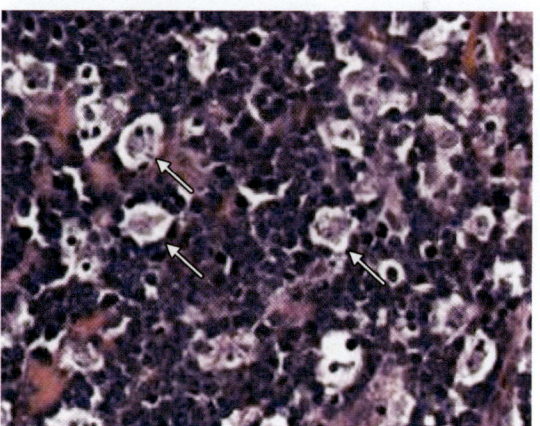

ESSENTIAL THROMBOCYTHEMIA

○ Characterized by massive proliferation of megakaryocytes and platelets. Symptoms include bleeding and thrombosis.

○ Blood smear shows markedly increased number of platelets, which may be large or otherwise abnormally formed (See figure) .

Praveen Kumar Gupta, Vandana Puri, Complete Review of Pathology & Hematology for NBE; 4th Edition

Praveen Kumar Gupta, Vandana Puri, Complete Review of Pathology & Hematology for NBE; 4th Edition

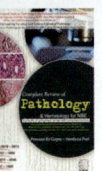

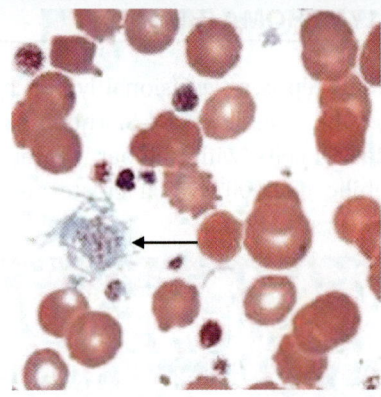

○ Erythromelalgia may occur

MYELOFIBROSIS

○ Obliteration of bone marrow with **fibrosis** due to increases fibroblast activity. Often associated with massive splenomegaly and "**teardrop**" RBCs.

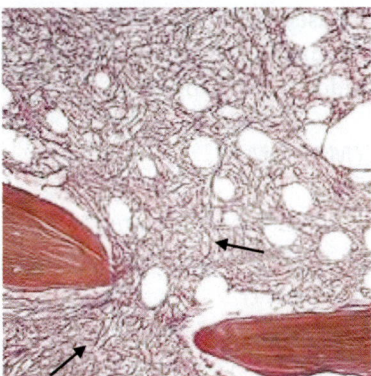

Fibrosis

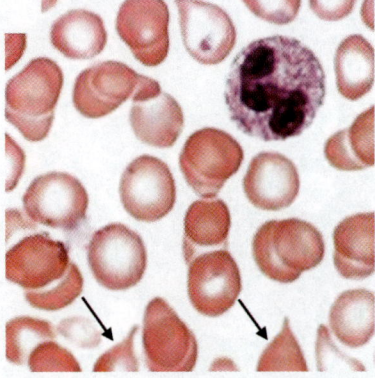

Teardrop

"Bone marrow is crying because it's fibrosed and is a dry tap."

SMALL CELL (OAT CELL) CARCINOMA

Location: Central

Characteristics: Undifferentiated → very aggressive. May produce ACTH (Cushing syndrome), SIADH, or

Antibodies against presynaptic Ca2+ channels (Lambert-Eaton myasthenic syndrome) or neurons (Paraneoplastic myelitis, encephalitis, subacute cerebellar degeneration). Amplification of myc oncogenes common. Managed with chemotherapy +/– radiation.

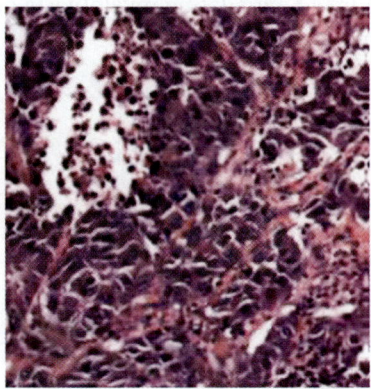

Histology: Neoplasm of neuroendocrine Kulchitsky cells → small dark blue cells. Chromogranin **A** ⊕, neuron-specific enolase ⊕.

SQUAMOUS CELL CARCINOMA

Location: Central

Characteristics: Hilar mass arising from bronchus; Cavitation; Cigarettes; hyperCalcemia (produces PTHrP).

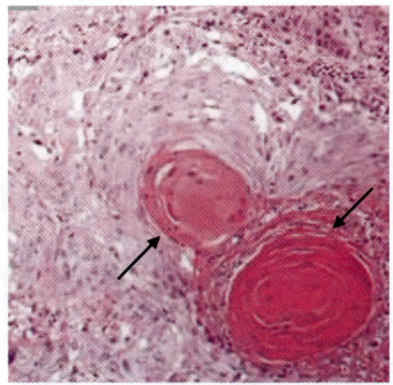

Fig. Keratin pearls

Histology: Keratin pearls and intercellular bridges.

LARGE CELL CARCINOMA

Location: Peripheral

Characteristics: Highly anaplastic undifferentiated tumor; poor prognosis. Less responsive to chemotherapy; removed surgically. Strong association with smoking.

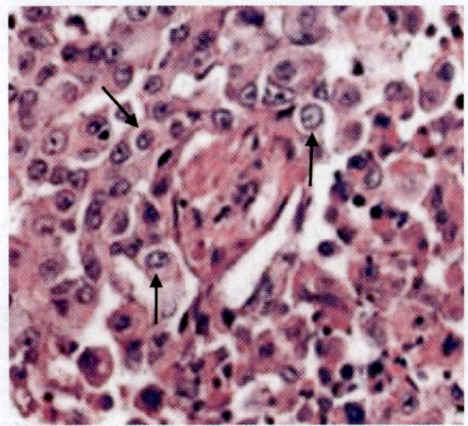

Fig. Pleomorphic giant cells

Histology: Pleomorphic giant cells

ARTERIOLOSCLEROSIS

- Most common.
- Affects small arteries and arterioles.
- **Two types:** Hyaline (thickening of vessel walls inessential hypertension or diabetes mellitus) and hyperplastic ("onion skinning" in severe hypertension with proliferation of smooth muscle cells).

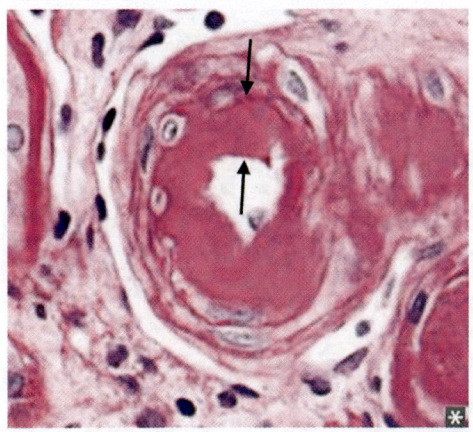

Fig. Hyaline arteriolosclerosis

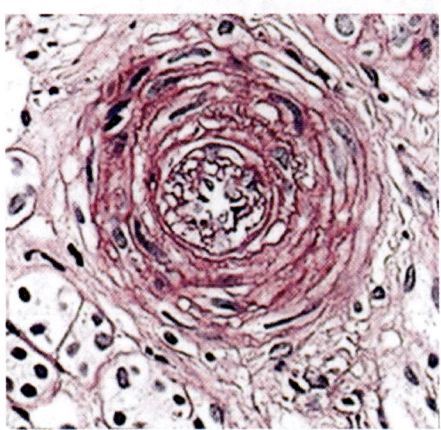

Fig. Onion skinning

ACUTE ENDOCARDITIS

- **It** is typically occurs due to a *high virulence organism* that can colonize a normal valve, such as *Staphylococcus aureus*.

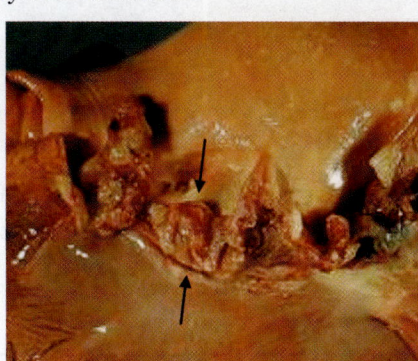

- Acute endocarditis produces large destructive vegetations (fibrin, platelets, bacteria, and neutrophils).
- The prognosis is poor, with mortality of 10–40%.

RHEUMATIC FEVER

- Most commonly heart valves involved: Mitral > Aortic >> Tricuspid (high-pressure valves affected most).

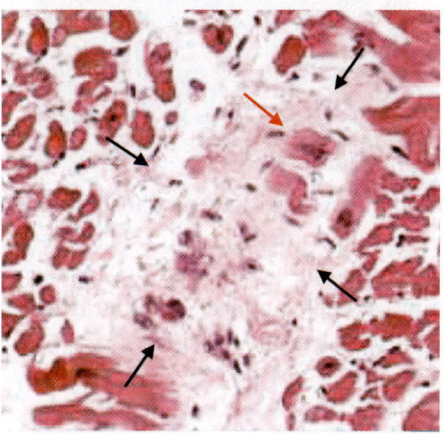

- Early lesion is mitral valve regurgitation; late lesion is mitral stenosis.
- It is Associated with Aschoff bodies (granuloma with giant cells [blue arrows in figure]), Anitschkow cells (enlarged macrophages with ovoid, wavy, rod-like nucleus [red arrow in figure]).

BARRETT ESOPHAGUS

- Specialized intestinal metaplasia (Figure A)—replacement of non-keratinized stratified squamous epithelium with intestinal epithelium (non-ciliated columnar with goblet cells [stained blue in figure B]) in distal esophagus.

Praveen Kumar Gupta, Vandana Puri, Complete Review of Pathology & Hematology for NBE; 4th Edition

545

Praveen Kumar Gupta, Vandana Puri, Complete Review of Pathology & Hematology for NBE; 4th Edition

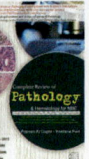
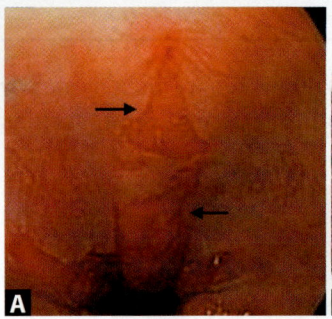
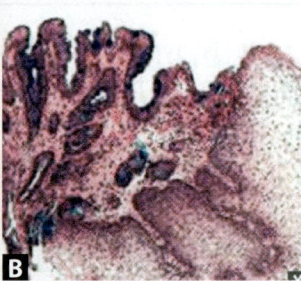

○ Due to chronic gastroesophageal reflux (GERD).

○ Associated with increases risk of esophageal adenocarcinoma.

CELIAC DISEASE

○ Autoimmune-mediated intolerance of gliadin (gluten protein found in wheat) →malabsorption and steatorrhea.

○ Associated with HLA-DQ2, HLA-DQ8.

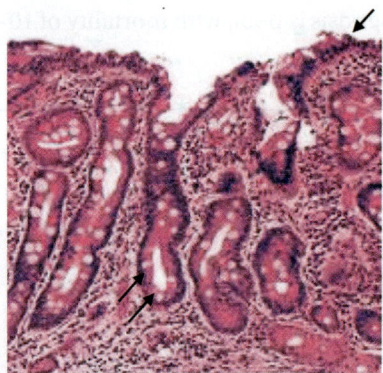

○ **Findings:** IgA anti-tissue transglutaminase (IgA tTG), anti-endomysial, anti deamidated gliadin peptide antibodies; villous atrophy (arrow in A shows blunting), crypt hyperplasia (double arrows in A), and intraepithelial lymphocytosis.

COLONIC POLYPS

○ Growths of tissue within the colon.

○ May be neoplastic or non-neoplastic.

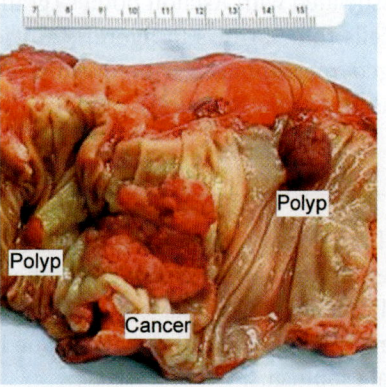

○ Grossly characterized as flat, sessile, or pedunculated (on a stalk) on the basis of protrusion into colonic lumen. Generally classified by histologic type.

ADENOMATOUS POLYPS

○ Neoplastic, via chromosomal instability pathway with mutations in APC and KRAS.

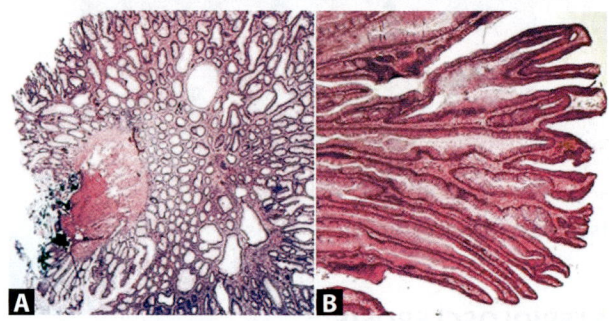

○ Tubular (Fig: A) histology has less malignant potential than villous (Fig B); tubulovillous has intermediate malignant potential.

○ Usually asymptomatic; may present with occult bleeding.

ALCOHOLIC HEPATITIS

○ Requires sustained, long-term consumption.

○ Swollen and necrotic hepatocytes with neutrophilic infiltration.

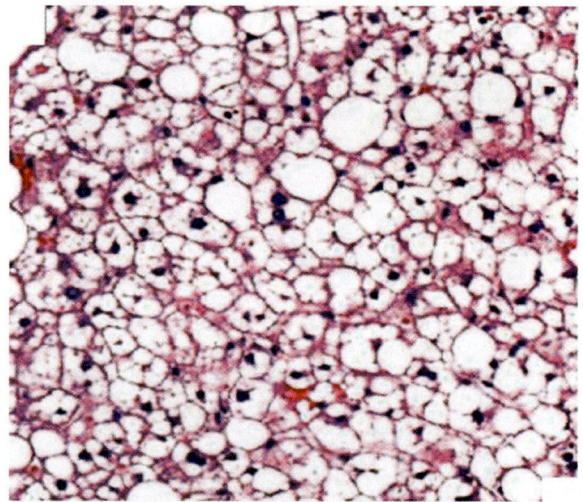

○ Mallory bodies seen (intracytoplasmic eosinophilic inclusions of damaged keratin filaments).

ALCOHOLIC CIRRHOSIS

○ Final and usually irreversible form.

○ Regenerative nodules surrounded by fibrous bands in response to chronic liver injury → portal hypertension and end-stage liver disease.

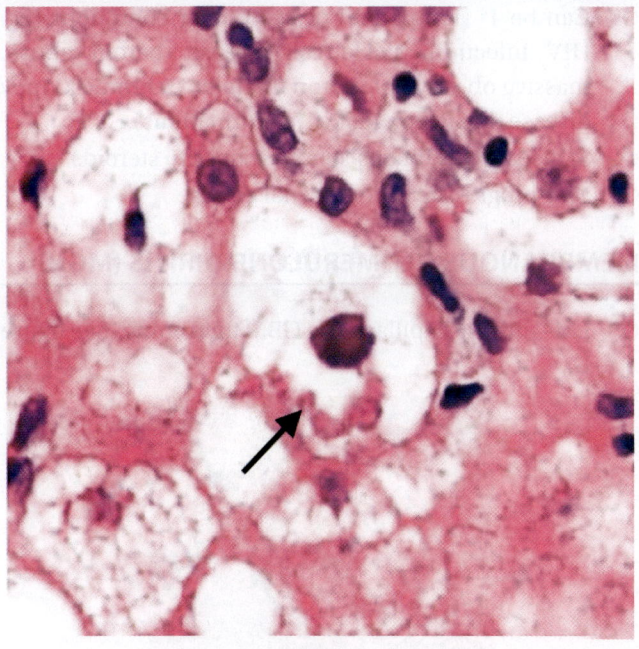

○ Sclerosis around central vein (arrows in figure) may be seen in early disease.

OLIGODENDROGLIOMA

○ Relatively rare, slow growing.
○ Most often in frontal lobes (fig A).
○ "Chicken-wire" capillary pattern.

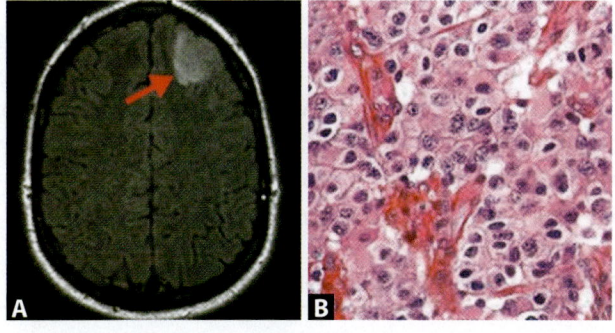

○ Oligodendrocyte origin.
○ "Fried egg" cells— round nuclei with clear cytoplasm (Fig B).
○ Often calcified

MENINGIOMA

○ Common, typically benign 1° brain tumor.
○ Most often occurs near surfaces of brain and in parasagittal region.
○ Extra-axial (external to brain parenchyma) and may have a dural attachment ("tail" Fig: A). Often asymptomatic; may present with seizures or focal neurologic signs.

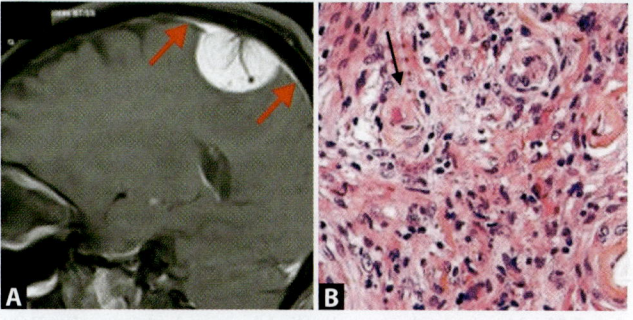

○ Resection and/or radiosurgery. Arachnoid cell origin.
○ Spindle cells concentrically arranged in a whorled pattern; psammoma bodies [Figure B] (laminated calcifications).

Medulloblastoma

○ Most common malignant brain tumor in childhood.
○ Commonly involves cerebellum (Fig: A).
○ Can compress 4th ventricle, causing non-communicating hydrocephalus.

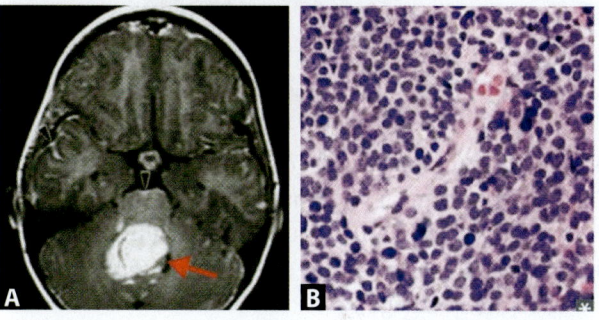

○ Can send "drop metastases" to spinal cord. Form of primitive neuroectodermal tumor (PNET).
○ Homer-Wright rosettes, small blue cells (Fig B).

MEMBRANOPROLIFERATIVE GLOMERULONEPHRITIS (MPGN)

○ Type I—subendothelial immune complex (IC) deposits with granular IF; "tram-track" appearance on PAS stain (See figure A) and HandE stain (See figure B) due to GBM splitting caused by mesangial in growth.

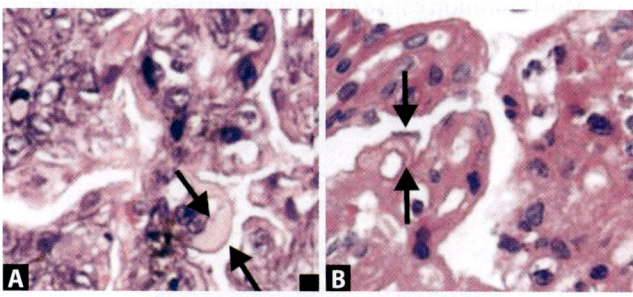

○ Type II—also called dense deposit disease.
○ MPGN is a nephritic syndrome that often copresents with nephrotic syndrome.

Praveen Kumar Gupta, Vandana Puri, Complete Review of Pathology & Hematology for NBE; 4th Edition

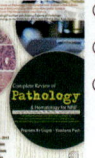

○ Type I may be 2° to hepatitis B or C infection.

○ May also be idiopathic.

○ Type II is associated with C3 nephritic factor (IgG antibody that stabilizes C3 convertase → persistent complement activation → decreases C3 levels).

MINIMAL CHANGE DISEASE (MCD) [LIPOID NEPHROSIS]

○ **LM:** Normal glomeruli (lipid may be seen in PCT cells).

○ **IF:** Θ.

○ **EM:** Effacement of foot processes (See figure C).

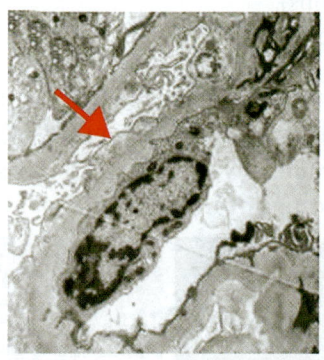

○ Most common cause of nephrotic syndrome in children. Often 1° (idiopathic) and may be triggered by recent infection, immunization, immune stimulus.

○ Rarely, may be 2° to lymphoma (e.g. cytokine-mediated damage).

○ 1° disease has excellent response to corticosteroids.

FOCAL SEGMENTAL GLOMERULOSCLEROSIS (FSGN)

○ **LM**—segmental sclerosis and hyalinosis (See figure D).

○ **IF**—often Θ, but may be ⊕ for nonspecific focal deposits of IgM, C3, C1.

○ **EM**—effacement of foot process similar to minimal change disease.

○ Most common cause of nephrotic syndrome in African Americans and Hispanics.

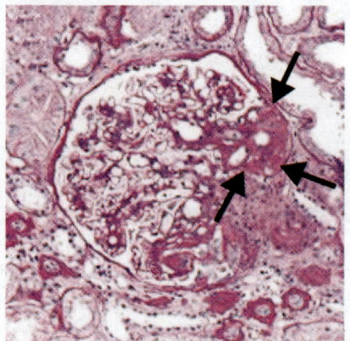

○ Can be 1° (idiopathic) or 2° to other conditions (eg, HIV infection, sickle cell disease, heroin abuse, massive obesity, interferon treatment, chronic kidney disease due to congenital malformations).

○ 1° disease has inconsistent response to steroids.

○ May progress to chronic renal disease

MEMBRANOUS GLOMERULONEPHRITIS (MGN)

○ LM—diffuse capillary and GBM thickening (See figure E).

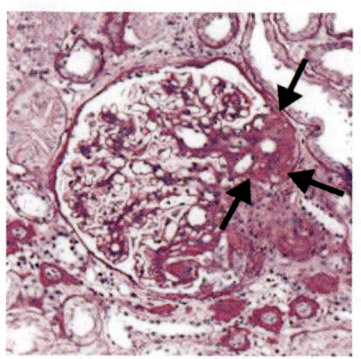

○ IF—granular as a result of immune complex deposition. Nephrotic presentation of SLE.

○ EM—"spike and dome" appearance with subepithelial deposits.

○ Most common cause of 1° nephrotic syndrome in Caucasian adults.

○ Can be 1° (eg, antibodies to phospholipase A2 receptor) or 2° to drugs (eg, NSAIDs, penicillamine, gold), infections (eg, HBV, HCV, and syphilis), SLE, or solid tumors.

○ 1° disease has poor response to steroids.

○ May progress to chronic renal disease.

GRANULOSA CELL TUMOR

○ Most common malignant stromal tumor.

○ Predominantly women in their 50s. Often produces estrogen and/or progesterone and presents with postmenopausal bleeding, sexual precocity (in pre-adolescents), and breast tenderness.

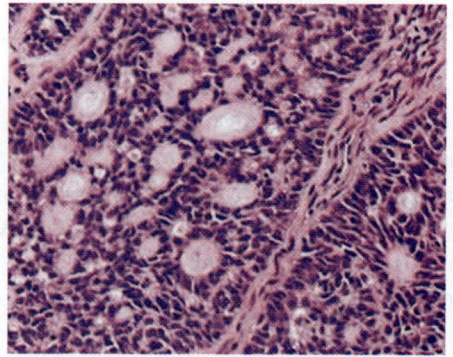

- Histology shows Call-Exner bodies (granulosa cells arranged haphazardly around collections of eosinophilic fluid, resembling primordial follicles).

DYSGERMINOMA

- Most common in adolescents.
- Equivalent to male seminoma but rarer. 1% of all ovarian tumors; 30% of germ cell tumors.

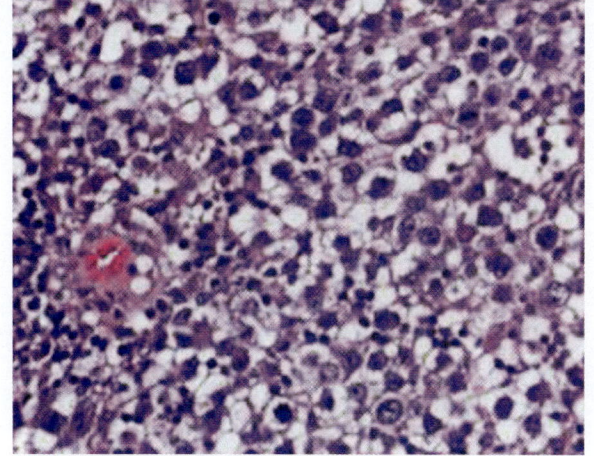

- Sheets of uniform "fried egg" cells.
- hCG, LDH = tumor markers.

YOLK SAC (ENDODERMAL SINUS) TUMOR

- Aggressive, in ovaries or testes and sacrococcygeal area in young children.
- Most common tumor in male infants.
- Yellow, friable (hemorrhagic), solid mass.

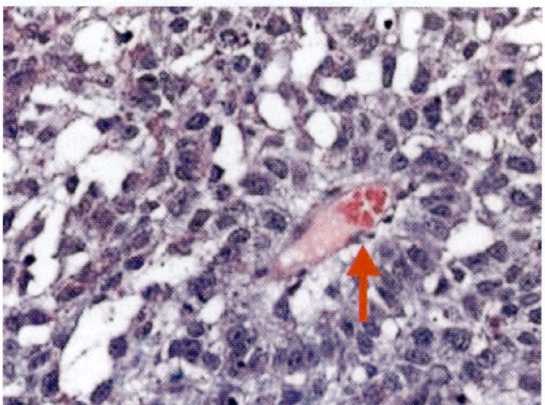

- 50% have Schiller-Duval bodies (resemble glomeruli).
- AFP = tumor marker.

DUCTAL CARCINOMA IN SITU

- Fills ductal lumen (black arrow in figure indicates neoplastic cells in duct; blue arrow shows engorged blood vessel).

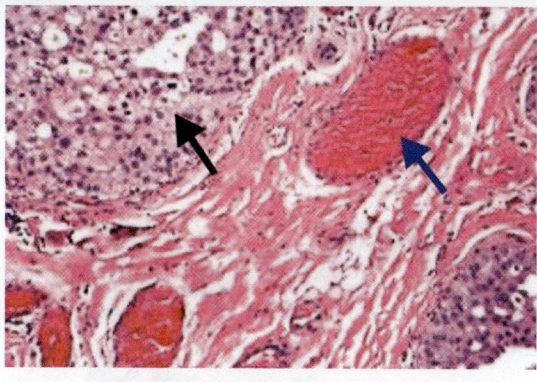
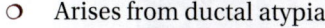

- Arises from ductal atypia.
- Often seen early as microcalcifications on mammography.
- Early malignancy without basement membrane penetration.

INVASIVE DUCTAL CARCINOMA

- Firm, fibrous, "rock-hard" mass with sharp margins and small, glandular, duct-like cells.
- Tumor can deform suspensory ligaments → dimpling of skin.

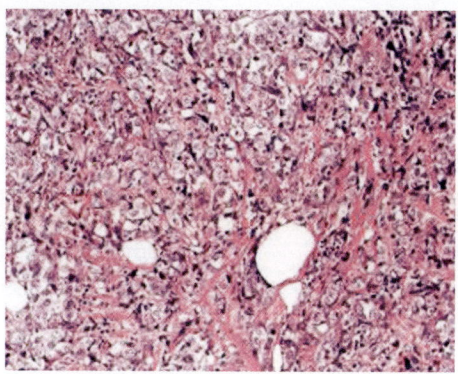

- Classic morphology: "stellate" infiltration.
- Most common (~ 75% of all breast cancers).

INVASIVE LOBULAR CARCINOMA

- Orderly row of cells ("single file" given in figure), due to decreases of E-cadherin expression.

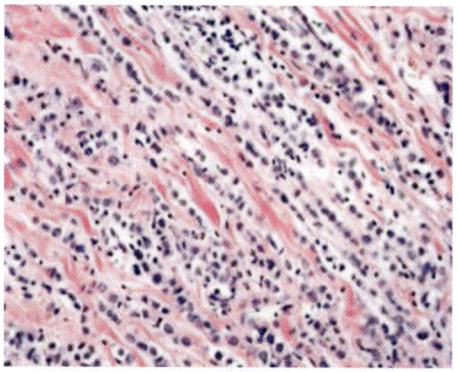

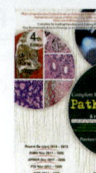

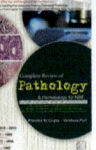

Praveen Kumar Gupta, Vandana Puri, Complete Review of Pathology & Hematology for NBE; 4th Edition

PAPILLARY CARCINOMA

○ Most common, excellent prognosis. Empty-appearing nuclei with central clearing ("Orphan Annie" eyes), psamMoma bodies, nuclear grooves (Papi and Moma adopted Orphan Annie).

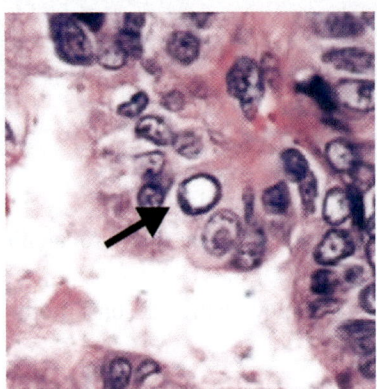

○ Increases risk with RET and BRAF mutations, childhood irradiation.

MEDULLARY CARCINOMA

○ From parafollicular "C cells"; produces calcitonin, sheets of cells in an amyloid stroma (stains with Congo red).

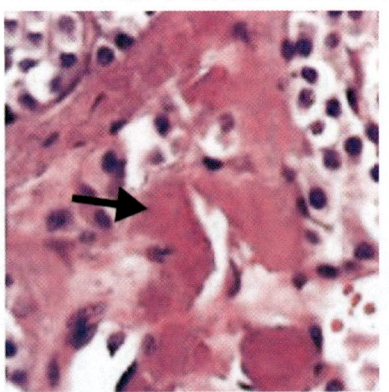

○ Associated with MEN 2A and 2B (RET mutations).

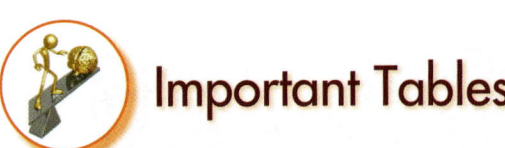

Important Tables

Table 1: Cytokines and cytokine receptors

Cytokine	Receptor	Cell Source	Cell Target	Biologic Activity
IL-1,		Monocytes/macrophages, B cells	All cells	• Explained in detail in text
IL-2		T cells[q]	T cells, B cells	• **T cell activation and proliferation[q],** • **B cell growth[q]**
IL-3		T cells	**Bone marrow progenitors[q]**	• **Hematopoietic progenitor stimulation.[q]**
IL-4		T cells		• **T_H2 differentiation and proliferation.[q]** • B cell Ig **class switching[q]**
IL-5		**T cells, mast cells & eosinophils**	**Eosinophils,[q] basophils[q]**	• **Eosinophil activation.[q]**
IL-6	**Gp130**	**Monocytes/macrophages, B cells**		• **Myeloma cell[q]** growth • **Osteoclast growth and activation.[q]** • T and B cell **differentiation** and **growth[q]**
IL-7		Bone marrow, **thymic epithelial cells[q]**		• Important for **T-cell development[q]**
IL-8	**CXCR1, CXCR2**	Monocytes/macrophages	**Neutrophils**	• **Neutrophil migration[q]** (*neutrophil chemotactic factor*) • **Stimulates angiogenesis.[q]** • **Suppresses hepatic precursor proliferation.[q]**
IL-9		T cells	Bone marrow progenitors	• **Induces mast cell proliferation and function[q]**
IL-10		Monocytes/ macrophages, T cells, B cells		• **Anti-inflammatory molecule[q]**

Cytokine	Receptor	Cell Source	Cell Target	Biologic Activity
IL-11	Gp130	Bone marrow stromal cells	Megakaryocytes,	• **Induces megakaryocyte colony formation**^{Q}
IL-12		Activated macrophages	T cells	• **Induces T_H1 T helper cell formation & lymphokine-activated killer cell formation.**^{Q}
IL-13		T cells (T_H2)		• **Inhibits macrophage proinflammatory cytokine production.**^{Q}
IL-14		T cells	B cells	• Induces B cell proliferation
IL-15		Monocytes/macrophages,	T cells	• T cell activation and proliferation. • **Promotes angiogenesis**^{Q}
IL-16	CD4	Mast cells,CD8+ T cells	CD4+ T cells,	• **Chemoattraction of CD4+ T cells,**^{Q} • **Inhibits HIV replication.**^{Q}
IL-17		CD4+ T cells		• **Neutrophil recruitment**^{Q}
IL-18		Keratinocytes, macrophages		• Upregulated **IFN production**^{Q}
IL-21		CD4 T cells	NK cells	• **Down-regulates NK cell activating molecules, NKG2D/DAP10**^{Q}
IL-23		Macrophages	T cells	• **Opposite effects of IL-12 (IL-17, -IFN)**^{Q}

Courtesy: Praveen Kumar Gupta, Vandana Puri, Complete Review of Pathology & Hematology for NBE; 4th Edition

Table 2: Type of modified macrophages

Modified Macrophages	Location
Adipose tissue macrophages	Adipose tissue
Monocyte	Bone Marrow/Blood
Kupffer cell	Liver
Sinus histiocytes	Lymph node
Alveolar macrophages (dust cell)	Pulmonary alveolus of Lungs
Tissue macrophages (Histiocyte) leading to Giant cells	Connective Tissues
Langerhans cell	Skin and Mucosa
Microglia	Central Nervous System
Hofbauer cell	Placenta
Intraglomerular mesangial cell	Kidney
Osteoclasts	Bone
Epithelioid cells	Granulomas
Red Pulp Macrophage (Sinusoidal lining cells)	Red pulp of Spleen
Peritoneal macrophages	Peritoneal cavity

Courtesy: Praveen Kumar Gupta, Vandana Puri, Complete Review of Pathology & Hematology for NBE; 4th Edition

Table 3: Types of giant cells

Variety	Characteristics
Physiological giant cells	Osteoclasts, syncytiotrophoblasts and megakaryocytes.
Langhan giant cell	Nuclei present in the periphery, in a **horse shoe** pattern. Seen is **tuberculosis.**^{Q}
Foreign body giant cell	• Nuclei are arranged randomly or haphazardly here. • Seen in granuloma formed by **foreign bodies** like sutures (intravenous drug abuse, talc) • Appears **refractile**^{Q} when viewed with polarized light
Touton giant cells	• Seen in **xanthomas, fat necrosis, xanthogranulomatous inflammation, dermatofibroma.**^{Q} • Formed by fusion of epithelioid cells • Contain a ring of nuclei surrounded by foamy cytoplasm.
Warthin-Finkeldey giant cells	Measles.^{Q}
Reed-Sternberg cells	**Hodgkin's lymphoma**^{Q}
Tumor giant cells^Q	Tumors e.g HCC

Courtesy: Praveen Kumar Gupta, Vandana Puri, Complete Review of Pathology & Hematology for NBE; 4th Edition

Table 4: Cancer predisposition syndromes and associated gene

Syndrome	Gene	Chr.	Inherit.	Tumors
Ataxia telangiectasia	*ATM*	11q22	AR	Breast
Bloom syndrome	*BLM*	15q26	AR	Acute Leukemia
Cowden syndrome	PTEN	10q23	AD	Breast, thyroid
Familial adenomatous polyposis	*APC*	5q21	AD	Intestinal adenoma, colorectal

Praveen Kumar Gupta, Vandana Puri, Complete Review of Pathology & Hematology for NBE; 4th Edition

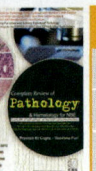

Praveen Kumar Gupta, Vandana Puri, Complete Review of Pathology & Hematology for NBE; 4th Edition

Syndrome	Gene	Chr.	Inherit.	Tumors
Familial melanoma	p16INK4	9p21	AD	Melanoma, pancreatic
Familial Wilms' tumor	WT1	11p13	AD	Kidney (pediatric)
Hereditary breast/ovarian cancer	BRCA1 BRCA2	17q21 13q12	AD	Breast, ovarian, colon, prostate
Her. diffuse gastric Ca	CDH1	16q22	AD	Stomach
Hereditary multiple exostoses	EXT1 EXT2	8q24	AD	Exostoses, chondrosarcoma
Hereditary retinoblastoma	RB1	13q14	AD	Retinoblastoma, osteosarcoma
Hereditary nonpolyposis colon cancer (HNPCC)	MSH2/6	2p16	AD	Colon, endometrial, ovarian, stomach, small bowel, ureter Ca
Hereditary papillary renal carcinoma	MET	7q31	AD	Papillary kidney
Juvenile polyposis	SMAD4	18q21	AD	Gastrointestinal, pancreatic
Li-Fraumeni Synd	TP53	17p13	AD	Sarcoma, breast
Multiple endocrine neoplasia type 1	MEN1	11q13	AD	Parathyroid, endocrine, pancreas, and pituitary
Multiple endocrine neoplasia type 2a	RET	10q11	AD	Medullary thyroid carcinoma, pheochromocytoma
Neurofibromatosis type 1	NF1	17q11	AD	Neurofibroma, neurofibrosarcoma, brain
Neurofibromatosis type 2	NF2	22q12	AD	Vestibular schwannoma, meningioma, spine
NBCCS (Gorlin syndrome)	PTCH	9q22	AD	Basal cell carcinoma, medulloblastoma, jaw cysts
Tuberous sclerosis	TSC	9q34 16p13	AD	Angiofibroma, renal angiomyolipoma
Von Hippel–Lindau	VHL	3p25	AD	Kidney, cerebellum, pheochromocytoma

Courtesy: Praveen Kumar Gupta, Vandana Puri, Complete Review of Pathology & Hematology for NBE; 4th Edition

Table 5: CD markers used for hematolymphoid neoplasms, location/characteristics

Hematological cells	Immunophenotyping Markers (on Flow Cytometry)
Blasts	**CD34,**[Q] tdt (Lymphoblasts), HLADR
RBC's	Glycophorin A
Megakaryocytic marker	**CD41,**[Q] **CD61**
WBC's	**CD 45**[Q] **(Leukocyte Common Antigen)**[Q]
Myeloid cells	**Anti- MPO,**[Q] CD13, CD33, CD14, CD117
B –cells	**CD19,**[Q] CD20, CD22, FMC7, CD23, **CD79 a,** CD79 b, S Ig, IgM
T-cells	**CD3,**[Q] CD2, CD5, CD7, CD8, TCR-α/β, **TCR-γ/δ**
NK cells	**CD16,**[Q] **CD56,**[Q] CD57
Plasma cells	**CD38,**[Q] **CD138,**[Q] kappa and Lambda light chains

Courtesy: Praveen Kumar Gupta, Vandana Puri, Complete Review of Pathology & Hematology for NBE; 4th Edition

CD Marker	Location/ Characteristics
CD1	**CD1a: Cortical thymocytes, dendritic cells (DCs), epidermal Langerhans cells**
	CD1b: Langerhans cells
	CD1c: **Thymocytes, B cells,** mantle zone, and umbilical cord.
	CD1d: Intestinal epithelium, kidney tubular epithelia, hepatocytes, and thymus
CD2	Thymocytes, T cells
CD3	Signaling component of **T cell receptor** (TCR) complex
CD4	A co-receptor for MHC Class II; also a receptor **used by HIV** to enter T cells
CD5	T cells, **thymocytes, and B cells, Seen in CLL,** Mantle cell lymphoma and T-cell lymphoma.
CD7	**Thymocytes,** some T cells
CD8	Co-receptor for **MHC Class I**
CD9	**Pre B cells,** eosinophils, basophils and platelets.
CD10	**Pre-B cells, germinal-center B** cells, ALL, **follicular B- cell lymphomas**
CD11c	Dendritic cells and **hairy cell leukemia** cells.
CD13	Myelomonocytic cells, AML, lymphoma and lymphocytic leukemia
CD14	**Macrophages** which binds to bacterial lipopolysaccharide.
CD16	Fc receptor for IgG on NK cells
CD19	Component of the **B-cell co-receptor**
CD20	Transmembrane protein found on **B cells**
CD21	**CR2,** mature B cells, **Receptor for complement (C3d) and Epstein-Barr virus (EBV).**

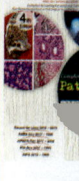

Praveen Kumar Gupta, Vandana Puri, Complete Review of Pathology & Hematology for NBE; 4th Edition

CD Marker	Location/ Characteristics
CD22	Inhibitory receptor for **B cell receptor (BCR) signaling**.
CD23	Mature B cells, monocytes, activated macrophages, Seen in **CLL**
CD24	**B lymphocytes**
CD25	High-affinity receptor for **IL-2; Hairy cell leukemias**
CD28	T-cells, **co-stimulatory effect on the T-cell.**
CD30	Present on **activated T and B cell**; Hodgkin disease, **anaplastic large cell lymphomas**.
CD31	**PECAM-1**, a cell adhesion molecule on platelets and endothelial cells
CD33	Immature **myeloid cells, AML blasts and mature monocytes.**
CD34	**Stem cell marker,** adhesion, found on hematopoietic precursors
CD38	**Plasma,** and B & T activated cells
CD40	Co-stimulatory protein found on APCs induces antibody **isotype switching in B cells.**
CD41	GpIIb/IIIa causes platelet aggregation, mutation causes **Glanzmann thrombasthenia.**
CD42	GpIb/V/IX causes platelet adhesion, deficiency results in **Bernard-Soulier Syndrome**
CD44	Matrix adhesion molecules
CD45	Leucocyte common antigen (LCA)
CD54	Intercellular adhesion molecule -1 **(ICAM-1)**
CD55	Complement decay-accelerating factor **(DAF)**
CD56	**NCAM** (neural cell **a**dhesion molecule) on NK Cells some T-lymphocytes
CD59	Membrane attack complex inhibition factor **(MACIF)**
CD61	Integrin αIIbβ3 (gpIIb/IIIa) on platelets; major role is in platelet aggregation.
CD62E	E-selectin
CD62L	L-selectin

CD Marker	Location/ Characteristics
CD62P	P-selectin
CD64	**Fc-gamma receptor 1 (fcyri)** on macrophages and monocytes.
CD68	Used as immunocytochemical marker for staining of monocytes/macrophages.
CD69	An early **activation marker on T cells and NK cells**.
CD71	**Transferrin receptor**, mediates cellular uptake of iron
CD72	Mediator of B-cell - T-cell interactions
CD 80 (B7-1) CD 86 (B7-2)	When bound to CD28 on T-cells, can provide the **co-stimulatory effect**. Causes up-regulation of a **high affinity IL-2 receptor** allowing T cells to proliferate.
CD91	**Low density lipoprotein (LDL)** receptor-related protein 1 (LRP1)
CD95	**Fas Receptor- receptor for Fas ligand**, an extrinsic apoptotic signal
CD103	**Hairy cell leukemia** (most specific)
CD106	VCAM-1
CD117	**c-kit,** the receptor for Stem Cell Factor, Myeloid marker
CD122	Beta subunit of IL-2 receptor
CD133	Hematopoietic and CNS stem cell marker, Astrocytoma proliferation
CD138	A plasma cell-surface glycoprotein, known as syndecan-1
CD141	**Thrombomodulin**
CD144	VE-Cadherin adhesion molecule on the **vascular endothelium**
CD209	DC-SIGN, C-type lectin receptor found on dendritic cell subsets
CD235a	**Glycophorin,** a protein on blood cells

Courtesy: Praveen Kumar Gupta, Vandana Puri, Complete Review of Pathology & Hematology for NBE; 4th Edition

Table 6: Mrphological differentiation of malaria parasites

	P. falciparum	*P. vivax*	*P. ovale*	*P. malariae*
Infected red cells	Normal size,[a] Maurer's clefts[b]	Enlarged; Schuffner's dots[c]	Enlarged; oval and fimbriated; Schuffner's dots[c]	Normal or microcytic; stippling not usually seen
Ring forms (early trophozoites)	Delicate; frequently 2 or more; accole forms;[d] small chromatin dot	Large, thick; usually single (occasionally 2 in cell; large chromatin dot)	Thick compact rings	Very small, compact rings

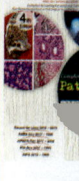

Falciparum Ring forms

Vivax Trophozoite

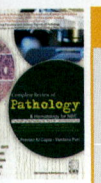

Praveen Kumar Gupta, Vandana Puri, Complete Review of Pathology & Hematology for NBE; 4th Edition

	P. falciparum	P. vivax	P. ovale	P. malariae
Later trophozoites	Compact, vacuolated; sometimes 2 chromatin dots	Amoeboid; central vacuole; light blue cytoplasm	Smaller than P. Vivax, slightly amoeboid	Band across cell; deep blue cytoplasm
Schizonts	18-24 merozoites filling 2/3 of cell	12-24 merozoites, irregularly arranged	8-12 merozoites filling 3/4 of cell	6-12 merozoites in daisy-head around central mass of pigment
Pigment	Dark to black clumped mass	Fine granular; yellow brown	Coarse light brown	Dark, prominent at all stages
Gametocytes	Crescent of sausage-shaped; diffuse chromatin; single nucleus	Spherical compact, almost fills cell; single nucleus	Oval, fills 3/4 of cell; similar to but smaller than P. vivax	Round; fills 1/2 to 2/3 of cell; similar to P. vivax but smaller, with no Schuffner's dots

Falciparum gametocyte

Courtesy: Praveen Kumar Gupta, Vandana Puri, Complete Review of Pathology & Hematology for NBE; 4th Edition

Types/ Patterns	Characteristics	Images
Coagulative necrosis (E.g. Infarction of all solid organs except CNS)	• **Most common type**[Q] • **Architecture** of dead tissues is **preserved** • **Mechanism:** Protein denaturation	Loss of nuclei pink cytoplasm Gross image of kidney showing coagulative necrosis — Microscopic finding showing coagulative necrosis (preserved cell outlines with loss of nuclei)
Liquefactive necrosis	• **Digestion** of the dead cells, resulting in **transformation of tissue into a liquid** viscous mass • Focal bacterial or, occasionally, fungal **infections** are seen; E.g. Necrosis in **CNS**[Q] • **Mechanism:** Enzymatic action.	Gross showing liquefactive necrosis Gross: Brain showing liquefactive necrosis — Liquefactive necrosis in the brain — Mic: Image shows dissolution of tissue
Gangrenous necrosis	• Commonly used term in clinical practice, but **not a specific pattern of cell death**[Q] • **Wet** gangrene (type of Liquefactive necrosis) and **Dry** gangrene (type of Coagulative necrosis)	Well demarcation between normal and abnormal — Intestine Dry gangrene — Wet gangrene

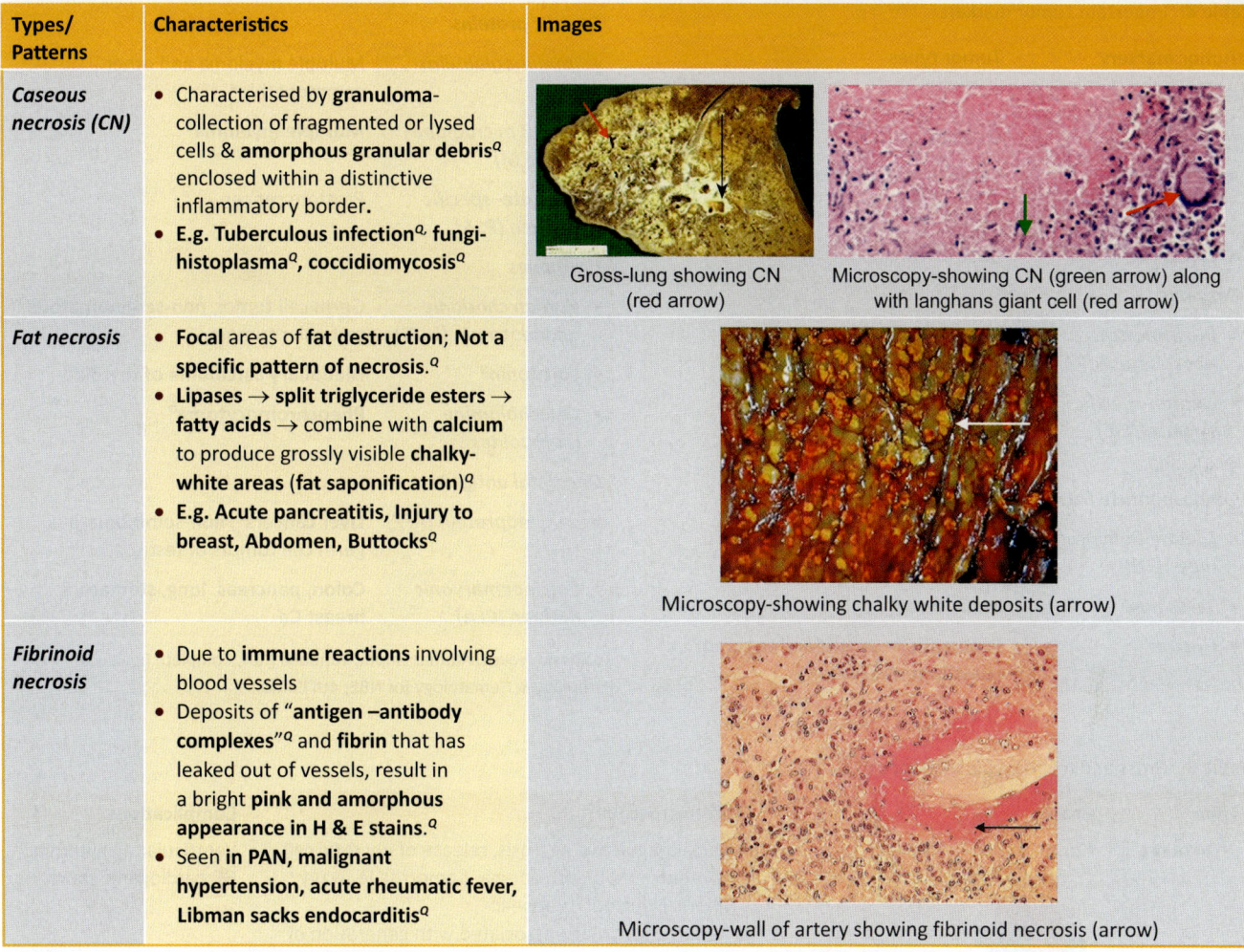

Types/ Patterns	Characteristics	Images
Caseous necrosis (CN)	• Characterised by **granuloma-**collection of fragmented or lysed cells & **amorphous granular debris**[Q] enclosed within a distinctive inflammatory border. • E.g. **Tuberculous infection**[Q], fungi-**histoplasma**[Q], **coccidiomycosis**[Q]	Gross-lung showing CN (red arrow) — Microscopy-showing CN (green arrow) along with langhans giant cell (red arrow)
Fat necrosis	• **Focal** areas of **fat destruction; Not a specific pattern of necrosis.**[Q] • **Lipases** → **split triglyceride esters** → **fatty acids** → combine with **calcium** to produce grossly visible **chalky-white areas (fat saponification)**[Q] • E.g. **Acute pancreatitis, Injury to breast, Abdomen, Buttocks**[Q]	Microscopy-showing chalky white deposits (arrow)
Fibrinoid necrosis	• Due to **immune reactions** involving blood vessels • Deposits of "**antigen –antibody complexes**"[Q] and **fibrin** that has leaked out of vessels, result in a bright **pink and amorphous appearance in H & E stains.**[Q] • Seen **in PAN, malignant hypertension, acute rheumatic fever, Libman sacks endocarditis**[Q]	Microscopy-wall of artery showing fibrinoid necrosis (arrow)

Courtesy: Praveen Kumar Gupta, Vandana Puri, Complete Review of Pathology & Hematology for NBE; 4th Edition

Table 7: Types of renal graft rejection: *(on the basis of the morphology & underlying mechanism)*

Features	Hyperacute rejection	Acute Rejection	Chronic Rejection
Time to occur	**Minutes to hours**[Q]	**Days** (months or even years)[Q]	**Months or even years**[Q]
Mechanism (Type of hypersensitivity)	• **Type 2 HSN:**[Q]due to preformed antibodies • Type 3 HSN	• **Type 4 HSN**-Cellular rejection[Q] • Type 2-mediated by anti-donor antibodies	• **Type 4-HSN** Cellular rejection[Q]
Histology	• **Neutrophillic infiltration**[Q] & thrombotic occlusion of capillaries • **Fibrinoid necrosis** occurs in arterial walls. Showing fibrin thrombi in glomerulus along with ischemic necrosis	In **cell-mediated rejection:** • Tubulo-interstitial pattern **(tubulitis)** • Vascular pattern **(endotheliitis)** In **antibody mediated rejection:** Inflammation of glomeruli & peritubular capillaries with **deposition of C4d**[Q] Showing C$_4$d deposition in peritubular capillaries	**Intimal thickening** with inflammation; Glomerulopathy; **peritubular capillaritis**[Q] **Interstitial fibrosis**[Q] & tubular atrophy

Courtesy: Praveen Kumar Gupta, Vandana Puri, Complete Review of Pathology & Hematology for NBE; 4th Edition

Praveen Kumar Gupta, Vandana Puri, Complete Review of Pathology & Hematology for NBE; 4th Edition

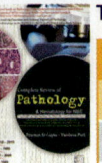

Praveen Kumar Gupta, Vandana Puri, Complete Review of Pathology & Hematology for NBE; 4th Edition

Table 8: Important tumor markers

Tumor markers	Tumor types
Glycoproteins	
• *CA-125*^{Q}	**Ovarian**^{Q} cancer
• *CA-19-9*^{Q}	**Colon** cancer, **pancreatic** cancer
• *CA-15-3*	**Breast**^{Q} cancer
• *CA 72-4*	**Gastric**^{Q} carcinoma
Enzymes	
• *Prostatic acid phosphatase (PAP)*	**Prostate cancer**^{Q}
• *Neuron-specific enolase(NSE)*	**Small-cell** cancer of lung, **Neuroblastoma**^{Q}
• *Alkaline phosphatase (ALP)*	**Osteosarcoma**^{Q}
• *Lactate Dehydrogenase (LDH)*	**Prostate Ca**^{Q}, **testicular tumors, Lymphoma, Ewing's sarcoma**^{Q}
• *Tyrosinase*	**Melanoma**^{Q}
• *Gastrin*	**Pancreatic neuroendocrine tumor (Gastrinoma, ZES)**^{Q}

Specific proteins	
• *Immunoglobulins (Ig)*	Multiple myeloma and other gammopathies
• *Beta 2 microglobulin*^{Q} *(β_2M)*	**Multiple myeloma**^{Q}
• *Prostate- specific antigen (PSA)*	Prostate cancer
Hormones	
• *Human chorionic gonadotropin (HCG)*	Germ cell tumor, **non-seminomatous**^{Q} testicular tumors
• *Calcitonin*^{Q}	**Medullary carcinoma of thyroid**^{Q}
• *Catecholamine metabolites*	**Pheochromocytoma**^{Q}
Oncofetal antigens	
• *α – Fetoprotein (AFP)*	**Liver cancers**^{Q}, **non-seminomatous** germ cell tumors of testis
• *Carcinoembryonic antigen (CEA)*^{Q}	**Colon, pancreas, lung, stomach & breast Ca**

Courtesy: Praveen Kumar Gupta, Vandana Puri, Complete Review of Pathology & Hematology for NBE; 4th Edition

Table 8: Gross and microscopic sequence of changes

Time	Gross	Light microscope	Complications
0–24 hours	None 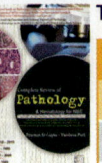 Occluded artery; Infarct; Dark mottling; pale with tetrazolium stain	• Early coagulative necrosis, release of necrotic cell contents into blood; edema, hemorrhage, wavy fibers. Neutrophils appear. • Reperfusion injury, associated with generation of free radicals, leads to hypercontraction of myofibrils through increases free calcium influx.	Ventricular arrhythmia, HF, cardiogenic shock
1–3 days	Hyperemia	• Extensive coagulative necrosis. Tissue surrounding infarct shows acute inflammation with neutrophils.	Post infarction fibrinous pericarditis
3–14 days	Hyperemic border; central yellow-brown softening—maximally yellow and soft by 10 days	• Macrophages, then granulation tissue at margins.	• Free wall rupture → tamponade; papillary muscle rupture → mitral regurgitation; interventricular septal rupture due to macrophage-mediated structural degradation

Time	Gross	Light microscope	Complications
2 weeks to several months	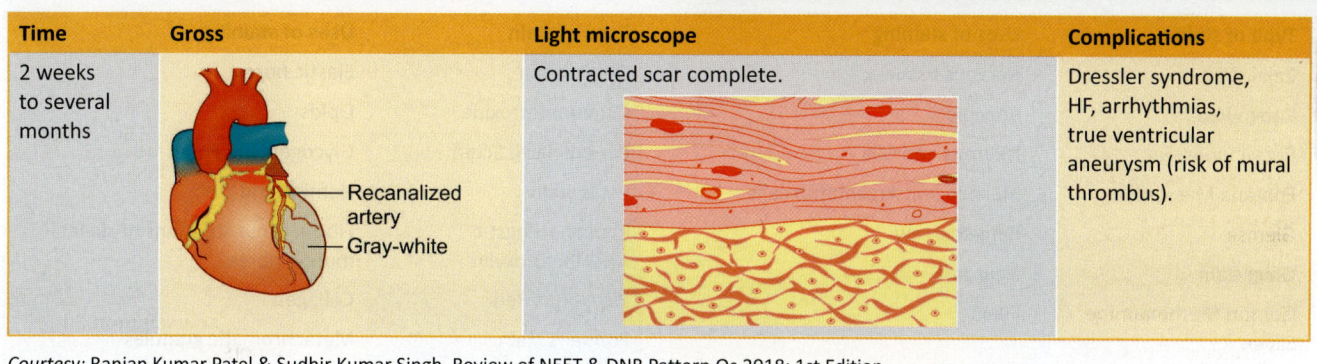 Recanalized artery / Gray-white	Contracted scar complete.	Dressler syndrome, HF, arrhythmias, true ventricular aneurysm (risk of mural thrombus).

Courtesy: Ranjan Kumar Patel & Sudhir Kumar Singh, Review of NEET & DNB Pattern Qs 2018; 1st Edition

Table 9: Pathological bodies

Inclusion bodies	Diseases
Asteroid body	Sarcoidosis and Sporotrichosis
Aschoff bodies	Rheumatic fever
Bodies of Arantius	Aortic valve nodules
Bollinger bodies	Fowl pox
Body of Highmore	Mediastinum testis
Babes Ernst granules	Corynebacterium diphtheria
Brassy body	Dark shrunken blood corpuscles in malaria
Civatte bodies	Lichen planus
Coccoid X bodies	Psittacosis
Citron bodies	Clostridium septicum
Creola bodies	Asthma
Call Exner bodies	Granulose theca cell tumour
Councilman bodies	Hepatitis
Chromatid bodies	Entamoeba histolytica pre-cyst
Donovan bodies	Granuloma inguinale
Ferruginous body	Asbestosis
Gamma gandy bodies	Congestive splenomegaly
Guarnieri bodies	Vaccinia
Henderson Peterson bodies	Molluscum contagiosum
Heinz bodies	G6PD deficiency
Hirano bodies	Alzheimer's disease
Keratin pearls	Squamous cell carcinoma
Lafora body	Myoclonic epilepsy
Leishman Donovan bodies	Kala – azar
Levinthal Coles, Lile bodies	Psittacosis
Lewis bodies	Parkinsonism
Mallory bodies	Primary biliary cirrhosis, Alcoholic hepatitis, Wilson's disease, Chronic cholestasis, Hepatocellular carcinoma
Michaelis Gutmann body	Malacoplakia

Inclusion bodies	Diseases
Miyagawa's corpuscles	Buboes from LGV
Mooser bodies	Endemic typhus
Moot bodies	Multiple myeloma
Owl – eye inclusions	CMV and herpes
Pick body	Pick's disease
Psammoma bodies	Papillary carcinoma of thyroid, serous cystadenoma of ovary, meningioma, mesothelioma
Reilly bodies	Hurler's syndrome
Rokitansky bodies	Teratoma
Ross's bodies	Syphilis
Rushton bodies	Odontogenic cyst
Russell bodies	Multiple myeloma
Sandstorm bodies	Parathyroid glands
Schaumann bodies	Sarcoidosis
Schiller Duval bodies	Yolk sac tumour
Sclerotic bodies	Chromoblastomycosis
Torres body	Yellow fever
Verocay bodies	Schwannoma
Warthin – Finkeldey giant cells	Measles
Winkler bodies	Syphilis
Zebra bodies	Metachromatic leukodystrophy

Courtesy: Ranjan Kumar Patel & Sudhir Kumar Singh, Review of NEET & DNB Pattern Qs 2018; 1st Edition

Table 10: Stains

Type of stain	Uses of staining
Acid Fast stain	Mycobacterial organisms
Alcian Blue	Mucins and Muco substances
Aldehyde Fuchsin	Pancreatic Islet Beta Cell granules
Alizarin Red S	Calcium
Bielschowsky stain	Reticular fibres, Neurofibrillary tangles and Senile plaques

557

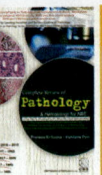

Praveen Kumar Gupta, Vandana Puri, Complete Review of Pathology & Hematology for NBE; 4th Edition

Type of stain	Uses of staining
Cajal stain	Nervous tissue
Congo Red	Amyloid
Cresyl Violet	Neurons and Glia
Fontana Masson's	Melanin and Argentaffin cells
Giemsa	Bone marrow
Golgi stain	Neurons
Gomori Methenamine Silver	Fungi
Gram Stain (Taylor's)	Bacteria
Hematoxylin and Eosin	Routine tissue sections
Luna stain	Elastin and Mast cells
Luxol Fast Blue	Myelin
Masson's Trichrome	Connective tissue and Collagen
Mucicarmine	Epithelial Mucin
Oil Red O	Lipid

Type of stain	Uses of staining
Orcein stain	Elastic fibres
Osmium tetroxide	Lipids
Periodic Acid Schiff	Glycogen and Fungi
Perl's stain	Hemisiderin
Phosphotungstic AcidHematoxylin	Fibrin, Cross striations of skeletal muscle fibres
Picrosirius Red	Collagen
Ponder's stain	Metachromatic granules
Reticulum Silver	Reticulum fibres
Safranin O	Mucin, Cartilage, Mast cells
Toluidine Blue	Mast cell granules
Verhoeff Vangleson	Elastic fibres
Von Kossa	Calcium salts

Courtesy: Ranjan Kumar Patel & Sudhir Kumar Singh, Review of NEET & DNB Pattern Qs 2018; 1st Edition

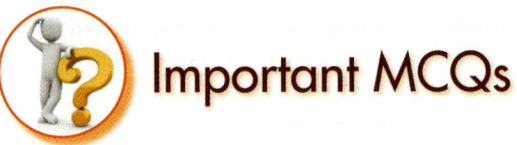 Important MCQs

1. **True about Metaplasia is?**
   a. Involves only epithelial cells
   b. Is irreversible
   c. Occurs at stem cells level
   d. Columnar is the most common type

2. **Antiapoptotic gene?**
   a. FLIP
   b. P53
   c. BAX
   d. BIM

3. **The RBCs with schizonts of P. Falciparum are not visible on peripheral blood smear due to which of the following reason?**
   a. Capillary adherence or sequestration of parasitized RBCs
   b. ADCC mediated RBC destruction
   c. Selective hemolysis of affected RBCs in spleen
   d. Cellular lysis due to hemozoin produced by the parasites Erythrocyte Changes in Malaria

4. **Primary granule of neutrophil has?**
   a. Proteinase 3
   b. Alkaline phosphatse
   c. Acid protease
   d. Lactoferrin

5. **Granulation tissue appear at the site of injury by**
   a. <24 hours
   b. 24–72 hours
   c. 48–96 hours
   d. 5–7 days

6. **Septic Shock is due to:**
   a. Vasodilatation
   b. Decreased Cardiac output
   c. Endothelial damage
   d. All of the above

7. **Nutmeg liver seen in**
   a. Alcoholic liver disease
   b. Chronic venous congestion
   c. Hepatoma
   d. Secondary carcinoma deposits in liver

8. **PRSS1 gene is on ?**
   a. Chr20q
   b. Chr 17p
   c. Chr 7q
   d. Chr1p

9. **BRCA1 is the most common gene mutated in familial breast cancer. This gene is located on which chromosome?**
   a. 13
   b. 17
   c. 20
   d. 21

10. **In Downs syndrome there is?**
    a. Translocation
    b. Mutations
    c. Paternal nondisjunction
    d. Maternal nondisjunction

11. **Rh incompatibility is an example of**
    a. Immune complex reaction
    b. Ag Ab reaction
    c. Delayed hypersensitivity
    d. Immediate type

12. **Type V hypersensitivity reaction is a subtype of:**
    a. Type I
    b. Type II
    b. Type III
    d. Type IV

Praveen Kumar Gupta, Vandana Puri, Complete Review of Pathology & Hematology for NBE; 4th Edition

13. Combined B & T cell immunodeficiency is/are seen in?

a. Severe Combined Immunodeficiency
b. Adenosine deaminase deficiency
c. Wiskott-Aldrich syndrome
d. Ataxia telangiectasia
e. DiGeorge syndrome

14. Lack of differentiation is called?

a. Anaplasia
b. Metaplasia
c. Dysplasia
d. Carcinoma

15. Most common gene involved in endometrial ca is?

a. PTEN
b. BRAF mutation
c. KRAS
d. Mismatch repair genes

16. The tumor suppressor gene p 53 induces cell cycle arrest at:

a. G2- M phase
b. S - G2phase
c. G1 - S phase
d. Go-phase

17. Most common malignancy in children?

a. Leukemia
b. Brain tumors
c. Neuroblastoma
d. Retinoblastoma

18. Translocation t(8;14) of c-MYC gene is seen in

a. Follicular lymphoma
b. Burkitt lymphoma
c. Mantle cell lymphoma
d. Diffuse large B cell lymphoma

19. Most common malignancy of blood is?

a. ALL
b. CL L
c. AML
d. CML

20. Marker of T -lymphocyte is?

a. CD8
b. CD20
c. CD19
d. CD45

21. Screening test for thalassemia

a. Alkali denaturation test
b. Kleihauer test
c. Hb electrophoresis
d. NESTROFT

22. Direct coomb's test detects-

a. Antigen in serum
b. Antibodies in RBC surface
c. Antigen in RBC surface
d. Antibodies in serum

23. Pancytopenia with hypocellular bone marrow seen in

a. Fanconi's anemia
b. Paroxysmal nocturnal hemoglobinuria
c. Hairy cell leukemia
d. Myelopthisis

24. The coronary artery most commonly involved in ath-erosclerosis

a. Left anterior descending artery
b. Left main coronary artery
c. Right coronary artery
d. Circumflex coronary artery

25. Characteristic histological finding in benign hypertension

a. Proliferative end arteritis
b. Necrotizing arteriolitis
c. Hyaline arteriosclerosis
d. Cystic medial necrosis

26. Onion skin thickening of arteriolar wall is seen in:

a. Atherosclerosis
b. Median calcific sclerosis
c. Hyaline arteriosclerosis
d. Hyperplastic arteriosclerosis

27. Commonest cause of right ventricular failure is:

a. Cor pulmonale
b. Pulmonary involvement
c. Endomyocardial fibrosi
d. Left ventricular failure

28. Which type of endocarditis has vegetation on both sides of the valves:

a. Infective endocarditis
b. Libman Sack'endocarditis
c. RF
d. None

29. ARDS is due to defect in?

a. Type 1 pneumocytes
b. Type 2 pneumocytes
c. Endothelial cells
d. Clara cells

30. Infraclavicular lesion of tuberculosis is known as:

a. Ghon's focus
b. Puhl's focus
c. Assmans focus
d. Simmon's focus

31. Most common cause for lung abscess?

a. Staph aureus
b. Staph pyrogen
c. Bacteroids
d. Klebsiella

32. Achalasia cardia:

a. Absence of nerves
b. Absence of muscles
c. Hypertrophy of nerves
d. None

33. MC site for stomach Ca:

a. Lesser curvature
b. Antrum
c. Greater curvature
d. Pylorus

34. Pipe stem appearance in barium enema is seen:

a. Crohns disease
b. Ulcerative colitis
c. Schistosomiasis
d. Carcinoma colon

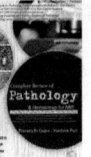

35. Most common hepatotoxin causing acute liver injury
a. Acetaminophen
b. Alcohol
c. Paracetamol
d. Halothane

36. Calciviridae is?
a. Hepatitis A
b. Hepatitis E
c. Hepatitis C
d. Hepatitis D

37. Hallmark of chronic hepatitis
a. Interface hepatitis
b. Ballooning degeneration of hepatocytes
c. Cholestasis
d. Periportal fibrosis and bridging fibrosis

38. Which one of the following tests is best for measuring glomerular function?
a. Blood urea
b. Serum creatinine
c. Creatinine clearance rate
d. Ultrasound of kidney

39. Mesangial deposits of Lambda light chain is seen in
a. Amyloidosis
b. FSGS
c. MPGN
d. Membranous nephropathy

40. Most common cause of nephrotic syndrome in children-
a. Membranous GN
b. Minimal change disease
c. PSGN
d. RPGN

41. Schiller- Duval bodies is seen in:
a. Choriocarcinoma
b. Embryonal cell Ca
c. Endodermal sinus tumour
d. Immature teratoma

42. Gleason's grading system is for -
a. Carcinoma testis
b. Carcinoma colon
c. Carcinoma thyroid
d. Carcinoma prostate

43. Molecular classification of breast cancer is based on?
a. Gene profiling
b. ER, PR, and HER-2 neu
c. Histology
d. Mutations

44. In hashimoto's disease serum antibodies are mainly against
a. Thyroid follicles
b. Thyroxine
c. Thyroglobulins
d. Iodine

45. Whipple's triad is diagnostic of:
a. Gastrinoma
b. Insulinoma
c. Somatostatinoma
d. Glucogonoma

46. Mechanisms responsible for chronic complications of Diabetes include all of the following except:
a. Non-enzymatic Glycosylation
b. Protein Kinase C activation
c. Disturbances in Polyol Pathways
d. Chronic Inflammation

47. The "Lepra cells" are:
a. histologically
b. Histiocytes
c. Lymphocytes
d. Neutrophils Plasma cells

48. Phagocytosis in brain is caused by:
a. Astrocytes
b. Microglia
c. Oligodendrocytes
d. Ependymal cells

49. Characteristic pathological feature of Parkinson's disease is presence of:
a. Lewy bodies
b. Babes nodule
c. Ncuro fibrillary tangle
d. Negri-bodies

50. The appearance of cobweb formation in CSF indicates
a. Pyogenic meningitis
b. Viral meningitis
c. Tuberculous meningitis
d. Fungal meningitis

51. CD 30 is/are marker for:
a. Anaplastic large cell lymphoma
b. Embryonal cell carcinoma
c. Squamous Cell Carcinoma
d. Seminoma
e. Hodgkin's lymphoma

52. Hodgkin lymphoma type that more commonly presents as fever of unknown origin
a. Nodular sclerosis
b. Mixed cellularity
c. Lymphocyte predominance
d. Lymphocyte depletion

53. Sea blue histiocytes are seen in
a. Chronic lymphoblastic leukemia
b. Chronic myeloid leukemia
c. Langerhan cell histiocytosis
d. Burkitt lymphoma

54. "Smudge cells" in the peripheral smear are characteristic of
a. Chronic myelogenous leukemia
b. Chronic lymphocytic leukemia
c. Acute myelogenous leukemia
d. Acute lymphoblastic leukemia

55. Following are the findings in sickle cell Anemia, except:
a. Fish mouth vertebra
b. Enlarged heart
c. Splenomegaly
d. Leukocytosis
e. Serum electrophoresis is done

560

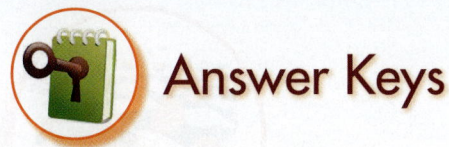

Answer Keys

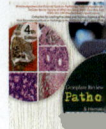

1.	c	**2.**	a	**3.**	a	**4.**	c	**5.**	b	**6.**	d	**7.**	b	**8.**	c	**9.**	b	**10.**	d
11.	b	**12.**	b	**13.**	a, b, c, d	**14.**	a	**15.**	a	**16.**	c	**17.**	a	**18.**	b	**19.**	a	**20.**	a
21.	d	**22.**	b	**23.**	a	**24.**	a	**25.**	c	**26.**	d	**27.**	a	**28.**	b	**29.**	a	**30.**	c
31.	a	**32.**	a	**33.**	b	**34.**	b	**35.**	a	**36.**	b	**37.**	d	**38.**	c	**39.**	a	**40.**	b
41.	c	**42.**	d	**43.**	a	**44.**	a	**45.**	b	**46.**	d	**47.**	b	**48.**	b	**49.**	a	**50.**	c
51.	a,b,e	**52.**	b	**53.**	b	**54.**	b	**55.**	None										

Praveen Kumar Gupta, Vandana Puri, Complete Review of Pathology & Hematology for NBE; 4th Edition

Pharmacology

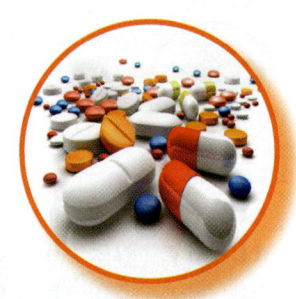

 Spotters

○ This is a **transdermal patch** and this route is for systemic use of drugs.

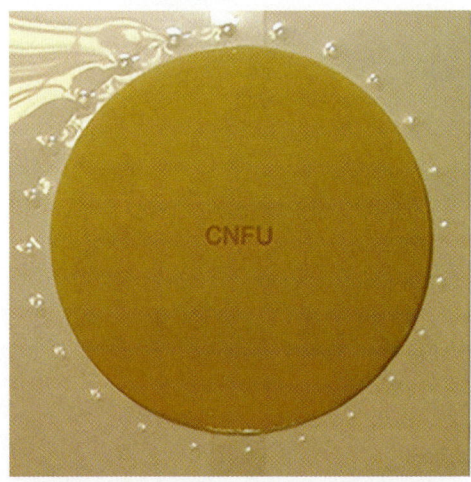

○ The drug in the picture are **suppositories** given by rectal route.

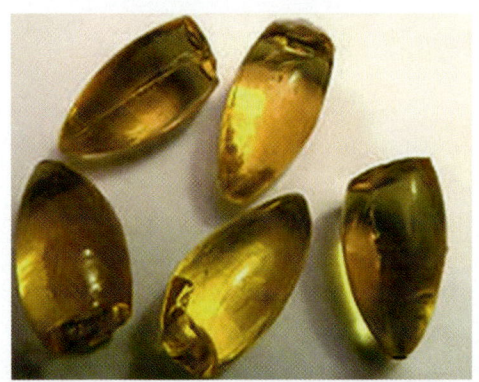

The features of the child suggestive of **fetal hydantoin syndrome** are

○ Facial cleft
○ Microcephaly

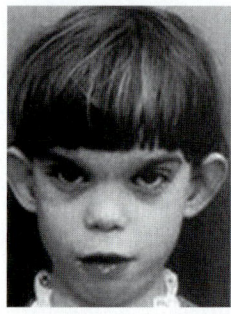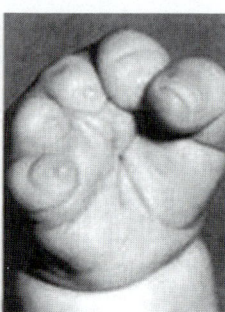

The features of the baby suggestive of **fetal alcohol syndrome** are

○ Small palpebral fissures
○ Thin vermilion border
○ Smooth philtrum

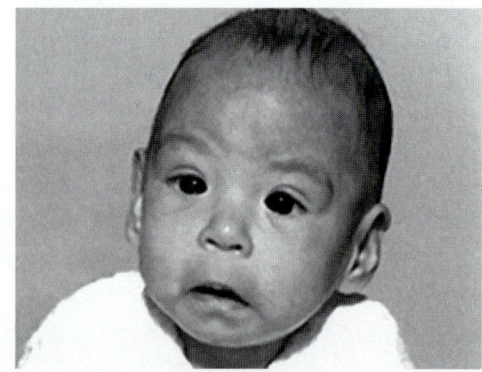

○ The given picture depicts **improvement of ptosis** and is suggestive of **tensilon test** for diagnosis of myasthenia gravis.

○ Though neostigmine can be used, the preferred drug for diagnosis is edrophonium due to its rapid and fast action.

○ The hexagonal stones in the picture are cysteine stones associated with **cystinuria**.

○ Acetazolamide alkalinizes urine and increases solubility of cysteine and decreases chances of stone formation.

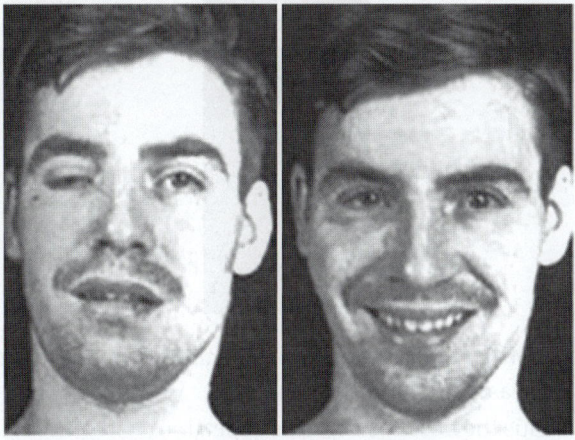

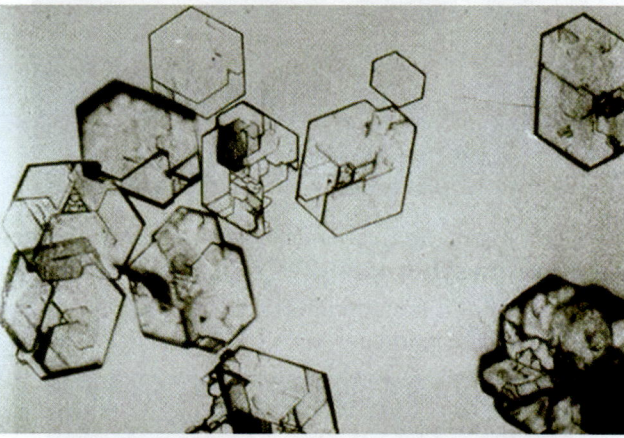

○ The device in the picture **epipen** contains epineprine for emergency self administration.

○ It can be used in anaphylaxis; in bee sting it's use as anaphylactic can be seen.

○ In cobra bite neostigmine is used.

○ In scorpion bite vasodilators like prazosin are used.

○ Envelope shaped stones in the picture are **calcium oxalate stones**.

○ These calcium stone formations can be treated by thiazides as they can increase calcium absorption and decrease it in urine.

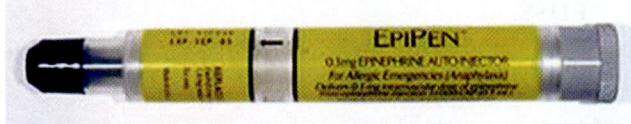

○ **Blue gray pigmentation**, as seen in the picture is characteristic of amiodarone, which is also known as **ceruloderma**.

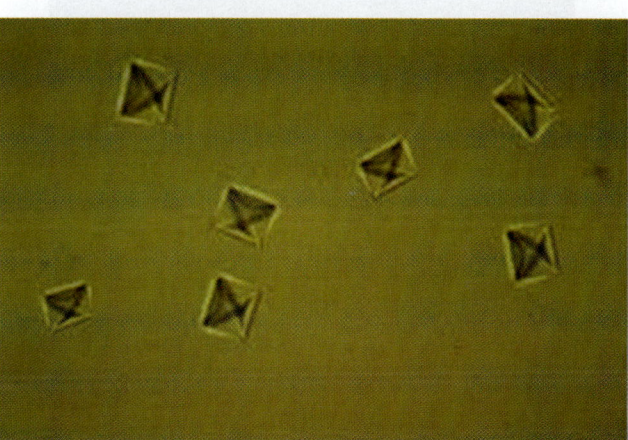

○ Massive **ascites** with dilated and prominent superficial veins of the abdomen are suggestive of cirrhotic ascites.

○ In cirrhotic ascites there is upregulation of aldosterone synthesis and hence it best responds to aldosterone antagonists like spironolactone.

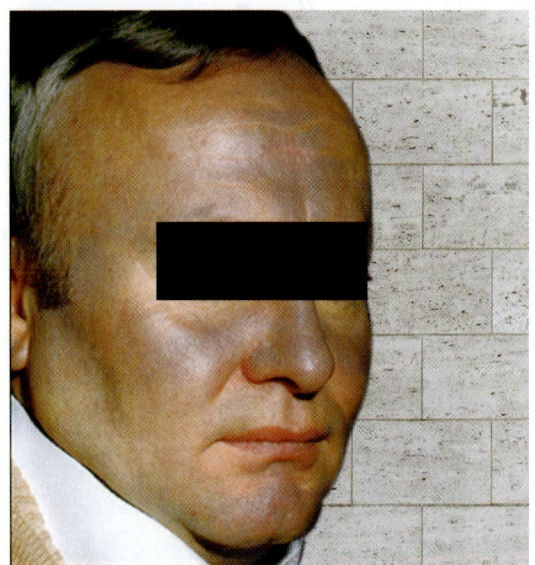

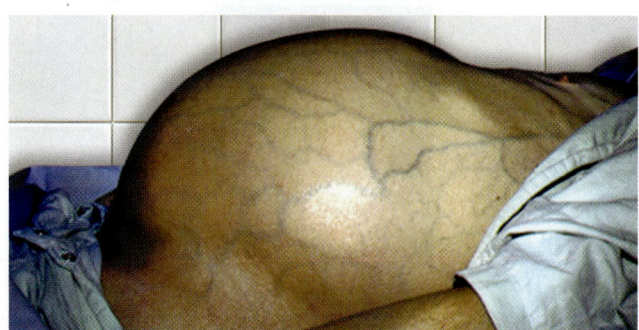

Ranjan Kumar Patel, Conceptual Review of Pharmacology for NBE; 3rd Edition

Ranjan Kumar Patel, Conceptual Review of Pharmacology for NBE; 3rd Edition

○ The female in the picture has **hirsutism** and **hyperplasia** of gums, which are characteristic of phenytoin.

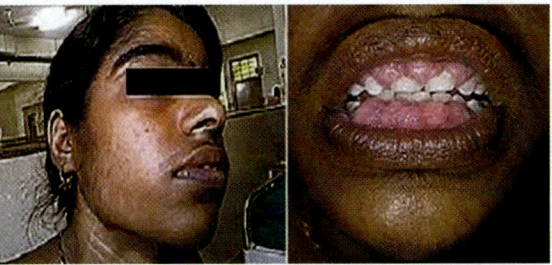

○ Lamotrigine and carbamazepine can cause **Steven Jhonson syndrome**.

○ To prevent it lamotrigine is started at low doses and then dose is gradually increased.

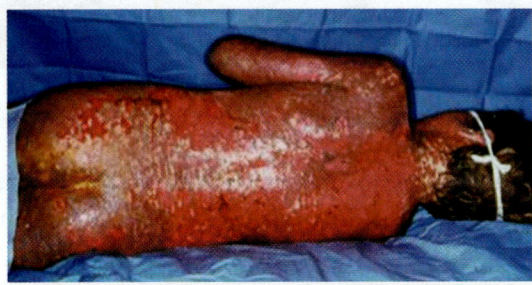

○ The procedure given in the picture is **ECT**.

○ Methohexital is a barbiturate anaesthetic agent that paradoxically causes seizures.

○ Hence it is the anaesthetic agent of choice in ECT.

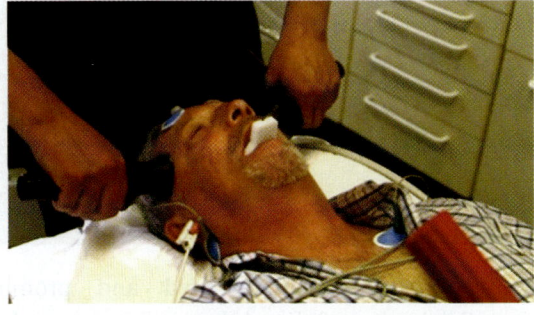

○ The female is having **acute dystonia** in the picture.

○ All the drugs in the options can cause acute dystonia but the risk is higher with potent typical antipsychotic like haloperidol.

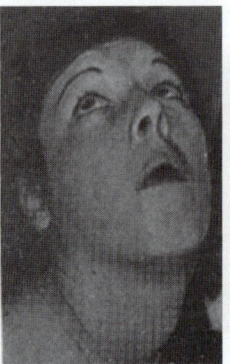

○ The stooping gait given in the picture is characteristic of **Parkinson's disease**.

○ Selegeline is the only drug that has inhibitory effect on neurodegeneration.

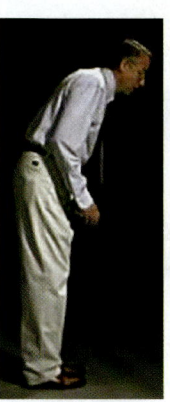

○ **MMSE test** is done for diagnosis of Alzheimer's disease.

○ Thus the best answer is donepezil.

MINI MENTAL STATE EXAMINATION (MMSE)

Name:

DOB:

Hospital Number:

One point for each answer   DATE:

○ The disability scale given in the picture is known as **EDSS**.

○ Drug with maximum effect on EDSS is mitoxantrone followed by natalizumab.

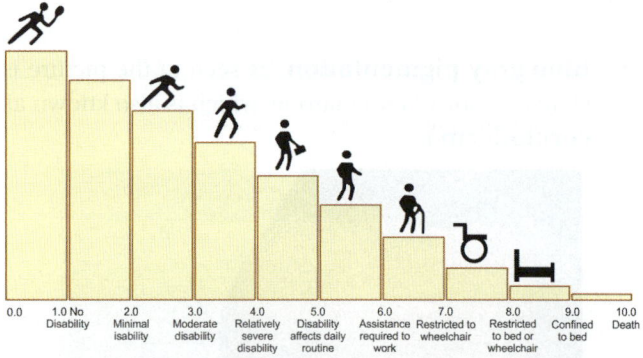

| 0.0 | 1.0 No Disability | 2.0 Minimal isability | 3.0 Moderate disability | 4.0 Relatively severe disability | 5.0 Disability affects daily routine | 6.0 Assistance required to work | 7.0 Restricted to wheelchair | 8.0 Restricted to bed or wheelchair | 9.0 Confined to bed | 10.0 Death |

○ The condition given in the picture is known as **green nail syndrome**, caused by pseudomonas.

○ Ceftazidime is the antibiotic of choice for pseudomonas infaction.

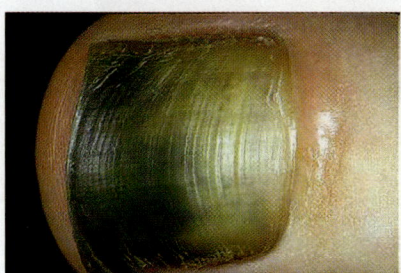

Ranjan Kumar Patel, Conceptual Review of Pharmacology for NBE; 3rd Edition

○ The white coloured discharge seen in the picture is specific for **gonorrhoea**.

○ Ceftriaxone is the drug of choice for gonorrhoea.

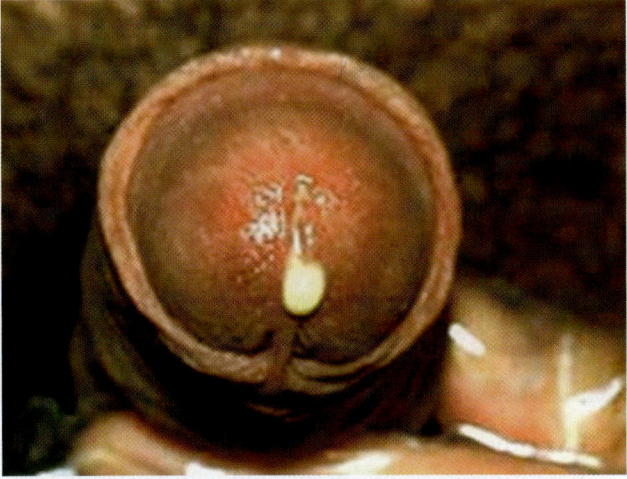

○ The condition given in the picture is **diphtheria**.

○ The drug of choice in diphtheria is erythromycin.

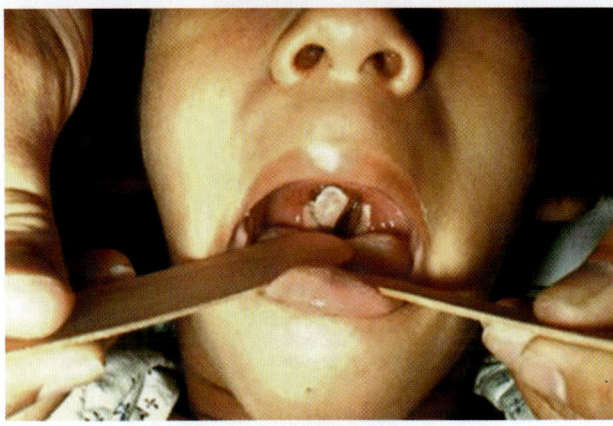

○ The blister packet given in the picture is used for **category III tuberculosis**.

○ It contains three drugs Isoniazid, Rifampicin and Pyrazinamide.

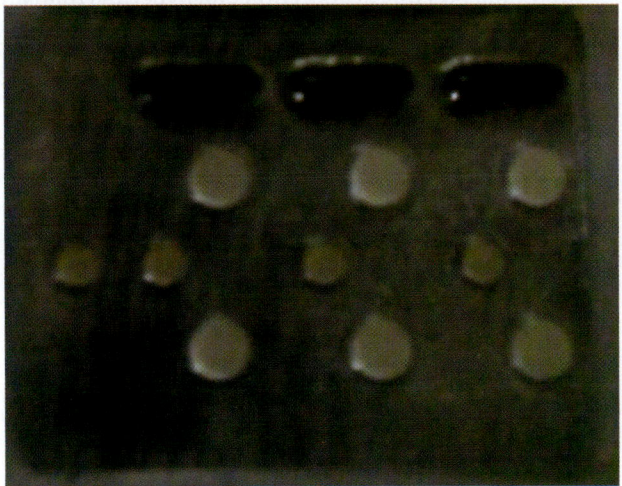

○ Patient on rifampicin should not be given **nevirapine** as it is metabolized by CYP3A4.

○ Rather efavirenz is substituted in its place in case of tuberculosis.

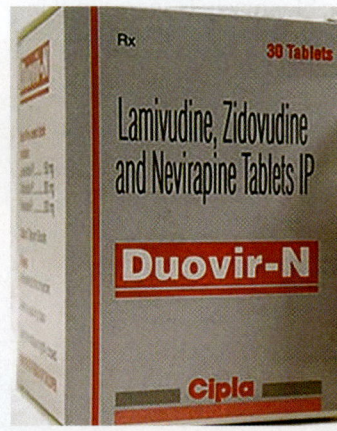

○ The kit in the picture is used for treatment of

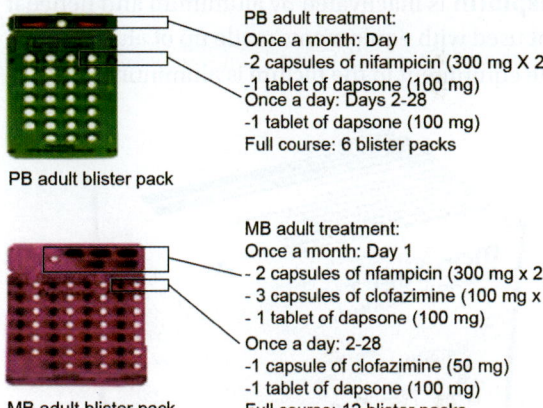

PB adult blister pack

PB adult treatment:
Once a month: Day 1
-2 capsules of nifampicin (300 mg X 2)
-1 tablet of dapsone (100 mg)
Once a day: Days 2-28
-1 tablet of dapsone (100 mg)
Full course: 6 blister packs

MB adult blister pack

MB adult treatment:
Once a month: Day 1
- 2 capsules of nfampicin (300 mg x 2)
- 3 capsules of clofazimine (100 mg x 3)
- 1 tablet of dapsone (100 mg)
Once a day: 2-28
-1 capsule of clofazimine (50 mg)
-1 tablet of dapsone (100 mg)
Full course: 12 blister packs

○ The picture depicts a patient of **giant cell tumor**, which presents as swelling near the joints with movement restrictions.

○ Denosumab has been approved in 2013 for treatment of giant cell tumor by FDA.

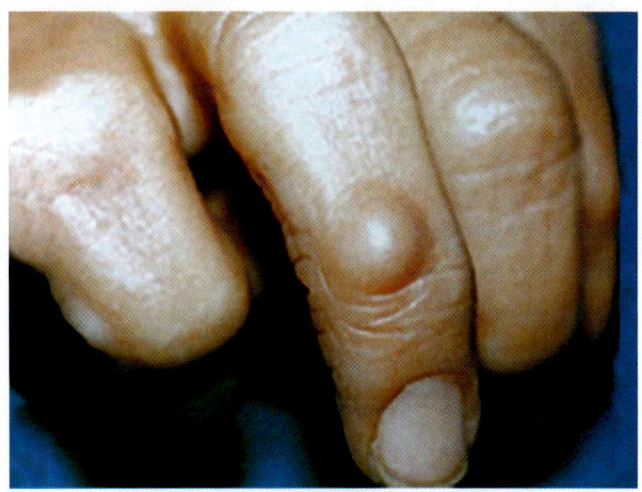

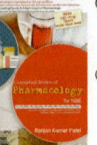

Ranjan Kumar Patel, Conceptual Review of Pharmacology for NBE; 3rd Edition

○ The streaks of hyperpigmentation seen on the back is called as **flagellate dermatitis**.

○ It is a common complication associated with bleomycin, as the enzyme bleomycin hydrolase to metabolize bleomycin is sparse in skin.

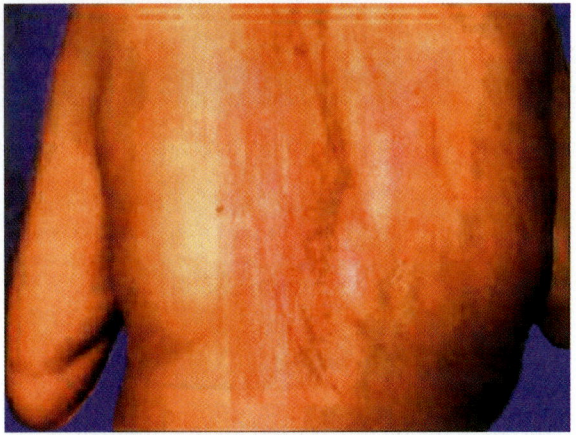

○ **Cisplatin** is inactivated by aluminum and hence it is not used with equipments made up of aluminum.

○ The equipment in the picture is aluminum needle.

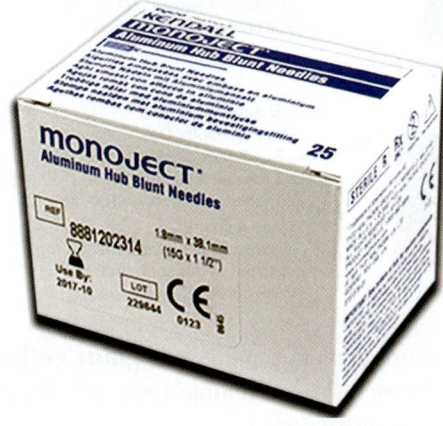

○ The drug in the picture **leucovorin** is used along with methotrexate and pemetrexed to prevent toxicity.

○ It is used to 5-FU to increase its sensitivity or anticancer effect.

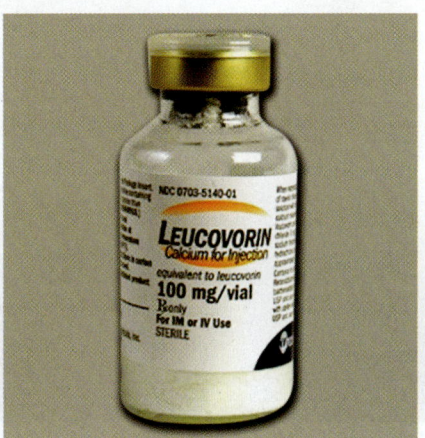

○ This is a case of **hand and foot syndrome**, which presents with desquamation and erythema of palms and soles.

○ Among the drugs in options, capecitabine commonly causes this side effect.

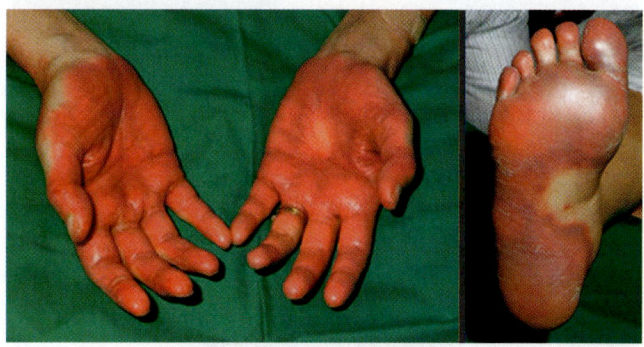

○ The drug in the picture, **mesna** is used to prevent hemorrhagic cystitis associated with ifosfamide and cyclophosphamide.

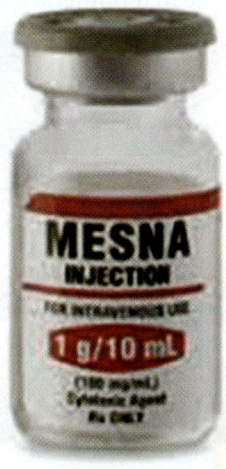

○ **Exopthalmos** in the picture is suggestive of hyperthyroidism.

○ Methimazole is the drug of choice for hyperthryroidism.

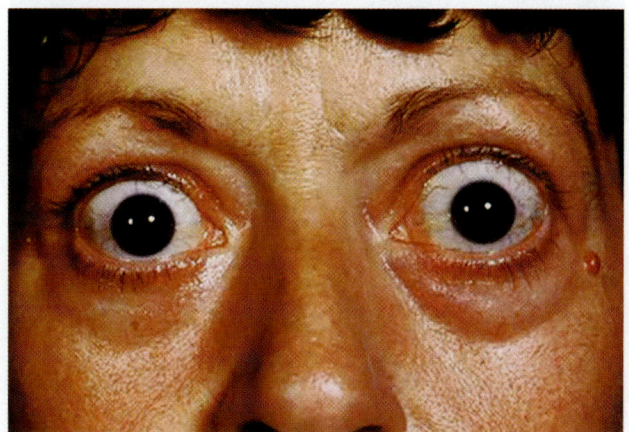

○ The picture depicts a case of **precocious puberty** for which GNRH agonists like goserelin is preferred by continuous administration.

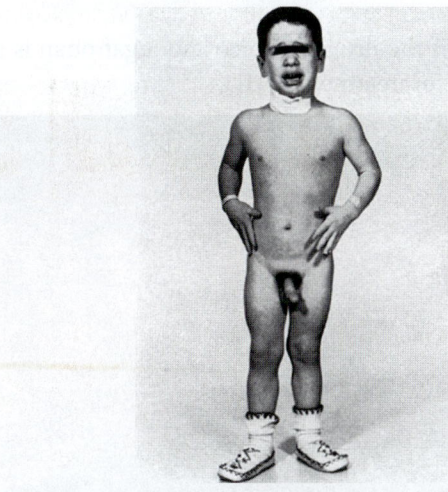

○ 2 tablets of **levonogesterol** given in the picture are used 12 hours apart for emergency contraception.

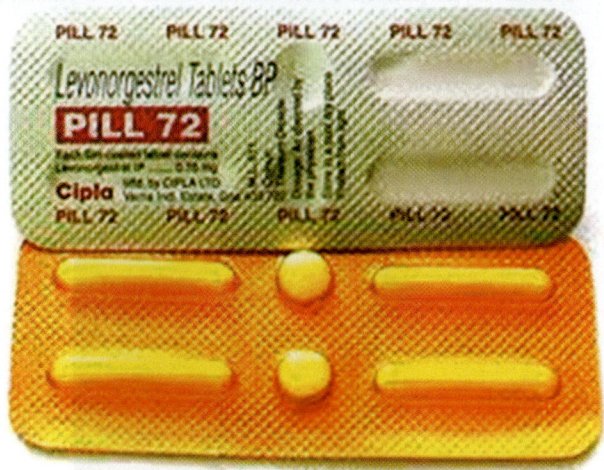

○ Ergotamine can cause severe peripheral **vasoconstriction and gangrene** in organs with end arteries like fingers.

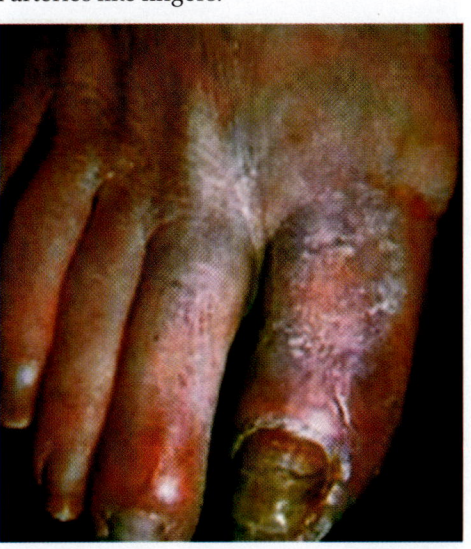

○ **Z deformity** given in the picture is seen with rheumatoid arthritis.

○ The best treatment option currently to prevent this is methotrexate plus an anti-TNF drug like infliximab.

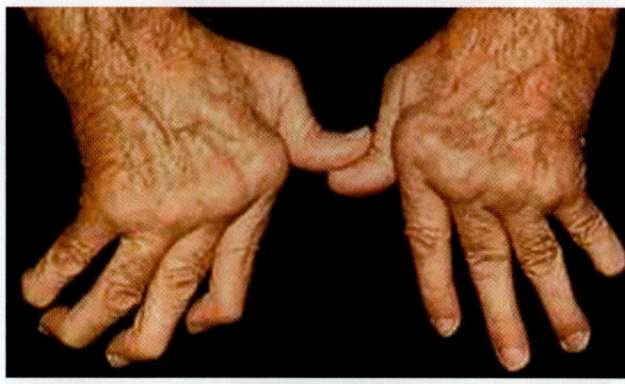

○ The device in the picture is a **dry powder inhaler**, which does not require coordination with inspiration. Rather the inspiratory drive pulls drug out of the device.

○ MDIs require coordination with inspiration.

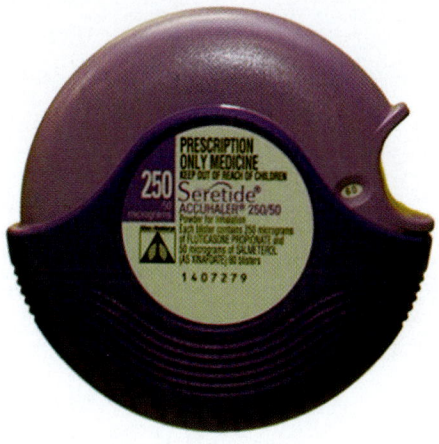

○ **Spacer** is a device that connects to the MDI and patient inhales drug from the spacer.

○ This causes lesser deposition of steroid in oropharyngeal cavity and hence lesser oropharyngeal candidiasis and systemic side-effects are seen.

○ This device makes it easier to use MDI in children.

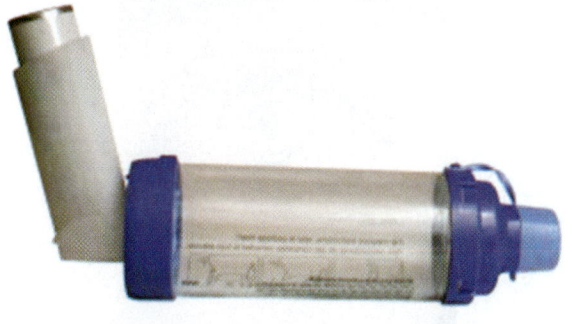

Ranjan Kumar Patel, Conceptual Review of Pharmacology for NBE; 3rd Edition

○ Bismuth can cause black **discoloration of tongue** stool.

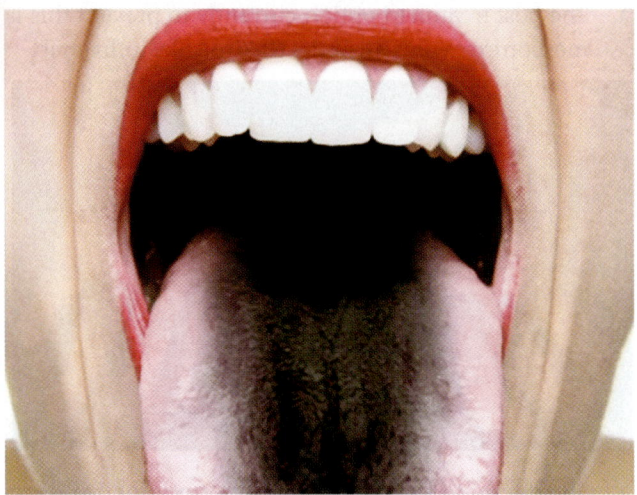

○ The kit given in the picture for rapid diagnosis of **H. pylori infection** in blood sample.

○ The antibiotics used in H. pylori are ampicillin, clarithromycin, metronidazole and tetracycline.

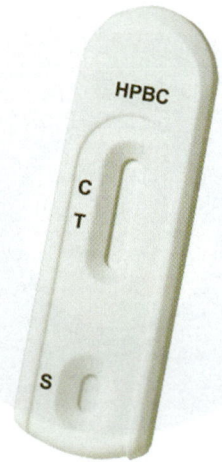

○ Cannabinoid receptor agonists like dronabinol and nabilone can cause conjunctival congestion known as **blood shot eyes**.

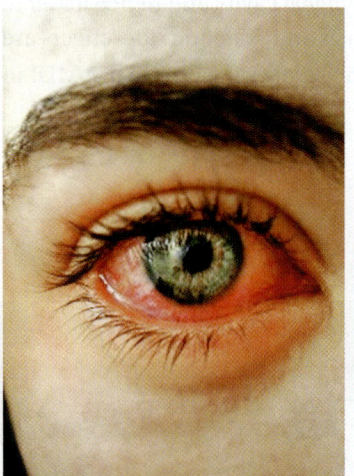

○ UFH can cross react to LMWH and hence in case of **HIT** none of these should be used.

○ However as fondaparinux does not cross react it can be used.

○ Lepirudin is the drug of choice and argatroban is an alternative for treatment of HIT.

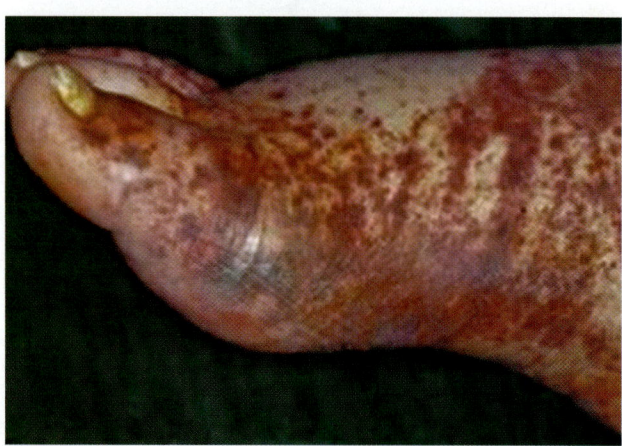

○ **Nasal hypoplasia** seen in the USG is a classical teratogenic feature of warfarin.

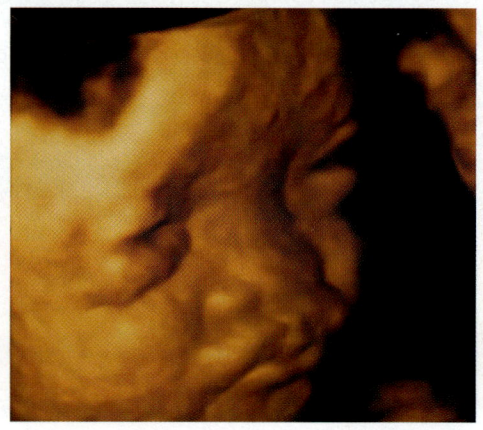

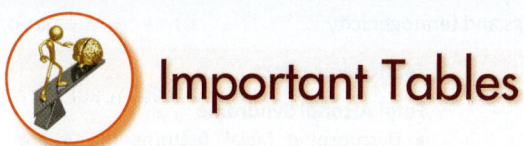

Important Tables

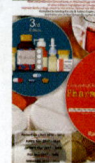

Ranjan Kumar Patel, Conceptual Review of Pharmacology for NBE; 3rd Edition

Table 1: Systemic routes of drug administration

Routes	Benefits	Drawbacks	Drugs
Oral	Cheapest Convenient Safest	First pass metabolism **Most variable absorption** due to various factors like lipid solubility, food intake, digestive enzymes,, etc.	Most drugs Remember: A drug with suffix tide or ase (e.g. Octreotide, Nesiritide, Asparginase etc) are peptides. Hence these are broken down in GIT and never given by oral route.
Sublingual	No first pass metabolism and faster effect as drug is absorbed directly into SVC Drug can be spitted out after desirable effect	Tooth discoloration and decay Cardiac side-effects	Nitroglycerine IDN Nifedipine Ephedrine Ergotamine Buprenorphine
Rectal	50% lesser first pass metabolism as from rectum 50% blood directly drains into IVC bypassing liver **Unpleasant and irritant drugs can be given**	Unreliable absorption	Diazepam for febrile seizures in children
Intravenous	100% bioavailability Fastest acting (Preferred in emergency) Irritants can be given Large volume can be given Peptides with high molecular weight are given	Increased chances of acute toxicity Drugs in oily medium cause hemolysis and hence are contraindicated	IV Drugs of choice Nicardipine: Hypertensive emergency Furosemide: Pulmonary edema Adenosine: PSVT Lorazepam: Status epilepticus
Intramuscular	Drugs in oily medium and irritants can be given Self-administration possible	Drugs in oily medium cause pain on injection NE is contraindicated as it can cause muscle necrosis due to potent vasoconstriction	IM Drugs of choice Adrenaline: Anaphylactic shock
Subcutaneous	Prolonged duration of action due to slow absorption	Irritants cannot be given as pain and necrosis can be seen	Insulin Contraceptives Adrenaline
Pulmonary	Faster effect due to rapid absorption by huge capillary network No first pass metabolism Local effect possible as in BA or COPD	Irritants can precipitate bronchospasm	Insulin (Exubera) Zanamivir Tobramycin SABA in BA Anticholinergics in COPD ICS
Transdermal	Longer duration of effect	Only lipid soluble drugs can be given	Nitroglycerine Fentanyl Scopolamine Nicotine Contraceptives HRT Clonidine
Intranasal	Rapid absorption and faster effect Ease of administration Preferred for peptides	Possible only for potent drugs Variable absorption	**Desmopressin** GnRH agonists Calcitonin Fentanyl

Courtesy: Ranjan Kumar Patel, Conceptual Review of Pharmacology for NBE; 3rd Edition

Ranjan Kumar Patel, Conceptual Review of Pharmacology for NBE; 3rd Edition

Table 2: Drugs banned and withdrawn

Drugs	Reason for ban or withdrawal
Astemizole Terfenadine Cisapride Tegaserod	QT prolongation
Fenfluramine	Cardiac valve defects Pulmonary hypertension
Gatifloxacin	Hyperglycemia
Letrozole banned in pregnancy	Teratogenicity Bone malformation Cardiac stenosis
Phenylpropanolamine	Stroke
Phenformin	Lactic acidosis
Nimesulide banned in children < 12 years	Hepatotoxicity
Refecoxib Valdecoxib	Myocardial infarction Stroke
Rimonabant	Depression Suicidal tendency
Rosiglitazone	Myocardial infarction Stroke
Sibutramine	Myocardial infarction Stroke
Troglitazone	Hepatic necrosis

Courtesy: Ranjan Kumar Patel, Conceptual Review of Pharmacology for NBE; 3rd Edition

Table 3: Important drug schedules in India

Schedule G	List of drugs that don't need prescription but requires a mandatory text on label "Caution: It is dangerous to take this preparation, except under medical supervision". E.g. antihistaminics.
Schedule H	List of drugs that can be sold only when a prescription is produced. Most drugs belong to this category.
Schedule P	It is about drug expiry period, i.e. maximum period till which drug can be used with intact potency.
Schedule W	List of drugs marketed under generic names only.
Schedule X	List of psychotropic drugs which need special license for manufacture and sale.
Schedule Y	Guidelines on clinical trials, import and manufacture of new drugs.

Courtesy: Ranjan Kumar Patel, Conceptual Review of Pharmacology for NBE; 3rd Edition

Table 4: Drugs and teratogenicity

Drug	Teratogenic effect
Alcohol	**Fetal Alcohol Syndrome** • Dysmorphic facial features (all 3 are required) ▪ Small palpebral fissures ▪ Thin vermilion border ▪ Smooth philtrum • Prenatal and/or postnatal growth impairment • Central nervous system abnormalities (1 required) ▪ Structural: head size < 10th percentile, significant brain abnormality on imaging ▪ Neurological ▪ Functional: global cognitive or intellectual deficits ▪ Functional deficits in at least three domains
Fluconazole	• Oral clefts • Abnormal facies • Cardiac abnormalities • Skull, long-bone, and joint abnormalities
ACE inhibitors	• **Fetal RAAS inhibition** followed by hypotension and reduced perfusion causes fetal-growth restriction and calvarium maldevelopment • Oligohydramnios causes pulmonary hypoplasia and limb contractures.
Leflunomide	• Hydrocephalus • Eye anomalies • Skeletal abnormalities
Chloramphenicol	• Gray baby syndrome
Nitrofurantoin	• Hypoplastic left heart syndrome • Microphthalmia/anophthalmia • Facial clefts • Atrial septal defects
Sulfonamides	• Anencephaly • Left ventricular outflow tract obstruction • Choanal atresia • Diaphragmatic hernia
Tetracycline	• Yellow discoloration of deciduous teeth • Bone growth abnormality
Fluoroquinolones	Cartilage growth defect
Cyclophosphamide	• Skeletal abnormalities • Limb defects • Cleft palate • Eye abnormalities
Methotrexate	Fetal methotrexate aminopterin syndrome • Craniosynostosis with "clover-leaf" skull • Wide nasal bridge • Low-set ears • Micrognathia • Limb abnormalities

Drug	Teratogenic effect
Trastuzumab	• Pulmonary hypoplasia • Skeletal abnormalities
Diethylsilbestrol	Vaginal adenosis, vaginal and cervical cancer in female fetus after 20+ years
Corticosteroids	Facial clefts
Lithium	Ebstein's anomaly
Isotretinoin	• Bilateral microtia • Anotia with stenosis of external ear canal • Flat, depressed nasal bridge and ocular hypertelorism • Cleft lip and palate
Thalidomide	• Phocomelia • Cranial nerve defects • Anorectal stenosis • Cardiac defects
Warfarin	• Stippling of the vertebrae and femoral epiphyses • Nasal hypoplasia with depression of the nasal bridge (saddle nose)
Valproate	• Neural tube defect • Cardiovascular defect
Phenytoin	**Fetal hydantoin syndrome** • Facial cleft • Microcephaly • IUGR • Hypertelorism • Triphalangeal thumb
Penicillamine	Loose skin

Courtesy: Ranjan Kumar Patel, Conceptual Review of Pharmacology for NBE; 3rd Edition

Table 5: Comorbidities

Associated Comorbidity with Hypertension	Drugs Preferred
DM CKD Scleroderma Nephrotic syndrome	ACEI/ARB
Angina Previous MI Hyperthyroidism Migraine Anxiety with somatic manifestations Essential tremor Atrial fibrillation and flutter Preoperative hypertension	Beta blockers
Osteoporosis	Thiazides
Raynaud's disease Cyclosporine induced hypertension	CCB
BPH Dyslipidemia	α_1 blockers

Courtesy: Ranjan Kumar Patel, Conceptual Review of Pharmacology for NBE; 3rd Edition

Table 6: Drug-induced ion abnormalities

Ion abnormality	Causative drugs
Hypokalemia	• Beta 2 agonists • Alpha blockers • Insulin • Theophylline/Caffeine • B12/Folic acid • Amphotericin B

	• Diuretics except K sparing ones
	  ■ CA inhibitors
	  ■ Loops
	  ■ Thiazides
	  ■ Osmotic diuretics
	• Penicillin
	• Fludrocortisone

Hyperkalemia	• Beta blockers (Nonselective)
	• Digoxin
	• Sch
	• Renin-angiotensin-aldosterone system (RAAS) inhibitors
	  ■ ACEI
	  ■ ARB
	  ■ Renin inhibitors
	  ■ Aldosterone antagonists
	• Amiloride/Triamterene
	• Trimethoprim
	• Pentamidine
	• Nonsteroidal anti-inflammatory drugs (NSAIDs)
	• Cyclosporine/Tacrolimus
	• Heparin

Hypomagnesemia	• PPI
	• Ethanol
	• Diuretics
	  ■ Loops
	  ■ Thiazides
	  ■ Osmotic
	• Pentamidine
	• Foscarnet
	• Cyclosporine
	• Aminoglycosides
	• Amphotericin B
	• Cetuximab

Hypermagnesemia	• Cathartics • Urologic irrigants • Antacids • Enemas • Laxatives • Lithium • Theophylline
Hyponatremia	• Chlorpropamide • Vincristine • Cyclophosphamide • Nicotine • Clofibrate • SSRI
	• NSAIDS • Oxytocin • TCA • Nicotine

Ranjan Kumar Patel, Conceptual Review of Pharmacology for NBE; 3rd Edition

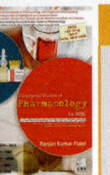

Ranjan Kumar Patel, Conceptual Review of Pharmacology for NBE; 3rd Edition

Ion abnormality	Causative drugs
Hypernatremia	• Bicarbonate • Steroids • Androgens • Estrogen • Lithium • Demeclocycline • Foscarnet • Expired tetracycline
Hypercalcemia	• Thiazides • Lithium • Vitamin D • Vitamin A intoxication • Aluminium intoxication • Theophylline • Estrogen • Tamoxifen
Hypocalcemia	• Bisphosphonates • Cisplatin • Foscarnet • Calcitonin • Loops • Glucocorticoids • Antiepileptics • PPI • PTU • Colchicine toxicity

Courtesy: Ranjan Kumar Patel, Conceptual Review of Pharmacology for NBE; 3rd Edition

Epilepsy	
Generalized • GTCS • Absence seizure Valproate • Myoclonic Seizure	
Partial	Carbamazepine
Lennox Gastaut Syndrome	Valproate
Infantile Spasm	ACTH
Infantile spasm with TS	Vigabatrin
Rolandic Epilepsy (Benign epilepsy of childhood)	Carbamazepine
Seizures in Pregnancy	$MgSO_4$
Seizures in Neonates	Phenobarbital
Dravet Syndrome (Severe myoclonic epilepsy of childhood)	Valproate
West Syndrome (Infantile spasm + MR)	ACTH
Status Epilepticus Lorazepam	

Courtesy: Ranjan Kumar Patel, Conceptual Review of Pharmacology for NBE; 3rd Edition

Table 7: Treatment of Specific Infections

Antifungal prophylaxis	
Induction chemotherapy of acute leukemia	Posoconazole

Post allo bone marrow transplant	Pre engrafment – Voriconazole Post engrafment – Posoconazole
Asymptomatic bacteriuria	Nitrofurantoin Or Amoxicillin
Biliary tract infections (Cholangitis or cholecystitis caused by E.coli, klebsiella etc.)	Ceftriaxone Or Piperacillin – Tazobactam
Brain abscess Subdural empyema	Ceftriaxone or cefotaxime + Metronidazole
Cervicitis Urethritis	Ceftriaxone + Azithromycin

ENT Infections	
Malignant otitis externa	Piperacillin + Tazobactam
Acute otitis media	Amoxicillin + Clavulanate
Mastoiditis	Acute – Cefotaxime or Ceftriaxone Chronic – Piperacillin + Tazobactam
Epiglottitis	Ceftriaxone or Cefotaxime

Febrile neutropenia	Stable patient – Ceftazidime Unstable patient – Piperacillin – Tazobactam Or Cefoperazone – Sulbactam
Neonatal meningitis Neonatal sepsis	Ampicillin + Gentamycin

Ocular infections	
Bacterial conjunctivitis	Gatifloxacin/Levofloxacin/ Moxifloxacin opthalmoligical solution
Bacterial keratitis	Moxifloxacin solution
Bacterial keratitis in contact lens users (pseudomonas)	Tobramycin or Gentamycin solution + Piperacilin or Ticarcillin solution
Fungal keratitis	Natamycin
Acanthamoeba keratitis	Chlorhexidine or Polyhexamethylenebiguanide + Hexamidine solution
Orbital cellulitis	Cloxacillin + Ceftriaxone + Metronidazole

Osteomyelitis (Acute)	Ceftriaxone
Prostatitis	Doxycycline Or Cotrimoxazole
Prosthetic joint infection	Ceftriaxone + Vancomycin
Pyelonephritis	Uncomplicated – Gentamicin or Amikacin Complicated – Piperacillin – Tazobactam Or Amikacin Or Cefoperazone – Sulbactam

Septic abortion	Ampicillin + Metronidazole
Diverticulitis	Mild – Amoxycillin + Clavulanate Moderate – Ceftriaxone + Metronidazole Severe – Meropenam
Infective endocarditis : Streptococcal or Enterococcal	Penicillin G or Ampicillin + Gentamycin
Infective endocarditis: Staphylococcal	Vancomycin
Liver Abscess	Amoxycillin – Clavulanate or Ceftriaxone + Metronidazole
Ludwig's angina Vincent's angina	Clindamycin Or Amoxicillin – Calvulanate
Lung abscess Empyema	Piperacillin – Tazobactam Or Cefoperazone – Sulbactam
Meningitis	Acute bacterial – Ceftriaxone Post neurosurgery – Meropenam + Vancomycin With basilar skull fracture – Ceftriaxone
Post-necrotizing pancre-atitis: infected pseudo-cyst or pancreatic abscess	Piperacillin – Tazobactam Or Cefoperazone – Sulbactam
Rhinosinusitis (Acute bacterial)	Amoxicillin – Clavulanate
Skin and soft tissue infection	
Cellulitis Furunculosis	Amoxicillin – Clavulanate Or Ceftriaxone
Necrotizing fasciitis	Piperacillin – Tazobactam Or Cefoperazone – Sulbactam + Clindamycin
Spontaneous bacterial peritonitis	Cefotaxime Or Piperacillin – Tazobactam Or Cefoperazone – Sulbactam
Secondary bacterial peritonitis due to intra-abdominal abscess or GI perforation	Piperacillin – Tazobactam Or Cefoperazone – Sulbactam

Courtesy: Ranjan Kumar Patel, Conceptual Review of Pharmacology for NBE; 3rd Edition

Table 8: Kinase inhibitors list

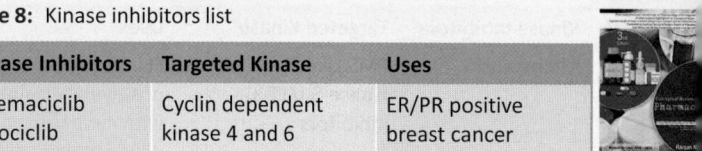

Kinase Inhibitors	Targeted Kinase	Uses
Abemaciclib Rivociclib Palbociclib	Cyclin dependent kinase 4 and 6	ER/PR positive breast cancer
Acalabrutinib	Bruton's tyrosine kinase	Ibrutinib resistant mantle cell lymphoma
Afatinib	EGFR > Her 2 tyrosine kinase	Non small cell cancer of lungs
Axitinib	VEGFR tyrosine kinase	Renal cell cancer
Imatinib – 1st generation	BCR-ABL tyrosine kinase	Drug of choice for CML GIST
Bosutinib Dasatinib 2nd generation Nilotinib Ponatinib – 3rd generation	BCR-ABL tyrosine kinase	Used for treatment of Imatinib resistant CML
Crizotinib	Anaplastic Lymphoma tyrosine Kinase (ALK)	ALK positive non-small cell cancer of lung
Ceritinib Brigatinib Alectinib Lorlatinib	Anaplastic Lymphoma tyrosine Kinase (ALK)	Ceritinib resistant ALK positive non-small cell cancer of lung
Cabozantinib	PAN tyrosine kinase	Medullary thyroid cancer RCC
Erlotinib	EGFR tyrosine kinase	Non-small cell cancer of lungs Pancreatic cancer
Gefitinib	EGFR tyrosine kinase	Non-small cell cancer of lungs
Ibrutinib	Bruton's tyrosine kinase	CLL Waldenstrom Macroglobulinemia Mantle cell lymphoma Marginal zone lymphoma
Idelalisib	Phosphoinositide-3 Kinase (PI3K)	Relapsed CLL Follicular B cell NHL Small lymphocytic lymphoma
Lapatinib	Her-2 tyrosine kinase	Trastuzumab resistant breast cancer
Lenvatinib	VEGFR tyrosine kinase	Renal cell carcinoma Medullary thyroid cancer

Ranjan Kumar Patel, Conceptual Review of Pharmacology for NBE; 3rd Edition

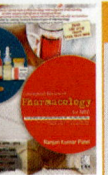

Ranjan Kumar Patel, Conceptual Review of Pharmacology for NBE; 3rd Edition

Kinase Inhibitors	Targeted Kinase	Uses
Midostaurin	FMS Like Tyrosine kinase-3 (FLT-3) inhibitors	FLT-3 mutation positive AML along with cytarabine and daunorubicin Mastocytosis Mast cell leukemia
Neratinib	HER 1, 2 and 4 tyrosine kinase	Trastuzumab resistant breast cancer
Osimertinib	EGFR tyrosine kinase	Non-small cell cancer of lung positive for EGFR T790M mutation
Pazopanib	VEGFR tyrosine kinase	Soft tissue sarcoma
Regorafenib	PAN tyrosine kinase	GIST
Ruxilotinib	Janus Kinase	Myelofibrosis
Sunitinib	VEGFR tyrosine kinase	Renal cell cancer GIST
Sorafenib	VEGFR tyrosine kinase	Hepatocellular carcinoma (DOC)
Trametinib Cobimetinib	MEK 1/2	Unresectable or metastatic malignant melanoma positive for V600E or V600K BRAF mutation
Vemurafenib Dabrafenib	BRAF tyrosine kinase	Unresectable or metastatic malignant melanoma positive for V600E BRAF mutation
Vandetanib	EGFR, VEGFR tyrosine kinases	Medullary thyroid cancer

Courtesy: Ranjan Kumar Patel, Conceptual Review of Pharmacology for NBE; 3rd Edition

Table 9: Other monoclonal antibodies

Monoclonal Antibodies	Target	Uses
Actoxumab	C. difficile toxin A	Prevention of C. difficile infection
Aducanumab	Beta-amyloid	Alzheimer's disease
Alemtuzumab	CD52	Low grade lymphoma Multiple sclerosis
Alirocumab Evolocumab	PCSK-9 receptor – Degrades LDL receptor	Familial hypercholesterolemia
Atezolizumab	PDL-1 (Programmed Death Ligand)	Urothelial carcinoma – Locally advanced or metastatic Non-small cell lung cancer – Metastatic

Monoclonal Antibodies	Target	Uses
Avelumab	PDL-1 (Programmed Death Ligand)	Metastatic Merkel cell carcinoma
Basiliximab Daclizumab	CD-25/IL-2 receptor	Acute graft rejection Multiple sclerosis
Belimumab	B Lymphocyte	SLE
Bezlotoxumab	C. difficile toxin B	Prophylaxis of pseudomembranous enterocolitis
Blinatumomab	Bispecific T cell Engager (BiTE)	Relapsed/Refractory ALL (Philadelphia chromosome negative)
Bolosozumab Romosozumab	Sclerostin	Osteoporosis
Brodalumab	IL-17 A receptor	Plaque psoriasis
Brentuximab Vedotin	CD 30	CLL
Bevacizumab	VEGFR	Renal Cell cancer Diabetic retinopathy
Cetuximab Panitumumab	EGFR	Head and neck cancer Colorectal cancer
Dartaumumab	CD 38	Multiple myeloma resistant to bortezomib plus lenalidomide
Denosumabw	RANK ligand	Metastatic osteolytic lesions Postmenopausal osteoporosis
Dinutuximab	GD-2 glycolipid	High risk neuroblastoma
Diridivumab	Hemagglutinin	Influenza
Dupilumab	IL-4	Atopic dermatitis
Durvalumab	PDL-1	Urothelial carcinoma – Locally advanced or metastatic
Eculizumab	Complement-5	PNH
Efungumab	Heat Shock Protein (HSP) of Candida	Invasive candidiasis treatment along with Amphotericin B
Elotuzumab	SLAMF 7 (Signalling Lymphocytic Activation Molecule Family member 7)	Multiple myeloma treatment in combination with lenalidomide and dexamethasone who received prior 1-3 therapies
Emicizumab-kxwh	Bispecific anti factor IX a and factor X antibody	Hemophilia A
Gemtuzumab Ozogamycin	CD 33	CD 33 Positive AML

Monoclonal Antibodies	Target	Uses
Girentuximab	Carbonic anhydrase 9 or G250 antigen expressed in clear cell RCC	Clear cell RCC
Guselkumab	IL-23	Plaque psoriasis
Idarucizumab	Dabigatran	Reversal of dabigatran's anticoagulant effect
Ipilimumab	CTLA-4	Malignant melanoma
Inotuzumab Ozogamycin	CD 22	Relapsed or refractory B cell ALL
Necitumumab	EGFR	Metastatic squamous non-small cell cancer of lung
Nivolumab Pembrolizumab	PD1 (Programmed Death 1) receptor	Malignant melanoma
Obiltoxaximab	Bacillus anthrax	Anthrax
Ocrelizumab	CD20	Rheumatoid arthritis Multiple sclerosis – RRMS and PPMS
Ofatumumab Obinutozumab	CD20	Rituximab resistant CLL
Olaratumab	PDGFR-alpha	Soft tissue sarcoma
Omalizumab	Ig E	Bronchial asthma
Otelixizumab Teplizumab	CD-3	Type I DM in children
Palivizumab	RSV	RSV prophylaxis
Rafivirumab	Rabies virus	Prophylaxis of rabies
Ramucirumab	VEGFR	Gastric cancer

Monoclonal Antibodies	Target	Uses
Ranibizumab	VEGFR	Choroidal neovascularization Macular edema Deafness associated with NF-II
Reslizumab	IL-5	Severe asthma
Rituximab	CD20	Mnemonic: CANT MIS Ritu C: CLL A: Autoimmune haemolytic anemia N: NHL T: TTP M: Multiple sclerosis I: ITP S: SLE Ritu: Rheumatic arthritis
Sarilumab Tocilizumab	IL-6	Rheumatoid arthritis
Secukinumab Ixekizumab	IL-17	Psoriasis
Siltuximab	IL-6	Multicentric Castleman's disease
Trastuzumab Pertuzumab	Her-2	Her-2 positive breast cancer
Ustekinumab	IL 12,23	Psoriasis
Vedolizumab	α4β7 integrin	Inflammatory bowel disease Ulcerative colitis Crohn's disease
Ziv-aflibercept	VEGFR, PLGFR	Colorectal cancer

Courtesy: Ranjan Kumar Patel, Conceptual Review of Pharmacology for NBE; 3rd Edition

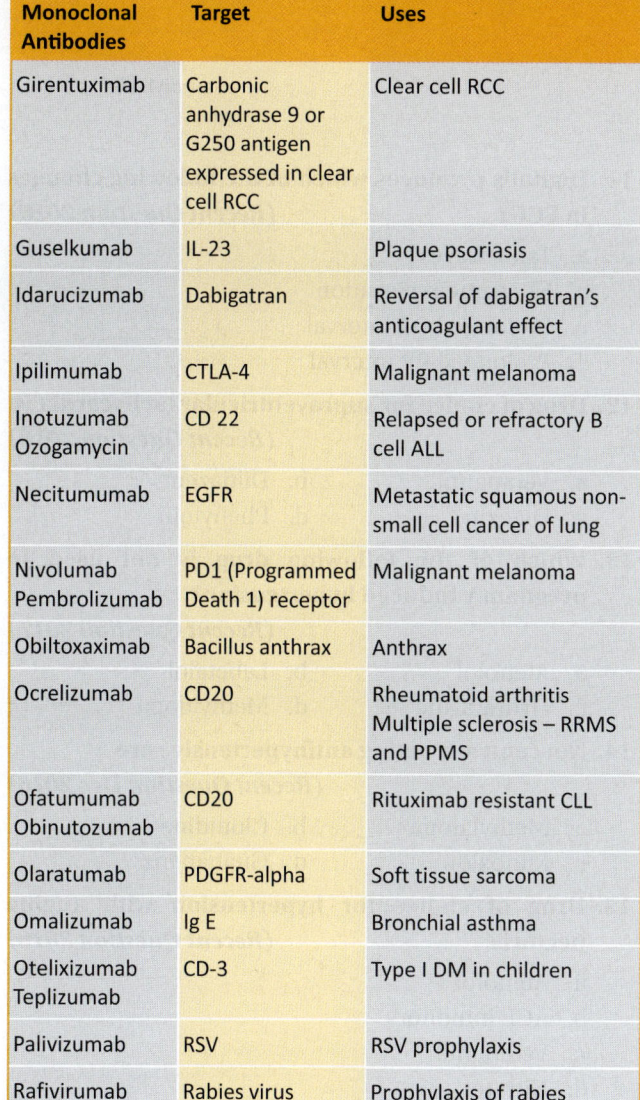

Ranjan Kumar Patel, Conceptual Review of Pharmacology for NBE; 3rd Edition

Important MCQs

Ranjan Kumar Patel, Conceptual Review of Pharmacology for NBE; 3rd Edition

1. **True about pKa is:**   *(Recent Question 2017)*
   a. pH at which ionized fraction of drug equals to unionized fraction
   b. pH at which ionized fraction of drug is more than unionized fraction
   c. pH at which ionized fraction of drug is less than unionized fraction
   d. pH at which ionized fraction of drug is twice unionized fraction

2. **Zero order kinetics is shown by all except:**
   (Recent Question 2016)
   a. High dose salicylates   b. Phenytoin
   c. Ethanol   d. Methotrexate

3. **Phase 1 clinical trial is for?**   *(AIIMS Nov 2015)*
   a. Pharmacokinetics   b. Dose
   c. Safety   d. Efficacy

4. **Which is most common drug studied for desensitization?**   *(Recent Question Dec 2016)*
   a. Penicillin   b. Allopurinol
   c. Isoniazid   d. Insulin

5. **Atropine is not given in which of the following case of poisoning:**   *(AIIMS Nov 2017)*
   a. Baygon   b. Parathion
   c. Endrin   d. TIK 20

6. **Neostigmine is used in the following except**
   (Recent Question 2016)
   a. Myasthenia gravis   b. Cobra bite
   c. Atony of bladder   d. Glaucoma

7. **The short acting anticholinesterase drug is**
   (Recent Question 2016)
   a. Edrophonium   b. Demecarium
   c. Dyflos   d. Ectothiophate

8. **Selective beta 2 blocker is**   *(Recent Question 2016)*
   a. Butoxamine   b. Betoxolol
   c. Esmolol   d. Bisoprolol

9. **Beta blockers are contraindicated in**
   a. Acute aortic dissection   *(Recent Question 2016)*
   b. Angina pectoris
   c. Post MI
   d. Sick sinus syndrome

10. **QT prolongation is caused by:**
    (Recent Question 2017)
    a. Quinidine   b. Omeprazole
    c. Lidocaine   d. Penicillin

11. **Digitalis produces which of the following changes in ECG?**   *(Recent Question 2016)*
    a. Tall T waves
    b. ST segment elevation
    c. Prolonged QT interval
    d. Prolonged PR interval

12. **Drug of choice for supraventricular tachycardia is**
    (Recent Question 2016)
    a. Verapamil   b. Diltiazem
    c. Digoxin   d. Phenytoin

13. **Which of the following drug is not used in pregnancy induced hypertension?**
    (Recent Question 2017)
    a. Atenolol   b. Labetalol
    c. Hydralazine   d. Methyldopa

14. **Not centrally acting antihypertensive are**
    (Recent Question Dec 2016)
    a. Methyl dope   b. Clonidine
    c. Minoxidil   d. Guanabenz

15. **Drug of choice for hypertension with angina pectoris**   *(Recent Question 2016)*
    a. Atenolol
    b. ACE inhibitors
    c. Verapamil
    d. Nitrates

16. **Drug(s) causing QT interval prolongation:**
    (PGI May 2017)
    a. Amiodarone   b. Cisapride
    c. Calcium gluconate   d. Magnesium therapy
    e. Ketoconazole

17. **All of the following drugs are used in myocardial infarction except**   *(WBPG 2015)*
    a. Fibrinolytics
    b. Plasminogen activator inhibitor
    c. Antithrombin
    d. Platelet inhibitor

18. **'Coronary steal' phenomenon is seen with?**
    (MHCET 2009)
    a. Verapamil   b. Diltiazem
    c. Nicorandil   d. Dipyridamole

19. **Drug of choice for severe rheumatic chorea is:**
    (Recent Question 2017)
    a. Valproate   b. Haloperidol
    c. Immunoglobulin   d. Diazepam

20. **Most common antiepileptic causing toxic epiderm necrosis** *(Recent Question Dec 2016)*
   a. Carbamazepine   b. Valproate
   c. Phenytoin   d. Gabapentine

21. **Which drug is contraindicated in pregnancy?** *(Recent Question 2016)*
   a. Phenytoin   b. Insulin
   c. Heparin   d. All

22. **Inverse agonist is:** *(Recent Question 2016)*
   a. Buspirone   b. β carboline
   c. Flumazenil   d. Zolpidem

23. **Which of the following mood stabilizer has antisuicidal effect?** *(AIIMS May 2017)*
   a. Lithium   b. Valproate
   c. Carbamezapine   d. Lamotrigine

24. **Drug used for Alzheimer's disease acting on NMDA receptor is** *(Recent Question Dec 2016)*
   a. Donepezil   b. Memantine
   c. Tacrine   d. Galantamine

25. **In alcohol withdrawal, drug of choice is** *(Recent Question 2016)*
   a. TFP   b. Chlormethazole
   c. Chlordiazepoxide   d. Buspirone

26. **Drug of choice for scrub typhus is:** *(AIIMS Nov 2017)*
   a. Doxycycline   b. Azithromycin
   c. Ciprofloxacin   d. Chloramphenicol

27. **Which of the following is not bacteriostatic:** *(Recent Question 2017)*
   a. Linezolid   b. Clindamycin
   c. Vancomycin   d. Erythromycin

28. **Broad spectrum antibiotic is** *(Recent Question 2016)*
   a. Erythromcycin   b. Streptomycin
   c. Tetracycline   d. All

29. **Anti TB drug associated with max ocular side-effects is** *(Recent Question Dec 2016)*
   a. Rifampicin   b. Isonizad
   c. Ethambutol   d. Pyrazinamide

30. **Which antiviral drug is used in both HIV and hepatitis B:** *(Recent Question 2017)*
   a. Aciclovir   b. Abacavir
   c. Emtricitabine   d. Enfuvirtide

31. **Amphotericin B acts on** *(Recent Question 2017)*
   a. Cell membrane   b. Cell wall
   c. Nucleus   d. Cytoplasm

32. **Most effective drug in severe falciparum malaria** *(AIIMS Nov 2014)*
   a. Quinine   b. Cholorquine
   c. Artesunate   d. Mefloquine

33. **Double Platin based therapy is used for**
   a. Wilm's tumor   *(Recent Question Dec 2016)*
   b. Hodgkin's lymphoma
   c. Non-hodgkin's lymphoma
   d. Lung cancer

34. **Which antineoplastic is cell cycle s phase inhibitor** *(Recent Question Dec 2016)*
   a. Vincristine   b. 5FU
   c. Paclitaxel   d. Cyclophosphamide

35. **Rituximab is antibody against?** *(Recent Question 2016)*
   a. CD20   b. VEGF
   c. EGFR   d. IL-2

36. **Drug used safely in renal failure without change in dose** *(AIIMS Nov 2016)*
   a. Linagliptin   b. Sitagliptin
   c. Vildagliptin   d. saxagliptin

37. **HbAIC is decreased most by?** *(Recent Question 2016)*
   a. Biguanides   b. Sulfonylureas
   c. Thiazolidinediones d. Acarbose

38. **Which insulin is never mixed with other insulins?** *(Recent Question 2016)*
   a. Lente   b. Aspart
   c. Lispro   d. Glargine

39. **Fastest acting antithyroid drugs** *(Recent Question 2016)*
   a. Iodides of Na/ K   b. Propylthiuracil
   c. Methimazole   d. Nitrates

40. **Drug that decreases size of prostate is** *(AIIMS Nov 2017)*
   a. Tamsulosin   b. Sildenafil
   c. Finasteride   d. Flutamide

41. **Which of the following is glucocorticoid inhibitor:** *(Recent Question 2017)*
   a. Metyrapone   b. Mapracorat
   c. Mitotane   d. Miltefosine

42. **Orally active anti-diabetic drug used in type-1 DM** *(TNPG 2015)*
   a. Acarbose   b. Taragliptins
   c. Glimipride   d. Amylin analogues

43. **Drug of choice for acute migraine is** *(Recent Question 2016)*
   a. Sumatriptan   b. Ergot alkaloids
   c. Ondansetron   d. Ketanserin

44. **Which of the following anti rheumatic drug acts by increasing extracellular adenosine?** *(AIIMS May 2017)*
   a. Hydroxychloroquine b. Leflunomide
   c. Methotrexate   d. Azathioprine

Ranjan Kumar Patel, Conceptual Review of Pharmacology for NBE; 3rd Edition

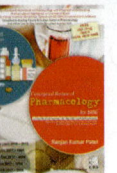

Ranjan Kumar Patel, Conceptual Review of Pharmacology for NBE; 3rd Edition

45. **Which drug is not used for acute bronchial asthma** *(Recent Question 2016)*
    a. Salmeterol
    b. Formeterol
    c. Salbutamol
    d. Corticosteroids

46. **The drug that produces least inhibition of CYP450 is** *(AIIMS May 2016)*
    a. Omeprazole
    b. Rabeprazole
    c. Lansoprazole
    d. Pantoprazole

47. **Proton pump inhibitors are most effective when they are given** *(Recent Question 2016)*
    a. After meals
    b. Shortly before meals
    c. Along with H_2 blockers
    d. During prolonged fasting periods

48. **Antidote of fibrinolytic drug is** *(AIIMS May 2017)*
    a. Heparin
    b. Epsilon aminocaproic acid
    c. Protamine
    d. Alteplase

49. **Which is not an antiplatelet drug ?** *(Recent Question Dec 2016)*
    a. Aspirin
    b. Streptokinase
    c. Clopidogrel
    d. Ticlopidine

50. **Which of the following has proved antithrombotic property** *(Recent Question 2016)*
    a. Gelatin
    b. Dextran 40
    c. Dextran 100
    d. Hexastarch

 ## Answers Keys

1.	a	2.	d	3.	a	4.	a	5.	c	6.	d	7.	a	8.	a	9.	d	10.	a
11.	d	12.	a	13.	a	14.	c	15.	a	16.	a,b, e	17.	b	18.	d	19.	c	20.	a
21.	a	22.	b	23.	a	24.	b	25.	c	26.	a	27.	c	28.	c	29.	c	30.	c
31.	a	32.	c	33.	d	34.	b	35.	a	36.	a	37.	b	38.	d	39.	a	40.	c
41.	a	42.	a	43.	a	44.	c	45.	a	46.	d	47.	b	48.	b	49.	b	50.	b

Microbiology

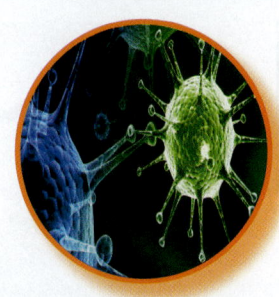

 **Spotters**

○ **Bug:** H influenzae
○ **Media Used for Isolation:** Chocolate agar

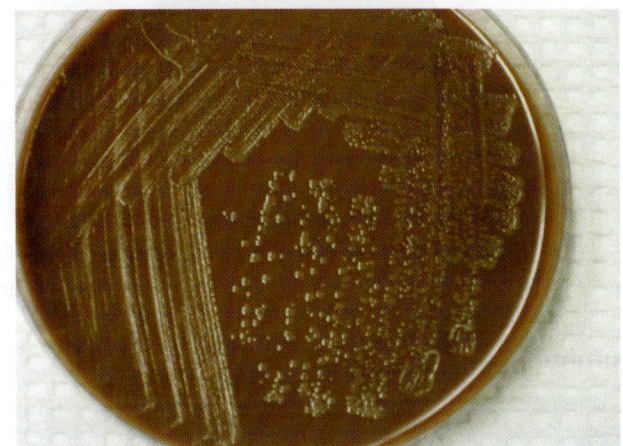

○ Media Contents/Other: Factors V (NAD+) and X (haematin)
○ Bug: N gonorrhoeae, N meningitidis
○ Media Used for Isolation: **Thayer-Martin agar**

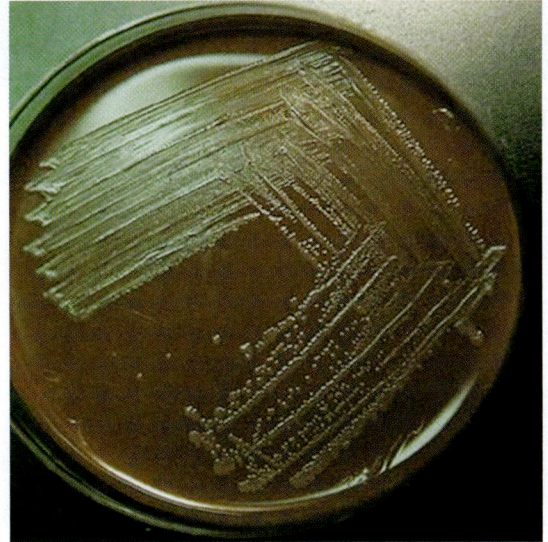

○ **Media Contents/Other:** Selectively favours growth of Neisseria by inhibiting growth of gram ⊕ organisms with **V**ancomycin, gram ⊖ organisms except Neisseria with **T**rimethoprim and **C**olistin, and fungi with **N**ystatin.

Mnemonics: Very **T**ypically **C**ultures *Neisseria*

○ **Bug:** B pertussis
○ **Media Used for Isolation: Bordet:** Gengou agar (Bordet for Bordetella), Regan-Lowe medium

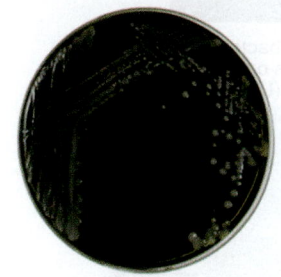

Fig. 1: Regan-Lowe medium   **Fig.** Bordet- Gengou agar (Bordet for Bordetella)

○ **Media Contents/Other:** Potato extract Charcoal, blood, antibiotic
○ **Bug:** C. diphtheriae
○ **Media Used for Isolation:** Tellurite agar, Löffler medium

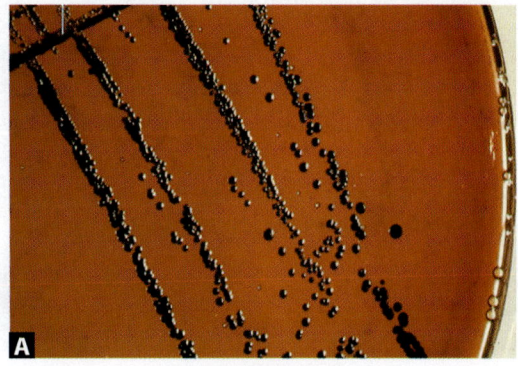

Tellurite agar

Malathi Murugesan, Microns Microbiology Simplified; 1st Edition

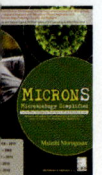

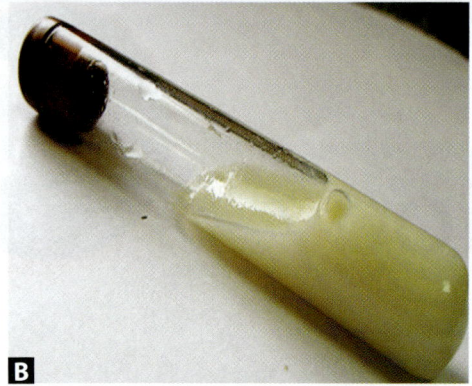

Löffler medium

- **Bug:** M tuberculosis
- **Media Used for Isolation:** Löwenstein-Jensen agar

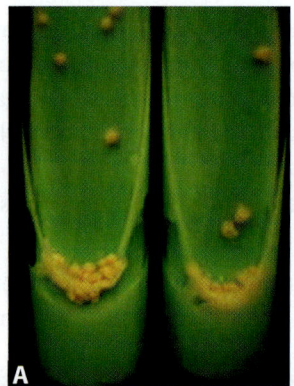

Colonies of Mycobacterium tuberculosis on Lowenstein-Jensen (LT) Medium

- **Bug:** M pneumoniae
- **Media Used for Isolation:** Eaton agar

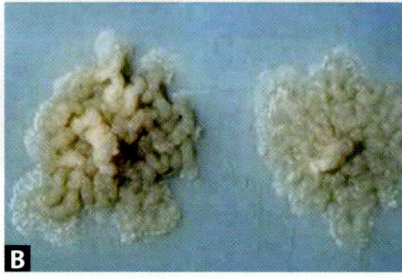

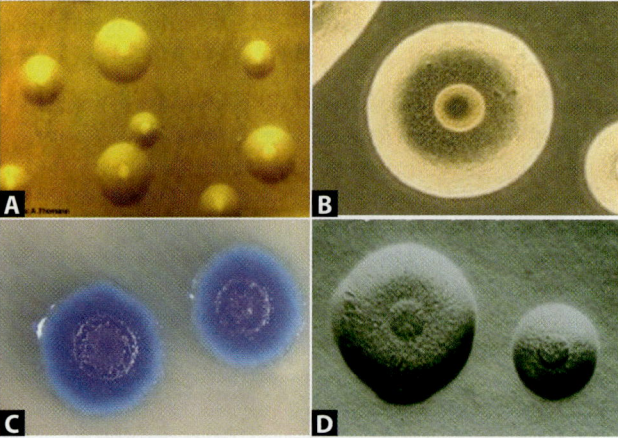

- **Media Contents/Other:** Requires cholesterol
- **Bug:** E. coli
- **Media Used for Isolation:** Eosin–methylene blue (EMB) agar

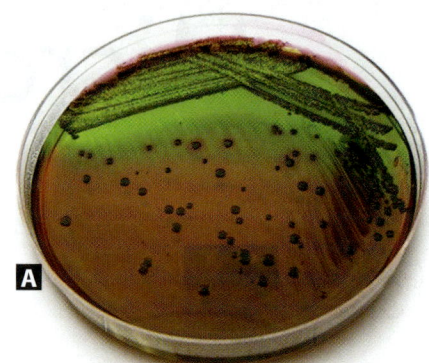

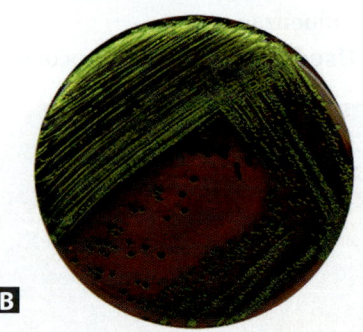

- Media Contents/Other: Colonies with green metallic sheen

Tumbling Motility: Listeria

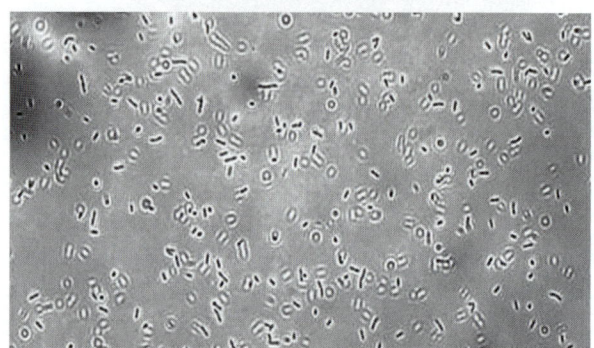

Gliding Motility: Mycoplasma

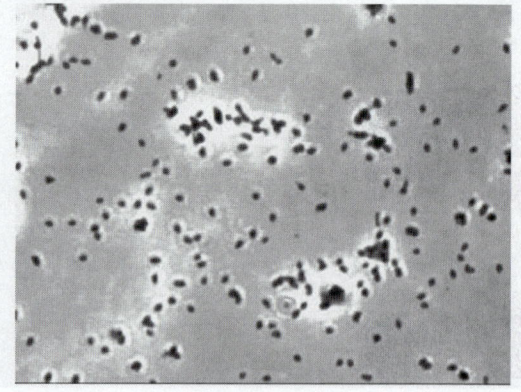

Darting Motility: Vibrio Cholerae, Campylobacter

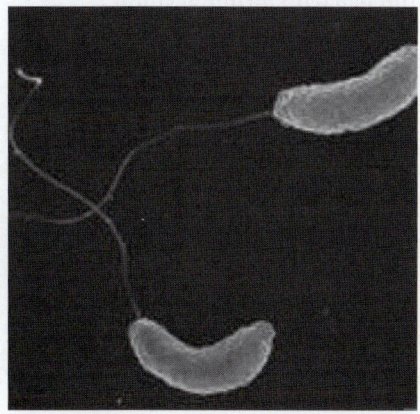

Swarming Motility: Proteus, Clostridium tetani

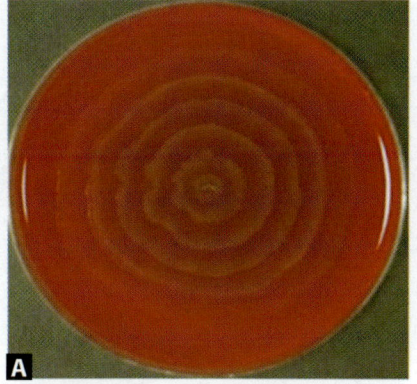

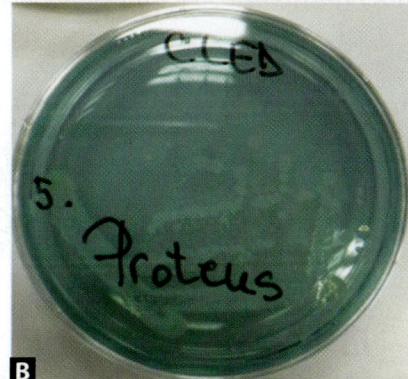

Corkscrew, Lashing, Flexion, Extension: Spirochete

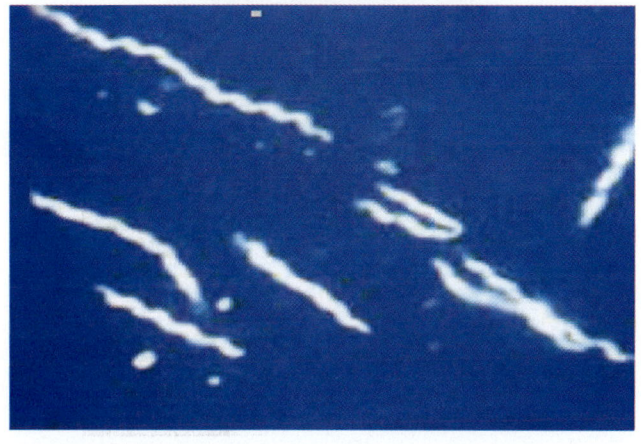

Diphyllobothrium Lactum: Operculated eggs in stool

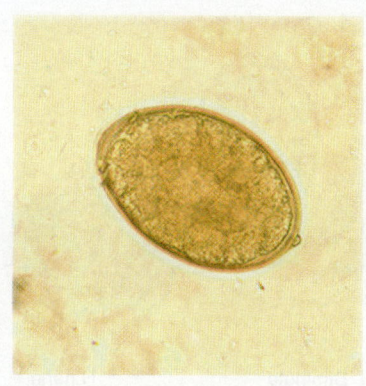

Hymenolepis Nana: Egg smaller, bile non stained and has polar filament.

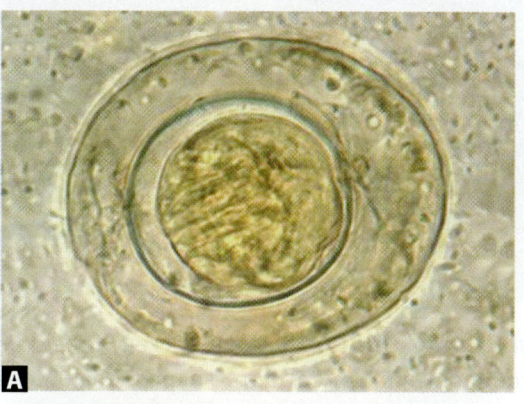

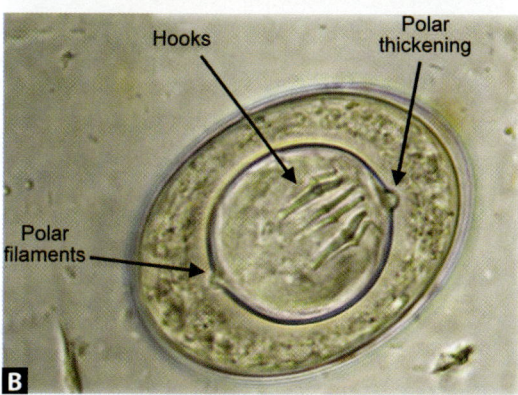

Hymenolepis Diminuta: Detection of Egg in stool; Egg larger and lack of polar filament.

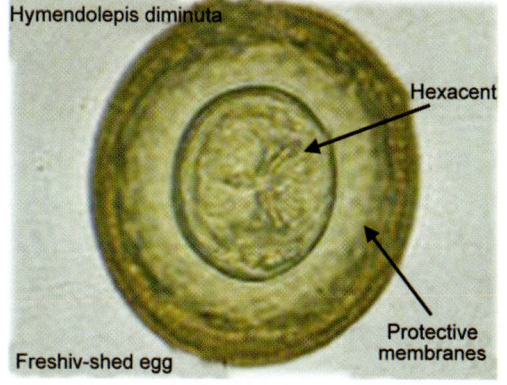

Malathi Murugesan, Microns Microbiology Simplified; 1st Edition

Malathi Murugesan, Microns Microbiology Simplified; 1st Edition

H.NANA Vs H. DIMINUTA

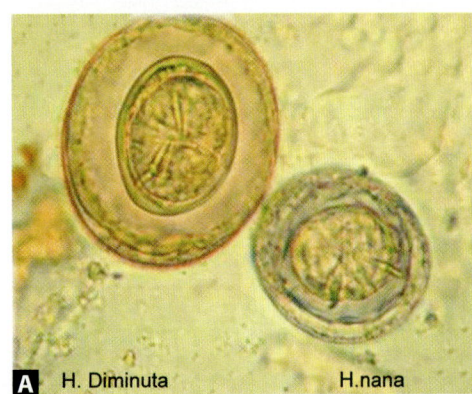

A   H. Diminuta   H.nana

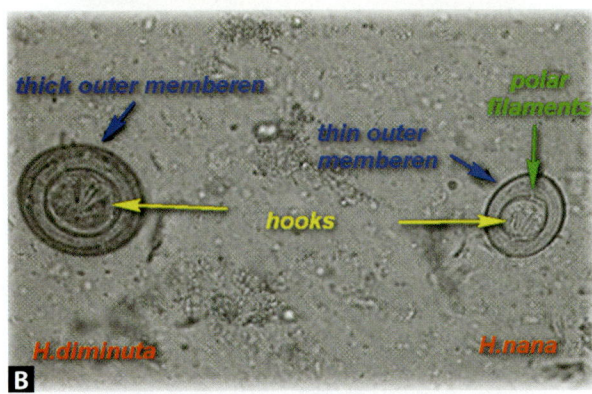

B

Dipylidium Caninum: Eggs in packets, Proglottid has two common genital pore, Barrel shaped Proglottid.

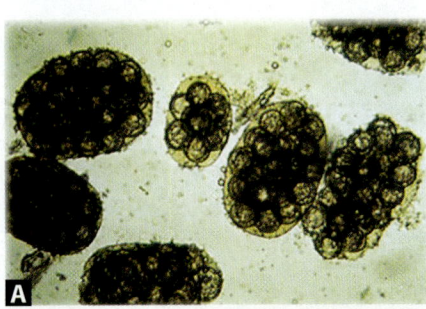

A

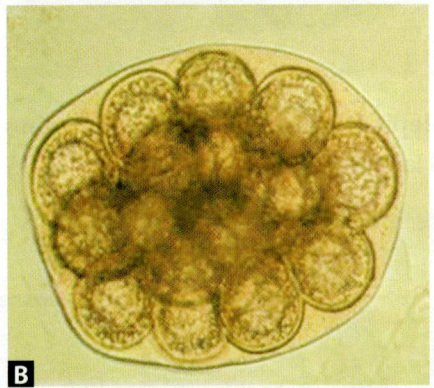

B

Schistosoma Hematobium: Schistosoma haematobium egg with terminal spine

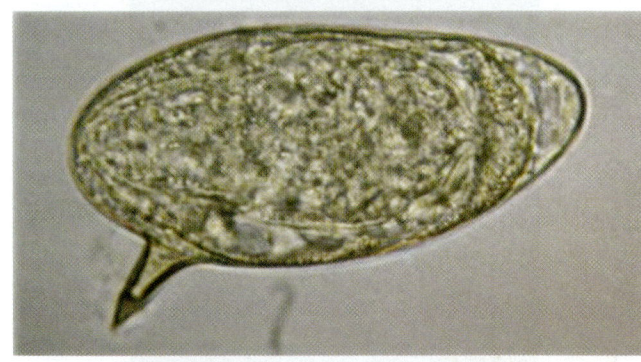

Schistosoma Mansoni: Egg has lateral spine (feces), eggs of S. mansoni are acid fast.

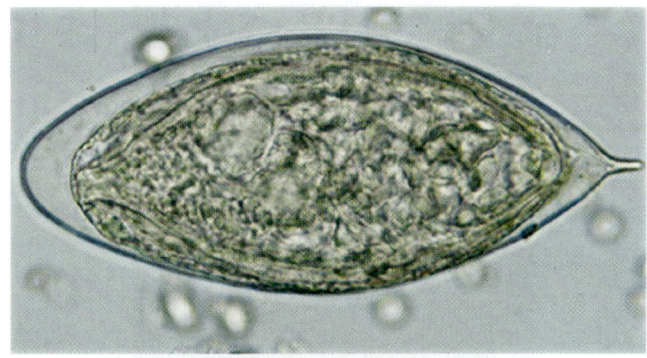

Schistosoma Japonicum: Egg with nubby spine

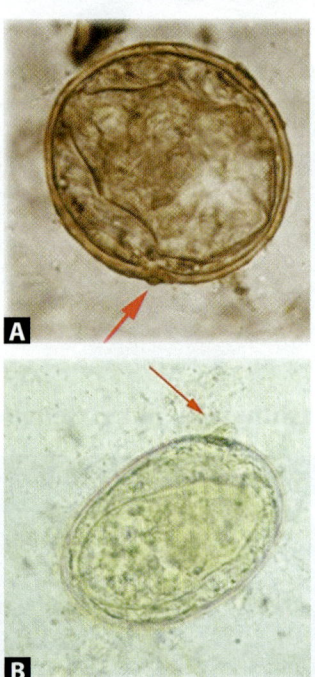

A

B

Fasciola Hepatica: Operculated eggs in stool

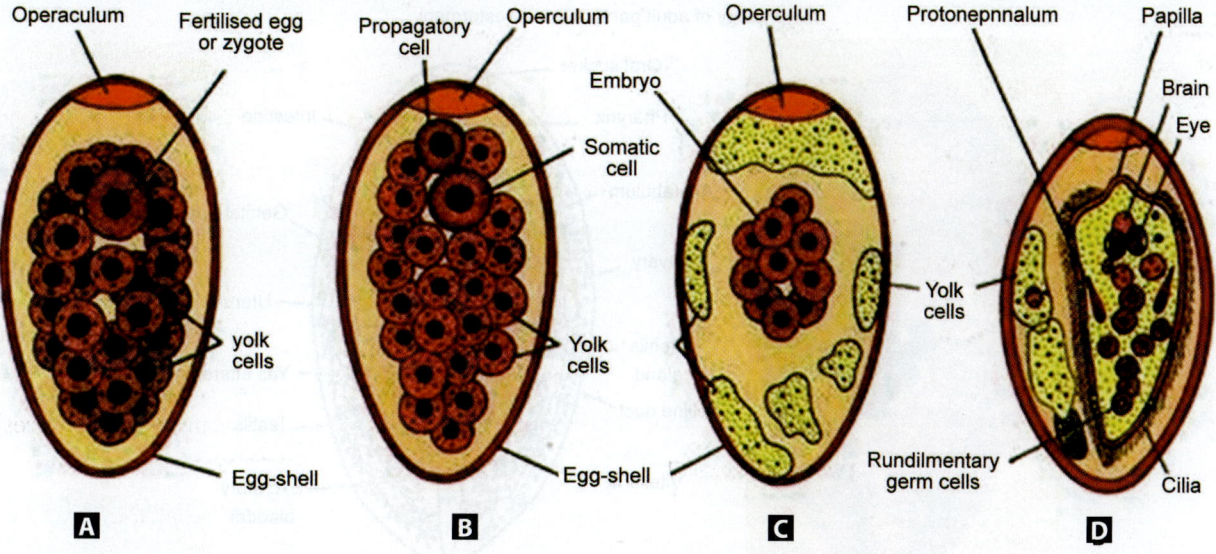

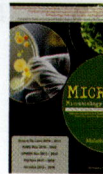

Malathi Murugesan, Microns Microbiology Simplified; 1st Edition

Operaculum — Fertilised egg or zygote — yolk cells — Egg-shell **A**

Propagatory cell — Operculum — Yolk cells — Egg-shell **B**

Operculum — Embryo — Somatic cell — Yolk cells — Rundilmentary germ cells **C**

Protonepnnalum — Papilla — Brain — Eye — Yolk cells — Cilia **D**

Figs 3A to D: *Fasciola hepatica*. Early stages of development. **A.** Fertilised egg; **B.** Two cell stage; **C.** Many cell stage; **D.** Miracidium in capsules

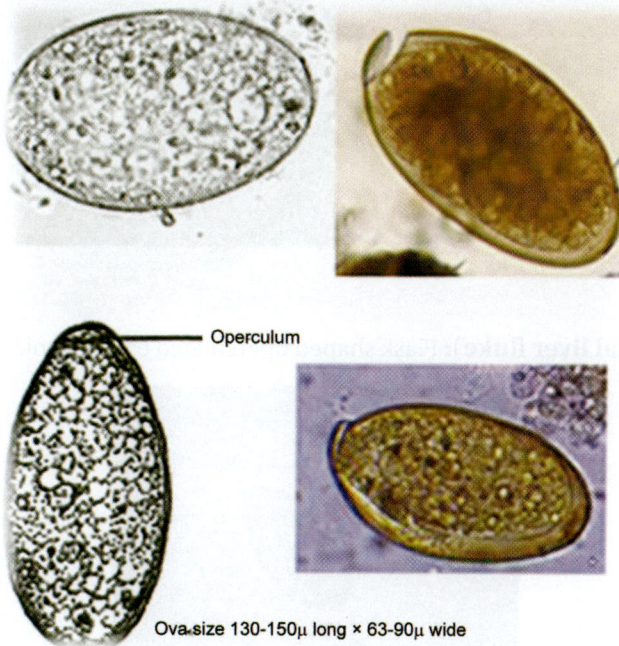

Operculum

Ova size 130-150µ long × 63-90µ wide

Fasciola Buski: Operculated eggs in stool

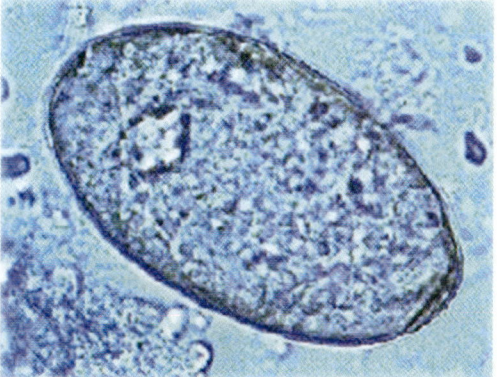

Malathi Murugesan, Microns Microbiology Simplified; 1st Edition

Paragonimus Westermani (Lung Fluke): Operculated eggs in early morning, deeply coughed sputum

Morphology of adult paragonimus westermani

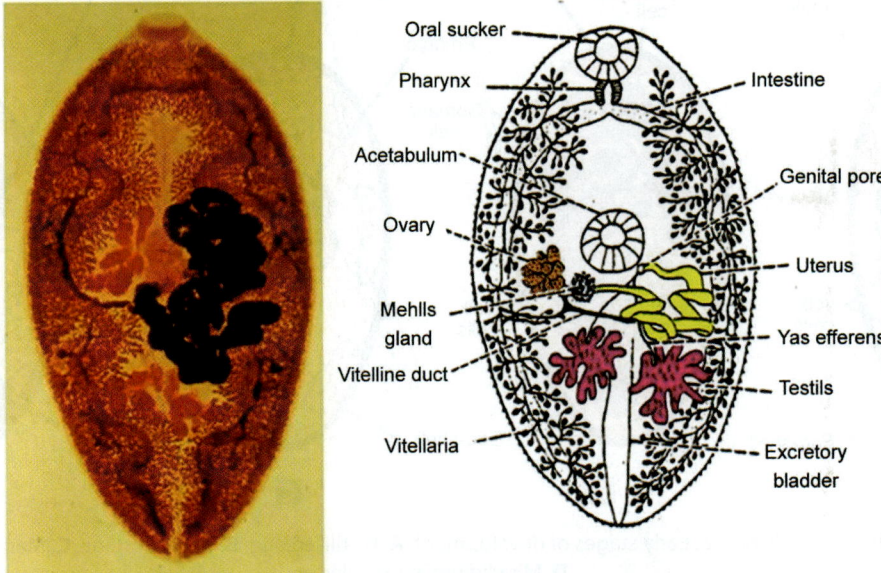

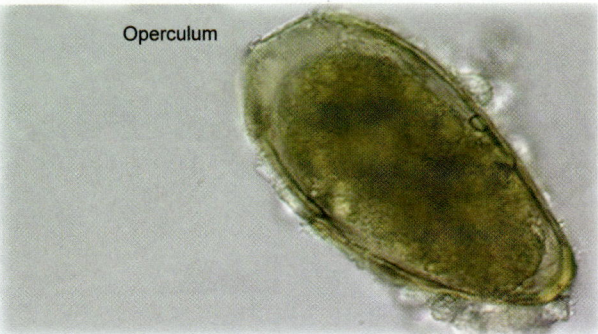

Clonorchis Sinensis (Oriental liver fluke): Flask shaped operculated egg in stool.

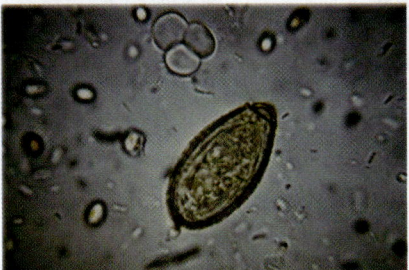

Varicella-Zoster virus (HHV-3)

- **Route of transmission:** Respiratory secretions
- **Clinical significance:** Varicella-zoster chickenpox (A), shingles (B), encephalitis, pneumonia. Most common complication of shingles is post-herpetic neuralgia.

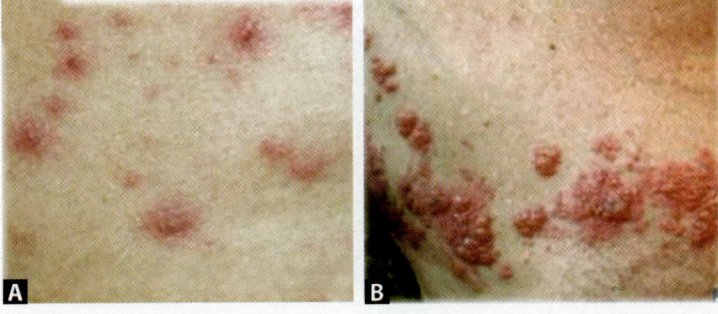

Notes: Latent in dorsal root or trigeminal ganglia; CN V1 branch involvement can cause herpes zoster ophthalmicus.

Epstein-Barr Virus (HHV-4)

Route of transmission: Respiratory secretions, saliva; aka "kissing disease," (common in teens, young adults)

Clinical significance: Mononucleosis—fever, hepatosplenomegaly, pharyngitis, and lymphadenopathy (especially posterior cervical nodes **(A).** Avoid contact sports until resolution due to risk of splenic rupture. Associated with lymphomas (e.g., endemic Burkitt lymphoma), nasopharyngeal carcinoma (especially Asian adults), lymphoproliferative disease in transplant patients.

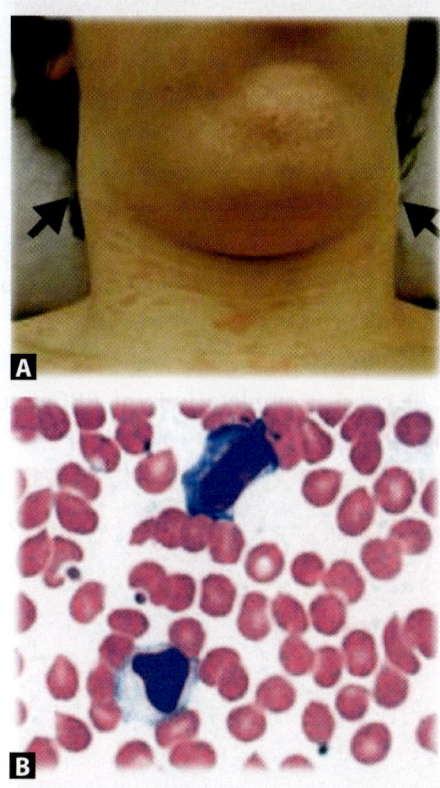

Notes: Infects B cells through CD21. Atypical lymphocytes on peripheral blood smear(B)—not infected B cells but reactive cytotoxic T cells. ⊕ Monospot test—heterophile antibodies detected by agglutination of sheep or horse RBCs. Use of amoxicillin in mononucleosis can cause characteristic maculopapular rash.

Human Herpes Virus 8

Route of transmission: Sexual contact

Clinical significance:

○ Kaposi sarcoma (neoplasm of endothelial cells).
○ Seen in HIV/AIDS and transplant patients.

○ Dark/ violaceous plaques or nodules
○ Representing vascular proliferations.

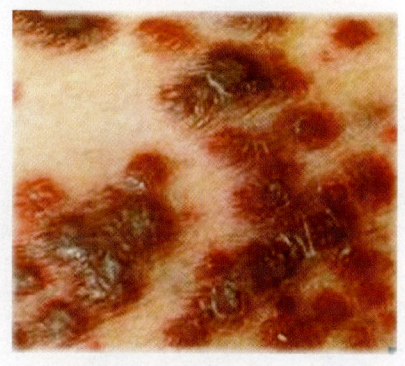

Notes: Can also affect GI tract and lungs.

HSV Identification

○ Viral culture for skin/genitalia.
○ CSF PCR for herpes encephalitis.
○ Tzanck test—a smear of an opened skin vesicle to detect multinucleated giant cells commonly seen in HSV-1, HSV-2, and VZV infection. PCR of skin lesions is currently test of choice. Intranuclear eosinophilic Cowdry inclusions also seen with HSV-1, HSV-2, VZV.

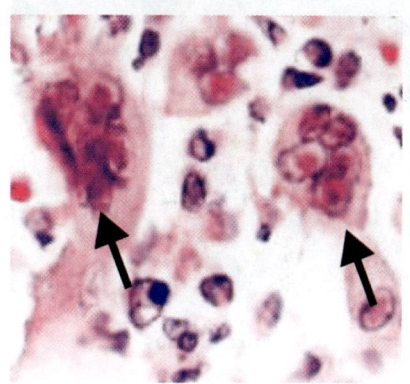

Nocardia

○ Aerobe
○ Acid fast (weak)

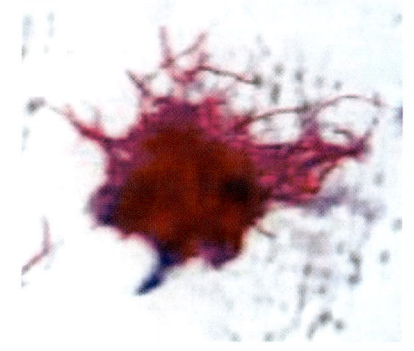

Malathi Murugesan, Microns Microbiology Simplified; 1st Edition

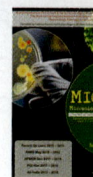

Malathi Murugesan, Microns Microbiology Simplified; 1st Edition

Actinomyces

- Anaerobe
- Not acid fast

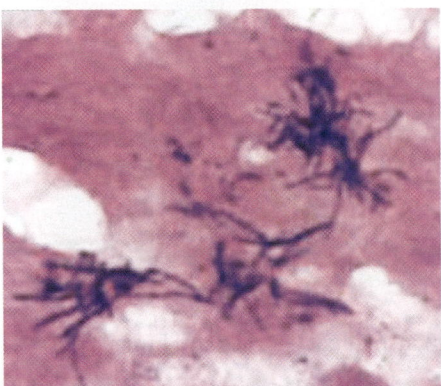

Silver Stain

- Pneumocystis jirovecii,
- Legionella,
- Helicobacter pylori

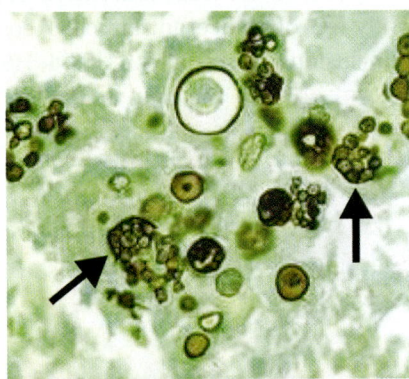

Coccidioides

Gonococci

- No polysaccharide capsule
- No maltose metabolized
- No vaccine due to antigenic variation of pilus proteins

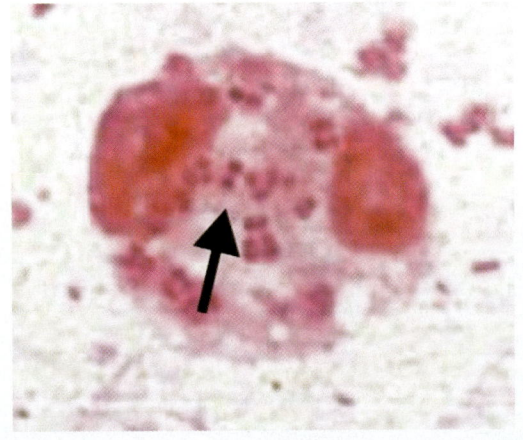

- Sexually or perinatally transmitted

α-hemolytic bacteria

- Gram ⊕ cocci. Partial reduction of hemoglobin causes greenish or brownish color without clearing around growth on blood agar.

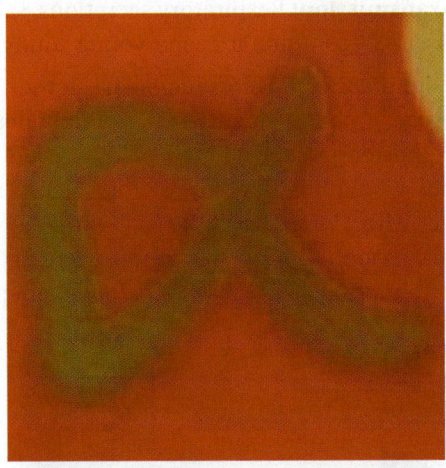

- Include the following organisms:
  - Streptococcus pneumoniae (catalase ⊖ and optochin sensitive)
  - Viridans streptococci (catalase ⊖ and optochin resistant)

β-hemolytic bacteria

- Gram ⊕ cocci. Complete lysis of RBCs clear area surrounding colony on blood agar.

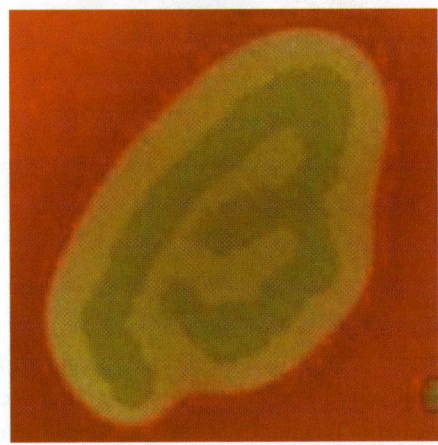

- Include the following organisms:
  - Staphylococcus aureus (catalase and coagulase ⊕)
  - Streptococcus pyogenes—group A strep (catalase ⊖ and bacitracin sensitive)
  - Streptococcus agalactiae—group B strep (catalase ⊖ and bacitracin resistant)

Klebsiella

- Gram ⊖ rod; intestinal flora that causes lobar pneumonia in alcoholics and diabetics when aspirated. Very mucoid colonies caused by abundant polysaccharide capsules.

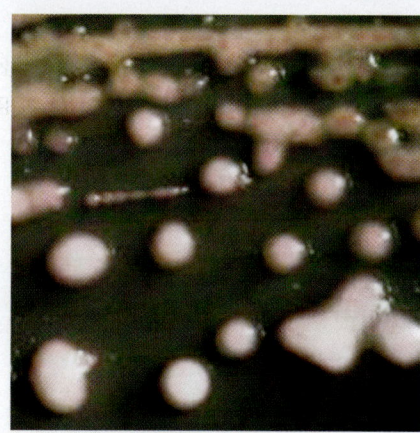

○ Dark red "currant jelly" sputum (blood/mucus).

Histoplasmosis

○ Macrophage filled with Histoplasma (smaller than RBC).

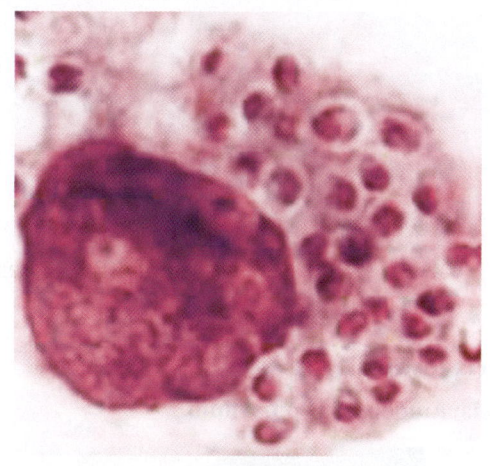

○ Histo hides (within macrophages) Bird (e.g., starlings) or bat droppings.

Blastomycosis

○ Broad-based budding of Blastomyces (same size as RBC).

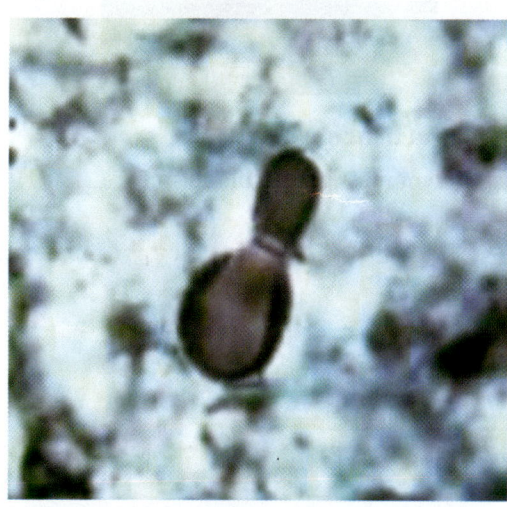

○ Forms granulomatous nodules

Coccidioidomycosis

○ Spherule (much larger than RBC) filled with endospores of Coccidioides.

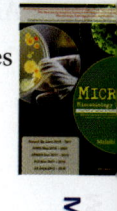

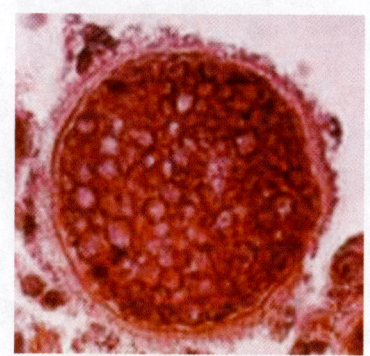

Paracoccidioidomycosis

○ Budding yeast of Paracoccidioides with "captain's wheel" formation (much larger than RBC).

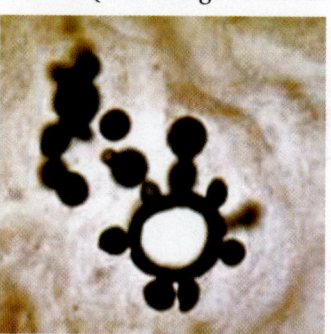

Candida albicans

○ Dimorphic; forms pseudohyphae and budding yeasts at 20°C.

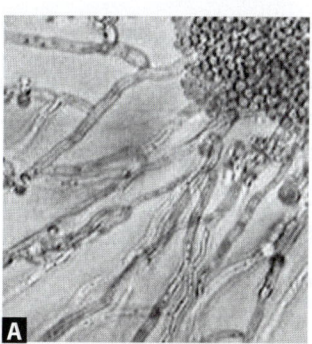

Pseudohyphae

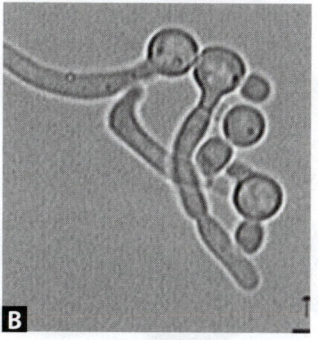

Germ tubes

○ Germ tubes at 37°C.

Malathi Murugesan, Microns Microbiology Simplified; 1st Edition

Malathi Murugesan, Microns Microbiology Simplified; 1st Edition

Aspergillus fumigatus

○ Septate hyphae that branch at 45° Acute Angle.

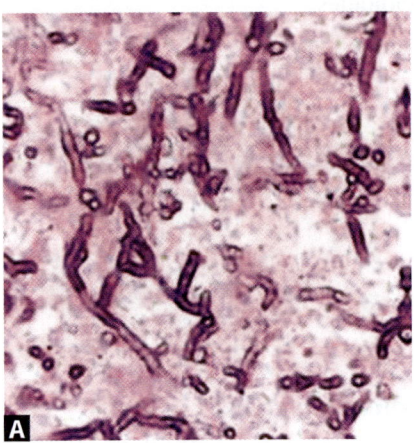

Acute angle

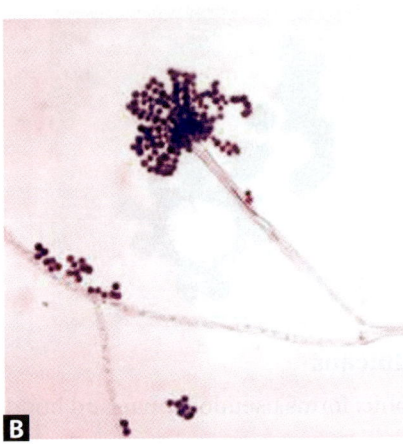

Conidiophore

○ Produces conidia in radiating chains at end of conidiophore

Mucor and Rhizopus spp.

○ Irregular, broad, non-septate hyphae branching at wide angles.

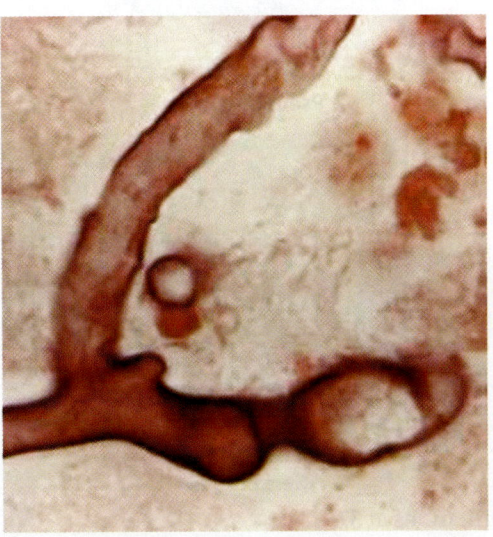

Pneumocystis jirovecii

○ Disc-shaped yeast seen on methenamine silver stain of lung tissue.

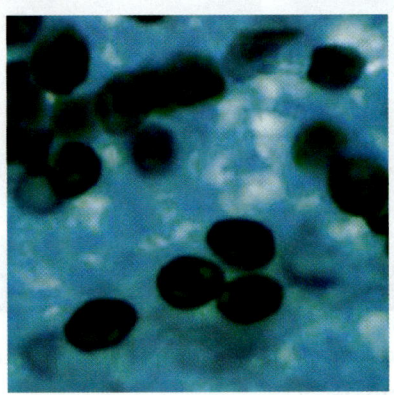

Toxoplasma Gondii

Diagnosis: Serology, biopsy (tachyzoite)

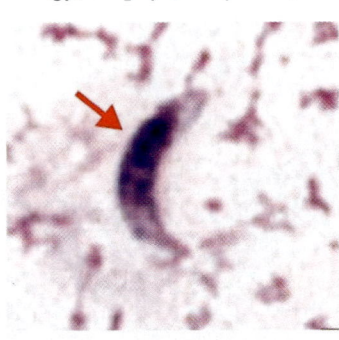

Naegleria fowleri

Diagnosis: Amoebas in spinal fluid

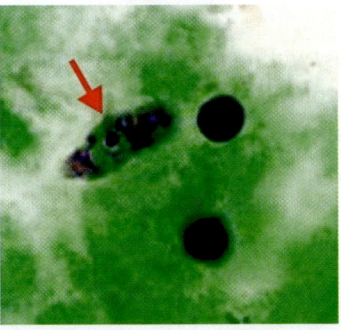

Trypanosoma brucei

Diagnosis: Trypomastigote in blood smear

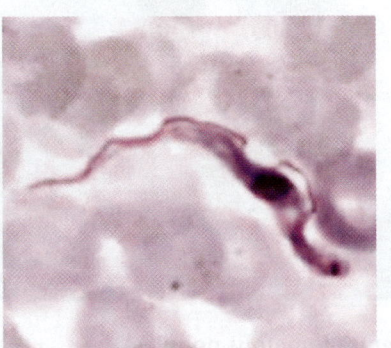

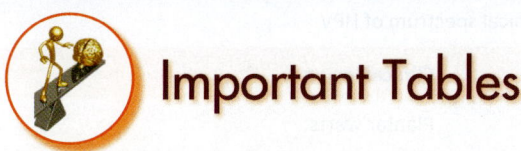

Important Tables

Malathi Murugesan, Microns Microbiology Simplified; 1st Edition

Table 1: Official and common names of Herpesvirus

Official name	Common name
Herpesvirus type 1	HSV – 1 – Herpes simplex virus 1
Herpesvirus type 2	HSV – 2 – Herpes simplex virus 2
Herpesvirus type 3	Varicella Zoster virus
Herpesvirus type 4	Epstein Barr virus
Herpesvirus type 5	Cytomegalovirus
Herpesvirus type 6	Human B cell lymphotropic virus
Herpesvirus type 7	R K virus
Herpesvirus type 8	Rhadinovirus

Courtesy: Malathi Murugesan, Microns Microbiology Simplified; 1st Edition

Table 2: Stages of Hemoflagellates

Amastigotes and Promastigotes	Leishmania
Amastigote	Trypanosoma cruzi
Epimastigotes and Trypomastigotes	Trypanosoma brucei and cruzi

Courtesy: Malathi Murugesan, Microns Microbiology Simplified; 1st Edition

Table 3: Lab diagnosis of Taenia infections

Taenia solium	Taenia saginata
• Intestinal taeniasis– diagnosed by demonstration of gravid proglottids in the feces; • As eggs are morphologically similar with *T.saginata* it does not help in confirmatory diagnosis	• Intestinal taeniasis– diagnosed by demonstration of gravid proglottids in the feces; • As eggs are morphologically similar with *T.saginata* it does not help in confirmatory diagnosis
• Neurocysticercosis– diagnosed by imaging methods like CT and MRI which shows the number, site and stage of cysticerci (calcifications) • CT is best method • Serodiagnosis like ELISA helps to identify the antibodies in serum and CSF • Postmortem diagnosis by demonstration of cysticerci in the brain biopsy tissue	*Eggs of both Taenia saginata and solium can be differentiating by acid fast staining*
	Eggs of *T. saginata* are acid fast
	Eggs of *T. solium* are non acid fast
Treatment: • Praziquantel • Niclosamide • Albendazole • ***Praziquantel is the ideal DOC + needs to be given with steroids to avoid inflammatory reactions caused by dead cysticerci***	*Treatment:* • Praziquantel • Niclosamide

Courtesy: Malathi Murugesan, Microns Microbiology Simplified; 1st Edition

Table 4: Organism and culture appearances

Culture appearance	Organism
Golden yellow colonies	Coagulase positive staphylococci
White colonies/Oil paint	Coagulase negative staphylococci
Glossy colonies	Avirulent streptococci
Spidery colonies/Sunray	Actinomyces
Jet black colonies	Salmonella
Satellitism	H. Influenza
School of fish/Rail track	H. ducreyi
Stormy fermentation	Gl. Perfringens
Thumb print/Aluminium paint/Bisected pearl/ Mercury drops	Bordetella
Fried egg colonies	Mycoplasma
Draughtsman/Carom coin	Pneumococci
Fish in stream/Swarm of gnats	V. Cholerae

Courtesy: Ranjan Kumar Patel & Sudhir Kumar Singh, Review of NEET & DNB Pattern Qs 2018; 1st Edition

Table 5: Fever causing organisms

Fever	Organism
Shanghai fever	Pseudomonas
Undulant/Malta fever	Brucella
Brazilian purpuric fever	Haemophilus aegyptius
Haverhill/Rat bite fever	Streptobacillus moniliformis
Soduku	Spirillum minus
Cat scratch disease	Bartonella henslae
Oraya fever/Carrion's disease	Bartonella bcilliformis
Goal fever/Epidemic thypus	R. prowazekii
Weil's disease	Leptospira

Courtesy: Ranjan Kumar Patel & Sudhir Kumar Singh, Review of NEET & DNB Pattern Qs 2018; 1st Edition

Table 6: Classification of Virus

DNA Virus

DNA virus	Virion	Nuclei acid
Parvo virus B-19	Naked	SS (–)
Papilloma virus, JC virus, BK virus, Polyoma virus	Naked	ds circular (+/–)
Adeno virus	Naked	ds (+/–)
Hepatitis B virus	Enveloped	ds with ss (+/–) circular
HSV – I, II, EBV, CMV, VZV	Enveloped	ds (+/–)
Variola, Molluscum contagiosum	Complex coats	ds (+/–)

Malathi Murugesan, Microns Microbiology Simplified; 1st Edition

RNA Virus

RNA virus	Virion	Nuclei acid
Polio, Coxsackie, Entero, Rhino, Hepatitis A virus	Naked	SS (+)
Astrovirus	Naked	SS (+)
HEV, Norwalk	Naked	SS (+)
Rota, Reo, Orbivirus	Naked	ds segmented (+/−)
Rubella	Enveloped	SS (+)
HCV, HGV, Yellow fever, Dengue fever	Enveloped	SS (+)
Lassa fever virus	Enveloped	SS segmented (−)
Corona virus	Enveloped	SS (+)
HIV − 1, 2, HLTV − 1, 2, Slow viral group	Enveloped	SS diploid (+)
Influenza − A, B, C	Enveloped	SS segmented (−)
Hanta virus, Sandfly fever virus	Enveloped	SS segmented (−)
Bornavirus	Enveloped	SS
Rabies, Vesicular stomatitis virus	Enveloped	SS (−)
Parainfluenza, RSV, Mumps, Rubeola, New Castle virus	Enveloped	SS (−)
Marburg virus, Ebola virus	Enveloped	SS (−)

Courtesy: Ranjan Kumar Patel & Sudhir Kumar Singh, Review of NEET & DNB Pattern Qs 2018; 1st Edition

Table 7: Clinical spectrum of HPV

HPV type	Clinical lesion
1, 4	Plantar warts
2, 4, 26, 27, 29	Common warts
3, 10, 28, 41	Flat warts
5, 8	Epidermodysplasia verruciformis
6, 11	Anogenital condylomas, Laryngeal papillomas Intraepithelial neoplasia
7	Hand warts
9, 12, 14, 15, 17, 19 − 25, 36, 46, 47	Epidermodysplasia verruciformis
13, 32	Oral focal epithelial hyperplasia
16, 18, 30, 31, 33, 35, 39, 45, 51, 52, 56	High grade dysplasia, CA genital mucosa, CA Larynx and Oesophagus
34, 40, 42, 44, 53 − 55, 58, 59, 61, 62, 64, 66, 69	Intraepithelial neoplasia
75, 77	Common warts in organ transplant patients
37	Keratocanthoma

Courtesy: Ranjan Kumar Patel & Sudhir Kumar Singh, Review of NEET & DNB Pattern Qs 2018; 1st Edition

Table 8: Parasites − Life cycles

Parasite	Definitive host	Intermediate host	Infective form
Protozoa			
Entamoeba histolytica	Human	−	Mature quadrinucleate cyst
Naegleria fowleri	Human		Amoeboid form of trophozoites
Acanthamoeba culbertsoni	Human		Trophozoites, Cyst
Giardia lamblia	Human		Mature cyst
Trichomonas vaginalis	Male/Female		Trophozoites
Trypanosoma brucei gambiense	Human	Tsetse fly	Metacyclic trypomastigote
Trypanosoma brucei rhodesiense	Human	Tsetse fly	Metacyclic trypomastigote
Trypanosoma cruzi	Human	Reduviid bug	Metacyclic trypomastigote
Leishmania donovani	Human	Phlebotomus sandfly	Promastigote
Plasmodium	Female anopheles mosquito	Human	Sporozoites
Babesia	Ixodid ticks	Human	Sporozoites
Toxoplasma gondii	Cats (Enteric cycle)	Human (Exoenteric cycle)	Tissue containing tissue cyst and oocyst
Isospora belli	Human		Sporulated oocyst
Cryptos-poridium parvum	Human		Sporulated oocyst
Cyclospora cayetanensis	Human		Sporulated oocyst

Parasite	Definitive host	Intermediate host	Infective form
Sarcocystsis hominis	Human	Cattle	Oocyst in undercooked beef
Sarcocystis suihominis	Human	Pig	Oocyst in undercooked pork
Sarcocystis lindemani		Human	Ingestion of water with oocyst
Balantidium coli	Pig	Human	Cyst
Cestodes			
Diphyllobothrium latum	Man	Fresh water eldman	Third stage plerocercoid larva
		Fresh water fish	
Spirometra	Dog, Cat	Cyclops	Third stage plerocercoid larva
		Snakes, Frogs, Fishes	
Taenia saginata	Human	Cattle	Cysticercus bovis
Taenia solium	Human	Pig	Cysticercus cellulosae
Cysticercosis	Human	Human	Egg of T.solium
Echinococcus granulosus	Dog, Wolf, Jackal, Fox	Sheep, Cattle	Ingestion of water contaminated with eggs
Hymenolepis nana	Human		Ingestion of water contaminated with eggs
Dipylidium caninum	Dogs, Cats	Flea	Ingestion of flea harbouring cysticercoids larva
Trematodes			
Schistosoma hematobium	Humans	Fresh water snails	Cercaria larva
Schistosoma mansoni	Humans	Fresh water snails	Fork tailed cercaria
Schistosoma japonicum	Humans	Fresh water snails	Fork tailed cercaria
Clonorchis sinensis	Human	Snail	Metacercaria larva
		Fish	
Fasciola hepatica	Sheep, Goat, Human	Snail	Metacercaria encysted on aquatic vegetation
		Aquatic plants	
Fasciolopsis buski	Man, Pigs	Snail	Metacercaria encysted on aquatic vegetation
		Aquatic plants	
Heterophyes	Humans, Cats, Dogs	Snails	Undercooked fishes containing metacercaria
		Fishes	
Gastrodiscoides hominis	Man, Pigs	Snails	Metacercaria encysted on aquatic vegetation
		Aquatic plants	
Paragonimus westermani	Man	Fresh water snail	Metacercaia encysted in crab or cray fish
		Fresh water crab/ Cray fish	
Nematodes			
Trichinella spiralis	Pig, Man		Encysted larva in striated muscles
Trichuris trichiura	Man		Embryonated eggs containing rhabditiform larvae
Strongyloides stercoralis	Man		Third stage filariform larvae
Ancylostoma duodenale	Man		Third stage filariform larvae
Enterobius	Man		Embryonated
Vermicularis			Eggs
Ascaris lumbricoides	Man		Embryonated eggs with rhabditiform larva
Wuchereria bancrofti	Man	Culex mosquito	Active motile third stage filariform larvae
Brugia malayi	Man	Mansonia	Active motile third stage filariform larvae
Brugia timori	Man	Anopheles	Active motile third stage filariform larvae
Loa loa	Man	Chrysops	Infective third stage larvae

Malathi Murugesan, Microns Microbiology Simplified; 1st Edition

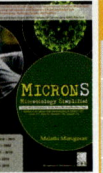

Malathi Murugesan, Microns Microbiology Simplified; 1st Edition

Parasite	Definitive host	Intermediate host	Infective form
Onchocerca volvulus	Human	Simulium flies	Infective third stage larvae
Dracunculus medinensis	Man	Cyclops	Infective third stage larvae
Angiostrongylus cantonensis	Rats	Molluscs, Slugs, Snails	Infective third stage larvae
Capillaria philippinensis	Birds	Fish	Fish containing third stage larvae
Gnathostomata spinigerum	Dog, Cat	Cyclops Fresh water fish and Frogs	Infective third stage larvae

Courtesy: Ranjan Kumar Patel & Sudhir Kumar Singh, Review of NEET & DNB Pattern Qs 2018; 1st Edition

Table 9: CD 4+ Count Associated with Disease in HIV + Patients

CD4+ Cell Count < 500/mm³

Pathogen	Presentation	Findings
Candida albicans	Oral thrush	Scrapable white plaque, pseudohyphae on microscopy
EBV	Oral hairy leukoplakia	Unscrapable white plaque on lateral tongue
Bartonella henselae	Bacillary angiomatosis	Biopsy with neutrophilic inflammation
HHV-8	Kaposi sarcoma	Biopsy with lymphocytic inflammation
HPV	Squamous cell carcinoma, commonly of anus (men who have sex with men) or cervix (women)	

CD4+ Cell Count < 200/mm³

Pathogen	Presentation	Findings
Histoplasma capsulatum	Fever, weight loss, fatigue, cough, dyspnea, nausea, vomiting, diarrhoea	Oval yeast cells within macrophages
HIV	Dementia	
JC virus (reactivation)	Progressive multifocal leukoencephalopathy	Non enhancing areas of demyelination on MRI
Pneumocystis jirovecii	*Pneumocystis* pneumonia	"Ground-glass" opacities on CXR

CD4+ cell count < 100/mm³

Pathogen	Presentation	Findings
Aspergillus fumigatus	Haemoptysis, pleuritic pain	Cavitation or infiltrates on chest imaging
Candida albicans	Esophagitis	White plaques on endoscopy; yeast and pseudohyphae on biopsy
CMV	Retinitis, esophagitis, colitis, pneumonitis, encephalitis	Linear ulcers on endoscopy, cotton wool spots on fundoscopy Biopsy reveals cells with intranuclear (owl eye) inclusion bodies
Cryptococcus neoformans	Meningitis	Encapsulated yeast on India ink stain or capsular antigen ⊕
Cryptosporidium spp.	Chronic, watery diarrhoea	Acid-fast oocysts in stool
EBV	B-cell lymphoma (eg, non-Hodgkin lymphoma, CNS lymphoma)	CNS lymphoma—ring enhancing, may be solitary (vs *Toxoplasma*)
Mycobacterium avium intracellulare, Mycobacterium avium complex	Nonspecific systemic symptoms (fever, night sweats, weight loss) or focal lymphadenitis	
Toxoplasma gondii	Brain abscesses	Multiple ring-enhancing lesions on MRI

Courtesy: Ranjan Kumar Patel & Sudhir Kumar Singh, Review of NEET & DNB Pattern Qs 2018; 1st Edition

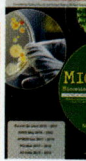

Table 10: Major histocompatibility complex (MHC) I and II

	MHC I	MHC II
Loci	HLA-**A**, HLA-**B**, HLA-**C** MHC I loci have 1 letter	HLA-**DP**, HLA-**DQ**, HLA-**DR** MHC II loci have 2 letters
Binding	TCR and CD8	TCR and CD4
Structure	1 long chain, 1 short chain	2 equal-length chains
Expression	All nucleated cells, APCs, platelets Not on RBCs	APCs
Function	Present **endogenously** synthesized **antigens** (e.g., viral or cytosolic proteins) to **CD8+ cytotoxic T cells**	Present **exogenously** synthesized **antigens** (e.g, bacterial proteins) to CD4+ helper T cells.
Antigen Loading	Antigen peptides loaded onto MHC I in RER after delivery via TAP (Transporter associated with antigen endosome processing)	Antigen loaded following release of invariant chain in an acidified
Associated proteins	β2-microglobulin Invariant chain	Invariant chain

Courtesy: Ranjan Kumar Patel & Sudhir Kumar Singh, Review of NEET & DNB Pattern Qs 2018; 1st Edition

Malathi Murugesan, Microns Microbiology Simplified; 1st Edition

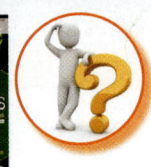

Malathi Murugesan, Microns Microbiology Simplified; 1st Edition

Important MCQs

1. Side chain theory for antibody production is proposed by *(Recent Pattern 2017)*
   a. Robert Koch
   b. Paul Ehrlich
   c. Elie Metchnikoff
   d. Louis Pasteur

2. Whitmore bacillus is
   a. Hemophilus influenza
   b. Burkholderia pseudomallei
   c. Corynebacterium pseudotuberculosis
   d. Burkholderia mallei

3. Temperature used for Pasteurisation is: *(Recent Pattern 2018)*
   a. 72°C for 20 min   b. 63°C for 30 min
   c. 100°C for 10min   d. 94°C for 20 min

4. Blood spill in operation theatre is cleaned with:
   a. Chlorine compound   *(Recent Pattern 2017)*
   b. Phenolic compound
   c. Quartnery ammounium compounds
   d. Alcoholic compounds

5. Simple basal media is: *(Recent Pattern July 15)*
   a. Simple nutrient agar
   b. Alkaline peptone water
   c. Glucose broth
   d. Blood agar

6. Advantage of CLED agar over MacConkey agar is:
   a. Supports the growth of Gram positive bacteria
   b. Prevent the swarming of Proteus
   c. Differentiates LF and NLF
   d. Helpful in diagnosis of UTI

7. Recombinant DNA technology is useful in all of the following except:
   a. Vaccine production   b. ELISA – antigen
   c. Transgenic animals   d. Southern blot

8. Staphylococcal pathogenicity is indicated by- *(Recent pattern Nov 2015)*
   a. Coagulase positivity   b. Hemolysis
   c. Lipoteichoic acid   d. Endotoxin

9. All are true about Streptococcus, except- *(AIIMS May 2010, 2011)*
   a. Streptodornase cleaves DNA
   b. Streptolysin O is active in reduced state
   c. Streptokinase is produced from serotype A, C, K
   d. Pyrogenic toxin A is plasmid mediated

10. In a school child had abscess on lower leg. Swab taken revealed Gram-positive b-hemolytic streptococci, and these were bacitracin sensitive. School physician observed that similar organism was isolated from throats of many other children. Which of the following is true statement with regards to this patient- *(AIIMS Nov 2015)*
    a. Difference in surface protein can differentiate the pathogenic bacteria from the pharyngeal culture bacteria
    b. Component C carbohydrate can differentiate the pathogenic bacteria from the throat culture bacteria
    c. MEG 3 positive are throat culture streptococci
    d. Depending on the M protein the cutaneous pathogenic bacteria can be differentiated from the pharyngeal culture bacteria

11. Regarding ASO titer all are seen except- *(AIIMS Nov 2009)*
    a. ASO can be increased in school children
    b. Maybe negative in poststreptococcal glomerulo-nephritis
    c. ASO titer included in major criteria in Jones criteria
    d. May not be elevated in 20% cases of carditis

12. Most severe form of conjunctivitis in neonates is caused by: *(Recent Pattern 2018)*
    a. Chlamydia trachomatis
    b. Staphylococcus aureus
    c. Neisseria gonorrhea
    d. Streptococcus agalactiae

13. Elek's gel precipitation test is seen in- *(Recent Pattern Aug 2013)*
    a. Clostridium   b. Corynebacterium
    c. Bacteroides   d. Campylobacter

14. Schick test is for- *(Recent Pattern 2012)*
    a. Susceptibility to diphtheria
    b. Susceptibility to tetanus
    c. Susceptibility to scarlet fever
    d. Susceptibility to RF

15. Best method of diagnosis for Clostridium difficile *(AIIMS Nov 2017)*
    a. Pure strain isolation from culture
    b. Immunofluorescence
    c. Toxin detection by ELISA
    d. Toxin gene detection by PCR

Malathi Murugesan, Microns Microbiology Simplified; 1st Edition

16. Most important serotype of *E. coli* causing Hemolytic Uremic Syndrome:

(Recent Pattern July 2016)

   a. O157: H7 of EHEC   b. O107: H7 of EIEC
   c. O157: H7 of ETEC   d. O109: H7 of EAEC

17. True about Widal test: *(Recent Pattern Dec 2016)*

   a. Anti-O antibody persists longer
   b. O antigen of S.paratyphi is used
   c. H-antigen is most immunogenic
   d. Felix tube is used for O agglutination

18. Burkholderia cepacia is intrinsically resistant to:

(Recent Pattern 2018)

   a. Ciprofloxacin   b. Ceftriaxone
   c. Polymyxin B   d. Ampicillin

19. The factor which promotes virulence of M. tuberculosis:

   a. Wax D   b. Cord factor
   c. Muramyl dipeptide   d. Mycolic acid

20. Which of the following is photochromogenic-

(Recent Pattern Dec 2014)

   a. M. kansasii   b. M. scrofulaceum
   c. M. intracellulare   d. M. avium

21. Urine LAM is used for diagnosis of:

(AIIMS Nov 2017)

   a. Mycobacterium tuberculosis
   b. Mycobacterium leprae
   c. Mycoplasma
   d. Listeria monocytogenes

22. Most sensitive test in syphilis:

(Recent Pattern Dec 2016)

   a. VDRL   b. TPHA
   c. RPR   d. FTA – ABS

23. Urease breath test is used for which organism:

   a. Haemophilus influenzae *(Recent Pattern 2018)*
   b. Campylobacter jejuni
   c. Helicobacter pylori
   d. Ureaplasma urealyticum

24. Lipschutz bodies are seen in:

(Recent Pattern Dec 2016)

   a. Hodgkin's disease   b. Viral hepatitis
   c. Herpes   d. Influenza

25. What is integrated temperate phage genome?
(Recent Pattern July 2016)

   a. Prophage   b. Telophage
   c. Transphage   d. Metaphage

26. Congenital varicella zoster infection causes:
(Recent Pattern July 2016)

   a. Microcephaly   b. Limb hypoplasia
   c. IUGR   d. All of the above

27. Herpes zoster multiply in: *(Recent Pattern 2018)*

   a. Dorsal root ganglion
   b. Peripheral nerve
   c. Epithelium of skin
   d. Pharyngeal epithelial cells

28. A neonate presented with periventricular calcification on CT brain; Best method of diagnosis of etiological agent is: *(AIIMS Nov 2017)*

   a. Biopsy   b. CSF
   c. Blood   d. Urine

29. Which influenza strain, not of human origin and can cause pandemic? *(Recent Pattern Dec 2016)*

   a. H1N1   b. H2N2
   c. H5N1   d. H9N1

30. Acute hemorrhagic fever with renal involvement is caused by: *(Recent Pattern Jul 2016)*

   a. KFD   b. Yellow fever
   c. Hanta fever   d. JE

31. Diagnosis of Dengue fever can be made earliest by:

   a. Viral culture *(Recent Pattern Jul 2015)*
   b. NS -1 antigen detection
   c. IgG antibody detection
   d. Nucleic acid test

32. Zika virus is associated with:

   a. Guillian-Barre syndrome
   b. Macrocephaly
   c. Genital defects
   d. Dysplasia

33. Crimean Congo hemorrhagic fever is transmitted by:

   a. Mosquito
   b. Tick
   c. Sandfly
   d. Rodent

34. Which of the following does not indicate Hepatitis B replication: *(Recent Pattern July 2016)*

   a. HBsAg   b. HBeAg
   c. HBV DNA   d. Viral copies

35. True about HCV is: *(Recent Pattern July 2016)*

   a. Most common mode of transmission is by needle puncture
   b. Diagnosis is established by viral isolation from blood
   c. Chances of perinatal transmission are directly correlated with degree of maternal viremia
   d. Associated with polyarteritis nodosa (PAN)

36. Cryoglobulinemia is associated with:

(Recent Pattern 2018)

   a. HAV   b. HBV
   c. HCV   d. HDV

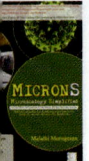

Malathi Murugesan, Microns Microbiology Simplified; 1st Edition

37. There are 3 to 5% healthy hepatitis B carriers in India who are asymptomatic. They have the risk of developing HCC in future because:

(AIIMS Nov 2017)

   a. They are unable to mount inflammation against the virus.
   b. Virus can integrate with host DNA and form complementary DNA
   c. There is a risk of elevation of transaminases
   d. Liver parenchymal cells are in a state of high proliferation

38. Which of the following is included in AIDS related complex? *(Recent Pattern 2018)*

   a. Vaginal candidiasis   b. Invasive Ca cervix
   c. Cyclospora infection   d. Herpes zoster virus

39. Mean transformation time for HIV to AIDS is:

(Recent Pattern 2018)

   a. 7.5 years   b. 10 years
   c. 15 years   d. 12 years

40. Acute Primary Amoebic meningoencephalitis true is *(Recent Pattern 2017)*

   a. Meningitis caused by acanthamoeba species is acute in nature
   b. Diagnosis is by demonstration of trophozoite in CSF
   c. Caused by feco-oral transmission
   d. More common in tropical climate

41. A 15 year old girl residing in a village recently returned from a vacation visiting her friends in another village. she complained of severe headache and fever, was diagnosed as a case of pyogenic meningitis and admitted to the hospital. She died 5 days later. Which of the following organism should be considered in the diagnosis?

   a. Entamoeba histolytica   *(AIIMS 2017)*
   b. Naegleria fowleri
   c. Toxoplasma gondii
   d. Falciparum malaria

42. Espundia is caused by   *(Recent pattern 2018)*

   a. *L.donovani*   b. *L.tropica*
   c. *L.mexicana*   d. *L.braziliensis*

43. Consumption of uncooked pork is likely to cause which of the following helminthic diseases:

(AIIMS 2017)

   a. Taenia saginata   b. Taenia solium
   c. Hydatid cyst   d. Trichuris trichura

44. All the following spread by auto infection except?

   a. Taenia solium   *(Recent pattern 2018)*
   b. Strongyloides stercoralis
   c. Hymenolepis nana
   d. Hymenolepis diminuta

45. The cause of larva currens: *(Recent pattern 2017)*

   a. Strongyloides stercoralis
   b. Necator americanus
   c. Ankylostoma duodenale
   d. H.nana

46. Cutaneous larva migrans is due to:

   a. Ancylostoma braziliensis *(Recent pattern 2017)*
   b. Wucheria bancrofti
   c. Brugia malayi
   d. Dracunculus medinensis

47. Latex agglutination study of the antigen in CSF helps in the diagnosis of *(Recent Pattern Jul 2016)*

   a. Cryptococcus   b. Candidiasis
   c. Aspergillosis   d. Histoplasmosis

48. 1, 3 beta D-glucan is helpful for identification of:

(AIIMS Nov 2017)

   a. Invasive candidiasis b. Rhizopus
   c. Cryptococcus   d. Mucormycosis

49. First chemical barrier encountered by micro-organism for common exposed sites:

(AIIMS 2017)

   a. Lysozyme   b. Acidic pH
   c. Skin   d. Lactose

50. All are mononuclear-macrophage, except:

(Recent Pattern 2017)

   a. Histiocytes   b. Microglia
   c. Kupffer cells   d. B-cells

51. Which of the following features is not shared between 'T Cells' and 'B Cells': *(AIIMS 2017)*

   a. Positive selection during development
   b. Class 1 MHC expression
   c. Antigen specific receptors
   d. All of the above

52. Activator of alternative complement pathway:

(Recent Pattern 2017)

   a. Antigen-antibody complex
   b. Mannose-binding lectin
   c. Microbial surface polysaccharide
   d. All of the above

53. Antigen-antibody precipitation is maximally seen in which of the following: *(AIIMS 2017)*

   a. Excess of antibody
   b. Excess of antigen
   c. Equivalence of antibody and antigen
   d. Antigen Hapten interaction

54. Indirect coomb's test detect: *(Recent Pattern 2017)*

   a. Incomplete antibody bound to RBC
   b. Free antibody
   c. Free agglutinable RBCs
   d. None Of the above

55. Passive cutaneous anaphylaxis detects:

(Recent Pattern 2018)

a. Heterocytotropic antibody
b. Wheal and flare response
c. Atopy
d. Delayed type hypersensitivity

56. Prausnitz kustner [PK] reaction is which type of hypersensitivity: *(Recent Pattern 2017)*

a. Type 1   b. Type 2
c. Type 3   d. Type 4

57. SCID which is true: *(Recent Pattern 2017)*

a. Adenosine deaminase deficiency
b. Decreased circulating lymphocytes
c. NADPH oxidase deficiency
d. C1 esterase deficiency

58. CD59 deficiency leads to: *(Recent Pattern 2017)*

a. Hereditary angioneurotic odema
b. Paroxysmal nocturnal hemoglobinuria
c. Chediak Higashi syndrome
d. Job syndrome

Answers Keys

1.	b	2.	b	3.	b	4.	a	5.	a	6.	a	7.	d	8.	a	9.	d	10.	d
11.	c	12.	c	13.	b	14.	a	15.	c	16.	a	17.	c	18.	c	19.	b	20.	a
21.	a	22.	d	23.	c	24.	c	25.	a	26.	d	27.	a	28.	b	29.	c	30.	c
31.	b	32.	a	33.	b	34.	a	35.	c	36.	c	37.	b	38.	b	39.	b	40.	b
41.	b	42.	d	43.	b	44.	d	45.	a	46.	a	47.	a	48.	a	49.	c	50.	d
51.	a	52.	c	53.	c	54.	b	55.	a	56.	d	57.	a	58.	b				

Forensic Medicine & Toxicology

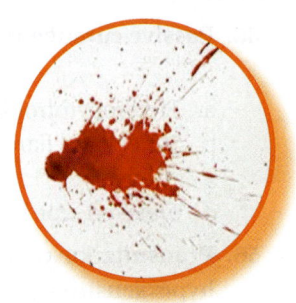

 Spotters

1. Male skull Vs female skull

Features	Male skull	Female skull
Muscle ridges, glabella. Zygomatic arch	More prominent	Less prominent
Forehead	Steeper, less rounded	Vertical, round
Mastoid process	Large, round, blunt	Small, smooth, pointed
Fronto nasal junction	Distinct angulation	Smoothly curved
Palate	Large, u-shaped	Small, parabolic
Orbits	Square, rounded margins, small	Rounded, sharp margins, large
Condylar facet	Long, narrow	Small, broad
Foramen magnum	Relatively large, long	Small, round
Cranial capacity	More capacious (1450–1550cc)	Less capacious (1300–1350cc)

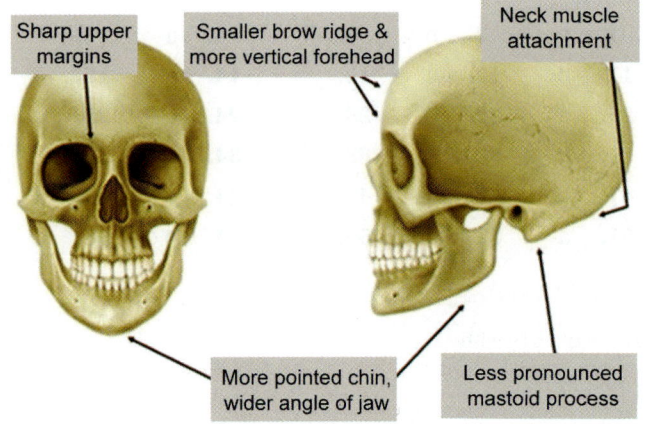

Sharp upper margins
Smaller brow ridge & more vertical forehead
Neck muscle attachment
More pointed chin, wider angle of jaw
Less pronounced mastoid process

Fig. Female skull

2. Male pelvis Vs female pelvis

Features	Male pelvis	Female pelvis
Shape	Deep funnel	Flat bowl
Pelvic brim	Heart shaped	Circular or elliptical
Greater sciatic notch	Smaller, narrower, deeper	Large, wide, shallow
Sub pubic angle	V-shaped 70-75˚	U-shaped 90-100˚
Obturator foramen	Large, oval with base upwards	Small, triangular with apex forwards
Ischial tuberosity	Inverted	Everted
Sacroilial articulation	Large extends to 2 – 3 vertebrae	Small extends to 2- 2 vertebrae
Sacrum	Long narrow, even curvature	Short wide, upper half straight, lower half curve forward.

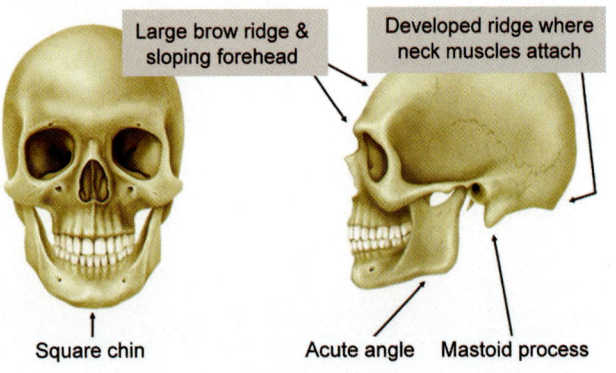

Large brow ridge & sloping forehead
Developed ridge where neck muscles attach
Square chin
Acute angle
Mastoid process

Fig. Male skull

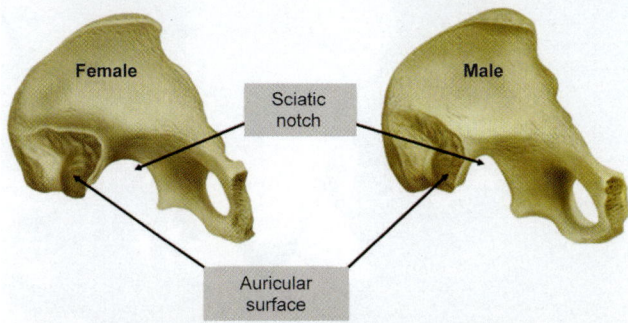

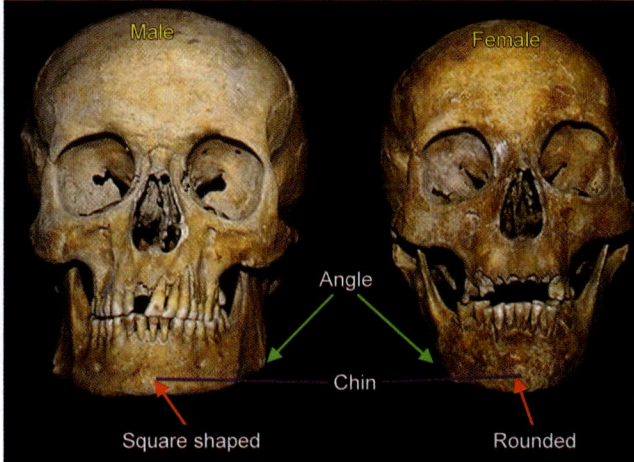

3. Male mandible Vs female mandible

Features	Male	Female
Appearance	Large, prominent muscle markings	Small Not prominent muscle markings
Chin	Square shaped	Rounded
Angle of body with ramus	Less obtuse < 125 degree	More obtuse > 125 degree
Angle of mandible	Everted	Inverted

4. Instrument use in autopsy

Names	Uses
Enterotome	For opening the intestines these large scissors are used. To do so the bulb end of the blade is inserted into the lumen (the hollow inside) of the gut, and it is smoothly stripped down the length of the intestine. The internal blade is prevented by the blunt bulb from perforating the gut from the inside.
Skull chisel	Generally chisel is used to finish the separation of the top of the calvarium from the lower skull, once scoring the calvarium (the vault-like part of the skull that holds the brain) with the vibrating saw or hand saw is done. Thus exposing the brain and its coverings (meninges).
Hagedorn needle	Hagedorn needle (Sailmaker's needle) is a large needle with an eye for sewing up the body after the autopsy is finished. The stitching procedure is similar to that used on the outer covering of baseballs.
Rib cutters	Appear like small pruning shears and are used to cut through the ribs before lifting off the chest plate. Much less expensive pruning shears from a hardware store is actually been used by some prosectors.
Scalpel	It has longer handle therefore can be reached deeper into the body cavities and can also be distinguished easily from the surgeon's scalpel. It is usually of 22 size and disposable blade, which is the largest commonly available.
Toothed forceps	Teeth on toothed forceps "pickups" provide strength in gripping during removal of heavy organs. In surgical pathology, use of toothed forceps is not adviced as teeth can increase the risk of cross contamination between specimens.
Scissors	For opening hollow organs (such as the gallbladder) and trimming of tissues, these are otherwise considered unremarkable scissors. In case of blunt dissection, scissors can also be used. In cutting "opening" motion is used instead of more familiar "closing" motion.
Bone saw	This is rarely used hand saw nowadays often by pathologists where fear of infection from aersols thrown up is much more due to vigorously vibrating saw. Though the hand saw is very slow-going compared to the vibrating saw, this can be used to saw through the skull.
Hammer with hook	To separate the calvarium from the lower skull, the hammer is used with the chisel. The hook is with the hammer is handy in pulling the calvarium away.
Breadknife	This is also known as "long knife," and is used to cut the solid organ smoothly into slices for the purpose of examination, display and photography of the cut surfaces. Particularly facile prosectors perform almost all of the soft tissue dissections (including stripping the gut from the mesentery and opening the heart chambers) with the help of large, unlikely-looking blade. Example includes—a disposable blade. Models of breadknife with permanent, re-sharpenable blades are also available.

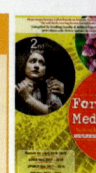

J Magendran, New SARP Series for NEET/NBE/AI Forensic Medicine Nothing Beyond for PGMEE; 2nd Edition

EXTRA EDGE

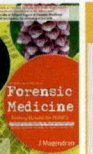

Names	Uses
Vibrating saw	Also known as "Stryker saw". For most prosectors faced with removing the brain, vibrating saw is the instrument of choice. The blade in vibrating saw reciprocates rapidly with small amplitude, which prevents the saw from cutting soft tissues, notably the prosector's hand. The disadvantage of vibrating saws over the hand saw is that they throw up more potentially infectious aerosols.

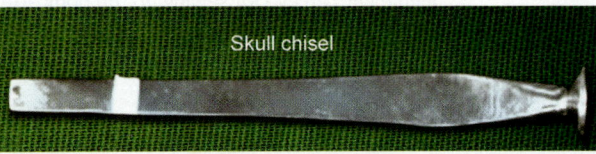
Skull chisel

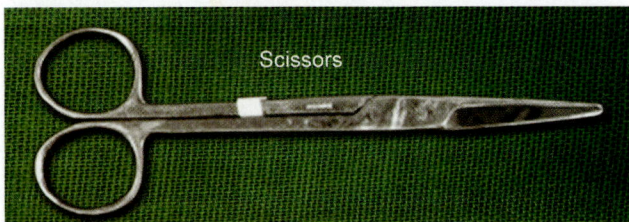
Scissors

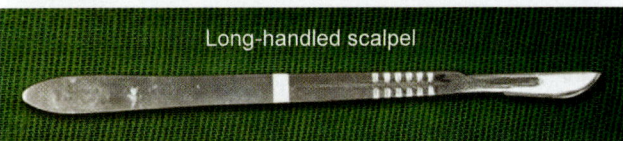
Long-handled scalpel

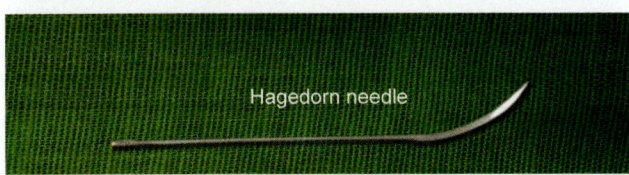
Hagedorn needle

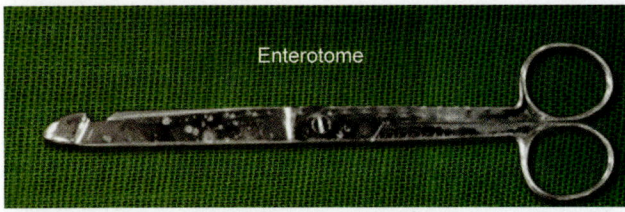
Enterotome

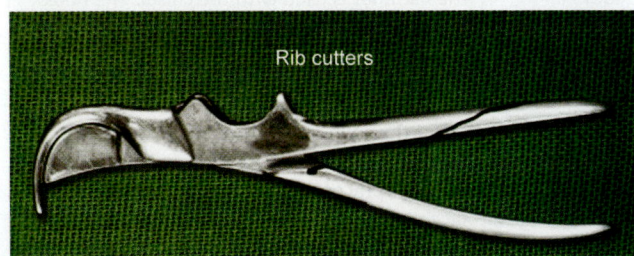
Rib cutters

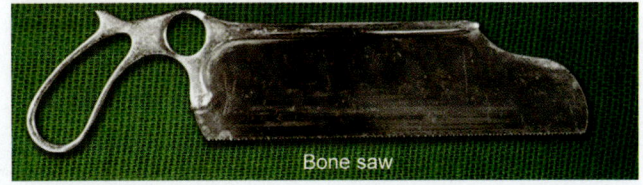
Bone saw

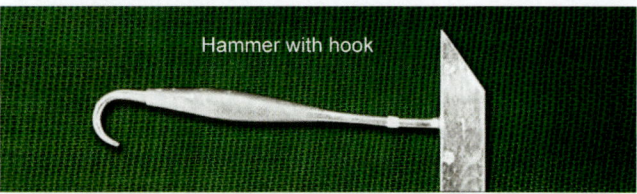
Hammer with hook

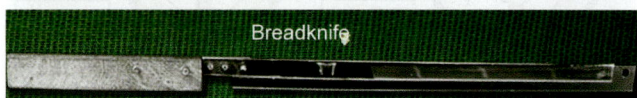
Breadknife

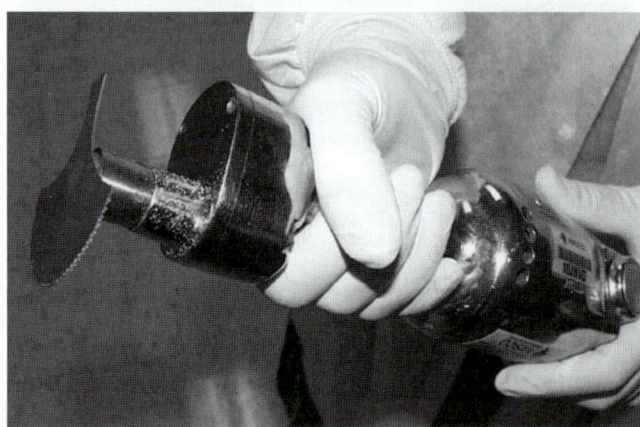

5. Livor mortis

- Suggilation, vabices, hypostasis, staining, darkening of death.
- Livor mortis can be seen as early as **30 minutes** after death. Since lividity results from the heart stopping, it may begin appearing antemortem in decedents who die as a result of cardiac failure. This stains the surrounding tissue. Lividity **usually becomes fixed 6-8 hours after death.**

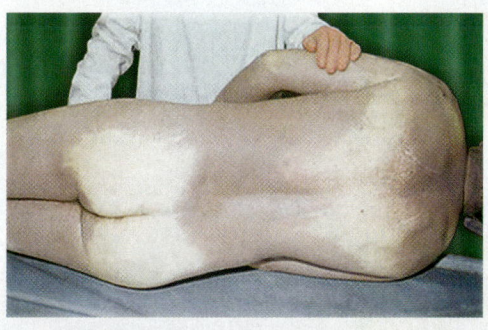

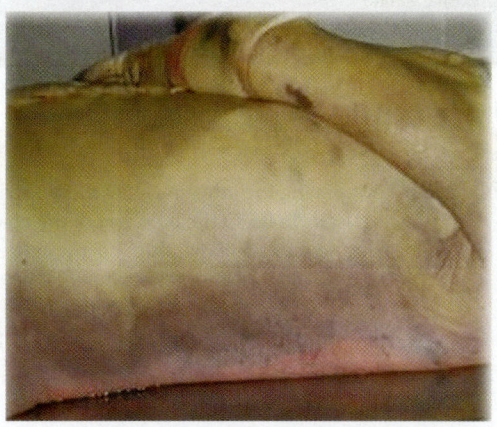

J Magendran, New SARP Series for NEET/NBE/AI Forensic Medicine Nothing Beyond for PGMEE; 2nd Edition

6. Pallor mortis

- Defined as "**Paleness of Death'**.
- Tone of the body
  - Happens **15-20 minute** after death
  - Happens due to lack of capillary circulation in the body.
  - Can't be used to determine time of death except if the body is found still with colour.

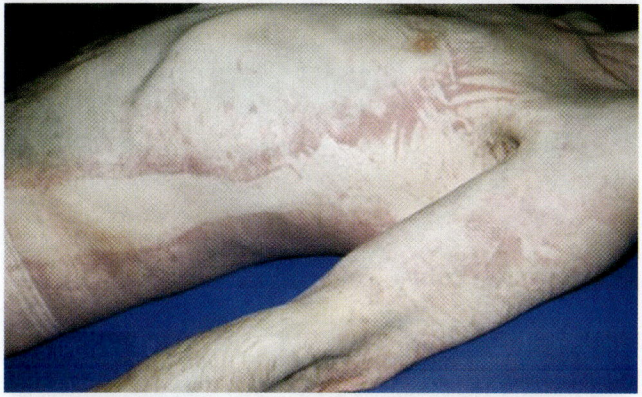

7. Rigor mortis

- A chemical change causes muscle mass to become rigid; looks like body is frozen in place (fixed).
- Small muscles go into rigor first.
- Rigor usually occurs from head to toe.

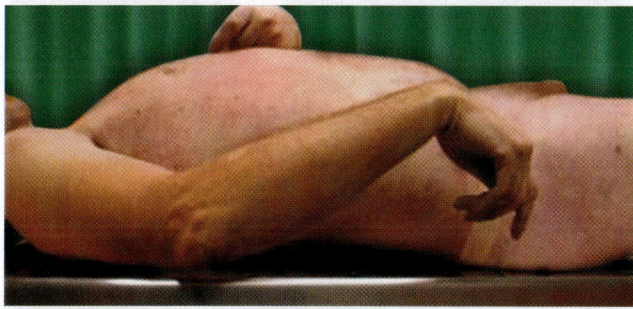

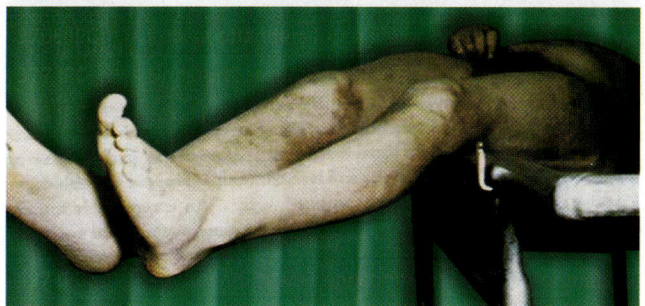

8. Abrasion

- Destruction of the skin, which usually involves the superficial layers of the skin.
- Slight bleeding, heal rapidly and no scar formation.
- Abrasion given idea about the direction of force.
- Patterned abrasions are helpful to find out the causative weapon.
- Age of injury can be determined.

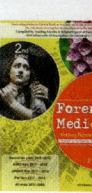

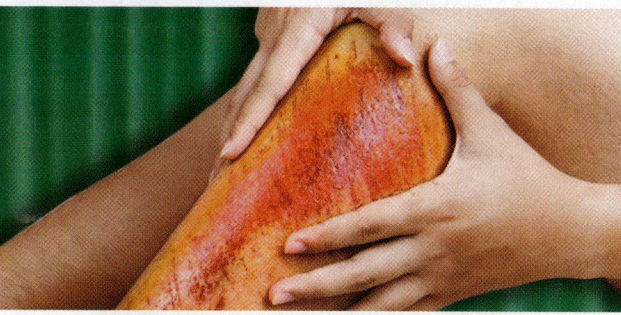

9. Contusion

- Contusion is the extravasation of blood under the skin due to rupture of blood vessels, usually capillaries, as a result of blunt force injury.
- Present not only in the skin, but also in internal organ-lung, brain or muscle.

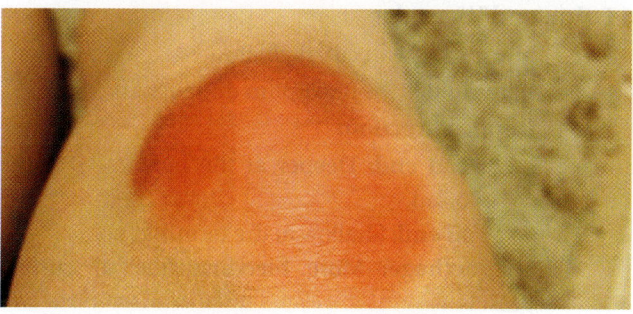

Differential diagnosis of Contusion

Postmortem Lividity

- Postmortem lividity (one of the early changes after death) appears as patches and merge together.
- Such patches of lividity resembles contusion

Artificial Bruise/Pseudo Bruise

- Certain irritant substance and plant juices are applied on the skin to mimic artificial bruise.
- These substances induce inflammation and vesication to simulate bruise.
- Artificial bruises are produced to make false allegations of assault.

J Magendran, New SARP Series for NEET/NBE/AI Forensic Medicine Nothing Beyond for PGMEE; 2nd Edition

10. Laceration

- Irregular shape.
- Irregularand uneven margins
- Contused edges
- Floor of laceration shows following features:-
    - Tissue bridges
    - Crushed
    - Less hemorrhage
    - Foreign particle like mud may be seen embedded in the wound, which give clue about the scene of crime.

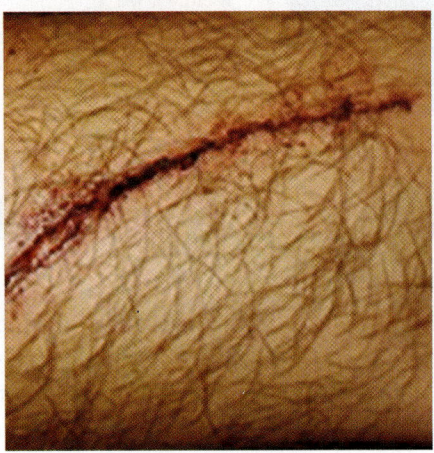

11. Incised Wound

- **Margins:** Clean cut, regular
- **Length:** It is the maximum dimensions
- **Depth/Direction:**
    - **Head end:** Deeper at the beginning of the wound.
    - **Tail end:** Shallow at the termination
- **Hemorrhage:** More bleeding due to cutting vessels.

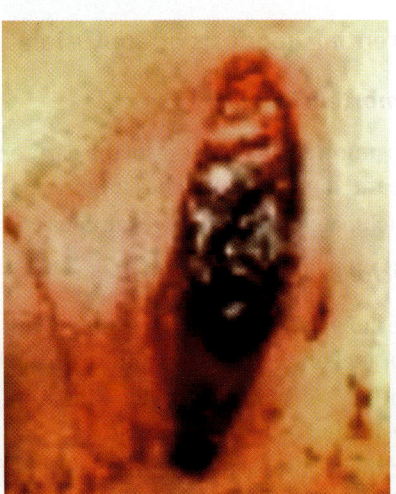

12. King cobra

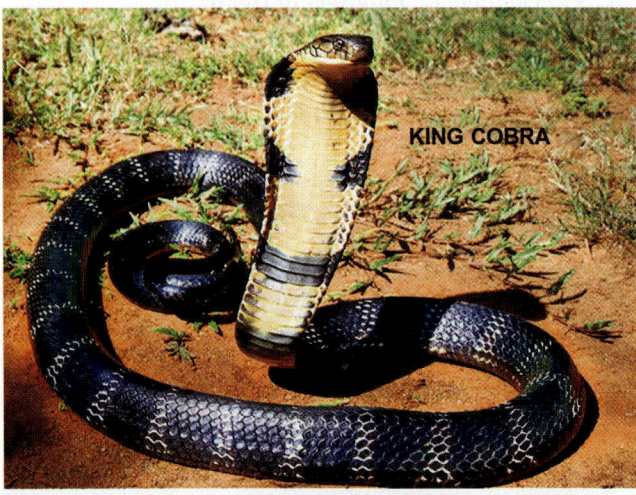

KING COBRA

13. Common cobra

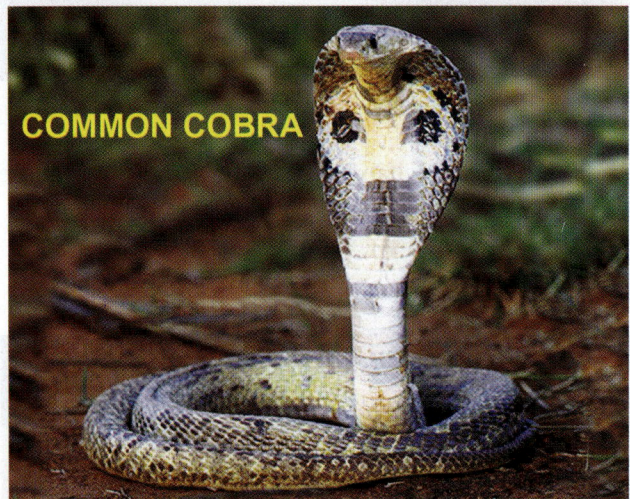

COMMON COBRA

14. Russels vipers

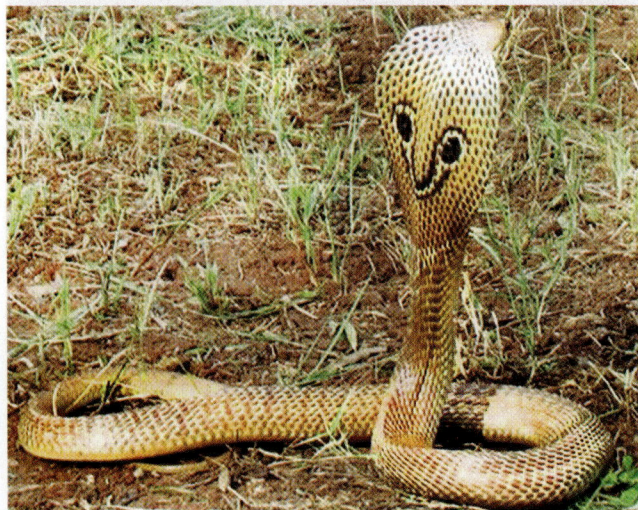

J Magendran, New SARP Series for NEET/NBE/AI Forensic Medicine Nothing Beyond for PGMEE; 2nd Edition

15. Saw scaled viper

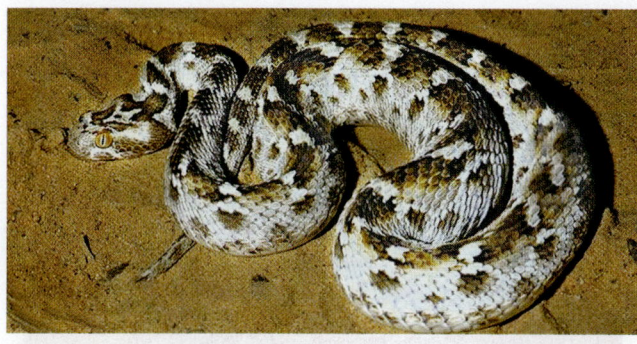

16. Copper sulphate

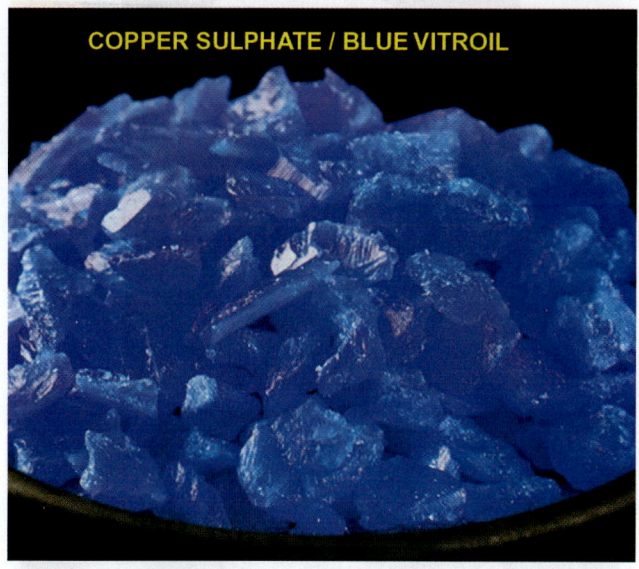

COPPER SULPHATE / BLUE VITROIL

17. Lead tetroxide

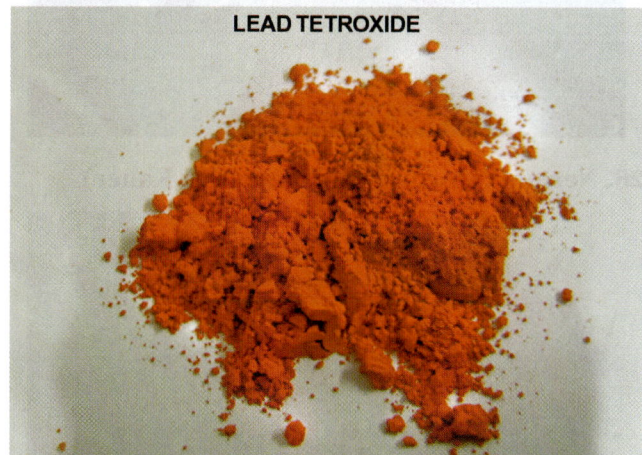

LEAD TETROXIDE

18. White phosphorus

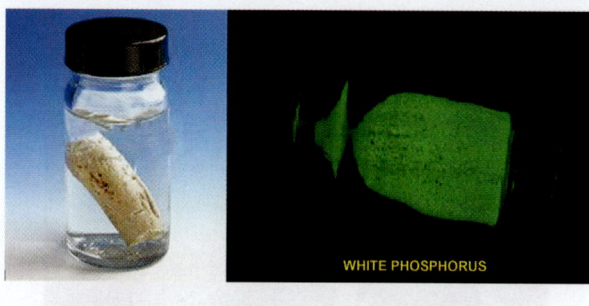

WHITE PHOSPHORUS

19. Washerwoman hand

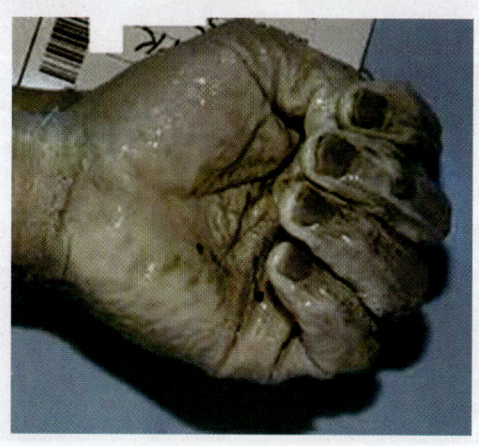

20. Adipocere

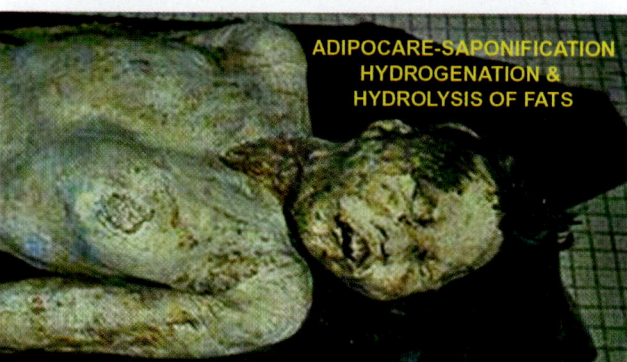

ADIPOCARE-SAPONIFICATION HYDROGENATION & HYDROLYSIS OF FATS

21. Mummification

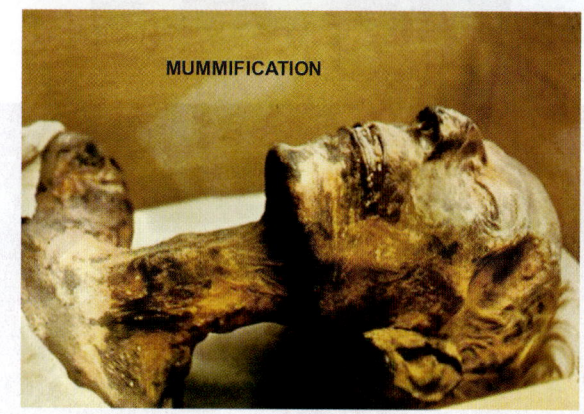

MUMMIFICATION

J Magendran, New SARP Series for NEET/NBE/AI Forensic Medicine Nothing Beyond for PGMEE; 2nd Edition

J Magendran, New SARP Series for NEET/NBE/AI Forensic Medicine Nothing Beyond for PGMEE; 2nd Edition

22. Calotropis

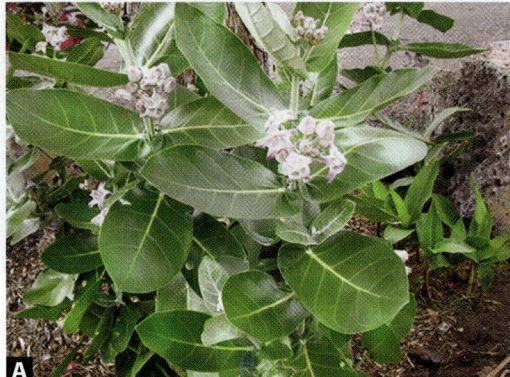

A

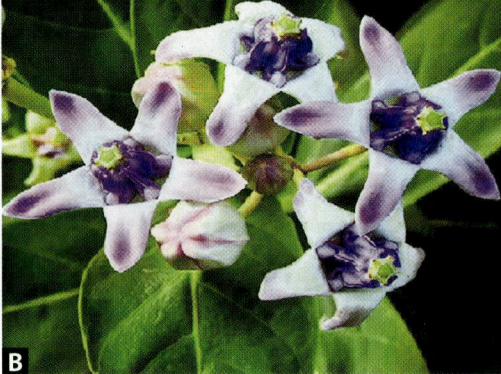

B

23. Capsicum annum

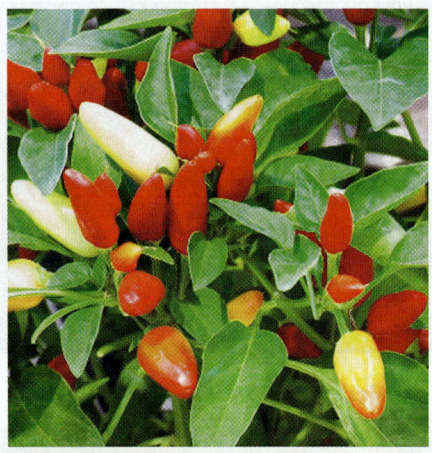

24. Amanita Phalloides

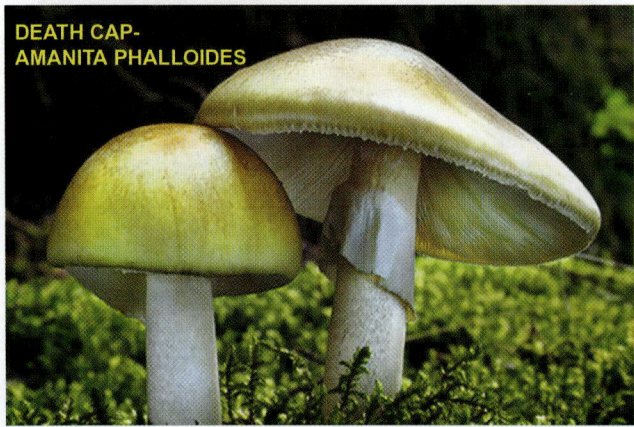

DEATH CAP-
AMANITA PHALLOIDES

25. Dutra alba

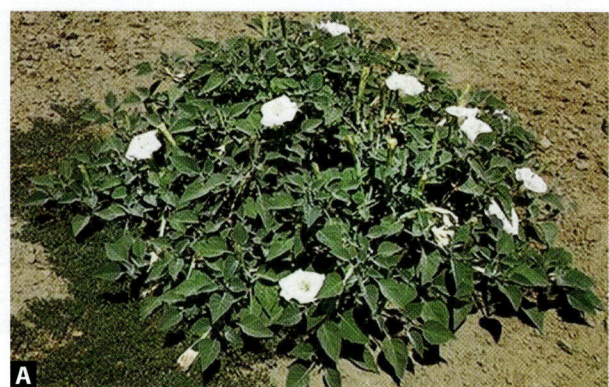

A

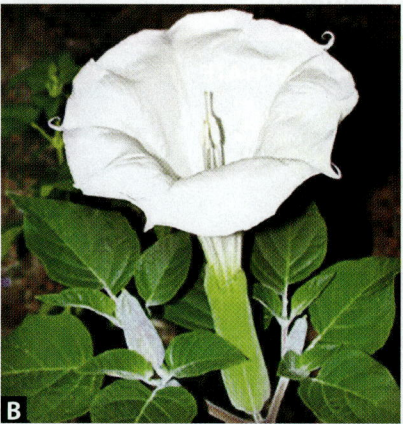

B

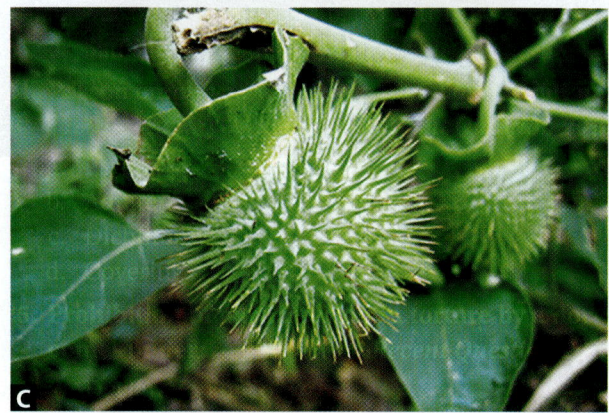

C

26. Nerium Odorum (Pink Oleander, Kaner)

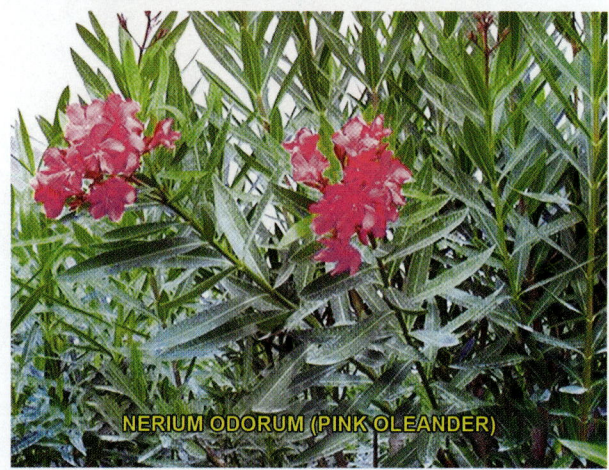

NERIUM ODORUM (PINK OLEANDER)

27. Strychnos Nux Vomica, Poison Nut, Quaker Buttons

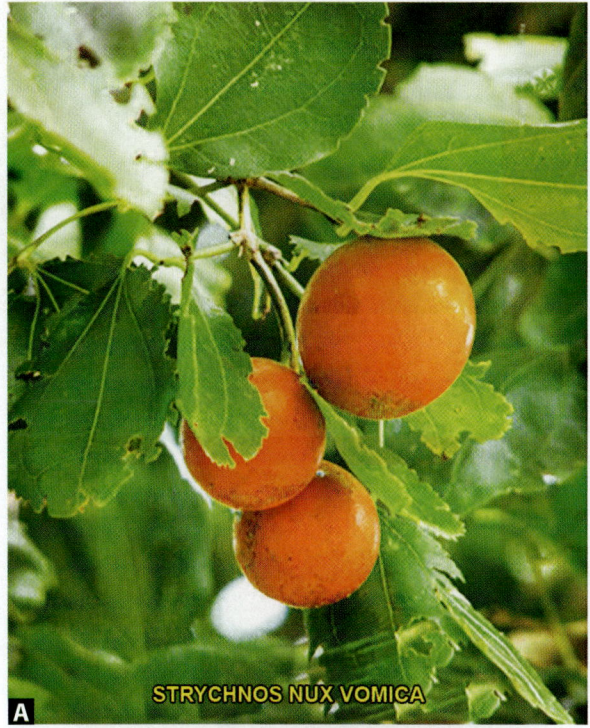

STRYCHNOS NUX VOMICA

A

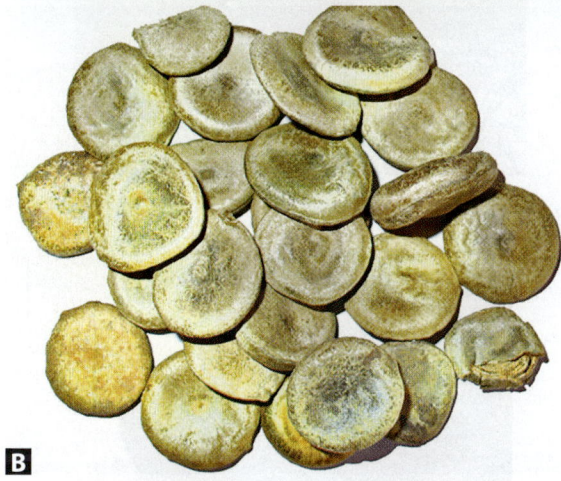

B

28. Poisonous Mushroom – Amanita muscaria

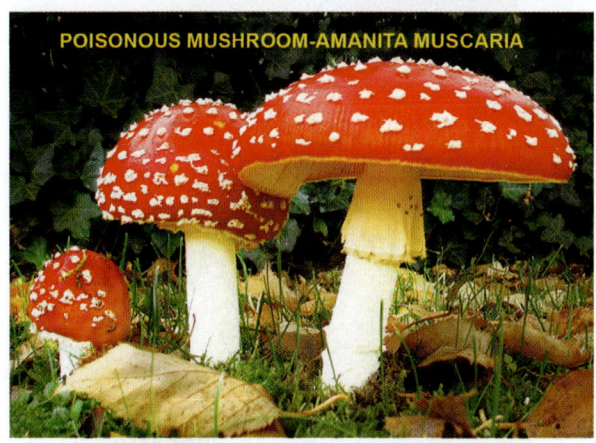

POISONOUS MUSHROOM-AMANITA MUSCARIA

29. Poppy (Opium) Capsule

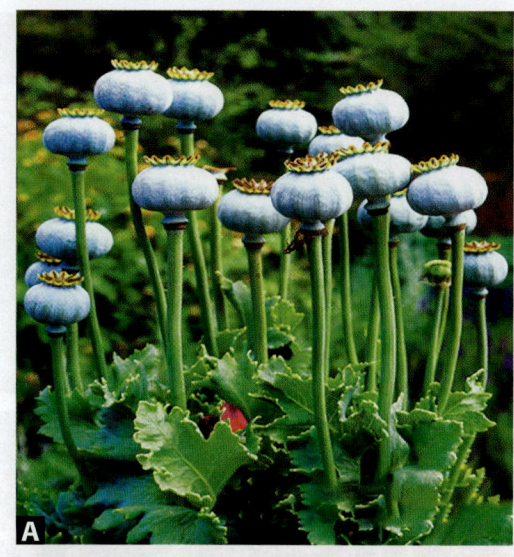

A

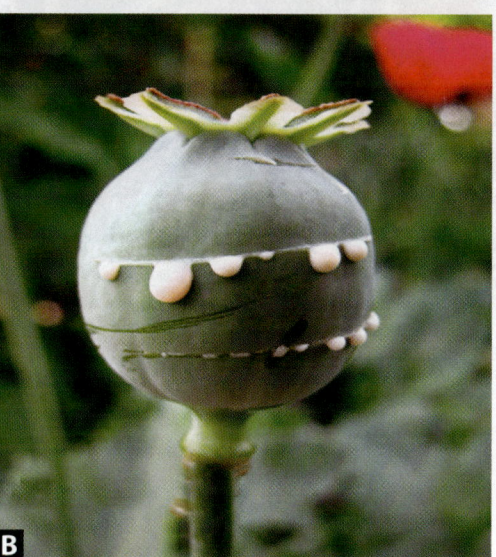

B

30. Croton Tiglium (Jamalgota)

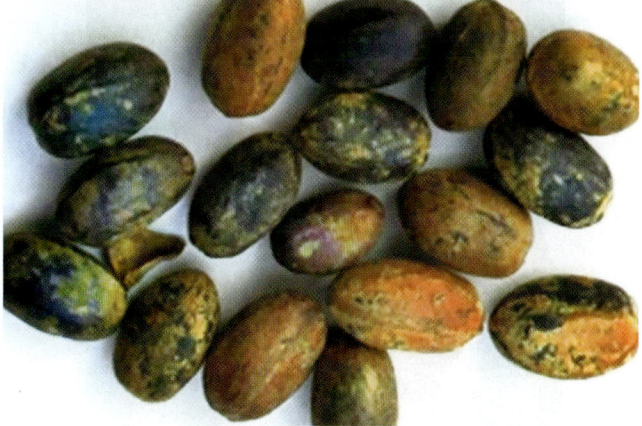

CROTON TIGLIUM

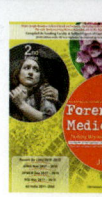

J Magendran, New SARP Series for NEET/NBE/AI Forensic Medicine Nothing Beyond for PGMEE; 2nd Edition

J Magendran, New SARP Series for NEET/NBE/AI Forensic Medicine Nothing Beyond for PGMEE; 2nd Edition

31. Ricinus Communis Seeds

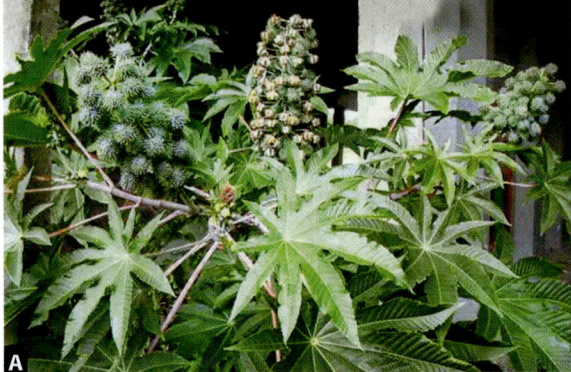

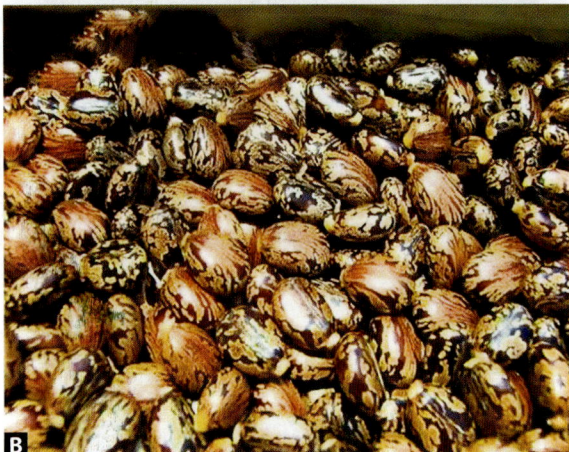

32. Semicarpus Anacardium

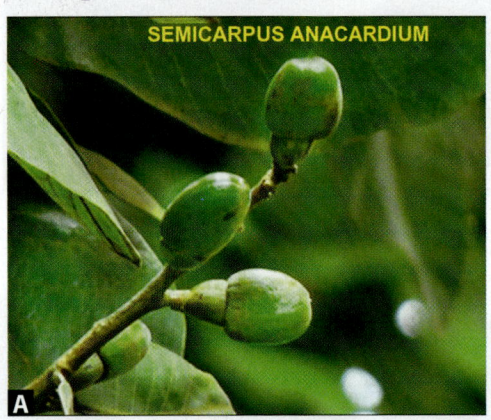

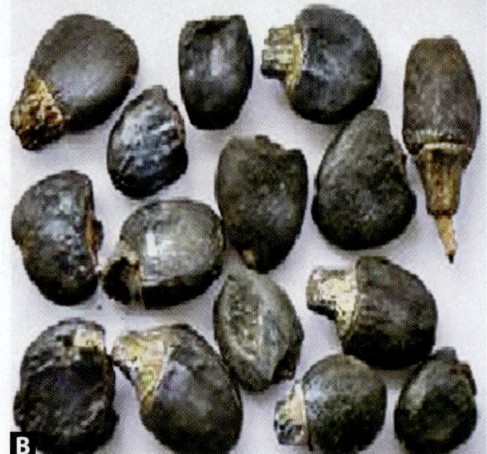

33. Bansdola

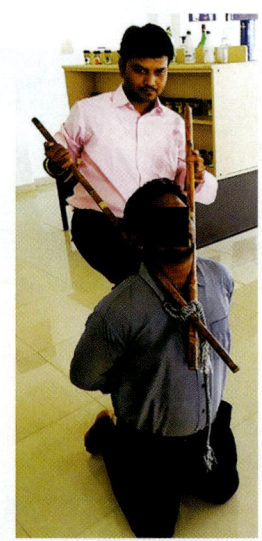

34. Smothering

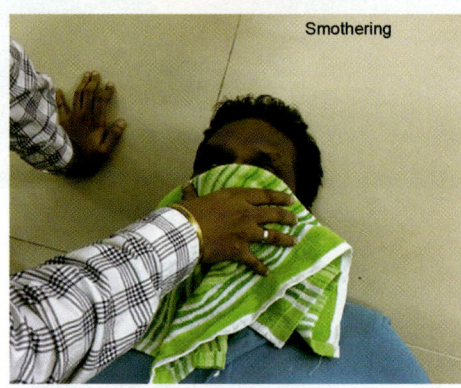

35. Burking

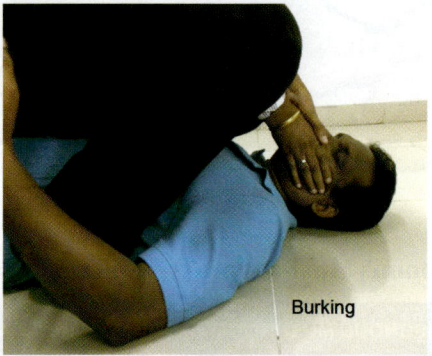

34. Mugging

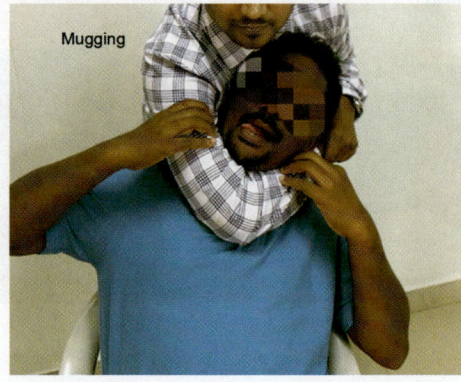

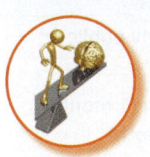

Important Tables

Table 1: Indian penal code (1860)

34 IPC	Equal responsibility in a crime with common intent
44 IPC	Injury
Criminal responsibility	
82 IPC	No criminal responsibility below 7 years
83 IPC	No criminal responsibility between 7 to 12 years
84 IPC	No criminal responsibility of insane
85 IPC	No criminal responsibility of forcible drinking
86 IPC	Criminal responsibility of voluntary drinking
Consent	
87 IPC	Act not intended to cause death or grievous hurt with consent of person
88 IPC	Act done in good faith with consent of person
89 IPC	Act done in good faith on a child under 12 years
90 IPC	Invalidity of consent if given under fear of injury or under misconception
91 IPC	Excludes acts which are offences independently of harm caused
92 IPC	Act done in good faith without consent of person
93 IPC	Communication made for benefit of person
166B IPC	Punishment for non treating of a victim of rape by a person in charge of a hospital, public or private, whether run by the Central Government, the State Government, local bodies or any other person (1 year imprisonment)
172 IPC	Punishment for avoiding summons (1 month SI)
173 IPC	Punishment for intentionally preventing serving of summons (6 months SI)
174 IPC	Punishment for intentionally avoiding order by a public servant (1 month SI)
Perjury	
191 IPC	Perjury
192 IPC	Fabricating evidence
193 IPC	Punishment for perjury (7 years imprisonment)
194 IPC	Punishment of perjury leading to capital punishment (life imprisonment or 10 years RI)
195 IPC	Punishment of perjury leading non-capital punishment (life imprisonment or 7 years imprisonment)
False certificate	
197 IPC	Issuing false certificates
198 IPC	Using false certificates
Related to evidences	
175 IPC	Punishment for intentionally omitting to produce any legally bound document (1 month SI)
176 IPC	Punishment for intentionally omitting to inform a legally bound subject (1 month SI)

178 IPC	Punishment for refusing oath when duly required (6 months SI)
179 IPC	Punishment for refusing to answer a authorized public servant (6months SI)
180 IPC	Punishment for refusing to sign a self statement (3 months SI)
181 IPC	Punishment for making false statement on oath or affirmation to public servant (3 years imprisonment)
182 IPC	Punishment for furnishing false information to a public servant with an intent to cause public servant to use his lawful power to injury of another person (6 months imprisonment)
199 IPC	Making false statement in an declaration receivable as evidence in court of law
201 IPC	Disappearance of evidence (7 years imprisonment)
202 IPC	Intentionally omitting to provide information of a legally bound offence (6 months imprisonment)
203 IPC	Giving false evidence about an offence committed (2 years imprisonment)
212 IPC	Harbouring or concealing an known offender (5 years imprisonment)
228A IPC	Disclosure of identity of the rape victim (upto 2 years imprisonment)
268 IPC	Public nuisance
Transmission of fatal infections	
269 IPC	Negligent act causing spread of disease dangerous to life (6months imprisonment)
270 IPC	Malignant act causing spread of disease dangerous to life (2 years imprisonment)
274 IPC	Adulteration of drugs (6 months imprisonment)
276 IPC	Selling adultered drugs (6 months imprisonment)
276 IPC	Selling a drug as a different drug (6 months imprisonment)
284 IPC	Rash or negligent act with any poisonous substance as to endanger human life (6 months imprisonment)
294 IPC	Obscene acts and songs (3 months punishment)
Offences causing death	
299 IPC	Culpable homicide
300 IPC	Murder
302 IPC	Punishment for murder (death or imprisonment for life)
303 IPC	Murder by life convict (death punishment)
304 IPC	Culpable homicide not amounting to murder (imprisonment for life or 10 years imprisonment)
304A IPC	Rash or negligent act causes death of another person (2 years imprisonment) – medical negligence

J Magendran, New SARP Series for NEET/NBE/AI Forensic Medicine Nothing Beyond for PGMEE; 2nd Edition

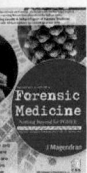

J Magendran, New SARP Series for NEET/NBE/AI Forensic Medicine Nothing Beyond for PGMEE; 2nd Edition

304B IPC	Dowry death (7 years imprisonment)
305 IPC	Abatement of suicide of child or insane person (death, life imprisonment)
306 IPC	Abetment of suicide (10 years imprisonment)
307 IPC	Attempt to murder (10 years imprisonment)
308 IPC	Attempt to commit culpable homicide (3-7 years imprisonment)
309 IPC	Attempting to commit suicide (1 year SI) – no more offence

Criminal abortion

312 IPC	Criminal abortion with consent (3 years imprisonment and if woman is quick 7 years imprisonment)
313 IPC	Criminal abortion without consent (10 years imprisonment)
314 IPC	Criminal abortion leading to death (10 years imprisonment and if act is done with her consent then he is punished with life imprisonment)
315 IPC	Intentionally preventing a child from being born or causing its death after being born alive (10 years imprisonment)
316 IPC	Causing death of a quick unborn child amounts to culpable homicide (10 years imprisonment)

Offence against children

317 IPC	Exposure and abandonment of child under twelve years, by parent or person having care of it (upto 7 years)
318 IPC	Concealment of birth (2 years imprisonment)

Offices causing bodily injuries

319 IPC	Hurt
320 IPC	Grievous hurt
321 IPC	Voluntarily causing hurt
322 IPC	Voluntarily causing grievous hurt
323 IPC	Punishment for voluntarily causing hurt (upto 1 year)
324 IPC	Hurt by means of dangerous weapon (3 years imprisonment)
325 IPC	Voluntarily causing grievous hurt (7 years imprisonment)
326 IPC	Voluntarily causing grievous hurt by dangerous weapon (10 years imprisonment)
326A IPC	Vitriolage (7 years imprisonment)
326B IPC	Attempting vitriolage (5 years imprisonment)
328 IPC	Voluntarily causing hurt by administration of a poison (10 years imprisonment)
330 IPC	Torture - Voluntarily causing hurt to extort confession, or to compel restoration of property (imprisonment upto 7 years)
331 IPC	Torture - Voluntarily causing grievous hurt to extort confession, or to compel restoration of property (imprisonment upto 10 years)
332 IPC	Voluntarily causing hurt to any public servant (3 years imprisonment)

333 IPC	Voluntarily causing grievous hurt to any public servant (10 years imprisonment)
334 IPC	Voluntary causing hurt on provocation (1 month imprisonment or fine up to ₹ 500 or both)
335 IPC	Voluntary causing grievous hurt on provocation (4 years imprisonment or up to ₹ 2000 fine or both)
337 IPC	Causing hurt to any person by rash or negligent act (6months of imprisonment)
338 IPC	Causing grievous hurt to any person by doing rash or negligent act (2 years of imprisonment)

Restraint

339 IPC	Wrongful restraint
340 IPC	Wrongfull confinement
341 IPC	Punishment for wrongful restraint (upto 1 month)
342 IPC	Punishment for wrongful confinement (1 years imprisonment)
343 IPC	Punishment for wrongful confinement for 3 days (2 years imprisonment)
344 IPC	Punishment for wrongful confinement for 10 days (3 years imprisonment)

Assault

351 IPC	Assault
352 IPC	Punishment for assault or criminal force otherwise than on grave provocation (upto 3 months)
353 IPC	Assault or criminal force to deter public servant from discharge of his duty (upto 2 years imprisonment)
354 IPC	Outraging modesty of woman (1 years imprisonment)
354C IPC	Voyeurism (1 year imprisonment first time and 3 years subsequently)
354D IPC	Stalking (3 years imprisonment first time and 5 years subsequently)
358 IPC	Assault or criminal force on grave provocation (upto 1 month)

Kidnapping

359 IPC	Kidnaping
360 IPC	Person conveying any person beyond limits of India without his consent is said to have kidnapped that person from India
361 IPC	Kidnapping from lawful guardianship
362 IPC	Abduction
363 IPC	Punishment for kidnapping (7 years imprisonment)
363A IPC	Kidnapping a minor for employment or begging (10 years imprisonment and if he maims a minor life imprisonment)
364 IPC	Kidnapping to put in danger of being murdered (life imprisonment or 10 years RI)
364A IPC	Kidnapping for ransom, etc.
365 IPC	Kidnapping to be secretly and wrongfully confined (7 years imprisonment)
366 IPC	Kidnapping any woman to compel to marry against her will or forced for illicit intercourse (10 years imprisonment)

366A IPC	Inducing a minor girl for illicit intercourse (10 years imprisonment)
366B IPC	Importing girls under 21 years of age from outside India or from J and K for illicit intercourse (10 years imprisonment)
367 IPC	Kidnapping or abducting in order to subject person to grievous hurt, slavery, etc. (10 years imprisonment)
369 IPC	Kidnapping or abducting child under ten years with intent to steal from its person (7 years imprisonment)
Minors protections	
372 IPC	Selling minor for purposes of prostitution, etc. (10 years imprisonment)
373 IPC	Buying minor for purposes of prostitution, etc. (10 years imprisonment)
374 IPC	Unlawful compulsory labour (1 years imprisonment)
Sexual offences	
375 IPC	Rape
376 (i) IPC	Punishment for rape (not less than 10 years upto life)
376 (ii) IPC	Punishment for Rape by specific people, certain situations (not less than 10 years upto life) Ex. Custodial Rape, Acquaintance Rape
376 (iii) IPC	Punishment for rape on Girl below 16 years (not less than 20 years upto life)
376A IPC	Rape resulting in death or persistent vegetative state (20 years upto life)
376AB IPC	Punishment for Rape on Girl below 12 years (not less than 20 years upto life or death)
376B IPC	Sexual intercourse with wife during separation (not less than 2 year upto 7 years)
376C IPC	Rape by seduction or induction by a person in authority (not less than 6 years upto 10 years)
376D IPC	Gang rape (20 years upto life)
376DA IPC	Gang Rape on Girl below 16 years (upto life)
376DA IPC	Gang Rape on Girl below 12 years (upto life or death)
376E IPC	Repeat offenders (upto life or death)
377 IPC	Unnatural sexual offences (upto 10 years)
493 IPC	Sexual intercourse with a woman by deceitfully making her believe that they are married (10 years imprisonment)
494 IPC	Second marriage in lifetime of spouse is void (7 years imprisonment)
497 IPC	Adultery (5 years imprisonment but only for male)
498 IPC	Kidnapping of another person's wife for illicit intercourse (2 years imprisonment)
498A IPC	Cruelty to a woman for dowry (3 years imprisonment)
506 IPC	Criminal intimidation (2 years imprisonment and intimidation involves threat to cause death, grievous hurt or destruction of property by fire or impute chastity of woman then 7 years imprisonment)
507 IPC	Criminal intimidation by an anonymous communication (2 years imprisonment)
509 IPC	Insulting modesty of woman (1 years SI)
510 IPC	Misconduct in public by a drunken person (imprisonment upto 24 hours)
511 IPC	Attempt to commit any offence (one-half of longest term of imprisonment provided for that offence)

Courtesy: Ranjan Kumar Patel & Sudhir Kumar Singh, Review of NEET & DNB Pattern Qs 2018; 1st Edition

Table 2: Types of punishments/tortures

Terms	Meaning
Autoerotic hanging	Victim's usually young males (with masochism or trans vest ism) enhance sexual pleasure by compressing the blood vessels of neck by any means
Lynching	When several persons acting jointly and illegally over power an individual and hang him
Mugging (choke holding)	Strangulation of victim's neck against the forearm
Garrotting	Victim is attacked from back without warning and strangled by throwing a ligature over the neck and tightening it quickly
Spanish windlass	It is a type of garrotting. It used to be the official mode of execution in Spain. In this an iron callar around the neck was tightened by a screw for stangling
Bansdola	Neck is compressed between two sticks or hard objects
Throttling	Manual strangulation effected by hand
Burking method of smothering used by Burk and Hare and traumatic asphyxia	Burk used to sit on chest covering with one hand the mouth and nostril and pushing up the jaw with other hand and Hare used to pull him round the room by feet
Smothering	Asphyxia caused by mechanical occlusion of external are passage
Chocking	Asphyxia caused by mechanical occlusion of enternatare passage
Gaging	Chocking by preventing air entry through mouth and nostril by filling cloth etc in mouth
Cafe coronary	Accidental chocking by bolus of food obstructing larynx. Death is mostly due to asphyxia or less commonly due to reflex cardiac arrest caused by stimulation of laryngeal nerve endings
Overlying (compression suffocation)	Compression of chest prevents breathing. It occurs when mother shares a bed with infant

Courtesy: Ranjan Kumar Patel & Sudhir Kumar Singh, Review of NEET & DNB Pattern Qs 2018; 1st Edition

J Magendran, New SARP Series for NEET/NBE/AI Forensic Medicine Nothing Beyond for PGMEE; 2nd Edition

J Magendran, New SARP Series for NEET/NBE/AI Forensic Medicine Nothing Beyond for PGMEE; 2nd Edition

Table 3: Antidotes

Poisons	Antidotes
Acids	B-aminoproprionitrile
Alpha adrenergics	Phentolamine
Amantins	Benzyl penicillin
Arsenic	Dimercaprol, unithiol
Benzodiazepines	Flumazenil
Beryllium	Aurintricarboxylic acid, sodium salicylate
Beta adrenergics	Propranolol
Beta blockers	Glucagon, isoprenaline
Botulism	Guanidine
Carbon monoxide	Hyperbaric oxygen, tocopherol
Central anticholinergics	Physostigmine
Chloroquine	Diazepam
Cholinergic agents	Atropine
Copper	Penicillamine, trientine
Coumarin derivatives	Vitamin k
Cyanide	Amyl nitrite, dicobalt edetate,
	Hydroxocobalamine, sodium nitrite, sodium thiosulphate
Cyanide, CO, H$_2$S	Oxygen
Digitalis	Digoxin specific antibody fragments
Ergotism	Sodium nitroprusside
Heparin	Protamine sulphate
Insulin	Glucose
Iron, Aluminium	Desferrioxamine
Isoniazid	Pyearidoxine
Lead, Mercury	Succimer
Malignant hyperthermia	Dantrolene
Mercury	N-acetylpenicillamine
Methanol, Ethylene alcohol	Ethanol, 4-methylp yearazole
Opiates	Naloxone
Organic peroxides	Ascorbic acid
Organophosphates	Oximes
Oxalates, Fluorides	Calcium salts
Paracetamol	Acetyl cysteine, methionine
Peripheral anticholinergics	Neostigmine
Radioactive metals	Pentetic acid
Thallium	Potassium hexacyanoferrate

Courtesy: Ranjan Kumar Patel & Sudhir Kumar Singh, Review of NEET & DNB Pattern Qs 2018; 1st Edition

Table 4: Recommended emergency antidotes

Activated charcoal	Amyl nitrate	Antivenin
Glucagon's	Flumenazil	Calcium chloride
Leucovorin	Fomepizole	Calcium gluconate gel
Methylene blue	Folic acid	Desferrioxamine
N-acetyl cysteine	Ethanol	Digoxin immune fab
Naloxone	Physostigmine	Polyethylene glycol
Sodium nitrite	Sodium thio sulphate	Pralidoxime
Vitamin K	Succimer	Sodium bicarbonate

Courtesy: Ranjan Kumar Patel & Sudhir Kumar Singh, Review of NEET & DNB Pattern Qs 2018; 1st Edition

Table 5: Odour present in poisoning

Rotten eggs odor	Hydrogen sulphide
Garlic odor	Arsenic poisoning, Aluminium phosphide, Parathion, White phosphorus
Fishy odor	Zinc phosphide poisoning
Burnt rope odor	Cannabis
Bitter almond odor	Cyanide poisoning
Sweet or Fruity	Ethanol, Chloroform, Nitrites
Acrid	Paraldehyde, Chloral hydrate
Kerosene	Organophosphates
Coal gas	Carbon monoxide
Shoe polish	Nitrobenzene

Courtesy: Ranjan Kumar Patel & Sudhir Kumar Singh, Review of NEET & DNB Pattern Qs 2018; 1st Edition

Table 6: Poison and post-mortem staining

Poison	Post-mortem staining
Phosphorus, copper	Yellow or dark brown
Carbon monoxide	Cherry red
Nitrites, Aniline, Chlorates	Chocolate or copper brown
Hydrogen cyanide	Pink/Bright red
Opium	Black
Hydrogen Sulphide	Bluish green
Clostridium perfringens Septicemia	Bronze or green brown

Courtesy: Ranjan Kumar Patel & Sudhir Kumar Singh, Review of NEET & DNB Pattern Qs 2018; 1st Edition

Table 7: Poisons and tests

Tests	Poisons
Trinders's test	Salicylates
Ferric chloride test	Phenol, Phenothiazines, Salicylates
Lee Jones Test	Cyanide (Blue color)

Contd...

Tests	Poisons
Qualitative desferrioxamine color test	Iron
Meixner test, meizer test	Amatoxin (Mushroom)
Isonitrile test	Carbon tetrachloride, Chloroform
Litmus test	Corrosives
Marqui's test	Opium
Marsh test	Arsenic
Tensilon test	Botulism

Courtesy: Ranjan Kumar Patel & Sudhir Kumar Singh, Review of NEET & DNB Pattern Qs 2018; 1st Edition

Table 8: Peculiar effects of bullets

Ricochet bullet	Before striking the target, Bullet strikes an intervening object and rebounds to the target
Yawning bullet	Travel in irregular fashion, produce a key hole entry wound
Dum dum bullet	A jacketed bullet with nose cut off
Souvenir bullet	Left in the body for some time and covered with dense fibrous tissue
Tandem/piggy back bullet	Two bullets ejected one after other, first one failed to leave and ejected by the next one.
Frangible bullet	Fragments at the site of impact
Mushroom bullet	Expands upon impact and thus produces more serious wound
Crime bullet/exhibit bullet	Bullet found in the body

Contd...

Tracer bullet	Projected that are bullet with a small p yerotechnic charge in their base
Test bullet	Test fired bullet

Note: Wounding power of bullet is directly related to the kinetic energy at the moment of impact (Depends mainly on the velocity of the bullet).

Courtesy: Ranjan Kumar Patel & Sudhir Kumar Singh, Review of NEET & DNB Pattern Qs 2018; 1st Edition

Table 9: Viscera preserved routinely in case of suspected poisoning
- Stomach and contents
- Small intestine (Upper 30 cm) and contents
- Liver (200–300 gm)
- One half of the each kidney
- Blood (30 ml)
- Urine(30 ml)

Additional Viscera to be Preserved

Viscera	Poison
Heart	Strychnine, digitalis, oleander
Brain	Opiates, co, cyanide, anesthetics
Spinal cord	Strychnine
CSF	Alcohol
Vitreous	Alcohol, chloroform
Skin	Hypodermic injection marks
Bone, nail	Arsenic, antimony, thallium
Fat	Insecticides, pesticides

Courtesy: Ranjan Kumar Patel & Sudhir Kumar Singh, Review of NEET & DNB Pattern Qs 2018; 1st Edition

J Magendran, New SARP Series for NEET/NBE/AI Forensic Medicine Nothing Beyond for PGMEE; 2nd Edition

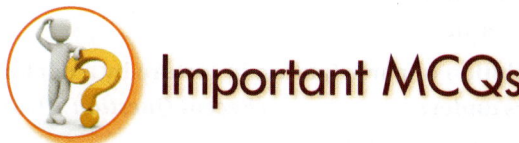

Important MCQs

1. **According to Transplantation of Humans Act, all of the following specialist are authorized for pronouncing brain death except:** *(AIIMS 2016)*
   a. Neurosurgeon
   b. Doctor performing the liver transplant
   c. Doctor attending the patient
   d. RMP in charge of the hospital

2. **All of the following is true about Kevorkian sign except:** *(JIPMER 2017)*
   a. Persist even after 3 years of death
   b. Appear within minutes of death
   c. Visualized using ophthalmoscope
   d. Cattle tracking sign

3. **Hasse's rule is for:** *(Recent Question 2016)*
   a. Fetal age
   b. Fetal sex
   c. Race
   d. Height

4. **First bone to ossify:** *(AIIMS 2017)*
   a. Scaphoid
   b. Lunate
   c. Capitate
   d. Pisiform

5. **Pelvis alone helps in:** *(Recent Question 2016)*
   a. 95% sex determination
   b. 90% sex determination
   c. 75% sex determination
   d. 50% sex determination

6. **UV rays examination is done for:** *(Recent Question 2015)*
   a. Faded tattoo
   b. Blood stains
   c. Hair examination
   d. None of the above

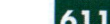

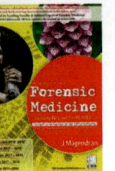

J Magendran, New SARP Series for NEET/NBE/AI Forensic Medicine Nothing Beyond for PGMEE; 2nd Edition

7. **The 'knot' in judicial hanging is placed at:**
   (AIIMS 2006) (Recent Question 2016)
   a. Behind the neck
   b. Side of the neck
   c. Below the chin
   d. Choice of hangman

8. **Hyoid bone fracture is most commonly seen in?**
   (Recent Question 2015)
   a. Hanging
   b. Gagging
   c. Throttling
   d. Choking

9. **Emphysema aquosum is associated with?**
   a. Dry drowning   *(Recent Question 2013,15)*
   b. Wet drowning
   c. Immersion syndrome
   d. Secondary drowning

10. **Paltauf's haemorrhages are seen in:**
    (Recent Question 2013)
    a. Brain
    b. Lungs
    c. Heart
    d. Liver

11. **Incised looking lacerated wound site is?**
    (Recent Question 2014)
    a. Forehead
    b. Hand
    c. Thorax
    d. Abdomen

12. **Ladder tears seen in:**   *(Recent Question 2015)*
    a. Carotid arteries
    b. SVC
    c. Descending aorta
    d. IJV

13. **Marshall's triad is seen in:** *(Recent Question 2013)*
    a. Explosive injury
    b. Gunshot injury
    c. Drowning injury
    d. Lightning injury

14. **Miner's cramps are associated with:**
    (Recent Question 2014)
    a. Heat collapse
    b. Heat cramps
    c. Sunstroke
    d. Heat exhaustion

15. **Match the following:**   *(AIIMS 2017)*

Poison	Common name
• Cocaine	• Purple haze
• LSD	• White lady
• Abrus	• Hunan Hand
• Capsicum	• Gunchii

   a. 1 = a, 2 = b, 3 = c, 4 = d
   b. 1 = b, 2 = a, 3 = d, 4 = c
   c. 1 = d, 2 = a, 3 = b, 4 = c
   d. 1 = c, 2 = d, 3 = a, 4 = b

16. **Least toxic form of lead is:** *(Recent Question 2015)*
    a. Lead acetate
    b. Lead oxide
    c. Lead carbonate
    d. Lead sulphide

17. **Abdominal colic pain is a feature of which poisoning:**   *(Recent Question 2016)*
    a. Opium addiction
    b. Arsenic poisoning
    c. Mercuric poisoning
    d. Lead poisoning

18. **Cyanide poisoning antidote:**   *(AIIMS 2016)*
    a. Sodium nitrite
    b. Sodium thiosulfate
    c. Sodium bicarbonate
    d. Sodium gluconate

19. **St Anthony fire disease is:**
    (Recent Question 2015)
    a. Opioid poisoning
    b. Cannabis poisoning
    c. Ergot poisoning
    d. Dhatura poisoning

20. **Quod hanc means:**   *(Recent Question 2014)*
    a. Medically impotent
    b. Legally impotent
    c. Impotent towards all women
    d. Impotent towards a particular woman

21. **Nullity of marriage is considered in?**
    a. Adultery in first 7 years   *(Recent Question 2016)*
    b. Infertility of husband
    c. Assault in first 7 years
    d. Age > 55 years

22. **Disclosure of name of rape victim punishable under:**   *(AI 2012; AIIMS 2013)*
    a. Sec. 304-A IPC
    b. Sec. 354 IPC
    c. Sec. 376 IPC
    d. Sec. 228-A IPC

23. **Sexual asphyxia is seen in cases of:**
    (AIIMS 2006; Recent Question 2013,15)
    a. Masochism
    b. Voyeurism
    c. Sadism
    d. Fetishism

24. **Person employed without medical qualification in medical field:**   *(Recent Question 2016)*
    a. Perjury
    b. Adultery
    c. Dichotomy
    d. Covering

25. **Prohibition of participation in torture by a doctor comes under:**   *(Recent Question 2015)*
    a. Declaration of Tokyo
    b. Declaration of Helsinki
    c. Declaration of Oslo
    d. Declaration of Geneva

26. **Criminal responsibility of insane in India is defined in:**   *(AIIMS 2017)*
    a. McNaughten's rule
    b. Curren's rule
    c. Durham's rule
    d. American law institute test

27. **Section 84 IPC**   *(Recent Question 2016)*
    a. Criminal responsibility of mentally ill
    b. Criminal responsibility of Alcoholic
    c. Criminal responsibility of dying person
    d. Criminal responsibility of Accident victim

28. A physician punishable for medical negligence for infecting a normal healthy person with HIV +ve needle under section *(AIIMS 2017)*

   a. 166 B IPC   b. 202 IPC

   c. 203IPC   d. 269 IPC

29. 23 years female was cheated in name of marriage & a man was in contact with her belongs to: *(Recent Question 2016)*

   a. Sec. 492   b. Sec. 493

   c. Sec. 494   d. Sec . 495

 **Answers Keys**

1.	b	2.	a	3.	a	4.	c	5.	a	6.	a	7.	b	8.	c	9.	b	10.	b
11.	a	12.	c	13.	a	14.	b	15.	b	16.	d	17.	d	18.	a	19.	c	20.	d
21.	a	22.	d	23.	a	24.	d	25.	a	26.	a	27.	a	28.	d	29.	b		

J Magendran, New SARP Series for NEET/NBE/AI Forensic Medicine Nothing Beyond for PGMEE; 2nd Edition

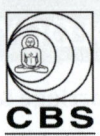

CBS EXAM BOOKS 2018

Where Knowledge meets the Innovation

CBS — Dedicated to Education

Most comprehensive Colored book on Pathology Fully Updated with Robbin's 10th Edition Includes Recent Updates of WHO 2015 Lung, WHO 2016 Male Genital System & WHO 2017 CNS/ Hematopoietic classifications

Compiled by Leading Faculties and Subject Experts of Pathology

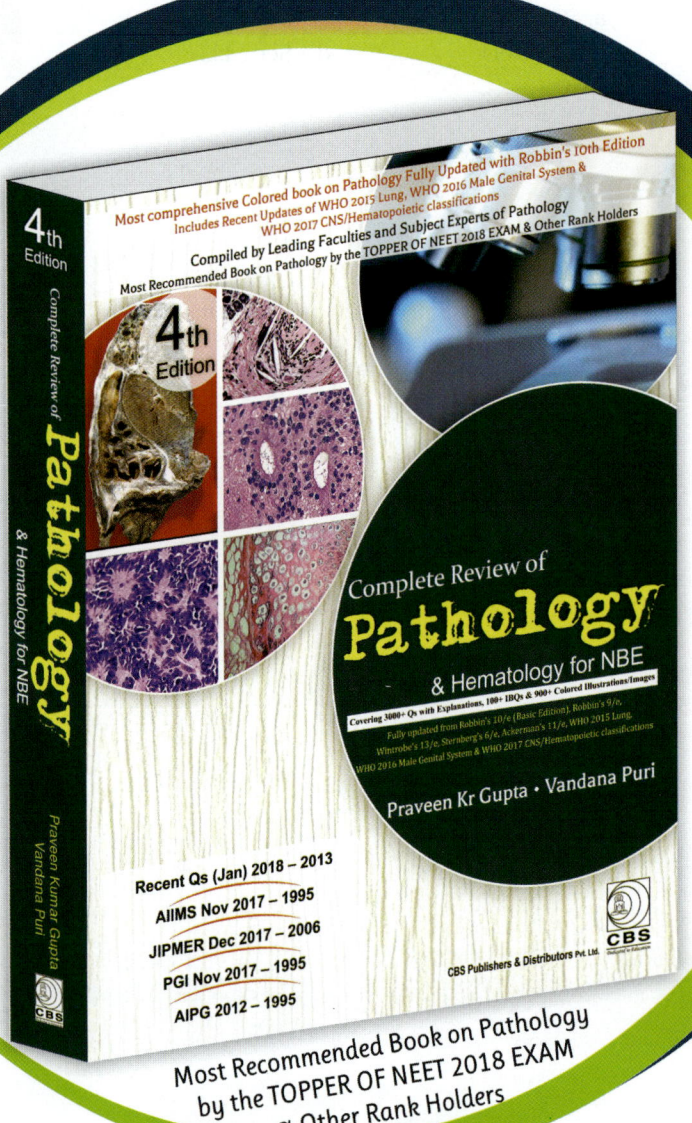

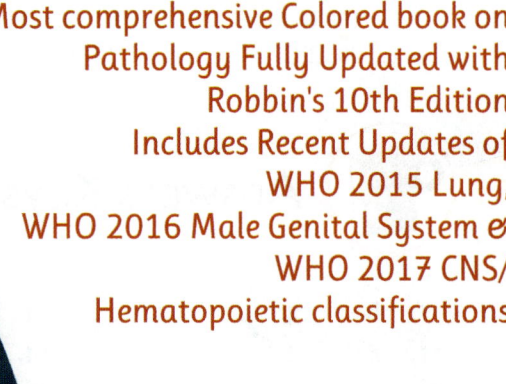

Authors
Praveen Kr Gupta
Vandana Puri

4/e, 2018   **Pages: 812**

MRP ₹ 950/-

Salient Features

- Chapter-wise Synopsis with Image-based Qs for Integrated Approach
- More than 3500 Explained Qs with References covering All National level exams (AI, DNB, AIIMS, PGI, UPSC, JIPMER)
- All Qs given Topic-wise & Sub topic-wise
- 500+ High yield Tables, Illustrations and Mnemonics for quick memorization
- The most Important Topics for PGMEE compiled in Annexures for Quick Revision
- Fully Colored Layout with Latest Updates, Key Points, High yield facts
- Separate chapters on Recent advances, miscellaneous topics like soft tumors, oral cavity, etc. are included

Above books available at **All Medical Book Stores of India**

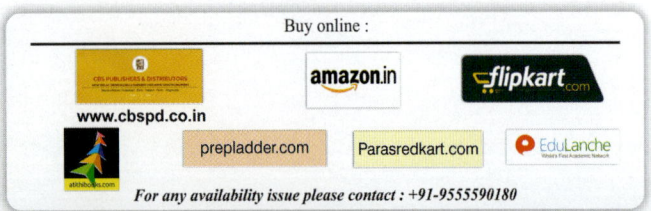

Buy online :

www.cbspd.co.in

amazon.in   flipkart.com

prepladder.com   Parasredkart.com   EduLanche

For any availability issue please contact : +91-9555590180

Win Assured Complimentary Books

Simply Join our CBS Exam Books FB Page & Register Yourself

facebook.com/cbspgmeexambooks

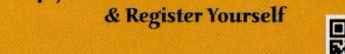

CBS Publishers & Distributors Pvt. Ltd.
• New Delhi • Bengaluru • Chennai • Kochi • Kolkata • Mumbai • Pune • Hyderabad • Nagpur • Patna • Vijayawada

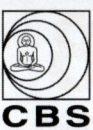

CBS EXAM BOOKS 2018
Where Knowledge meets the Innovation

Most comprehensive Colored book on Pharmacology with Clinical Correlations given in all the chapters highlighted as conceptual Boxes. All details of drugs are covered in clinical boxes.

This book is Compiled by Leading Faculty & Subject Expert of Pharmacology

Author
Ranjan Kumar Patel

3/e, 2018

Pages: 670

MRP ₹ 895/-

Salient Features

- New Chapter added on complete Anesthesia
- Chapter-wise Synopsis with Image-based Qs (Integrated Approach)
- More than 3200 Explained Qs with References covering All National level exams (AI, DNB, AIIMS, PGI, JIPMER, NIMHANS)
- All Qs are given Topic-wise & Subtopic-wise
- 300 New Qs Added from Most Recent Exams of Nov/Dec 2016
- 100+ Conceptual, 50+ Clinical boxes and 100+ Illustrations
- 100+ Image-based Qs from all Recent Exams

Above books available at **All Medical Book Stores of India**

Buy online :

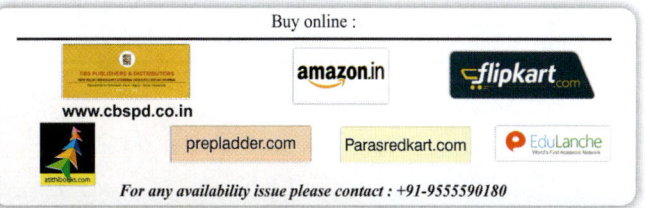

www.cbspd.co.in

amazon.in

flipkart.com

prepladder.com

Parasredkart.com

EduLanche

For any availability issue please contact : +91-9555590180

Win Assured* Complimentary Books

Simply Join our CBS Exam Books FB Page & Register Yourself

facebook.com/cbspgmeexambooks

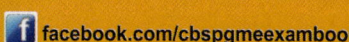
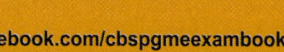

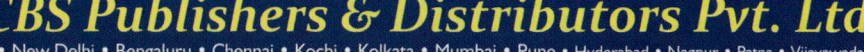

CBS Publishers & Distributors Pvt. Ltd.
• New Delhi • Bengaluru • Chennai • Kochi • Kolkata • Mumbai • Pune • Hyderabad • Nagpur • Patna • Vijayawada

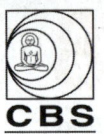

CBS EXAM BOOKS 2018

Where Knowledge meets the Innovation

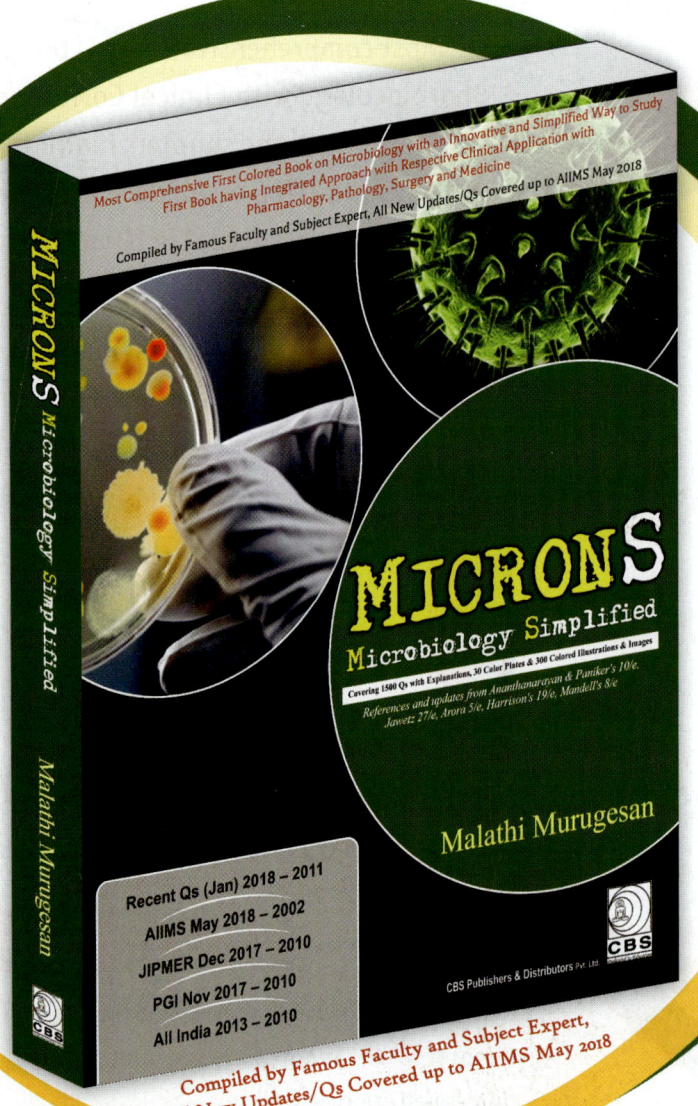

Most Comprehensive First Colored Book on Microbiology with an Innovative and Simplified Way to Study

First Book having Integrated Approach with Respective Clinical Application with Pharmacology, Pathology, Surgery and Medicine

Author
Malathi Murugesan

10 Reasons to Refer MICRONS

S. no.	Features	MICRONS	Other Books on Microbiology
1	Authored by leading faculty of various institutes	Yes	No
2	Simplified and Lucid approach to the subject	Yes	No
3	Integrated approach with other subjects like Pharmacology, Pathology, Surgery & Medicine	Covered throughout the book	Not covered extensively
4	Special emphasis on Mycology and Parasitology (trending topics in PGMEE)	Given	Not given
5	Enriched with latest updates about BMW rules 2016, Zika virus, Ebola virus, MERS-CoV, recent updates in vaccines	Covered	Not covered
6	Important points from PGMEE perspective highlighted	Done	Not done
7	Questions covered till May 2018	Covered	Not covered
8	Separate section on Infectious Diseases developed with reference from Harrison's 19/e and Mandell's Infectious Diseases	Given	Not given
9	Special emphasis on Antimicrobial susceptibility	Given	Not given
10	Strong facebook/online support for queries	Yes	No

1/e, 2018

Pages: 550

MRP ₹ 895/-

Above books available at **All Medical Book Stores of India**

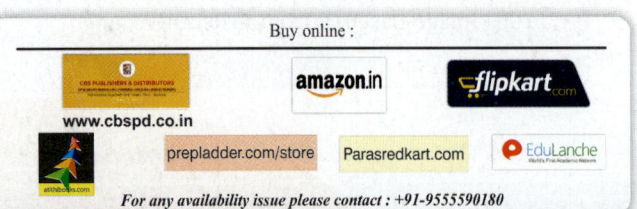

Buy online :

www.cbspd.co.in

prepladder.com/store   Parasredkart.com

For any availability issue please contact : +91-9555590180

Win Assured* Complimentary Books

Simply Join our CBS Exam Books FB Page & Register Yourself

 facebook.com/cbspgmeexambooks

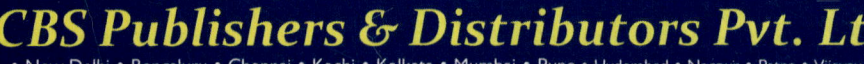

CBS Publishers & Distributors Pvt. Ltd.

• New Delhi • Bengaluru • Chennai • Kochi • Kolkata • Mumbai • Pune • Hyderabad • Nagpur • Patna • Vijayawada

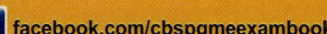